Comprehensive Surgical Management of Congenital Heart Disease

Comprehensive Surgical Management of Congenital Heart Disease

Richard A Jonas MD
Professor of Surgery, Harvard Medical School
Boston, Massachusetts, USA

with

James DiNardo MD
Peter C Laussen MBBS
Robert Howe CCP
Robert LaPierre CCP
Gregory Matte CCP

Illustrated by Rebekah Dodson

HODDER ARNOLD
AN HACHETTE UK COMPANY

First published in Great Britain in 2004 by
Arnold, part of Hodder Education, an Hachette UK Company,
338 Euston Road, London NW1 3BH

http://www.hoddereducation.com

British Library Cataloguing in Publication Data
A catalogue record for this book is available from the British Library

Library of Congress Cataloging-in-Publication Data
A catalog record for this book is available from the Library of Congress

ISBN 978 0 340 80807 8

7 8 9 10

Commissioning Editor: Joanna Koster
Development Editor: Sarah Burrows
Project Editor: Anke Ueberberg
Production Controller: Deborah Smith
Cover Design: Lee-May Lim

Typeset in 10/12 pt Minion by Macmillan Publishing Solutions
Printed and bound in the UK by MPG Books, Bodmin, Cornwall
Text printed on FSC accredited material

FSC **Mixed Sources**
Product group from well-managed forests and other controlled sources
www.fsc.org Cert no. SA-COC-1565
© 1996 Forest Stewardship Council

To my loving wife Katherine and three wonderful children, Andrew, Michael and Nicole-Sofia.
Without their commitment, support and encouragement this book could not have been written.

Contents

About the author

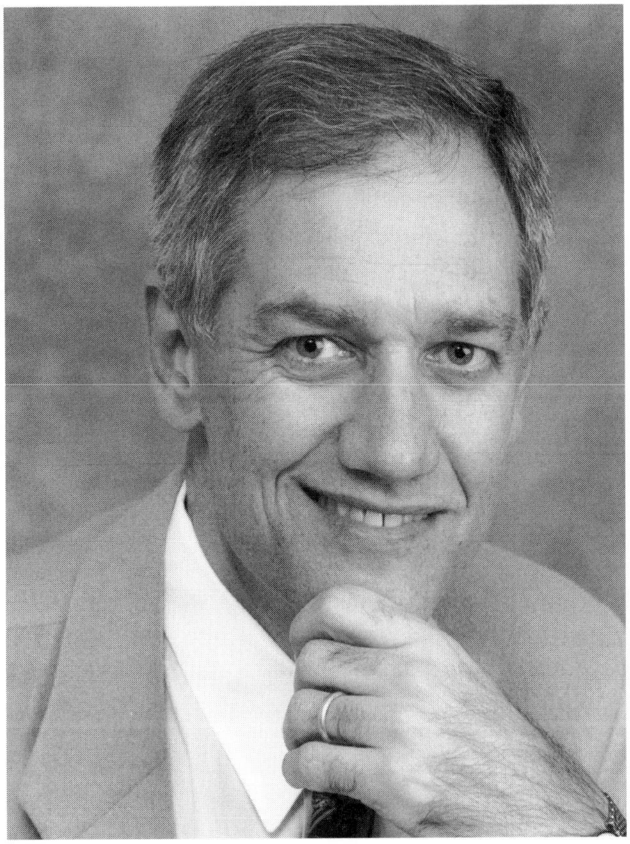

Dr Richard Jonas was born in Adelaide, South Australia. He was educated at St Peter's College and attended the University of Adelaide Medical School. He undertook his general surgical training at the Royal Melbourne Hospital and subsequently his cardiothoracic surgical training at Royal Children's Hospital in Melbourne, Australia, and Green Lane Hospital in Auckland, New Zealand. After fellowships at the Brigham and Women's Hospital and Children's Hospital Boston he was appointed to the Department of Surgery at Harvard Medical School in 1984. In 1994 Dr Jonas was appointed to the William E Ladd Chair of Surgery at Harvard Medical School and became the Cardiovascular Surgeon in Chief at Children's Hospital Boston. In 2004 he became Co-director of the Children's National Heart Institute in Washington DC. He is currently president of the American Association for Thoracic Surgery.

Dr Jonas has a busy clinical practice undertaking approximately 300 complex congenital reconstructive procedures each year. He is responsible for training cardiothoracic surgery residents and also maintains active NIH-supported laboratory and clinical research programs in addition to his administrative responsibilities. He has helped in the development of international cardiac surgical programs, particularly in Shanghai, China, and more recently has been invited to direct the development of the cardiac program for a new children's hospital in Iraq. Dr Jonas lives in Washington DC with his wife Katherine, daughter Nicole-Sofia and sons Andrew and Michael.

Previous books:

Kirklin JW, Barratt-Boyes BG (associate authors: Blackstone EH, **Jonas RA**, Kouchoukos NT). *Cardiac Surgery: Morphology, Diagnostic Criteria, Natural History, Techniques, Results and Indications*. New York: Churchill Livingstone, 1992.

Castaneda AR, **Jonas RA**, Mayer JE, Hanley FL. *Cardiac Surgery of the Neonate and Infant*. New York: WB Saunders, 1994.

Jonas RA, Elliott MJ (eds). *Cardiopulmonary Bypass in Neonates, Infants and Small Children*. London: Butterworth-Heinemann, 1994.

Jonas RA, Newburger JW, Volpe JJ (eds). *Brain Injury and Pediatric Cardiac Surgery*. London: Butterworth-Heinemann, 1995.

Preface

January 1983 was an extremely important month for the field of congenital heart surgery and by sheer serendipity was also a very important month for me personally. In that very month I took up a fellowship position at Harvard Medical School and Children's Hospital Boston to undertake further training in congenital heart surgery. In that same month, Bill Norwood, who was working at Boston Children's at the time, published the first report of successful surgical palliation of hypoplastic left heart syndrome, the last major challenge still facing congenital heart surgeons. Also that month Bill Norwood and Aldo Castaneda performed the world's first successful neonatal arterial switch procedures without any fanfare and in front of an unsuspecting and subsequently astounded OR team including myself. These two seminal events signified that congenital heart surgery had evolved to the point where the goal of corrective surgery as early in life as possible had been realized. This goal had been actively promoted by my mentor in New Zealand, Sir Brian Barratt-Boyes, as well as by Aldo Castaneda and Bill Norwood for many years. When they began the journey towards that goal in the 1970s the mortality risk for many primary corrective procedures was enormously high. Today most neonatal procedures can be performed with a mortality risk of little more than 1 to 2% and even the Norwood procedure can often be undertaken with a mortality risk of less than 10%.

This book chronicles the developments that underlie the astounding change in outlook that has occurred for babies with congenital heart disease over the two decades since Castaneda and Norwood pushed the field into the neonatal era. Unlike multi-authored textbooks of congenital heart surgery, this book is unashamedly selective. It represents the distillation of nine years of surgical training with several of the world's greatest surgical mentors as well as 20 years' experience with the superb surgical team in Boston. It does not pretend to be encyclopedic but is nevertheless a comprehensive attempt to describe what is important in the management of neonates, infants, children and adults with congenital heart disease. And yet in spite of the fact that this book represents a single surgeon's insights and experiences there is an honest attempt to compare the results, outcomes and approaches with a selection of the most important alternative approaches published in the literature.

The book is organized in three sections. The background section describes the rationale for early corrective surgery and provides practical information regarding surgical methods and materials. It also includes enormously valuable information provided by my friends and colleagues Jim DiNardo and Peter Laussen about the support that is required for the anesthetic and ICU management that are essential components of a successful congenital heart program.

The second section of the book focuses on cardiopulmonary bypass and includes a chapter on hardware options by Bob Howe, Bob LaPierre and Greg Matte from the superb perfusion team at Children's Hospital. This section has allowed me to review much of the clinical and laboratory research that I undertook in Boston over the 20 years I was there and have continued in Washington DC at the Children's National Heart Institute. It reflects a personal interest in the refinement of techniques of cardiopulmonary bypass particularly as they apply to optimal care of the neonate and infant. Once again, this approach has resulted in a review that is not exhaustive in its coverage of the outstanding investigative work undertaken by many groups other than the author's own. However it does chronicle the remarkable advances that have occurred in this area which have undoubtedly contributed to the dramatically improved results of surgery for congenital heart disease that are observed today.

The final section of the book covers individual congenital anomalies and is also not all-inclusive in that it does not cover areas such as tumors of the heart or acquired pediatric anomalies such as Kawasaki's disease. It also does not cover all possible treatment options such as cardiac transplantation where I did not consider myself to be expert in the field. These areas are well covered in several currently available multi-authored textbooks of cardiac surgery.

Despite the enormous advances that have been made in the field of surgery for congenital heart disease much of what we do continues to be based on little or no hard data. Many opportunities remain for enthusiastic young people to focus their curiosity. The development of multi-institutional databases and registries to accelerate clinical research studies such as the efforts by the Congenital Heart Surgeons' Society and STS Nomenclature and Coding Committee, ongoing laboratory research studies and the individual efforts of congenital cardiovascular teams around the world will undoubtedly further improve the outlook for children born today and in the future with congenital heart disease.

Richard Jonas
2004

Acknowledgements

Without question the most enjoyable aspect of writing this book was the opportunity to work closely with the book's artist, Rebekah Dodson. Becky and I had worked closely on previous projects including the Castaneda textbook published by WB Saunders and several articles published in the surgical atlas *Operative Techniques in Thoracic and Cardiovascular Surgery*. Rather remarkably however we did not see each other in person over the entire two and a half year period that the book was written and all illustrations were drawn. This was achieved through the miracle of the Internet using whiteboard networking which allowed both of us to view a draft of a figure and make corrections on that figure which could be saved and printed. Needless to say however these many conversations at the end of a day in the operating room often were not confined to the figures alone but also enhanced my education regarding the deficiencies of the Boston Red Sox, the history and politics of medical illustration and many other topics about which Becky is a fountain of knowledge. The stunning beauty and meticulous consistency of the figures that have resulted from Becky's efforts stand as a testament to her skill as an artist and her insights into the complexities of congenital cardiac morphology.

Laura Young, my assistant for the 20 years that I worked in Boston and who continues to support me in Washington DC, also contributed an enormous amount of effort and energy in the production of this book. Much of this book was written during long distance travel to many different parts of the world. Laura was meticulous in collating files that arrived electronically at unpredictable times and in unpredictable sequence and coordinated the overall production process with Becky Dodson and the publishing team in London.

Not only did I have outstanding assistance at the US end in the production of this book but also at the London end. Ms Jo Koster assembled a truly spectacular team of young women including Anke Ueberberg, Sarah Burrows, and Debbie Smith. The core team from Arnold was ably assisted by copyeditor Anne Waddingham and proofreader Clare Freeman. It was a remarkable experience to work with a team that collaborated so closely, effectively and efficiently. I should also thank Nick Dunton from Arnold who initially approached me with the idea for this book.

I would like to thank my co-authors Jim DiNardo, who wrote Chapter 4 on anesthetic management, Peter Laussen, who wrote Chapter 5 on ICU management and Robert Howe, Robert LaPierre and Gregory Matte who wrote Chapter 6 on hardware options for cardiopulmonary bypass. I had the pleasure to work with my co-authors in the clinical arena for many years and knew that they could be relied upon to produce outstanding contributions to this book. I was not disappointed.

This book represents the distillation of the author's experience and exposure to multiple surgical groups and mentors. My initial interest and enthusiasm to enter the field of cardiothoracic surgery was stimulated by Mr D'Arcy Sutherland, chief of cardiothoracic surgery at the Royal Adelaide Hospital in Adelaide, South Australia. D'Arcy subsequently accepted me as his registrar at Royal Children's Hospital in Melbourne when he was the director there in 1979. Not only did D'Arcy accept me as his registrar but simultaneously he recruited a promising young staff surgeon from New Zealand who had recently completed his training in Boston, namely Roger Mee. It was a remarkable experience to work with two of the world's outstanding surgeons at one of the world's great children's hospitals in 1979 to 1980. Fortunately I had come to the Royal Children's Hospital in Melbourne with a strong foundation from my general surgical training at the Royal Melbourne Hospital. Particularly inspirational at the Melbourne was the vascular surgery group including Mr DG 'Scotty' Macleish who led the group including Brian Buxton, now Chief of Cardiothoracic Surgery at the Austin Hospital, Peter Field, now Chief of Vascular Surgery at the Royal Melbourne, and James Tatoulis, now Chief of Cardiothoracic Surgery at the Royal Melbourne. At Green Lane Hospital in Auckland, New Zealand, Sir Brian Barratt-Boyes had a remarkably different style from the relaxed and congenial D'Arcy Sutherland. Sir Brian was an incredible fund of knowledge with a truly encyclopedic understanding of everything that had ever been written on a given topic. He was also a spectacular technical surgeon who could perform a homograft aortic valve replacement with remarkable ease and fluidity. In addition to the mentoring I received in New Zealand from Sir Brian it was a great pleasure to work with the other members of the New Zealand team, particularly Alan Kerr who was also closely involved in the congenital surgery at Green Lane. At the Brigham and Women's Hospital Larry Cohn and Jack Collins introduced me to the superb efficiency and productivity of a major US teaching hospital. They subsequently arranged for my rotation for a fellowship at

Children's Hospital with Aldo Castaneda and William Norwood. Drs Castaneda and Norwood were a remarkable yin and yang of surgical approach. That harmonious balance produced an incredibly productive and innovative atmosphere at Children's Hospital in the early 1980s. I consider myself very lucky to have been a part of that.

Over the 20 years that I was at Children's Hospital Boston I had the opportunity to work with many gifted, intelligent and capable colleagues in the multiple areas that make up a cardiovascular program. Without the teamwork and selfless dedication of these many individuals this book would never have resulted. In fact the team at Children's worked in such a closely collaborative spirit that it is truly impossible to select out individuals to acknowledge but nevertheless I do thank each and every one of my former colleagues at Children's Hospital for allowing me to be a part of a truly outstanding team effort.

In addition to my clinical responsibilities in Boston and now in Washington, I have over the years enjoyed the opportunity to work with a number of international groups including the group at the Shanghai Children's Medical Center where I worked in conjunction with Project Hope. I thank Dr Ding Wen Xiang and Dr Chen Shu Bao and their many colleagues including Drs Su, Liu, Cao, Zhu, Xu and Yan for their dedication and efforts in improving surgical outcomes for children in China. In Szeged, Hungary, I enjoyed the opportunity to collaborate with Dr Marta Katona and her group. More recently I have worked closely with Drs Lulu Abu Shaban, Babu Uthaman, Mustafa Al Obandi and their colleagues in Kuwait, Dr Shahraban Abdulla in Dubai and Drs Hajar and Rachel Hajar in Qatar.

On the research side it has been an honour to work with so many talented and gifted colleagues and once again it is difficult to single out individuals to thank. However in the clinical investigation group Drs Jane Newburger, David Bellinger, David Wypij and Joe Volpe were always enormously supportive and helpful of our efforts to develop clinical trials. Dr John Kirklin and Dr Eugene Blackstone were inspirational in their meticulous clinical research efforts on behalf of the Congenital Heart Surgeons' Society. My collaboration with them subsequently led to my participation in the second edition of their great textbook which was an enormously valuable experience and allowed me the opportunity to get to know very well these two giants of academic surgery. In the laboratory at Children's Hospital our grants manager Mary Littlefield, our office manager Kathy Milligan and our laboratory fellows have always been an inspiration through their hard work and innovative ideas.

It was a pleasure to work with so many diligent and talented young clinical fellows within the cardiothoracic training programs at Harvard Medical School as well as those at the University of Massachusetts and Boston University, and today to work closely with trainees from George Washington University and the combined military cardiothoracic surgery training program. These young people have made incredibly important contributions to this book by allowing me the privilege of presenting much of what is written here at regular teaching rounds as well as through our less formal discussions during the many hours we stand together each day in the operating room.

Finally I want to thank Ned Zechman, the inspirational CEO of Children's National Medical Center as well as Peter Holbrook, Mark Batshaw and Gerard Martin for their persistent and ultimately successful efforts in luring me to join the Children's National Heart Institute in Washington DC. It has been an exciting experience to become a part of such an enthusiastic team committed to improving the care of both children and adults with congenital heart disease.

List of abbreviations

ALCAPA	anomalous left coronary artery from the pulmonary artery
Ao	aorta
AMP	adenosine monophosphate
AP	anteroposterior
APC	aortopulmonary collateral
AR	aortic regurgitation
AS	aortic stenosis
ASD	atrial septal defect
ATP	adenosine triphosphate
AV	atrioventricular
CoA	aortic coarctation
CPAP	continuous positive airway pressure
CPB	cardiopulmonary bypass
CS	coronary sinus
CT	computed tomography
C-TGA	corrected transposition of the great arteries
CVR	coronary vascular reserve
d-TGA	dextro-transposition of the great arteries
DHCA	deep hypothermic circulatory arrest
DKS	Damus-Kaye-Stansel procedure
DOLV	double outlet left ventricle
DORV	double outlet right ventricle
DPF	differential pathway factor
DPT	diastolic perfusion time
ECG	electrocardiography
ECMO	extracorporeal membrane oxygenation
EEG	electroencephalography
EF	ejection fraction
$ETCO_2$	end-tidal carbon dioxide
FFP	fresh frozen plasma
FiO_2	fraction of inspired oxygen
FRC	functional residual capacity
HCM	hypertrophic cardiomyopathy
HLHS	hypoplastic left heart syndrome
IAA	interrupted aortic arch
ICU	intensive care unit
IQ	intelligence quotient
IVC	inferior vena cava
IVS	intact ventricular septum
LA	left atrium
LAD	left anterior descending
LAP	left atrial pressure
LBB	left bundle branch
LCC	left coronary cusp
L–R	left to right
LMCA	left main coronary artery
LPA	left pulmonary artery
l-TGA	levo-transposition of the great arteries
LVOT	left ventricular outflow tract
MCA	middle cerebral artery
MPA	main pulmonary artery
MRI	magnetic resonance imaging
MV	mitral valve
NEC	necrotizing enterocolitis
NIRS	near infrared spectroscopy
NYHA	New York Heart Association (classification)
PA	pulmonary artery
PaO_2	arterial oxygen partial pressure
PAPVC	partial anomalous pulmonary venous connection
PDA	patent ductus arteriosus
PEEP	positive end-expiratory pressure
PFO	patent foramen ovale
PGE1	prostaglandin E1
PS	pulmonary stenosis
PTFE	polytetrafluoroethylene
PV	pulmonary vein
PVR	pulmonary vascular resistance
Q_p	total pulmonary blood flow
Q_s	total systemic blood flow
RA	right atrium
RAP	right atrial pressure
RBB	right bundle branch
RCA	right coronary artery
RCC	right coronary cusp
REV	*reparation a l'etage ventriculaire*
R–L	right to left
RPA	right pulmonary artery
RSV	respiratory syncytial virus
RV	right ventricle
RVOT	right ventricle outflow tract
SaO_2	arterial oxygen saturation
ScO_2	cerebral oxygen saturation
SVC	superior vena cava
SVR	systemic vascular resistance
TAP	transannular patch

TAPVC	total anomalous pulmonary venous connection
TCD	transcranial Doppler
TEE	transesophageal echocardiography
TGA	transposition of the great arteries
TGV	transposition of great vessels
TOF	tetralogy of Fallot
t-PA	tissue plasminogen activator
TV	tricuspid valve
VACTERL	vertebral abnormalities, anal atresia, cardiac abnormalities, tracheoesophageal fistula and/or esophageal atresia, renal agenesis and dysplasia and limb defects
VAD	ventricular assist device
VATS	video-assisted thoracoscopic surgery
VAVD	vacuum assisted venous drainage
VSD	ventricular septal defect

SECTION 1

Background

1

Why early primary repair?

THE EARLY YEARS OF CARDIAC SURGERY

The first successful surgical procedure for congenital heart disease was performed by Dr Robert E Gross at Children's Hospital Boston in 1938 (Figure 1.1). The patient was seven years old when Dr Gross ligated her patent ductus arteriosus[1] (Figure 1.2). In 1945 Dr Gross undertook the first repair of coarctation in the United States shortly after Craaford had described his success in Sweden.[2,3] Writing in his landmark textbook *The Surgery of Infancy and Childhood* in 1953[4] Gross stated: 'From laboratory observations on aortic anastomoses in growing pigs, it has been found that it is possible for the lumen to enlarge reasonably well with the increase in size of the growing animal, but in some instances it lags behind somewhat. Hence, in a human baby, we generally prefer to carry along with treatment by medical means, and then to perform aortic resection and anastomosis later in childhood when there is more reasonable promise that the pathway will be large enough to be adequate during adult life.'

The development of the heart-lung machine and of open cardiac procedures for congenital heart disease introduced a number of new reasons, in addition to growth, why surgeons in the early years of surgery for congenital heart disease recommended delaying surgery well beyond the neonatal period and infancy. Early heart-lung machines had multiple deleterious effects that were particularly dangerous for the young infant. The priming volume for early circuits was usually several liters, which necessitated exposure of an infant to what was effectively a massive blood transfusion of homologous blood (Figures 1.3 and 1.4). The inflammatory mediators such as bradykinin and complement[5] that were released in large quantities as part of the 'systemic inflammatory response' to bypass were particularly problematic for the neonate and young infant who have a propensity to greater vascular permeability and tissue edema than the older child.[6,7]

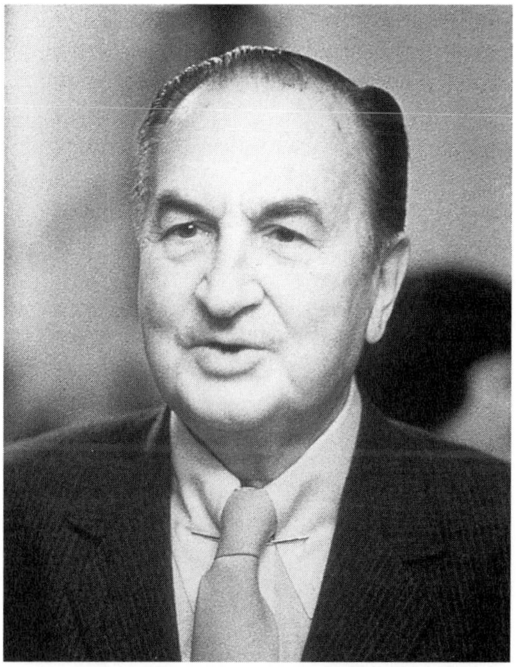

Figure 1.1 *Dr Robert E Gross was the second William E Ladd Professor of Surgery at Harvard Medical School and Children's Hospital Boston. In 1938 he was Dr Ladd's chief resident when he was the first to successfully ligate a patent ductus arteriosus.*

Anesthesia for babies was in its infancy and intensive care units appropriate for young babies did not exist. Diagnosis of heart disease was dependent on the invasive technique of cardiac catheterization which often led to its own complications. Surgeons did not have microvascular instrumentation or the knowledge of delicate surgical techniques necessary to perform repairs involving the fragile tissues of the newborn or young infant. For all these reasons every attempt was made to manage the child medically and to defer surgery until the

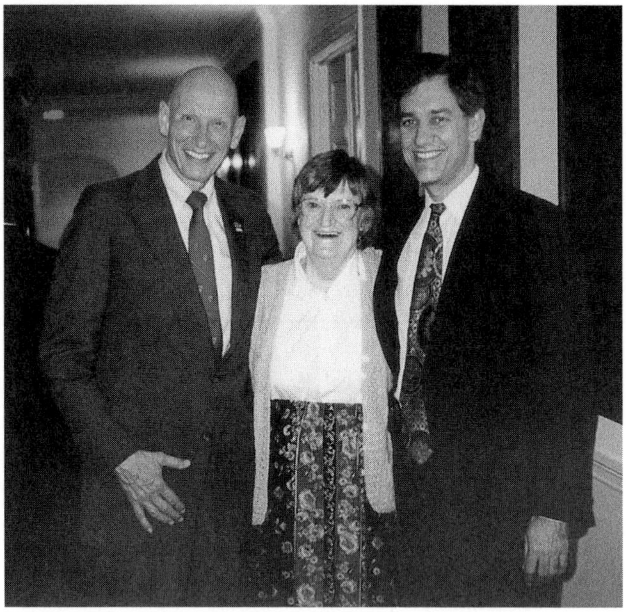

Figure 1.2 *In 1995 Dr Gross' first patient to survive ductal ligation attended the Robert E Gross memorial lecture presented by Dr Alex Haller, also a pioneer in pediatric surgery, like Dr Gross. The author is on the patient's left with Dr Haller on her right.*

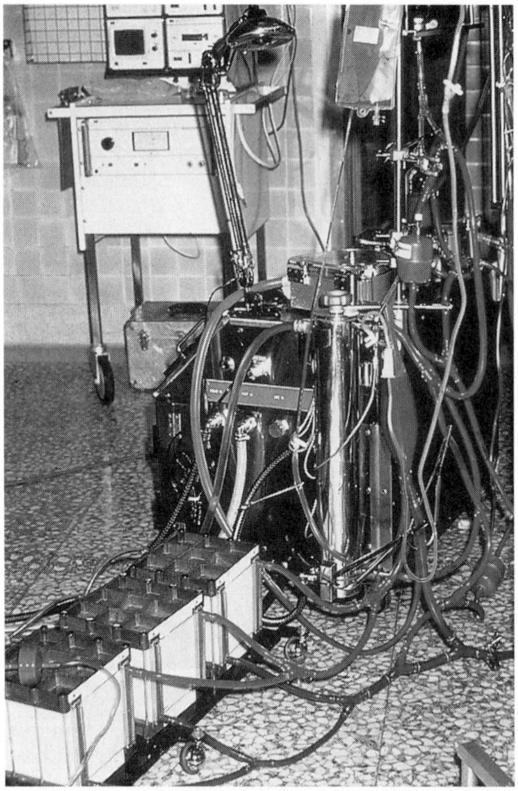

Figure 1.3 *Early membrane oxygenators had a priming volume of several liters. This oxygenator was used at St Vincent's Hospital, Melbourne, Australia in the mid 1970s.*

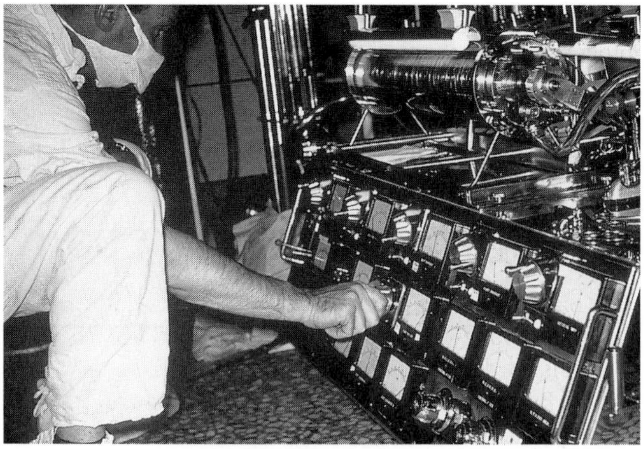

Figure 1.4 *Early oxygenators such as this disc oxygenator used at the Royal Adelaide Hospital, South Australia in the 1960s by Mr D'Arcy Sutherland had a priming volume of several liters. Early oxygenators were particularly injurious to neonates and young infants.*

child was considered to be better able to withstand the stresses of surgery. And for the child who could not be managed medically, a number of ingenious *palliative* surgical procedures were developed.

PALLIATIVE SURGICAL PROCEDURES: THE TWO-STAGE APPROACH TO CONGENITAL HEART DISEASE

The pathophysiology of congenital heart disease is limited to three main problems. There may be a volume load in which one or both ventricles must pump more than the usual amount of blood. This is most commonly because of excessive pulmonary blood flow resulting from a septal defect. There may be a pressure load for one or both ventricles. This is usually secondary to obstruction to outflow from the affected ventricle. Finally there may be cyanosis which may be secondary to reduced pulmonary blood flow but also may be because of inadequate mixing between two parallel circulations as in transposition of the great arteries. Early procedures were designed to palliate but not cure these problems, thereby allowing the child to grow to an age and size at which 'curative' surgery was thought to carry a lesser risk.

Systemic to pulmonary arterial shunts

A systemic to pulmonary arterial shunt reduces cyanosis by increasing pulmonary blood flow. Although this is a conceptually simple procedure, it nevertheless carries a number of important challenges for the surgeon. Most importantly the size of the shunt must be appropriate for the size of the child. But since the goal of the procedure is to achieve growth of the child, what may be large enough for the child at the time of the procedure may not be large enough in the future. On the other hand if the shunt is too large it will impose a volume load on one or both ventricles so the child will have traded the problems of cyanosis for the secondary problems associated with a volume load, most notably congestive heart failure with associated failure to thrive.

THE BLALOCK–TAUSSIG SHUNT

The Blalock–Taussig shunt was a marvelous technical innovation introduced by the surgeon Alfred Blalock working with his cardiologist Helen Taussig at Johns Hopkins in 1947.[8] Blalock was able to connect the subclavian artery directly to the pulmonary artery to increase pulmonary blood flow. Blalock had discovered, perhaps without realizing it, that the size of the subclavian artery happened to be appropriate for supplying enough but not too much pulmonary blood flow. Furthermore it had growth potential and could therefore sustain the child for many years. But in these early years which predated the development of vascular surgery and certainly predated microvascular surgery, the procedure was technically demanding for many surgeons, particularly working with small babies. Unless the anastomosis was constructed perfectly there was a high risk of shunt thrombosis. This led others to seek a technically simpler procedure with a higher probability of patency.

WATERSTON SHUNT

The Waterston shunt is an anastomosis between the ascending aorta and the right pulmonary artery.[9] It is performed through a right thoracotomy with a side-biting clamp applied to both vessels. But the size of the anastomosis is critical. It was very common for this shunt to result in excessive pulmonary blood flow. With growth there is frequently distortion of the pulmonary arteries.

POTTS SHUNT

The Potts shunt is an anastomosis between the descending aorta and the left pulmonary artery.[10] It is performed through a left thoracotomy with a side-biting clamp applied to both vessels. The Potts shunt has all the disadvantages of the Waterston shunt and in addition is very difficult to take down.

MODIFIED BLALOCK (PTFE INTERPOSITION) SHUNT

The modified Blalock shunt was introduced by deLeval as a technically simpler version of the classic shunt described by Blalock.[11] The original approach recommended by deLeval was through a left thoracotomy. The left subclavian artery is much easier to expose than the right. A polytetrafluroethylene (PTFE: Goretex, Impra) tube graft between 4 and 6 mm in diameter is anastomosed to the left subclavian artery and the left pulmonary artery. The left subclavian artery is said to limit flow to an appropriate amount and by using a larger graft the child is able to grow without becoming excessively cyanosed. Modifications of this shunt are presently the most popular systemic to pulmonary artery shunt (see Chapter 20).

Pulmonary artery banding

By far the commonest congenital heart anomaly is a VSD. A VSD results in a volume load for both ventricles. If the defect is large and the pulmonary resistance is low, the child is likely to have symptoms of congestive heart failure including failure to thrive. The high pressure and high flow in the pulmonary arteries will eventually lead after a year or two to irreversible damage to the pulmonary microcirculation, i.e. pulmonary vascular disease.

In 1950 Muller and Dammann described surgical application of a band around the main pulmonary artery to reduce the pressure and flow in the lungs.[12] As with shunts a band has the problem that it does not allow growth so that what may be an appropriate degree of band tightness for an infant will be too tight for the older child. Thus the child will become increasingly cyanosed with growth. Banding also leads to scarring of the main pulmonary artery that can lead to permanent distortion at the origins of the right and left pulmonary arteries and/or distortion of the pulmonary valve.

Atrial septectomy

Although cyanosis is usually secondary to reduced pulmonary blood flow it can also be a result of transposition physiology (see Chapter 15). Unless there is a patent ductus or septal defect to allow mixing of the parallel pulmonary and systemic circulations, the child will die from cyanosis. In 1950 Blalock and Hanlon described an ingenious procedure that allowed removal of a large part of the atrial septum to create an ASD for a child with transposition.[13] The procedure is performed through a right thoracotomy. The right pulmonary artery is snared. A side-biting clamp is applied that includes the right atrial free wall anterior to the septum as well as left atrium posterior to the septum. Incisions are made anterior and posterior to the septum which can then be pulled through the partially opened clamp.

With the advent of the Rashkind balloon septosotomy in 1966 it was rarely necessary to perform this procedure.[14,15]

DISADVANTAGES OF THE TWO-STAGE APPROACH

Pathology secondary to palliative surgery

All of the palliative surgical procedures carry a risk of morbidity and mortality, no matter how skilled and experienced the surgical team. The Waterston shunt, the Potts shunt and pulmonary artery bands are notorious for causing pulmonary artery distortion. But even a perfect Blalock shunt requires dissection of the right or left pulmonary artery, which is followed by adventitial scarring. Even if a stenosis cannot be seen it is very likely that the vessel wall compliance is decreased in the region of dissection and anastomosis.

All of the palliative procedures result in some degree of intrapericardial scarring which can obscure important cardiac landmarks including the coronary arteries. If a thoracotomy is performed there is a cosmetic disadvantage from the additional skin scar but more importantly there may be scoliosis later in life. Palliative procedures are also an additional cost for the family both financially and emotionally.

Pathology secondary to continuing presence of congenital heart disease

Because palliative procedures do not correct but simply palliate congenital cardiac pathology, there will be ongoing deleterious consequences of the abnormal circulation. Most importantly the transition from fetal to neonatal to mature physiology is unable to proceed in the usual fashion which has consequences for all organ systems of the body. On the other hand early primary repair creates a physiologically normal circulation which allows normal maturation of the individual.

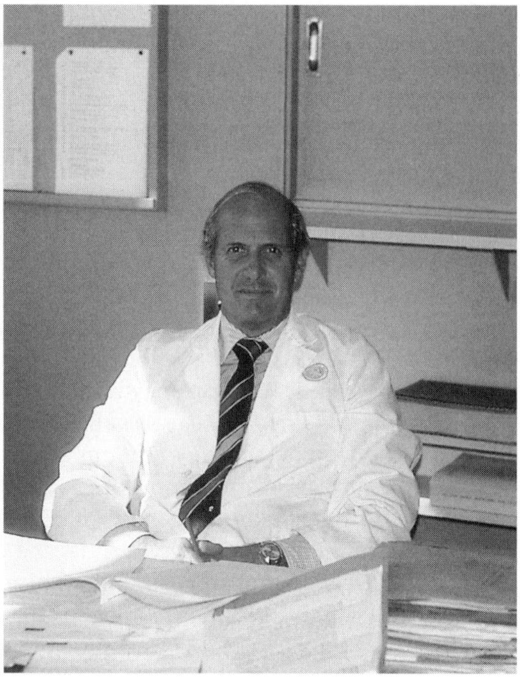

Figure 1.5 *Sir Brian Barratt-Boyes demonstrated in Auckland, New Zealand during the late 1960s that primary correction of congenital heart anomalies during infancy could be performed with a low mortality if exposure to cardiopulmonary bypass was minimized.*

ADVANTAGES OF EARLY PRIMARY REPAIR

The advantages of early primary repair were apparent from the earliest years of open heart surgery. Open heart surgery did not begin with the introduction of the heart-lung machine. Inflow occlusion with hypothermia was introduced at the University of Minnesota in 1953[16] but suffered from the important disadvantage that the time for intracardiac exposure was limited and was therefore not suitable for delicate repairs in small infants. However, a dramatic demonstration of the advantages of early repair was provided by C Walton Lillehei's cross-circulation operations in 1952 and 1953.[17,18] Using a parent as the 'oxygenator' it was possible to correct a number of congenital anomalies in infants with remarkably low morbidity and mortality and excellent long-term results. But after a support adult suffered brain injury the technique fell into disrepute and attention was focused on open heart surgery conducted with cardiopulmonary bypass. For the next two decades, through the 50s and 60s, the standard of care evolved to the two-stage approach with initial palliation and repair later in life.

In 1972 Brian Barratt-Boyes (Figure 1.5) astounded the world with his reports of successful primary repair in infancy of a wide range of congenital cardiac anomalies.[19] Both he and subsequently Castaneda (Figure 1.6) at Children's Hospital Boston[20,21] were able to achieve remarkable results in spite of the still relatively primitive state of cardiopulmonary bypass. They minimized exposure of the child to the deleterious effects of bypass by employing the technique of deep hypothermic circulatory arrest (see Chapter 9).

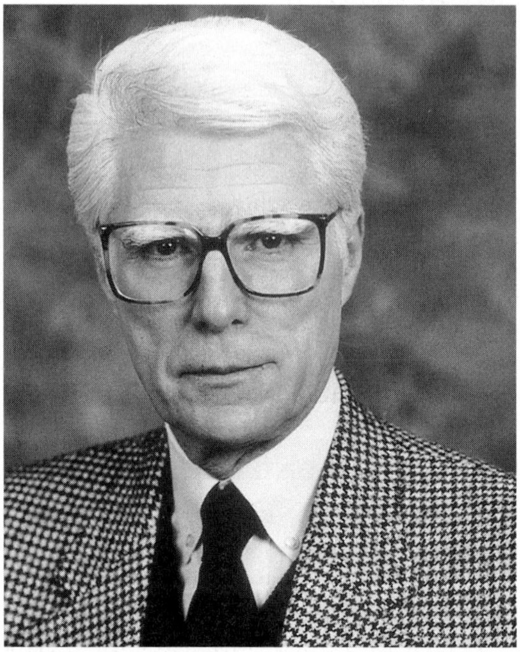

Figure 1.6 *Dr Aldo Castaneda was the third William E Ladd Professor of Surgery at Harvard Medical School and Children's Hospital Boston. Dr Castaneda, like Barratt-Boyes, popularized the concept of primary repair of congenital heart disease during infancy using deep hypothermic circulatory arrest.*

Over the next 10–15 years controversy raged regarding whether primary repair should become the standard of care for all cardiac anomalies. An important landmark occurred at the First World Congress of Pediatric Cardiac Surgery in Bergamo, Italy in 1988. Dr John Kirklin, a longtime and very vocal opponent of early primary repair entitled his keynote address 'The movement of cardiac surgery to the very young'.[22] He essentially conceded that, for many anomalies, early primary repair was as good an approach, or better, than the traditional two-stage approach. Two major events had changed his mind. One was the introduction of prostaglandin E1 in the late 1970s. The ability to maintain ductal patency in neonates allowed for preoperative stabilization, accurate diagnosis and subsequent successful repair of many complex anomalies that until that time had carried an exceedingly high mortality. Subsequently the introduction of the neonatal arterial switch procedure by Castaneda and Norwood in Boston demonstrated an important fact.[23] Although the operative mortality of the neonatal procedure was somewhat higher than the alternative Senning procedure (which was usually performed at several months of age), if one enrolled all patients with transposition from birth, an approach of early repair resulted in lower total mortality. Deaths from palliative procedures and deaths in the interval period before the Senning procedure exceeded the difference in operative mortality between the two procedures.[24]

SPECIFIC ADVANTAGES OF PRIMARY REPAIR FOR THE PATIENT

Advantages of primary repair for the heart

To fully appreciate the advantages for the heart of early repair versus an approach of palliation it is necessary to have a thorough understanding of the transition that occurs between the fetal circulation and the neonatal circulation and subsequent maturation.[25] Knowledge of the transitions in cardiopulmonary circulation is also helpful in understanding the embryological background for many of the simpler anomalies such as patent ductus (failure of normal ductal closure), coarctation (excessive ductal closure) and ASD (failure of normal foramen ovale closure).

FETAL CIRCULATION

Before birth the fetus must obtain oxygen and other nutrients from the placenta. The fetal circulation diverts blood from the lungs to the placenta through several mechanisms (Figure 1.7). Firstly the lungs themselves must have a high intrinsic vascular resistance. In part this is achieved by the collapsed state of the lungs but more importantly the resistance vessels, the pulmonary arterioles are heavily muscularized with the muscle extending far further peripherally than in mature lungs.[26]

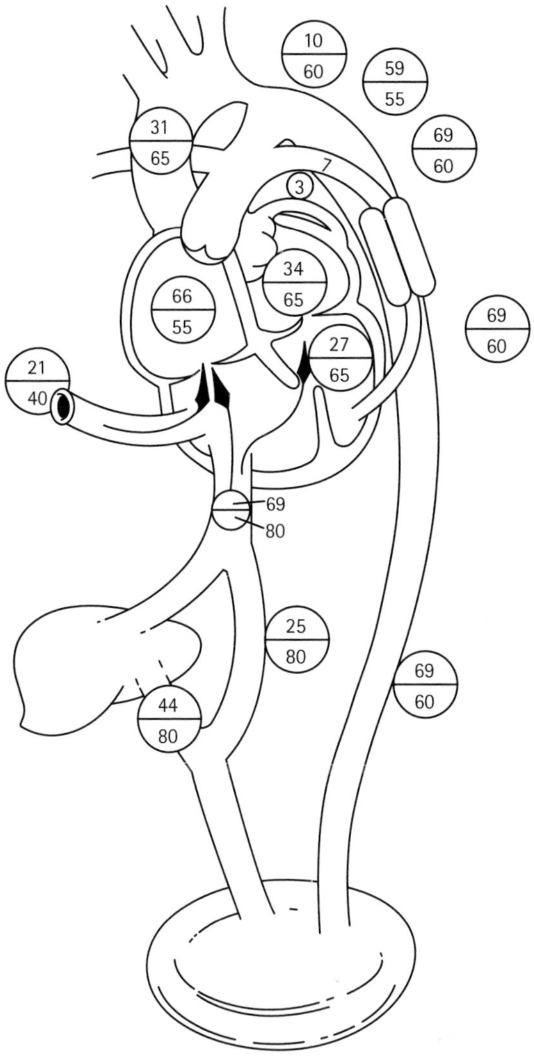

Figure 1.7 *Dr Abe Rudolph, formerly director of the catheterization laboratory at Children's Hospital Boston, while working in San Francisco, made an enormously important contribution to the understanding of congenital heart disease by his laboratory studies of the fetal circulation in lambs. Upper figures within the circles represent percentages of blood flow through the various components of the fetal circulation; lower figures represent oxygen saturation values (%). (Modified from ref. 27.)*

Because blood exiting from the right ventricle cannot easily enter the pulmonary circulation because of its high resistance, it tends to pass through the patent ductus and from there is preferentially directed into the descending aorta. From there it passes through the right and left common iliac arteries, the right and left internal iliac arteries and from there into the umbilical arteries into the placenta. Because the right ventricle is pumping to the systemic circulation there is no difference in pressure in the right ventricle relative to the left ventricle.

The transfer of oxygen across the placental membrane from maternal to fetal blood would be a very inefficient process if the hemoglobin in the fetus were the same as the mother's. The fetus has fetal hemoglobin which picks up oxygen much more avidly than mature hemoglobin and will not deliver oxygen unless the tissue oxygen level is much lower. Thus in a sense the fetus is by mature standards in a state of chronic hypoxia. The arterial oxygen saturation in the aorta is no more than 60–65%.[27] It is important to remember this fact when making decisions for the early postnatal child.

Blood returns to the fetus through the single umbilical vein. It passes through the ductus venosus to the inferior vena cava and is mainly directed by the foramen ovale across the atrial septum to the left atrium. Thus the most highly oxygenated blood will be pumped by the left ventricle to the coronary arteries and the carotid and subclavian arteries to supply the heart and the brain.

Venous blood returning from the brain passes down the superior vena cava and is preferentially directed to the right ventricle. From there it returns to the descending aorta and can either supply the abdominal organs or return to the placenta.

NORMAL TRANSITIONAL CIRCULATION

Following birth expansion of the lungs results in an immediate reduction in pulmonary vascular resistance. More blood passes into the lungs from the right ventricle and the left atrial pressure increases. The greater pressure in the left atrium relative to the right atrium which is now receiving less blood in the absence of placental return results in closure of the foramen ovale. The ductus venosus and ductus arteriosus close over the next few days through a combination of smooth muscle contraction and thrombosis with subsequent fibrosis. The pulmonary resistance continues to fall rapidly in the first days of life as smooth muscle in the pulmonary arterioles regresses.

As the pressure in the pulmonary arteries decreases the pressure in the right ventricle also decreases towards the adult level of 20–25% of left ventricular pressure.

CARDIAC MATURATION AFTER BIRTH

During the first year of life there is a continuing transition of the cardiopulmonary and vascular anatomy and physiology towards the mature state. For example fetal hemoglobin is gradually replaced by adult hemoglobin. Pulmonary resistance continues to fall. The right ventricle, which is the same thickness as the left ventricle at birth (reflecting the fact that both ventricles worked at the same pressure until ductal closure) becomes relatively thinner than the left ventricle which is rapidly increasing in thickness and total mass.[28] This is achieved by a combination of hyperplasia (new myocytes) and hypertrophy (enlargement of myocytes with increased levels of the contractile proteins myosin and actin) in the left ventricle.[29] The exact age at which cardiac myocytes lose the ability to divide is unclear but may be in the range of the first week or two to perhaps as late as three months.[30]

As new muscle develops in the immature individual it is accompanied by the development of new coronary blood vessels through the process of angiogenesis. Older individuals lose the ability to produce an appropriate increase in coronary vascular cross-sectional area and therefore have a reduced myocardial perfusion reserve if there is hypertrophy in response to a continuing pressure or volume load.[31]

In the same way that fetal hemoglobin changes to adult hemoglobin through the assembly of different isoforms of the constituents of the complex hemoglobin molecule, likewise there are changes in the constituent isoforms of myosin as maturation proceeds. A return to fetal isoforms within cardiac myosin signals a pathological state of muscular hypertrophy which can occur in response to an excessive pressure load or other disease states.[32] Volume loading of a ventricle also necessitates production of new muscle to maintain stable wall stress. The dilation of the ventricle which occurs secondary to a volume load will result in thinning of the ventricular wall unless new muscle is formed.

FAILURE OF NORMAL CARDIAC MATURATION WITH PALLIATED CIRCULATION

Because palliative surgical procedures do not correct the underlying abnormal anatomy and physiology there is likely to be a failure of the normal transitions described above which can have long-term deleterious consequences for the individual. The most common example is failure to close a large VSD as is the case with a child with tetralogy of Fallot who receives a shunt or the child with complete atrioventricular canal who receives a band. Right ventricular pressure will remain at systemic level. The right ventricle must hypertrophy to the same degree as the left ventricle which has long-term implications for myosin isoform adaptation and development of the coronary microcirculation. The relative shapes of the ventricles are affected: instead of the right ventricle adopting its usual crescent shape wrapped around the left ventricle, it will be rounder. This has important implications for the tricuspid valve which is distinguished from the mitral valve by having chordal attachments arising from the ventricular septum. The abnormal direction of pull of the septal chords can contribute to the development of tricuspid valve regurgitation. Now the ventricle will be both pressure and volume loaded.

Advantages of primary repair for the lungs

Primary repair in the neonatal period reduces both pressure and flow in the pulmonary circulation to normal. This allows for the normal transition of the pulmonary vasculature that occurs throughout the first year of life.[33] Pulmonary resistance decreases as the thick medial smooth muscle found in the neonate regresses. Within just the first month of life the ratio of wall thickness to external diameter reaches the 'adult' level of 6%.[34] Pulmonary growth in the first years of life involves development of new alveoli accompanied by new vessel development. This alveolar phase of lung development involves the formation of secondary septa in the original terminal saccules along with deposition of elastin.[35] There is some dispute about the duration of this phase with some authors concluding that alveolarization is complete by 24 months[35] while others have suggested that adult numbers of alveoli are not reached until eight years of age.[33,36] However, if perfusion remains abnormal during this period because of failure to establish a normal circulation, then lung development is likely to be abnormal.

PULMONARY VASCULAR DISEASE

Failure to reduce pulmonary artery pressure and flow in the first year or two of life introduces a risk that pulmonary vascular disease will develop. Initially this is seen as a failure of the normal regression of medial smooth muscle.[37] In time the intima will respond to the shear stress caused by the increased flow and pressure with thickening and fibrosis. As there is further progression there will be necrosis within vessel walls, medial fibrosis, formation of new vessels and occlusion of vessels.[38] Physiologically the child will progress from a state where the pulmonary vascular resistance is elevated but responds to oxygen and nitric oxide to a state where there is no change in pressure or flow with inspiration of these agents. In general a child is considered inoperable if the pulmonary resistance is greater than three quarters of systemic resistance and is fixed. This will usually correspond to a fixed resistance of greater than 12–15 Wood units. From this point the child will become progressively more cyanosed because of decreasing pulmonary blood flow until death occurs secondary to the complications of long-standing cyanosis. If the child was initially pink with a left to right shunt, the transition from pink to blue is termed Eisenmenger's syndrome.

Palliative procedures are designed to protect the lungs from the development of vascular disease. A pulmonary artery band should be tightened to reduce pressure to less than 50% systemic pressure at which level vascular disease is unlikely. However, migration of a band distally is not an uncommon problem, particularly if the band is applied through a left thoracotomy. It is difficult to fix the right side of the band. Also the anatomy of the pulmonary bifurcation, i.e. the fact that the right pulmonary artery emerges at a right angle to the main pulmonary artery quite a bit proximal to the origin of the left pulmonary artery, places the origin of the right pulmonary artery at risk of impingement by the band. If the origin of the right pulmonary artery is severely narrowed by the band more flow is directed into left pulmonary artery which is now at risk of developing vascular disease. Thus the child will have an underdeveloped right pulmonary artery and right lung and vascular disease in the left lung.

A similar complication as that seen with a migrated pulmonary artery band was not uncommon with Potts and Waterston shunts. There is a tendency for the anastomosis to not lie directly on the posterior wall of the ascending aorta in the case of the Waterston shunt. The proximal right pulmonary artery is twisted to the right and becomes severely stenosed or occluded. This reduces flow into the left lung which will become hypoplastic. All of the flow from the shunt is directed into the right lung which is at significant risk of developing vascular disease.

Even the classic Blalock shunt is not immune from the risk of causing vascular disease. If the shunt is constructed with absorbable suture at the anastomosis there can be excessive growth resulting in excessive pressure and flow and ultimate development of vascular disease.

Advantages of primary repair for the brain

BRAIN DEVELOPMENT IN THE FIRST YEAR OF LIFE

There is an enormous increase in the size and complexity of the human brain during the first year of life which risks being compromised by abnormal cardiovascular physiology.[39] The human neonatal brain weighs 350 g, while the adult brain weighs 1400 g. Much of this growth occurs during the first year of life with brain weight increasing to 500 g by three months, 660 g by six months and 925 g by one year of age.[40] Although there is little evidence that neurons are added after birth, there is a large increase in the number of glial cells, the size and complexity of the neurons, the amount of myelin and the number and complexity of neuronal connections. The primary visual cortex, for example, increases in thickness until the sixth postnatal month when it attains values observed in adults. However, in other cortical areas there is a long and variable increase in cortical thickness that approaches maturity around 10 years after birth.[41]

The number of synaptic connections increases tremendously in the first year of life. In the visual cortex, for example, there is a gradual increase in synaptic density during late gestation and in early postnatal life.[41] However, between two and four months postnatally there is a steep increase during which time the number of synapses doubles. After one year of age, however, there is a decline in synaptic density until adult values (50–60% of maximum) are attained at about 11 years of age (Figure 1.8).

Positron emission tomography has demonstrated that cerebral metabolic activity parallels the rise and decline in the number of synapses in human frontal cortex suggesting that the exuberant synapses are metabolically active. In newborns there is little metabolic activity in the cerebral cortex though there is substantial subcortical activation. Over the first three to four years of life, cortical metabolic rate increases until it reaches a level which is twice that seen in adults. After four years of age metabolic activity decreases until adult levels are reached at around 15 years.

There are important maturational changes in high energy phosphate metabolism in the first weeks of life. ATP synthesis catalysed by creatine kinase increases about four times in the rat brain in the narrow timeframe between 10 and 15 days of postnatal age.[42] This allows the maturing animal to mobilize energy stores more rapidly from phosphocreatine and may

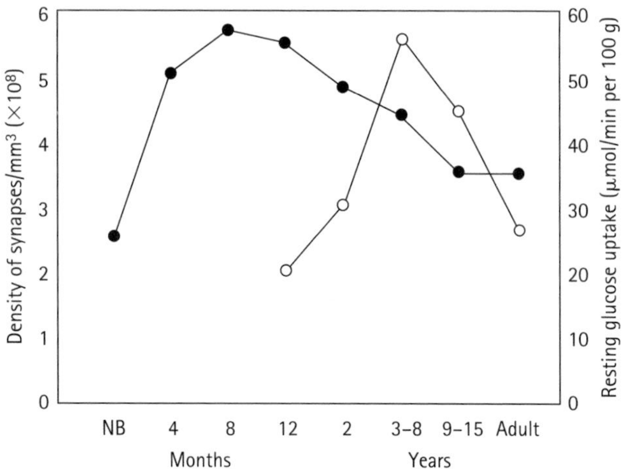

Figure 1.8 *Synaptic density in the human visual cortex (black circles) increases rapidly in the first year of life. Beyond one to two years of age the density of synapses decreases. The white circles illustrate resting glucose uptake in the occipital cortex. (Adapted from Zigmond MJ, Bloom FE, Landis SC, Roberts JL, Squire LR (eds).* Fundamental Neuroscience. *San Diego, Academic Press, 1999, p 1315, with permission from Elsevier.)*

protect against energy 'surges' in response to excitotoxic hypoxic–ischemic stresses that occur during birth.[43–45] The limited number of synapses and limited energy stores of the neonate during delivery bring to mind the protective strategy of shipping a new computer with the components not yet wired together and the battery uncharged.

EFFECTS OF CYANOSIS AND CONGESTIVE HEART FAILURE

There are few hard data demonstrating the effects of chronic cyanosis or chronic congestive heart failure on cerebral development. Newburger et al[46] studied the cognitive outcome in children with transposition who had undergone physiological correction at various ages. She was able to demonstrate that there was a correlation between older age at repair and worse outcome, presumably secondary to the effects of chronic cyanosis.

Chronic congestive cardiac failure is usually manifest in children as failure to thrive. Presumably this has a significant impact on the organ which is maturing most rapidly in the first year of life, i.e. the brain.

In contrast to the effects of chronic cyanosis the effects of acute severe hypoxia on the brain have been well documented. Hypoxic–ischemic brain injury has been well studied in the newborn, usually in the setting of birth asphyxia.[45] Hypoxic-ischemic brain injury results in the release of massive quantities of glutamate and other neurotransmitters. The excitation of neurons in the setting of limited energy substrates can result in cell death which has been labelled 'excitotoxicity'. In the developing brain the areas at greatest risk of injury from excitotoxicity probably correspond to areas of greatest synaptic development and density.[47]

Other advantages of primary repair for the patient: risk of death

The principal argument stated by those who oppose an approach of primary repair is that the risk is too great. In fact studies such as the Congenital Heart Surgeon's study of the management of transposition have demonstrated that the mortality risk of an initial palliative procedure combined with the risk of an interval period of medical treatment combined with the risk of the corrective procedure is greater than the risk of a corrective procedure alone.[24] In the case of surgery for transposition cited the early mortality risks of the definitive procedures appeared to favor an atrial level repair. However, a complete and inclusive analysis demonstrated conclusively the survival advantage of the arterial switch strategy. It is important to use current statistics when comparing different approaches and not to use historical controls because the mortality risk of all procedures both open and closed have improved tremendously over the last 10–15 years.

ADVANTAGES OF PRIMARY REPAIR FOR THE FAMILY

Consider two scenarios: the young family, perhaps with their first child, is told that their child has tetralogy of Fallot. The parents are told to take the child home and that surgery will be undertaken later in the first year of life. However, they are warned that there is a chance that the child might have a cyanotic spell, particularly if the child is allowed to become upset, which could result in death or brain damage unless the parents seek medical care immediately. The parents live in great fear that the slightest cry may signify the onset of a spell and are extremely overprotective towards the child. When the child does begin to have spells a few weeks later a shunt is undertaken. The child requires multiple follow-up visits and is scheduled for a subsequent corrective operation a year later. The parents worry constantly about the operation which is finally undertaken at 18 months of age.

In the second scenario an approach of early primary repair is recommended. Following diagnosis in the neonatal period surgery is scheduled for four weeks of age, which allows the parents time to make the necessary logistical arrangements. By five weeks the child is home with a normal circulation. The parents are reassured that there is no further risk of a cyanotic spell and are able to treat the child normally.

Having a child with a congenital heart problem is a great stress for young families. One need only look at the incidence of divorce in this setting to appreciate the magnitude of the problem.[48] It is essential that caregivers focus on the whole family unit rather than only considering the child.

ADVANTAGES OF PRIMARY REPAIR FOR SOCIETY: ECONOMICS

The traditional two-stage approach requires a period of medical treatment and observation before the palliative procedure, two surgical procedures and an interval period of medical palliation. The combined costs have been documented to be approximately double the cost of primary repair.[49]

CONCLUSIONS

An approach of complete repair in the neonatal period or early infancy of all congenital cardiac anomalies which have no probability of spontaneous resolution is preferred. There is no evidence in the current era of any survival advantage when a palliative procedure is employed to defer definitive surgical repair. There are multiple advantages for the patient's development in having as normal a circulation as possible as early in life as possible. There are many secondary advantages of early primary repair for the patient's family as well as for society in general.

REFERENCES

1. Gross RE, Hubbard JP. Surgical ligation of a patent ductus arteriosus. Report of first successful case. *JAMA* 1939; **112**:729–731.
2. Crafoord C, Nylin G. Congenital coarctation of the aorta and its surgical treatment. *J Thorac Surg* 1945; **14**:347–361.
3. Gross RE. Surgical correction for coarctation of the aorta. *Surgery* 1945; **18**:673–678.
4. Gross RE. *The Surgery of Infancy and Childhood.* Philadelphia, WB Saunders, 1953.
5. Kirklin JK, Westaby S, Blackstone EH, Kirklin JW, Chenoweth DE, Pacifico AD. Complement and the damaging effects of cardiopulmonary bypass. *J Thorac Cardiovasc Surg* 1983; **86**:845–857.
6. Harake B, Power GG. Thoracic duct lymph flow. A comparative study in newborn and adult sheep. *J Dev Physiol* 1986; **8**:87–95.
7. Rosenthal SM, LaJohn LA. Effect of age on transvascular fluid movement. *Am J Physiol* 1975; **228**:134–140.
8. Blalock A, Taussig HB. The surgical treatment of malformations of the heart in which there is pulmonary stenosis or pulmonary atresia. *JAMA* 1945; **128**:189–202.
9. Waterston DJ. Treatment of Fallot's tetralogy in children under one year of age. *Rozhl Chir* 1962; **41**:181.
10. Potts WJ, Smith S, Gibson S. Anastomosis of the aorta to a pulmonary artery. *JAMA* 1946; **132**:627–631.
11. de Leval MR, McKay R, Jones M, Stark J, MacCartney FJ. Modified Blalock-Taussig shunt. Use of subclavian artery orifice as flow regulator in prosthetic systemic-pulmonary artery shunts. *J Thorac Cardiovasc Surg* 1981; **81**:112–119.
12. Muller WH, Dammann JF. The treatment of certain congenital malformations of the heart by the creation of pulmonic stenosis to reduce pulmonary hypertension and excessive pulmonary blood flow: A preliminary report. *Surg Gynecol Obstet* 1952; **95**:213.
13. Blalock A, Hanlon CR. The surgical treatment of complete transposition of the aorta and the pulmonary artery. *Surg Gynecol Obstet* 1950; **90**:1–15.
14. Rashkind WJ, Miller WW. Creation of an atrial septal defect without thoracotomy. A palliative approach to complete transposition of the great arteries. *JAMA* 1966; **196**; 991–992.
15. Rashkind WJ, Miller WW. Transposition of the great arteries. Results of palliation by balloon atrioseptostomy in thirty-one infants. *Circulation* 1968; **38**:453–462.
16. Lewis FJ, Taufic M. Closure of atrial septal defects with the aid of hypothermia: Experimental accomplishments and the report of the one successful case. *Surgery* 1953; **33**:52–59.
17. Warden HE, Cohen M, Read RC, Lillehei CW. Controlled cross circulation for open intracardiac surgery. *J Thorac Surg* 1954; **28**:331.
18. Lillehei CW, Cohen M, Warden HE, Ziegler NR, Varco RL. The results of direct vision closure of ventricular septal defects in eight patients by means of controlled cross circulation. *Surg Gynecol Obstet* 1955; **101**:446.
19. Barratt-Boyes BG, Neutze JM, Harris EA. *Heart Disease in Infancy.* Edinburgh, Churchill Livingstone, 1973.
20. Castaneda AR, Lamberti J, Sade RM, Williams RG, Nadas AS. Open-heart surgery in the first three months of life. *J Thorac Cardiovasc Surg* 1974; **68**:719–731.
21. Castaneda AR, Jonas RA, Mayer JE, Hanley FL. *Cardiac Surgery of the Neonate and Infant.* Philadelphia, WB Saunders, 1994.
22. Kirklin JW. The movement of cardiac surgery to the very young. In Crupi G, Parenzan L, Anderson RH (eds). *Perspectives in Pediatric Cardiology.* Mt Kisco, NY, Futura Publishing Co, 1989, pp 3–22.
23. Castaneda AR, Norwood WI, Jonas RA, Colan SD, Sanders SP, Lang P. Transposition of the great arteries and intact ventricular septum: Anatomical repair in the neonate. *Ann Thorac Surg* 1984; **5**:438–443.
24. Norwood WI, Dobell AR, Freed MD, Kirklin JW, Blackstone EH. Intermediate results of the arterial switch repair. A 20-institution study. *J Thorac Cardiovasc Surg* 1988; **96**:854–863.
25. Rudolph AM. The changes in the circulation after birth. Their importance in congenital heart disease. *Circulation* 1980; **41**:343–359.
26. Haworth SG, Sauer U, Buhlmeyer K, Reid L. Development of the pulmonary circulation in ventricular septal defect: a quantitative structural study. *Am J Cardiol* 1977; **40**:781–788.
27. Rudolph AM. Changes in the circulation after birth. In Rudolph AM (ed). *Congenital Diseases of the Heart.* Chicago, Year Book Medical Publishers, 1974.
28. Emery JL, Mithal A. Weights of cardiac ventricles at and after birth. *Br Heart J* 1961; **23**:313.
29. Zak R. Development and proliferative capacity of cardiac muscle cells. *Circ Res* 1974; **35**:17–26.
30. Anversa P, Olivetti G, Loud AV. Morphometric study of early postnatal development in the left and right ventricular myocardium of the rat. I. Hypertrophy, hyperplasia and binucleation of myocytes. *Circ Res* 1980; **46**:495–502.
31. Flanagan MF, Fujii AM, Colan SD, Flanagan RG, Lock JE. Myocardial angiogenesis and coronary perfusion in left ventricular pressure overload hypertrophy in the young lamb: Evidence for inhibition with chronic protamine administration. *Circ Res* 1991; **68**:1458–1470.
32. Izumo S, Nadal-Ginard B, Mahdavi V. Protooncogene induction and reprogramming of cardiac gene expression produced by pressure overload. *Proc Natl Acad Sci USA* 1988; **85**:339–342.

33. Reid LM. Lung growth in health and disease. *Br J Dis Chest* 1984; **78**:113–134.
34. Haworth SG. Pulmonary vascular development. In Long WA (ed). *Fetal and Neonatal Cardiology.* Philadelphia, WB Saunders, 1990, pp 51–63.
35. Burri PH. Postnatal development and growth. In Crystal RG, West JB, Barnes PJ, et al (eds). *The Lung.* New York, Raven Press, 1991, pp 677–687.
36. Inselman LS, Mellins RB. Growth and development of the lung. *J Pediatr* 1981; **98**:1–15.
37. Heath D, Edwards JE. The pathology of hypertensive pulmonary vascular changes in the pulmonary artery with special reference to congenital cardiac septal defect. *Circulation* 1958; **18**:533–547.
38. Rabinovitch M, Keane JF, Norwood WI, et al. Vascular structure in lung tissue obtained at biopsy correlated with pulmonary hemodynamic findings after repair of congenital heart defects. *Circulation* 1984; **69**:655–667.
39. Castaneda AR, Jonas RA, Mayer JE, Hanley FL. *Cardiac Surgery of the Neonate and Infant.* Philadelphia, WB Saunders, 1994, pp 8–18.
40. Afifi AK, Bergman RA. *Basic Neuroscience.* Baltimore, Urbain & Schwartzberg, 1986.
41. Albert MS, Diamond AD, Fitch RH, Neville HJ, Rapp PR, Tallal PA. Cognitive development. In Zigmond MJ, Bloom FE, Landis SC, Roberts JL, Squire LR (eds). *Fundamental Neuroscience.* San Diego, Academic Press, 1999, p 1315.
42. Holtzman D, Olson J, Zamvil S, Nguyen H. Maturation of potassium stimulated respiration in rat cerebral cortex slices. *J Neurochem* 1982; **39**:274–276.
43. Meldrum B. Protection against ischemic neuronal damage by drugs acting on excitatory neurotransmission. *Cerebrovasc Brain Metab Rev* 1990; **2**:27–57.
44. Olney JW, Ho OL, Rhee V. Cytotoxic effects of acidic and sulphur-containing amino acids on the infant mouse central nervous system. *Exp Brain Res* 1971; **14**:61–76.
45. Volpe JJ. Hypoxic ischemic encephalopathy: Basic aspects and fetal assessment. In Volpe JJ (ed). *Neurology of the Newborn.* Philadelphia, WB Saunders, 1987, pp 160–195.
46. Newburger JW, Silbert AR, Buckley LP, Fyler DC. Cognitive function and age at repair of transposition of the great arteries in children. *N Engl J Med* 1984; **310**:1495–1499.
47. Greenamyre T, Penney JB, Young AB, Hudson C, Silverstein FS, Johnston MV. Evidence for transient perinatal glutamatergic innervation of globus pallidus. *J Neurosci* 1987; **7**:1022–1030.
48. Silbert AR, Newburger JW, Fyler DC. Marital stability and congenital heart disease. *Pediatrics* 1982; **69**:747–750.
49. Ungerleider RM, Kanter RJ, O'Laughlin M, et al. Effect of repair strategy on hospital cost for infants with tetralogy of Fallot. *Ann Surg* 1997; **225**:779–783.

2

Surgical technique

INTRODUCTION

Surgery for congenital heart disease requires a wide range of strengths, skills and knowledge of techniques which are rarely written about in text books or journals. There is no question that certain individuals can master the necessary skills more easily than others but fundamentally they are skills that can be taught and learned.

There are emotional and psychological challenges in all surgical specialties but congenital heart surgery presents its own special challenges. It is heart-breaking to witness the shock of discovery of severe life-threatening cardiac disease in any newborn. But to be a part of the same experience with a childless couple who may have tried for years to achieve pregnancy, endured the stresses of pregnancy and then have to confront major surgery for their child is doubly painful. It is said that the death of a child is the single greatest tragedy that anyone can face in a lifetime. The congenital heart surgeon bears witness to the truth of these words many times in a career. On the other hand there is no greater reward than to be able to save a child from the certain death threatened by a serious congenital cardiac malformation. It is this fact, and the fundamental knowledge that one has made every possible effort to do one's best for every child, that allows the congenital cardiac surgeon to carry the weight of those who do not survive.

Congenital cardiac surgery offers not only emotional and psychological challenges but also physical ones. A wide range of patient size is encountered. In the same day the surgeon may deal with the tiny structures and fragile tissues in a 450 g preterm infant and later be confronted by a 400 pound (180 kg) adult with a history of multiple previous operations. Thus there is a need to be able to 'shift gears' and to transition from the delicacy of the eye surgeon to the brute strength of the orthopedic surgeon. The reoperative procedure in the adult may take many hours and demand physical stamina and endurance as well as strength. Muscle strength and stamina are not things that just happen. No matter how busy a surgeon's schedule, there must be time to maintain physical fitness.

Many congenital surgical procedures must be performed under time pressure. Application of the aortic cross clamp starts the clock ticking and requires that the procedure be completed within two to three hours at most. Thus the surgeon must carefully plan and sequence the procedure so that it is completed within this timeframe. The surgeon must aim for a meticulously correct procedure and be self-critical of the result. On the other hand the time limit must be respected and may require that reasonable compromises be accepted. There is no question that the aphorism 'perfect is the enemy of good' must be understood and practiced by every congenital cardiac surgeon.

Congenital cardiac surgery requires an ability to multitask. While there are many others in the room who are responsible for critically important tasks, it is ultimately the surgeon who must tell the family if the child has not survived and it is the surgeon to whom the family has directly entrusted their child. Thus the surgeon must constantly monitor the performance of all team members, particularly those who are inexperienced. The surgeon must monitor the status of the patient, the perfusion conditions, keep track of ischemic time, plan the next steps in the procedure as well as focus on meticulous performance of the task at hand whether that be dissection, cannulation or suturing. This requires practice in hearing what one is not listening to and seeing what one is not looking at.

GENERAL SETUP

Room temperature

One of the first things the visitor to the cardiac operating room notices is the low temperature. Hypothermia is an essential part of brain, heart and spinal cord protection during periods of reduced blood flow, such as cross-clamp periods and low flow cardiopulmonary bypass. It is important to remember that the surgical team should be aiming to keep the myocardial temperature at less than 10°C during the cross-clamp period and during circulatory arrest or low flow the brain temperature should be maintained at less than 15°C. Surface cooling before bypass is almost certainly useful. Therefore the room temperature should be maintained at less than 17–18°C until all clamps have been released and the patient is being rewarmed at full flow. Hyperthermia following ischemia should be assiduously avoided as it has been shown to exacerbate reperfusion injury.[1]

Lighting

Intense lighting is an often unrecognized source of heat. The yellowish light from tungsten sources contains very much more infrared heat than halogen sources which have an obvious blue hue. The limited spotlight of a halogen headlight reduces tissue heating relative to dependence on large overhead lights. The limited area that is illuminated by a headlight also improves visualization for the surgeon by reducing glare from areas other than the direct field of view of the surgeon. One only needs to witness how obsessional the radiologist is about switching off all other light sources when viewing an X-ray to be reminded of the importance of reducing distracting sources of light. Congenital cardiac surgery should always be performed with a headlight.

Magnification

Magnification with surgical loupes is an essential part of almost every congenital cardiac procedure. Many surgeons prefer expanded field 3.5 × loupes with a relatively long focal length of 48–51 cm (19 or 20 in). If all members of the surgical team are wearing loupes they are able to keep their heads at a distance from the field and yet have improved vision relative to the naked eye. No matter how good one's vision is without loupes, it will be better with magnification. And as time marches on and presbyopia develops, loupes become even more essential.

In addition to improving vision, loupes are an important aid to optimal use of the surgical headlight. The field of vision through the loupes must be carefully and accurately aligned with the spotlight at the beginning of the procedure. This will ensure that there is accurate lighting of the surgical field of view throughout the procedure.

Headlight video camera

Modern miniaturized video cameras mounted on the headlight are very useful for the congenital cardiac surgeon. Since almost all congenital cardiac surgery is in a sense 'minimally invasive' in that the cardiac incisions must be limited, it is often difficult for all members of the team to be able to follow the progress of the procedure. Use of a video camera allows not only the second and first assistant to view details of the anatomy they might not otherwise be able to see, but in addition the nurses, perfusion technician and anesthesia team can see at a glance what phase of the procedure is in progress.

Instruments

There is a misconception that surgery on small patients should be performed using small instruments. While it is true that many of the instruments used for congenital cardiac surgery need to be delicate, they should not necessarily be short. They need to be long enough to allow three pairs of hands – the surgeon and two assistants – to simultaneously work within a limited incision. On the other hand the depth of the surgical field in neonates and infants is very much less than the depth that the adult surgeon is used to. This is an important advantage for the surgeon in that it allows the hand to be stabilized on the chest wall. Congenital cardiac surgeons can use time in the dentist's chair profitably by analysing the methods by which dentists and hygienists stabilize their hands without leaning on the jaw. As with dental instruments, most of the movement of instruments used by the congenital cardiac surgeon should be controlled by the fine muscles of the hand and not by the forearm and shoulder girdle muscles. Microvascular instruments, such as the Castro-Viejo needle holder are specifically designed to be controlled by the fingers rather than by the arms and are therefore ideal (Figure 2.1).

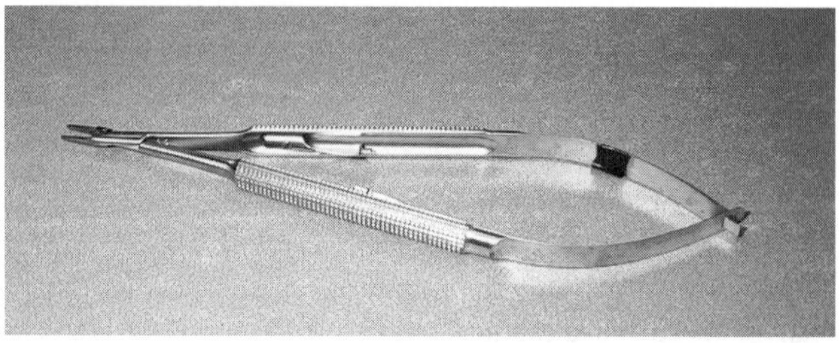

Figure 2.1 *Microvascular instruments such as the Castro-Viejo needle holder are particularly useful for delicate neonatal congenital cardiac procedures. These instruments are designed to be controlled by the fingers rather than by the arms.*

INCISIONS

Primary median sternotomy

The median sternotomy is used for the overwhelming majority of congenital cardiac surgical procedures. It has many advantages. Relative to most other surgical incisions it has less postoperative pain, particularly in young children who have very flexible bones and elastic ligaments. Opening the sternum requires hinging of the ribs at the costovertebral joints which is part of the normal motion of the ribs with respiration. Unlike adults, children rarely complain of back, neck or interscapular pain following a sternotomy. The incision does not require stretching, cutting or tearing of any muscles unlike so many other incisions. The blood supply of the bone is excellent in children so that healing is usually rapid and complete. Sternal osteomyelitis is almost unheard of in young children even following purulent mediastinitis. Fortunately the latter is relatively rare.

The skin incision used for a standard median sternotomy should be individualized according to the procedure which is to be performed. For example, the Norwood procedure with a Blalock shunt involves work on the great vessels and right subclavian artery so that the incision should extend up to the sternal notch. On the other hand the lower end of the incision can be limited and does not need to extend to the bottom of the xiphoid process. For the majority of intracardiac procedures, however, the top end of the skin incision can be limited to end some distance below the sternal notch. This is an important cosmetic consideration since the major disadvantage of the standard incision is the fact that it can be seen in a visually important area of the body. By limiting the upper end of the incision it is possible to conceal the incision with most clothing.

It is critically important that the bone incision be exactly in the midline. The width of the sternum varies tremendously between children and it may be very narrow. If the incision is made off midline there is a real risk that the sternal wires will cut through the delicate cartilaginous bone resulting in an unstable sternum and poor healing. An unstable sternum will increase the risk of mediastinal infection. Unlike adults where infection can precipitate instability of the sternum, in children sternal instability is much more often the result of an off-midline incision or poor wiring technique and infection is secondary.

Minimally invasive sternotomy

There are a number of options to improve the cosmetic appearance of the standard sternotomy incision. It has not been possible to prove that minimally invasive incisions reduce pain or speed convalescence.[2] Our preference has been to limit the incision in the sternum to the lower half or two thirds leaving the manubrium at least intact. The sternum is sufficiently flexible in children that there seems to be little or no advantage in 't-ing' off the incision to one or other side. The skin incision can be limited to as short as 3.5–4 cm and can be kept entirely below the level of the nipples. While this limited incision allows for safe closure of septal defects we generally do not use it for more complex procedures.

Reoperative sternotomy

Reopening a sternal incision can be done safely as long as it is carefully planned and executed. Planning begins with the preoperative studies which should document the distance between the back of the sternum and cardiac structures. The surgical team should also have knowledge about the status of the femoral and iliac vessels. This knowledge may be available from the preoperative catheterization or simply from careful palpation of the femoral pulses and observation for evidence of previous cutdown incisions. At least one groin should be prepped into the surgical field. Injury to the right heart can generally be dealt with easily by cannulating the femoral artery and placing a pump sucker in the injured structure. On the other hand injury to the aorta is a serious problem and must be avoided. Even emergency cannulation of the femoral vessels after an aortic injury has occurred will not be helpful because blood pumped into the arterial system from any cannulation site will simply exit via the site of aortic injury. Certain anomalies carry a higher risk of injury to the aorta, most notably d-transposition of the great arteries. The preoperative catheterization should include lateral images which have a sufficiently large frame size to show both the sternal wires and images of the aorta. This may require a long sequence to allow the levo phase of a right heart injection to outline the aorta. If the aorta is close to the posterior table of the sternum and particularly if there is obvious adhesion which will be apparent because of absence of relative movement between the two structures, then femoral cannulation is required of both the femoral artery and vein before the sternotomy is begun. The child should be cooled on femoral bypass before the bone is cut in the vicinity of the aorta.

If the preoperative studies demonstrate that a right heart structure is very close or adherent to the sternum, at a minimum the femoral artery should be cannulated before the bone is cut. It is often wise to cannulate a femoral vein also with a thin-walled cannula, such as the Biomedicus cannula. The cannula should be advanced to the level of the right atrium to allow good decompression of the right heart. If the femoral arteries are occluded bilaterally it may be necessary to use an external iliac artery. Rather than following the femoral vessels up under the inguinal ligament it is preferable to use an iliac fossa retroperitoneal approach. It should be exceedingly rare that axillary artery cannulation is required. Carotid artery cannulation is not recommended other than in the most extreme situations because there is a risk that cerebral blood flow will be compromised.

The previous skin scar is usually excised and the sternal wires are cut and removed. The xiphoid process is divided and the linea alba is opened to allow a plane to be developed behind the lower end of the sternum. Rake retractors are used to elevate the lower end of the sternum off the heart and to provide a counter pressure to the oscillating sternal saw. Short segments of bone are cut through sequentially up to but not through the posterior table which is then divided with heavy scissors while visualizing the space behind the sternum. Electrocautery is now used again to develop space more cephalad. If a conduit is known to be close to the left side of the sternum it may be advisable to free up only the right half of the sternum until the retractor is placed. However ultimately dissection should extend to the pleural cavities bilaterally. This will allow the pleural cavities to be drained at the completion of the procedure but more importantly it allows the heart to be moved around more freely, thereby improving exposure without having to retract the chambers of the heart itself with undue force.

When the bone incision has been completed and the sternal retractor is in place dissection is begun using the electrocautery. Dissection should be begun in the space between the diaphragm and the inferior surface of the heart which is almost always a free space. Grasping the diaphragm with forceps and moving it up and down helps to identify the correct plane. The space is traced rightwards until the right atrium is identified. Sufficient inferior right atrial free wall is cleared to allow placement of at least one venous cannula.

The focus of dissection should now shift to the aorta. Once again a sufficient area is cleared to allow safe cannulation. In fact it may be the surgeon's choice to proceed with cannulation at this stage. The remainder of the dissection can proceed during the cooling phase of bypass. Decompression of the right atrium allows dissection in this area to proceed more rapidly and safely.

Sternal closure

The sternum is closed with wires of an appropriate gauge for the child's size. If the sternum is very narrow it may be advisable to place the wires through the costal cartilage to increase the depth of the bite. Ischemic necrosis caused by the encircling wires is rarely if ever seen. On the other hand wires with an inadequate depth of bite will often cut through the thin and delicate bone of the child's sternum.

If there is hemodynamic instability or ongoing bleeding that is difficult to control it may be wise to leave the sternum open. This situation most commonly arises in neonates but rarely beyond infancy. If hemodynamic instability is severe and the surgical team has determined that there is no remediable anatomic cause, it may even be advisable to stent open the sternum. This can be done with the malleable Logan Bow used for cleft palate surgery though there are many innovative alternatives, such as a partial syringe. An Esmarch latex patch is sutured to the skin edges with continuous nylon. Betadine ointment is applied to the edges of the patch. An iodoform-impregnated adhesive plastic drape is then placed widely over the surgical site covering both the Esmarch patch and the exiting chest tubes, monitoring lines and temporary pacemaker wires.

Posterolateral thoracotomy

A posterolateral thoracotomy is used for repair of coarctation but little else in the modern era. Today shunts and bands are placed through a sternotomy approach and a patent ductus is ligated through ports using a video-assisted approach.

The thoracotomy for coarctation repair should be in the third or fourth space but never the fifth. It is mainly a posterior rather than a lateral incision so that it should not be necessary to divide any of the serratus anterior. Only a small amount of the trapezius should be divided and none of the erector spinae.

The thoracotomy incision should be closed with absorbable pericostal sutures to avoid intercostal muscle compression by a permanent suture. The ribs should not be pulled together so tightly that they overlap. The muscle layer is closed with a running absorbable suture, such as Vicryl followed by a subcutaneous and subcuticular layer. In small, sick neonates it is occasionally advisable to close the thick skin of the back with interrupted nylon sutures because this area is prone to breaking down, presumably because of its less-good blood supply and the fact that the child is lying on the incision.

DISSECTION

The blood supply of the child's mediastinum is remarkably profuse. The advantage for the surgeon is that healing is rapid and risk of infection is low. However the disadvantage is that bleeding can be troublesome. Bleeding can be reduced by accurate dissection in the less vascular planes that almost always exist between structures, no matter how many previous procedures. There is probably no single skill in the field of congenital surgery which seems to be as innate as the ability to see these tissue planes. Surgical mentors when comparing notes about a trainee are apt to make the statement 'he or she can "see" the planes'. Nevertheless the ability to find the planes can be learned over time. And, most importantly, skill can be developed in using electrocautery for dissection.

Electrocautery

Electrocautery is an essential tool for the congenital cardiac surgeon. Every surgeon will learn to find a blend of cutting and coagulation current that suits his or her dissecting style. The blend will need to be varied depending on the tissue characteristics. For example, the woody edematous planes that are found in the child who has had a bidirectional Glenn shunt are best developed with a predominantly coagulation current with appropriate counter traction developed between the surgeon and assistant to open the plane. A strong coagulation current is often useful when taking lung adhesions down because very vascular adhesions will have developed, particularly to the heart itself but also to the chest wall. However once the pericardial cavity has been entered it is often best to change to sharp dissection with curved tip Metzenbaum scissors. The curved tip is used to gently push the planes apart and to develop the adhesions which can then be cut.

Electrocautery carries a risk of injury to nerves, particularly the phrenic nerve, if it is used indiscriminately. Care must be taken to reduce the strength of the current when dissecting close to the phrenic. It may be advisable to use sharp dissection when very close to the nerve. However when adhesions are very dense and vascular, injury to nerves can occur despite the most meticulous care in dissection.

PLANNING THE SEQUENCE OF AN OPERATION

Congenital cardiac procedures often involve complex three-dimensional reconstruction. By carefully planning the sequence of the operation the surgeon can optimize the exposure and the efficiency of the procedure. Lack of planning is usually very obvious. It is very easy to 'paint oneself into a corner' from which point the only way out is to take down some of the work that has already been done. Take for example the reconstruction for truncus arteriosus. After the pulmonary arteries have been harvested from the truncus by transecting the trunk one could then choose to reanastomose the aorta. But a better approach is to perform the distal anastomosis of the homograft while the aorta is divided. The exposure of the homograft to pulmonary artery bifurcation is immeasurably better when the surgeon does not have to work over and behind the aorta. And of course the homograft must have been selected, thawed and rinsed by the time it is needed so this should have been done at an earlier phase of the procedure.

Another example of sequencing which can shorten ischemic time is the repair of coarctation with hypoplastic arch. If a reverse subclavian flap is to be constructed to deal with the arch then this should be done before ligating the duct. The distal aortic clamp is applied across the isthmus and the reverse subclavian flap is performed first while the distal aorta is perfused by the patent duct. Subsequently the clamps are moved to allow the duct to be ligated and divided and the coarctation to be resected and repaired by direct anatomosis.

Walking oneself through the steps of an operation before the procedure itself should be an essential part of any procedure by any surgeon, no matter how experienced. The planning phase will also allow a decision to be made about the critically important issue of cannulation for cardiopulmonary bypass.

CANNULATION AND VENTING

Mediastinal or peripheral?

Central cannulation is preferred for the vast majority of congenital cardiac procedures. The use of femoral or iliac cannulation has been discussed above in the setting of the reoperative sternotomy.

Arterial cannulation

There is no 'routine' site for cannulation of the ascending aorta for congenital surgical procedures. The surgeon should always think about how the arterial cannula can be sited to optimize exposure. For example for an arterial switch procedure it is important to place the cannula as distally as possible though there is no advantage in cannulating the arch as clamp placement might compromise innominate artery flow. In repair of interrupted aortic arch it is important to place the cannula on the right side of the ascending aorta opposite the site of the planned anastomosis. The tip of the cannula will then project into the arch and will not 'back-wall' which can result in swings in arterial line pressure. In fact the small size of the ascending aorta in neonates and infants means that it is often useful to place the cannula in such a way that it will project into the arch rather than back-walling in the ascending aorta. Furthermore a small rubber ring cut from a tourniquet should be placed on the cannula and adjusted to set the tip at an appropriate depth according to the size of the aorta. For an aorta that is no more than 5–6 mm in diameter the depth will be set at 2.5–3 mm. The small size of the aorta also means that the construction of the aortic purse-string suture is very important. As shown in Figure 2.2, a small diamond-shaped purse-string should be placed. The longer axis should never lie transversely as this will increase the risk that when the purse-string is tied down it may stenose the aorta.

The different models and brands of arterial cannula that are available are discussed in Chapter 6. Some specific, unusual arterial cannulation situations, such as for interrupted aortic arch and hypoplastic left heart syndrome, are discussed in the respective chapters.

Venous cannulation

SINGLE VENOUS RIGHT ATRIAL CANNULA

A single venous cannula is placed within the right atrium for cooling to deep hypothermia for circulatory arrest and is also often used when the procedure will be limited to the left heart and there are no septal defects, e.g. resection of a subaortic membrane. It can be used for continuous bypass for neonates and small infants who do have septal defects when the majority of the procedure is extracardiac, such as the arterial switch procedure. When the cannula is well placed it is even possible to perform intracardiac procedures, such as VSD closure for infant tetralogy repair with bypass ongoing, by relying on the competence of the tricuspid valve. There are both advantages and disadvantages with a single right atrial cannula.

Advantages

Apart from its simplicity one of the most important advantages of the single venous cannula is that it is highly unlikely that there will be unidentified venous obstruction during the bypass run. The surgeon is able to monitor the adequacy of venous drainage very easily by observing the degree of

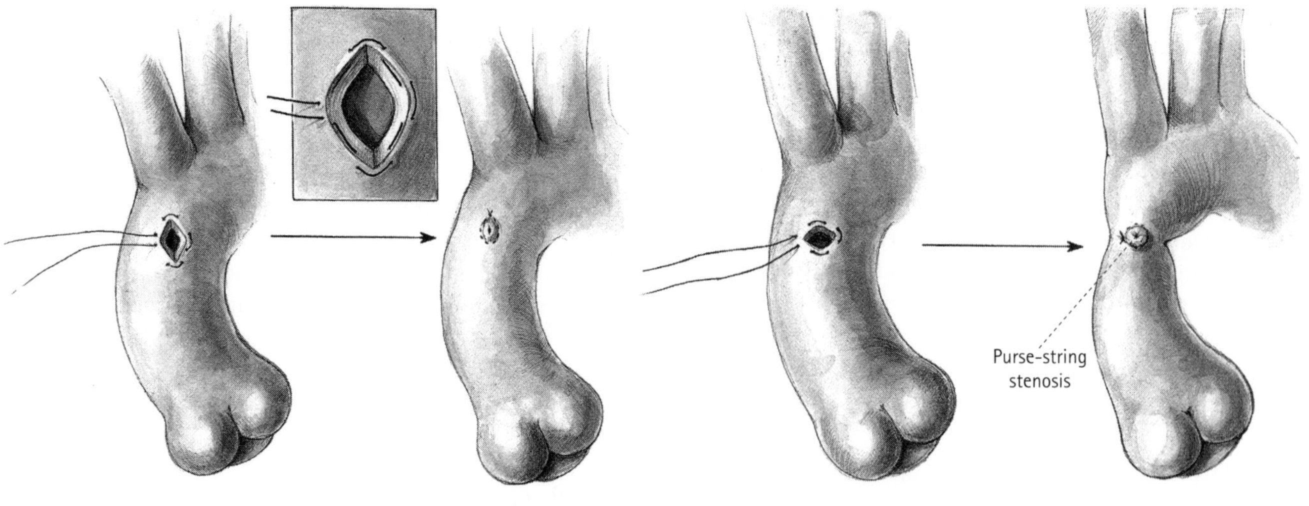

Figure 2.2 *A four-bite, diamond-shaped purse-string is used for arterial cannulation of the ascending aorta. The long axis of the diamond should lie in the long axis of the aorta. If the purse-string lies transversely there is a risk that a stenosis will be created.*

distention of the right atrium. If there is an ASD present the cannula will serve as both the venous cannula as well as a left heart vent.

Direct caval cannulation of the cavae causes an intimal injury that can be the site of thrombosis and if the purse-string is excessively large can result in stenosis of the cava. Caval cannulation necessitates dissection of the cavae and placement of tourniquets unless vacuum-assisted drainage (VAVD) is used. VAVD introduces its own set of risks. All of these problems are avoided by use of a single venous cannula.

Disadvantages

Entrainment of air into the venous line is one of the most important disadvantages of a single venous cannula. A large amount of air will break the siphon and require that the venous line be refilled (this can be done by the perfusionist by retrograde pumping after disconnecting the cannula from the venous line but must be done very carefully). Excessive air in the venous line also increases the risk that air emboli will pass through the oxygenator though the emboli should subsequently be removed by the arterial line filter. However if the tricuspid valve is not congenitally abnormal and has not been distorted by surgery it is usually possible to avoid or minimize this problem. Some surgeons find that a right-angle cannula placed in the right atrial appendage is the best method for avoiding the cannula tip passing through the tricuspid valve and taking air, while others use a straight cannula also inserted through the appendage with the tip sitting at the SVC orifice.

A single venous cannula allows blood to enter the right heart and can allow more rapid rewarming of the myocardium than is seen with double venous cannulation. Since lower systemic temperatures are usually used in children than in adults this is less of a problem than it is with adult surgery.

CAVAL CANNULATION WITH TOURNIQUETS

Caval cannulation can be achieved with two straight cannulas placed through the right atrium or by direct cannulation of the SVC and IVC. Direct caval cannulation is generally preferred if the surgical approach is through the right atrium. It is important for the surgeon to understand that one or other cannula can be partially or even completely obstructed with little apparent change in hemodynamics. Obstruction can occur because too large a cannula has been selected and the side holes are occluded against the caval wall. If the cannula is twisted or wedged the end hole may also occlude. This happens not uncommonly in neonates and small infants. The monitored perfusion pressure may actually rise and the venous saturation may also rise as the perfusate is redirected to the upper or lower half of the body, depending on which cannula has been occluded. These changes are likely to reassure rather than warn the surgical team that there is a problem. Even a central venous catheter may show no change as the tip is often below the caval tourniquet. The only warning sign may be that the perfusionist reports that volume is being lost from the circuit and that venous return is decreased. The surgeon should constantly look for changes in the relative venous saturations in the two cannulas. The blood returning from an obstructed cannula is usually much darker than normal. Careful study of the transparent plastic 'Y' where the two venous flows come together usually allows the reduced flow coming from the obstructed cannula to be seen. It is remarkable how minor an adjustment of the cannula is often required to correct the problem, emphasizing that the problem can also be caused by very little movement of the cannulas.

BILATERAL SVCs, BILATERAL HEPATIC VEINS

There are many options for venous cannulation available for children with complex venous anatomy. The method of cannulation should be individualized depending on the relative sizes of the cavas and the presence or absence of a communicating innominate vein. For example if there is a small left SVC and a left innominate vein is present, it is reasonable to place a tourniquet around the left SVC and use dual venous cannulation of the SVC and IVC. If the left SVC is as large as the right SVC and the procedure is simple, such as ASD closure, it is reasonable to place a pump sucker in the coronary sinus to drain the left SVC. If the procedure is more complex and the child is larger, a third venous cannula can be placed directly in the left SVC in addition to the right SVC and the IVC. Occasionally if there is a separate large hepatic vein and two SVCs, the surgeon may choose to use four venous cannulas Y'd together to the venous line.

VENOUS CANNULATION FOR THE BIDIRECTIONAL GLENN SHUNT

Experience with the Senning and Mustard procedures in neonates demonstrated that it was possible to rewarm the patient after an atrial diversion procedure using the same venous cannulation site as was used for cooling, i.e. the original right atrial appendage which is now part of the pulmonary venous atrium. Blood from the SVC and IVC must pass through the pulmonary circulation before entering the venous cannula to return to the pump. It is probably useful to occasionally inflate the lungs to reduce pulmonary resistance during this phase of the perfusion. While this technique works reasonably for the atrial switch procedures it introduces an important risk if it is used for the bidirectional Glenn shunt (or hemi-Fontan procedure). In this situation only blood returning from the upper body and most importantly the brain must pass through two resistance beds. Thus flow is likely to redistribute to be predominantly through the lower body. Therefore a right-angle cannula should be placed to drain the SVC system whenever there is a bidirectional Glenn-type circulation. This applies not only to the rewarming phase of the Glenn procedure itself but also to the cooling phase of the subsequent Fontan procedure. We generally prefer to place the cannula in the left innominate vein so that it does not interfere with manipulation of the SVC as required during the bidirectional Glenn procedure. The cannula should be small enough to allow flow to pass around it from the internal jugular vein opposite to the side the cannula is directed (Figure 2.3).

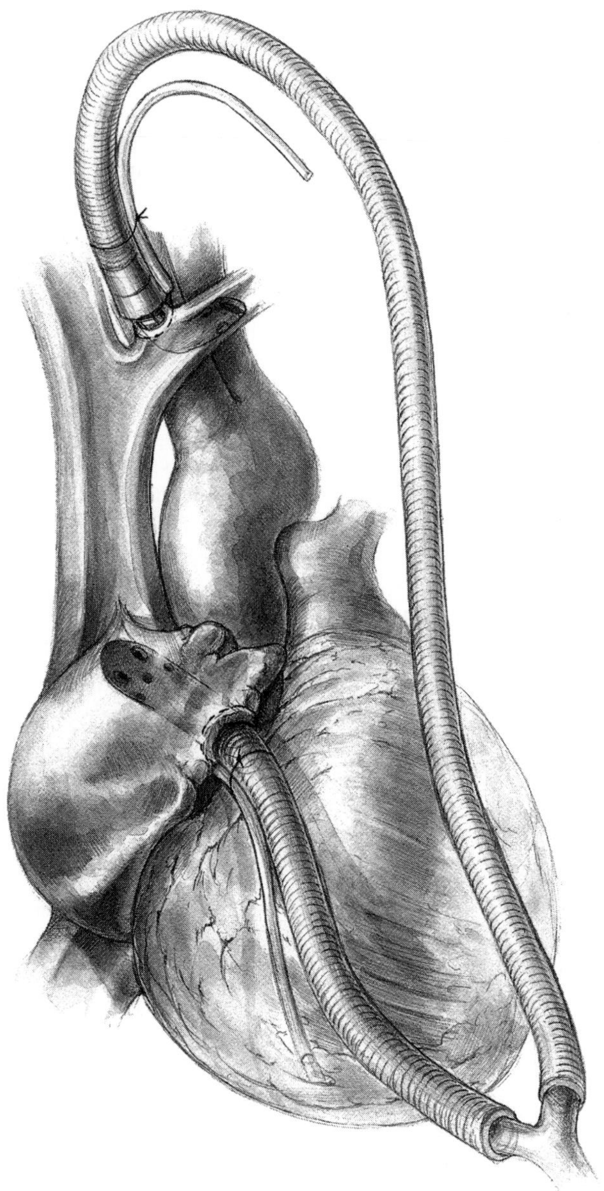

Figure 2.3 *Two venous cannulas are placed for a bi-directional Glenn shunt. The right-angle cannula in the left innominate vein should be small enough to allow flow to pass around it from the internal jugular vein opposite to the side the cannula is directed.*

Left heart venting

It is critically important that the congenital surgeon understands principles of left heart venting and yet this is a topic that is rarely written about or discussed. Left heart distention for only a few seconds causes injury to the myocardium and is probably one of the most important causes of postoperative low cardiac output. It is much less well tolerated by the neonate than in adults and older children. Left heart distention also causes pulmonary edema and is probably a frequent cause of so-called 'post-pump lung'. If the situation should arise that the surgeon becomes acutely aware of unanticipated left heart distention, it is essential to immediately reduce pump flow and thereby reduce perfusion pressure and to immediately decompress the left heart through one of the methods discussed below.

There are many more potential causes of left heart distention in patients with congenital cardiac disease relative to adults with acquired cardiac disease. The most important cause is that left heart return is often increased because of cyanosis or the presence of major aortopulmonary collateral vessels. While normal 'bronchial' return is only 3% of the cardiac output, it can easily be as much as 50% in the patient with massive collateralization. An unrecognized patent ductus can be a source of increased left heart return. A patent aortopulmonary shunt also increases left heart return. Aortopulmonary window, truncus arteriosus and anomalous coronary artery from the pulmonary artery are other anomalies where the surgeon must carefully guard against left heart distention. Finally aortic regurgitation is a unique cause of left heart distention in that it is upstream to a competent valve (mitral) from the left atrium. Thus the method for venting must be to drain the left ventricle itself while all the other causes can be dealt with by left atrial or pulmonary artery venting.

WHEN IS VENTING NECESSARY?

As long as the left ventricle is able to eject the left heart return coming into it, there is not likely to be injury to the ventricle or the lungs. However at the onset of bypass the ionized calcium level drops acutely secondary to both hemodilution as well as the chelating effects of citrate in blood used in the pump prime, thereby reducing myocardial contractility. Hypothermia will slow the heart and reduce its ability to eject the left heart return. The surgeon needs to carefully monitor how well the ventricle is coping and should make a judgment as to when to place a left heart vent. Although some surgeons place a vent while the heart is beating and the aorta is not cross-clamped, this is not recommended, particularly if the heart is beating vigorously. There is a real risk that air will be entrained into the left heart through the incision in the left atrium or through the vent cannula as it is introduced. It is safer to wait until either the heart has fibrillated or the cross clamp has been applied. However distention may occur before the heart has fibrillated. The surgeon needs to watch the main pulmonary artery as the best guide to left heart distention because it is usually difficult to see the degree of left ventricular distention directly and it is usually not possible in young patients to insert a Swan–Ganz catheter. If the pulmonary artery is becoming tense and the heart has not fibrillated, the pump flow must be immediately reduced and the cross clamp applied. Pump flow is returned to normal. While the cardioplegia is being infused a vent can be inserted through the right superior pulmonary vein into the left atrium or across the mitral valve into the left ventricle. It is important to place the purse-string for the vent adjacent to the atrial septum, i.e. close to Sondergard's groove so that the vent enters tangentially through the atrial septum. This will reduce the risk of bleeding if the same site is subsequently used for a left atrial monitoring line.

ALTERNATIVE METHODS OF VENTING

It is important to appreciate that the pulmonary artery is directly connected to the left heart and is a potential site of left heart decompression. Although it is rare to insert a vent cannula into the pulmonary artery, it is common to have the pulmonary arteries open, e.g. in tetralogy of Fallot repair or during performance of the arterial switch procedure, truncus repair etc. Thus a left atrial vent may not be necessary so long as the operation is sequenced such that the pulmonary arteries remain at least partially open until left heart contractility has been re-established. In repair of tetralogy this can also be achieved by not completing the ventricular end of a transannular patch until the heart is beating reasonably vigorously because, in the absence of the pulmonary valve, the right ventricle is a reasonable site for venting.

The presence of either a ventricular or an atrial septal defect increases the options for left heart venting. For example, sequencing the arterial switch procedure so as to leave the ASD open until late in the procedure allows the left heart to be vented by a single right atrial cannula. This will avoid an annoying return of blood through the divided main pulmonary artery during the procedure, which is how the left heart return will choose to vent itself if the ASD is closed and a separate vent is not placed.

VASCULAR ANASTOMOSES

It is rare for the congenital cardiac surgeon to have to perform vascular anastomoses to 1 or 1.5 mm vessels, such as are regularly faced by coronary surgeons. On the other hand vessels are often very fragile and must be brought together under some degree of tension. Vascular anastomoses in children must allow for growth. While there are many different methods for constructing vascular anastomoses that work well for individual surgeons, the following are some principles that have been found to be useful.

End to end, slide plasty and end to side anastomoses

There are clearly important differences between anastomoses which are end to end versus end to side. The end to side anastomosis should incorporate principles of the patch plasty as described below because it involves critically important heel and toe sites. The slide plasty is a useful variation on a direct end to end anastomosis. It allows a narrow segment of vessel to be incorporated in the anastomosis and avoids a circumferential anastomosis which reduces the risk that the anastomosis will be purse stringed. The anastomotic area is actually larger than the adjoining vessel and probably has better growth potential. It is often applied in the setting of a coarctation associated with arch or isthmus hypoplasia (Figure 2.4).

Interrupted or continuous (running) suture?

Traditional surgical dogma would suggest that an interrupted suture technique should be used to permit growth and yet few congenital surgeons use anything other than running sutures. There are several reasons. Firstly it has been found from clinical experience, e.g. with the neonatal

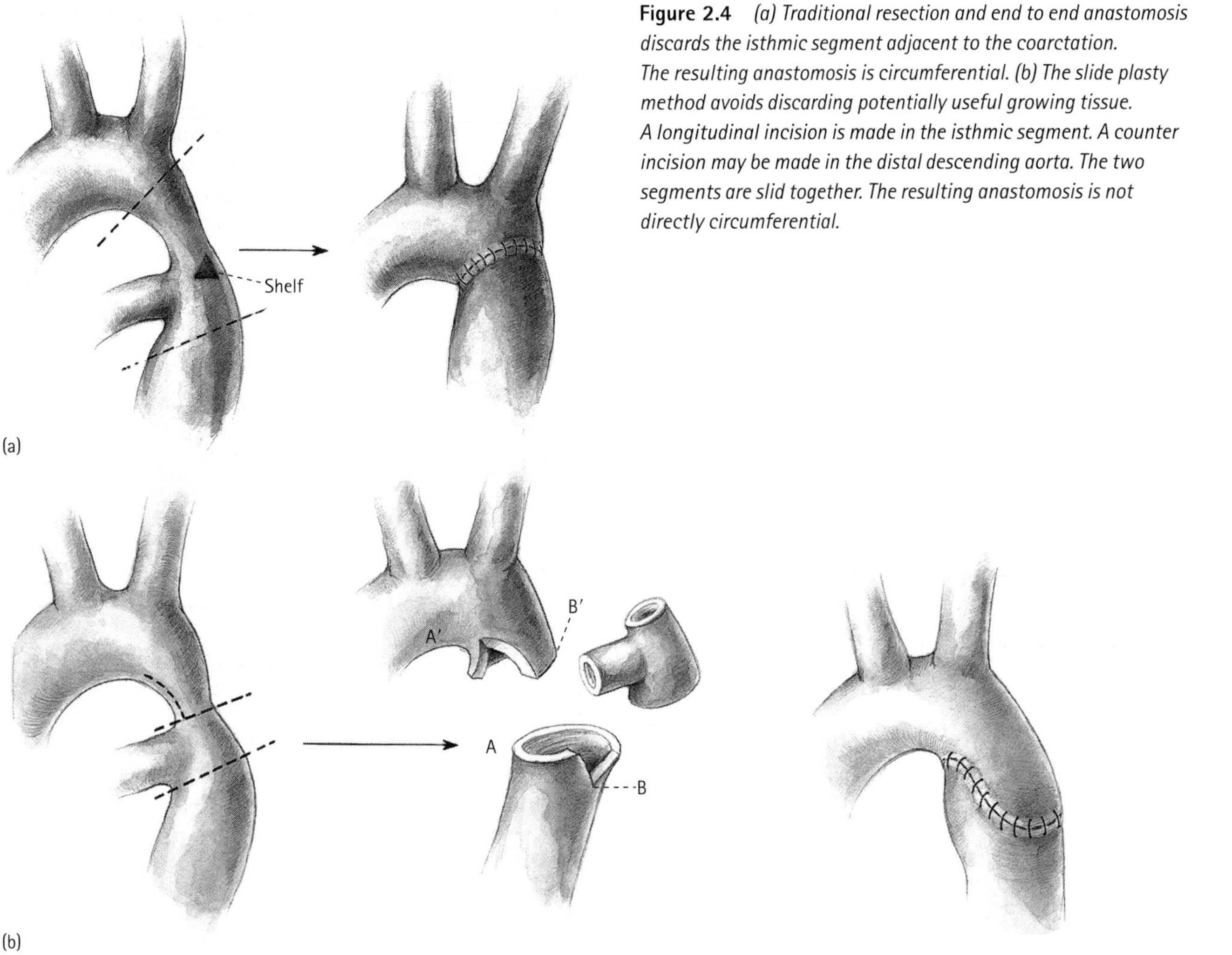

Figure 2.4 *(a) Traditional resection and end to end anastomosis discards the isthmic segment adjacent to the coarctation. The resulting anastomosis is circumferential. (b) The slide plasty method avoids discarding potentially useful growing tissue. A longitudinal incision is made in the isthmic segment. A counter incision may be made in the distal descending aorta. The two segments are slid together. The resulting anastomosis is not directly circumferential.*

arterial switch procedure, that anastomoses do grow despite a running anastomosis. The suture is actually a spiral and like a spring it stretches out straight as the vessels enlarge. Whether it is fracture of fine 6/0 and 7/0 polypropylene sutures that permits growth, as claimed by many surgeons, is unproven. Clinical experience has also demonstrated that excessive tension on an anastomosis is a far more important cause of anastomotic stenosis than the suture technique.

A continuous suture technique is more hemostatic than an interrupted technique. This is particularly true if the anastomosis is under some degree of tension. By placing multiple bites before the anastomosis is drawn together, the tension on each suture bite is reduced according to the principle of the block and tackle. The sailor raising a heavy sail is able to do so only because the tension on the rigging is reduced by a factor equal to the number of loops through the pulley (Figure 2.5). In the ame way, as the surgeon pulls the multiple preliminary bites of an anastomosis together, there is less tendency for multiple small tears to occur at each bite because of the reduced tension on each bite. The anastomosis is therefore more hemostatic.

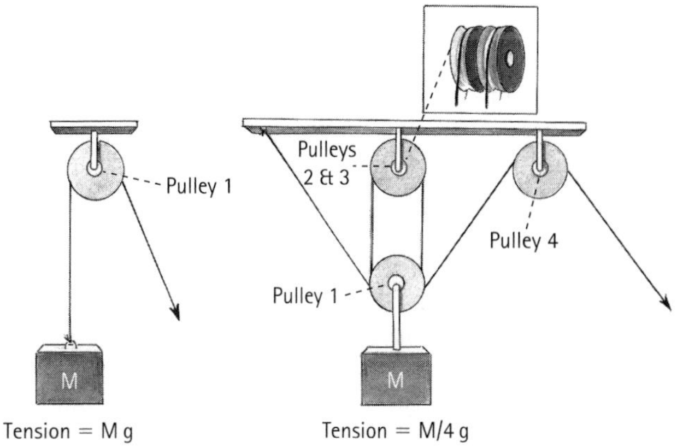

Figure 2.5 *The block and tackle principle is helpful in reducing the tension on individual suture bites when a continuous running suture technique is employed. The figure illustrates that with a single pulley (left, analogous to an interrupted suture technique) the tension on the single strand is equal to the weight being lifted. When there are four strands with four pulleys (right, analogous to a running suture technique) the tension on each suture is reduced to one quarter of the mass being lifted.*

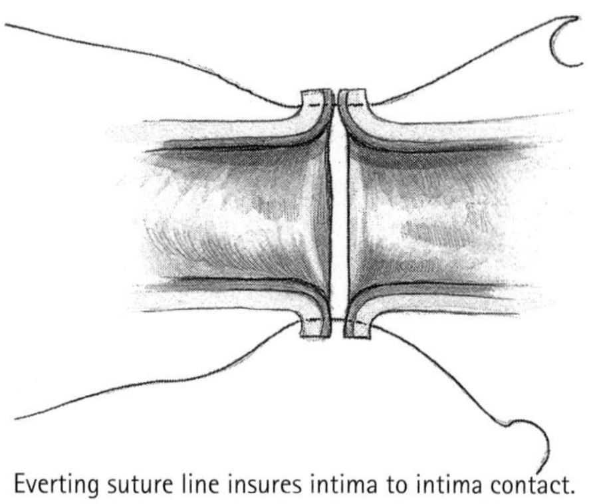

(a) Everting suture line insures intima to intima contact. Suturing must be done from the outside

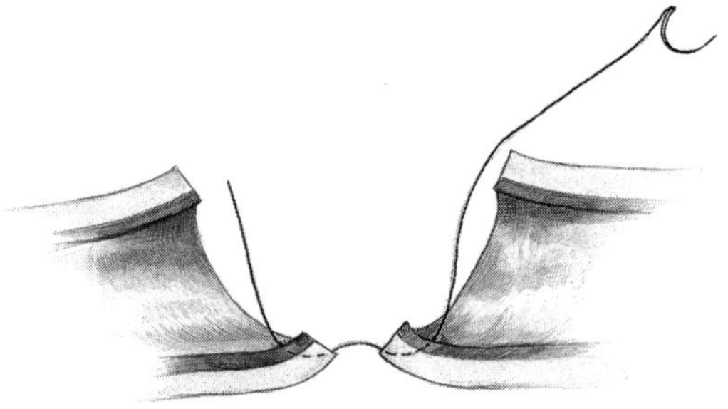

Deep bite on intima, shallow bite on adventitia

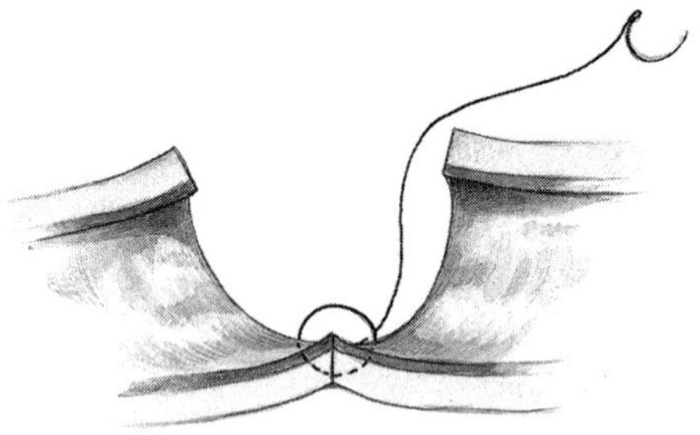

(b) Satisfactory intima to intima contact

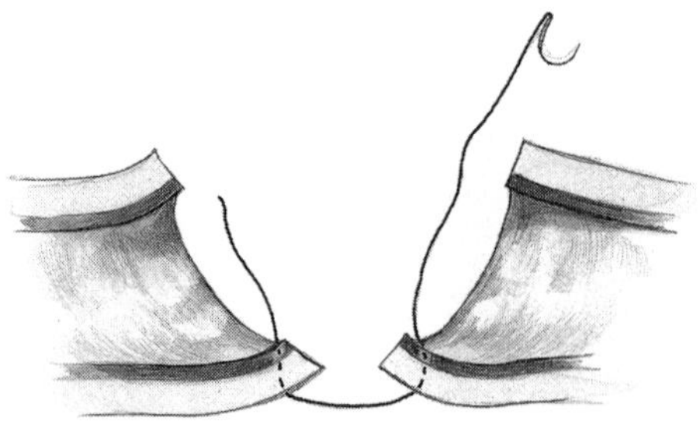

Poor technique for inverting suture line

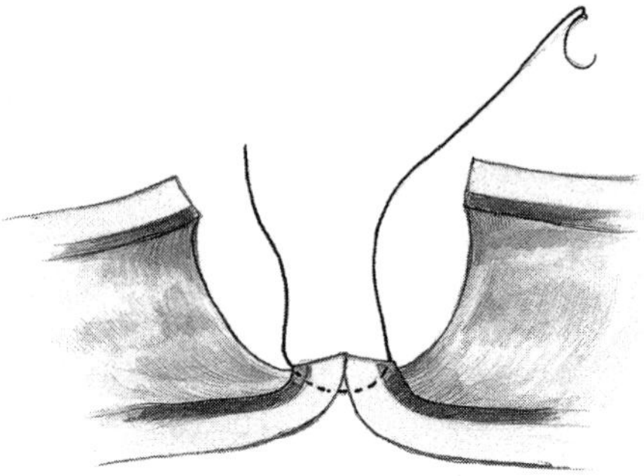

(c) Shallow intima bites expose media and adventitia in lumen

Figure 2.6 *(a) Ideally vascular anastomoses should be constructed in an everting fashion so that intima to intima contact is optimized. (b) Satisfactory intima to intima contact can be achieved with an internal inverting suture line so long as deep bites are taken on the intima with shallow bites on the adventitia. (c) If shallow bites are taken on the intima with deep bites on the adventitia then media and adventitia will be exposed within the lumen of the vessel undergoing anastomosis.*

A continuous suture technique is very much faster than an interrupted technique and allows for a reduced ischemic time. However it is important to appreciate that the width of spacing of the suture bites determines the degree of possible purse-stringing of the anastomosis. Very wide bites will gather the tissue together and narrow the anastomosis.

Inverting or everting suture?

Traditional dogma suggests that all vascular anastomoses should be constructed so as to evert the adventitia and allow intima to intima contact within the lumen of the anastomosis (Figure 2.6a). It is the intima after all that produces prostacyclin and has other properties that minimize platelet adhesion and initiation of the coagulation cascade. An everting suture line can be achieved by suturing from the outside of the vessel with either an over and over whip stitch or with a continuous horizontal mattress suture. However this is not practical in many situations, e.g. it is often necessary to suture the back wall of an anastomosis from within the lumen with the surgeon sewing forehand towards himself or herself. Therefore a technique must be used that minimizes exposure of media and adventitia in the lumen despite using an internal inverting suture. Figure 2.6b demonstrates how this is achieved. The surgeon should take larger bites of intima relative to the depth of bite of adventitia when performing an inverting suture. This technique is also advisable though not as important when performing an external everting suture.

POINTS OF TRANSITION FROM INVERTING TO EVERTING

If the surgeon has sutured the back wall of an anastomosis towards him/herself as an inverting suture using a forehand stitch, and then the front wall as an everting suture also forehand towards him/herself, there will be two points of transition where the vessel walls must cross one another (Figure 2.7). These are important potential sites of bleeding. If it will be very difficult to reaccess these sites, such as the coronary button anastomoses in the arterial switch procedure, it is wise to reinforce them before moving on. At a minimum the

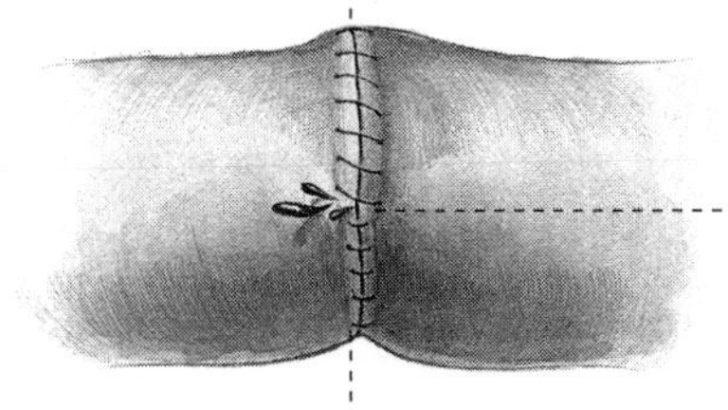

Figure 2.7 *The point of transition between an everting and inverting suture line is an important potential site for bleeding. Points of transition should be reinforced with additional interrupted sutures if they are not likely to be readily accessible later in the procedure.*

surgeon should make a mental note as to where these sites are throughout the reconstruction and return to them first if bleeding is a problem. Another option is to avoid such points of transition, which can be achieved in a number of ways, e.g. mattressing these points and suturing backhand for one or other leg.

How deep, how wide?

It is useful to analyse how the depth and spacing of sutures influences the physical forces holding the anastomosis together.[3] As Figure 2.8 illustrates, deeper bites increase the vector of force holding the anastomosis together, i.e. the vector running in the longitudinal direction of the vessels being anastomosed. On the other hand wider spacing reduces the needed vector of force. As discussed above the greater number of bites resulting from closer spacing also reduces the tension on each bite according to the block and tackle effect as well as reducing the purse-stringing effect of a continuous suture. Thus in general it is worth remembering the maxim 'deeper and closer' albeit remembering that excessively deep sutures will result in a bunching up of tissue at the anastomosis which may increase the risk of stenosis.

MISMATCHED VESSELS

It is common to have to perform end to end anastomoses between vessels of very different diameter. A mismatch of less than 2:3 can be managed using differential suture spacing (Figure 2.9a) for the larger versus smaller vessel. The larger vessel must be gathered by placing sutures more widely apart relative to the spacing in the smaller vessel. This should be done uniformly around the vessel to achieve a symmetrical taper though it is sometimes wise to aim for maximal gathering where the suture line can be reaccessed most easily, rather than, for example, on the back wall in a difficult area.

If the mismatch between vessels is greater than 2:3, e.g. 1:2, it may be advisable to create a dog-ear at a strategically

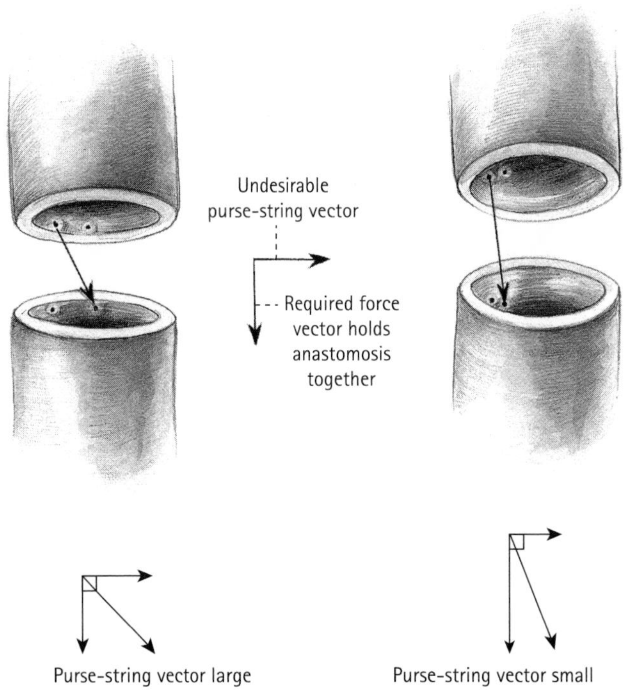

Figure 2.8 *Widely spaced shallow sutures reduce the force vector which holds the two vessels together at an anastomosis. Deeper bites placed more closely together will result in a more secure hemostatic anastomosis.*

unimportant point in the anastomosis (Figure 2.9b). For example, in the setting of an arterial switch procedure, the dog-ear should be away from coronary buttons.

Absorbable or nonabsorbable suture

The advantages of different suture materials are discussed in Chapter 3. In general, however, nonabsorbable polypropylene suture is preferred over absorbable because of its low surface drag. This results in tension distributing itself evenly throughout the anastomosis. Loose suture loops are probably the most common cause of important anastomotic bleeding. It is essential for the assistant who is following the suture to pull it up with an appropriate amount of tension. Before tying the suture the surgeon must tension it for several seconds to eliminate any residual slackness. If necessary a nerve hook should be used to eliminate loose loops by pulling them through.

PATCH PLASTY TECHNIQUE

The patch plasty is one of the most frequently used techniques in the congenital cardiac surgeon's armamentarium. It is used to enlarge stenotic and hypoplastic structures in such a way as to retain growth potential. Figure 2.10 illustrates the principle, i.e. the circumference of the structure in question

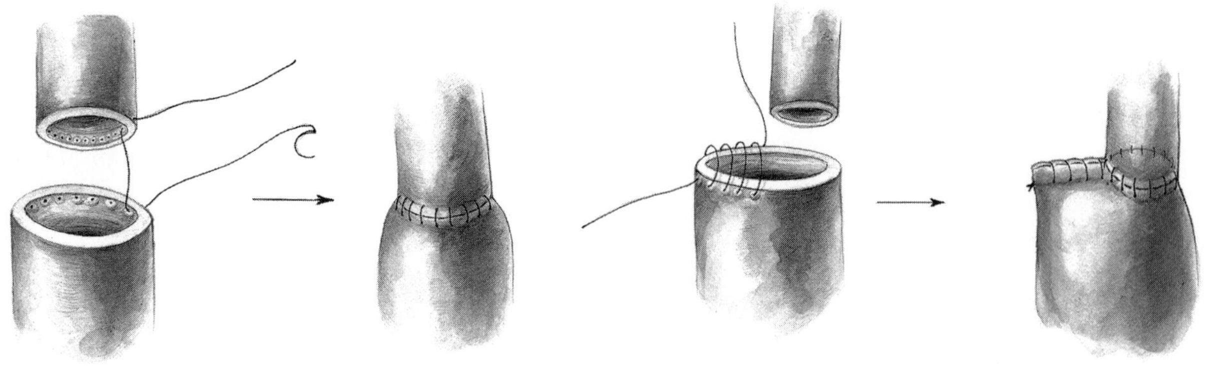

Figure 2.9 *(a) Differential suture spacing allows anastomosis of a larger to a smaller vessel. The larger vessel must be gathered by placing sutures more widely apart relative to the spacing in the smaller vessel. (b) If the mismatch between vessels undergoing end to end anastomosis is greater than 2:3, it may be advisable to create a dog-ear at a strategically unimportant point in the anastomosis.*

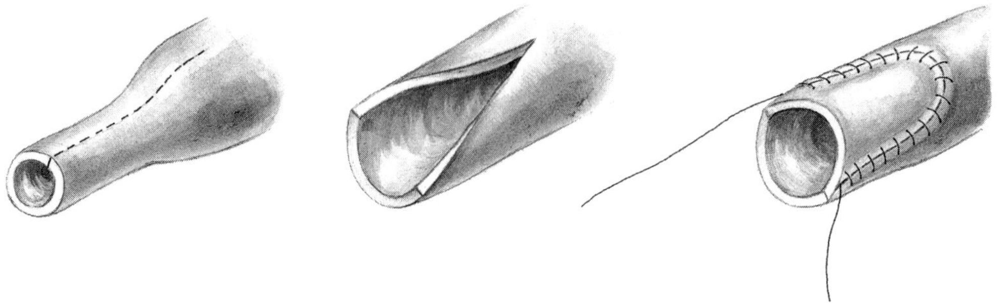

Figure 2.10 *The patch plasty is a frequently used technique for enlarging a stenotic structure. The toe of the patch must be rounded to avoid a stenosis at the toe of the patch.*

is enlarged by the width of the patch. It is important to remember that the factor π is involved. What may seem like a large patch will only increase the diameter of the vessel by one third of the patch width. Furthermore unless the toe and heel of the patch are carefully constructed there is a real risk that the structure will actually be narrowed at these points. This principle also applies to the heel and toe of an end to side anastomosis.

Differential suture spacing for heels and toes

This is one of the most important technical principles in congenital cardiac surgery. The principle is very familiar to any individuals with a military background who have spent time on the parade ground practicing marching drills or to those with a mechanical interest who have spent time disassembling the differential gear driving a rear-wheel-drive car axle. As a platoon of soldiers wheels to the right or left or as a car turns a corner, the inside column of soldiers or the inside wheel covers much less ground than the outer column or outer wheel. It is fascinating to watch how surgical trainees have an innate desire to recreate this form of spacing when suturing around the curve of the heel or toe of a patch which is being placed into a linear incision in a vessel or a ventricle. This form of spacing is guaranteed to create a stenosis (Figure 2.11). The vessel will be purse-stringed as the suture is drawn tight. The surgeon must strive to create exactly the opposite spacing as he comes around the heel or toe. The patch itself must be cut relatively square and never in a pointed diamond shape. Sutures should be spaced very close in the vessel at the apex of the incision. In contrast the spacing of sutures in the patch should be very much wider. At the apex itself the ratio of patch to vessel spacing may be as great as 3:1 or 4:1 with a gradually decreasing ratio as the suture line reaches the sides, as distinct from the end of the patch (Figure 2.11b). Trainees must be constantly reminded that the patch is being used to enlarge the vessel: therefore take wider bites on the patch than on the vessel.

Creating patches with depth

In certain situations it is necessary to construct structures with depth, for example, the hood supplementing the anastomosis of a homograft conduit to the right ventricle or a valve cusp for the aortic valve. This can be achieved by careful design of the patch shape and by an extreme degree of differential suture ratio (Figure 2.12). Basically the patch must be gathered to create the shape of a sailboat's spinnaker by very wide spacing on the patch with much narrower spacing on the right ventricle.

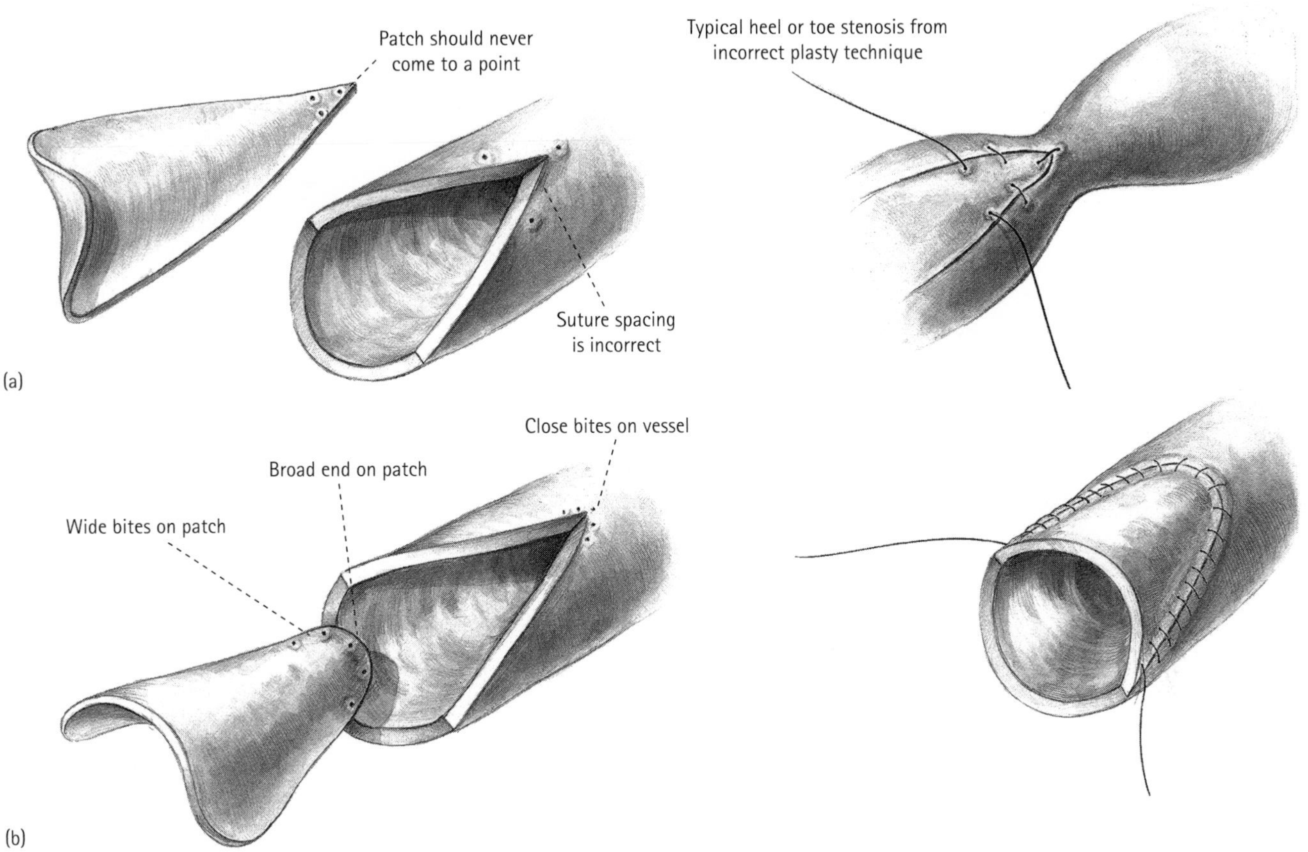

Figure 2.11 *(a) Incorrect technique for patch plasty. The patch has been cut to come to a sharp point. The differential spacing of sutures is the opposite of the required technique. Sutures have been placed widely on the stenotic vessel and close together at the toe of the patch. When the patch is tied into position a stenosis will result. (b) The correct technique for patch plasty: the patch has been cut with a blunt rounded end. Sutures have been placed closely on the vessel at the apex of the incision and widely on the patch.*

MINIMIZING AIR EMBOLISM

Most congenital cardiac procedures result in air being introduced into the cardiac chambers. However elimination of air is more easily accomplished than in adults for several reasons. Most importantly the small size of the cardiac chambers means that the volume of air which is involved is relatively small. Furthermore the most difficult problem with adults is that large volumes of air are often trapped in the pulmonary veins of emphysematous lungs that do not collapse during the procedure. The lungs in children usually collapse completely so that the veins do not conceal air that is released late.

Transesophageal echocardiography (TEE) is useful in educating surgeons as to how effective they have been in eliminating air from the heart. Several maneuvers have been found to be useful. The left heart can be filled with saline either directly from a syringe or through a left heart vent. At the same time the cardioplegia site in the ascending aorta is widely opened to allow air to vent. Blood can be used to fill the left heart if a single venous cannula is in use. By raising the venous pressure by temporarily retarding venous return, blood will pass through the lungs into the left heart where it will displace air as long as there is an open vent site, such as the cardioplegia needle site in the ascending aorta. Blood can also be delivered into the left heart by inflation of the lungs though one must be careful to prevent the subsequent negative pressure created as the lungs relax drawing air back into the left heart. The patient's position can be moved by rolling the table and changing from reverse Trendelenburg to regular Trendelenburg while at the same time gently milking blood and air from the appropriate chambers. Following clamp release the cardioplegia needle site in the aorta should be allowed to bleed freely. Like the TEE, this is a useful quality control maneuver for the surgeon. Ideally little or no air should be seen or more importantly heard to exit from the venting site. Finally the heart should be allowed to eject for at least several minutes before coming off bypass. Ventilation also should be started some time before weaning from bypass to displace any air which may have been trapped in the lungs.

Although considerable effort should be used to eliminate air from the left heart it is important to remember that air can easily pass through the lungs from the right heart. Thus every effort should be made to eliminate air from the right heart as well as the left. If air embolism does occur, for example, into the coronary arteries, adequate time should be allowed for

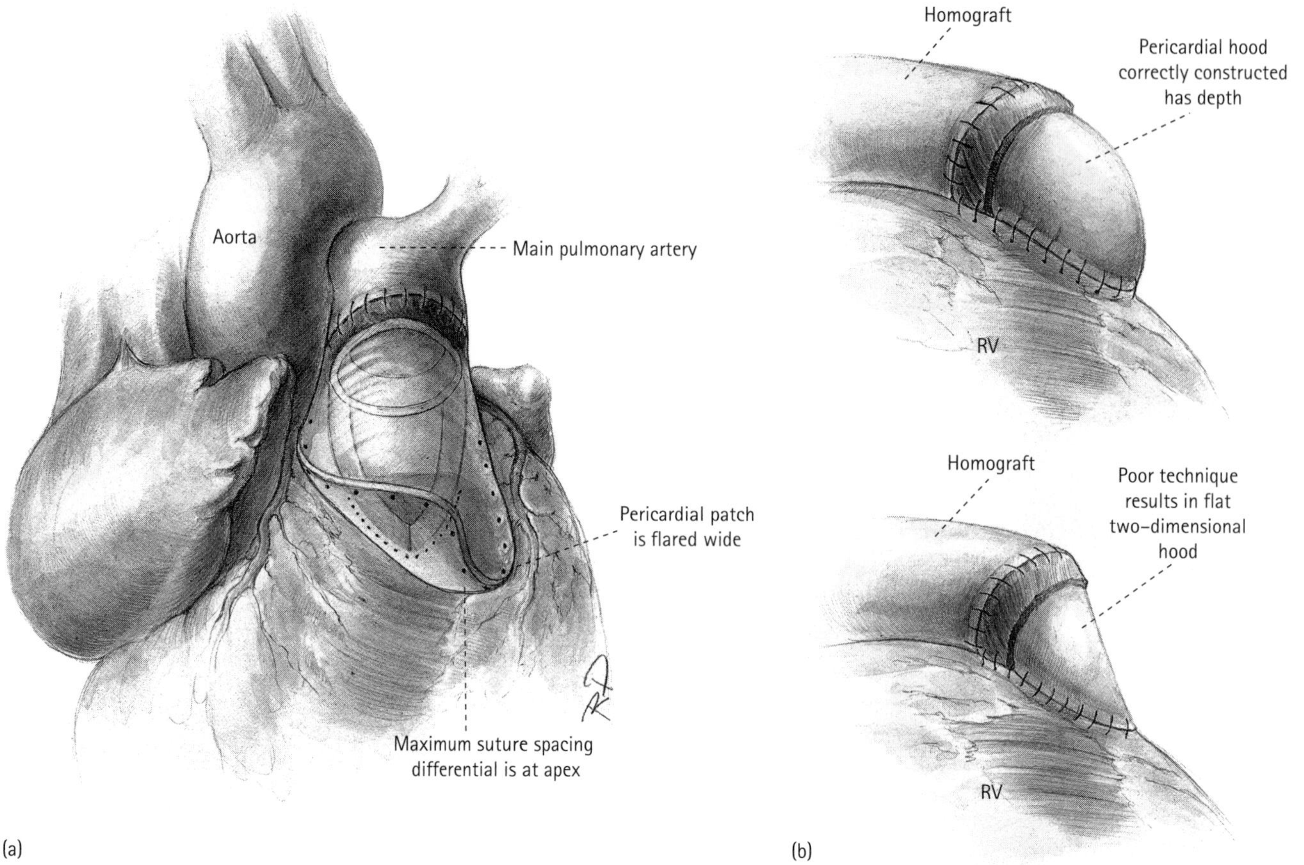

Figure 2.12 *(a) The hood which is used to supplement the proximal anastomosis of a homograft to the right ventricle is a good example of a patch which must be sutured in a fashion to create depth. This is achieved by flaring the lower end of the patch when it is cut to shape. The sutures are placed so as to gather the patch aggressively, particularly as the apex of the incision is rounded. Very wide bites are taken at this point on the patch with much closer bites on the ventricle. (b) A correctly constructed pericardial hood has depth while poor technique will result in a flattened two dimensional hood which may stenose the anastomosis internally.*

the heart to recover before coming off bypass. Pulsatile ejection and a higher perfusion pressure seem to be useful in encouraging air to pass through systemic vascular beds.

HEMOSTASIS

Surgeons have a tendency to attribute post-operative bleeding to poor management of coagulation and it is indeed true that a coagulopathy will eventually be present in any patient who has required massive transfusion. Clearly the key is to avoid the initial bleeding which causes the need for transfusion. There are many important factors under the surgeon's control that will prevent that initial bleeding.

Dissection in the correct plane

As discussed above it is important for the surgeon to recognize the avascular or at least minimally vascular plane that exists between most structures even after multiple previous operations. Dissection should be limited to this plane. When vessels are encountered they must be effectively cauterized with the coagulation current. Large raw areas, such as the undersurface of the chest wall in a reoperation, must be extensively cauterized.

Suture technique

Needle holes in natural tissue will usually seal in a short time if the correct technique has been used. It is important to turn the needle in the curve of the needle and not to drag it through the tissue, particularly in fragile vessels, such as small pulmonary arteries. Choice of a smaller needle, e.g. the BV1 rather than an RB2 6/0 Prolene will leave smaller holes that bleed less. Suture lines that are under tension have a greater tendency to bleed. Tension should be minimized by wide mobilization of the structures being sutured. Persistent needle hole bleeding should stimulate a search for distal obstruction, e.g. the distal arch reconstruction for hypoplastic left heart syndrome if there is persistent bleeding from the proximal neoaorta.

Needle holes in PTFE are often a problem. They can be dealt with by using fine prolene sutures placed as horizontal

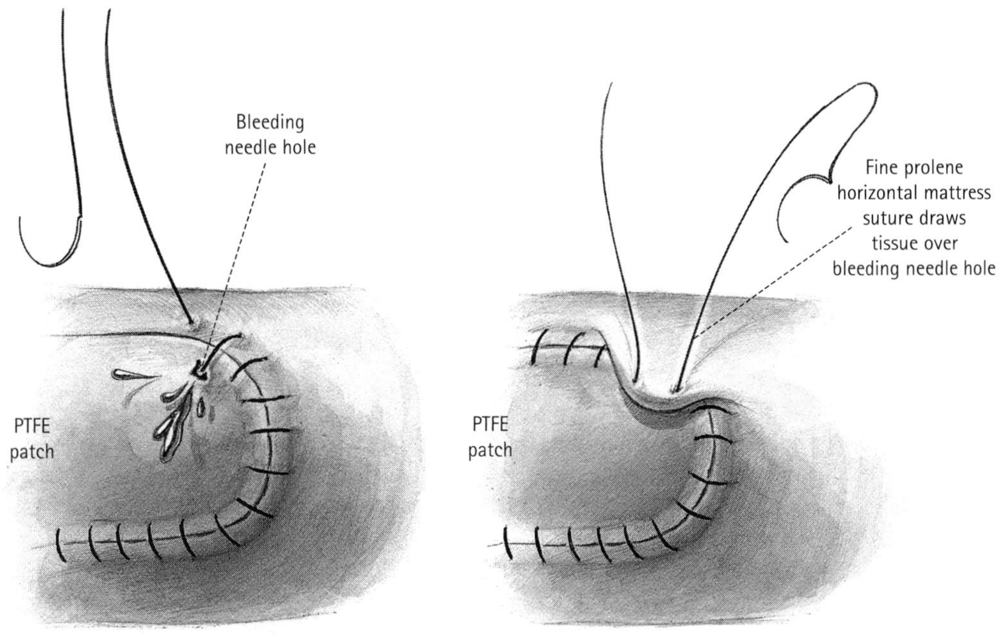

Figure 2.13 *Bleeding needleholes can be troublesome when PTFE is sutured. Bleeding may occur in spite of the use of PTFE sutures. A helpful technique to control bleeding is to draw tissue over the needle holes with fine prolene horizontal mattress sutures.*

mattress sutures to draw adjacent adventitial tissue over each hole (Figure 2.13). The bites in the PTFE should be partial thickness.

Excessive hemodilution

Hemodilution dilutes not only red cells but also coagulation factors. The surgeon who complains that the blood is like water often has him or herself to blame. Aiming for a perfusate hematocrit of 30% is almost certainly preferable to a lower hematocrit not only for its greater oxygen carrying capacity but also because it means less dilution of coagulation factors and platelets. Less hemodilution does not necessarily translate to greater use of blood products. In a randomized trial of hematocrit 20% versus 30% there was no difference in the total usage of blood and products between the two groups because there was less postoperative bleeding in the high hematocrit group.[4]

Hemodilution is caused by factors other than the initial selected hematocrit. Irrigation fluid is a common source that is often allowed to enter the cardiotomy suckers. Cardioplegia should be vented to the wall suction and not allowed to enter the venous cannula. If crystalloid is diluting the perfusate it should be aggressively removed during bypass by conventional ultrafiltration.

Protamine administration

Protamine reactions are almost unheard of in neonates and infants and are very rare in older children. Therefore the protamine should be administered over two to three minutes and definitely not over a period of more than five minutes. Longer periods of protamine administration can result in transfusion of bank blood in relatively large quantities which can begin the vicious cycle of bleeding and transfusion.

Packing

Individual surgeons will have their own preference regarding the optimal hemostatic packing material. Gel foam soaked in bovine thrombin is very effective though there is a small risk of inducing antibodies which may prove troublesome in theory at a future operation. The packing should be timed carefully so that it is placed just as the protamine infusion is completed. For the next 10–15 minutes there should be a honeymoon period of good coagulation. The surgical team should work hard and fast at this time to take advantage of this temporary phase of excellent coagulation. The packing should be left undisturbed adjacent to deep suture lines initially for at least 10 minutes while the more superficial layers are dealt with.

Coagulation factors and platelets

In neonates and young infants it is usually wise to administer both platelets and cryoprecipitate following a major procedure such as an arterial switch. More information about transfusion, including emphasis on the importance of calcium management, is given in Chapter 4.

Aprotinin

There is no question that aprotinin infused during bypass and postoperatively can reduce postoperative bleeding, particularly in neonates and infants. It is important to understand that this comes at the price that unwanted clotting can also occur and in fact does. Shunt thrombosis after a Norwood operation is a life-threatening event as is coronary thrombosis after an arterial switch. On the other hand an experienced surgical team can almost always manage bleeding without too much difficulty. We do not use aprotinin for the arterial switch but we do recommend it for most other neonatal procedures, such as truncus repair and interrupted aortic arch.

Antifibrinolytic agents

Epsilon amino caproic acid (Amicar) and tranexamic acid are useful agents which are not quite as effective as aprotinin in controlling post-pump bleeding. They suffer from the same disadvantages as aprotinin in that they may cause unwanted postoperative clotting, e.g. thrombosis of the Fontan baffle pathway or the Fontan fenestration. They are often useful in a reoperative setting but should not be necessary for most primary procedures. If a surgical team finds that they are essential they should closely examine the other factors described above as it is likely that they will be able to improve some other aspect of their hemostasis management.

Reoperation

Reoperation for bleeding should be exceedingly rare after a primary congenital cardiac procedure, i.e. an incidence of 1% or less. It is difficult to specify specific volumes of blood loss that should be an indication for reoperation. Probably the most useful indication is that the volume of chest tube output is increasing after three or four hours rather than decreasing. Evidence of hemodynamic compromise with a falling arterial pressure and rising atrial pressures together with echocardiographic evidence of clot or blood around the heart should also stimulate the ICU and surgical team to consider reopening the chest. Reoperation can be safely undertaken in many circumstances in the ICU so long as appropriate equipment is available and it is not anticipated that a complex surgical intervention will be required to deal with ongoing bleeding.

REFERENCES

1. Shum-Tim D, Nagashima M, Shinoka T et al. Postischemic hyperthermia exacerbates neurologic injury after deep hypothermic circulatory arrest. *J Thorac Cardiovasc Surg* 1998; **116**:780–792.
2. Laussen PC, Bichell DP, McGowan FX, Zurakowski D, DeMaso DR, del Nido PJ. Postoperative recovery in children after minimum versus full-length sternotomy. *Ann Thorac Surg* 2000; **69**:591–596.
3. Rubenstein C, Russelll WJ. Wound closure and suturing patterns: A vector analysis of suture tension. *Aust NZ J Surg* 1992; **62**:733–737.
4. Jonas RA, Wypij J, Roth SJ et al. The influence of hemodilution on outcome after hypothermic cardiopulmonary bypass: results of a randomized trial in infants. *J Thorac Cardiovasc Surg*, in press.

3

Biomaterials for congenital cardiac surgery

INTRODUCTION

One of the most important basic principles of surgery for congenital heart disease is that operations should be designed to incorporate growth potential. This can usually be achieved by careful use of in-situ tissues, creation and subsequent sliding or rotation of autologous flaps as well as transfer of free autologous flaps. However situations arise where autologous tissue is not available and a choice must be made between the various biomaterials that are available. This chapter will review the properties, advantages and disadvantages of a number of biomaterials used in various applications for congenital cardiac surgery.

PATCHES AND BAFFLES

There are numerous situations where patches are employed in congenital cardiac surgery. The most common application is closure of a septal defect. However patch enlargement of hypoplastic structures such as the small infundibulum, main pulmonary artery or branch pulmonary arteries in tetralogy is also frequently necessary.

The term 'baffle' is used to denote a patch which directs blood from one chamber to another chamber or great artery, for example, the intraventricular baffle constructed as part of the Rastelli procedure for correction of transposition with VSD and pulmonary stenosis. Unlike the term as applied in common usage, such as sound baffles or baffles in storage tanks, a baffle in a congenital heart operation should totally seal and separate the blood inside the baffle from the blood outside. A baffle often has a complex three-dimensional shape and therefore imposes stringent demands on the material employed in terms of need for elasticity and conformability.

Pericardium

AUTOLOGOUS PERICARDIUM

Autologous pericardium is one of the most useful materials for application as a patch or baffle. It has several advantages including the fact that it is immediately available, sterile, nonimmunoreactive and free. Autologous pericardium can be used in its fresh state, either pedicled or as a free graft, or it can be used as a free graft after fixation with glutaraldehyde. Whether fixed or unfixed pericardium has the important advantage that there is minimal bleeding through suture holes. Although the pericardium itself will thicken and fibrose over time there is little adjacent fibrous reaction such as is seen with Dacron.

Glutaraldehyde treatment of autologous pericardium

Treatment of pericardium with 0.6% glutaraldehyde (Polyscientific, Bay Shore, NY) results in cross-linking of collagen molecules and strengthens the pericardium as well as fixing its shape and reducing its elasticity. Aldehyde fixation is the same process that is used in tanning animal hides to make leather. The pericardium should be clipped to cardboard to prevent shrinkage and to ensure that the edges are not rolled (Figure 3.1). The duration of exposure to glutaraldehyde determines the degree of fixation and can be varied according to the planned use of the patch. Usually between 15 and 30 minutes is appropriate. The patch should then be removed from its cardboard backing and should be thoroughly rinsed in the same way that a porcine valve is rinsed to remove residual glutaraldehyde.

There are several benefits derived from fixing pericardium. The patch can be cut and shaped with the expectation that when it is exposed to pressure it will retain approximately the same shape and size. Despite fixation pericardium retains a

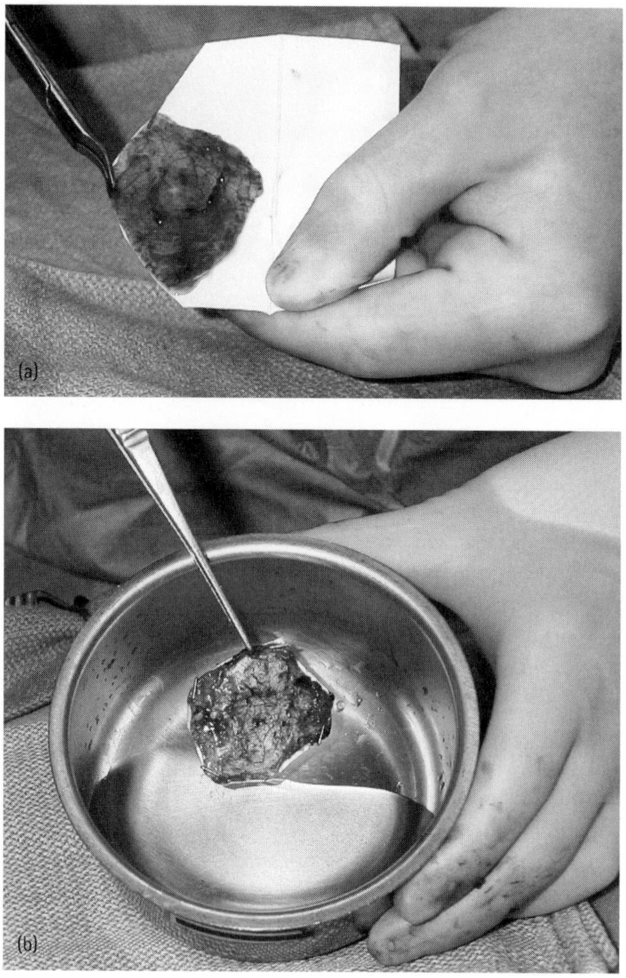

Figure 3.1 *Autologous pericardium treated with glutaraldehyde is one of the most frequently used biomaterials for reconstructive congenital cardiac surgery. The anterior pericardium is harvested. (a) The pericardium is clipped to cardboard with surgical clips. (b) The pericardium is fixed in 0.6% glutaraldehyde for 15–30 minutes. The glutaraldehyde must be thoroughly rinsed from the pericardium before implantation.*

degree of elasticity and conformability that allows it to be shaped into complex baffles with almost no risk of kinking and infolding. The edges of fresh pericardium tend to roll and are difficult to suture unless held under tension. Most importantly over the longer term the risk of aneurysmal dilation is reduced by fixation, particularly if the patch will be exposed to systemic pressure.

The disadvantages of fixation of pericardium are relatively minor. Over the longer term glutaraldehyde fixation can predispose to a mild degree of calcification. The fact that the size of the patch is fixed may be a disadvantage if there is hope that the patch might enlarge with time, thereby giving the appearance of growth. Finally glutaraldehyde is toxic and should be handled with care and in such a way that the surgical team is not exposed to its fumes. It is important to color the solution with a dye such as methylene blue so that it is not confused with crystalloid solutions and inadvertently irrigated into the surgical field.

Fresh pericardium

Fresh, untreated pericardium is difficult to handle and over the longer term can both shrink as well as stretch. There is evidence from its use to construct conduits that there can be an impressive degree of enlargement[1] though aneurysmal dilation is also seen. It should not be used in larger children or adults when it will be exposed to systemic pressure. Fresh pericardium has been used as an in-situ patch, for example to supplement the pulmonary venous atrium in the Senning procedure[2] or to enlarge the pulmonary veins for congenital pulmonary vein stenosis.[3] There is no clear evidence that there is any advantage in using in situ or pedicled pericardium relative to its use as a free graft.

Cryopreserved allograft (homograft) pericardium

Allograft pericardium is collected by tissue banks from cadavers and after antibiotic treatment is cryopreserved using the same process used for storage of valves. Allograft pericardium has several disadvantages relative to autologous pericardium. There is a risk of viral transmission (HIV, hepatitis B and C), it is not immediately available in that it requires thawing and rinsing and it is expensive. It has the handling disadvantages of fresh autologous pericardium. Over the longer term it is probable that it has a risk of calcification despite the absence of glutaraldehyde treatment most likely because of immune factors. It should be used with great caution if it will be exposed to systemic pressure.

GLUTARALDEHYDE TREATED XENOGRAFT PERICARDIUM

Pericardium harvested from cows (bovine) and horses (equine) and treated with glutaraldehyde has been a popular patching material in Japan. It has the advantages of being rapidly available off the shelf (after rinsing the glutaraldehyde) and has essentially no risk of disease transmission. However the combination of a powerful immune response to the xenograft tissue (probably the residual cellular debris in particular) as well as the effect of the aldehyde results in a severe degree of calcification often in as short a time as a few months.

Cryopreserved allograft (homograft) arterial wall

Allograft arterial wall is excellent material for patch plasty enlargement of stenotic vessels. It is usually quite hemostatic and conforms nicely to irregular contours. It has several disadvantages however. It can transmit viral disease, it is very expensive ($2000+) and it requires time for thawing and rinsing (about 20 minutes). Allograft pulmonary artery wall is often unpredictable as to the size it will stretch to when under pressure. There is a risk of calcification particularly for aortic allografts though this risk appears to be less with patches of allograft than for allograft tube-graft conduits.

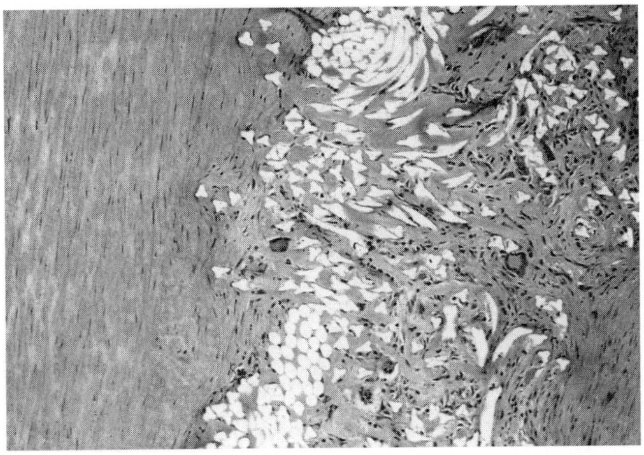

Figure 3.2 *Dacron stimulates an aggressive inflammatory response with subsequent fibrosis. This is helpful in closing small peri-patch VSDs, for example, but is a problem for Dacron conduits.*

Dacron

Dacron (polyethylene terephthalate) is a synthetic polymer that was developed by the DuPont company in the 1950s during the period immediately following the Second World War when there was an explosion of knowledge in the field of plastics technology. It was soon recognized that Dacron was more stable and resistant to degradation when in a biologic milieu than some of its polymer cousins such as Nylon and Ivalon.[4–7] Ivalon was widely used in the early years of congenital surgery as a patching material for closure of septal defects. It often broke down after several years and required surgical replacement for the recurrent septal defect that resulted.

Although Dacron is stable and retains much of its strength even after many years of implantation it does stimulate a fairly aggressive inflammatory response with subsequent fibrosis (Figure 3.2). The fibrous tissue can be more firmly anchored to the patch if a 'velour' form of Dacron is used. Dacron velour has loops of fiber that project either on one side of the basic knit or weave ('knitted single velour' or 'woven single velour') or on both sides ('double velour'). A patch of Dacron used for closure of a VSD will become overgrown with fibrous tissue within a few weeks to months. For the majority of VSDs this is probably an advantage as the fibrosis will help to seal the wrinkles and irregularities and even the suture holes that initially cause tiny multiple residual VSDs. These small defects are readily detected by color Doppler. Serial studies demonstrate that these hemodynamically insignificant defects gradually close when a Dacron patch has been used. In contrast we have the impression that when less reactive materials such as pericardium and PTFE are used for VSD closure there is more likely to be long-term persistence of small residual VSDs. On the other hand if a Dacron patch lies closely adjacent to a semilunar valve, the fibrosis is a disadvantage so that Dacron should probably be avoided in this setting.

Another disadvantage of Dacron is that it is much less elastic and conformable than biologic materials such as pericardium and homograft arterial wall. Although this does not present a problem when it is used as a flat patch for simple septal defect closure, it is a problem when it is used for construction of a complex baffle. This is particularly true in smaller children where the wall tension in a small diameter baffle is not sufficient to straighten out any inward kinks. Furthermore the fibrosis within a small diameter baffle will soon result in baffle stenosis. For these reasons we are careful to avoid Dacron for baffle construction in small children and particularly in neonates and infants. This is true for both the Dacron velour flat patch material as well as crimped segments of tube graft with or without Hemashield treatment (see below).

ePTFE (Goretex, Impra)

Teflon, like Dacron, is a synthetic polymer. Microporous expanded polytetrafluoroethylene (ePTFE) is a form of Teflon in which the polymer is arranged as a lattice of nodes interconnected by filaments. During its development in the early 1970s many variations of internodal spacing (pore size) were tested, with the conclusion that a pore size of 20–30 μm was optimal for healing.[8] PTFE was developed specifically for use as a biomaterial. The advantages of pores in allowing ingrowth and anchoring of a fibrous pseudointima had been learned from development of Dacron vascular grafts (see below). It was subsequently found that PTFE had the useful property of allowing water vapor to pass through it while water does not. Thus PTFE is now widely used for clothing and footwear because of its ability to 'breathe'.

PTFE stimulates less of a fibrous reaction than Dacron. This is useful in some situations and a disadvantage in others. In the setting of standard VSD closure this may mean that there is a higher probability of persistence of small peri-patch residual VSDs. However it is an advantage for baffles. It is also an advantage for construction of the hood which is used to supplement the anastomosis of a homograft conduit to the right ventricle. PTFE is more conformable than Dacron particularly when the newer 'stretch' form is used. Thus it is our preferred material for pulmonary artery patch plasty if a biologic material is not available. However if the patch will be exposed to high pressure there is likely to be a significant problem with needle-hole bleeding. Although PTFE suture can reduce this problem it certainly does not eliminate it. The technique for controlling bleeding through PTFE needle holes is described in Chapter 2.

VALVED AND NONVALVED CONDUITS

There are a number of situations in congenital cardiac surgery where a tube-like connection must be established using a conduit. The paradigm is a conduit between the right ventricle and the pulmonary artery bifurcation for tetralogy of

Fallot with pulmonary atresia where there is complete failure of development of the main pulmonary artery. Conduits were also a popular method for establishing connection between the systemic venous circulation and the pulmonary arteries in the early development of the Fontan procedure and for a time were also placed between the apex of the left ventricle and the descending aorta for complex left ventricular outflow tract obstruction. More recently the extracardiac conduit modification of the Fontan operation has re-emerged as a popular option. Many of the conduits used today in congenital cardiac surgery were originally developed for the management of acquired vascular disease though the earliest clinically applied vascular tube graft was the aortic allograft developed by Robert Gross in Boston for the management of coarctation.

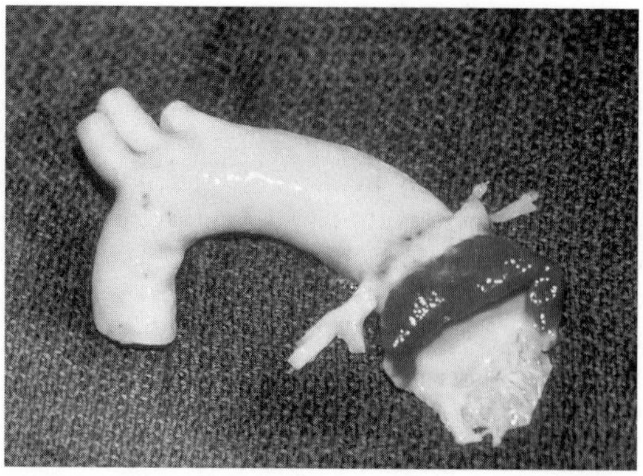

Figure 3.3 *Robert E Gross, working at Children's Hospital Boston, pioneered the use of aortic allografts (homografts) which were first used for thoracic aortic replacement following resection of coarctation. Ross and Barratt-Boyes subsequently applied aortic allografts for aortic valve replacement and as right ventricle to pulmonary artery conduits.*

History of the development of nonvalved vascular tube grafts

ALLOGRAFT BLOOD VESSELS

In the early 1900s, Carrel pioneered the use of transplanted allograft (homograft) arteries and veins as vascular substitutes in an experimental setting using canine models.[9–11] He developed a number of surgical techniques and instruments that remain in use today. However it was not until the development of antibiotics in the 1940s that Carrel's ideas could be applied clinically.

Crafoord working in Sweden in 1944 was the first to undertake successful repair of a coarctation clinically,[12] followed shortly thereafter by Gross at Children's Hospital Boston.[13] Gross was concerned that although the elasticity of the aorta would allow resection and direct anastomosis in most cases of coarctation, this was not universally so. He needed a safe arterial substitute and, like Carrel, looked to a nonvalved aortic allograft (Figure 3.3). In laboratory studies investigating methods of preparation and storage of aortic allografts, Gross found that some methods of storage frequently resulted in catastrophic failure (i.e. death from rupture of the allograft). Nine of 12 dogs that received abdominal aortic allografts that had been frozen to -72°C (the temperature of 'dry ice' – CO_2) without a cryoprotective agent died within two weeks of surgery when the allograft ruptured. In contrast, none of the 25 allografts that had been stored in a balanced salt solution at 4°C ruptured.[14]

During the decade that ensued many aortic allografts were implanted for coarctation with no widely known reports of failure, although undoubtedly aneurysms, aorto left bronchial fistulas, and rupture occurred sporadically.[15,16] Subsequently, arterial allografts were applied to other peripheral vascular problems such as abdominal aortic aneurysm and iliac and femoral arterial occlusive disease. This clinical experience in the early 1950s suggested that there was a higher risk of aneurysm formation or thrombosis with allografts from peripheral muscular arteries such as the femoral artery than there was when proximal, more elastic arteries, such as the ascending aorta, were used. In addition, the logistical and legal problems of collection and storage led to general dissatisfaction with allografts.[17,18]

SYNTHETIC VASCULAR GRAFTS

The Dacron tube graft

As described above Dacron is a synthetic polymer that was developed in the 1950s. DeBakey in Houston was one of the first to recognize that a tube graft could be constructed from fabric woven or knitted from Dacron and then sealed by blood clot. His mother was a seamstress and helped him to roll a flat sheet of Dacron and to sew a longitudinal seam to construct one of the first fabric vascular tube grafts. He used these early tube grafts to replace the abdominal aorta of adult patients with aneurysms with remarkable success. However early tube grafts had a tendency to kink. This problem was reduced by crimping the Dacron by chemical or heat treatment of the graft, though this did weaken the fibers somewhat. Knitting machines were developed which eliminated the seam.

Sterling Edwards, another pioneer in the field of vascular surgery emphasized in an early report that it was the porosity of fabric tubes that gave them a paradoxical advantage over nonporous alternatives.[19] A totally impervious conduit, such as a Silastic tube, showed progressive accumulation of pseudointima, forming an inert capsule (both inner and outer) with no adhesion of that capsule to the prosthesis, much like the thick nonadherent capsule surrounding a pacemaker generator.[20]

Wesolowski and coworkers pursued the relationship between synthetic conduit porosity and healing with a wide range of laboratory studies.[21,22] In 1961 they concluded that optimal healing occurred with a water porosity of 5000 ml/cm^2 per minute at a pressure of 120 mmHg. Most of the higher porosity *knitted* Dacron grafts currently in use have a porosity of approximately 2000 ml/cm^2 per minute. In the nonheparinized patient undergoing peripheral vascular surgery this high porosity can be controlled at the time of implantation by preclotting the graft with the patient's own blood. This is not adequate for the fully heparinized patient undergoing cardiac surgery. Numerous attempts were made beginning in the 1960s to achieve temporary porosity control with biologic sealants other than the patients own fibrin clot. However, early investigators had persistent problems with cracking and separation of sealant materials.[23–25]

An alternative approach to biologic sealants for temporary porosity control was to use less porous fabric. This led to the introduction of woven fabric tubes with a baseline porosity of 100–250 ml/cm^2 per minute, such as the Cooley Veri-Soft graft (Meadox Medical, Newark, NJ). Because acceptable blood loss in the heparinized patient requires a porosity of less than 50 ml/cm^2 per minute, even these grafts require preclotting. Another technique that was popular before the development of sealed grafts was to bake these moderate-porosity, woven tube grafts after soaking them in heparinized blood or albumin. To avoid the need for any graft preparation, very tightly woven, very low porosity grafts, such as the Cooley Lo-Por graft (Meadox Medical, Newark, NJ), were introduced. Such grafts have a baseline porosity of approximately 50 ml/cm^2 per minute. They are difficult to handle because of their rigidity and difficulty with needle penetration. In addition, Edwards' and Wesolowski's predictions about the healing of such grafts proved to be correct.[19,21] These grafts accumulate a poorly adherent, thick pseudointima with areas of hemorrhagic dissection between the luminal surface of the graft and the pseudointima. Although this may not be of clinical significance in a large-diameter (greater than 20 mm) straight tube graft (e.g. one used for replacement of an abdominal aortic aneurysm), it is certainly significant in smaller grafts, particularly when placed in growing children (Figure 3.4).

It was Sauvage et al who introduced the concept of adding velour internally, externally, or both. Sauvage correctly believed that velour would encourage fibrous and vascular ingrowth and thus anchor the pseudointima. This prevents repeated episodes of dissection leading to thickening of the pseudointima.[26–28] Velour loops also have the advantage that they decrease the porosity of the fabric, but only to a limited degree. Therefore, the search continued for a suitable technique of incorporating a biologically degradable component within the graft.

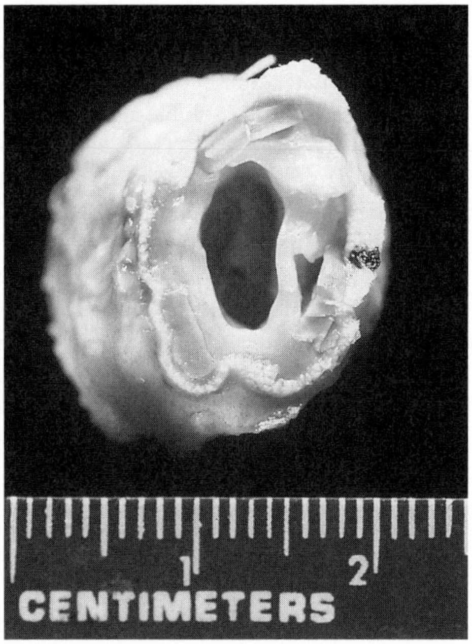

Figure 3.4 *Small diameter Dacron tube grafts rapidly become obstructed by the pseudointima which accumulates. In very low porosity grafts the pseudointima is poorly anchored to the Dacron and tends to dissect.*

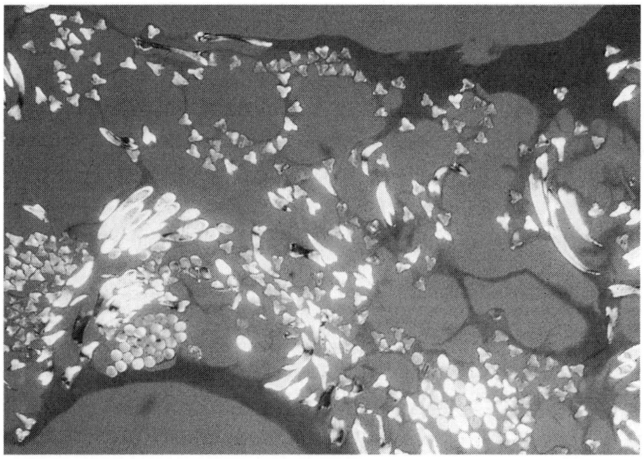

Figure 3.5 *The Hemashield process allows temporary porosity control of high porosity Dacron using a resorbable biological sealant (aldehyde cross-linked collagen). The figure illustrates unimplanted Hemashield treated Dacron showing the sealant material.*

Biologic sealants for Dacron grafts

Wesolowski studied the 'sealant' concept with a number of materials, including aldehyde cross-linked collagen.[29] He determined from this work that delayed resorption of the absorbable component (such as strongly cross-linked collagen) actually accelerated pseudointima formation and graft occlusion.

However collagen can be loosely cross-linked by using formaldehyde rather than glutaraldehyde. This is the basis of the Hemashield process (Meadox Medical, Newark, NJ) that currently is commercially available in the United States (Figure 3.5). Laboratory studies using subcutaneous implants of treated Dacron in rats, as well as circulatory implants in sheep, have suggested that this material has little effect on the normal healing process of the Dacron graft though there is still the usual inflammatory response and fibrosis as is seen with untreated Dacron. Studies have confirmed excellent porosity control to less than 10 ml/cm^2 per minute.[30,31] The Hemashield process is also very effective in controlling bleeding through suture needle holes.

Another approach similar to the Hemashield process is to use the tropocollagen subunits of collagen as found in gelatin (Gelweave, Vascutek/Sulzer Carbomedics, Austin, TX). Tropocollagen is highly water soluble and has been used as a plasma expander for many years. The collagen subunits are weakly cross-linked using aldehyde. The degree of cross-linking can be controlled by chemically converting some of the amino groups that take part in the cross-link to carboxyl groups. Laboratory studies undertaken at Children's Hospital Boston suggest that this approach like the Hemashield process does not significantly impede the normal healing process of knitted Dacron grafts.[32]

A number of researchers continue to pursue the concept of a composite fabric in which one of the yarns incorporated in the weave is bioresorbable. Careful assessment must be made of the rate of decay of fabric strength; the fabric must have sufficient long term strength to resist aneurysm formation.[33–35]

Expanded PTFE (Goretex, Impra) tube grafts

ePTFE, as noted above, is a form of Teflon in which the polymer is arranged as a lattice of nodes interconnected by filaments. Early clinical implants used for aortic or iliac artery replacement had a tendency toward aneurysmal dilation. This was overcome by the addition of an external PTFE wrap or by increasing the thickness of the graft wall. In its current commercial form, this material (known as Gore-Tex or Impra) has proved to be considerably more successful than Dacron as a small (<7 mm internal diameter) arterial prosthesis. PTFE conduits have the same disadvantages as PTFE patches particularly persistent needle-hole bleeding (which is only partially overcome by the use of PTFE suture in the fully heparinized patient) and the difficulty of conforming this material to the irregular course sometimes required for cardiac reconstructive purposes. The new 'stretch' form of PTFE has much less of a tendency to kink relative to standard PTFE and is therefore preferred for baffles and complex patches. It is important to note that PTFE manufactured for use as a conduit should not be used within the heart in a situation where the external surface will be exposed to blood, e.g. for the intraatrial baffle constructed for a modified Fontan procedure. This surface is not designed to contact blood and may be thrombogenic. Internal baffles should be constructed from the form of PTFE specifically designated for use as a cardiovascular patch.

Endothelial lining of synthetic prostheses

To improve the long-term patency of small caliber conduits a number of centers undertook research investigating the seeding of endothelial cells onto Dacron or PTFE grafts. Humans do not endothelialize synthetic conduits (in contrast to many laboratory animals such as dogs). Endothelial cells can be mechanically or enzymatically debrided from a suitable dispensable autologous blood vessel. The cells are then suspended in the patient's blood which is used to preclot the prosthesis. Cell culture techniques can be used to increase the number of cells. Despite promising early results, these techniques present logistic difficulties.[36] In addition, there is emerging doubt that even if endothelial cells remain viable when bonded directly to synthetic material many important functions such as their antithrombogenic properties, including the synthesis of prostacyclin, may not be preserved in this setting. Attention is currently being directed at the role of the basement membrane in facilitating normal endothelial cell function. The future may lie with tissue engineering techniques to develop the entire vessel architecture using autologous cells.

BIOLOGIC GRAFTS OTHER THAN ARTERIAL ALLOGRAFTS

A number of vascular xenografts have been described since Carrel first reported the use of frozen and formalin-preserved arterial xenografts as arterial substitutes.[10] Rosenberg and associates[37] described the treatment of bovine carotid arteries with ficin to remove the antigenicity of the smooth muscle followed by collagen cross-linking with dialdehyde starch. Although this graft is useful as a subcutaneous arteriovenous fistula for hemodialysis, its susceptibility to thrombosis and aneurysm formation has limited its application for other vascular procedures.

Human umbilical vein treated with glutaraldehyde and incorporated within a mesh of Dacron was popular for a time and initially functioned as well as saphenous vein for above knee, femoropopliteal bypass. With longer periods of implantation however there was an increasing risk of aneurysmal degeneration, thrombosis, and false aneurysm formation at the sites of anastomoses.[38]

Vascular tube grafts as conduits for congenital cardiac surgery

AORTIC AND PULMONARY ALLOGRAFT CONDUITS

Although the first reports of successful clinical implantation of a conduit for congenital heart disease was Klinner's description of the use of an autologous pericardial tube in 1964[39] and Rastelli's report from the Mayo Clinic in 1965,[40] the first conduits used regularly for cardiac reconstructive procedures were aortic allografts placed between the right ventricle and pulmonary artery for tetralogy of Fallot with pulmonary atresia. Because adequate pericardium often is not available in these patients and because of the hemodynamic advantages of incorporating a valve in the conduit, Ross and Somerville introduced the concept of a valved, aortic allograft conduit in Britain in 1966[41] (see Figure 3.3). Unlike Gross's allograft conduits for coarctation, Ross included the aortic valve with the aortic root and ascending aorta, thus re-creating the valved right ventricular outflow tract. Ross's allografts were collected from cadavers, generally within 24–48 hours of death. After dissection the allografts were treated with an antibiotic solution for a few days and were then stored in either a balanced salt solution or in tissue culture medium at 4°C for up to four weeks.

When allografts were introduced in the United States as either a right ventricle to pulmonary artery conduit or as an aortic valve replacement, at least two important changes to

Ross's original method were made. First, instead of a weak antibiotic solution to 'sterilize' the allografts, high-power irradiation was employed. Instead of being stored in a balanced salt solution, with or without tissue culture medium at 4°C, many allografts were freeze dried. These techniques, particularly in combination, led to death of cells and severe damage to the collagen within the valve leaflets. Although Ross had observed calcification in the wall of this conduit, valve leaflet calcification had been extremely rare.[41,42] In contrast, stenosis rapidly developed in the valve of the irradiated, freeze-dried allograft, and therefore, allografts fell into general disrepute in the United States until they were rediscovered in the mid-1980s[43] (see below).

Current methods of allograft collection and preparation

The organization of regional organ and tissue banks has facilitated the collection of allografts. Most donors in the United States when homografts were reintroduced in the mid-1980s were brain-dead (but heart-beating) multiple-organ donors. The collection was undertaken in the sterile setting of an operating room. Following a rapid increase in demand for a wide range of allograft sizes by the late 1980s, homograft collection expanded to include cadavers, as has been the practice in Britain, New Zealand, and other countries since the 1960s. In the early 1990s the FDA declared that allografts were to be treated as implantable devices necessitating strict quality controls for the tissue banks and commercial interests responsible for homograft preparation. This resulted in a reduction in the number of organizations undertaking homograft preparation in the United States.

Allografts stored at 4°C gradually lose cellular viability and tissue integrity and are discarded within four to six weeks of collection. This presents a major logistic problem, particularly in the management of smaller children, where the number of appropriate size donors is limited. Major advances in cryopreservation technology currently allow the preservation of many cells, such as sperm and red cells, and even complete embryos, which can be preserved possibly indefinitely. Whereas Gross used an uncontrolled rate of freezing to the temperature of dry ice (−72°C), current practice involves a controlled rate of freezing to the temperature of liquid nitrogen (−196°C). In addition, a cryoprotectant such as dimethyl sulfoxide (DMSO) also helps to prevent formation of intracellular ice crystals during the freezing process. The specific antibiotics employed can also influence the long-term performance of allografts. Studies by Armiger and associates in the 1980s[44] suggested that a combination of cefoxitin, lincomycin, polymyxin B, vancomycin, and amphotericin (CLPVA) was optimal for facilitating ongrowth and ingrowth of recipient cells into the leaflets of the allograft valve. Subsequent studies by companies responsible for preparation of homografts in the US resulted in modification of this antibiotic mixture in an attempt to maximize cellular viability, although this increases the risk of persistent bacterial contamination, necessitating discarding of the allograft. Changes in the antibiotic formulation may have been responsible at least in part for cases of serious sepsis that have occurred with implantation of allograft tissue other than valves and conduits. Fortunately serious sepsis has not been observed with cardiac allograft tissue.

Cellular viability and long-term allograft performance

A longstanding controversy has centered on the importance of continuing viability of donor cells in the maintenance of allograft durability. The point of view espoused by Barratt-Boyes for many years has been that the allograft is primarily a collagenous skeleton and that donor cellular viability is unimportant. Preservation of the mucopolysaccharide ground substance, as well as the ultrastructure of collagen and elastin during preparation, is considered important. Appropriate preparation is also important to encourage both ongrowth and ingrowth of recipient cells onto the valve leaflets.[44] This lappet of tissue at the critical hinge area of the valve is important for leaflet durability. The usual mechanism of failure of allografts is rupture of the leaflets in the hinge area, resulting in valvar regurgitation. In the case of aortic allografts, the conduit wall almost always becomes heavily calcified, so it is unlikely that viability of cells could influence the durability of conduit function. In the case of pulmonary allografts, calcification of the arterial wall is less common and, when present, usually less pronounced relative to aortic allografts.[45] This may be related to both the fact that the arterial wall of the pulmonary allograft is thinner (60% of aortic allograft thickness) and as well as the fact that the elastin concentration is less, as elastin tends to be the nidus for calcification. At least three laboratory studies have suggested that pulmonary allografts harvested from immature animals and implanted into growing animals can increase in size with time.[45–47] Whether this represents growth secondary to viable cells or to simple dilatation remains unknown.

An alternative to the collagenous skeleton theory is the theory supported by O'Brien et al from Brisbane, Australia for many years.[48,49] O'Brien believes that continuing viability of donor fibroblasts is important for the maintenance and continuing synthesis of collagen. In an anecdotal case in which a valve was retrieved 10 years after implantation, they were able to demonstrate by chromosome studies that donor cells were viable. Others have argued that this does not confirm a functional role for any remaining viable donor cells.[45] There is little disagreement that the majority of endothelial cells become necrotic during the collection, preparation and storage procedures. Yankah and associates[50,51] quantitated the percentage of viable endothelial cells in a rat model and found that all endothelial cells were dead within five days of harvesting.

If the importance of cellular viability is accepted, then modifications must be made to the harvesting, preparation and storage methods to guarantee maximal cell viability. This was the stimulus for modification of the antibiotic solution to sterilize the valve before cryopreservation. Cryopreservation itself must be carefully controlled to maximize cellular viability. When this is done properly long-term viability will be much enhanced relative to that with simple storage at 4°C.

In the most recent work examining the durability of homografts the importance of cellular viability has been questioned. In fact Schoen et al have suggested that the cellular material in allografts is the focus of calcification.[52] Therefore a new process has been developed (Synergraft, Cryolife, Kennesaw, GA) that removes cells in the hope that this will reduce failure secondary to calcification. Clinical implants are presently being undertaken but long-term data are not yet available.

Role of rejection in determining allograft durability

Until the widespread application of cryopreserved allografts in the mid-1980s most allografts used clinically were non-viable, so immune reactions to cellular elements were irrelevant. Collagen is a ubiquitous protein that does not stimulate an immune response per se, and fibroblasts, in contrast to endothelial cells, do not express class II antigens, which are important in the rejection response. After the introduction of cryopreserved 'viable' allografts, attention was directed at the potential role of immune mechanisms in damaging allograft durability. In a series of elegant experiments, Yankah and coworkers[51] demonstrated that implantation of a viable aortic allograft in the abdominal aorta of inbred species of rats resulted in accelerated rejection of skin grafts from the same donor species. This has led some centers to use short-term immunosuppression in patients after allograft valve insertion. However, this does not seem to be justified until a more formal clinical study has conclusively demonstrated significant benefits of such an approach. The introduction of acellular allografts will of course eliminate the need to consider immunosuppression.

Mode of failure of allograft conduits

Failure of allografts implanted in children as conduits is most commonly a result of outgrowth of the conduit. Longitudinal growth can result in lengthening and narrowing. Aggressive calcification can protrude into the lumen and the valve leaflets may become rigid and stenotic and even calcified. There may be compression by the sternum of the proximal anastomosis. Experience with the Ross procedure in which large allograft conduits are placed in the orthotopic position and there is little or no risk of compression has revealed a disappointing tendency for some allograft conduits to rapidly shrink to a size that is markedly smaller than the original implant size. It is suspected that this may be immune mediated though there are no data to support this hypothesis.[53]

Catastrophic failure of allograft conduits used for cardiac reconstruction has not yet been reported. However, based on the clinical experience of vascular surgeons during the 1950s, it seems likely that with more widespread application of this biologic material, there will be occasional very late (decades) failure by allograft rupture or the formation of pseudoaneurysms or conduit to bronchus fistulas.[15,54,55] This may be more likely with pulmonary homografts. When applied in a situation where it will be exposed to pressure equal to or greater than systemic pressure, a pulmonary allograft conduit can show rapid dilatation.[45–47] Because the pulmonary valve itself lacks a fibrous annulus, there is a significant risk of pseudoaneurysm formation at the proximal anastomosis. In fact, such pseudoaneurysms necessitated two reoperations among the first 100 pulmonary allografts inserted at Children's Hospital in Boston between 1985 and 1989 and have been seen regularly since, sometimes following balloon dilation. Also, rupture of a pulmonary allograft exposed to systemic pressure as part of the reconstruction for a neonate with hypoplastic left heart syndrome was seen early in the experience though this was in the setting of sepsis. Nevertheless it would seem prudent to limit the use of pulmonary allografts to sites where the predicted intra-allograft pressure will be substantially subsystemic. In addition, any child receiving an allograft conduit must be carefully followed for life for early detection of the potential complications described.

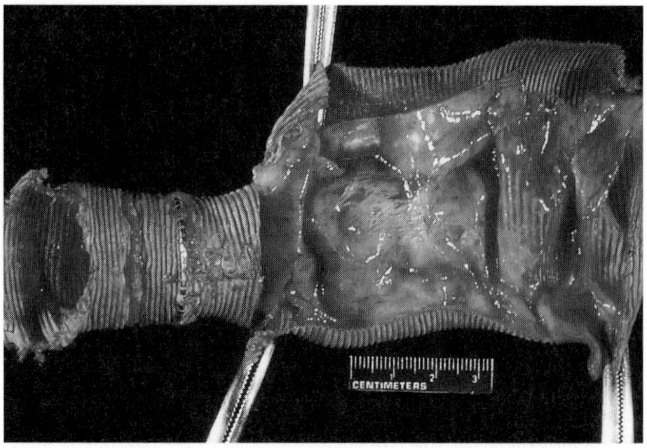

Figure 3.6 *Low porosity Dacron conduits containing a glutaraldehyde treated porcine valve were introduced in the early 1970s. These conduits failed rapidly in children because of a combination of pseudointima formation on the low porosity Dacron as well as calcification of the glutaraldehyde treated xenograft valve.*

BIOPROSTHETIC CONDUITS

In the early 1970s, very low porosity, woven Dacron valved conduits became available.[56] Such conduits were combined with the glutaraldehyde-treated pig valve as pioneered by Carpentier et al.[57] The immense logistic advantages of such conduits, which could be stocked in a complete range of sizes, proved attractive, and during the ensuing decade many thousands of these Hancock and Carpentier-Edwards conduits were implanted.

Within just five years, reports of the unsatisfactory performance of these conduits appeared (Figure 3.6).[58,59] As could have been predicted from Wesolowski's studies in 1963, a thick pseudointima frequently accumulated rapidly. In addition, others noted that glutaraldehyde tanning of pig valves resulted in rapid calcification in children[60,61] (see below). Thus, a combination of pseudointima formation and valve stenosis resulted in a less than 50% freedom from conduit replacement within nine years of implantation even in larger children. They were also far too rigid and large to be successfully applied in neonates and small infants. There was a risk that the stent supporting the valve would compress the left main coronary artery. In their favor, however, it should be noted once they had been successfully implanted the mode of failure of these conduits was only very rarely catastrophic. Simple monitoring of the systolic murmur and right ventricular hypertrophy on the electrocardiogram allowed for elective replacement of these conduits, which easily shelled out of their covering of pseudoadventitia, at very low risk.

Addition of a valve to the conduit appeared to accelerate pseudointima formation,[62] and thus one response to the problem was a more liberal use of nonvalved conduits. However, by this time the superior long-term results of Ross and others using allografts became widely appreciated,[63,64] and in the mid-1980s the allograft once again became the conduit of first choice for cardiac reconstruction in the United States.

Over the last decade bovine jugular veins containing a valve have been developed by Brown[65] for use as cardiac conduits and are now commercially available in Europe (Contegra, Medtronic, Minneapolis, MN).[66] These grafts are fixed with glutaraldehyde to cross-link the collagen. An anticalcification process is also applied. There is presently little long-term information.

Recently some groups have begun to explore the possibility of using unstented xenograft aortic valves (e.g. Medtronic Freestyle, Medtronic, Minneapolis, MN) for right ventricle to pulmonary artery connection. Because these xenografts are treated with glutaraldehyde it is very likely that they will suffer from accelerated calcification when used in children less than 18–20 years of age. No long-term information is available.[67]

Another xenograft option more specifically designed for children and treated with a proprietary anticalcification process has not proven satisfactory in one early report.[68] One other option is the use of a PTFE conduit containing a glutaraldehyde treated bovine pericardial valve.[69] Perhaps some of the newer anticalcification processes will be helpful but this is yet to be demonstrated.

MANAGEMENT OF THE STENOTIC CONDUIT

As described above conduits become stenotic for a number of reasons. The lifespan is determined by how many of these factors are present and most importantly by the original size of the conduit and the rate of growth of the child. On occasion it is possible to gain an extra year or two by balloon dilation of a stenotic allograft usually in combination with stent placement.[70] Placement of a stent across the proximal anastomosis will result in free regurgitation. Stents in this location are also vulnerable to sternal compression and may fragment and embolize. There is also a risk of compression of the left main coronary artery, the course of which should be identified in relation to the planned site of placement of the stent before it is deployed.

Surgical replacement of the obstructed RV-PA conduit

Surgical management of the stenotic conduit is a common operation that can be performed today at very low risk. It is useful to image the conduit by angiography relative to the sternal wires at the time of catheterization when balloon dilation and stenting may be performed. It is usually then possible to follow the gradient across the conduit by Doppler and to avoid a second catheterization before the surgery. The exact indications for conduit replacement remain poorly defined and will remain so until more sophisticated analyses of right ventricular function are available. Hopefully MRI will enable this in the near future. In general today conduit replacement is recommended if right ventricular pressure is estimated to be more than about two thirds left ventricular pressure. Dilation of the right ventricle, diminished function, evidence by imaging of severe narrowing or the presence of symptoms may direct earlier replacement.

A careful decision must be made regarding the use of femoral bypass for conduit change. Most large centers do not use femoral bypass routinely though the femoral vessels must be assessed at least by palpation and should be prepped into the field. Following the reoperative sternotomy (Chapter 2) the right atrium is cannulated usually with a single venous cannula and the arterial cannula is introduced into the ascending aorta. The aorta is not cross-clamped and the heart is allowed to beat throughout the procedure usually at a mild level of hypothermia such as 30°C. It is important to be aware of the presence of septal defects including a patent foramen ovale. If these are present there is a risk that air or calcific debris can be introduced into the systemic circulation. Under these circumstances it may be advisable to cross clamp the aorta.

The stenotic conduit is usually excised and is replaced in a fashion similar to insertion of a first-time conduit (see Chapter 2). However another option is to filet open the previous conduit and to perform a patch plasty enlargement. A variation of this approach can also be used when the original conduit has been a Dacron conduit which is usually surrounded by an external fibrous 'peel'. This is particularly appealing if the conduit was a tightly woven conduit which will lift out easily from its bed of fibrous tissue. Dacron conduits treated with collagen impregnation such as the Hemashield process are more densely incorporated and less suitable for a patch plasty approach. The fibrous peel is opened longitudinally and enlarged with a patch plasty using PTFE or Dacron. Long-term results reported with this approach have been encouraging though it should be reserved for the same circumstances where a nonvalved conduit might be used.[71]

WHEN CAN A NONVALVED CONDUIT BE USED?

It is probably inadvisable to use a nonvalved conduit in situations where the pulmonary vascular resistance is elevated such as in the neonate and young infant although there are a few reports of successful application even in this situation using a nonvalved connection, e.g. for the repair of truncus arteriosus.[72] It is also an advantage to have a valve within the conduit if the pulmonary arteries are hypoplastic or distorted, e.g. by previous shunts. When the pulmonary arteries are of normal size and resistance a nonvalved conduit appears to be well tolerated; after all the physiology is the same as that for a transannular patch after repair of tetralogy with pulmonary stenosis. It is also important to recognize that allograft valves within conduits usually become incompetent within a few months to years of implantation.

THE FUTURE: AUTOGRAFTS AND TISSUE ENGINEERING

The growth potential of tubular segments of arterial autograft in children has been confirmed over many years by experience with renovascular reconstruction using segments of iliac artery.[73,74] Furthermore, the potential for a relatively narrow strip of autologous tissue to provide appropriate growth when incorporated as a small part of the circumference of an otherwise nongrowing tube has been observed in a number of reconstructive cardiac procedures, including the Mustard and Norwood procedures. These observations led us to incorporate a strip of free arterial autograft as part of a conduit, the rest of which is constructed of pericardium. Appropriate growth was confirmed in 10-month-old lambs over 12 months.[75] A clinical implant, consisting of a longitudinal strip of free aortic autograft on an aortic allograft, has been inserted and has also demonstrated satisfactory growth.

Autologous pericardium formed into a valved conduit has been described by Kreutzer et al. The intermediate term results are very encouraging.[1] However as with allografts the pericardial valve becomes incompetent within a few months of implantation.

Finally tissue engineering methods have been used to develop a 'living skin equivalent' which has been an important advance in the treatment of extensive skin loss caused by burns. Using cell culture methods, the layers of the dermis are built up, resulting in skin that is histologically and functionally similar to normal skin. Concerted efforts are currently under way to fabricate a living blood vessel equivalent as well as a semilunar valve employing the same technology.[76] This approach should prove to be the answer to the longstanding problem of identifying the ideal conduit for children.

VALVES

Emphasis on valvuloplasty techniques

The palliative nature of valve replacement in both adults and children has become widely appreciated since the 1980s. More recently this has come to include the Ross operation which was widely believed in the early 1990s to be a panacea for aortic valve disease. Unfortunately this has not proven to be the case.[77,78] The development of transesophageal echocardiography, including color Doppler and 3D reconstruction, has facilitated not only an improved understanding of mechanisms of valve dysfunction but also an appreciation of techniques that can be successfully applied to repair both semilunar and atrioventricular valves.[79,80] Nevertheless, as is discussed in Chapter 17, situations arise where valve repair is not possible and under these circumstances a decision must be made regarding the most appropriate valve replacement option.

Biologic valves

ALLOGRAFTS

The history of the development of allografts as conduits has been described above. The aortic valve was first implanted as an allograft orthotopic valve replacement in 1962 by Barratt-Boyes in New Zealand[81] and independently by Ross in London.[82] The technique they described involved insertion of the valve within the patient's own aortic root, termed a 'subcoronary freehand implant'.

Technique of subcoronary freehand implantation of aortic allograft

The allograft should be thawed and rinsed. The allograft mitral valve should be trimmed to within 4 or 5 mm from the aortic valve leaflets. It is also important to thin the allograft ventricular septal muscle that lies below the right and noncoronary cusps of the allograft aortic valve. There must be sufficient muscle left to allow secure suturing but not so much that it will bulge into the outflow tract and contribute to a residual gradient.

Two suture lines are required. The lower suture line is facilitated by inverting the valve within itself. When the valve has been everted back to its normal state the second more cephalad suture line is constructed. Scallops are cut in the two coronary sinuses to allow the coronary arteries to remain in situ. The commissural posts must be aligned exactly to avoid regurgitation with careful judgment to allow for subsequent closure of the aortotomy. This technique is not suitable for the adult patient with a small aortic root and is rarely feasible in children.

Technique of aortic allograft insertion as a root replacement

An alternative technique for aortic allograft implantation which can be used in children is to place the valve as a complete aortic root replacement. A circumferential suture line attaches the allograft root to the left ventricular outflow tract and the distal anastomosis is performed to the ascending aorta. The coronary arteries are implanted as buttons. Although care must be taken to ensure that the lower suture line is hemostatic and that there no distortion or kinking of the coronary arteries, aortic root replacement requires considerably less skill and judgment than the freehand subcoronary implant technique originally described by Barratt-Boyes and Ross. It was this technique that became very popular for aortic valve replacement in the US in the late 1980s.[83]

Results of aortic allograft valve replacement

The excellent hemodynamic characteristics of this valve reported by Barratt-Boyes and Ross have been confirmed in many reports.[84] In addition, there appears to be virtually no risk of thromboembolism, even in the absence of anticoagulants. Freedom from the need for anticoagulants during early childhood and through the child-bearing years is an obvious important advantage. The valve is also silent, and in many countries it can be obtained without great logistic difficulty at a reasonable cost for harvesting and processing. Like any biologic material that is not wholly viable, there is eventual tissue deterioration resulting in failure of the valve leaflets, usually adjacent to the hinge areas. Barratt-Boyes and coworkers reported the rate of freedom from significant valve incompetence in adults to be 78% at 10 years.[84] O'Brien and associates reported a 100% rate of freedom from valve failure owing to tissue deterioration at 10 years in 192 valves that were stored by cryopreservation and inserted in adults.[48] Results in children have been far less satisfactory, particularly in children less than three or four years of age. Aggressive calcification can occur within a few months resulting in early failure through stenosis or regurgitation.[85]

Allograft availability

When there was a sudden increase in interest in allograft aortic valve replacement in the United States beginning in the mid-1980s, regional organ banks had difficulty coping with the demand. This was particularly true with respect to small pediatric sizes which were mainly to be used as conduits. Studies at Children's Hospital Boston confirmed satisfactory structural integrity of allografts collected up to 48 hours after donor death, which meant that collection no longer needed to be confined to brain-dead, heart-beating organ donors in whom sterile collection was undertaken in the operating room as part of a multiple-organ harvest.[86] Extending collection to cadaver hearts helped to improve the availability of valves in pediatric sizes. Also the pulmonary allograft began to be used with increasing frequency initially because of the shortage of aortic allografts. Although the pulmonary allograft is a satisfactory substitute for the patient's own pulmonary valve, it is not advisable to use it as an aortic valve replacement. This is particularly true if the physician is considering aortic root replacement with the pulmonary root and valve.[87,88]

Allografts used in locations other than the aortic valve position

Various attempts have been made over the years to use allograft valves as atrioventricular valve replacements.[89,90] The mitral valve, including the papillary muscles, has been used as an implant but has generally failed because of shortening and fibrosis of the subvalvar support apparatus. Aortic allograft valves have been mounted on a stent and placed in the mitral position but have soon failed, because in the absence of glutaraldehyde treatment, allograft tissue is not strong enough to withstand the stresses resulting from stent mounting.[91] In addition, the normal aortic valve must withstand only aortic diastolic pressure, whereas the mitral valve must withstand left ventricular systolic pressure.

PULMONARY AUTOGRAFT: THE ROSS PROCEDURE

In 1967 Ross described the use of the patient's own pulmonary valve as an aortic valve replacement.[92] In Ross's original description of the procedure the pulmonary root was inserted into the aortic position as a subcoronary freehand implant using the same technique that had been described originally by Ross and Barratt-Boyes for insertion of an aortic allograft. With this method the autograft is supported by the aortic sinuses of Valsalva. The pulmonary autograft like the aortic allograft may also be placed as an aortic root replacement with reimplantation of the coronary arteries. The right ventricular outflow tract must be reconstructed, generally using a pulmonary allograft. Details of the technique are described in Chapter 18, as part of the description of the Ross/Konno procedure.

Results of the Ross procedure

There was considerable enthusiasm for the Ross procedure for aortic valve replacement in children in the early 1990s. The autograft has the important advantage that it will grow and because it is viable and not subject to rejection, valve leaflet integrity is maintained probably for life. However some important problems began to emerge during the latter half of the 1990s.[77,93,94] Most importantly it was found that the neoaortic root had a tendency in some children to dilate excessively with consequent regurgitation of the valve. Children whose original problem was aortic regurgitation are particularly prone to this problem. Attempts to fix the annulus by placement of a band of Dacron have not eliminated dilation of the sinuses of Valsalva but in some cases have resulted in creation of subaortic stenosis. Another disappointing finding has been that the pulmonary allograft used for reconstruction often becomes stenotic and requires replacement surgically. This occurs even when the original pulmonary allograft has been large, perhaps even adult size. It is possible that immunologic factors cause what appears to be rapid shrinking of some allografts.[53,95] Gerosa and associates also have described a disappointing high incidence of bacterial endocarditis in the autografts over the very long-term from Ross's original series.[96] This is surprising in view of the known viability of the autograft and its excellent hemodynamic characteristics.

Bioprosthetic valves

Bioprosthetic valves can be defined as a biologic valve modified with prosthetic material in some way such as being supported by a stent. Many varieties of bioprosthetic valves have been marketed since the 1970s. The most popular initially were porcine aortic valves treated with glutaraldehyde to cross-link collagen, followed by mounting of the valve in a plastic or metal stent. These valves did not have good hemodynamics and in the smaller sizes which might have been used for children had unacceptable gradients. Stent-mounted porcine valves have been superseded in the main by stent-mounted pericardial valves, usually bovine pericardium fixed with glutaraldehyde. An early version of the bovine pericardial valve was the Ionescu-Shiley valve which had a high rate of failure because of tearing of the tissue.[97] Changes in the design of the stent and the technique of mounting of the pericardium in the stent have resulted in improved durability in adults. Nonstent-mounted porcine valves have been introduced in various forms over the last few years, e.g. the Toronto SPV and the Medtronic Freestyle valve. These are glutaraldehyde-fixed porcine valves which are more user friendly for implantation using variations of the subcoronary freehand technique described above for aortic allograft insertion. These valves have very much better hemodynamics than stent-mounted valves because of their greater effective orifice area.

Unfortunately, bioprosthetic valves are uniformly unsuitable for pediatric implantation because of their susceptibility to accelerated calcification.[60,98] The exact mechanism is not clear, although it is related in part to the accelerated calcium metabolism of children, who are in the process of ossifying cartilage. It appears that after 20–25 years of age, accelerated calcification is less of a problem. In addition to the accelerated calcium metabolism of childhood another factor contributing to the rapid calcification of bioprostheses is glutaraldehyde treatment. It may be possible to decrease glutaraldehyde-induced calcification by the use of agents such as ethanol to extract phospholipids from the valve tissue.[99]

Various proprietary treatments, e.g. 'Xenologic Treatment' by Edwards (Irvine, CA) and 'No-React' by Shellhigh Inc (Milburn, NJ) are said to reduce calcification of xenograft fixed tissue though the long-term effectiveness in children is unclear.

Mechanical valves

The first widely used mechanical valve, the caged ball design typified by the Starr-Edwards valve generally was not suitable for pediatric use. This is a high-profile valve which, when placed in the mitral position, for example, projects into the left ventricular outflow tract.[100] In the aortic position in a small aortic root, it is likely to have very poor hemodynamics, as blood must pass between the ball and the ascending aortic wall. The Bjork-Shiley tilting-disk valve was successfully applied for many years as a pediatric aortic or mitral valve replacement.[101,102] The valve had a low profile and could be rotated within its sewing ring, which was an important advantage. In small infant and neonatal hearts, there is often only one position where the disk occluder will move completely freely. The Bjork-Shiley valve was removed from the market in the United States in 1988 because of a small but important incidence of outlet strut fracture.[103]

Following the removal of the Bjork-Shiley valve from the market, the St Jude medical valve became and has in general remained the valve of first choice for pediatric implantation. This bileaflet valve has excellent hemodynamic characteristics, although it is inferior to the aortic allograft.[104] There is a small but real incidence of thromboembolism even when there is careful control with anticoagulants (which is certainly recommended, using sodium warfarin (Coumadin) for both aortic and mitral valve replacement). The inability to rotate the valve within the sewing ring was an important disadvantage of the St Jude valve in its original form. This has been addressed in more recent models such as the 'Regent valve rotatable'. The patent for the St Jude valve expired in approximately 2000 so that a number of alternative bileaflet pyrolytic carbon valves have appeared on the market, e.g. On-X (Medical Carbon Research Institute, Austin, TX), CarboMedics (Sulzer CarboMedics Inc, Austin, TX).[105]

THE 'COMPOSITE CONDUIT' FOR AORTIC ROOT AND ASCENDING AORTA REPLACEMENT

Bileaflet carbon valves are available incorporated within a woven Dacron tube graft. The St Jude valve is supplied within a woven Dacron tube graft sealed with the Hemashield process while the Carbomedics valve is available with the Gelweave process. The composite conduit is useful for replacement of the dilated aortic root and ascending aorta with associated aortic regurgitation. The coronary arteries are mobilized on buttons of aortic wall and are implanted into the orthotopic sites on the conduit. It is important to use a hand held cautery unit to cut the graft material to ensure that there is no fraying of the edges. In the pediatric setting the composite conduit is most commonly applied for patients with Marfan's syndrome. The Ross procedure must not be performed in this situation since the genetic mutation affects the collagen in the pulmonary root as well as the aortic root. It is our feeling that the aortic valve should be replaced in children whose aortic root requires replacement because of dilation irrespective of the competence of the aortic valve. Although success has been reported by David and others with valve-preserving procedures for adult patients with Marfan's syndrome,[106] it is likely that children with Marfan's syndrome have a more severe form of the disease and are therefore more likely to have progressive aortic valve regurgitation if the valve is preserved. If the aortic root must be replaced during infancy because of massive dilation of the root and ascending aorta it may be necessary to use an aortic homograft since the smallest diameter graft is 20 mm bonded to a 19 mm valve. However homografts in the aortic position in infants can fail very rapidly because of accelerated calcification so every attempt should be made to use a composite Dacron prosthesis rather than a homograft if at all possible.

SIZES OF MECHANICAL VALVES FOR INFANTS AND NEONATES

One advantage of the aortic allograft, in addition to those already described, is that, in theory, it is available in an infinite range of sizes, with the internal diameter ranging from about 6–25 mm. This is not the case for mechanical valves. It is simply not commercially viable for a company to manufacture small size valves for pediatric implantation because of the small number used worldwide. The Bjork-Shiley valve was previously manufactured to a minimum annular diameter of 17 mm. This was the most commonly used valve in a series of 25 infant mitral valve replacements at Children's Hospital Boston from 1973 to 1987.[107] The minimum size of the St Jude valve is 19 mm though this measurement includes the sewing ring. The company has introduced a modified sewing ring form of the 19 mm valve ('Hemodynamic Plus') which is marketed as a 17 mm valve. The Carbomedics company has also introduced modifications in the sewing ring of their 19-mm prosthesis. By using a very thin sewing ring, this valve can be reclassified as a 16- or 18-mm valve, although the hemodynamic performance is the same as that for the 19-mm valve because the same leaflets are employed. The very thin sewing ring does not mold as well to the irregular contours of the infant heart, so the risk of paravalvular leak may be increased using this valve. Furthermore, the leaflets of the Carbomedics valve project farther from the valve housing than those of the St Jude valve. The fact that the two leaflets in the St Jude valve hinge almost entirely within the valve ring is an important advantage in the pediatric setting. Even when the valve is inserted within a small chamber such as the small left atrium of the young infant for mitral valve replacement, it is rare to have a problem with restriction of leaflet movement.

SUTURES

Absorbable versus nonabsorbable

Nonabsorbable polypropylene suture (e.g. Prolene, Ethicon, Somerville, NJ) is by far the most widely used suture for congenital cardiac surgery. Its most important characteristic is its low tissue drag. Not only does this allow the suture to be drawn through delicate tissue without cutting suture 'slits' but more importantly it allows tension to be redistributed throughout a long running suture evenly, eliminating slightly loose loops which would otherwise result in bleeding. Although there are a few reports of laboratory studies demonstrating an advantage for absorbable sutures for the growth of anastomoses,[108] this is probably not the case in the human so long as very light grade nonabsorbable suture is used. In the experience at Children's Hospital Boston with the neonatal arterial switch procedure which involves a large number of growing suture lines which have been performed for many years with 6/0 and 7/0 polypropylene the incidence of anastomotic stenosis has been exceedingly small.[109]

There are some situations where the greater tissue drag of absorbable sutures such as Maxon or polydiaxanone (PDS) is an advantage. The anastomosis of the superior vena cava to the right pulmonary artery as part of the bidirectional Glenn shunt has a marked tendency to purse-string if polypropylene is used. This can be overcome by interrupting the suture line at either end or even by using an interrupted technique though this has important disadvantages as described in Chapter 2. Our preferred method to avoid purse-stringing is to use an absorbable monofilament suture such as Maxon (US Surgical/Davis and Geck).

Monofilament versus braided

Polypropylene is a monofilament suture. Its monofilament construction contributes to its low tissue drag. However monofilament sutures in general and specifically polypropylene handle poorly for tying and other surgical maneuvers. Monofilaments have a 'memory' meaning that they tend to stay in the coiled shape that they were packaged in. This problem has been reduced but not eliminated by packaging in long multi-packs. However another option is to use a braided multifilament suture such as braided polyester, e.g. Ethibond, Tevdek. These sutures have little or no memory and tie much more securely than polypropylene. Tissue drag has been reduced by coating the suture with Teflon though this increases the risk of suture throws undoing unless each throw is carefully set into place. Another disadvantage of a multifilament suture is the higher risk of bacteria being wicked into the interstices of the suture where they can be difficult to eliminate. Thus the monofilament nature as well as the strength of stainless steel wire make this the ideal material for sternal closure. Sternal wires are also useful radiological markers for the sternum when a reoperation is planned. Cardiologists should open the aperture for their cineangiograms to include the sternal wires on the lateral view. This will assist the surgeon in planning the reoperative sternotomy.

Monofilament absorbable versus braided absorbable

Polyglactin (Vicryl, Dexon) is a widely used absorbable suture that is braided. Polydioxanone (PDS) is also absorbable but is a monofilament. There is another important difference between these two sutures. Vicryl is absorbed by an acute inflammatory response within a few weeks. Polydioxanone is absorbed by hydrolysis, i.e. it slowly dissolves over several months. Histological examination of these different sutures reveals multiple acute inflammatory cells surrounding Vicryl while there is a chronic inflammatory response surrounding PDS. Not surprisingly there is subsequently more fibrosis surrounding Vicryl. This may be the explanation for the result of a laboratory study examining tracheal anastomoses in growing lambs undertaken at Childrens Hospital Boston. There was a significantly greater luminal area in anastomoses constructed with PDS versus those constructed with Vicryl.[110]

PTFE suture

PTFE suture is marketed as a means of decreasing the problem of needle-hole bleeding from PTFE patches and conduits. It achieves this goal principally by the smaller diameter of the needles to which it is swaged. These very thin needles can be difficult to work with in reoperative situations. The suture itself has low tissue drag so that it can be difficult to tie securely.

Importance of suture grade and needle selection

The surgeon should always select the finest suture that will securely hold structures together. Finer sutures result in less fibrosis at the suture line which probably facilitates growth. Appropriate needle selection is also important. Smaller gauge needles leave smaller holes and result in less bleeding. This can be important in neonatal procedures such as the arterial switch and Stage I Norwood procedure. We mostly use a small 3/8 circle needle (BV1, Ethicon) and 6/0 or 7/0 prolene for these procedures rather than the larger half-circle RB2 needle.

PLEDGETTS

Pledgetts should be used far less frequently in pediatric surgery than they are in surgery for acquired heart disease in adults. The epicardium and endocardium are very much stronger than in elderly adults. This is also true of the adventitia of the great vessels. Most importantly the small size of structures means that the wall tension is very much less than in adults so there is less risk that tissues will tear. Pledgetts also can obscure the source of bleeding. Nevertheless there are situations where use of very small Teflon or pericardial pledgetts is advisable, e.g. for VSD closure using an interrupted technique in neonates and infants and for reinforcement of the valve resuspension as part of the traditional repair of complete atrioventricular canal.

REFERENCES

1. Kreutzer C, Kreutzer GO, De C Mayorquim R et al. Early and late results of fresh autologous pericardial valved conduits. *Semin Thorac Cardiovasc Surg Pediatr Card Surg Annu* 1999; **2**:65–76.
2. Corno AF, Laks H, George B, Williams RG. Use of in situ pericardium for surgical relief of pulmonary venous obstruction following Mustard's operation. *Ann Thorac Surg* 1987; **43**:443–444.
3. Najm HK, Caldarone CA, Smallhorn J, Coles JG. A sutureless technique for the relief of pulmonary vein stenosis with the use of in situ pericardium. *J Thorac Cardiovasc Surg* 1998; **115**:468–470.
4. Deterling RA, Bhonslay SB. An evaluation of synthetic materials and fabrics suitable for blood vessel replacement. *Surgery* 1955; **38**:71.
5. Edwards WS, Tapp JS. Chemically treated nylon tubes as arterial grafts. *Surgery* 1955; **38**:61.
6. Sauvage LR, Wesolowski SA. The healing and fate of arterial grafts. *Surgery* 1955; **38**:1090.
7. Vorheese AD, Jaretzki A, Blakemore AH. The use of tubes constructed from Vinyon "N" cloth in bridging arterial defects: A preliminary report. *Ann Surg* 1952; **135**:332.
8. Campbell CD, Goldfarb D, Detton DD, Roe R, Goldsmith K, Diethrich EB. Expanded polytetrafluroethylene as a small artery substitute. *Trans Am Soc Artif Intern Organs* 1974; **20**:86–90.
9. Carrel A. Heterotransplantation of blood vessels preserved in cold storage. *J Exp Med* 1907; **9**:226.
10. Carrel A. Results of the transplantation of blood vessels, organs, and limbs. *JAMA* 1908; **51**:1662.
11. Carrel A. Ultimate results of aortic transplantations. *J Exp Med* 1912; **15**:389.
12. Crafoord C, Nylon G. Congenital coarctation of the aorta and its surgical treatment. *J Thorac Surg* 1945; **14**:347.
13. Gross RE, Hufnagel CA. Coarctation of the aorta: Experimental studies regarding its surgical correction. *N Engl J Med* 1945; **233**:287.
14. Gross RE, Bill AH, Pierce EC. Methods for preservation and transplantation of arterial grafts. *Surg Gynecol Obstet* 1949; **88**:689.
15. Hagland LA, Sweetman WR, Wise RA. Rupture of an abdominal aortic homograft with ileal fistula. *Am J Surg* 1959; **98**:746.
16. Oldham KT, Johansen K, Winterscheid L, Larson EB. Remembrance of things past: aortobronchial fistula 15 years after thoracic aortic homograft. *West J Med* 1983; **139**:225–228.
17. Brock L. Long-term degenerative changes in aortic segment homografts, with particular reference to calcification. *Thorax* 1968; **23**:249–255.
18. Meade JW, Linton RR, Darling RC, Menendez CV. Arterial homografts. A long term clinical follow-up. *Arch Surg* 1966; **93**:392–399.
19. Edwards WS. The effect of porosity in solid plastic artery grafts. *Surg Forum* 1957; **8**:446.
20. Andrade JD. Interfacial phenomena and biomaterials. *Med Instrum* 1973; **7**:110–119.
21. Wesolowski SA. The healing of vascular prostheses. *Surgery* 1965; **57**:319.
22. Wesolowski SA, Fries CC, Karlson KE et al. Porosity: Primary determinants of ultimate fate of synthetic vascular grafts. *Surgery* 1961; **50**:91.
23. Bascom JU. Gelatin sealing to prevent blood loss from knitted arterial grafts. *Surgery* 1961; **50**:504.
24. Humphries AW, Hawk WA, Cuthbertson AM. Arterial prosthesis of collagen impregnated Dacron tulle. *Surgery* 1961; **50**:947.
25. Jordan GL, Stump MM, Allen J et al. Gelatin impregnated prosthesis implanted into porcine thoracic aorta. *Surgery* 1963; **53**:45.
26. Holub DA, Trono R, Klima T et al. Macroscopic, microscopic, and mechanical analyses of prototype double velour vascular grafts. *Bull Tex Heart Inst* 1978; **5**:365.
27. Mitchell RS, Miller CD, Bilingham ME et al. Comprehensive assessment of the safety, durability, clinical performance, and healing characteristics of a double velour knitted Dacron arterial prosthesis. *Vasc Surg* 1980; **14**:197.
28. Sauvage LR, Berger K, Wood SJ, Nakagawa Y, Mansfield PB. An external velour surface for porous arterial prostheses. *Surgery* 1971; **70**:940–953.
29. Wesolowski SA, Fries CC, Domingo RT et al. The compound prosthetic vascular graft: A pathologic survey. *Surgery* 1963; **53**:19.
30. Jonas RA, Schoen FJ, Levy RJ, Castaneda AR. Biological sealants and knitted Dacron: Porosity and histological comparisons of vascular graft materials with and without collagen and fibrin glue pretreatments. *Ann Thorac Surg* 1986; **41**:657–663.
31. Jonas RA, Schoen FJ, Ziemer G, Britton L, Castaneda AR. Biological sealants and knitted Dacron conduits: Comparison of collagen and fibrin glue pretreatments in circulatory models. *Ann Thorac Surg* 1987; **44**:283–290.

32. Jonas RA, Ziemer G, Schoen FJ, Britton L, Castaneda AR. A new sealant for knitted Dacron prostheses: Minimally cross-linked gelatin. *J Vasc Surg* 1988; **7**:414–419.
33. Bowald S, Busch C, Eriksson I. Absorbable material in vascular prostheses. A new device. *Acta Chir Scand* 1980; **146**:391–395.
34. Galletti PM, Ip TK, Chiu TH, Nyilas E, Trudeli LA, Sasken H. Extending the functional life of bioresorbable yarns for vascular grafts. *Trans Am Sac Artif Intern Organs* 1984; **30**:399–400.
35. van der Lei B, Darius H, Schror K, Nieuwenhuis P, Molenaar I, Wildevuur CR. Arterial wall regeneration in small caliber vascular grafts in rats. *J Thorac Cardiovasc Surg* 1985; **90**:378–386.
36. Shindo S, Takagi A, Whittemore AD. Improved patency of collagen-impregnated grafts after in vitro autogenous endothelial cell seeding. *J Vasc Surg* 1987; **6**:325–332.
37. Rosenberg N, Gaughran ERL, Henderson J. The use of segmental arterial implants prepared by enzymatic modification of heterologous blood vessels. *Surg Forum* 1956; **6**:242.
38. Dardik H, Dardik II. Successful arterial substitution with modified human umbilical vein. *Ann Surg* 1976; **183**:252–258.
39. Klinner W. Indikationsstellung und operative Technik für die Korrektur der Fallotschen Tetralogie. *Langenbecks Arch Klin Chirurgie* 1964; **308**:40.
40. Rastelli GC, Ongley PA, Davis GD et al. Surgical repair for pulmonary valve atresia with coronary-pulmonary artery fistula: Report of case. *Mayo Clin Proc* 1965; **40**:521.
41. Ross DN, Somerville J. Correction of pulmonary atresia with a homograft aortic valve. *Lancet* 1966; **2**:1446.
42. Saravalli OA, Somerville J, Jefferson KE. Calcification of aortic homografts used for reconstruction of the right ventricular outflow tract. *J Thorac Cardiovasc Surg* 1980; **80**:909–920.
43. Ciaravella JM, McGoon DC, Danielson GK, Wallace RB, Mair DD, Ilstrup DM. Experience with the extracardiac conduit. *J Thorac Cardiovasc Surg* 1979; **78**:920–930.
44. Armiger LC, Gavin JB, Barratt-Boyes HG. Histologic assessment of orthotopic aortic valve leaflet allografts: Its role in selecting graft pretreatment. *Pathology* 1983; **15**:67–73.
45. Allen MD, Shoji Y, Fujimura Y et al. Growth and cell viability of aortic versus pulmonic homografts in the systemic circulation. *Circulation* 1991; **84** (suppl):III 94–99.
46. Kadoba K, Armiger LC, Sawatari K, Jonas RA. Mechanical durability of pulmonary allograft conduits at systemic pressure: Angiographic and histological study in lambs. *J Thorac Cardiovasc Surg* 1993; **105**:132–141.
47. Molina JE, Edwards J, Bianco R et al. Growth of fresh frozen pulmonary allograft; conduit in growing lambs. *Circulation* 1980; **80**:183–190.
48. O'Brien MF, Stafford EG, Gardner MAH, Pohlner PG, McGiffin DC. A comparison of aortic valve replacement with viable cryopreserved and fresh allograft; valves, with a note on chromosomal studies. *J Thorac Cardiovasc Surg* 1987; **94**:812–823.
49. O'Brien MF, Stafford G, Gardner M et al. The viable cryopreserved allograft. aortic valve. *J Card Surg* 1987; **2**:153–167.
50. Yankah AC, Hetzer R. Procurement and viability of cardiac valve allografts. In Yankah AC, Hetzer R, Miller DC et al (eds). *Cardiac Valve Allografts 1962–1987*. New York, Springer-Verlag, 1988, p. 23.
51. Yankah AC, Wottge HU, Muller-Rucholtz W. Prognostic importance of viability and a study of a second set allograft valve: An experimental study. *J Card Surg* 1988; **3**:263–270.
52. Mitchell RN, Jonas RA, Schoen FJ. Pathology of explanted cryopreserved allograft heart valves: comparison with aortic valves from orthotopic heart transplants. *J Thorac Cardiovasc Surg* 1998; **115**:118–127.
53. Wells WJ, Arroyo H Jr, Bremner RM, Wood J, Starnes VA. Homograft conduit failure in infants is not due to somatic outgrowth. *J Thorac Cardiovasc Surg* 2002; **124**:88–96.
54. DeWeese MS, Fry WJ. Small-bowel erosion following aortic resection. *JAMA* 1962; **179**:142.
55. Gerber A, Rubaum N. Gastrointestinal hemorrhage due to rupture of an aortic homograft. *Calif Med* 1966; **105**:377.
56. Bowman FO, Hancock WD, Malm JR. A valve containing Dacron prosthesis. *Arch Surg* 1974; **107**:724–728.
57. Carpentier A, Lemaigre G, Robert L, Carpentier S, Dubost C. Biological factors affecting long-term results of valvular heterografts. *J Thorac Cardiovasc Surg* 1969; **58**:467–483.
58. Alfieri O, Blackstone EH, Kirklin JW, Pacifico AD, Bargeron LM. Surgical treatment of tetralogy of Fallot with pulmonary atresia. *J Thorac Cardiovasc Surg* 1978; **76**:321–335.
59. Bailey WW, Kirklin JW, Bargeron LM, Pacifico AD, Kouchoukos NT. Late results with synthetic valved external conduits from venous ventricle to pulmonary arteries. *Circulation* 1976; **56**:73–79.
60. Geha AS, Laks H, Stansel HC et al. Late failure of porcine valve heterografts in children. *J Thorac Cardiovasc Surg* 1979; **78**:351–364.
61. Williams DB, Danielson GK, McGoon DC, Puga FJ, Mair DD, Edwards WD. Porcine heterograft valve replacement in children. *J Thorac Cardiovasc Surg* 1982; **84**:446–450.
62. Fiore AC, Peigh PS, Robison RJ, Glant MD, King H, Brown JW. Valved and nonvalved right ventricular pulmonary arterial extracardiac conduits. *J Thorac Cardiovasc Surg* 1983; **86**:490–497.
63. Shabbo FP, Wain WH, Ross DN. Right ventricular outflow reconstruction with aortic homograft conduit: Analysis of the long term results. *Thorac Cardiovasc Surg* 1980; **28**:21–25.
64. Kay PH, Ross DN. Fifteen years' experience with the aortic homograft: The conduit of choice for right ventricular outflow tract reconstruction. *Ann Thorac Surg* 1985; **40**:360–364.
65. Scavo VA, Turrentine MW, Aufiero TX, Sharp TG, Brown JW. Valved bovine jugular venous conduits for right ventricular to pulmonary artery reconstruction. *ASAIO J* 1999; **45**:482–487.
66. Breymann T, Thies WR, Boethig D, Goerg R, Blanz U, Koerfer R. Bovine valved venous xenografts for RVOT reconstruction: results after 71 implantations. *Eur J Cardiothorac Surg* 2002; **21**: 703–710.
67. Schmid FX, Keyser A, Wiesenack C, Holmer S, Birnbaum DE. Stentless xenografts and homografts for right ventricular outflow tract reconstruction during the Ross operation. *Ann Thorac Surg* 2002; **74**:684–688.
68. Pearl JM, Cooper DS, Bove KE, Manning PB. Early failure of the Shelhigh pulmonary valve conduit in infants. *Ann Thorac Surg* 2002; **74**:542–548.
69. Allen BS, El-Zein C, Cuneo B, Cava JP, Barth MJ, Ilbawi MN. Pericardial tissue valves and Gore-Tex conduits as an alternative for right ventricular outflow tract replacement in children. *Ann Thorac Surg* 2002; **74**:771–777.
70. Powell AJ, Lock JE, Keane JF, Perry SB. Prolongation of RV-PA conduit life span by percutaneous stent implantation. Intermediate-term results. *Circulation* 1995; **92**: 3282–3288.
71. Cerfolio RJ, Danielson GK, Warnes CA et al. Results of an autologous tissue reconstruction for replacement of obstructed extracardiac conduits. *J Thorac Cardiovasc Surg* 1995; **110**:1359–1366.

72. Barbero-Marcial M, Tanamati C. Alternative nonvalved techniques for repair of truncus arteriosus: Long-term results. *Semin Thorac Cardiovasc Surg Pediatr Card Surg Annu* 1999; **2**:121–130.
73. Kent KC, Salvatierra O, Reilly LM, Ehrenfeld WK, Goldstone J, Stoney RJ. Evolving strategies for the repair of complex renovascular lesions. *Ann Surg* 1987; **206**:272–278.
74. Novick AC, Stewart BH, Straffon RA. Autogenous arterial grafts in the treatment of renal artery stenosis. *J Urol* 1977; **118**:919–922.
75. Sawatari K, Kawata H, Armiger LC, Jonas RA. Growth of composite conduits utilizing longitudinal arterial autograft in growing lambs. *J Thorac Cardiovasc Surg* 1992; **103**:47–51.
76. Sodian R, Hoerstrup SP, Sperling JS et al. Early in vivo experience with tissue-engineered trileaflet heart valves. *Circulation* 2000; **102**:III22–29.
77. Walker T, Heinemann MK, Schneider W, Wehrmann M, Bultmann B, Ziemer G. Early failure of the autograft valve after the Ross procedure. *J Thorac Cardiovasc Surg* 2001; **122**:187–188.
78. Laudito A, Brook MM, Suleman S et al. The Ross procedure in children and young adults: a word of caution. *J Thorac Cardiovasc Surg* 2001; **122**:147–153.
79. Marx GR, Sherwood MC. Three-dimensional echocardiography in congenital heart disease: a continuum of unfulfilled promises? No. A presently clinically applicable technology with an important future? Yes. *Pediatr Cardiol* 2002; **23**:266–285.
80. Bacha EA, Satou GM, Moran AM et al. Valve-sparing operation for balloon-induced aortic regurgitation in congenital aortic stenosis. *J Thorac Cardiovasc Surg* 2001; **122**:162–168.
81. Barratt-Boyes BG. Homograft aortic valve replacement in aortic incompetence and stenosis. *Thorax* 1965; **19**:131.
82. Ross DN. Homograft replacement of the aortic valve. *Lancet* 1962; **2**:487.
83. Hopkins RA. Left ventricular outflow tract obstruction. In Hopkins RA (ed) *Cardiac Reconstructions with Allograft Valves*, New York, Springer-Verlag, 1989.
84. Barratt-Boyes BG, Roche AH, Subramanyan R, Pemberton JR, Whitlock RM. Long-term follow-up of patients with the antibiotic-sterilized aortic homograft valve inserted freehand in the aortic position. *Circulation* 1987; **75**:768–777.
85. Clarke DR. Invited letter concerning: accelerated degeneration of aortic allografts in infants and young children. *J Thorac Cardiovasc Surg* 1994; **107**:1162–1164.
86. Kadoba K, Armiger L, Sawatari K, Jonas RA. The influence of time from donor death to graft harvest on conduit function of cryopreserved aortic allografts in lambs. *Circulation* 1991; **84** (suppl II) 100–111.
87. Kadoba K, Armiger LC, Sawatari K, Jonas RA. Mechanical durability of pulmonary allograft conduits at systemic pressure. *J Thorac Cardiovasc Surg* 1993; **105**:132–141.
88. Koolbergen DR, Hazekamp MG, de Heer E et al. Structural degeneration of pulmonary homografts used as aortic valve substitute underlines early graft failure. *Eur J Cardiothorac Surg* 2002; **22**:802–807.
89. Giannelly RE, Angell WW, Stinson E et al. Homograft replacement of the mitral valve. *Circulation* 1968; **38**:664.
90. Sievers HH, Lange PE, Yankah AC et al. Allogenous transplantation of the mitral valve. An open question. *Thorac Cardiovasc Surg* 1985; **33**:227.
91. Maxwell L, Gavin JB, Barratt-Boyes BG. Uneven host tissue ongrowth and tissue detachment in stent mounted heart valve allografts and xenografts. *Cardiovasc Res* 1989; **23**:709–714.
92. Ross DN. Replacement of aortic and mitral valves with a pulmonary autograft. *Lancet* 1967; **2**:956.
93. Elkins RC, Lane MM, McCue C. Ross operation in children: late results. *J Heart Valve Dis* 2001; **10**:736–741.
94. Elkins RC, Lane MM, McCue C, Chandrasekaran K. Ross operation and aneurysm or dilation of the ascending aorta. *Semin Thorac Cardiovasc Surg* 1999; **11**:50–54.
95. Raanani E, Yau TM, David TE, Dellgren G, Sonnenberg BD, Omran A. Risk factors for late pulmonary homograft stenosis after the Ross procedure. *Ann Thorac Surg* 2000; **70**:1953–1957.
96. Gerosa G, McKay R, Ross DN. Replacement of the aortic valve or root with a pulmonary autograft in children. *Ann Thorac Surg* 1991; **51**:424.
97. Butany J, Vanlerberghe K, Silver MD. Morphologic findings and causes of failure in 24 explanted Ionescu-Shiley low-profile pericardial heart valves. *Hum Pathol* 1992; **23**:1224–1233.
98. Sanders SP, Levy RJ, Freed MD et al. Use of Hancock porcine xenografts in children and adolescents. *Am J Cardiol* 1980; **46**:429.
99. Lee CH, Vyavahare N, Zand R et al. Inhibition of aortic wall calcification in bioprosthetic heart valves by ethanol pretreatment: biochemical and biophysical mechanisms. *J Biomed Mater Res* 1998; **42**:30–37.
100. Castaneda AR, Anderson RC, Edwards JE. Congenital mitral stenosis resulting from anomalous arcade and obstructing papillary muscles: Report of correction by use of ball valve prosthesis. *Am J Cardiol* 1969; **24**:237–240.
101. Attie F, Lopez-Soriano F, Ovseyvitz J et al. Late results of mitral valve replacement with the Bjork-Shiley prosthesis in children under 16 years of age. *J Thorac Cardiovasc Surg* 1986; **91**:754–758.
102. Iyer KS, Reddy S, Rao M, Venugopal P, Bhatia ML, Gopinath N. Valve replacement in children under twenty years of age. Experience with the Bjork-Shiley prosthesis. *J Thorac Cardiovasc Surg* 1984; **88**:217–224.
103. Blot WJ, Omar RZ, Kallewaard M et al. Risks of fracture of Bjork-Shiley 60 degree convexo-concave prosthetic heart valves: long-term cohort follow up in the UK, Netherlands and USA. *J Heart Valve Dis* 2001; **10**:202–209.
104. Emery RW, Nicoloff DM. St. Jude Medical cardiac valve prosthesis. *J Thorac Cardiovasc Surg* 1979; **78**:269–276.
105. Moidl R, Simon P, Wolner E. The On-X prosthetic heart valve at five years. *Ann Thorac Surg* 2002; **74**:S1312–1317.
106. David TE, Armstrong S, Ivanov J, Webb GD. Aortic valve sparing operations: an update. *Ann Thorac Surg* 1999; **67**: 1840–1842.
107. Kadoba K, Jonas RA, Mayer JE, Castaneda AR. Mitral valve replacement in the first year of life. *J Thorac Cardiovasc Surg* 1990; **100**:762–768.
108. Myers JL, Waldhausen JA, Pae WE Jr, Abt AB, Prophet GA, Pierce WS. Vascular anastomoses in growing vessels: the use of absorbable sutures. *Ann Thorac Surg* 1982; **34**:529–537.
109. Blume ED, Wernovsky G. Long-term results of arterial switch repair of transposition of the great vessels. *Semin Thorac Cardiovasc Surg Pediatr Card Surg Annu* 1998; **1**: 129–138.
110. Friedman E, Perez-Atayde AR, Silvera M, Jonas RA. Growth of tracheal anastomoses in lambs. Comparison of PDS and Vicryl suture material and interrupted and continuous techniques. *J Thorac Cardiovasc Surg* 1990; **100**:188–193.

4

Anesthesia for congenital heart surgery

JAMES A. DINARDO

INTRODUCTION

This chapter is intended to provide a general overview of the anesthetic care of children, particularly infants and neonates undergoing operative repair or palliation of congenital heart lesions. Individual chapters in Section 3 contain more specific information.

PHYSIOLOGY

An understanding of the physiology of congenital heart disease is an essential foundation for anesthetic management of the child undergoing congenital heart surgery.

Shunting

Shunting is the process whereby venous return into one circulatory system is recirculated through the arterial outflow of the same circulatory system. Flow of blood from the systemic venous atrium (RA) to the aorta produces recirculation of systemic venous blood. Flow of blood from the pulmonary venous atrium (LA) to the pulmonary artery (PA) produces recirculation of pulmonary venous blood. Recirculation of blood produces a physiologic shunt. Recirculation of pulmonary venous blood produces a physiologic left to right (L–R), whereas recirculation of systemic venous blood produces a physiologic right to left (R–L) shunt. A physiologic R–L or L–R shunt commonly is the result of an anatomic R–L or L–R shunt. In an anatomic shunt, blood moves from one circulatory system to the other via a communication (orifice) at the level of the cardiac chambers or great vessels. Physiologic shunts can exist in the absence of an anatomic shunt; transposition physiology being the best example.

Effective blood flow is the quantity of venous blood from one circulatory system reaching the arterial system of the other circulatory system. Effective pulmonary blood flow is the volume of systemic venous blood reaching the pulmonary circulation, whereas effective systemic blood flow is the volume of pulmonary venous blood reaching the systemic circulation. Effective pulmonary blood flow and effective systemic blood flow are the flows necessary to maintain life. Effective pulmonary blood flow and effective systemic blood flow are always equal, no matter how complex the lesions. Effective blood flow usually is the result of a normal pathway through the heart, but it may occur as the result of an anatomic R–L or L–R shunt.

Total pulmonary blood flow (Q_p) is the sum of effective pulmonary blood flow and recirculated pulmonary blood flow. Total systemic blood flow (Q_s) is the sum of effective systemic blood flow and recirculated systemic blood flow. Total pulmonary blood flow and total systemic blood flow do not have to be equal. Therefore, it is best to think of recirculated flow (physiologic shunt flow) as the extra, noneffective flow superimposed on the nutritive effective blood flow.

Calculation of $Q_p:Q_s$ (the ratio of total pulmonary blood flow to systemic blood flow) is greatly simplified when the determination is made using low inspired concentrations of oxygen. This allows the contribution of oxygen carried in solution ($PO_2 \times 0.003$) to be ignored. Failure to account for this component when determination of $Q_p:Q_s$ is made using an FiO_2 of 1.0 will introduce substantial (100%) error. If FiO_2 is low the determination of $Q_p:Q_s$ can be simplified to the following equation using just oxygen saturations:

$$Q_p:Q_s = \frac{SaO_2 - SsvcO_2}{SpvO_2 - SpaO_2}$$

where a = arterial, svc = superior vena cava, pv = pulmonary vein (assumed to be 98% in the absence of significant pulmonary disease) and pa = pulmonary artery.

From a practical point in the operating room with an $FiO_2 < 0.5$, $Q_p:Q_s$ can be calculated using a SVC saturation, a PA saturation, and a systemic saturation. A quick check for a residual ventricular septal defect can be done by comparing RA and PA saturations with an $FiO_2 < 0.5$ if no atrial level communication exists. A PA saturation more than 80% under these circumstances suggests the presence of a significant left to right shunt.

In any lesion where there is potential for a large $Q_p:Q_s$, it is possible for systemic cardiac output to be compromised. For a given systemic cardiac output an increase in $Q_p:Q_s$ will necessitate an increase in ventricular volume proportional to the $Q_p:Q_s$ increase. At some point systemic ventricular output will reach a maximum once reserves of heart rate, preload and contractility have been exhausted and increases in $Q_p:Q_s$ will occur at the expense of systemic cardiac output.

Intercirculatory mixing

Intercirculatory mixing is the unique situation that exists in transposition of the great vessels (TGV). This lesion is depicted in detail in Figure 4.1. In TGV, two parallel circulations exist due to the existence of atrioventricular concordance (RA–RV, LA–LV) and ventriculoarterial disconcordance (RV–aorta, LV–PA). This produces a parallel rather than a normal series circulation. In this arrangement, blood flow will consist of parallel recirculation of pulmonary venous blood in the pulmonary circuit and systemic venous blood in the systemic circuit. Therefore, the physiologic shunt or the percentage of venous blood from one system that recirculates in the arterial outflow of the same system is 100% for both circuits. Unless there are one or more communications between the parallel circuits to allow intercirculatory mixing, this arrangement is not compatible with life. In other words, one or more communications must exist so that effective pulmonary and systemic blood flow can be established.

An anatomic R–L shunt is necessary to provide effective pulmonary blood flow, whereas an anatomic L–R shunt is necessary to provide effective systemic blood flow. Effective pulmonary blood flow, effective systemic blood flow and the volume of intercirculatory mixing are always equal. Total systemic blood flow is the sum of recirculated systemic venous blood plus effective systemic blood flow. Likewise, total pulmonary blood flow is the sum of recirculated pulmonary venous blood plus effective pulmonary blood flow. Recirculated blood makes up the largest portion of total pulmonary and total systemic blood flow with effective blood flows contributing only a small portion of the total flows. This is particularly true in pulmonary circuit where the total pulmonary blood flow (Q_p) and the volume of the pulmonary circuit

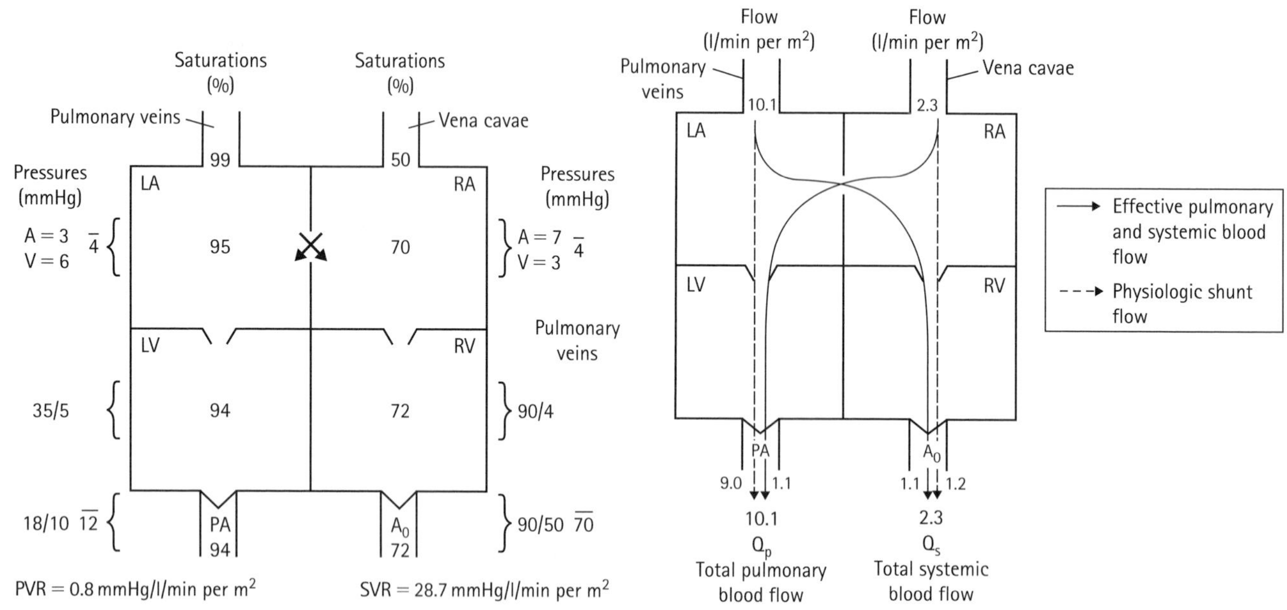

Figure 4.1 *Depiction of saturations, pressures and blood flows in complete transposition of the great vessels with a nonrestrictive atrial septal defect and a small left ventricular outflow tract gradient. Intercirculatory mixing occurs at the atrial level. Effective pulmonary and effective systemic blood flows are equal (1.1 l/min per m²) and are the result of a bidirectional anatomic shunt at the atrial level. The physiologic L–R shunt is 9.0 l/min per m²; this represents blood recirculated from the pulmonary veins to the pulmonary artery. The physiologic R–L shunt is 1.2 l/min per m²; this represents blood recirculated from the systemic veins to the aorta. It is apparent that total pulmonary blood flow (10.1 l/min per m²) is almost five times total systemic blood flow (2.3 l/min per m²) and that the bulk of pulmonary blood flow is recirculated pulmonary venous blood. In this depiction, pulmonary vascular resistance is low (approximately 1/35 of systemic vascular resistance) and there is a small (17 mmHg peak to peak) gradient from the left ventricle to the pulmonary artery. These findings are compatible with a high pulmonary blood flow depicted.*

(LA–LV–PA) is four to five times larger than the total systemic blood flow (Q_s) and the volume of the systemic circuit (RA–RV–Ao). The net result is production of transposition physiology, in which the pulmonary artery oxygen saturation is greater than the aortic oxygen saturation.

Arterial saturation (SaO_2) will be determined by the relative volumes and saturations of the recirculated systemic and effective systemic venous blood flows reaching the aorta. This is summarized in the following equation:

$$\text{Aortic saturation} = \frac{\text{(Systemic venous saturation)(recirculated systemic venous blood flow)} + \text{(pulmonary venous saturation)(effective systemic venous blood flow)}}{\text{Total systemic venous blood flow}}$$

This is illustrated in Figure 4.1 where

$$SaO_2 = \frac{(50)(1.2) + (99)(1.1)}{2.3} = 72\%$$

Obviously, the greater the effective systemic blood flow (intercirculatory mixing) relative to the recirculated systemic blood flow, the greater the aortic saturation. For a given amount of intercirculatory mixing and total systemic blood flow, a decrease in systemic venous or pulmonary venous saturation will result in a decrease in arterial saturation.

In TGA with intact ventricular septum (IVS) the anatomic mixing sites are usually a patent ductus arteriosus (PDA) and foramen ovale. Obviously, in TGA with ventricular septal defect intercirculatory mixing occurs predominantly at the ventricular level. The dynamics of intercirculatory mixing in TGA/IVS are complex. Anatomic shunting at the atrial level is ultimately determined by the size of the atrial communication and the cyclic pressure variations between the left and right atria. The volume and compliance of the atria, ventricles, and vascular beds in each circuit, as well as heart rate and phase of respiration all influence this relationship. Shunting is from the right atrium to the left atrium during diastole as the result of the reduced ventricular and vascular compliance of the systemic circuit. In systole, shunt is from the left atrium to the right atrium primarily because of the large volume of blood returning to the left atrium as a result of the high volume of recirculated pulmonary blood flow.

The direction of shunting across the PDA largely depends on the pulmonary vascular resistance and the size of the intra-atrial communication. When the resistance is low and the intra-atrial communication is nonrestrictive, shunting is predominantly from the aorta to the pulmonary artery via the PDA (effective pulmonary blood flow) and predominantly from the left to right atrium across the atrial septum (effective systemic blood flow). When resistance is elevated shunting across the PDA is likely to be bidirectional, which would in turn encourage bidirectional shunting across the atrial septum. When resistance is high and pulmonary artery pressure exceeds aortic pressure, shunting at the PDA will be predominantly from the pulmonary artery to the aorta. This will create reverse differential cyanosis – physiology wherein the preductal arterial saturation is lower than the postductal arterial saturation. This physiology is usually the result of a restrictive atrial communication producing left atrial hypertension and is associated with low effective blood flows (poor mixing) and hypoxemia. A balloon atrial septostomy can be lifesaving in this setting. Decompression of the left atrium promotes mixing at the atrial level and also reduces pulmonary vascular resistance and pulmonary artery pressure, promoting mixing at the PDA.

Single ventricle physiology

Single ventricle physiology is a term used to describe the situation wherein complete mixing of pulmonary venous and systemic venous blood occurs at the atrial or ventricular level and one ventricle then distributes output to both the systemic and pulmonary beds. As a result of this physiology:

- ventricular output is the sum of pulmonary blood flow (Q_p) and systemic blood flow (Q_s)
- the distribution of systemic and pulmonary blood flow is dependent on the relative resistances to flow (both intra and extracardiac) into the two parallel circuits
- oxygen saturations are the same in the aorta and the pulmonary artery.

This physiology can exist in patients with one well developed ventricle and one hypoplastic ventricle as well as in patients with two well formed ventricles.

In the case of a single anatomic ventricle there is often obstruction to either pulmonary or systemic blood flow as the result of obstruction to inflow and/or outflow from the hypoplastic ventricle. In this circumstance there must be a source of both systemic and pulmonary blood flow to assure postnatal survival. In some instances of a single anatomic ventricle a direct connection between the aorta and the pulmonary artery via a PDA is the sole source of systemic blood flow (hypoplastic left heart syndrome) or of pulmonary blood flow (pulmonary atresia with intact ventricular septum). This is known as ductal dependent circulation. In other instances of a single anatomic ventricle intracardiac pathways provide both systemic and pulmonary blood flow without the necessity of a PDA. This is the case in tricuspid atresia with normally related great vessels, a nonrestrictive ventricular septal defect and minimal or absent pulmonary stenosis.

In certain circumstances single ventricle physiology can exist in the presence of two well formed anatomic ventricles, such as:

- tetralogy of Fallot with pulmonary atresia where pulmonary blood flow is supplied via a PDA or aortopulmonary collaterals
- truncus arteriosus
- severe neonatal aortic stenosis and interrupted aortic arch; in both lesions a substantial portion of systemic blood flow is supplied via a PDA
- heterotaxy syndrome

Table 4.1 *Examples of single ventricle anomalies*

	Aortic blood flow from	Pulmonary artery blood flow from
Hypoplastic left heart syndrome	PDA	RV
Severe neonate aortic stenosis	PDA	RV
Interrupted aortic arch	LV (proximal) PDA (distal)	RV
Pulmonary atresia with intact ventricular septum	LV	PDA
Tetrology of Fallot with pulmonary atresia	LV	PDA, APCs
Tricuspid atresia, NRGA with pulmonary atresia	LV	PDA, APCs
Tricuspid atresia, NRGA with restrictive VSD and pulmonary stenosis	LV	LV through VSD to RV
Tricuspid atresia, NRGA with nonrestrictive VSD and no pulmonary stenosis	LV	LV through VSD to RV
Tricuspid atresia, d-TGA with nonrestrictive VSD and pulmonary atresia	LV through VSD to RV	PDA, APCs
Tricuspid atresia, d-TGA with nonrestrictive VSD and pulmonary stenosis	LV through VSD to RV	LV
Tricuspid atresia, d-TGA with nonrestrictive VSD and no pulmonary stenosis	LV through VSD to RV	LV
Tricuspid atresia, d-loop ventricles, l-TGA, subpulmonic stenosis	LV	LV through VSD to RV
Tricuspid atresia, l-loop ventricles, l-TGA, subaortic stenosis	LV through VSD to RV	LV
Truncus arteriosus	LV and RV	Aorta
DILV, NRGA	LV	LV through VSD to BVF
DILV, l-loop ventricles, l-TGA, restrictive BVF	LV through VSD to BVF, PDA	LV

APC = aortopulmonary collateral; BVF = bulboventricular foramen; DILV = double inlet right ventricle; d(l)-TGA = dextro (laevo) transposition of the great arteries; LV = left ventricle; NRGA = normally related great arteries; PDA = patent ductus arteriosus; RV = right ventricle; VSD = ventricular septal defect.

Despite the fact that patients with totally anomalous pulmonary venous return have complete mixing of pulmonary and systemic venous blood at the atrial level they do not manifest the other features necessary to create single ventricle physiology. This holds true as well for lesions in which a common atrial or ventricular chamber exists due to bidirectional (both L–R and R–L) anatomic shunting across a large defect (atrial septal or ventricular septal) and where there is no obstruction to ventricular outflow. Table 4.1, although not comprehensive, lists a number of the wide variety of single ventricle physiology lesions.

With single ventricle physiology the arterial saturation (SaO_2) will be determined by the relative volumes and saturations of pulmonary venous and systemic venous blood flows that have mixed and reach the aorta. This is summarized in the following equation:

$$\text{Aortic saturation} = \frac{\begin{array}{l}\text{(Systemic venous saturation)}\\ \text{(total systemic venous blood flow)}\\ + \text{(pulmonary venous saturation)}\\ \text{(total pulmonary venous blood flow)}\end{array}}{\begin{array}{l}\text{(Total systemic venous blood flow +}\\ \text{total pulmonary venous blood flow)}\end{array}}$$

This is illustrated in Figure 4.2 where:

$$SaO_2 = \frac{[(65)(3.3) + (98)(2.8)]}{(3.3 + 2.8)} = 80\%$$

From this equation, it is apparent that with single ventricle physiology, three variables will determine arterial saturation:

- The ratio of total pulmonary to total systemic blood flow ($Q_p:Q_s$) – a greater proportion of the mixed blood will consist of saturated blood (pulmonary venous blood) than of desaturated blood (systemic venous blood) when $Q_p:Q_s$ is high. Figure 4.5 demonstrates the increase in arterial saturation that occurs in complete mixing lesions with increases in pulmonary blood flow relative to systemic blood flow. Figure 4.3 also demonstrates that an arterial saturation approaching 100% is possible only with an extremely large $Q_p:Q_s$.
- Systemic venous saturation – for a given $Q_p:Q_s$ and pulmonary venous saturation, a decrease in systemic venous saturation will result in a decreased arterial saturation. Decreases in systemic venous saturation occur as the result of decreases in systemic oxygen delivery or increases in systemic oxygen consumption. Recall that systemic oxygen delivery is the product of systemic blood flow and arterial oxygen content. Arterial oxygen content, in turn, is dependent on the hemoglobin concentration and the arterial saturation.
- Pulmonary venous saturation – in the absence of large intrapulmonary shunts and/or V/Q mismatch pulmonary venous saturation should be close to 100% breathing room air. In the presence of pulmonary parenchymal disease, pulmonary venous saturation may be reduced. The V/Q mismatch component of pulmonary venous desaturation will be largely eliminated with an FiO_2 of 1.0 while the intrapulmonary shunt contribution will not be eliminated. For any given systemic venous saturation and $Q_p:Q_s$, a reduction in pulmonary venous saturation will result in a decreased arterial saturation.

The primary goal in the management of patients with single ventricle physiology is optimization of systemic oxygen delivery and perfusion pressure. This is necessary if end-organ

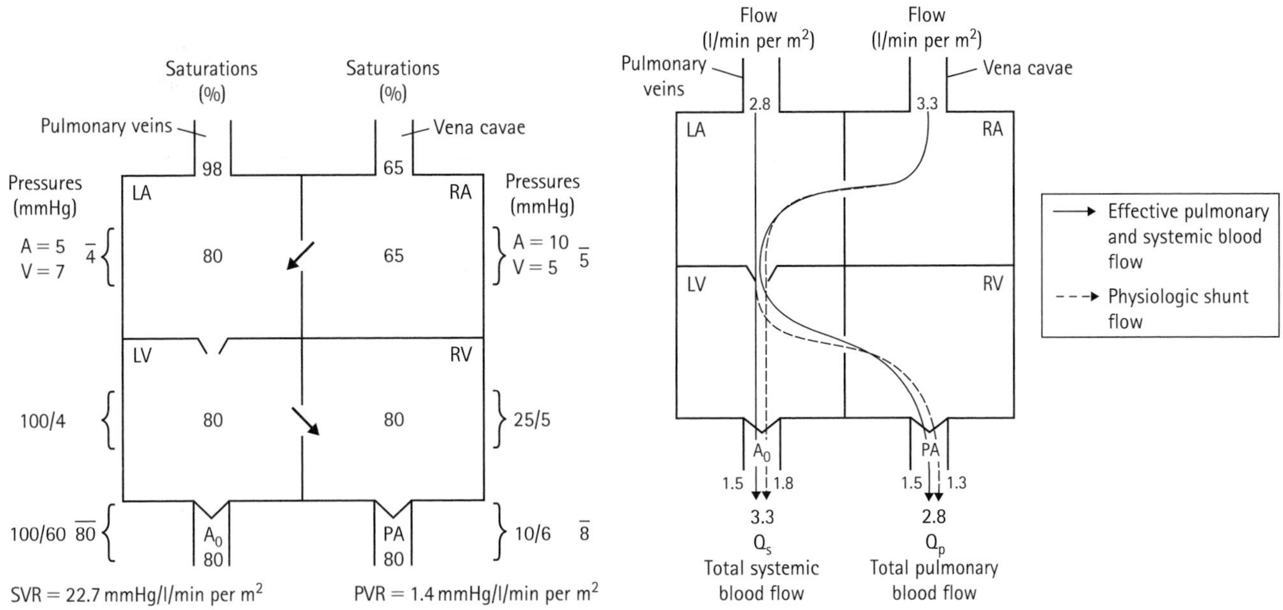

Figure 4.2 *Depiction of saturations, pressures and blood flows in tricuspid atresia with a mildly restrictive atrial septal defect, a small restrictive ventricular septal defect and mild pulmonic stenosis. Complete mixing or blending occurs at the atrial level. This complete mixing is the consequence of an obligatory physiologic and anatomic R–L shunting across the atrial septal defect. Effective pulmonary and effective systemic blood flow are equal (1.5 l/min per m²). Effective systemic blood flow occurs via a normal pathway through the heart. Effective pulmonary blood flow is the result of an anatomic R–L shunt at the atrial level and an anatomic L–R shunt at the ventricular level. This illustrates the concept that when complete outflow obstruction exists and there is obligatory anatomic shunting, a downstream anatomic shunt must exist to deliver blood back to the obstructed circuit. Q_p is 2.8 l/min per m² and is the sum of effective pulmonary blood flow (1.5 l/min per m²) and a physiologic and anatomic L–R shunt (1.2 l/min per m²) at the ventricular septal defect. Q_s is 3.3 l/min per m² and is the sum of effective systemic blood flow (1.5 l/min per m²) and a physiologic and anatomic R–L shunt (1.8 l/min per m²) at the atrial septal defect. In this depiction, there is a small pressure gradient at the atrial level and a large pressure gradient at the ventricular level. In addition there is a small additional gradient at the level of the pulmonic valve.*

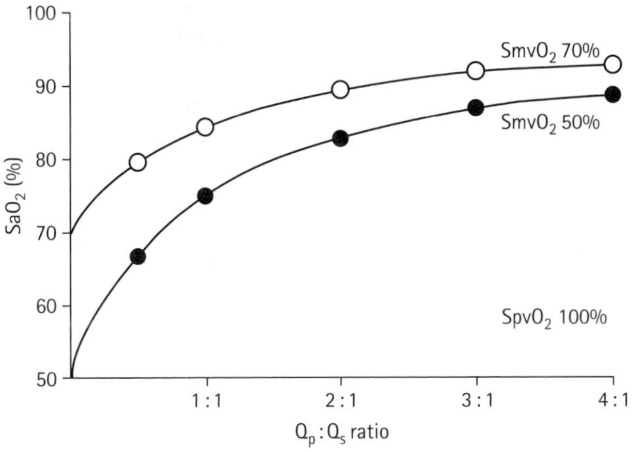

Figure 4.3 *Influence of the Q_p: Q_s ratio, mixed venous oxygenation saturation ($SmvO_2$) and pulmonary venous oxygen saturation ($SpvO_2$) on arterial oxygen saturation (SaO_2) in complete mixing lesions. Note that Q_p: Q_s ratios higher than 3 : 1 do not substantially increase arterial oxygen saturation. (From Rudolph AM:* Congenital Diseases of the Heart. *Chicago, Mosby Year Book, 1974, p 125, with permission.)*

(myocardial, renal, hepatic, splanchnic) dysfunction and failure are to be prevented. This goal is achieved by balancing the systemic and pulmonary circulations. The term 'balanced circulation' is used because both laboratory and clinical investigations have demonstrated that maximal systemic oxygen delivery (the product of systemic oxygen content and systemic blood flow) is achieved for a given single ventricle output when Q_p: Q_s is at or just below 1 : 1. This relationship is illustrated in Figure 4.4. Increases in Q_p: Q_s in excess of 1 : 1 are associated with a progressive decrease in systemic oxygen delivery because the subsequent increase in systemic oxygen content is more than offset by the progressive decrease in systemic blood flow. Decreases in Q_p: Q_s just below 1 : 1 are associated with a precipitous decrease in systemic oxygen delivery because the subsequent increase in systemic blood flow is more than offset by the dramatic decrease in systemic oxygen content.

Since Q_p: Q_s is not a readily measurable parameter in a clinical setting pulse oximetry is commonly used as surrogate method of assessing the extent to which a balanced circulation exists. An arterial saturation of 75–80% is felt to be indicative of a balanced circulation. It is important to point out, however, that an arterial saturation of 75–80% is indicative of a Q_p: Q_s at or near 1 : 1 only if the pulmonary venous

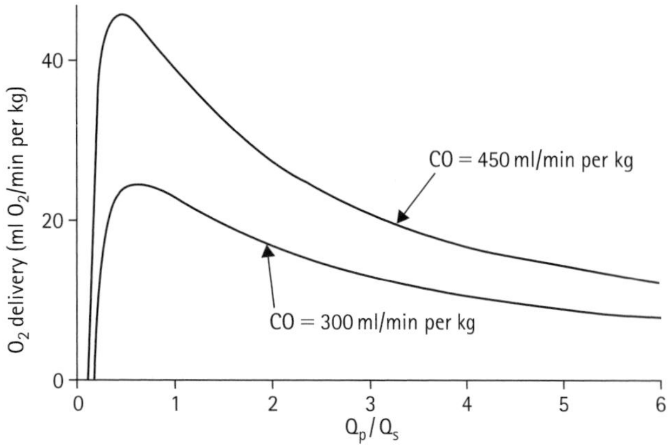

Figure 4.4 *Systemic oxygen delivery versus Q_p/Q_s in a patient with single ventricle physiology. For a range of cardiac outputs (CO), systemic oxygen delivery peaks at or near a $Q_p:Q_s$ just under 1.0.*

saturation is 95–100% and the mixed venous saturation is 50–55%. In fact, based on these assumptions, the equation used to calculate $Q_p:Q_s$ in patients with univentricular physiology:

$$= \frac{SaO_2 - SmvO_2}{SpvO_2 - SaO_2}$$

where a = arterial, pv = pulmonary vein and mv = mixed veins, can be simplified to

$$\frac{25}{(95 - SaO_2)}.$$

In this simplified equation $SpvO_2$ is assumed to be 95% (low FiO_2) and the A–V O_2 saturation difference is assumed to be 25%.

Unfortunately, an arterial saturation of 75–80% can exist at the extremes of $Q_p:Q_s$ depending on pulmonary and systemic venous saturation. Specifically, in the presence of a high $Q_p:Q_s$ it is possible for there to be inadequate systemic oxygen delivery (systemic venous desaturation, a wide A–V O_2 difference, metabolic acidosis) in the presence of what is considered to be an adequate arterial saturation of 75–80%. In addition, clinically unrecognized episodes of pulmonary venous desaturation ($SpvO_2$ less than 90%) further confound assessment of $Q_p:Q_s$ based on SaO_2.[1]

Control and manipulation of pulmonary vascular resistance and subsequently of $Q_p:Q_s$ is accomplished most reliably through ventilatory interventions. Clinically, both hypercarbia to achieve a pH of 7.35–7.40 and an 17% FiO_2 can be utilized to increase resistance and reduce $Q_p:Q_s$.[2–4] Hypercarbia ($PaCO_2$ of 40–55 torr) can be obtained via alveolar hypoventilation or via increased inspired carbon dioxide (3% $FiCO_2$). At our institution hypercarbia is reliably obtained utilizing hypoventilation without use of inspired carbon dioxide. Care is taken to assure adequate tidal volumes with maintenance of functional residual capacity so as not to induce intrapulmonary shunting and V/Q mismatch resulting in inadvertent hypoxemia. An appropriate degree of hypercarbia can be obtained with a tidal volume of 10–15 ml/kg, a positive end expiratory pressure of 3–5 cmH_2O and a respiratory rate of 4–8 breaths per minute. Lower rates are required as the infant cools and metabolic rate decreases.

Myocardial ischemia

Patients with congenital heart disease are more at risk for the development of subendocardial ischemia than is commonly appreciated. In some congenital lesions abnormalities in the coronary circulation predispose to the development of myocardial ischemia but in many others ischemia occurs in the presence of normal coronary arteries secondary to myocardial oxygen supply/demand imbalance.

Subendocardial perfusion is largely determined by coronary perfusion pressure, which is the mean aortic diastolic pressure minus the ventricular end-diastolic pressure. In addition the time interval available for perfusion (predominately diastole) is critical. As a result, the relationship between heart rate, diastolic blood pressure and ventricular end-diastolic pressure will determine whether subendocardial ischemia occurs. These factors as they apply to patients with congenital heart disease are considered below.

AORTIC DIASTOLIC PRESSURE

Subendocardial perfusion in a ventricle with systemic pressure occurs predominately in early diastole. In normal children subendocardial some perfusion of the pulmonary or right ventricle can occur in systole as well as in diastole because pulmonary ventricular systolic pressure is low. However, in many congenital lesions systolic pressure in both ventricles is systemic and in some cases the pulmonary ventricle may have suprasystemic pressures. As a result perfusion of both ventricles may be dependent on the rapid increase in early diastolic flow.

Aortic diastolic pressure which is normally low in neonates and infants is further compromised in single ventricle physiology lesions because these lesions promote diastolic runoff of aortic blood into the lower resistance pulmonary circuit. The subgroup of patients with ductal dependent systemic blood and patients with truncus arteriosus are particularly at risk for excessive aortic diastolic runoff. Coronary perfusion is further compromised in patients with aortic atresia because the coronary ostia are perfused retrograde through the diminutive ascending aorta.

SUBENDOCARDIAL PRESSURE

Subendocardial pressure is elevated and subendocardial perfusion is compromised in the presence of an elevated ventricular end-diastolic pressure. Elevated end-diastolic pressure may be the result of impaired diastolic function (both reduced ventricular compliance and impaired ventricular relaxation),

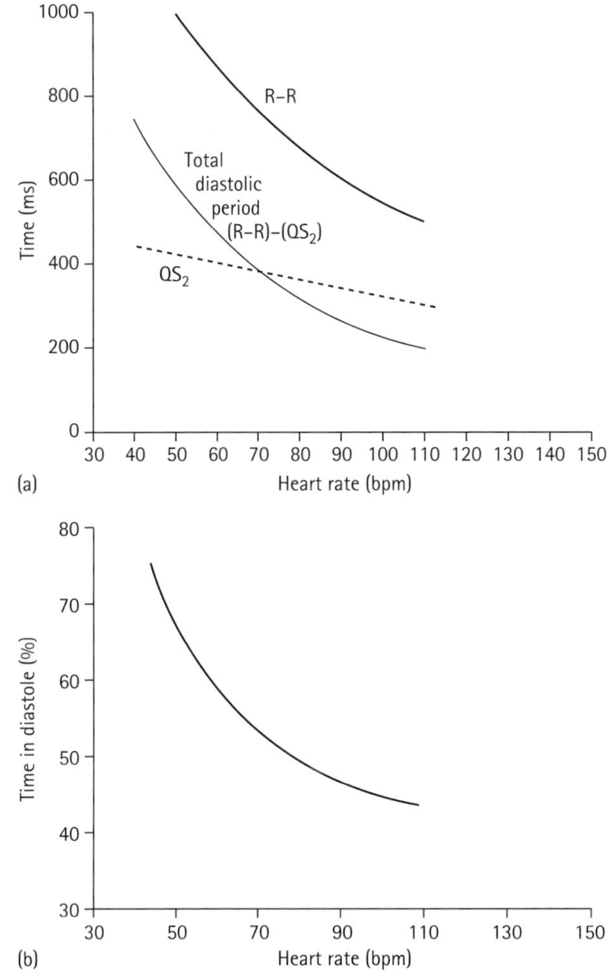

Figure 4.5 *(a) Increases in heart rate cause decreases in length of each cardiac cycle (R–R interval). Decreases in length of systole (QS_2) with increases in heart rate are far less dramatic than decreases in length of diastole (R–R)–(QS_2). (b) Percent of each cardiac cycle (R–R interval) spent in diastole at various heart rates. Small changes in heart rate are seen to cause large decreases in percent of time spent in diastole. (From Boudoulas H: Changes in diastolic time with various pharmacologic agents.* Circulation *1979:* ***60****:165, with permission.)*

impaired systolic function, increased ventricular end-diastolic volume, or a combination of all three. For example, elevated ventricular end-diastolic pressure occurs as the result of the ventricular volume overload which accompanies single ventricle lesions, lesions with a high $Q_p : Q_s$, and regurgitant AV and semilunar valve lesions. The ventricular hypertrophy which accompanies pressure overload lesions is particularly detrimental to subendocardial perfusion. Pressure overload induced ventricular hypertrophy reduces ventricular compliance and elevates ventricular end-diastolic pressure. In addition, the extravascular compressive forces which accompany a high external pressure workload further compromise myocardial perfusion by reducing transmural coronary vascular reserve (the ratio of hyperemic myocardial blood flow to baseline myocardial blood flow).

HEART RATE

As illustrated in Figure 4.5 the duration of diastole diminishes geometrically as heart rate increases while the duration of systole remains relatively constant. As a direct consequence of this the time available for diastolic coronary artery perfusion or diastolic perfusion time falls geometrically as heart rate increases. Consequently, a higher diastolic pressure is necessary to maintain subendocardial perfusion at higher heart rates. The obvious corollary is that subendocardial perfusion is more likely to be maintained in the presence of a low diastolic blood pressure if the heart rate is slower. In an infant with hypoplastic left heart syndrome and an aortic diastolic pressure of 25 mmHg a heart rate of 130–140 bpm may well be tolerated without evidence of subendocardial ischemia whereas it is unlikely that a heart rate of 170–180 bpm will be tolerated at the same diastolic pressure. In patients with pressure induced ventricular hypertrophy tachycardia can induce subendocardial ischemia in presence of a normal aortic diastolic blood pressure and unobstructed coronary arteries.[5]

ANATOMIC CORONARY ARTERY LESIONS

Anatomic coronary artery abnormalities complicate the management of patients with a number of congenital cardiac lesions such as pulmonary atresia with intact ventricular septum, Kawasaki's Disease, anomalous left coronary artery from the pulmonary artery and Williams syndrome. These coronary abnormalities will be addressed in detail Section 3.

PRE-CARDIOPULMONARY BYPASS ANESTHETIC MANAGEMENT

General considerations

Hemodynamic stability and avoidance of hypercyanosis prior to initiation of cardiopulmonary bypass (CPB) is dependent on prompt and efficient induction of anesthesia, placement of monitoring lines and preparation of the child for surgery. The time interval from induction of anesthesia until surgical preparation and draping of the patient generally does not exceed 45–60 minutes. During this interval the heating/cooling blanket under the patient is set at 42°C, and the ambient room temperature is elevated to 20°C. It is not our routine practice to make use of warming lights. Once preparation begins the room temperature is reduced to 10°C and the heating/cooling blanket is set at 30°C. When deep hypothermic CPB is to be utilized ice bags are placed around the child's head after preparation and draping. We strive to reduce the patient's core temperature to 30–32°C just prior to the initiation of CPB. This strategy requires close observation of the progression of the operative procedure as excessive cooling can predispose to dysrhythmias (bradycardia, ventricular irritability) and hypotension.

Maintenance caloric requirements in the awake neonate/infant are 100 cal/kg body weight per day or 4 cal/kg per hour.

This caloric requirement can be met with glucose 25 g/kg per day or 1 g/kg per hour. From a practical point of view this glucose requirement can be met with 10% dextrose (1 g/ml) run at the maintenance volume replacement rate of 4 ml/kg per hour. Ten percent dextrose run at half this rate (2 ml/kg per hour) is usually sufficient to meet the caloric requirements of an anesthetized infant while avoiding both the hyper- and hypoglycemia that can be detrimental to neurologic outcome particularly following deep hypothermic circulatory arrest (DHCA). It is our practice to discontinue dextrose infusions prior to commencement of CPB as the associated neuroendocrine response to CPB generally produces mild hyperglycemia. Some patients receive nutritional support as part of medical stabilization prior to surgery. We discontinue high calorie total parenteral nutrition and intralipid therapy and replace it with a 10% dextrose infusion several hours prior to transport to the operating room. Continued administration of these high calorie infusions makes intraoperative serum glucose management problematic. In these patients higher dextrose infusion rates may be necessary pre-CPB to avoid rebound hypoglycemia.

As with all pediatric patients meticulous care must be directed toward airway management. Children with high pulmonary blood flow particularly those with interstitial pulmonary edema have surprisingly poor lung compliance necessitating higher than expected airway pressures. Care must be taken not to insufflate the stomach with air during mask ventilation. The relatively large occiput of small children will cause the head to flex forward, placement of a small roll under the neck or shoulders will allow the head to remain in the neutral position. Placement of an oral airway in neonates and infants will greatly facilitate mask ventilation by pulling the large tongue away from the pharyngeal wall. In children less than 10–12 years old nasal endotracheal tubes are utilized in our institution as they provide better stability intra- and postoperatively. In patients with high venous pressure such as those with a bidirectional Glenn shunt or Fontan nasal endotracheal tubes must be passed cautiously as substantial nasal bleeding can be initiated. Uncuffed endotracheal tubes with a leak at or near 25 cmH_2O are generally used in children under eight years of age. Consideration is given to use of a cuffed endotracheal tube in patients where poor pulmonary compliance secondary to lung water, chest wall edema, or abdominal distention are anticipated to compromise minute ventilation. In these patients temporary inflation of the cuff will allow higher airway pressures to be utilized as needed.

Premedication

Premedication prior to induction can be used to facilitate a number of objectives. In older children it can be used to alleviate anxiety prior to an intravenous or inhalation induction. In younger children, premedication eases separation of the child from the parents. In infants judicious premedication alone or in combination with inhaled nitrous oxide can greatly simplify placement of an intravenous catheter in an otherwise struggling infant. We commonly use midazolam 1.0 mg/kg orally in infants and younger children who have not had prior cardiac surgery. In children over one year who have undergone prior operative procedures we commonly use oral ketamine 7–10 mg/kg in combination with midazolam 1.0 mg/kg. These children are remarkably tolerant to midazolam as the result of either heightened anxiety or previous intra- and postoperative exposure to benzodiazepines. In circumstances where premedication is deemed important and the child will not take oral medication the intramuscular route can be used. Ketamine 2–3 mg/kg and glycopyrrolate (10 μg/kg) alone or in combination with midazolam 0.1 mg/kg works well.

Induction of anesthesia

No one anesthetic technique is suitable for all patients with congenital heart disease. The patient's age, cardiopulmonary function, degree of cyanosis, and emotional state all play a role in the selection of an anesthetic technique. Intravenous administration of induction agents clearly affords the greatest flexibility in terms of drug selection and drug titration and allows prompt control of the airway. Intravenous induction is the preferred technique in patients with severely impaired ventricular systolic function and in patients with systemic or suprasystemic pulmonary artery pressures. Most neonates and infants are candidates for intravenous inductions not as the result of any inherent contraindications to other forms of induction but due to the pathophysiologic conditions likely to exist in patients presenting for cardiac surgery at this age.

Mask induction of anesthesia with sevoflurane or halothane can be accomplished safely in children without severe cardiorespiratory compromise. However, reduced pulmonary blood flow in cyanotic patients will prolong the length of induction and the interval during which the airway is only partially controlled. In addition, in these patients even short intervals of airway obstruction or hypoventilation may result in dramatic hypoxemia.

Intravenous induction in infants and neonates is usually accomplished using a high dose synthetic narcotic technique in combination with pancuronium. The vagolytic and sympathomimetic effects of pancuronium counteract the vagotonic effect of synthetic opioids. In patients with a low aortic diastolic blood pressure and a high baseline heart rate consideration should be given to use of one of the muscle relaxants which do not affect heart rate such as vecuronium or cis-atracurium. In older children with mild to moderately depressed systolic function lower doses of a synthetic opioid can be used in conjunction with etomidate (0.1–0.3 mg/kg). The myocardial depressive and vasodilatory effects of propofol and thiopental make them unsuitable as induction agents except in patients with simple shunt lesions (atrial septal defect) in whom cardiovascular function is preserved.

An alternative to intravenous induction in infants and neonates with difficult peripheral intravenous access is intramuscular induction with ketamine (3–5 mg/kg), succinylcholine (5 mg/kg), and glycopyrrolate (10 μg/kg).

Glycopyrrolate is recommended to reduce the airway secretions associated with ketamine administration and to prevent the bradycardia which may accompany succinylcholine administration. This technique provides prompt induction and immediate control of the airway with tracheal intubation and is useful in circumstances where it is anticipated that initial intravenous access will have to be obtained via the external jugular vein, femoral vein, or internal jugular vein. This technique is hampered by the fact that the short duration of action of succinylcholine limits the period of patient immobility. An alternative technique combines intramuscular ketamine (4–5 mg/kg), glycopyrrolate (10 μg/kg) and rocuronium (1.0 mg/kg). This technique is hampered by the longer time interval until attainment of adequate intubating conditions and the longer duration of action of rocuronium as compared to succinylcholine.[6]

Maintenance of anesthesia

Anesthesia is generally maintained using a synthetic opioid (fentanyl or sufentanil) based technique. These opioids may be used alone in high doses (25–100 μg/kg fentanyl or 2.5–10 μg/kg sufentanil) or in low to moderate doses (5–25 μg/kg fentanyl or 0.5–2.5 μg/kg sufentanil) in combination with an inhalation agent (generally isoflurane or sevoflurane) or a benzodiazepine (generally midazolam). The high dose technique is particularly useful in neonates and infants. Patients in this age group presenting for surgery as a rule have significant ventricular pressure and/or volume overload. In addition many of these patients have tenuous subendocardial and systemic perfusion secondary to runoff into the pulmonary circulation and the low diastolic blood pressure which accompanies it. Given the limited contractile reserve available in the immature myocardium it is not surprising that the myocardial depressive and systemic vasodilatory effects of inhalation agents and the synergistic vasodilatory effects of benzodiazepines and opioids may be poorly tolerated in this patient group.

Maintenance of anesthesia during CPB is important. Light anesthesia particularly during cooling and rewarming may lead to elevated SVR requiring a reduction in pump flow rate which compromises both somatic perfusion and the efficiency of cooling and rewarming. In addition, light anesthesia and subclinical shivering due to inadequate neuromuscular blockade are avoidable causes of increased systemic oxygen consumption. Increased systemic oxygen consumption during CPB will be manifest as a lower than acceptable venous saturation (less than 65%) at what should be an adequate CPB flow rate for the patient. Furthermore, for a membrane oxygenator at or near its maximum flow capacity a low venous saturation may result in a lower than acceptable arterial saturation on CPB. Maximum flow capacity is defined as the maximum volume of blood with a hemoglobin level of 12% at a temperature of 37°C that can enter the oxygenator with a saturation of 65% and leave with a saturation of at least 95%. In an effort to reduce CPB prime volume the smallest membrane oxygenator compatible with the anticipated CPB flow rates is usually chosen and these membrane oxygenators are often operating close to their maximum flow capacity particularly during rewarming.

High dose synthetic narcotic anesthesia (specifically sufentanil 30 μg/kg) has previously been demonstrated to provide better attenuation of the neuroendocrine stress response and lower morbidity and mortality following neonatal cardiac surgery than halothane morphine anesthesia.[7] While it is appealing to link this attenuation of plasma epinephrine, norepinephrine, glucose, cortisol, adrenocortical hormone and lactate to improved outcome, more recent investigations call this association into question. In two studies no correlation between the dose of fentanyl or plasma fentanyl levels and the magnitude of the neuroendocrine response could be demonstrated nor could any correlation between the magnitude of the neuroendocrine response and outcome be demonstrated.[8,9] The neuroendocrine stress response is only one arm of the much larger systemic inflammatory response initiated by surgery and CPB. This response involves the complement system, monocyte and macrophage activation, and ultimately endothelial cell activation and initiation of the leukocyte–endothelial cell adhesion cascade. Efforts to improve outcome by attenuating stress response will likely require a multifaceted approach directed toward this process.

Lower doses of opioid in conjunction with an inhalation agent or benzodiazepine are suitable for older patients with better cardiovascular reserve and less severe pathophysiology. In fact, carefully selected patients (over one year old, no pulmonary hypertension, benign past medical history) undergoing simple atrial or ventricular septal defect closure are candidates for immediate tracheal extubation in the operating room or in the intensive care unit within two to three hours.[10] Remifentanil is a new synthetic opioid with a very short half-life (three to four minutes) as a result of its metabolism by nonspecific plasma esterases. The context sensitive half-life of remifentanil is constant meaning that half-life is largely independent of infusion duration. Its short half-life dictates delivery as a bolus (0.5–1.0 μg/kg) followed by a continuous infusion (0.25–1.0 μg/kg per minute). This drug is useful in circumstances where the hemodynamic stability of high dose opioid anesthesia is desirable for short, clearly defined intervals. Remifentanil provides poor postoperative analgesia given its rapid termination of effect and therefore administration of a longer acting opioid is often necessary.

Monitoring

ELECTROCARDIOGRAPHY AND BLOOD PRESSURE

Once the patient is brought into the operating room, routine monitors are placed prior to induction of anesthesia. A five-lead electrocardiograph with leads II and V_5 displayed allows rhythm and ischemia monitoring. A noninvasive automated blood pressure cuff and a pulse oximeter probe are placed on the child. Intra-arterial access is obtained following induction;

however, many neonates who have been medically stabilized in the ICU preoperatively will have an arterial catheter in place. Generally, percutaneous arterial access can be accomplished in even the smallest neonates. Radial and femoral arteries are the sites most commonly utilized. Posterior tibial and dorsalis pedis arteries may be used as well; however, these sites suffer from the limitation that they often do not reflect central aortic pressure during and immediately following hypothermic CPB in neonates and infants. Brachial arteries are not used given the high risk of distal limb ischemia. Consideration is given to any previous or proposed surgical procedure which may compromise the reliability of ipsilateral upper extremity intra-arterial pressure monitoring such as a Blalock-Taussig shunt, modified Blalock-Taussig shunt, subclavian artery patch repair of aortic coarctation, or sacrifice of an aberrant subclavian artery. During coarctation repair or during procedures performed on the distal aortic arch or aortic isthmus compromise of distal aortic blood flow as well as the potential for compromise of left upper extremity blood flow necessitates right upper extremity blood pressure monitoring. Previous catheterization procedures particularly those of an interventional nature may result in femoral or iliac artery occlusion. On occasion, surgical access (cutdown) to a peripheral artery is necessary.

Umbilical artery catheters which are in situ are used short-term. They are generally replaced with a peripheral arterial catheter in the ICU or operating room and removed. Ultimately blood pressure monitoring consists of an intra-arterial catheter and an upper and lower extremity noninvasive blood pressure cuff. Detection of residual coarctation or aortic arch/isthmus obstruction is generally accomplished via comparison of upper and lower extremity blood pressures using an arterial catheter and a noninvasive blood pressure cuff.

SYSTEMIC OXYGEN SATURATION

Oxygen saturation monitoring is accomplished with pulse oximeter probes on both an upper and a lower extremity; these can be placed in pre- and postductal locations if the physiology warrants.

END TIDAL CARBON DIOXIDE

End tidal carbon dioxide ($ETCO_2$) monitoring is routinely employed with the caveat that the difference between $PaCO_2$ and $ETCO_2$ will vary as physiologic dead space varies, and that in some circumstances the difference may be large (>10–15 torr). Any acute reduction in pulmonary blood flow (decreased cardiac output, pulmonary embolus, increased intracardiac right to left shunting) will increase this gradient. More specifically, children having had a bidirectional Glenn tend to have a large $PaCO_2$–$ETCO_2$ gradient related to increased physiologic dead space. An increased portion of the lung in these patients is ventilated but not perfused (zone 1, alveolar pressure > pulmonary artery pressure > pulmonary venous pressure) because of the low pulmonary artery driving pressure (SVC pressure). In patients with single ventricle physiology (most commonly those with hypoplastic left heart syndrome or truncus arteriosus) who are overcirculated (high $Q_p:Q_s$) prior to initiation of CPB, the right pulmonary artery may be partially or completely occluded by the surgeon to mechanically limit pulmonary blood flow. This maneuver dramatically increases physiologic dead space and as a result $ETCO_2$ will vastly underestimate $PaCO_2$.

CENTRAL VENOUS PRESSURE

Percutaneous central venous access offers numerous advantages and can be reliably obtained even in small neonates with sufficient technical skill and attention to detail. The preferred access sites in our institution are the internal jugular and femoral veins. Four French 5 cm double lumen catheters are available for use in neonates and infants, five French 5 cm double lumen catheters are available for use in young children and 6–9 French catheters are available for use in older children. Central venous access is not without risks, particularly in neonates and infants, and therefore the decision to place a percutaneous central venous catheter must involve consideration of the relative risks and benefits.

The advantages are:

- central venous pressure monitoring
- infusion site for vasoactive and intropic agents
- infusion site for blood products and intravascular volume replacement
- sampling of SVC blood for measurement of SVC oxygenation saturation to determine the adequacy of cardiac output and to determine $Q_p:Q_s$ (internal jugular)
- cardiac rhythm analysis (detection of cannon A-waves may accompany loss of atrial-ventricular synchrony)
- detection of inadequate SVC drainage leading to cerebral venous hypertension during CPB (internal jugular).

The disadvantages are the risk of:

- pneumothorax (internal jugular)
- hematoma with vascular or tracheal compression/displacement
- thoracic duct injury (left internal jugular)
- air embolus
- internal jugular and/or SVC thrombosis (a devastating complication in patients being staged to a single ventricle repair)
- femoral vein thrombosis (this complicates access for subsequent diagnostic and interventional catheterization procedures)
- infection which may predispose to subsequent venous thrombosis.

The risk of thrombosis and infection can be reduced by maintaining a heparin infusion (2 units/hour) through the central line lumens postoperatively and by removing the lines as soon as possible (one to two days).

At our institution many neonates and infants are managed prior to CPB without central venous lines. Transthoracic intracardiac lines (RA, LA, PA) placed by the surgeon prior to termination of CPB can be used for pressure monitoring, infusion of vasoactive and inotropic agents, and blood product and volume replacement. In older children particularly those undergoing re-operation with adhesion of the aorta or RV to PA conduit to the sternum large bore central venous catheters are used in conjunction with a readily available rapid infusion system. In these children transthoracic intracardiac lines while suitable for pressure monitoring and infusion of drugs are too long and are of insufficient caliber to serve as adequate conduits for rapid volume replacement.

TEMPERATURE

Rectal, esophageal and tympanic membrane temperatures are monitored for all CPB cases. Equilibration of rectal temperature with tympanic and esophageal temperature serves as the best index of homogenous somatic cooling and rewarming. Rectal temperature lags behind esophageal and tympanic membrane temperature during both cooling and rewarming. Both esophageal and tympanic membrane are core temperature monitoring sites and temperature changes at these sites generally mirror brain temperature changes. However, individual patient's esophageal and tympanic membrane temperatures have been shown to both over- and underestimate brain temperature by as much as 5°C during cooling and rewarming.[11] This observation underscores the importance of providing an adequately long period of core cooling prior to commencement of low-flow CPB or DHCA. The likelihood that target brain temperature (15–18°C) will be reached is greatly increased if core cooling is utilized to bring tympanic, esophageal, and rectal temperatures to this target temperature.

NEAR INFRARED SPECTROSCOPY (NIRS)

This is an evolving technology which holds promise as a real-time, online monitor of cerebral tissue oxygenation. Laboratory work utilizing NIRS technology to investigate cerebral tissue oxygenation in a neonatal piglet model of DHCA and CPB is abundant and reviewed elsewhere.[12,13] Clinical investigations utilizing NIRS devices in neonates/infants are limited and both normal and critical values for cerebral oxygenation have yet to be determined. Nonetheless, it is clear that the technology has an emerging role in detecting cerebral deoxygenation and in guiding appropriate corrective interventions.[14–17]

This technology is based on the physical principle that light of an appropriate wavelength passing through a solution of a colored compound (chromophore) will be absorbed by the compound. As a result of this absorption the intensity of the light emerging from the solution will be lower than the intensity of the light projected into the solution. This principle through application of the Beer–Lambert equation:

$$\log\left(\frac{I_o}{I}\right) = c\alpha d$$

which allows quantification of the concentration (c) of a chromophore if the emergent light intensity (I) is measured and the following are known:

- extinction coefficient (α), a constant which describes the absorption characteristics of a particular chromophore at a given wavelength of light
- thickness of the solution (d)
- incident light intensitoy (I_o).

NIRS technology is particularly suited to analysis of cerebral tissue oxygenation because wavelengths of light in the near infrared range (650–900 nm) contain photons capable of penetrating tissue far enough to reach the cerebral cortex and because the peak absorption spectra of the chromophores best suited to reflect tissue oxygenation – oxyhemoglobin (HbO_2), deoxyhemoglobin (Hb) and oxidized cytochrome aa_3 (CytOx) reside in this wavelength range. CytOx is a very valuable measurement of neuronal oxygen delivery because this intracellular (mitochondrial) chromophore is the last enzyme in the respiratory chain. As such the CytOx signal provides direct information about tissue oxygenation that may not be provided by HbO_2 under conditions of hypothermia and alkalosis. Specifically, it is conceivable that a high HbO_2 results from conditions that produce a higher affinity of oxygen for hemoglobin with poor offloading to tissue.

NIRS technology is also particularly suited to use in neonates and infants because the thin skull and small head allow light to be transmitted through one side of the head and detected on the other side, a technique known as transmission spectrometry. In children and adults reflectance technology is necessary due to the thicker skull and larger head. All commercially available NIRS devices utilize reflectance technology. With this technology the transmission and detection optodes are placed a few centimeters (3–6 cm) apart on the same side of the head. There are in fact two closely placed (1–2 cm apart) detection optodes. The more proximal optode receives light which passes primarily through extracranial tissue (skin, bone) while the distal optode receives light which also passes through brain tissue. The difference between the two signals represents light passing through brain tissue.

At present three types of NIRS technology exist:

- continuous wave (cwNIRS)
- time-domain (tdNIRS)
- frequency-domain (fdNIRS).

While tdNIRS and fdNIRS instruments allow absolute quantification of cerebral HbO_2, Hb and CytOx, cwNIRS allows only relative quantification (change from an unknown baseline). Currently only cwNIRS devices are commercially available. While fdNIRS devices may become commercially available soon it is unlikely that tdNIRS devices will be marketed given the complexity of this technology.

The limitations of NIRS technology can be summarized as follows:

- cwNIRS does not currently allow determination of absolute attenuation ($I_o - I$). This is the result of the inability of the technology to quantify how much attenuation is due to light absorption and how much is due to light which is lost to detection through scattering. cwNIRS technology is based on the assumption that the quantity of scattering remains constant and that changes in attenuation will be the result of changes in absorption. Thus while absolute attenuation remains unknown, *changes* in attenuation from an arbitrary baseline can be measured. Spatially resolved spectrometry (SRS) is an enhancement of cwNIRS which directly estimates absorption and scattering using several detection optodes housed in a single source to obtain multi-distance measurements of optical attenuation. tdNIRS and fdNIRS devices allow accurate quantification of both light absorption and light scattering.

- cwNIRS does not allow direct determination of *d* – the optical path length, the distance the light travels through tissue between the transmission optode and the detector optode. Scattering of light in tissue causes the light to travel a path longer than a straight line path. The relationship between the straight line path length (largely the distance between the transmitter and receiver optodes) and the actual path length is defined as the differential pathway factor (DPF). tdNIRS and fdNIRS devices which are capable of measuring actual path length have been used to determine the DPF used in cwNIRS devices. DPF is tissue specific and in addition varies with wavelength, hematocrit, between neonates/infants and adults, and with pathologic states such as cerebral edema. Despite this the DPF used in cwNIRS devices is assumed to be a near constant. DPF is generally assumed to be 4.99 in the neonatal brain meaning that light travels 4.99 times further than the straight line path. This assumed value for DPF allows *changes* in chromophore concentration to be quantified.
- all NIRS technology has difficulty clearly delineating the CytOx signal. There is significant crosstalk between CytOx and hemoglobin such that measured CytOx is highly dependent on hematocrit.[18] In addition, unlike HbO_2 and Hb CytOx has a broad peak absorption spectrum. As a result characterization of the signal requires multiple wavelengths and complicated algorithms.
- cerebral oxygen saturation (ScO_2) as measured by all NIRS technology is the combined oxygen saturation of an uncertain mix of arterioles, capillaries and venules. Traditional pulse oximetry differs in this respect from NIRS because it is capable of isolating and measuring the arteriole component by gating measurements to pulsatility. It has been previously assumed that ScO_2 represented contributions of cerebral arterial and venous blood in a ratio of 25 : 75 with the contribution of capillary blood felt to be negligible. More recent data suggest that in children the average ratio is 15 : 85. The issue is further complicated by the fact that there is significant variability in the ratio (from 0 : 100 to 40 : 60) between patients.[19]

TRANSCRANICAL DOPPLER

The role of transcranial Doppler (TCD) monitoring in the care of pediatric cardiac surgical patients is evolving. TCD allows measurement of cerebral blood flow velocity as well as detection of cerebral microemboli and is a technology ideally suited to use in neonates and infants.[20] The thin skull of neonates/infants combined with a low frequency ultrasonic transducer allows transmission of ultrasonic energy into brain tissue with little signal attenuation. Placement of a 2 MHz pulsed wave Doppler probe over the temporal bone allows the ultrasonic signal to be aligned parallel to the proximal (M1) segment of the middle cerebral artery (MCA). The ability of pulsed wave Doppler to be gated to a specific depth allows determination of blood flow velocity in the MCA just distal to the takeoff of the anterior cerebral artery. This pulsed wave Doppler interrogation yields a velocity spectrum in the MCA for each cardiac cycle. The accuracy of this velocity determination is dependent on cos θ, the angle between the interrogating ultrasound beam and the blood flow vector. Accuracy is highest when the ultrasound beam and blood flow vector are parallel to each other ($\theta = 0°$ or 180°). No flow can be detected when the ultrasound beam and blood flow vector are perpendicular to each other ($\theta = 90°$ or 270°). As long as θ is under 20° the velocity assessment will be acceptable (6% underestimation of true velocity).

Integration of the area under the velocity spectrum yields the time-velocity integral (TVI) in units of cm per cardiac cycle. The product of vessel TVI and vessel cross-sectional area (units of cm^2) is flow (units of cm^3 per cardiac cycle). If it is assumed that MCA cross-sectional area remains constant then there is a linear relationship between TVI and MCA blood flow. However, MCA vasoconstriction with flow held constant will yield an increased TVI (increased peak and mean velocity) while MCA dilation with flow held constant will yield a reduced TVI (decreased peak and mean velocity). Obviously, interpretation of TCD velocity data becomes more complicated if flow and resistance both vary. Use of systolic (V_S), mean (V_M), and diastolic (V_D) velocities to generate the pulsatility index $PI = (V_S - V_D)/V_M$ and the resistance index $RI = (V_S - V_D)/V_S$ aid in this analysis.

Clinical investigations of cerebral blood flow velocity have been conducted,[21,22] however, normal TCD velocity values in various patient subgroups (cyanotic versus noncyanotic, age, following DHCA), and under various CPB conditions (hematocrit, flow, pressure, acid-base status, temperature) have yet to be determined. TCD determination of cerebral blood may prove useful as a continuous surveillance monitor for detection of inadequate flow or obstructed cerebral venous drainage during CPB.

Cerebral microemboli produce transient increases in reflected Doppler energy as compared to the background

Doppler spectra. These high intensity transient signals can be counted by the TCD microprocessor and displaced as microembolic events per hour. Due to their higher reflective capacity gaseous emboli can be detected over a greater distance than particulate emboli and as a result have a higher sample velocity length (the product of emboli duration and velocity). At present, cerebral emboli detection with TCD requires the constant attention of a skilled observer because TCD technology alone lacks sufficient sensitivity and specificity to distinguish between gaseous brain emboli, particulate brain emboli and artifacts. Enhancements of TCD technology including multi-frequency Doppler and multi-gate Doppler are expected to improve artifact rejection while automation of sample velocity length determination may allow differentiation of particulate and gaseous microemboli. Clinically, TCD emboli detection is being investigated as a tool to refine post-CPB de-airing routines and to reduce the number of cannulation and perfusion related iatrogenic embolic events.[23,24]

TRANSESOPHAGEAL ECHOCARDIOGRAPHY

Transesophageal echocardiography (TEE) technology has progressed to the point where a 7.5 MHz multi-plane probe is available for intraoperative use in neonates and infants. These probes possess continuous wave Doppler, pulse wave Doppler, color Doppler and M-mode capability. While this technology is capable of providing a wealth of information it should be pointed out that it is not a substitute for comprehensive surgical assessment as there exists a definable incidence of both functional and structural discrepancies between TEE and operative findings.[25] Although intraoperative TEE can be performed safely in the smallest patients (2.8–3.5 kg) caution must be exercised as the presence of the probe in the esophagus has been observed to cause: tracheal and bronchial compression with compromise of ventilation, inadvertent tracheal extubation, right main stem bronchial intubation, esophageal perforation, aortic arch compression with loss of distal perfusion, and compression of the left atrium resulting in left atrial hypertension or compromise of ventricular filling.[26,27] In particular, ante- or retroflexion of the probe must be performed with caution in small patients.

It has been demonstrated that intraoperative TEE has a major impact on post-CPB decision making (such as return to CPB to repair residual lesions) in approximately 15% of cases when it is used nonselectively.[28] We use intraoperative TEE selectively (about 30% of CPB cases) most commonly in cases involving repair of a semilunar or AV valve, complex ventricular outflow tract reconstructions, and for delineation of complicated anatomy which can not be completely delineated with transthoracic echocardiography preoperatively.[29] In the subset of patients undergoing valve repair and outflow tract reconstruction TEE provides the best immediate assessment of the adequacy of the operative procedure and if necessary directs its revision. TEE is not helpful in assessment of residual arch obstruction following stage 1 repairs as this area is poorly visualized. While detection of retained intracardiac air is certainly facilitated by use of intraoperative TEE it remains to be determined what role the technology will play in improving cardiac de-airing algorithms particularly in neonates/infants.

The role of TEE in the detection of residual ventricular septal defects following repair of both simple and complex defects deserves some discussion. Residual defects less than 3 mm are detectable by TEE but generally do not require immediate reoperation as they are hemodynamically insignificant. The majority (75%) of these small defects is not present at the time of hospital discharge as determined by transthoracic echocardiography.[30] Residual defects of more than 3 mm detected by TEE require immediate reoperation only if they are associated with intraoperative hemodynamic (elevated left atrial and/or pulmonary artery pressure in the presence of good ventricular function) and oximetric ($Q_P:Q_S$ greater than 1.5:1 or RA to PA oxygen saturation stepup with FiO_2 of 0.50 or less) evidence that they are significant. Given this it can be argued that in a setting where routine assessment of left atrial and pulmonary artery pressure and intracardiac oxygen saturation is possible, in the operating room TEE is not necessary in order to detect significant residual defects.

Cannulation and commencing cardiopulmonary bypass

Continuous surveillance of the surgical field by the anesthesiologist is imperative during the cannulation process. This is the only way in which transient periods of arterial desaturation and hypotension that may occur during dissection, placement of purse-string sutures, and cannulation can be differentiated from impending hemodynamic decompensation requiring treatment. As an example, transient loss of the arterial wave form may occur during placement and positioning of the arterial cannula in small children due to impingement on the posterior aortic wall. Failure to recognize the temporary and benign nature of this process can lead to unnecessary and potentially deleterious treatment with vasoactive agents. During placement of venous cannulas blood loss may require judicious volume replacement. Volume replacement via the arterial cannula requires communication between surgeon, anesthesiologist, and perfusionist if iatrogenic complications such as air embolization and over-pressurization of the arterial line are to be avoided. In some circumstances synchronized cardioversion may be necessary to terminate a poorly tolerated supraventricular tachycardia induced during venous cannulation.

As CPB commences the anesthesiologist should assess the adequacy of venous drainage. The head should be checked for evidence of venous engorgement or cyanosis. If an internal jugular line is in place the transduced pressure in the SVC should be displayed. Any pressure greater than 1–2 mmHg requires reassessment of SVC drainage. The conclusion that a high SVC pressure is the result of the catheter tip being kinked or contained in a clamp is one of exclusion. Deterioration in cerebral oxygenation by NIRS or cerebral blood flow velocity by TCD should also alert the team to the possibility of impaired cerebral venous drainage.

Arterial inflow should be assessed as well. Nonexistent or extremely low (less than 10 mmHg) mean arterial pressure in conjunction with a high arterial perfusion line pressure as CPB commences at normal flow rates may herald impingement of the arterial cannula on the posterior aortic wall or less likely an aortic dissection. Misdirection of the arterial cannula into the subclavian or innominate artery will yield a high arterial perfusion line pressure in conjunction with an abnormally high pressure with wider than normal pulsations in the ipsilateral radial artery and an abnormally low pressure in the contralateral radial artery. A large discrepancy between right and left hemisphere cerebral oxygenation as assessed by NIRS, a large discrepancy between right and left hemisphere cerebral blood flow velocity as assessed by TCD, or detection of unilateral facial edema, coldness, otorrhea or rhinorrhea all suggest unilateral cerebral overperfusion.

POST-CARDIOPULMONARY BYPASS ANESTHETIC MANAGEMENT

Detailed discussion of post-CPB management is provided in Chapter 5. The following is intended to be an overview.

Preparation

An organized approach is taken to preparing for termination of CPB so that a smooth transition is ensured. There should be communication between the surgeon and anesthesiologist regarding anticipated difficulties terminating CPB. If residual lesions are likely to exist their effect on hemodynamics should be anticipated and a plan to determine their severity formulated.

Rewarming

Target brain temperature at the end of rewarming on CPB is 35–36°C. Slow core rewarming will allow this target temperature to be reached without inducing cerebral hyperthermia as it is detrimental to neurological outcome following DHCA.[31] If cerebral hyperthermia is to be avoided at no point in the rewarming process should rectal, esophageal, or tympanic membrane temperature exceed target brain temperature. Slow core rewarming also ameliorates temperature afterdrop following termination of CPB by promoting more homogenous somatic rewarming.

Anesthesia and muscle relaxation

Awareness is unlikely to exist during systemic hypothermia but may occur during rewarming. Some provision for amnesia must be made during rewarming particularly in older children. Inhalation agents used during CPB must not be relied upon as the brain concentrations of these agents are unpredictable during the transition from CPB to partial CPB to termination of CPB. A benzodiazepine administered as rewarming commences is a reliable method of amnesia. Provision of muscle relaxation and adequate depth of anesthesia are necessary to reduce systemic oxygen consumption. This is particularly important in patients with single ventricle physiology where for a given cardiac output and Q_p: Q_s a low mixed venous oxygen saturation will compromise systemic saturation.

Ventilation

Ventilation immediately prior to and following termination of CPB must be managed carefully. Commencement of ventilation should be coordinated with the surgical team. Visualization of the lungs by the anesthesiologist is critical during this juncture. Ventilation and held inspiration may be called for to aid in de-airing the heart. Pulmonary compliance may be compromised as a consequence of the systemic inflammatory response particularly in neonates and infants. Metered dose tracheal instillation of a β_2 agonist such as albuterol will generally improve the air trapping which accompanies this inflammatory response. There should be a low threshold for tracheal instillation of saline and endotracheal suctioning to remove secretions as well. This is particularly important in patients with small endotracheal tubes as these tubes can easily become occluded. Ventilation by hand is generally necessary until compliance is optimized.

The ventilator should be set to provide the minimum pressure necessary to achieve the desired tidal volume and I:E ratios of 1:3 to 1:4 may be necessary to minimize the effect of varying alveolar time constants and prevent air trapping. The minute ventilation necessary to achieve a desired $PaCO_2$ post-CPB is generally higher than that needed pre-CPB secondary to the higher metabolic rate associated with normothermia.

Pacing

Epicardial pacing may be necessary to optimize cardiac output. Bradycardia with the resultant requirement for an increase in stroke volume to maintain cardiac output is generally poorly tolerated immediately post-CPB particularly in patients with impaired diastolic function and those with volume overload lesions. In general asynchronous (nonsensing) pacing is used post-CPB to avoid electromagnetic interference from electrocautry. If the SA node rate is slow and AV node conduction is intact, atrial pacing (AOO) should be provided as activation of ventricular contraction via the native conduction system provides optimal ventricular synchrony. When both SA and AV node dysfunction exist, AV sequential pacing (DOO) will be necessary and the optimal AV interval will need to be determined. At pacing rates of 150–170 bpm this interval will likely be 100–120 ms in duration. An alternative to AV sequential pacing, when AV nodal block or a very prolonged AV interval exists in the presence of normal SA node function, is AV universal pacing (DDD). This mode will allow tracking (sensing) of the atrial rate with subsequent ventricular sensing and pacing to a set maximum rate at which point the pacemaker will produce Wenkebach type block. The disadvantage of this mode of pacing is that it is susceptible to electromagnetic interference.

Inotropic support

The decision to initiate inotropic support to facilitate separation from CPB must be individualized. Many patients undergoing repair of simple atrial and ventricular septal defects will not require any inotropic support. Most infants and neonates given the complexity of their repairs and their immature myocardium benefit from inotropic support to separate from CPB. First line inotropic therapy at our institution is dopamine 3–10 μg/kg per minute. This drug is infused directly into a surgically placed LA line also used for pressure monitoring or into a percutaneously placed central venous line. Direct infusion into the LA line allows immediate titration of the infusion rate without the necessity of a carrier solution. Epinephrine 0.05–0.3 μg/kg per minute is used as a second line inotropic agent.

Milrinone delivered as a bolus of 0.5 μg/kg followed by an infusion of 0.5–1.0 μg/kg per minute is a useful agent in patients in whom inotropic support and systemic vasodilation is desired. The loading dose of milrinone can cause profound systemic vasodilation and hypotension in adults but is remarkably well tolerated by children. Nonetheless it should be infused over 15–20 minutes. An alternative approach is to deliver a loading of milrinone while rewarming on CPB. A larger loading is utilized (0.75–1.0 μg/kg) to compensate for the larger volume of distribution. The subsequent vasodilation can be compensated for by increasing pump flows which may in turn promote more homogenous somatic rewarming.

Termination

Termination of CPB is accomplished after the heart has been de-aired, ventilation has been resumed, electrolyte (particularly calcium and potassium) homeostasis has been achieved, and adequate myocardial contractility, rate and rhythm have been established. A coordinated effort between surgeon, perfusionist, and anesthesiologist is then directed toward allowing the heart to fill and eject as venous drainage into the CPB reservoir is reduced and finally terminated.

VOLUME INFUSION

Volume infusion following termination of CPB is guided by both visualization of heart size and by analysis of intracardiac pressures and systemic blood pressure. Because volume can initially be delivered intravenously or via the arterial cannula communication between the surgeon, anesthesiologist, and perfusionist is necessary. The end point of volume infusion is optimization of pre-load recruitable stroke work. Volume infusion should result in an increase in blood pressure with little or no elevation in atrial pressures. If further infusion of volume results in an increase in heart size and elevation of left and/or right atrial pressure with no increase in blood pressure then it can be assumed that preload is optimized. Further volume infusion at this point is likely to distend the heart, elevate ventricular end-diastolic pressure and wall stress, and compromise subendocardial perfusion.

Infusion of citrated blood products or albumen can produce transient reductions in serum ionized calcium particularly in neonates and infants who have limited ability to mobilize calcium acutely. This acute hypocalcemia can produce dramatic reductions in myocardial contractility and vascular tone particularly when volume is infused centrally. Transient hypocalcemia is largely transfusion rate related and can be avoided by judicious volume infusion of citrated products (1–2 ml/kg per minute). Despite this, administration of calcium gluconate (10–30 mg/kg) may be necessary if filling pressures rise and blood pressure declines in response to what would be expected to be a preload enhancing volume infusion.

HEMOSTASIS

Protamine administration in children is rarely accompanied by reactions. Nevertheless it should be delivered slowly over three to five minutes. The surgeon and the perfusionist are made aware of its delivery so that the use of cardiotomy suction can be discontinued allowing the CPB circuit to remain heparinized.

Hemostasis following termination of CPB and protamine administration can be problematic for a number of reasons. Many of the surgical procedures involve long suture lines in high pressure vessels. In addition portions of the suture line such as the posterior aortic wall may be concealed making detection and control of the bleeding site challenging. Pre-existing and acquired coagulation deficiencies may be present as well.

Cyanosis has been implicated in the genesis of coagulation and fibrinolytic defects particularily in patients where secondary erythrocytosis produces a hemocrit greater than 60%. The vast majority of studies investigating the effects of cyanosis on hemostasis have been conducted in chronically cyanotic adults and children over one year old. Thrombocytopenia and qualitative platelet defects are common and are positively correlated with the level of erythrocytosis and arterial oxygen desaturation.[32] Defects in bleeding time, clot retraction and platelet aggregation to a variety of mediators have all been described. The importance of erythrocytosis in the genesis of these quantitative and qualitative defects is underscored by the observation that multiple therapeutic phlebotomies using either plasma or isotonic saline to replace whole blood and reduce hematocrit to the 50–60% range results in improvement of platelet count and platelet aggregation.[33] In addition shortened platelet survival time has been reported. Reduced survival time was weakly positively correlated with the level of erythrocytosis and arterial oxygen desaturation.[34] More recently, a baseline deficit in platelet GpIb receptors has been reported in cyanotic children.[35] These receptors play a pivotal role in inducing platelet aggregation and adhesion via von Willebrand factor. Prolonged prothrombin and thromboplastin times and low levels of fibrinogen and factors II, VII, IX, X, XI and XII have also been reported in association with cyanosis.[32] Coagulation factor abnormalities appear to occur with lower frequency than platelet defects but the full extent of coagulation factor abnormalities is unknown because this issue has been incompletely studied.

Chronic disseminated intravascular coagulation has been proposed as an additional mechanism leading to a coagulopathic state in cyanotic heart disease. While evidence of accelerated ongoing thrombin generation and fibrinolysis has been detected in cyanotic versus noncyanotic patients, chronic disseminated intravascular coagulation has not been substantiated.[36] It is likely that poor cardiac output rather than cyanosis per se is a risk factor for the condition.

Hypofibrinogenemia is known to exist in a substantial number of neonates pre-CPB and is a consistent finding in all neonates post-CPB.[37] Post-CPB hypofibrinogenemia is a consistent finding in older children as well. Loss of the highest molecular weight multimers of von Willebrand factor have also been identified in children with congenital heart disease.[38,39] Loss of these multimers appears to occur with greater frequency in children with cyanosis although this association has not been rigorously investigated.[39]

Platelets undergo an age-dependent maturation process and the platelets of neonates/infants are less reactive than those of children.[40] Platelets in the neonate are hyporeactive to thrombin (a very potent platelet agonist), epinephrine/ADP, collagen, and thromboxane A_2. Given the different receptors involved in these activation processes it has been suggested that this platelet hyporeactivity is the result of a relative defect in a shared signal transduction pathway. These defects are more prominent in low birth weight and preterm infants, a subset of patients more commonly seen in busy pediatric cardiac centers. In addition, the platelets of cyanotic neonates and infants are hyporeactive compared to the platelets of noncyanotic neonates and infants.

Dilutional coagulopathies may exist. The extent to which dilution of coagulation factors is present depends on the size of the patient, the extent of pre-existing factor deficiencies, and the volume and composition of the CPB pump prime. Dilution of coagulation factors in neonates/infants is less likely if the CPB pump prime consists of whole blood or reconstituted whole blood (packed red blood cells and fresh frozen plasma). Significant dilution of coagulation factors is likely if an asanguineous colloid or crystalloid prime is used. Dilution of coagulation factors and red cells can be mitigated by use of conventional or modified ultrafiltration.

In small patients platelet functional defects induced by CPB are overshadowed by the presence of CPB induced dilutional thrombocytopenia. Dilutional thrombocytopenia is a problem in neonates and infants given the relatively large CPB pump prime volumes and the absence of platelets in all prime solutions except fresh, unrefrigerated whole blood. Whole blood stored for more than a day at 4°C is devoid of platelets.

At our institution, where refrigerated whole blood (less than one week old) is used to prime a 300 ml CPB circuit for infants and neonates (2–5 kg), we have consistently found a 50–80% immediate post-CPB reduction in preoperative platelet count. Obviously the largest reductions are seen in the smallest patients undergoing the longest procedures.

COMPONENT THERAPY

Because fresh whole blood with functional platelets is rarely available, therapy for treatment of post-CPB coagulopathies requires component therapy. We prefer to use packed red cells in conjunction with component therapy (platelets, cryoprecipitate). This strategy allows efficient correction of coagulopathies and anemia using small volumes. This is particularly important in small patients where transfusion volume is constrained and dilutional anemia can accompany component therapy.

Platelet transfusions of 0.5–1.0 unit/kg may be necessary to normalize the post-CPB platelet count (250–600 K/ml) in neonates/infants. Since platelets are suspended in fresh frozen plasma (FFP), platelet transfusions in these patients also provide a substantial FFP transfusion. The minimum volume of FFP suspension for 1 unit of platelets is 20 ml (concentrated platelets) while the usual volume is 40 ml. As such a 2-unit platelet transfusion would provide a 4 kg patient with a 10–20 ml/kg FFP transfusion. It has been observed in children that FFP transfusion following platelet transfusion is not effective in restoring hemostasis and may in fact exacerbate bleeding while cryoprecipitate transfusion following platelet transfusion is effective in restoring hemostasis.[41] This is most likely due to the fact that the deficiencies which exist after platelet transfusion are not addressed by FFP because FFP has already been given as part of the platelet transfusion. Additional FFP transfusion after platelet transfusion in infants and neonates will likely induce a dilutional thrombocytopenia.

Cryoprecipitate contains fibrinogen, factor VIII/von Willebrand factor and factor XIII. One unit of cryoprecipitate (20–30 ml) contains 150 mg of fibrinogen and 80–120 units of factor VIII/von Willebrand factor. This quantity of fibrinogen is comparable to what would be found in 75 ml of FFP. This quantity of factor VIII/von Willebrand factor is comparable to what would be found in 80–120 ml of FFP. Obviously in small patients where volume constraints limit transfusion cryoprecipitate is a much more efficient source of fibrinogen and factor VIII/von Willebrand factor.

Cryoprecipitate 0.5 units/kg is transfused for bleeding which persists following normalization of platelet count. Transfusion of cryoprecipitate is generally believed to correct the hypofibrinogenemia that exists following termination of CPB. Data from our institution demonstrates that hypofibrinogenemia following platelet transfusion is uncommon given the whole blood CPB prime and the FFP transfusion which accompanies platelet transfusion. The clinical effectiveness of cryoprecipitate may be related to the transfusion of factor VIII/von Willebrand factor. It is now appreciated that surgical hemostasis is dependent on and initiated by formation of an initial platelet thrombus in a severed arteriole. This process involves platelets, vascular endothelium, integrin and nonintegrin adhesion receptors and their ligands. Wall shear rates in severed arterioles are high (1700 per second) and tethering, translocation and stable arrest of platelets leading to platelet adhesion and aggregation in arterioles requires at least three platelet receptors (GPIb, GPIa/IIb, GPIIIa/IIb and all three ligands (fibrinogen, collagen, von Willebrand factor).

ANTIFIBRINOLYTIC AGENTS

The continued generation of thrombin during CPB despite heparinization is largely responsible for induction of ongoing fibrinolysis. Adjuvant therapy to improve hemostasis post-CPB is directed toward use of antifibrinolytic agents. Sequential cleavage of fibrin by the serine protease plasmin is responsible for fibrinolysis. Plasmin is the activated form of plasminogen. Plasminogen contains lysine binding domains or kringles which allow it to bind to the lysine residues on fibrin. Fibrin bound plasminogen is subsequently cleaved to plasmin by tissue plasminogen activator (t-PA). t-PA also contains lysine binding domains which allows binding to fibrin. Free t-PA is capable of converting fibrin bound plasminogen to plasmin but t-PA bound to fibrin lysine residues stimulates activation of plasminogen to plasmin by two orders of magnitude. The lysine analogues tranexamic acid and ε-aminocaproic acid inhibit fibrinolysis by binding to plasminogen, thus rendering it incapable of binding to the lysine residues on fibrin, and by reducing the rate of conversion of plasminogen to plasmin by t-PA. Aprotinin is a broad spectrum serine protease inhibitor with particular affinity for plasmin. As such aprotinin is a potent inhibitor of fibrinolysis even at low doses.

In addition to its antifibrinolytic effect, aprotinin possesses other properties that ameliorate the effects of CPB on the hemostatic and inflammatory systems. Thrombin, a serine protease is the main effector protease of the coagulation cascade and arguably the most important physiologic platelet agonist. It has now been established that thrombin activation of platelets occurs via G-protein coupled protease activated receptors (PARs). Human platelets express PAR1 and PAR4. PARs are essentially receptors that carry their own tethered ligand. Thrombin recognizes and binds to the NH_2-terminal extracellular domain of PAR1 and PAR4. Subsequent proteolysis by thrombin results in exposure of a new NH_2-terminus that binds intramolecularly to the body of the receptor producing transmembrane signaling. This PAR1 ligand-receptor coupling mediates platelet activation at physiologic thrombin concentrations. Aprotinin blocks thrombin proteolysis of PAR1 and as a result prevents thrombin induced platelet activation. Aprotinin does not, however, inhibit platelet activation via epinephrine, ADP or collagen.[42,43] While aprotinin inhibition of kallikrein particularly at high doses undoubtedly plays a role in attenuating systemic inflammatory response syndrome, recent evidence suggests that multi-level inhibition of the leukocyte–endothelial cell adhesion cascade by aprotinin plays a more important role.[42,43] There is some suggestion that that this attenuation of systemic inflammatory response syndrome may result in improved postoperative myocardial function.[44]

In adults, the pharmacokinetics of aprotinin and both tranexamic acid and ε-aminocaproic acid have been elucidated and dose regimens to establish desired plasma levels determined.[45–47] In children, such determinations are more complicated given the large variability in patient size, type of operative procedure, age related distribution and elimination kinetics, CPB prime volume and the use of ultrafiltration. There are anecdotal reports of adverse thrombotic events such as shunt thrombosis and premature fenestration closure associated with use of lysine analogues and aprotinin in children. However, to date there exists little objective evidence to accurately quantify the risk of such events with use of these agents. A study at our institution demonstrated that use of tranexamic acid was not a risk factor in the genesis of premature fenestration closure in patients who had the Fontan procedure.[48]

ε-Aminocaproic acid

The pharmacokinetics of ε-aminocaproic acid in children has been studied in a group of eight patients ranging in age from five months to four years and in weight from 7.2–18.9 kg with CPB prime volumes of 650–850 ml. It was concluded that a bolus of 75 mg/kg over 10 minutes, 75 mg/kg in the CPB prime, and a continuous infusion of 75 mg/kg per hour following the bolus would be needed to maintain a constant therapeutic plasma concentration of ε-aminocaproic acid (>130 μg/ml).[49] In adults an ε-aminocaproic acid loading infusion of 50 mg/kg given over 20 minutes and a maintenance infusion of 25 mg/kg per hour would be needed to maintain the same target concentration.[45]

Tranexamic acid

With tranexamic acid in adults, a bolus dose of 12.5 mg/kg over 30 minutes, 1 mg/kg in the CPB prime, and a continuous infusion of 6.5 mg/kg per hour should result in a constant therapeutic plasma concentration of 53 μg/ml.[46] Preliminary data suggest that this dose would be inadequate in children. At Children's Hospital Boston we utilize tranexamic acid for reoperative procedures in a dose of 100 mg/kg as a bolus over 30 minutes, 100 mg/kg in the CPB prime, and a continuous infusion of 10 mg/kg per hour following the bolus. This dose has been demonstrated to be clinically effective.[50] In older patients a dose reduction is clearly indicated.

Aprotinin

Aprotinin is dosed in kallikrein inhibition units (KIU). A KIU is defined as the quantity of aprotinin which produces 50% inhibition of two kallikrein units. Aprotinin is packaged to contain 10 000 KIU/ml which is equivalent to 1.4 mg/ml. Clear demonstration of the efficacy of aprotinin in pediatric cardiac surgical patients has been problematic given the large numbers of uncontrolled variables (age, weight, procedure type, CPB prime volume and composition, ultrafiltration use) in the different study groups.[51] In adults, dosing on a per kilogram basis provides more consistent plasma aprotinin levels than a fixed dose regiment.[47] However, preliminary data from one group demonstrate a positive linear relationship between plasma aprotinin concentration and weight when aprotinin is dosed on a per kilogram basis in children less than 30 kg. Dosing on a per square meter basis would be expected to produce more consistent aprotinin concentrations in this patient group. In fact the efficacy (reduced time in the operating room, reduced use of autologous blood products, reduced mediastinal drainage) of a per square meter high dose aprotinin protocol (1.7×10^6 KIU/m^2 as a bolus and in the CPB prime, 4×10^5 KIU/m^2 per hour as a continuous infusion) has been demonstrated compared with placebo and a low dose protocol in re-operative patients with a mean age of 2.7 years.[52] At our institution aprotinin is rarely used for primary operative procedures and is used selectively in older high risk reoperative patients.

TRANSPORTATION TO THE INTENSIVE CARE UNIT

Transport from the operating room to the ICU requires meticulous attention to detail and preparation, particularly because it often involves moving a critically ill infant receiving inotropic and vasoactive infusions down multiple corridors and on at least one elevator. It should be an orderly process directed by the anesthesiologist. Care must be taken to avoid inadvertent tension on or disconnection of the patient's numerous monitoring and drainage catheters as the patient is moved from the operating table to the transport bed. The ICU team should receive a preliminary report on the patient well in advance of transport and should be notified again as the patient leaves the operating room. Once the patient reaches the ICU comprehensive report by nursing, anesthesia and surgery staff is given to the ICU staff.

The following is a checklist of items necessary prior to transport:

- oxygen tank full with enough reserve volume to safely make the trip
- infusion pumps and transport monitor with charged batteries
- full complement of resuscitation drugs
- airway equipment (laryngoscope, endotracheal tube, oral airway, mask)
- blood products or other volume anticipated to be needed during transport or in the ICU; products should be checked and labeled
- open line immediately available for volume or drug infusion; this line should be separate from the one used for inotropic agents
- chest and mediastinal tubes draining freely
- patient medical record, radiographs, anesthesia and perfusion records.

The patient should be hemodynamically stable and hemostasis established before transport is initiated. We generally transport with ECG, pulse oximetry and arterial pressure displayed on a transport monitor. At all points in the transfer process these three parameters must be displayed on either the transport or operating room monitor. Left and right atrial and pulmonary artery pressures are generally not monitored during transport. The transducers for these catheters are left in the operating room ready to be immediately reconnected in the event of a deterioration in hemodynamic status prior to transport.

The transition from the ventilator to the transport bag must be managed carefully. Close observation of hemodynamics, oxygen saturation, and chest wall movement are necessary to assure that the dynamics of ventilation provided by the ventilator are replicated as closely as possible with the transport bag. For patients who can be transported with an FiO_2 of 1.0 we use a Jackson-Rees system with bags ranging in size from 0.5–2 liters. For patients who need to be transported on room air we use an appropriately sized self inflating Laerdal bag which is not connected to an oxygen cylinder. The patient's hemodynamics and systemic oxygen saturation should be stable for at least five minutes while ventilated with the transport bag before leaving the operating room. This is particularly important for patients with single ventricle physiology in whom precise control of ventilation is being used to balance circulation.

REFERENCES

1. Taeed R, Schwartz SM, Pearl JM et al. Unrecognized pulmonary venous desaturation early after Norwood palliation confounds Gp : Gs assessment and compromises oxygen delivery. *Circulation* 2001; **103**:2699–704.
2. Ramamoorthy C, Tabbutt S, Kurth CD et al. Effects of inspired hypoxic and hypercapnic gas mixtures on cerebral oxygen saturation in neonates with univentricular heart defects. *Anesthesiology* 2002; **96**:283–8.
3. Tabbutt S, Ramamoorthy C, Montenegro LM et al. Impact of inspired gas mixtures on preoperative infants with hypoplastic left heart syndrome during controlled ventilation. *Circulation* 2001; **104**:1159–64.
4. Jobes DR, Nicolson SC, Steven JM, Miller M, Jacobs ML, Norwood WI, Jr.: Carbon dioxide prevents pulmonary overcirculation in hypoplastic left heart syndrome. *Ann Thorac Surg* 1992; **54**:150–1.
5. Rajappan K, Rimoldi OE, Dutka DP et al. Mechanisms of coronary microcirculatory dysfunction in patients with aortic stenosis and angiographically normal coronary arteries. *Circulation* 2002; **105**:470–6.
6. Kaplan RF, Uejima T, Lobel G et al. Intramuscular rocuronium in infants and children: a multicenter study to evaluate tracheal intubating conditions, onset, and duration of action. *Anesthesiology* 1999; **91**:633–8.

7. Anand KJ, Hickey PR. Halothane-morphine compared with high-dose sufentanil for anesthesia and postoperative analgesia in neonatal cardiac surgery. *N Engl J Med* 1992; **326**:1–9.
8. Gruber EM, Laussen PC, Casta A et al. Stress response in infants undergoing cardiac surgery: a randomized study of fentanyl bolus, fentanyl infusion, and fentanyl-midazolam infusion. *Anesth Analg* 2001; **92**:882–90.
9. Duncan HP, Cloote A, Weir PM et al. Reducing stress responses in the pre-bypass phase of open heart surgery in infants and young children: a comparison of different fentanyl doses. *Br J Anaesth* 2000; **84**:556–64.
10. Laussen PC, Reid RW, Stene RA et al. Tracheal extubation of children in the operating room after atrial septal defect repair as part of a clinical practice guideline. *Anesth Analg* 1996; **82**:988–93.
11. Stone JG, Young WL, Smith CR et al. Do standard monitoring sites reflect true brain temperature when profound hypothermia is rapidly induced and reversed? *Anesthesiology* 1995; **82**:344–51.
12. Sakamoto T, Hatsuoka S, Stock UA et al. Prediction of safe duration of hypothermic circulatory arrest by near-infrared spectroscopy. *J Thorac Cardiovasc Surg* 2001; **122**:339–50.
13. Nollert G, Jonas RA, Reichart B. Optimizing cerebral oxygenation during cardiac surgery: a review of experimental and clinical investigations with near infrared spectrophotometry. *Thorac Cardiovasc Surg* 2000; **48**:247–53.
14. Kurth CD, Steven JM, Nicolson SC. Cerebral oxygenation during pediatric cardiac surgery using deep hypothermic circulatory arrest. *Anesthesiology* 1995; **82**:74–82.
15. du Plessis AJ, Newburger J, Jonas RA et al. Cerebral oxygen supply and utilization during infant cardiac surgery. *Ann Neurol* 1995; **37**:488–97.
16. Kurth CD, Steven JL, Montenegro LM et al. Cerebral oxygen saturation before congenital heart surgery. *Ann Thorac Surg* 2001; **72**:187–92.
17. Austin EH, 3rd, Edmonds HL, Jr., Auden SM et al. Benefit of neurophysiologic monitoring for pediatric cardiac surgery. *J Thorac Cardiovasc Surg* 1997; **114**:707–15, 717; discussion 715–16.
18. Sakamoto T, Jonas RA, Stock UA et al. Utility and limitations of near-infrared spectroscopy during cardiopulmonary bypass in a piglet model. *Pediatr Res* 2001; **49**:770–6.
19. Watzman HM, Kurth CD, Montenegro LM, Rome J, Steven JM, Nicolson SC. Arterial and venous contributions to near-infrared cerebral oximetry. *Anesthesiology* 2000; **93**:947–53.
20. Babikian VL, Feldmann E, Wechsler LR et al. Transcranial Doppler ultrasonography: year 2000 update. *J Neuroimaging* 2000; **10**:101–15.
21. Gruber EM, Jonas RA, Newburger JW, Zurakowski D, Hansen DD, Laussen PC. The effect of hematocrit on cerebral blood flow velocity in neonates and infants undergoing deep hypothermic cardiopulmonary bypass. *Anesth Analg* 1999; **89**:322–7.
22. Zimmerman AA, Burrows FA, Jonas RA, Hickey PR. The limits of detectable cerebral perfusion by transcranial Doppler sonography in neonates undergoing deep hypothermic low-flow cardiopulmonary bypass. *J Thorac Cardiovasc Surg* 1997; **114**:594–600.
23. Rodriguez RA, Cornel G, Weerasena NA, Pham B, Splinter WM. Effect of Trendelenburg head position during cardiac deairing on cerebral microemboli in children: a randomized controlled trial. *J Thorac Cardiovasc Surg* 2001; **121**:3–9.
24. Borger MA, Feindel CM. Cerebral emboli during cardiopulmonary bypass: effect of perfusionist interventions and aortic cannulas. *J Extra Corpor Technol* 2002; **34**:29–33.
25. Chaliki HP, Click RL, Abel MD. Comparison of intraoperative transesophageal echocardiographic examinations with the operative findings: prospective review of 1918 cases. *J Am Soc Echocardiogr* 1999; **12**:237–40.
26. Stevenson JG. Incidence of complications in pediatric transesophageal echocardiography: experience in 1650 cases. *J Am Soc Echocardiogr* 1999; **12**:527–32.
27. Muhiudeen-Russell IA, Miller-Hance WC, Silverman NH. Unrecognized esophageal perforation in a neonate during transesophageal echocardiography. *J Am Soc Echocardiogr* 2001; **14**:747–9.
28. Randolph GR, Hagler DJ, Connolly HM et al. Intraoperative transesophageal echocardiography during surgery for congenital heart defects. *J Thorac Cardiovasc Surg* 2002; **124**:1176–82.
29. McGowan FX, Jr., Laussen PC. Con: transesophageal echocardiography should not be used routinely for pediatric open cardiac surgery. *J Cardiothorac Vasc Anesth* 1999; **13**:632–4.
30. Yang SG, Novello R, Nicolson S et al. Evaluation of ventricular septal defect repair using intraoperative transesophageal echocardiography: frequency and significance of residual defects in infants and children. *Echocardiography* 2000; **17**:681–4.
31. Shum-Tim D, Nagashima M, Shinoka T et al. Postischemic hyperthermia exacerbates neurologic injury after deep hypothermic circulatory arrest. *J Thorac Cardiovasc Surg* 1998; **116**:780–92.
32. Colon-Otero G, Gilchrist GS, Holcomb GR, Ilstrup DM, Bowie EJ. Preoperative evaluation of hemostasis in patients with congenital heart disease. *Mayo Clin Proc* 1987; **62**:379–85.
33. Maurer HM, McCue CM, Robertson LW, Haggins JC. Correction of platelet dysfunction and bleeding in cyanotic congenital heart disease by simple red cell volume reduction. *Am J Cardiol* 1975; **35**:831–5.
34. Waldman JD, Czapek EE, Paul MH, Schwartz AD, Levin DL, Schindler S. Shortened platelet survival in cyanotic heart disease. *J Pediatr* 1975; **87**:77–9.
35. Rinder CS, Gaal D, Student LA, Smith BR. Platelet-leukocyte activation and modulation of adhesion receptors in pediatric patients with congenital heart disease undergoing cardiopulmonary bypass. *J Thorac Cardiovasc Surg* 1994; **107**:280–8.
36. Levin E, Wu J, Devine DV, Alexander J, Reichart C, Sett S, Seear M. Hemostatic parameters and platelet activation marker expression in cyanotic and acyanotic pediatric patients undergoing cardiac surgery in the presence of tranexamic acid. *Thromb Haemost* 2000; **83**:54–9.
37. Kern FH, Morana NJ, Sears JJ, Hickey PR. Coagulation defects in neonates during cardiopulmonary bypass (see comments). *Ann Thorac Surg* 1992; **54**:541–6.
38. Gill JC, Wilson AD, Endres-Brooks J, Montgomery RR. Loss of the largest von Willebrand factor multimers from the plasma of patients with congenital cardiac defects. *Blood* 1986; **67**:758–61.
39. Turner-Gomes SO, Andrew M, Coles J, Trusler GA, Williams WG, Rabinovitch M. Abnormalities in von Willebrand factor and antithrombin III after cardiopulmonary bypass operations for congenital heart disease. *J Thorac Cardiovasc Surg* 1992; **103**:87–97.
40. Michelson AD. Platelet function in the newborn. *Semin Thromb Hemost* 1998; **24**:507–12.
41. Miller BE, Mochizuki T, Levy JH et al. Predicting and treating coagulopathies after cardiopulmonary bypass in children. *Anesth Analg* 1997; **85**:1196–202.
42. Landis RC, Haskard DO, Taylor KM. New antiinflammatory and platelet-preserving effects of aprotinin. *Ann Thorac Surg* 2001; **72**:S1808–13.

43. Landis RC, Asimakopoulos G, Poullis M, Haskard DO, Taylor KM. The antithrombotic and antiinflammatory mechanisms of action of aprotinin. *Ann Thorac Surg* 2001; **72**:2169–75.
44. Wippermann CF, Schmid FX, Eberle B et al. Reduced inotropic support after aprotinin therapy during pediatric cardiac operations. *Ann Thorac Surg* 1999; **67**:173–6.
45. Butterworth J, James RL, Lin Y, Prielipp RC, Hudspeth AS. Pharmacokinetics of epsilon-aminocaproic acid in patients undergoing aortocoronary bypass surgery. *Anesthesiology* 1999; **90**:1624–35.
46. Dowd NP, Karski JM, Cheng DC et al. Pharmacokinetics of tranexamic acid during cardiopulmonary bypass. *Anesthesiology* 2002; **97**:390–9.
47. Nuttall GA, Fass DN, Oyen LJ, Oliver WC, Jr., Ereth MH. A study of a weight-adjusted aprotinin dosing schedule during cardiac surgery. *Anesth Analg* 2002; **94**:283–9.
48. Casta A, Gruber EM, Laussen PC et al. Parameters associated with perioperative baffle fenestration closure in the Fontan operation. *J Cardiothorac Vasc Anesth* 2000; **14**:553–6.
49. Ririe DG, James RL, O'Brien JJ et al. The pharmacokinetics of epsilon-aminocaproic acid in children undergoing surgical repair of congenital heart defects. *Anesth Analg* 2002; **94**:44–9.
50. Reid RW, Zimmerman AA, Laussen PC, Mayer JE, Gorlin JB, Burrows FA. The efficacy of tranexamic acid versus placebo in decreasing blood loss in pediatric patients undergoing repeat cardiac surgery. *Anesth Analg* 1997; **84**:990–6.
51. Pouard P. Review of efficacy parameters. *Ann Thorac Surg* 1998; **65**:S40–3; discussion S43–4, S74–6.
52. D'Errico CC, Shayevitz JR, Martindale SJ, Mosca RS, Bove EL. The efficacy and cost of aprotinin in children undergoing reoperative open heart surgery. *Anesth Analg* 1996; **83**:1193–9.

5

Pediatric cardiac intensive care

PETER C. LAUSSEN

INTRODUCTION

Over the past two decades there have been substantial improvements in the mortality and morbidity associated with the management of congenital heart disease. Many factors have been responsible, including improvements in surgical procedures and techniques, modifications to cardiopulmonary bypass and advances in diagnostic and interventional cardiology. Equally important has been the development of specialized pediatric cardiac intensive care units for the preoperative management of these complex and challenging patients who range in age from preterm neonates to adults.

The cardiac intensive care unit has a pivotal role in a multidisciplinary and collaborative pediatric and congenital cardiovascular program. Because of the wide variation in patient demographics and the heterogeneous and complex nature of many congenital cardiac defects, it is essential these patients be managed by an experienced, knowledgeable and dedicated team of physicians and nurses. The range of anatomic defects and the significant pathophysiologic derangements that accompany congenital heart disease means that care should be 'proactive' rather than 'reactive'. An experienced team will be able to anticipate a particular clinical course, perceive an evolving clinical picture, and intervene or change management strategies early in the perioperative period. In addition, the intensive care team must develop strong relationships with cardiac surgeons and cardiologists to ensure appropriate planning and collaboration for patient management.

Optimal intensive care management requires not only an understanding of the subtleties of complex congenital cardiac anomalies but also knowledge of pharmacologic and mechanical support of the circulation, the specific effects of cardiopulmonary bypass on endothelial function and the systemic inflammatory response, an appreciation of immature organ systems and the transitional circulation of the neonate, an appreciation of respiratory physiology and the significance of cardiorespiratory interactions, as well as general intensive care management such as ensuring adequate nutrition and treatment of sepsis.

Many of the postoperative management problems after congenital cardiac surgery are quite different from those experienced in the adult cardiac intensive care unit (ICU) following surgery for acquired heart disease. For example, neonates, infants and young children are not able to communicate their level of distress and discomfort. Congenital cardiac intensivists often must rely on indirect clinical evidence from autonomic responses to stress, such as hypertension and tachycardia, and make careful judgements as to the level of pain relief or sedation. Pediatric patients are more likely to receive neuromuscular blocking agents to facilitate synchronization with mechanical ventilation and to prevent inadvertent dislodgement of invasive monitoring catheters, the endotracheal tube and chest tubes.

DEMOGRAPHICS

A thorough understanding of the anatomy and morphology of complex congenital heart defects is essential for the successful management of patients with complex congenital heart disease. This is particularly critical when establishing a diagnosis and planning surgical intervention. Equally important for the successful perioperative management in the ICU is a thorough understanding of the pathophysiology of various defects. This includes not only the preoperative pathophysiology associated with defects, but also the potential alteration in pathophysiology related to surgical repair and/or development of complications in the postoperative period.

Probably the most significant change in approach to the management of congenital heart disease over the past two decades has been the emphasis on early surgical intervention to repair specific defects in the neonate or infant. As discussed in Chapter 1, the underlying premise is that early intervention to correct cyanosis, volume or pressure loads on the myocardium and treat pulmonary hypertension will enhance subsequent growth and development. Such an approach is now the standard of care for the treatment of congenital heart disease, and as a result, the demographic makeup of patients in the ICU has changed substantially (Figure 5.1). In the early 1970s few neonates underwent cardiac surgical procedures and only a small percentage of these neonates had surgical repair using cardiopulmonary bypass. Early palliation or deferred surgery was the usual approach and repair was undertaken in older children. Over the next decade and by the mid-1980s, there was a substantial change in approach such that surgery in neonates and infants was established.

The trend toward early repair in neonates and infants has continued over the past decade. Approximately 50% of all patients undergoing cardiac surgery at Children's Hospital Boston currently are less than one year of age and approximately 20% are neonates (Figure 5.2). Of interest, however, is the wide spectrum of ages that are now presenting for cardiac surgery and managed within the intensive care unit. Many congenital cardiac defects are corrected but not cured, and as such, patients who were operated upon 10 or 15 years ago are now presenting for additional surgical procedures either because of residual defects or the development of progressive complications, such as valve regurgitation or stenosis and recurrence of obstruction to pulmonary or systemic outflow tracts.

Despite the change in patient demographics over the past two decades, the mortality associated with congenital heart surgery has continued to decline. This is illustrated in Figure 5.3. The current early surgical mortality at Children's Hospital Boston for all patients irrespective of diagnosis, surgical technique or modes of treatment in the cardiac ICU is approximately 1.5%. Along with the substantial decrease in mortality, however has been a substantial increase in the costs related to management of these patients. As mortality has declined, an important focus in the ICU is the provision of efficient and cost-effective care, and in particular efforts to

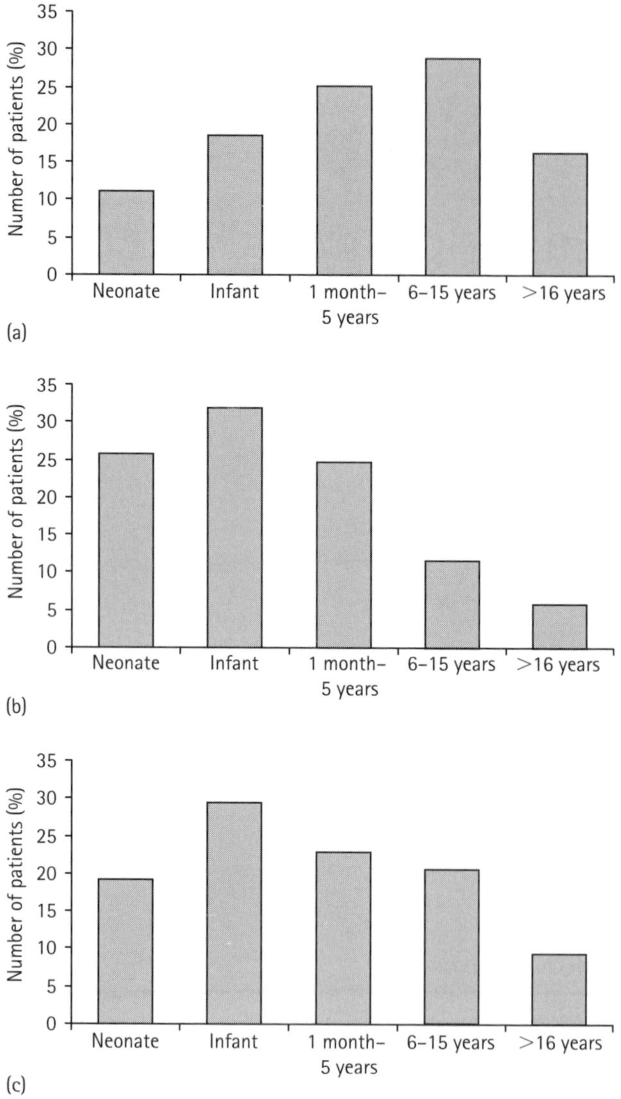

Figure 5.1 *The change in the age range of patients admitted to the cardiac intensive care unit following cardiac surgery at Children's Hospital Boston, over a two-decade period: (a) 1977, (b) 1987 and (c) 1997.*

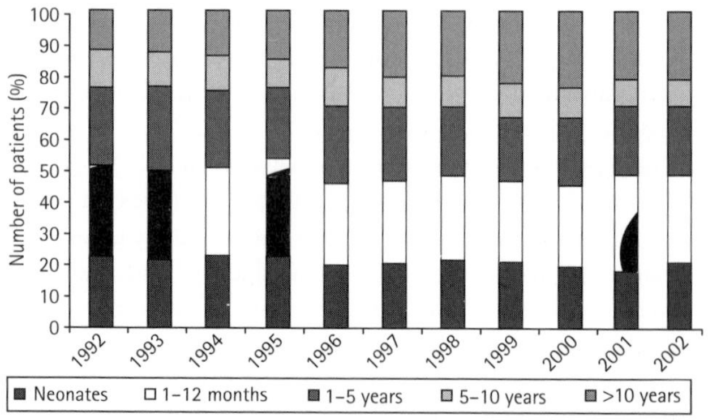

Figure 5.2 *The age ranges of patients undergoing cardiac surgery and admitted to the cardiac intensive care unit at Children's Hospital Boston over the past 10 years.*

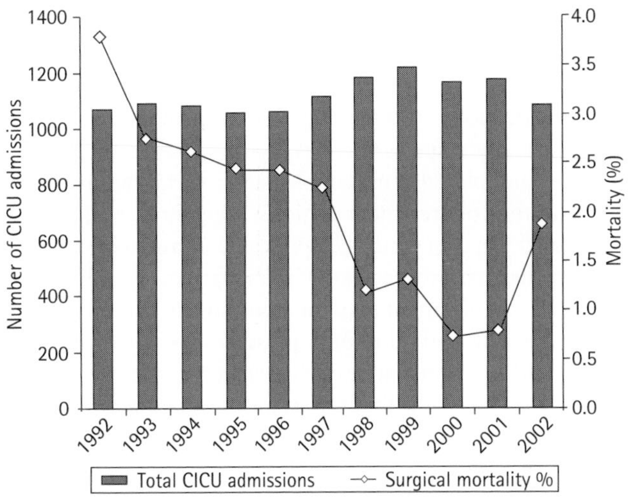

Figure 5.3 *The mortality in the cardiac intensive care unit (CICU) of patients undergoing congenital heart surgery over the past decade at Children's Hospital Boston.*

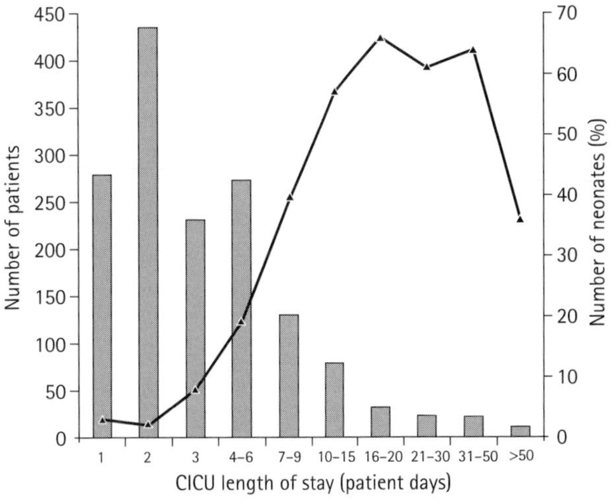

Figure 5.4 *The length of stay in the cardiac intensive care unit (CICU), Children's Hospital Boston. As the length of stay increases, so does the percentage of patients who are neonates.*

decrease the length of intensive care stay as well as total hospital stay.

Management of the critically ill neonate with congenital heart disease is a major focus within the congenital cardiac ICU. While neonates account for approximately 20% of all admissions to the cardiac ICU at Children's Hospital Boston, they account for over 40% of the length of stay. The median length of stay for all patients with congenital heart disease managed in the cardiac ICU is between two and four days; however, as the length of stay in the ICU increases, so does the percentage of these patients as neonates (Figure 5.4). Therefore, a thorough appreciation of the limited cardiorespiratory reserve and immature organ systems, along with the pathophysiology of congenital heart disease, response to surgery, and complications related to cardiopulmonary bypass in neonates is essential.

New challenges for management in the pediatric cardiac intensive care unit are at the extremes of patient size and age. Improvements in surgical techniques and cardiopulmonary bypass management have resulted in extension of successful reparative procedures to preterm and very low birth weight neonates. These patients pose additional considerations of organ immaturity along with technical considerations for surgical repair which can have a substantial impact on their management in the ICU. At the other end of this spectrum, older patients and adults with long standing congenital heart disease and pathophysiology are an increasing population of patients managed in the congenital cardiac ICU. Longstanding pathophysiologic derangements often mean these patients have limited reserve and may have significant end organ dysfunction that compromises postoperative recovery. Because of the unique and complex nature of their underlying defects and pathophysiology, these adults are often best managed within pediatric cardiovascular centers where the expertise to manage specific congenital heart defects is readily available.

PREOPERATIVE MANAGEMENT

The preoperative condition of a newborn with congenital heart disease often has a significant impact on postoperative recovery. For example, a newborn with systemic ventricular outflow tract obstruction may present with circulatory collapse from severe heart failure and pulmonary hypertension as the ductus arteriosus closes, and develop significant end organ injury as a consequence, including brain injury, renal failure, necrotizing enterocolitis, coagulopathy and sepsis. The development of fetal echocardiography is having a significant impact in the early diagnosis and management of congenital heart disease.[1–4] A fetus with significant structural heart disease can be delivered in a high-risk obstetrical unit, and after initial stabilization, be transferred to a cardiac ICU soon after birth. In addition, early interventions such as balloon dilation of an atrial septum in patients with transposition of the great arteries (TGA) or restrictive atrial septum in hypoplastic left heart syndrome (HLHS), can all be conducted in a controlled and timely fashion before the newborn develops significant low cardiac output state and end organ injury.

NICU or CICU?

The development of specialized programs for children with cardiac disease has been affirmed by the American Academy of Pediatrics in a recent policy statement that provides guidelines for pediatric cardiovascular centers. In particular, the academy recognized that interaction between medical and surgical disciplines is essential to provide high quality therapeutic outcomes for infants with congenital and acquired heart disease.[5] While in many centers newborns with congenital heart disease are managed within a neonatal ICU (NICU), it is our preference for newborns with significant heart disease to be transferred to the specialized cardiac ICU (CICU) where subsequent management by cardiology and cardiac surgery staff can be expedited.

In addition, many congenital defects require specific interventions and close monitoring to ensure adequate systemic perfusion. As an example, the critical balance between systemic and pulmonary blood flow in newborns with single ventricle disease such as hypoplastic left heart syndrome is extremely important to ensure adequate systemic perfusion. Physicians and nursing staff within a dedicated pediatric cardiac ICU are in general more comfortable managing newborns with lower arterial oxygen saturation levels (i.e. less than 85%). As part of the understanding of the underlying cardiac defect and physiology, it is essential that an appropriate range of oxygen saturation levels be maintained; often it is preferable for patient to be cyanosed and well perfused as opposed to well saturated and in shock. While the causes of a lower than normal oxygen saturation may be pulmonary venous desaturation from parenchymal lung disease, as is more commonly the case in neonatal and pediatric intensive care units, in the cardiac intensive care environment the newborn with structural heart disease may have lower than normal oxygen saturation because of abnormalities in intracardiac shunting or mixing, and alterations in cardiac output or oxygen delivery that have substantially lowered the mixed venous oxygen saturation.

The ability to appreciate the numerous factors that could contribute to altered cardiorespiratory interactions according to the patient's underlying anatomy and physiology is critical. It may necessitate additional diagnostic imaging with echocardiography or magnetic resonance imaging (MRI), or urgent intervention in the cardiac catheterization laboratory or cardiac operating room. The knowledge and experience of physicians and nurses within a subspecialized pediatric cardiac intensive care unit is essential to not only perceive the evolving clinical pictures described above, but also to expedite intervention by cardiac surgeons and cardiologists.

The heterogeneous range of complex cardiac defects, along with the wide spectrum of patient demographics as previously mentioned, place significant demands on the congenital cardiac intensive care unit. Physicians and nurses working in this environment need to have experience not only in critical care but also cardiology, cardiac surgery, and anesthesia. The full range of treatment modalities should be immediately available, including respiratory support with conventional mechanical ventilation and high frequency oscillatory ventilation, the spectrum of inotropic and vasoactive support, mechanical support of the circulation, and renal support strategies. The response to management strategies must be continually re-evaluated and adjusted when necessary. Clinical examination is key, along with frequent evaluation of hemodynamic variables and the electrocardiogram (ECG) and laboratory data. While early interventions and changes in management strategies may be necessary, equally as important is to know when a patient is in a stable condition and wait for anticipated recovery once treatment has been optimized.

The parents and families of children with congenital heart disease are often well informed nowadays with regards to anatomy and management options. In particular, the internet provides access to a wide range of information and opinions. In many respects this has changed the culture within the ICU, and placed considerable demands on staff to discuss the extremes of treatment options, sometimes even in circumstances that may not be applicable to a specific patient. Parents have more access to information, as well as an increasing involvement in discussions during clinical rounds. These are new and additional pressures for physicians and nurses within the pediatric cardiac critical care environment, and further highlight the importance of maintaining a high level of knowledge and experience by staff to ensure coherent treatment plans.

Preoperative clinical status

An accurate assessment of the cardiac output throughout the perioperative period in a patient with congenital heart disease should be a focus of management in the ICU. The maintenance of adequate cardiac output is important, because low output is associated with longer duration of mechanical ventilatory support, ICU stay, and hospital stay, all of which can increase the risk of morbidity and/or mortality.[6] Data from physical examination, routine laboratory testing, bedside hemodynamic monitoring, echocardiography and occasionally bedside cardiac output determination typically are sufficient to manage patients optimally. As a general guide, if patients are not progressing as expected and low output persists, cardiac catheterization should be performed to investigate and exclude the possibility of undiagnosed or residual structural defects.

Determinants of cardiac output

A preoperative volume or pressure load may have a significant impact on postoperative myocardial dysfunction and cardiac output.

NEONATAL CARDIORESPIRATORY PHYSIOLOGY

The determinants of myocardial performance, as described for the adult heart, are usually valid for children with congenital heart disease provided consideration is given to the immature respiration and myocardium. The neonate can respond suddenly to physiologically stressful circumstances; this may be expressed as rapid changes in pH, lactic acid, glucose, and temperature.[7]

Neonates and infants have limited physiologic reserve. The mechanical disadvantage of an increased chest wall compliance and reliance on the diaphragm as the main muscle of respiration limits ventilatory capacity. The diaphragm and intercostal muscles have fewer type 1 muscle fibers, i.e. slow contracting, high oxidative fibers for sustained activity, and this contributes to early fatigue when the work of breathing is increased. The neonate has a reduced functional residual capacity (FRC) secondary to an increased chest wall compliance (FRC being determined by the balance between chest wall and lung compliance). Closing capacity is also increased in newborns, and therefore oxygen reserve is reduced, and in conjunction with the increased basal metabolic rate and oxygen consumption two to three times adult levels, neonates and infants are at risk for hypoxemia. When the work of breathing increases, such as with parenchymal lung disease, airway obstruction, cardiac failure or increased pulmonary blood flow, a larger proportion of total energy expenditure is required to maintain adequate ventilation. In addition, the neonate has diminished nutrient reserves in terms of fat and carbohydrate, which must be factored into care. Infants with congestive heart failure therefore fatigue readily and fail to thrive.

Cardiorespiratory interactions are significant in neonates and infants. Ventricular interdependence means that a relative increase in right ventricle end-diastolic volume and pressure results in a leftward shift of the ventricular septum and diminished diastolic compliance of the left ventricle. Therefore, a volume load from an intracardiac shunt or valve regurgitation, and a pressure load from ventricular outflow obstruction or increased vascular resistance, may cause biventricular dysfunction.

A schematic comparison of length–tension relationships between the mature and immature myocardium is demonstrated in Figure 5.5. The immature myocardium generally has a higher resting filling pressure for a given end-diastolic volume, and the neonate in particular can readily develop pulmonary edema in the event of excessive fluid administration. Only 30% of the myocardial mass in the neonate comprises contractile tissue, compared with 60% in mature myocardium; the time to achieve full maturation is variable and dependent on the loading charactersistics, but in general a relatively normal proportion of contractile tissue is attained within the first year of life. The stroke volume is relatively fixed and the myocardium less compliant because of the reduced contractile tissue, and an increase in cardiac output is primarily heart-rate dependent. This is particularly critical post-cardiotomy and post-cardiopulmonary bypass when the myocardium may be edematous and relatively stiff; end-diastolic and atrial filling pressures are higher and a sinus tachycardia may be important for maintaining cardiac output. In addition, neonates have a lower velocity of shortening, a diminished length-tension relationship and a reduced ability to respond to afterload stress.[8–12] While at rest the fractional shortening of the immature myocardium during contraction is similar to that of mature myocardium, the mechanical limitation imposed by reduced contractile tissue means that there is diminished reserve. For example, if the neonatal myocardium is exposed to a significant volume load that causes stretch of myofibrils from an increase in end-diastolic volume, the length-tension relationship is shifted such that intrinsic contractility is impaired and early signs of cardiac failure ensue.

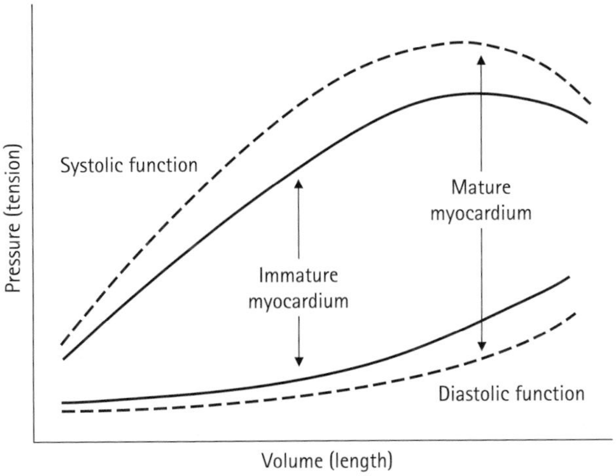

Figure 5.5 *Differences between the resting length–tension relationship of the mature and immature myocardium. Note the mature myocardium develops greater active tension than that of the immature myocardium.*

The cytoplasmic reticulum and T-tubular system are also underdeveloped and the neonatal heart is dependent on the trans-sarcolemmal flux of extracellular calcium both to initiate and sustain contraction. Calcium is therefore an effective short-term inotropic agent following cardiotomy in the newborn and infant, and calcium-channel blocking drugs must be used with extreme caution in patients less than one year of age.

VOLUME OVERLOAD

Causes of volume overload of the ventricles include an intracardiac left to right shunt, semilunar and atrioventricular valve regurgitation, and aortopulmonary artery connections. A typical pressure–volume loop for a volume-loaded ventricle is shown in Figure 5.6.[13,14] It is important to appreciate patients can have a volume load and be cyanosed or fully saturated, have one or two ventricles, or one or two separate outflow tracts, but whatever the anatomical defect causing the volume load, the clinical picture includes congestive heart failure and pulmonary hypertension (Table 5.1). The end-diastolic volume is increased, and the end-systolic pressure–volume line displaced to the right indicating reduced contractility. The volume load on the systemic ventricle and increased end-diastolic pressure contributes to increased lung water and pulmonary edema by increasing pulmonary venous and lymphatic pressures. Compliance of the lung is therefore decreased, and airway resistance increased secondary to small airway compression by distended vessels.[15–17] Lungs may feel stiff on hand ventilation and deflate slowly.

Besides cardiomegaly on chest radiograph, the lung fields are usually hyperinflated. Ventilation/perfusion mismatch contributes to an increased alveolar to systemic arterial oxygen ($A\text{–}aO_2$) gradient, and dead space ventilation.[18] Minute ventilation is therefore increased, primarily by an increase in respiratory rate. Pulmonary artery and left atrial enlargement may compress mainstem bronchi causing lobar collapse.

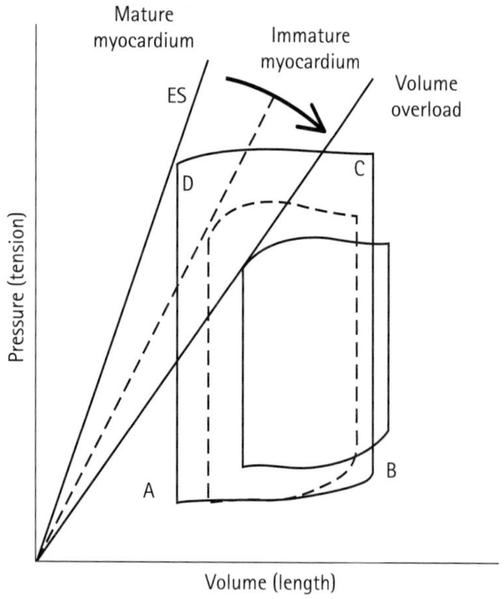

Figure 5.6 *Comparison of pressure–volume loops between the mature and immature ventricle with a volume load. The end-systolic pressure–volume line (ES), an index of contractility, is displaced downwards and to the right in the immature and volume-loaded heart. ES = end-systolic pressure volume line; A = end diastole; B = onset of isovolumetric contraction; C = onset of ventricular ejection; D = end-systole.*

Table 5.1 *Defects or surgical procedures contributing to volume overload*

	Acyanotic	Cyanotic
Two ventricles	ASD VSD CAVC DORV	TGA/VSD PA/VSD
Single ventricle		TA ± TGA HLHS DORV/MA Norwood procedure BT shunt
Aortopulmonary connection	PDA truncus arteriosus AP window	PA/MAPCA

ASD = atrial septal defect; VSD = ventricular septal defect; CAVC = complete atrioventricular canal; DORV = double outlet right ventricle; TGA = transposition of the great arteries; PA = pulmonary atresia; TA = tricuspid atresia; MA = mitral atresia; HLHS = hypoplastic left heart syndrome; BT = Blalock-Taussig; PDA = patent ductus arteriosus; MAPCA = multiple aortopulmonary collateral arteries; AP = aortopulmonary.

The time course over which irreversible ventricular dysfunction develops is variable, but if surgical intervention to correct the volume overload is undertaken within the first two years of life, residual dysfunction is uncommon.[14] The amount of volume overload is also critical. For example, a patient who has a dilated and poorly functioning ventricle with related atrioventricular valve or semilunar valve regurgitation is likely to demonstrate reduced systolic ventricular function following cardiotomy. Preoperative management with diuretic drugs, vasodilators and inotrope support may be effective in decreasing the volume load prior to surgery and possibly improve ventricular function. However, if there is little clinical improvement with medical management, surgical intervention should not be delayed. In general, corrective cardiac surgery should not be deferred to allow a patient to reach a certain weight (not defined) or until chronic respiratory symptoms improve (such as recurrent infection and wheezing). In most circumstances recovery of growth potential will not occur until the volume load on the ventricle and pulmonary circulation has been corrected.

If the increase in pulmonary blood flow and pressure continues, structural changes occur within the pulmonary vasculature, until eventually pulmonary vascular resistance (PVR) becomes persistently elevated.[19–21] The time course for developing pulmonary vascular obstructive disease depends on the amount of shunting, but changes may be evident by four to six months of age in some lesions, e.g. complete atrioventricular canal defect, and transposition of the great arteries with a ventricular septal defect (VSD). The progression is more rapid when both the volume and pressure load to the pulmonary circulation is increased, such as with a large VSD. When pulmonary flow is increased in the absence of elevated pulmonary artery pressure, as with an atrial septal defect (ASD), pulmonary hypertension develops much more slowly, if at all.

PRESSURE OVERLOAD

A typical pressure–volume loop from a chronic pressure load on the ventricle is shown in Figure 5.7.[14] The end-diastolic pressure is elevated, and the end-systolic pressure–volume line displaced to the left reflecting increased contractility and hyperdynamic state. Maintenance of preload, afterload and normal sinus rhythm is important to prevent a fall in cardiac output or coronary hypoperfusion. As the time course to develop significant ventricular dysfunction is longer in patients with a chronic pressure load compared with a chronic volume load, symptoms of congestive heart failure are uncommon unless the obstruction is severe and prolonged.

MYOCARDIAL FUNCTION

Factors that influence ventricular performance include myocardial fiber length (preload), the load or impedance imposed upon the contracting heart (afterload), and the contractile state of the muscle determined by the activation and rapidity of crossbridge formation within the myocyte (contractility) independent of preload or afterload. Along with heart rate, these factors determine cardiac output and systemic perfusion. As for adults, the adequate delivery of oxygen is fundamental for cellular and end organ function, particularly at times of stress such as during exercise, illness, or following surgery. An additional stress for the immature myocardium, particularly with associated congenital heart disease, is the need to meet the requirements for adequate

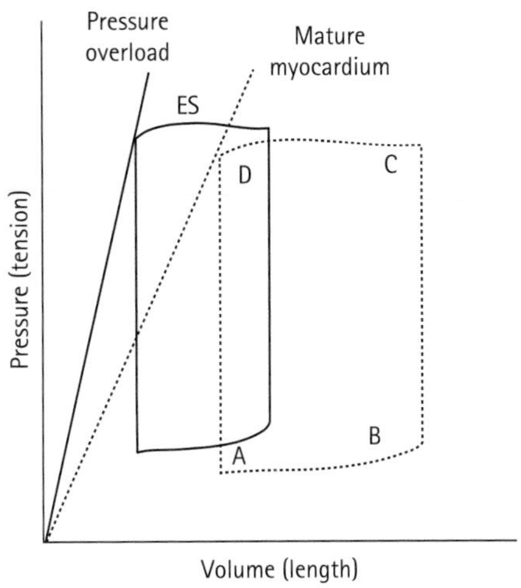

Figure 5.7 *Comparison of pressure–volume loops between the mature myocardium and pressure overloaded state. The end-systolic pressure–volume line is displaced to the left reflecting myocardial hypertrophy and increased contractility (hyperdynamic state). ES = end-systolic pressure–volume line; A = end diastole; B = onset of isovolumetric contraction; C = onset of ventricular ejection; D = end-systole.*

growth and development in newborns and infants in whom the basal metabolic rate is increased two to eightfold when compared with an adult.

Congestive heart failure

Symptom and signs consistent with congestive heart failure in a neonate or infant are indicated in Table 5.2. While there may be similar symptoms of congestive heart failure in patients with congenital versus acquired heart disease, the pathophysiologic basis for clinical symptoms may be quite different. Congestive heart failure occurs in children with congenital heart disease, as in adults, when myocardial function is depressed and end-diastolic volume increased. This is expressed as congestive symptoms of dyspnea with pulmonary edema or peripheral edema. However, congestive heart failure symptoms also appear in congenital heart disease when there may be increased ventricular output and only moderately elevated preload. Chest radiograph findings with congestive heart failure include cardiomegaly, air-trapping and hyperinflation (secondary to extrinsic compression of small airways by dilated pulmonary vasculature), increased vascular markings particularly in the perihilar region, and, in more severe cases, pulmonary edema when the ability of the lymphatic channels to drain the excessive lung water has been overwhelmed.

POSTOPERATIVE MANAGEMENT

The initial assessment following cardiac surgery begins with review of the operative findings. This includes details of the operative repair and cardiopulmonary bypass (CPB), particularly total CPB or myocardial ischemia times, concerns about myocardial protection, recovery of myocardial contractility, typical postoperative systemic arterial and central venous pressures, findings from intraoperative transesophageal echocardiogram, if performed, and vasoactive medication requirement. This information will guide subsequent examination, which should focus on the quality of the repair or palliation plus a clinical assessment of cardiac output. In addition to a complete cardiovascular examination, a routine set of laboratory tests should be obtained, including a chest radiograph, 12- or 15-lead electrocardiogram, blood gas analysis, serum electrolytes and glucose, an ionized calcium level, complete blood count and coagulation profile.

Table 5.2 *Symptoms and signs of cardiac failure in a neonate and infant*

Failure to thrive	Poor feeding pattern Food intolerance Emesis Diaphoresis
Increased respiratory work	Tachypnea Chest wall retraction Flaring of ala nasi Grunting Wheezing
Low cardiac output	Tachycardia Gallop rhythm Cardiomegaly Poor extremity perfusion Hepatomegaly Oliguria Weight gain Peripheral edema Altered conscious state

Monitoring

The level of bedside monitoring that is appropriate for each patient depends upon his/her cardiac diagnosis, the type of repair or palliation, and anticipated requirements for hemodynamic and respiratory data. All patients should have continuous monitoring of their heart rate and rhythm by ECG, systemic arterial blood pressure (invasive or noninvasive), pulse oximetry (SpO_2), and respiratory rate.

Breath-to-breath end-tidal carbon dioxide monitoring is also routine in mechanically ventilated patients to monitor for possible disconnection, misplacement or obstruction of the endotracheal tube. It is also a useful indicator for acute changes in pulmonary blood flow. The normal arterial to end-tidal carbon dioxide difference should be less than 5–10 mmHg. If there is a sudden decrease in pulmonary blood flow – for example, an acute obstruction of a modified Blalock-Taussig shunt – the end-tidal carbon dioxide will fall immediately. A wide arterial to end-tidal carbon dioxide difference could also indicate an increase in dead space ventilation, secondary to air-trapping for example, in addition to a reduction in pulmonary blood flow.

Arterial oxygen saturation monitoring can be performed in one of three ways:

- by pulse oximetry, which yields a peripheral oxygen saturation (SpO_2)
- by co-oximetry, which is a direct measurement of the oxygen saturation of arterial blood (i.e. the SaO_2)
- by calculation from the PaO_2 measured in an arterial blood gas sample.

Although the SpO_2 is the easiest and least invasive technique to use, it has important limitations, including greater inaccuracy with significant hypoxemia (e.g. SaO_2 less than 70%) and dependence on good peripheral perfusion.[22] In patients for whom the accuracy of systemic oxygen saturation data matters the most, co-oximetry is the preferred technique. Continuous oxygen saturation monitoring is mandatory in patients who are expected to have intracardiac mixing, right to left intracardiac shunting and hypoxemia after surgery. Significant reductions in arterial oxygen saturation must be detected immediately, so interventions can be performed if necessary. For example, in a patient whose pulmonary blood flow is dependent upon a systemic to pulmonary artery shunt, a sudden fall in oxygen saturation could indicate shunt thrombosis (which would also be supported by a concurrent fall in end-tidal carbon dioxide). An urgent surgical or catheter directed intervention may be required to restore shunt flow if thrombosis occurred.

The monitoring of central venous pressure is routine for many patients following cardiac surgery, except those who undergo the least complex procedures. For example, we do not routinely place a central venous line in patients undergoing thoracic procedures, such as coarctation of the aorta, vascular ring and patent ductus arteriosus (PDA) ligation, nor in patients undergoing cardiotomy with a short period of mildly hypothermic CPB, such as an atrial septal defect repair.

Intracardiac or transthoracic left atrial and pulmonary artery catheters are often used to monitor patients after complex reparative procedures. Pulmonary artery catheters are particularly useful in the management of patients with the following postoperative problems:

- a residual lesion producing an intracardiac left to right shunt (see below)
- residual right ventricle outflow tract obstruction, since a catheter 'pullback' can be performed to measure the RV to PA pressure gradient
- pulmonary hypertension, thereby allowing rapid detection of pressure changes and assessment of the response to interventions.

The mean PA pressure in nonpostoperative pediatric patients after the neonatal period varies between 10 and 20 mmHg[23] and, while often elevated initially after CPB and cardiac surgery, the mean pressure should be less than 25 mmHg. A mean PA pressure of more than 25 mmHg may be expected in patients with pulmonary hypertension prior to surgery. However, a more helpful measure of pulmonary hypertension other than the absolute pressure is the relationship of the PA pressure to the systemic blood pressure. Generally, the mean PA pressure should be less than 50% of the mean systemic blood pressure. If it is greater than 50% of systemic pressure, a complete assessment of the etiology and clinical status is necessary. This includes an assessment of RV function, preload to the LV and cardiac output, and reactivity of the pulmonary vascular bed (see below).

Left atrial catheters are especially helpful in the management of patients with ventricular dysfunction, coronary artery perfusion abnormalities, and mitral valve dysfunction. The mean LA pressure is typically 1–2 mmHg greater than mean RA pressure, which varies between 1 and 6 mmHg (average 3 mmHg) in pediatric patients undergoing cardiac catheterization.[24] In postoperative patients, mean LA and RA pressures are both often greater than 6–8 mmHg; however, they should be less than 15 mmHg.[25] The compliance of the RA is greater than that of the LA, so pressure elevations in the RA are typically less pronounced.[26]

Pressure wave form and oxygen saturation data from these catheters can provide a comprehensive profile of cardiac function. Causes of artefactual readings must be excluded when interpreting an elevated pressure. This is particularly important if the pressure is elevated in isolation, or the measurement is not consistent with concurrent clinical findings. Before reacting to an elevated pressure, it is always prudent to check the position of the transducer in relation to the heart (preferably zeroed at the mid-thoracic level), evalute the waveform to make sure the catheter is in the correct chamber and not immediately adjacent to a valve, and if possible turn off infusions running through the catheter. Finally, the exact position of all catheters must be determined on the initial postoperative chest radiograph, because unintended catheter tip placement can produce artefactual readings. For example, a left atrial catheter may be inadvertently wedged in one of the pulmonary veins so that the pressure measured is more a reflection of pulmonary pressure rather than true left atrial pressure.

Possible causes of abnormally elevated left atrial pressure are listed in Table 5.3. In addition to pressure data, intracardiac catheters in the RA (or a percutaneously placed central venous pressure catheter), LA, and PA can be used to monitor the oxygen saturation of systemic venous or pulmonary venous blood. Table 5.4 lists the causes of abnormally elevated or reduced RA, LA, and PA oxygen saturations. The RA oxygen saturation in children at rest with a normal cardiac output and no intracardiac shunting is 69–87% (mean 78%) in room air.[27] Following reparative surgery, patients with no intracardiac shunts and an adequate cardiac output may have a mild reduction in RA oxygen saturation to approximately 60%. However, a RA oxygen saturation of only 50% does not necessarily indicate low cardiac output. For example, if a patient has complete mixing and a SaO_2 of 75%, and the arteriovenous (AV) oxygen difference is normal at 25%, this indicates appropriate oxygen delivery and extraction. Elevated RA oxygen saturation is often due to left to right shunting at the atrial level (e.g. from the LA, from an anomalous pulmonary vein, or from a LV-to-RA shunt). Blood in the LA is normally fully saturated with oxygen. The two chief causes of reduced LA oxygen saturation are an atrial level right to left shunt and pulmonary venous desaturation from abnormal gas exchange.

The PA oxygen saturation is the best representation of the 'true' mixed venous oxygen saturation, because all sources of systemic venous blood should be thoroughly combined as they are ejected from the RV. This saturation is useful in the identification of residual left to right shunts following repair of VSD(s). The absolute valve of the PA oxygen saturation, as opposed to the 'stepup' in oxygen saturation from RA (lower) to PA (higher), is a better predictor of a significant postoperative residual shunt. In patients following tetralogy of Fallot or VSD repair, a PA oxygen saturation more than 80% within 48 hours of surgery with supplemental oxygen at a fractional inspired oxygen concentration (FiO_2) of less than 0.5 has been shown to be a sensitive indicator of a significant left to right shunt ($Q_p/Q_s > 1.5$) one year after surgery.[28,29] Determination of the PA oxygen saturation can be misleading in patients with systemic to pulmonary artery collaterals, because flow from these vessels into the pulmonary arteries can increase the oxygen saturation thereby falsely suggesting an intracardiac left to right shunt.

Table 5.3 *Causes of an elevated left atrial pressure after cardiotomy*

- Increased ventricular end-diastolic pressure:
  - decreased ventricular systolic or diastolic function
  - myocardial ischemia
  - systemic ventricular hypertrophy
- Mitral or tricuspid valve disease
- Semilunar valve disease
- Large left to right intracardiac shunt
- Chamber hypoplasia
- Intravascular or ventricular volume overload
- Cardiac tamponade
- Arrhythmia:
  - tachyarrhythmia
  - complete heart block

Low cardiac output state

RESIDUAL DEFECTS

A thorough understanding of the underlying cardiac anatomy, surgical findings and surgical procedures is essential because this will direct the initial postoperative evaluation and examination. Residual lesions may be evident by auscultation, intracardiac pressures and waveforms, and oxygen saturation data. For example, a large v-wave on the left atrial waveform may indicate significant residual mitral valve regurgitation. A stepup of the right atrial to pulmonary artery oxygen saturation of more than 10% may indicate a significant intracardiac shunt across a residual VSD. If there are significant concerns for important residual lesions that are compromising cardiac output and ventricular function, further evaluation with echocardiography and/or cardiac catheterization should be considered. Imaging of the heart may be difficult immediately after surgery because of limited transthoracic access and acoustic windows. During transthoracic echocardiography, it is important that hemodynamics be closely observed, because inadvertent pressure applied with the transducer may adversely affect filling pressures and mechanical ventilation. Similarly, vigorous antegrade flexion of a transesophageal echocardiography probe may alter left atrial filling or compromise ventilation by partial obstruction of a main stem bronchus.

SURGICAL PROCEDURE

While surgery may be routine for many uncomplicated defects, such as ASD closure, the approach for more complex intracardiac repairs may cause specific postoperative problems. For example, if a ventriculotomy is performed to close

Table 5.4 *Causes of abnormal right atrial, left atrial, or pulmonary artery oxygen saturation*

Location	Elevated	Reduced
Right atrium	Atrial level left to right shunt Anomalous pulmonary venous return Left ventricular to right atrial shunt Increased O_2 content Catheter tip position (e.g. near renal veins)	Increased VO_2 (e.g. low cardiac output) Decreased SaO_2 with a normal AV O_2 difference Anemia Catheter tip position (e.g. near coronary sinus)
Left atrium		Atrial level right to left shunt Decreased PvO_2 (e.g. parenchymal lung disease)
Pulmonary artery	Significant left to right shunt Small left to right shunt with incomplete mixing of blood Catheter tip position (e.g. PA 'wedge')	Increased O_2 extraction (e.g. low cardiac output, fever) Decreased SaO_2 with a normal AV O_2 difference Anemia

CO = cardiac output; PA = pulmonary artery; AV = arteriovenous; VO_2 = oxygen consumption; PvO_2 = pulmonary vein oxygen tension; SaO_2 = arterial oxygen saturation.

the VSD in a patient with tetralogy of Fallot, right ventricle dyskinesia and poor contraction may be apparent. On the other hand, if a transatrial approach had been used to close the VSD in the same patient, the risk for atrioventricular valve injury or dysrhythmias such as junctional ectopic tachycardia and heart block may be increased. Often unexpected findings or technical difficulties at the time of surgery means that modifications to the approach or procedure are necessary. A difficult procedure may lead to a longer time on CPB or additional traction on cardiac structures.

Failure to secure adequate hemostasis may expose the patient to significant volumes of tranfused blood products, and if there is inadequate drainage via chest drains placed at the time of surgery, the risk for cardiac tamponade is significant. This may be an acute event, but more commonly it is evident by progressive hypotension with a narrow pulse width, tachycardia, an increase in filling pressures and reduced peripheral perfusion with possible evolving metabolic acidosis. This is primarily a clinical diagnosis and treatment (i.e. opening of the sternum) should not be delayed while waiting for possible echocardiographic confirmation.

Pericardial and sternal closure following cardiac surgery may restrict cardiac function and can interfere with efficient mechanical ventilation. This is particularly important for neonates and infants in whom considerable capillary leak and edema may develop following CPB, and in whom cardiorespiratory interactions have a significant impact on immediate postoperative recovery. In the operating room, mediastinal edema, unstable hemodynamic conditions and bleeding are indications for delayed sternal closure, although it may also be considered semi-electively for patients in whom hemodynamic or respiratory instability are anticipated in the immediate postoperative period (e.g. following a Norwood procedure for HLHS). Urgent reopening of the sternum in the ICU following surgery is associated with higher mortality compared with leaving the sternum open in the operating room, and successful sternal closure can be achieved for most patients by postoperative day four with a low risk for surgical site infection.[30,31]

CARDIOPULMONARY BYPASS AND MYOCARDIAL ISCHEMIA

The effects of prolonged CPB relate in part to the interactions of blood components with the extracorporeal circuit, and development of a systemic inflammatory response. This is magnified in children due to the large bypass circuit surface area and priming volume relative to patient blood volume. Humoral responses include activation of complement, kallikrein, eicosinoid and fibrinolytic cascades; cellular responses include platelet activation and an inflammatory response with an adhesion molecule cascade stimulating neutrophil activation and release of proteolytic and vasoactive substances.[32,33]

The clinical consequences may include increased interstitial fluid and generalized capillary leak and potential multi-organ dysfunction. Total lung water is increased with an associated decrease in lung compliance and increase in A-aO_2 gradient. Myocardial edema results in impaired ventricular systolic and diastolic function. A secondary fall in cardiac output by 20–30% is common in neonates in the first 6–12 hours following surgery, contributing to decreased renal function and oliguria.[25] Sternal closure may need to be delayed due to mediastinal edema and associated cardiorespiratory compromise when closure is attempted. Ascites, hepatic congestion and bowel edema may affect mechanical ventilation, cause a prolonged ileus and delay feeding. A coagulopathy post-CPB may contribute to delayed hemostasis.

Over recent years, numerous strategies have evolved to limit the effect of this endothelial injury resulting from the systemic inflammatory response. Of these, the most important strategy is limiting both the time spent on bypass and use of deep hypothermic circulatory arrest (DHCA). This is clearly dependent, however, upon surgical expertise and experience, and in certain situations DHCA is necessary to effect surgical repair. Hypothermia, steroids and aprotinin (a serine protease inhibitor) are important pre-bypass measures to limit activation of the inflammatory response. Attenuating the stress response, the use of antioxidants such as mannitol, altering prime composition to maintain oncotic pressure and ultrafiltration during rewarming or immediately after bypass are also used to limit the clinical consequences of the inflammatory response. As a direct result of these advances, the clinical features noted above now have less of an impact on postoperative recovery.

Myocardial ischemia from inadequate coronary perfusion is often an underappreciated event in the postoperative pediatric patient. Nevertheless, there are a number of circumstances in which ischemia may occur, compromising ventricular function and cardiac output. Myocardial ischemia may occur intraoperatively because of problems with cardioplegia delivery or insufficient hypothermic myocardial protection, and from intracoronary air embolism. In the ICU setting, mechanical obstruction of the coronary circulation is usually the cause of myocardial ischemia rather than coronary vasospasm. Examples include extrinsic compression of a coronary artery by an outflow tract conduit or annulus of a prosthetic valve, and kinking or distortion of a transferred coronary artery button. While ECG changes may indicate ischemia (ST segment abnormalities), a sudden increase in left atrial pressure or sudden onset of a dysrhythmia such as ventricular fibrillation or complete heart block may be an earlier warning sign.

ALTERED CONTRACTILITY

Because decreased myocardial contractility occurs frequently after reparative or palliative surgery with CPB, pharmacologic enhancement of contractility is used routinely in the ICU. Tables 5.5 and 5.6 contain a list of commonly used vasoactive drugs in the pediatric cardiac intensive care unit. Before initiating treatment with an inotrope, however, the patient's intravascular volume status, serum ionized calcium level and cardiac rhythm should be considered. Inotropic agents

Table 5.5 *Vasoactive agents: noncatecholamines*

Agent	Doses (i.v. μg/kg per minute)	Peripheral vascular effect	Cardiac effect	Conduction system effect
Nitroprusside	0.5–5	Cyclic GMP: NO donor Direct acting systemic and pulmonary vasodilator	Decreased afterload	Reflex tachycardia
Nitroglycerin	0.5–10	Cyclic GMP: NO donor Primarily venodilator ± pulmonary vasodilation Enhance coronary vasoreactivity after aortic cross clamping	Decreased preload Decreased afterload Reduces myocardial work related to change in wall stress	Minimal
Milrinone	25–50 μg/kg loading dose 0.25–1.0 maintenance	Cyclic AMP Phosphodiesterase III inhibitor Systemic and pulmonary vasodilator	Contractility: weak Lusitropy: diastolic relaxation	Minimal tachycardia
Prostaglandin E1	0.01–0.05	Cyclic AMP Systemic and pulmonary vasodilation Maintain patency ductus arteriosus	Decreased afterload	Reflex tachycardia
Prostacyclin	0.005–0.02	Cyclic AMP Systemic and pulmonary vasodilation	Decreased afterload	Reflex tachycardia
Vasopressin	0.003–0.002 U/kg/min	Potent vasoconstrictor	No direct effect	None known

NO = nitric oxide.

enhance cardiac output more effectively if preload is adequate, so intravenous colloid or crystalloid administration should be given if preload is low. If hypocalcemia (normal serum ionized calcium levels are 1.14–1.30 mmol/l)[34] is detected, supplementation with intravenous calcium gluconate or calcium chloride is appropriate, because calcium is a potent positive inotrope itself, particularly in neonates and infants.[35]

Dopamine is usually the first-line agent to treat either mild (10–20% decrease in normal mean arterial blood pressure for age) or moderate (20–30% decrease in normal mean arterial blood pressure for age) hypotension. This sympathomimetic agent promotes myocardial contractility by elevating intracellular Ca^{2+}, both via direct binding to myocyte β_1-adrenoceptors and by increasing norepinephrine levels. Dopamine is administered by a constant infusion because of its short half-life, and usual starting doses for inotropy are 5–10 μg/kg per minute. At a dose greater than 5 μg/kg per minute, dopamine should be infused through a central venous catheter to avoid superficial tissue damage should extravasation occur. The dose is titrated to achieve the desired systemic blood pressure, although some patients, especially older children and adults, may develop an undesirable dose-dependent tachycardia.

If a patient does not respond adequately to dopamine at 10–15 μg/kg per minute or has severe hypotension (more than 30% decrease in mean arterial blood pressure for age), treatment with epinephrine should be considered. Epinephrine should be given exclusively via a central venous catheter and can be added to dopamine at a starting dose of 0.05–0.1 μg/kg per minute, with subsequent titration of the infusion to achieve the target systemic blood pressure. At high doses (i.e. 0.5 μg/kg per minute or more), epinephrine can produce significant renal and peripheral vasoconstriction, tachycardia and increased myocardial oxygen demand. Patients with severe ventricular dysfunction who require persistent or escalating doses of epinephrine greater than 0.1 μg/kg per minute may benefit from opening of the sternum and/or should be evaluated for the possibility of mechanical circulatory support with a ventricular assist device (VAD) or extracorporeal membrane oxygenation (ECMO) (see below).

A combination of epinephrine at low doses (e.g. less than 0.1 μg/kg per minute) or dopamine with an intravenous afterload reducing agent such as nitroprusside or milrinone is frequently beneficial to support patients with significant ventricular dysfunction accompanied by elevated afterload. Epinephrine is preferred to the equally potent inotrope norepinephrine because it generally is well tolerated in pediatric patients and causes less dramatic vasoconstriction. Norepinephrine is a direct acting α-agonist, primarily causing intense arteriolar vasoconstriction, but it also has positive inotropic actions. At doses of 0.01–0.2 μg/kg per minute, it can be considered in patients with severe hypotension and low systemic vascular resistance (SVR) (e.g. 'warm' or 'distributive' shock), inadequate coronary artery perfusion or inadequate pulmonary blood flow with a systemic to pulmonary artery shunt.

LOW PRELOAD

The diagnosis of insufficient preload is usually made by monitoring the mean atrial pressure or central venous pressure. The most common cause in the ICU is hypovolemia

Table 5.6 *Vasoactive agents: catecholamines*

Agent	Dose range (μg/kg per minute)	Peripheral vascular effect				Cardiac effect		Comment
		α	β_2	DA_1	DA_2	β_1	β_2	
Phenylephrine	0.1–0.5	3+	0	0		0	0	Systemic vasoconstrictor, increased SVR
								No inotropy
Isoproterenol	0.05–0.5	0	3+	0		3+	3+	Strong inotropic and chronotropic agent; peripheral vasodilator, reduces preload; pulmonary vasodilator. Limited by tachycardia and oxygen consumption
Norepinephrine	0.05–0.5	3+	0	0		2+	0	Systemic vasoconstrictor, increased SVR
								Moderate inotropy
Epinephrine	0.05–0.1	1–2+	1–2+	0		2–3+	2+	Increase contractility
		3+	0	0		3+	3+	β_2 effect with lower doses: vasodilation
								Tachycardia
	0.2–0.5							α effect with higher doses: vasoconstriction
Dopamine	2–4	0	0	2+	2+	0	0	Renal and splanchnic vasodilator
	5–10	0	2+	2+	2+	1–2+	1+	Increase contractility, tachycardia
	>10	2–3+	0	0	0	1–2+	2+	α effect with higher doses: vasoconstriction
Dobutamine	2–10	1+	2+	0		3+	1–2+	Increase contractility
								Systemic vasodilator: decreased SVR
								Less chronotropy and arrhythmias at lower doses; chronotropic advantage compared with dopamine may not be apparent in neonates
Fenoldopam	0.1–0.5	0	0	2+	0	0	0	Renal and splanchnic vasodilation at lower doses; may provide renal protection during CPB, exposure to contrast during angiography and cyclosporine toxicity
	0.5–2.0							Systemic vasodilation at higher doses: decreased SVR
								Limited chonotropy
								No inotropy

SVR = systemic vascular resistance; DA = dopaminergic receptor.

secondary to blood loss from postoperative bleeding. Initially after surgery and CPB, the filling pressures may be in the normal range or slightly elevated, but this often reflects a centralized blood volume secondary to peripheral vaso- and venoconstriction following hypothermic CPB. As the patient continues to rewarm and vasodilate in the ICU, considerable intravenous volume may be necessary to maintain the circulating blood volume. There may also be considerable third-space fluid loss in neonates and small infants who manifest the most significant systemic inflammatory response following CPB. The 'leaking' of fluid into serous cavities (e.g. ascites) and the extracellular space (progressive anasarca) requires that these patients receive close monitoring and volume replacement to maintain the circulating blood volume. Patients with a hypertrophied or poorly compliant ventricle, and those with lesions dependent on complete mixing at the atrial level, also often require additional preload in the early postoperative period.

HIGH AFTERLOAD

Elevated afterload in both the pulmonary and systemic circulations frequently follows surgery with CPB.[36] Excessive afterload in the systemic circulation is caused by elevated systemic vascular resistance and typically produces both diminished peripheral perfusion and low urine output. The extremities are often cool and may have a mottled appearance. Core hyperthermia may be apparent because of an inability to dissipate heat.

Treatment of elevated SVR includes recognizing and improving conditions that exacerbate vasoconstriction (e.g. pain, hypothermia) and administering a vasodilating agent. A vasodilator, which can be either a phosphodiesterase inhibitor (e.g. milrinone) or a nitric oxide donor (such as nitroglycerin, nitroprusside), is frequently added to an inotropic agent such as dopamine to augment cardiac output.[37–41] As previously noted, neonates, who tolerate increased afterload less well than older infants and children, appear to derive particular benefit from afterload reduction therapy. Afterload reduction with vasodilating agents should be used with caution in patients who have a relatively fixed stroke volume because of residual outflow obstruction, or a severely hypertrophied and stiff ventricle. In this circumstance, the maintenance or increase in cardiac output depends upon an appropriate heart rate response. If excessively tachycardiac, myocardial work will be increased and coronary perfusion possibly compromised; a short-acting beta-blocking agent, such as esmolol, could be administered concurrently with a vasodilator in this circumstance. It is important to note that simply relying on extremity temperature may be misleading; simply escalating treatment to ensure warm extremities when there are no other related clinical signs or biochemical derangements consistent with diminished cardiac output may be unnecessary. Further, the value of extremity temperature as a sign of low cardiac output varies with age. In the neonate and infant with immature myocardium, afterload stress is not well tolerated and instituting early systemic vasodilation is often beneficial to increase output and perfusion. This is not the case in older children and adolescents, who, like adults, have a higher resting afterload; starting a vasodilator simply on the basis of cool extremities may cause significant hypotension and coronary ischemia.

DYSRHYTHMIA OR LOSS OF ATRIOVENTRICULAR SYNCHRONY

An ECG is an essential component of the initial postoperative evaluation because the ICU team must identify whether the patient is in sinus rhythm early in the recovery period. If the rhythm cannot be determined with certainty from a surface 12- or 15-lead ECG, temporary epicardial atrial pacing wires, if present, can be used with the limb leads to generate an atrial ECG.[31] Temporary epicardial atrial and/or ventricular pacing wires are routinely placed in most patients to allow mechanical pacing should sinus node dysfunction or heart block occur in the early postoperative period. Because atrial wires are applied directly to the atrial epicardium, the electrical signal generated by atrial depolarization is significantly larger and thus easy to distinguish compared with the P wave on a surface ECG. The administration of adenosine to induce transient atrioventricular nodal block during a continuous atrial ECG may be useful to determine the morphology of the P wave; an external pacemaker must also be immediately available because of the risk for sustained heart block.

Sinus tachycardia, which is common and often secondary to medications (e.g. sympathomimetics), pain and anxiety, or diminished ventricular function, must be distinguished from a supraventricular, ventricular, or junctional tachycardia. Any of these tachyarrhythmias can lower cardiac output by either compromising diastolic filling of the ventricles or depressing their systolic function.[42] The treatment of a specific tachyarrhythmia can be very difficult when the cardiac output is also compromised. It may not be possible to reduce inotrope support because of hypotension, yet for an automatic atrial tachycardia, such as ectopic atrial tachycardia, this may be necessary as part of the treatment. Inducing mild hypothermia (35°C) is also useful on occasions to lower the heart rate and enhance the effect of the antiarrhythmic drug or to allow external pacing. Close collaboration with an electrophysiologist is recommended. If the tachyarrhythmia persists despite antiarrhythmic drugs and correction of possible underlying causes, such as biochemical disturbances, evaluation in the catheterization laboratory may be necessary, and radiofrequency used to ablate an arrhythmic focus in some circumstances. If the circulation is significantly compromised, mechanical support of the circulation should also be considered until the dysrhythmia has been controlled. A detailed discussion of postoperative dysrhythmias and their treatment is available elsewhere.[43]

The cardiac output of neonates and young infants is more heart rate-dependent than the cardiac output of children and adults.[44] Therefore, bradycardia is important to diagnose and treat to optimize the cardiac output of the youngest patients. High-grade second-degree heart block and third-degree (or complete) heart block can diminish output from either bradycardia or loss of atrioventricular synchrony or both. Patients at particular risk of traumatic third-degree heart block include those undergoing major left ventricular outflow tract reconstructions with myomectomy, those with l-looped ventricles, and those with large single or multiple VSD(s) in the superior portion of the interventricular septum. Third-degree block is transient in approximately one third of cases. If it persists beyond postoperative day 9–10, it is unlikely to resolve, and a permanent pacemaker is indicated.[45]

METABOLIC DERANGEMENT

Hypocalcemia may contribute to hypotension secondary to impaired contractility, particularly in the neonate, as noted previously. A low serum calcium level should be monitored in patients with DiGeorge syndrome, especially in patients with defects such as an interrupted aortic arch and truncus arteriosus. Other causes of hypocalcemia include chelation of calcium during administration of plasma and blood products, and increased losses during a sustained diuresis. Calcium acts as an effective short-term inotrope in the neonate and infant, and in older patients with a mature myocardium, its effect is primarily as a short-acting vasopressor.

Hypomagnasemia is also a cause for dysrhythmias and low output state during the immediate postoperative period, and has been related to longer duration of mechanical ventilation and ICU stay.[46]

Hyperlactatemia in the postoperative period may reflect an inadequate cardiac output and systemic hypoperfusion, and monitoring lactate levels may be a useful method to follow the response to treatment.[47] Particular sources of lactate in the neonate and infant are the brain and gut, and persistent hyperlactatemia despite treatment directed at improving cardiac output could indicate ongoing injury in these tissues and further investigation may be warranted. Alternatively, a persistent hyperlactatemia may also reflect delayed clearance and metabolism by the liver if splanchnic and hepatic perfusion is limited by a low cardiac output state.

Temperature instability during the immediate postoperative period is common, particularly in neonates and infants after prolonged CPB and complex surgical repair. Because of the large body surface area to mass ratio in neonates and infants, a 2–3°C reduction in core temperature may occur following CPB, during chest closure and transport to the CICU. This does not need to be corrected quickly in most cases. Hypothermia could contribute to a prolonged coagulopathy in the immediate postoperative period and if hemostasis is difficult to secure, rewarming to normothermia is indicated. Hypothermia is also a useful treatment for patients with certain tachyarrhythmias, such as junctional ectopic tachycardia.

In contrast to hypothermia, core hyperthermia should be avoided where possible and treated promptly if it does occur. Hyperthermia must be corrected particularly in patients who have undergone a period of deep hypothermic circulatory arrest because of the risk for secondary neurologic injury following a period of ischemia/reperfusion. Hyperthermia may be secondary to the inflammatory response induced by CPB, and also may be a response to low cardiac output state. Peripheral vasoconstriction limits the ability of the body to dissipate heat, thereby contributing to hyperthermia, as well as causing an increase in the afterload stress on the myocardium, an increase in pulmonary vascular resistance and centralizing the circulating blood volume. Treatment of hyperthermia includes the use of antipyretic drugs, topical cooling, cooling blankets (either circulating cold water or forced cold air) and possible administration of peripheral vasodilators.

MECHANICAL SUPPORT OF THE CIRCULATION

Mechanical assist devices can play an important role by providing short-term circulatory support to enable myocardial recovery. They can also provide longer-term support for the patient awaiting cardiac transplantation. Although a variety of assist devices are available for adult-sized patients, ECMO is the predominant mode of support for children.

Extracorporeal membrane oxygenation

Currently, over 300 children per year who receive ECMO for cardiac support are reported to the Extracorporeal Life Support Registry (ELSO) in the USA, with the majority of patients placed on ECMO following cardiac surgery.[48] While over 50% of these patients are decannulated from ECMO, the overall survival to discharge has only been between 35 and 40% of reported cases over the past decade (Table 5.7). Critical appraisal of indications and techniques is required if the success rate for cardiac ECMO is to increase to levels currently achieved in neonates with meconium aspiration syndrome (approximately 90%). At Children's Hospital Boston, we have utilized ECMO to support the circulation in now over 230 patients. Neonates comprise 41% of all our cardiac ECMO, with a current survival rate to discharge of 51%. The pediatric group (infants through to 16 years), comprises 55% of our total experience with an improved survival rate to discharge of 59%.

Substantial institutional variability in patient selection for ECMO makes comparison of published experience difficult.[49–53] Centers with an efficient and well-established ECMO service are more likely to utilize this form of support in patients with low cardiac output. Furthermore, surgical technique and bypass management are additional confounding factors which make comparisons of the use and indications for ECMO between institutions difficult to interpret. Nevertheless, this form of mechanical support can be demonstrated to be life saving, and it can be argued that it should be available at all centers where congenital heart surgery is performed.

Table 5.7 *Cumulative ELSO Registry data through January 2003*

	Survived ECMO (%)	Survived to discharge (%)
Neonatal		
Respiratory	86	78
Cardiac	57	38
ECPR	63	41
Pediatric		
Respiratory	62	55
Cardiac	56	39
ECPR	49	38
Adult		
Respiratory	53	46
Cardiac	40	31
ECPR	48	33

ECMO = extracorporeal membrane oxygenation; ELSO = Extracorporeal Life Support Organization; ECPR = external cardiopulmonary resuscitation.

Table 5.8 *Typical indications for extracorporeal membrane oxygenation*

Inadequate oxygen delivery

Low cardiac output

- chronic (cardiomyopathy)
- acute (myocarditis)
- weaning from cardiopulmonary bypass
- preoperative stabilization
- progressive postoperative failure
- pulmonary hypertension
- refractory arrhythmias
- cardiac arrest

Profound cyanosis

- intracardiac shunting and cardiovascular collapse
- acute respiratory failure exaggerated by underlying heart disease
- congenital heart disease, complicated by other newborn indications for ECMO such as meconium aspiration syndrome, primary pulmonary hypertension of the newborn, pneumonia, sepsis, respiratory distress syndrome

Support for intervention during cardiac catheterization

ECMO INDICATIONS

General indications and contraindications for ECMO support of the circulation in patients with congenital heart disease are listed in Tables 5.8 and 5.9.

Preoperative stabilization

ECMO may be useful for critically ill neonates prior to cardiac surgery, thereby enabling preoperative stabilization and limiting end-organ dysfunction prior to repair. Indications include severe low output state (e.g. critical aortic stenosis), pulmonary hypertension (e.g. obstructed totally anomalous pulmonary venous return) and severe hypoxemia (e.g. transposition with pulmonary hypertension).

Table 5.9 *Relative contraindications for extracorporeal membrane oxygenation*

- Endstage, irreversible or inoperable disease
- Family, patient directives to limit resuscitation
- Significant neurologic or end-organ impairment
- Uncontrolled bleeding within major organs
- Extremes of size and weight
- Inaccessible vessels during cardiopulmonary resuscitation

Failure to wean from CPB

Patients who fail to wean from cardiopulmonary bypass may be connected directly to an ECMO circuit in the operating room and brought to the intensive care unit in the hope of recovering myocardial function. These children typically have poorer survival rates for many reasons, including severity and complexity of disease, as well as increased bleeding. A critical decision for utilizing ECMO in this circumstance is whether the patient is a suitable candidate for cardiac transplantation if there is no significant recovery of function.

Post-cardiotomy

In general, ECMO appears to be most effective as a therapeutic option for patients who have a period of relative stability after reparative cardiac surgery, but then develop progressive myocardial or respiratory failure, or have a sudden cardiac arrest. This typically occurs during the first 24 hours after surgery and subsequent survival may be better in this group of patients following a period of myocardial rest and decompression. Our current survival rate for this group at Children's Hospital Boston is 64%.

Bridge to transplantation

While ECMO can be used to resuscitate the circulation and prevent end-organ dysfunction while awaiting potential myocardial recovery, it may also be used as a bridge to transplantation.[54] However, with limitations relating to donor availability and the potential complications while on ECMO, in particular bleeding, end-organ dysfunction and sepsis, the decision to proceed with listing for transplantation should be made early during the ECMO run. If there is no discernible recovery of myocardial function after 48–72 hours on ECMO support, transplant evaluation should be completed for appropriate patients.[53] Our current median waiting time on ECMO after listing for transplantation is six days for all patients, and we have been able to successfully bridge 55% of our patients to transplant. However, there are important age and size differences, with older children and adolescents being much more likely to survive a successful ECMO bridge to transplantation.

Resuscitation

The rapid deployment of ECMO during active cardiopulmonary resuscitation (CPR) in a pulseless circulation remains a contentious issue. The underlying premise is that survival following a sudden cardiac arrest and standard resuscitation in children is poor irrespective of the resuscitation setting.[55,56] Therefore a number of pediatric institutions have developed a rapid response system to provide early deployment and cannulation for ECMO.[57–59] A rapid response ECMO system was started at Children's Hospital Boston in 1996. Through January 2003, over 150 patients have been placed on ECMO with an overall survival to discharge rate of 57%. Of these patients, 52% were placed on ECMO during active CPR (rapid response system), and 55% of these patients have been successfully discharged from hospital.

The ability to efficiently and rapidly support the circulation or respiration in patients following cardiac surgery (and in children with cardiac disease in general) has improved our ability to salvage a group of children that previously would most likely have died. It is the utility of this type of support that has been an additional factor in the continued decline in surgical mortality over recent years.

We have utilized the rapid deployment system during cardiopulmonary arrest and resuscitation at a variety of locations throughout the hospital, including the ICU, cardiac catheterization laboratory, emergency department and noncardiac operating rooms. Typically, we now wait only five minutes (i.e. after one or two rounds of resuscitation medications) before determining that return of cardiovascular stability during CPR is unlikely and that ECMO should be deployed. An ECMO circuit is ready and carbon dioxide vacuumed at all times in the ICU, and can be crystalloid primed for use in 15 minutes. A neonatal membrane is used in this setup (size 0.8–1.5 m^2; appropriate for patients 2–15 kg). For older children and adults, a fresh circuit with a hollow-fiber membrane is used which takes little time to de-air and can be established within 15 minutes; once stable on ECMO, the hollow-fiber can be changed out for a conventional membrane if longer-term support is necessary. Blood products are added when they are available (typically after cannulation) and crystalloid is removed by direct withdrawal from the circuit into a syringe or by a volume-matched amount of ultrafiltration. Cardiac surgeons who are trained in cannulation techniques for open chest, groin or neck routes, and ECMO specialists and cardiac ICU physicians are immediately available inhouse 24 hours per day.

ECMO CANNULATION, STABILIZATION AND EVALUATION

Depending on the circumstances of hemodynamic decompensation (impending or actual cardiac arrest; nonoperated or postoperative cardiac patient) and surgeon preference, vascular access is obtained either by transthoracic approach with direct cannulation of the right atrium and aorta or peripherally through the neck or femoral vessels.

Medical support and resuscitation (i.e. airway stabilization with hand ventilation, intravascular volume replacement, catecholamine infusions, correction of electrolyte imbalance, sodium bicarbonate administration, arrhythmia suppression, cardiac pacing, core temperature cooling, and cardiac massage, etc.) are continued throughout the cannulation procedure and commencement of veno-arterial extracorporeal support until a stable circulation is achieved.

The ECMO circuit is a 'closed' circuit, which is an important distinction to a CPB circuit with cardiotomy suction used during cardiac surgery. There is very limited ability to handle any air in the venous limb of the ECMO circuit, and careful de-airing of both the arterial and venous cannulas is essential when connecting to the ECMO circuit. In our institution, blood flow is driven by a roller pump using a servoregulatory mechanism. This system permits high flow rates with minimal hemolysis and protects against entrainment of air. Priming volumes are determined by the surface area of the oxygenator membrane. The circuit is initially vacuumed with carbon dioxide to eliminate nitrogen which would lead to bubble formation after introduction of the saline priming solution. Normosol solution (Abbott Laboratories, Abbott Park, IL) is used to displace the carbon dioxide, and after the system has been de-bubbled, 5% albumin is added to decrease adsorption of fibrinogen to the circuit components during the subsequent blood priming. Guidelines for blood product priming components, equipment, and operational characteristics of the ECMO circuit according to patient size are displayed in Table 5.10. Table 5.11 shows guidelines for cannula size with respect to patient weight.

Following cannulation, the patient is connected to the ECMO circuit and the roller pump is adjusted to gradually achieve the desired flow rates of 100–150 ml/kg depending on the underlying cardiopulmonary physiology. Intracardiac and arterial blood pressures including waveform characteristics are noted. Usually, vasopressor infusions are used to maintain mean arterial blood pressure greater than 45 mmHg in neonates and greater than 60–70 mmHg in children and adults. A chest radiograph is obtained to check cannulas and line position as well as endotracheal tube and lung parenchymal status.

Elevated pre-membrane pressures (greater than 350 mmHg) at normal flows without change in post-membrane pressure, or evidence of blood to gas leak constitute membrane oxygenator dysfunction and may dictate oxygenator replacement. Extensive thrombus or consumptive coagulopathy with hypofribrinogenemia and thrombocytopenia constitute other indications for circuit replacement. When ECMO flow appears inadequate to meet the needs of the patient and limited venous drainage restricts additional flow, interpretation of arterial and atrial pressures may aid the formulation of a differential diagnosis (Table 5.12). Low flow states and/or significant hypotension require immediate analysis and intervention.

Assessing the adequacy of flow soon after initiation of ECMO is of paramount importance. Answering a checklist of questions facilitates this assessment.

Is the systemic ventricle adequately decompressed?

Venting the left atrium may be necessary to lower the left atrial pressure and decrease left ventricular wall stress thereby minimize ongoing myocardial injury. Adequate decompression can

Table 5.10 *ECMO circuit guidelines, Children's Hospital Boston*

Weight (kg)	2–15	16–20	21–35	36–60	>60	Stat (>15 kg)
Circuit	Neonatal	Pediatric	Pediatric	Adult	Adult	Stat
Membrane (m^2)	0.8–1.5	2.5	3.5	4.5	4.5	Optima
Prime						
5% albumin (ml)	50	100	100	100	100	100
Packed red blood cells (ml)	500	1000	1000	1500	1500	1000
Fresh frozen plasma (ml)	200	400	400	500	500	400
Cryoprecipitate (units)	2	3	3	4	4	3
Platelets (units)	2	4	4	6	6	6
Medications						
Heparin (units)	500	500	500	800	800	500
THAM (ml)	100	200	300	300	300	200
Calcium gluconate (mg)	1500	3000	3000	4000	4000	3000
Flows						
Minimum (ml/min)	100	200	250	300	600	500
Maximum (l/min)	1.8	4.5	5.5	6.5	6.5 (ea)	8.0
Sweep gas range (l/min)	1–4.5	2–8	2–11	2–13	2–13	0.5–20
Membrane volume (ml)	174	455	575	665	1330	260
Circuit volume (ml)	580	1500	1600	2500	3200	1000

* Add 100 units heparin for noromosol cannulations; THAM = tris-hydroxymethyl aminomethane.

Table 5.11 *Extracorporeal membrane oxygenation cannula size according to patient weight*

Weight (kg)	Venous (Fr)	Arterial (Fr)
2–4	8–14	8–10
5–15	15–19	12–15
16–20	19–21	15–17
21–35	21–23	17–19
36–60	23–25	19–21
60+	23–29	21

be assessed early by echocardiography, and signs of pulmonary edema. If not decompressed, strategies include placing a vent in the left atrium by direct placement via the atrial appendage or pulmonary veins through an open chest, or by a transcatheter approach in the catheterization laboratory[60] or augmenting ventricular ejection by judicious use of inotropic agents.

Is the perfusion pressure and flow adequate?

This can be determined by an assessment of perfusion pressure, patient color and appearance, the presence of an acidosis and whether or not there is adequate clearance of lactate, and whether the cannulas are appropriately sized and positioned. Hypotension with mean arterial blood pressure less than 30 mmHg in neonates or less than 50 mmHg in larger children and adults requires prompt evaluation and treatment.

Is hemostasis achieved?

This is not uncommonly a problem in the immediate postoperative period. Prompt control of bleeding has a direct influence on subsequent outcome. Tamponade physiology will affect venous return, circuit line pressure and ECMO flows; mediastinal re-exploration may be necessary to evacuate clot and control bleeding. In addition to surgical exploration, replacement of coagulation factors and use of antifibrinolytics must be considered (e.g. aminocaproic acid bolus 100 mg/kg followed by infusion 30 mg/kg per hour; an alternative for persistent post-cardiotomy bleeding may be aprotinin 30 000 iu/kg bolus and 10 000 iu/kg per hour for six hours). Initial guidelines include transfusion of packed red blood cell to maintain the hematocrit at greater than 35%, cryoprecipitate to keep serum fibrinogen more than 150 mg/dl and concentrated platelet transfusions to maintain the platelet count above 100 000/mm^3. A heparin bolus (30 units/kg) is usually given at the time of cannulation followed by infusion (20–30 units/kg per hour) adjusted to maintain an activated clotting time (ACT) of 180–200 s.

Are there specific considerations based on underlying pathology?

The management of an aortopulmonary shunt is critical in patients with single ventricle physiology. Systemic and pulmonary flow should be balanced by either partially clipping the shunt or using high ECMO flows. On ECMO, circuit flows up to 200 ml/kg minute or more are usually necessary to maintain adequate systemic perfusion while accounting for runoff into the pulmonary circulation through the shunt. Although partial temporary narrowing of the shunt may be advisable in some circumstances, it is unwise to completely occlude the only source of pulmonary blood flow to the pulmonary endothelium. It is possible to bypass the membrane oxygenator in patients following the Norwood procedure with a Blalock shunt without lung disease if higher flows are maintained and the shunt is patent.[61] This maneuver simplifies the circuit and may permit less use of heparin. ECMO, thus, effectively becomes a ventricular assist device.

Table 5.12 *Assessment of low flow states during extracorporeal membrane oxygenation*

Problem	Observations	Treatment options
Inadequate oxygen delivery and organ perfusion	Tachycardia, mottled skin, cool extremities, poor capillary refill, hypotension, oliguria, metabolic acidosis, hyperlactatemia, rising serum creatinine and liver function tests	Check cannula position Increase ECMO flow Increase native cardiac output
Inadequate ECMO flow: Circuit chatters, bladder collapses, inadequate venous return or high post membrane pressures	*Atrial pressures normal:*	
	Venous cannula malposition	Reposition venous cannula
	Venous cannula too small	Replace or add second venous cannula
	Venous thrombus formation	Surgical removal of thrombus or thrombolysis
	Excessive runoff through aorto-pulmonary shunt	Narrow shunt, embolize collaterals
	Atrial pressures low:	
	Bleeding	Surgical exploration, administer coagulation factors and blood, antifibrinolytics, reduce heparin
	Systemic vasodilation	Treat sepsis, administer vasoconstrictors
	Atrial pressures high:	
	Tamponade	Surgical exploration, evacuation of blood and clot
	Left ventricular overdistension	Place vent in left atrium, support ejection with catecholamine
	Aortic regurgitation	Reposition aortic cannula, assess need for aortic valve replacement
	Membrane pressure high:	
	Arterial cannula malposition	Reposition cannula
	Arterial cannula too small	Replace or add second arterial cannula (bifemoral arterial cannulation)

Problems related to cannula placement and adequacy of venous drainage must be considered in patients with single-ventricle physiology and complex venous anatomy, such as heterotaxy syndrome or possible vessel occlusion from prior catheterizations, and in patients with a cavopulmonary connection. The site of cannulation will be affected by vessel patency, and the underlying physiology might influence the number of venous cannulas used. For example, patients with a superior cavopulmonary anastomosis (bidirectional Glenn shunt) as the primary source of pulmonary blood flow frequently require separate venous drainage of the SVC and IVC, unless there is congenital interruption of the infra-hepatic IVC with drainage of lower body blood to the azygous vein. In the latter case a single venous cannula in the SVC might be sufficient. On the other hand, placement of a cannula in the SVC may be detrimental in patients with bidirectional Glenn shunt physiology because of the potential for reduced cerebral venous drainage, and therefore decreased cerebral perfusion. This is also a concern for patients with Fontan physiology; while it may be possible to achieve adequate drainage with a venous cannula placed in the Fontan baffle, in our experience, an additional SVC catheter is often necessary to achieve the desired or necessary flows on ECMO.[62]

Is there adequate end-organ perfusion?

Once stable flows and perfusion have been achieved, the ventricles decompressed and hemostasis secured, potential end-organ injury should be evaluated. For patients who have long-standing cyanotic heart disease, it may be preferable to start ECMO using a lower oxygen concentration (closer to room air) to attenuate the potential ischemic/refusion injury and potential for oxygen free radical injury. Neurologic protection must be considered. For patients placed on ECMO during active resuscitation, mild hypothermia (34°C) should be maintained for the first 12–24 hours on ECMO to prevent secondary neurologic injury. Assessment with head ultrasound, EEG or computerized tomography should be considered early; muscle relaxants should not be given and sedation minimized to allow an appropriate daily clinical assessment. In addition, renal function, liver function, risk for sepsis and possible gut ischemia should be frequently evaluated.

Residual cardiac defects

If a patient fails to wean from ECMO or there is delay in anticipated recovery of myocardial function, the possibility of a residual surgical problem must always be considered. This is usually difficult to diagnose by echocardiography alone, and cardiac catheterization (i.e. diagnostic or interventional) should be considered.

DAILY MANAGEMENT

The daily management of a patient on ECMO or other forms of extracorporeal life support requires a meticulous assessment of cardiorespiratory function, end-organ perfusion and injury, evolving complications such as bleeding or sepsis, and the mechanics of the ECMO circuit.[63]

Following ECMO cannulation and initial resuscitation, high flow rates (100–200 ml/kg per minute depending on the underlying pathophysiology) are used to 'rest' the heart and decompress the ventricle(s). However, in contrast to the concept of 'resting the lungs' for patients who are placed on ECMO for respiratory failure and lung injury, it is important that the heart regain contractile function and conduction as soon as possible to maintain a workload and avoid involution of the myocardial mass. For this reason inotropic support may be reintroduced earlier in cardiac patients compared with those on ECMO purely for respiratory support. Atrioventricular synchrony should be established as soon as possible. This may be achieved with external pacing if necessary. It is very important that dysrhythmias on ECMO be treated promptly. While it may be possible to maintain adequate systemic perfusion and ECMO flows, the heart may overdistend in the presence of certain dysrhythmias, in particular ventricular fibrillation, and this may cause irreversible myocardial injury.

Transient endothelial dysfunction is common after ECMO is established, identical to the injury resulting from CPB, and causes an elevated pulmonary vascular resistance and ventilation-perfusion abnormalities.[64] Permitting or promoting the heart to eject some blood into the pulmonary circulation while on ECMO may help endothelial recovery and prevent pulmonary hypertension when weaning from ECMO. It is important to remember that the pulmonary venous blood entering the left ventricle and ejected into the coronary circulation may be significantly desaturated, and this could cause myocardial ischemia or delay myocardial recovery. For this reason, mechanical ventilation is continued on cardiac ECMO to ensure pulmonary venous blood is well saturated. Ventilator settings are adjusted primarily according to lung compliance, which may reflect the degree of pre-existing cardiac-related or parenchymal lung disease. Tidal volumes of 7–9 ml/kg with peak inspiratory pressures not exceeding 25–28 cmH_2O and FiO_2 of 0.3–0.4 are usually maintained in patients with normal lung compliance. Changes in ventilator settings are guided by physical examination, an assessment of compliance based on hand ventilation and lung volumes, and the appearance of the lung fields on daily chest radiographs.

Fluid retention and body wall edema is very common in cardiac patients on ECMO because of endothelial dysfunction and capillary leak associated with reperfusion injury and inflammatory response,[65] changes in oncotic pressure depending on the priming solution, or decreased urine output secondary to alterations in perfusion and the influence of antidiuretic hormone, renin-angiotensin, and atrial natriuretic factor production.[66] Diuretic therapy is started early to achieve a negative fluid balance and treat anasarca as soon as possible; fluid overload is one of the most important factors that will determine eventual successful weaning from cardiac ECMO and longer-term survival. Furosemide bolus (1 mg/kg) followed by continuous infusion (0.2–0.3 mg/kg per hour) is usually the first choice to induce a diuresis, provided adequate renal perfusion has been achieved with ECMO flow and there has not been a significant or irreversible renal injury prior to starting ECMO. Chlorothiazide (10 mg/kg per dose every 12 hours) is added if the response to furosemide is suboptimal. Modified ultrafiltration is utilized in the setting of excessive fluid retention despite maximal diuretic therapy and circulatory support. Suspension of ultrafiltration is advisable in the setting of low atrial pressures with hypotension and frequent circuit shutdown due to low volume or pressure sensing within the bladder, at least until hemodynamics stabilize.

Neurologic assessment, although difficult in patients on ECMO, must be performed regularly. Abrupt changes in heart rate, blood pressure, skin perfusion, and pupillary size could indicate seizure activity in paralysed patients. Concerning findings should be promptly evaluated by cranial ultrasound, head CT scan, or electroencephalography because changes or abnormalities will impact the decision to continue ECMO support. Sedation and analgesia must also be continually reassessed. Muscle relaxation is advisable in unstable patients, but can be used intermittently as needed once the patient and ECMO flows are stable enough to allow neurologic evaluation. Parenteral nutritional support should be initiated within one to two days after establishing ECMO, although may be deferred if the ECMO course is likely to be relatively short, i.e. less than four days, and it is anticipated enteral nutrition can be introduced soon after discontinuing ECMO. Patients receiving mechanical support are at high risk for nosocomial infection, especially from skin flora with a direct portal of entry through catheters, chest sites, and open or closed sternotomy wounds. Patients with unexplained hemodyamic instability, coagulopathy, and elevated white blood cell count or fever should be pan-cultured and broad spectrum antibiotic cover initiated.

WEANING FROM ECMO

The strategies for weaning from cardiac ECMO are often quite different to those used to wean patients who are on ECMO for respiratory support. A thorough understanding of the underlying cardiac physiology, cardiorespiratory interactions and an appreciation for the expected range of oxygen saturations is important. Because of the high risk of complications and substantial mortality in cardiac patients associated with the duration of mechanical circulatory support beyond one week, consideration as to when and how to wean cardiac patients from ECMO should begin soon after cannulation once circulatory stability has been established. The disease process and circumstances resulting in hemodynamic failure or cardiac arrest may influence the expected duration of mechanical support. For example, patients who fail to separate from cardiopulmonary bypass after cardiac surgery due to severe pulmonary hypertension usually respond to a period of 24–48 hours on ECMO with inhaled nitric oxide therapy and inotropic support of the right heart. Similarly, patients who have a low cardiac output state or suffer cardiac arrest after cardiac surgery may have residual defects that allow rapid weaning and decannulation soon after reoperation. The likelihood of recovery of ventricular function should be decided within the first 48–72 hours so that cardiac transplantation status can be ascertained. ECMO instituted for catheter intervention or arrhythmia ablation procedures may be discontinued within hours of patient cannulation.[67] In contrast, patients with severe cardiomyopathies or those awaiting heart transplantation may require mechanical assistance for a much longer period. Patients with severe bronchiolitis due to respiratory syncytial virus complicating repair of congenital heart disease on CPB typically require two to three weeks of ECMO support for respiratory failure.

For patients with structurally normal hearts who require ECMO support for respiratory illness, the ability to wean is dependent on resolution of the primary pulmonary process, often with little need for support of the myocardium beyond moderate inotropic support, fluid and electrolyte management, and nutritional support. Once lung compliance and gas exchange have normalized, improvement of the lungs on chest radiograph is apparent, and a stable circulation with sufficient negative fluid balance has been achieved, the patient is sedated, paralysed and fully ventilated and the ECMO circuit clamped.

Patients requiring cardiovascular support with ECMO are partially weaned within the first 48 hours in order to assess myocardial function by echocardiography and hemodynamic evaluation. An acceptable PaO_2 obtained while the ECMO circuit is clamped, will vary substantially according to the underlying anatomy and pathophysiology. If transthoracic cannulation was used and problems with bleeding were encountered during the ECMO run, the mediastinum may require exploration prior to or during the weaning process. If only a short period of reconditioning of the myocardium is anticipated, the patient is frequently sedated and paralysed, dopamine infusion is increased to 5–10 μg/kg per minute, intravascular volume status is optimized, and ventilator settings are adjusted according to lung compliance and expected arterial oxygen saturation. ECMO flow is decreased by 25–50% over a period of several hours until the circuit is clamped. Volume is infused to achieve appropriate preload. Echocardiographic assessment of ventricular systolic function, valvar function, systemic and pulmonary outflow obstruction, and location and direction of intracardiac shunts is useful prior to weaning, as well as if there is a change in hemodynamics after the circuit has been clamped. Arterial blood gases, serum lactate levels and systemic (mixed) venous saturation are important guides to the stability of the circulation, ventilation and adequacy of perfusion after the circuit has been clamped. Decannulation from ECMO is undertaken once the patient has maintained a stable circulation and acceptable gas exchange for a period of up to four hours.

Ventricular assist devices

The experience with VADs in children remains relatively small primarily due to technical considerations and concerns regarding suitability of children with congenital heart disease for univentricular support. In adults, VAD support is useful as a bridge to transplantation and allows for recovery of end-organ function, elimination of edema, improvement in nutrition and provides rehabilitation of critically ill patients. An important component of these benefits is the ability of the device to allow for ambulation which cannot be accomplished currently with ECMO and centrifugal VADs. The main problem in adapting the VAD devices used for adult patients are size limitations and flow requirements; the risk for thromboembolic complications increases with lower flow.

Of the reported VAD use in pediatric patients, most have been left ventricular support (LVAD), which has been particularly beneficial in patients with an ischemic myocardium secondary to an anomalous left coronary artery from the pulmonary artery, and for retraining the 'unprepared' left ventricle in patients with d-TGA and intact ventricular septum after an arterial switch procedure.[68] Survival reported to date is similar to that achieved with cardiac ECMO.

Ventricular assist devices have a number of advantages. The circuit is simple in design, takes less time to prime, and requires little technical assistance once established. It may more effectively decompress the LV and pulsatile flow is possible with some devices. Bleeding complications and platelet transfusion are often less in patients on VAD compared with ECMO. Because of the lower complications associated with VAD, patients may be supported for a longer period as a bridge to transplantation. While ECMO can be instituted via percutaneous cannulation, VAD requires cannulation through an open chest which is a major limitation to VAD in pediatric patients for short-term support, other than those post cardiotomy.

The primary indication for ventricular assist in pediatric patients are those with severe ventricular dysfunction and low cardiac output state, with the aim of supporting the circulation and reducing the load on the ventricle to allow recovery of myocardial function. As for ECMO after cardiac surgery, it is essential that primary technical failure of the procedure or residual defects be ruled out. In neonates and infants, isolated ventricular dysfunction is uncommon because of ventricular inter-dependence and problems with pulmonary hypertension. Univentricular support may therefore be ineffective.

Current ventricular assist devices can be classified as pulsatile or nonpulsatile. Nonpulsatile systems include either a centrifugal vortex pump or impella axial flow design. The Biomedicus centrifugal pump is the most commonly used nonpulsatile pump for pediatric patients, and while it is easier to prime, maintain and generally less heparin is required, it is only suitable for short-term use. Pulsatile support systems for children are under evaluation.[69,70] Pneumatically driven, they consist of a polyurethane housing with an integrated diaphragm which forms a continuous blood contact interior. The pediatric VAD incorporates polyurethane trileaflet valves with minimal pressure drop and low thrombotic risk in acute application. In the MEDOS-HIA ventricular support system, left ventricular devices are able to eject 10, 25, 60 and 80 ml stroke volumes. For right ventricular support the stroke volumes are reduced by 10% for each size, i.e. 9, 22.5, 54 and 72 ml. The electropneumatic drive unit is capable of operating two blood pumps independently, synchronously and asynchronously.

Intra-aortic balloon pump

Intra-aortic balloon pumps have been used with success in infants and children, although experience is limited.[71] Problems in pediatric patients include size constraints of the device and balloon, difficulty synchronizing the balloon inflation–deflation cycle with faster heart rates, and the increased elasticity of the aorta, which makes effective counterpulsation difficult.

PULMONARY HYPERTENSION

Mechanisms of pulmonary hypertension

Pulmonary hypertension can be defined as a mean pulmonary artery pressure greater than 25 mmHg after the first few weeks of life.[23] There are four basic mechanisms that underlie pulmonary hypertension:

- increased PVR
- increased pulmonary blood flow with normal PVR
- a combination of increased PVR and increased blood flow
- increased pulmonary venous pressure.

Elevated PVR can produce significant morbidity in several ways:

- by increasing the afterload or workload of the RV, it has the potential to cause RV dysfunction or failure and compromise cardiac output
- a sudden increase in PVR that leads to low cardiac output from RV failure is termed a pulmonary hypertensive crisis;[72] unless resolved quickly, such an episode can escalate to a life threatening event (e.g. cardiac arrest)
- in patients with anatomic communications between pulmonary and systemic circulations (e.g. atrial or ventricular septal defects), elevated PVR can generate a right to left shunt and cause severe hypoxemia.

The resistance to blood flow through the lungs is primarily due to the anatomy of small lung blood vessels (i.e. their diameter, number and length), but it is also affected by blood viscosity. The diameter of these vessels is determined by the quantity and tone (degree of constriction) of smooth muscle cells in their walls, and by the presence of any abnormal anatomic changes that create narrowing of the vessel lumen. In the first 24–48 hours of life, PVR is often labile because of ongoing changes in the vasculature accompanying the transition from fetal life (high PVR) to extrauterine life (low PVR), including closure of the ductus arteriosus.[73] For this reason, major reparative or palliative surgeries that require CPB are generally avoided within hours of birth, unless necessary to save the patient's life. After three to four weeks of age, the tone of small lung vessels in infants with no cardiac or pulmonary disease is ordinarily low, such that the PVR is only approximately 20% of the SVR. Much of this fall in PVR is due to vascular remodeling, with a reduction in the amount of smooth muscle in the walls of small lung vessels.[74,75] It is during this period of falling PVR that infants with a large VSD or PDA typically develop signs and symptoms of congestive heart failure from increasing Q_p/Q_s. These patients thus have pulmonary hypertension from increased pulmonary blood flow that is near or at systemic blood pressure in the setting of normal PVR.

Children with many forms of congenital heart disease are prone to develop perioperative elevations in PVR.[20,21] This may complicate the postoperative course, when transient myocardial dysfunction requires optimal control of right ventricular afterload.[72,76–78] Treatment strategies should focus on the underlying etiology, and should be continually re-evaluated not only from the stand point of the absolute PA pressure, but also the overall circulation and systemic perfusion. Rather than treat a specific or target PA pressure, the relationship of the PA pressure to the systemic artery pressure, along with the function of the right ventricle are critical.

Postoperative pulmonary vascular reactivity has been related not only to the presence of preoperative pulmonary hypertension and left to right shunts[20,77,79] but also to the duration of total CPB.[80,81] Treatment of postoperative pulmonary hypertensive crises has been partially addressed by surgery at a younger age, pharmacologic intervention and other postoperative management strategies. However, recent developments in vascular biology have offered new insights into the possible causes and correction of post-CPB pulmonary hypertension.

Several factors peculiar to CPB may raise PVR. CPB produces a generalized endothelial injury that includes the pulmonary vasculature and can generate a transient elevation in PVR. Structural damage to the pulmonary endothelium is demonstrable after CPB, and the degree of pulmonary hypertension is correlated with the extent of endothelial damage after CPB and inability to release nitric oxide. Transient pulmonary vascular endothelial cell dysfunction has been demonstrated in neonates and older children by documenting the transient loss of endothelium dependent vasodilation immediately after cardiopulmonary bypass.[64,82] Microemboli, pulmonary leukosequestration, excess thromboxane production, atelectasis, hypoxic pulmonary vasoconstriction and adrenergic events have also been suggested to play a role in postoperative pulmonary hypertension.[78,83] Over recent years, numerous strategies have evolved to limit the effect of this endothelial injury resulting from the systemic inflammatory response. Hemofiltration has become a technique commonly used to hemoconcentrate, and possibly remove inflammatory mediators including complement, endotoxin, and cytokines.[84,85] Reports indicate an improvement in systolic and diastolic pressure during filtration, and improved pulmonary function has also been noted with reduction in pulmonary vascular resistance and total lung water.[86,87] The duration of postoperative mechanical ventilation, and CICU and hospital stay has also been demonstrated to be reduced.[84,88] Commonly used hemofiltration techniques include 'modified ultrafiltration' whereby the patient's blood volume is filtered after completion of bypass,[88] 'conventional hemofiltration' whereby both the patient and circuit are filtered during rewarming on bypass, and more recently described 'zero-balance ultrafiltration' in which high volume ultrafiltration essentially washes the patient and circuit blood volumes during the rewarming process.[85] Although there is currently no prophylactic or therapeutic treatment that is specific for this multi-factorial and complex injury, clinical trials of investigational agents designed to reduce ischemia/reperfusion injury by inhibiting leukocyte–endothelial adhesion interactions or oxygen free radical production are ongoing.[89,90] Postoperatively, the most effective strategy to treat an elevated PVR secondary to the effects of CPB includes attenuation of the neuroendocrine stress response, maintaining a normal to alkalotic pH during mechanical ventilation, and optimizing cardiac output and RV function. Once the circulation, mechanical ventilation and gas exchange have all been optimized, it is important to be observant and wait until myocardial function and cardiac output improve sufficiently to establish and maintain a diuresis. This may not develop until the second or third postoperative day. As endothelial function recovers and lung water decreases, the PA pressure will usually start to fall. Nitric oxide may be of benefit to treat an increase in PVR following CPB, particularly if the PA pressure is greater than 25 mmHg and there are concerns for RV function. However, in our experience the response to nitric oxide for this indication is variable.

In some circumstances, an increase in PA pressure and PVR is relatively fixed because of distal pulmonary artery stenoses or hypoplasia; provided the right ventricle is functioning normally at this pressure and cardiac output is maintained, no additional intervention is necessary in the immediate postoperative period. For example, a patient with tetralogy of Fallot and pulmonary atresia with small distal pulmonary arteries who has undergone complete repair, may have an elevated and relatively fixed proximal or main PA pressure measured between 50% and 75% of systemic pressure because of a reduced total surface area or arborization of the pulmonary vascular bed. A fenestrated VSD patch or small ASD is sometimes left after this surgery to provide a 'pop-off' to the systemic circulation; the patient will be cyanosed but cardiac output maintained. Significant RV hypertrophy is common in patients who have proximal or distal branch pulmonary artery stenoses. Provided RV coronary perfusion has not been compromised during CPB, and an important coronary artery has not been damaged at the time of reconstruction of the RV outflow tract, systolic RV function is often well preserved in the immediate postoperative period, and a persistent increase in PA pressure is well tolerated. In some circumstances, the hypertrophied RV is hyperdynamic, and may contribute to a dynamic RV outflow gradient. On the other hand, signs of right ventricle restrictive physiology or diastolic dysfunction must be closely assessed (see later).

If patients who have a large, high-pressure left to right shunt are not surgically repaired or palliated in the first months or years of life, they are at significant risk of developing progressive, irreversible anatomic changes in their lung vasculature resulting in pulmonary vascular obstructive disease. These pathologic vascular changes have been described and graded by Heath and Edwards.[21] In addition to a large VSD (or multiple VSDs) and a large PDA, the other lesions commonly associated with pulmonary vascular obstructive disease are complete common atrioventricular canal defect (especially in patients with trisomy 21), truncus arteriosus, d-TGA with a large VSD, and specific types of single ventricle defects with no obstruction to pulmonary blood flow. The physiologic result of this diffuse vascular obstruction is pulmonary hypertension; when advanced, pulmonary vascular obstructive disease can cause right to left shunting (i.e. shunt flow reversal) and hypoxemia. These patients have progressed from an initial state of high pressure, high volume pulmonary blood flow with normal PVR, through an intermediate state of high pressure, high volume pulmonary blood flow with elevated PVR, to an irreversible, pathologic state of high pressure, reduced volume pulmonary blood flow with high PVR. Surgical repair of the cardiac defect(s) in patients with hypoxemia and high PVR often does not improve the patient's pulmonary hypertension and is associated with a high perioperative mortality rate.[91]

Pulmonary hypertension also occurs in pediatric cardiac patients who have elevated pulmonary venous pressure. This mechanism of pulmonary hypertension occurs in newborns with pulmonary venous obstruction (e.g. total anomalous pulmonary venous connection (TAPVC) with obstruction) or atrioventricular valve atresia in the pulmonary venous atrium *plus* an intact atrial septum (e.g. single ventricle with mitral atresia and intact atrial septum). Urgent decompression of the hypertensive pulmonary veins or pulmonary venous atrium is required for survival in these patients. Following decompression, pulmonary artery pressures typically begin falling within hours to a few days, because the pulmonary hypertension is due, at least in part, to discrete mechanical obstruction as opposed to a diffuse increase in vascular smooth muscle.[72] Older pediatric patients who have pulmonary hypertension because of a left sided obstructive lesion such as mitral valve stenosis, also tend to resolve their pulmonary hypertension with relief of the obstruction, although resolution can be delayed.

Treatment of elevated PVR

The intensity of treatment that is appropriate for a patient with elevated PVR depends upon several factors, including the patient's diagnosis, degree of cardiac and respiratory

Table 5.13 *Strategies to treat pulmonary hypertension*

Acute		
Reduce SNS stimulation	Increase depth of analgesia and sedation	
	Consider paralysis with nondepolarizing neuromuscular blocking drugs	
	Treat hypo- and hyperthermia	
	Low doses of vasoconstrictive agents if possible	
Lower pulmonary vascular resistance		
Gas exchange	Increased alveolar oxygen tension	
	Alkalosis/treat acidosis (metabolic or respiratory)	
	Hypocapnia	
Mechanical ventilation	Maintain FRC	
	Avoid hypo- or hyperinflation	
	Low mean intrathoracic pressure	
Vasodilating drugs		
Specific		Nitric oxide
Nonspecific	cGMP system	Nitroprusside
		Glycerol trinitrate
	cAMP system	PDE3 inhibitors
		Isoproterenol
		Prostacyclin I_2
		Prostaglandin E1
Chronic	Support RV function: diuretics and digoxin	
	Calcium channel blocking drugs	
	Chronic inhaled NO	
	Prostacyclin I_2 infusion	
	Phosphodiesterase type 5 inhibitor	
	Endothelin receptor blocking drugs	

SNS = sympathetic nervous system; FRC = functional residual capacity; NO = nitric oxide.

dysfunction, magnitude of elevation in PVR, likelihood of response to therapy, and prognosis. For example, a pulmonary artery pressure of 40/25 mmHg in a stable neonate with a systemic blood pressure of 70/45 mmHg who just underwent repair of obstructed TAPVC does not require aggressive treatment, because pulmonary hypertension in these patients early after repair is expected, is typically short-lived, and is unlikely to cause significant morbidity at this moderate level.[92] However, if this patient were hemodynamically unstable on large doses of intravenous inotropic agents and had a pulmonary artery pressure at or near systemic blood pressure, more aggressive maneuvers to reduce PVR would be appropriate. Treatment options for acute and chronic pulmonary hypertension are shown in Table 5.13.

In patients who have either normal or elevated PVR (except in cases where PVR is elevated and fixed), several factors will affect vascular smooth muscle tone and can therefore alter PVR. Among these factors, it is important to recognize those that can be manipulated in the ICU, because interventions to reduce PVR may improve patient recovery. Pain control with a fentanyl infusion and sedation with a short-acting (e.g. midazolam) or long-acting (e.g. lorazepam) benzodiazepine have been associated with reduced and less labile PVR in the postoperative period.[36] Attention to adequate analgesia and sedation for stressful or invasive procedures such as endotracheal tube suctioning is particularly important for minimizing acute increases in PVR. Because the pulmonary arteries constrict with alveolar hypoxia, avoiding low alveolar PO_2, for example by administering supplemental oxygen and/or manipulating the ventilator in mechanically ventilated patients to increase the alveolar oxygen tension, can decrease PVR.[93,94] Acidosis also causes pulmonary vasoconstriction, whereas alkalosis produces pulmonary vasodilation.[93] Based upon experimental studies, it appears that serum pH itself (as opposed to the $PaCO_2$) is the predominant factor influencing vascular tone, because generating an alkalosis by infusing a base solution (e.g. $NaHCO_3$) is as effective in lowering PVR as decreasing $PaCO_2$ to produce a respiratory alkalosis.[95,96] In practice, this finding translates into close monitoring of the arterial blood gas (ABG) and avoidance of low serum pH. The degree of lung inflation significantly impacts PVR, with PVR at a minimum when the lung is inflated at FRC. Parenchymal lung diseases, such as pneumonia, and restrictive airways disease can also increase PVR. Specific attention to the appearance of lung volumes and parenchymal abnormalities on the chest radiograph, chest physical examination findings, bedside pulmonary mechanics (e.g. tidal volumes, minute ventilation, and mean airway pressure), and ABG values should allow detection and guide treatment of these problems.

Several intravenous vasodilators, including the nitric oxide donors nitroprusside and glycerol trinitrate, the phosphodiesterase inhibitors amrinone and milrinone, the eicosanoids prostaglandins E1 and prostacyclin I_2, tolazoline and isoproterenol have been used to treat postoperative patients with elevated PVR. The chief limitation with these pharmacologic agents is that their vasodilatory effects are not specific to the pulmonary vasculature, so that vasodilation of the systemic vasculature and systemic hypotension may accompany reduction of pulmonary hypertension.

The agent with the most selectivity for vasodilating the pulmonary vasculature is the gas nitric oxide. When inhaled through a mechanical ventilator at concentrations of 80 parts per million (ppm), nitric oxide can relax constricted smooth muscle cells in small pulmonary vessels and lower PVR.[97] The selective effect of inhaled nitric oxide on the pulmonary vasculature is due to rapid uptake and inactivation by hemoglobin as nitric oxide diffuses from alveoli to the lumen of lung capillaries. The usefulness of inhaled nitric oxide for congenital heart disease patients with pulmonary hypertension has been documented in several populations.[98] Following surgery, nitric oxide reduces pulmonary hypertension in patients with obstructed TAPVC, mitral stenosis, large, pre-existing left to right shunts, and pulmonary hypertensive crises related to CPB. Nitric oxide has also improved both pulmonary hypertension and impaired gas exchange in patients who have undergone lung transplantation. Patients with a variety of other pulmonary vascular or parenchymal diseases, including persistent pulmonary hypertension of the newborn[99,100] acute respiratory distress syndrome[101] and acute chest syndrome in sickle cell disease[102] have also shown significant improvements in oxygenation from treatment with inhaled nitric oxide.

The continuous variables used to monitor the response to nitric oxide should be clearly defined. Clinical signs that could indicate a response to nitric oxide resulting in a fall in PA pressure and PVR, include an increase in peripheral oxygen saturation, fall in heart rate and improved systemic perfusion, and improvement in respiratory symptoms such as wheezing and tachypnea. The response to nitric oxide can also be assessed by direct PA pressure measurement if a catheter is in situ, and by echocardiographic findings such as change in flow across a PDA or ASD, the amount of tricuspid and pulmonary valve regurgitation, the flow pattern across the pulmonary veins and the function of the RV.

Despite the potential response in the circumstances outlined above, nitric oxide should not be used indiscriminately. For example, patients with a fixed increase in PVR because of anatomic or structural abnormalities to the pulmonary vasculature, rarely demonstrate a response. Nitric oxide has been reported to lower the trans-pulmonary gradient following the Fontan procedure,[103] but in our experience, the response is variable and often not clinically significant. Similarly, in patients with a superior vena cava–pulmonary artery connection (bidirectional Glenn procedure), it is uncommon to demonstrate a response to nitric oxide in the immediate postoperative period. Elevated PVR should be an uncommon clinical finding after this type of surgery; particularly as a low PVR (ideally less than 2 Woods units) is a selection criterion for surgery. Even those patients in the 'high risk' group with a PVR of more than 3 Woods units, usually do not have a PA pressure high enough in the immediate postoperative period (i.e. greater than 25 mmHg) to demonstrate an appreciable benefit from nitric oxide. If there is coexisting parenchymal lung disease, however, and the patients are more hypoxemic than expected (i.e. PaO_2 less than 30–35 mmHg), nitric oxide may be effective by improving ventilation/perfusion matching. Caution should be exercised when administering nitric oxide to patients with left ventricular outflow obstruction, such as preoperative obstructed TAPVR, mitral stenosis or critical aortic stenosis in the newborn, and to any patient with severe left ventricular dysfunction and pulmonary hypertension. Sudden pulmonary vasodilation may occasionally unload the right ventricle sufficiently to increase pulmonary blood flow and harmfully augment preload in a compromised left ventricle.[104,105] The attendant rise in left atrial pressure may produce pulmonary edema.[106]

If the underlying pulmonary hypertensive process has not resolved, then the tendency for an abrupt increase in pulmonary artery pressure may be hazardous when nitric oxide therapy is withdrawn or interrupted.[92,107,108] The other concerns for use of inhaled nitric oxide include the generation of methemoglobin following the reaction of nitric oxide with hemoglobin, and the generation of nitrogen dioxide when nitric oxide and oxygen combine. These levels must be closely monitored during therapy, particularly at high inspired oxygen concentrations.

Chronic pulmonary hypertension

Additional strategies for managing pulmonary hypertension in the immediate postoperative period, and in particular longer-term management are currently being investigated. It is important to support the right ventricle when the afterload is increased, and diuretics and digoxin may be beneficial. Longer-term inhaled nitric oxide for ambulatory therapy of pulmonary hypertension is possible with nitric oxide delivered via nasal cannulas,[109] although the dose of nitric oxide delivered in this fashion is imprecise. Because of the variable dose and risk for dislodging nasal cannulas, it is important patients receiving chronic nitric oxide therapy in this fashion do not demonstrate symptoms or signs of an acute rebound or increase in PVR when nitric oxide is suddenly discontinued. A long-term continuous infusion of prostacyclin, a potent vasodilator and antiproliferative agent, has been demonstrated to improve exercise tolerance in patients with chronic pulmonary hypertension,[110] although its utility in pediatric patients with persistent elevation of PVR after cardiac surgery has not been established. The phospodiesterase V enzyme is responsible for cyclic GMP hydrolysis in the pulmonary vasculature. A selective inhibitor, sildenafil, has been demonstrated to effectively attenuate pulmonary hypertension rebound after acute withdrawal of nitric oxide,[111] and is currently under investigation for longer-term treatment for pulmonary hypertension. Some patients may respond to a calcium channel blocking drug, such as verapamil,[112] although the use should be restricted to patients who have previously demonstrated reactivity of their pulmonary vasculature to either nitric oxide or oxygen, and preferably a dose-response should be established with a pulmonary artery catheter in situ. Endothelin (ET) may play a role in intimal proliferation and vasoconstriction, and circulating endothelin is increased in patients with primary pulmonary hypertension.[113] Bosentan, an ETA/ETB receptor antagonist, has been demonstrated to improve exercise capacity; the indications and utility in postoperative pediatric patients has not been established.[114]

AIRWAY AND VENTILATION MANAGEMENT

Altered respiratory mechanics and positive pressure ventilation may have a significant influence on hemodynamics following congenital heart surgery. Therefore, the approach to mechanical ventilation should not only be directed at achieving a desired gas exchange, but also be influenced by the potential cardiorespiratory interactions of mechanical ventilation and method of weaning.

Endotracheal tube

The narrowest part of the airway before puberty is below the vocal cords at the level of the cricoid cartilage, and the use of uncuffed endotracheal tubes (ETT) has been generally recommended. While a leak around the tubes at an inflation pressure of approximately 20 cmH_2O is desirable, a significant air leak may have a detrimental effect on mechanical ventilation and delivery of a consistent ventilation pattern. Examples include patients with extensive chest and abdominal wall edema following CPB and patients with labile PVR and increased Q_p/Q_s. If a significant air leak exists, lung volume, and in particular FRC, will not be maintained and fluctuations in gas exchange can occur. During the weaning process, a significant leak will also increase the work of breathing for some neonates and infants. In these situations, it is therefore preferable to change the endotracheal tubes to a larger size or to use a cuffed tube. An alternative strategy is to place a cuffed tube at the time of initial intubation, but leave the cuff deflated unless a significant leak becomes problematic. If the cuff is inflated the pressure and volume of air in the cuff must be checked regularly. We prefer to use a nasal approach to place the tubes rather than oral. The tube is easier to secure to the bridge of the nose, and less likely to move in the trachea and therefore perhaps less likely to cause irritation, inflammation and stenosis. Infants and small children generally find the nasal tube more comfortable and causes less gagging and irritability during the weaning process.

In certain circumstances, a smaller than expected endotracheal tube may be necessary. This is particularly the case in patients with other congenital defects such as Down's syndrome (trisomy 21). Tracheal stenosis may also occur in association with some congenital cardiac defects such as a pulmonary artery sling. Extrinsic compression of the bronchi may occur secondary to pulmonary artery and left atrial dilation. This may be suspected by persistent hyperinflation or lobar atelectasis.

Cardiorespiratory interactions

Cardiorespiratory interactions vary significantly between patients, and it is not possible to provide specific ventilation strategies or protocols that are appropriate for all patients. Rather, the mode of ventilation must be matched to the hemodynamic status of each patient to achieve the adequate cardiac output and gas exchange. Frequent modifications to the mode and pattern of ventilation may be necessary during recovery after surgery, with attention to changes in lung volume and airway pressure. Changes in lung volume have a major effect on PVR, which is lowest at FRC, while both hypoinflation or hyperinflation may result in a significant increase in PVR because of altered traction on alveolar septae and extra-alveolar vessels.[115]

Positive pressure ventilation influences preload and afterload on the heart (Table 5.14). An increase in lung volume and intrathoracic pressure decreases preload to both the right and left atria. The afterload on the pulmonary ventricle is increased during a positive pressure breath secondary to the changes in lung volume and increase in mean intrathoracic pressure. If this is significant or there is limited functional reserve, RV stroke volume may be reduced and end-diastolic pressure increased. This in turn may contribute to a low cardiac output state and signs of RV dysfunction including tricuspid regurgitation, hepatomegaly, ascites, and pleural effusions. In contrast to the RV, the afterload on the systemic ventricle is decreased during a positive pressure breath

Table 5.14 *The cardiorespiratory interactions of a positive pressure mechanical breath*

	Afterload	Preload
Pulmonary ventricle	*Elevated* Increase RVEDp Increase RVp Decrease antegrade PBF Increase PR and/or TR	*Reduced* Decreased RVEDV Decreased RAp
Systemic ventricle	*Reduced* Decrease LVEDp Decrease Lap Decrease pulmonary edema Increase cardiac output	*Reduced* Decrease LVEDV Decrease Lap

RVEDp = right ventricle end diastolic pressure; RVp = right ventricle pressure; RVEDV = right ventricle end diastolic volume; PBF = pulmonary blood flow; PR = pulmonary regurgitation; TR = tricuspid regurgitation; LVEDp = left ventricle end diastolic pressure; LVEDV = left ventricle end diastolic volume; Lap = left atrial pressure; Rap = right atrial pressure.

secondary to a fall in the ventricle transmural pressure. The systemic arteries are under higher pressure and not exposed to radial traction effects during inflation or deflation of the lungs. Therefore, changes in lung volume will affect LV preload, but the effect on afterload is dependent upon changes in intrathoracic pressure alone rather than changes in lung volume. Positive pressure ventilation and positive end-expiratory pressure (PEEP) therefore has a significant beneficial effect in patients with left ventricular failure.

Patients with LV dysfunction and increased end-diastolic volume and pressure can have impaired pulmonary mechanics secondary to increased lung water, decreased lung compliance and increased airway resistance. The work of breathing is increased and neonates can fatigue early because of limited respiratory reserve. A significant proportion of total body oxygen consumption is directed at the increased work of breathing in neonates and infants with LV dysfunction, contributing to poor feeding and failure to thrive. Therefore, positive pressure ventilation has an additional benefit in patients with significant volume overload and systemic ventricular dysfunction by reducing the work of breathing and oxygen demand.

Weaning from positive pressure ventilation may be difficult in patients with persistent systemic ventricular dysfunction. As spontaneous ventilation increases during the weaning process, changes in mean intra-thoracic pressure may substantially alter afterload on the systemic ventricle. Once extubated, the subatmospheric intra-pleural pressure generated means that the transmural pressure across the systemic ventricle is increased. This sudden increase in wall stress may contribute to an increase in end-diastolic pressure and volume, leading to pulmonary edema and a low output state. It may be difficult to determine which patients are likely to fail extubation because of ventricular failure; even a small amount of positive pressure as used during continuous positive airway pressure (CPAP) or pressure support modes of ventilation may be sufficient to reduce afterload and myocardial work. Inotropic agents, vasodilators and diuretics should be continued throughout the weaning process and following extubation to maintain stable ventricular function in these patients.

The use of PEEP in patients with congenital heart disease has been controversial. It was initially perceived not to have a significant positive impact on gas exchange, and there was concern that the increased airway pressure could have a detrimental effect on hemodynamics and contribute to lung injury and air leak. Nevertheless, PEEP increases FRC, enabling lung recruitment, and redistributes lung water from alveolar septal regions to the more compliant peri-hilar regions. Both of these actions will improve gas exchange and reduce PVR. PEEP should, therefore, be used in all mechanically ventilated patients following congenital heart surgery. However, excessive levels of PEEP can be detrimental by increasing afterload on the RV. Usually 3–5 cmH_2O of PEEP will help to maintain FRC and redistribute lung water without causing hemodynamic compromise.

Postoperative hypoxemia

Based on a thorough understanding of the anatomy and surgical procedure, the range of acceptable postoperative oxygen tensions should be anticipated for a particular defect. A patient who has undergone a complete two-ventricle repair should have an arterial oxygen saturation more than 95% following surgery. A lower than expected saturation in this circumstance usually reflects pulmonary venous desaturation secondary to intrapulmonary shunting or venous admixture.

Following certain procedures, patients may benefit from strategies that allow right to left shunting at the atrial level in the face of postoperative right ventricular diastolic dysfunction, i.e. elevated end-diastolic pressure. In this circumstance, an arterial saturation in the 75–85% range might be expected in the immediate postoperative period. As ventricular compliance improves or pulmonary vascular resistance decreases, the amount of shunting at the atrial level should decrease and arterial oxygen saturation increase. This particularly applies to neonates who undergo a right ventriculotomy to repair tetralogy of Fallot and truncus arteriosus, patients who may have elevated RV afterload because of postoperative pulmonary artery hypertension, and in neonates who may have a small tricuspid valve and a noncompliant RV following repair, such as following the arterial switch procedure and aortic arch reconstruction in newborns with transposition of the great arteries and interrupted aortic arch.

The concept of leaving a small atrial level communication has been extended to older patients with single ventricle physiology undergoing the modified Fontan operation. If an atrial septal communication or fenestration is left at the time of the Fontan procedure, the resulting right to left shunt helps to preserve cardiac output. These children have fewer postoperative complications.[116] It is better to shunt blood right to left, accept some decrement in oxygen saturation but maintain ventricular filling and cardiac output, than to have high oxygen saturation but low blood pressure and cardiac output.

Following procedures in which mixing of pulmonary and systemic blood remains, the arterial oxygen tension should be 35–45 mmHg and saturation in the 75–85% range. If the SaO_2 is lower than anticipated, there are a number of important causes which must be evaluated (Table 5.15). These include:

- a reduction in effective pulmonary blood flow, such as from pulmonary ventricle outflow tract obstruction or increased pulmonary artery resistance, an intra-cardiac right to left shunt across an ASD or VSD, or a decompressing vessel from the pulmonary artery to pulmonary vein
- a reduction in pulmonary venous oxygen saturation from an intrapulmonary shunt
- a reduction in mixed venous oxygen saturation, such as from reduced oxygen delivery secondary to a low cardiac output state or low hematocrit, or increased oxygen extraction in a febrile or hyper-metabolic state following surgery.

Table 5.15 *Factors contributing to a lower than anticipated oxygen saturation in patients with common mixing lesions*

Etiology	Considerations
Low FiO_2	Low dialed oxygen concentration Failure of oxygen delivery device
Pulmonary vein desaturation	Impaired diffusion Alveolar process: e.g. edema/infectious Restrictive process: e.g. effusion/atelectasis Intra-pulmonary shunt RDS Pulmonary AVM PA to PV collateral vessel(s)
Reduced pulmonary blood flow	Anatomic RV outflow obstruction Anatomic pulmonary artery stenosis Increased PVR Atrial level right to left shunt Ventricular level right to left shunt
Low dissolved oxygen content	Low mixed venous oxygen level Increased O_2 extraction: hypermetabolic state Decreased O_2 delivery: low cardiac output state Anemia

FiO_2 = fractional inspired concentration of oxygen; RDS = respiratory distress syndrome; PA = pulmonary artery; AVM = arteriovenous malformation; PV = pulmonary vein; RV = right ventricle; PVR = pulmonary vascular resistance; VSD = ventricular septal defect.

Table 5.16 *Factors contributing to the inability to wean from mechanical ventilation after congenital heart surgery*

Residual cardiac defects
- volume and/or pressure overload
- myocardial dysfunction
- arrhythmias

Restrictive pulmonary defects
- pulmonary edema
- pleural effusion
- atelectasis
- chest wall edema
- phrenic nerve injury
- ascites/hepatomegaly

Airway
- subglottic edema and/or stenosis
- retained secretions
- vocal cord injury
- extrinsic bronchial compression
- tracheo-bronchomalacia

Metabolic
- inadequate nutrition
- diuretic therapy
- sepsis
- stress response

Weaning from mechanical ventilation

Weaning from mechanical ventilation is a dynamic process that requires continued re-evaluation. While most patients following congenital cardiac surgery who have had no complications with repair or CPB will wean without difficulty, some patients with borderline cardiac function and residual defects may require prolonged mechanical ventilation and a slow weaning process.

The method of weaning varies between patients. Most patients can be weaned using either a volume- or pressure-limited mode by simply decreasing the IMV rate. Guided by physical examination, hemodynamic criteria, respiratory pattern and arterial blood gas measurements, the mechanical ventilator rate is gradually reduced. Patients with limited hemodynamic and respiratory reserve may demonstrate tachypnea, diaphoresis and shallow tidal volumes as they struggle to breathe spontaneously against the resistance of the endotracheal tube. The addition of pressure or flow triggered pressure support 10–15 cmH_2O above PEEP is often beneficial in reducing the work of breathing.

Numerous factors contribute to the inability to wean from mechanical ventilation following congenital heart surgery (Table 5.16). As a general rule, however, residual defects following surgery causing either a volume or pressure load must be excluded first by echocardiography or cardiac catheterization.

Pulmonary edema, pleural effusions and persistent atelectasis may delay weaning from mechanical ventilation. Residual chest and abdominal wall edema, ascites and hepatomegaly limit chest wall compliance and diaphragmatic excursion. Chest tubes and peritoneal catheters may be necessary to drain pleural effusions and ascites, respectively.

If atelectasis persists, bronchoscopy is often useful to remove secretions and to diagnose extrinsic compression from enlarged pulmonary arteries, a dilated left atrium or conduits. Upper airway obstruction from vocal cord injury (e.g. recurrent laryngeal nerve damage during aortic arch reconstruction), edema or bronchomalacia can also be evaluated.

Phrenic nerve injury can occur during cardiac surgery, either secondary to traction, thermal injury from electrocautery or direct transection as a complication of extensive aortic arch and pulmonary hilar disection, particularly for repeat operations. Diaphragmatic paresis (no motion) or paralysis (paradoxical motion), should be investigated in any patient who fails to wean.[117] Increased work of breathing on low ventilator settings, increased $PaCO_2$ and an elevated hemidiaphragm on chest radiograph are suggestive of diaphragmatic dysfunction. Ultrasonography or fluoroscopy is useful for identifying abnormal diaphragmatic movement.

Fluid restriction and aggressive diuretic therapy can result in metabolic disturbances and limit nutritional intake. A hypochloremic, hypokalemic metabolic alkalosis with secondary respiratory acidosis is a common complication from high dose diuretic use and can delay the ventilator weaning process. Diuretic therapy should be continually re-evaluated based on fluid balance, daily weight (if possible), clinical examination and measurement of electrolyte levels and blood urea nitrogen.

Chloride and potassium supplementation is essential to correct the metabolic alkalosis.

It is essential to maintain adequate nutrition, particularly as patients will be catabolic early following cardiac surgery and may have a limited reserve secondary to preoperative failure to thrive. Fluid restriction may limit parenteral nutrition, and enteral nutrition may be poorly tolerated from splanchnic hypoperfusion secondary to low cardiac output or diastolic pressure.

Sepsis is a frequent cause for failure to wean from mechanical ventilation in the ICU. Invasive monitoring catheters are a common source for blood infections. Beside blood culture surveillance and antibiotics, removing or replacing central venous and arterial catheters should be considered as soon as possible during an episode of suspected or culture proven sepsis.

The signs of sepsis may be subtle and nonspecific, and often broad spectrum intravenous (i.v.) antibiotic covereage is started before culture results are known. Signs to note in neonates and infants include temperature instability (hyper- or hypothermia), hypoglycemia, unexplained metabolic acidosis, hypotension and tachycardia with poor extremity perfusion and oliguria, increased respiratory effort and ventilation requirements, altered conscious state and leukocytosis with left shift on blood count.

Colonization of the airway occurs frequently in patients mechanically ventilated for an extended period, but may not require intravenous antibiotic therapy unless there is evidence of increased secretions with fever, leukocytosis, new chest radiograph abnormalities or detection of an organism on Gram stain together with abundant neutrophils. Urinary tract infection and both superficial and deep surgical site infections must also be excluded in patients with clinical suspicion of sepsis (i.e. sternotomy or thoracotomy wounds).

FLUID MANAGEMENT

Because of the inflammatory response to bypass and significant increase in total body water, fluid management in the immediate postoperative period is critical. Capillary leak and interstitial fluid accumulation may continue for the first 24–48 hours following surgery, necessitating ongoing volume replacement with colloid or blood products. A fall in cardiac output and increased antidiuretic hormone secretion contribute to delayed water clearance and potential pre-renal dysfunction, which could progress to acute tubular necrosis and renal failure if a low cardiac output state persists.

During bypass, optimizing the circuit prime hematocrit and oncotic pressure, attenuating the inflammatory response with steroids and protease inhibitors such as aprotinin, and the use of modified ultrafiltration techniques have all been recommended to limit interstitial fluid accumulation.[85,88,118] During the first 24 hours following surgery, maintenance fluids should be restricted to 50% of full maintenance, and volume replacement titrated to appropriate filling pressures and hemodynamic response.

Oliguria in the first 24 hours after complex surgery and CPB is common in neonates and infants until cardiac output recovers. While diuretics are commonly prescribed in the immediate postoperative period, cardiac output must also be enhanced with volume replacement and vasoactive drug infusions for these to be effective.

Furosemide 1–2 mg/kg intravenous eight-hourly is a commonly prescribed loop diuretic, but needs to be excreted into the tubular system before producing diuresis (ascending limb of Henle). Low cardiac output therefore reduces its efficacy. Bolus dosing may result in a significant diuresis over a short period, thereby causing changes in intravascular volume and possibly hypotension. A continuous infusion of 0.2–0.3 mg/kg per hour after initial bolus of 1 mg/kg often provides a consistent and sustained diuresis without sudden fluid shifts. Chlorothiazide 10 mg/kg intravenous or peroral 12 hourly is also an effective diuretic, particularly when used in conjunction with loop diuretics.

Peritoneal dialysis, hemodialysis and continuous venovenous hemofiltration provide alternate renal support in patients with persistent oliguria and renal failure.[119,120] Besides enabling water and solute clearance, maintenance fluids can be increased to ensure adequate nutrition. The indications for renal support vary, but include blood urea nitrogen greater than 100 mg/dl, life threatening electrolyte imbalance such as severe hyperkalemia, ongoing metabolic acidosis, fluid restrictions limiting nutrition, and increased mechanical ventilation requirements secondary to persistent pulmonary edema or ascites.

A peritoneal dialysis catheter may be placed into the peritoneal cavity at the completion of surgery or later in the ICU. Indications in the ICU include the need for renal support or to reduce intra-abdominal pressure from ascites that may be compromising mechanical ventilation. Drainage may be significant in the immediate postoperative period as third space fluid losses continue, and replacement with albumin and/or fresh frozen plasma may be necessary to treat hypovolemia and hypoproteinemia.

To enhance fluid excretion if oliguria persists, 'mini-volume dialysis' may be effective using 10 ml/kg of 1.5% or 2.25% dialysate over a 30–40 minute cycle. A persistent communication between the peritoneum, mediastinum and/or pleural cavities following surgery will limit the effectiveness of peritoneal dialysis and is a relative contraindication.

Arteriovenous hemofiltration or hemodialysis through double lumen femoral or subclavian vein catheters can be used effectively in neonates. Complications related to venous access, thrombosis and hemodynamic instability are potential complications that require close monitoring.

GASTROINTESTINAL PROBLEMS

Splanchnic hypoperfusion may be secondary to low cardiac output from ventricular dysfunction, or from low diastolic pressure in patients with systemic to pulmonary artery runoff. It often manifests as a persistent ileus or feed intolerance; gut ischemia or necrotizing enterocolitis (NEC) may also develop.

Besides splanchnic hypoperfusion, other causes of feeding intolerance include bowel edema following CPB, delayed gastric emptying secondary to opioids, gastroesophageal reflux, and small bowel obstruction secondary to malrotation, which is common with heterotaxy syndrome. Patients with limited ventricular function may be unable to increase their cardiac output sufficiently to meet the metabolic demand associated with oral feeding and the absorption of food. Coexisting problems such as tachypnea also restrict oral intake. To ensure adequate nutrition in these situations, placement of a transpyloric feeding tube should be considered.

As in adult ICUs, stress ulceration and gastritis occur in pediatric patients. Prophylaxis with H_2 receptor blocking drugs and/or antacids should be used in any patient requiring protracted hemodynamic and respiratory support. Early resumption of enteral nutrition is encouraged to reduce the risk of nosocomial pulmonary infection by preventing bacterial overgrowth.

Congenital heart disease may be an important predisposing factor to developing necrotizing enterocolitis. Cardiac defects with the potential for significant runoff from the systemic to pulmonary circulation, specifically hypoplastic left heart syndrome, aortopulmonary window, truncus arteriosis, and patients who had episodes of poor systemic perfusion, are more likely to develop NEC.[121] This supports the notion that one of the principal underlying mechanisms of NEC in patients with congenital heart disease is mesenteric ischemia. Of note, the feeding history or the type of feed, the use of indwelling umbilical catheters and cardiac catheterization has not correlated with the incidence of NEC.

Clinical signs of NEC include abdominal distention, feed intolerance, temperature and glucose instability, heme-positive or frank blood in the stool, abdominal guarding and tenderness. Abdominal radiography may demonstrate distention or an abnormal gas pattern, pneumatosis, portal air or intraperitoneal air consistent with perforation. Thrombocytopenia and leukocytosis are usually evident on blood examination. If NEC results in perforation or severe bowl ischemia, the neonate may develop sepsis syndrome with hypotension, third space fluid loss, poor perfusion and edema. Most cases of NEC can be successfully managed medically without surgical intervention, although the duration of hospitalization is significantly prolonged in those who develop NEC.[122] Initial treatment includes stopping enteral feeds, and initiating intravenous maintenance fluids and broad spectrum intravenous antibiotics. Hemodynamic support may be necessary, and occasionally laparotomy if perforation occurs or hemodynamic instability persists. The key to management, however, is to improve perfusion and oxygen delivery to the gut. Therefore, once hemodynamically stable without clinical signs of sepsis syndrome, early cardiac surgical intervention to improve splanchnic perfusion is preferable.

Factors contributing to postoperative liver dysfunction include complications during CPB secondary to low perfusion pressure or inadequate venous drainage, and persistent low cardiac output causing ischemic hepatitis. Patients following a Fontan procedure may be at particular risk because of hepatic venous congestion. Marked elevations in liver transaminases may begin within hours of surgery and remain elevated for two to three days before gradually returning to normal. Fulminant hepatic failure is uncommon.

STRESS RESPONSE

Stress and adverse postoperative outcome have been linked closely in critically ill newborns and infants undergoing surgery.[7,123,124] This is not surprising given their precarious balance of limited metabolic reserve and increased resting metabolic rate. Metabolic derangements such as altered glucose homeostasis, metabolic acidosis, salt and water retention, and a catabolic state contributing to protein breakdown and lipolysis are commonly seen following major stress in sick neonates and infants (Table 5.17). This complex of maladaptive processes may be associated with prolonged mechanical ventilation and ICU stay, as well as increased morbidity and eventual mortality.

In the early experience of CPB in neonates and infants, the use of high-dose opioid techniques as the basis for anesthesia, with continuation of this strategy into the immediate postoperative period to modulate the stress response, was perceived to be one of the few clinical strategies associated with a measurable reduction in morbidity and mortality.[125] To a large extent, this experience formed the basis of anesthesia management for not only neonates and infants, but also older children undergoing congenital cardiac surgery during the past decade.

Table 5.17 *Systemic response to injury*

Autonomic nervous system activation
- catechol release
- hypertension, tachycardia, vasoconstriction

Endocrine response
- anterior pituitary: increased ACTH, growth hormone
- posterior pituitary: increased vasopressin
- adrenal cortex: increased cortisol, aldosterone
- pancreas: increased glucagon, insulin resistance
- thyroid: increased/stable T4/3

Metabolic response
- protein catabolism
- lipolysis
- glycogenolysis/gluconeogenesis
- hyperglycemia
- salt and water retention

Immunologic responses
- cytokine production
- acute phase reaction
- granulocytosis

However, it is important to review the effect of anesthesia with respect to the surgical stimulus and the likelihood of ongoing or postoperative stresses. There are differences in the activation and magnitude of the stress response for patients undergoing cardiac surgery prior to CPB, and with the response seen in patients once exposed to a bypass circuit. More recently, studies in neonates, infants and children undergoing cardiac surgery have demonstrated attenuation of the *pre-bypass* endocrine and hemodynamic response to surgical stimulation with a variety of anesthetic techniques.[126–128] However, it is now recognized that the systemic inflammatory response triggered by CPB is also a potent stimulus for initiating the neuroendocrine stress response, and high doses of opioids do not have a consistent or substantial impact on modifying activation of this response.[126,129]

As mentioned, the morbidity and mortality associated with cardiac surgery in neonates and infants has fallen despite the inconsistent effects of opioids on modulation of the stress response. A reasonable conclusion would seem to be that high-dose opioid anesthesia followed by continuation into the immediate postoperative period specifically to attenuate the stress response has a less critical role in determining outcome than was previously reported. Opioids have an important role during anesthesia for cardiac surgery because of the hemodynamic stability they provide, but high doses are not necessary for all patients. In the ICU environment, opioids should be used to provide analgesia, sedation and comfort, but they are not muscle relaxants, nor anti-hypertensive agents. On the other hand, overdosing with opioids simply prolongs the duration of mechanical ventilation, delays establishing enteral nutrition, induces tolerance and acute withdrawal phenomena, and may prolong discharge from the ICU.

SEDATION AND ANALGESIA

Sedation is often necessary to improve synchronization with the ventilator and maintain hemodynamic stability. However, excessive sedation and/or withdrawal symptoms from opioids and benzodiazepines will impair the weaning process. The response to sedation needs to be continually evaluated during the weaning process.

Benzodiazepines

Benzodiazepines are the most commonly used sedatives in the ICU because of their anxiolytic, anticonvulsant, hypnotic and amnestic properties. While providing excellent conscious sedation, they may cause dose-dependent respiratory depression and result in significant hypotension in patients with limited hemodynamic reserve. Following chronic administration, tolerance and withdrawal symptoms are common.

Midazolam as a continuous infusion 0.05–0.1 mg/kg per hour is useful in children following congenital heart surgery.[130] It is short acting and water soluble, although if cardiac output and splanchnic perfusion are diminished, hepatic metabolism is reduced and drug accumulation may occur. Tachyphylaxis may occur within days of commencing a continuous infusion, and withdrawal symptoms of restlessness, agitation and visual hallucinations may occur following prolonged administration. A reversible encephalopathy has been reported following the abrupt discontinuation of midazolam and fentanyl infusions, characterized by movement disorders, dystonic posturing and poor social interaction.[131]

Both diazepam and lorazepam can be effectively used within the ICU with the advantage of longer duration of action. Prescribed on a regular basis, lorazepam may provide useful longer-term sedation, supplementing an existing sedation regimen and assisting with withdrawal from opioids.

Chloral hydrate is commonly used to sedate children prior to medical procedures and imaging studies.[132] It can be administered orally or rectally in a dose ranging from 50 to 80 mg/kg (maximum dose 1 g). Onset of action is within 15–30 minutes with a duration of action between two and four hours. Between 10 and 20% of children may have a dysphoric reaction following chloral hydrate, frequently becoming excitable and uncooperative. On the other hand, some children may become excessively sedated with respiratory depression and potential inability to protect the airway. The regular administration of chloral hydrate to provide sedation in the ICU is controversial. Administered intermittently, it can be used to supplement benzodiazepines and opioids, may assist during drug withdrawal and is useful as a nocturnal hypnotic when trying to establish normal sleep cycles. Repetitive dosing to maintain prolonged sedation is not recommended by the American Academy of Pediatrics and should be avoided in the ICU.[133]

Opioids

Opioid analgesics are the mainstay of pain management in the ICU, and in high doses may provide anesthesia. They also provide sedation for patients while mechanically ventilated and blunt hemodynamic responses to procedures such as endotracheal tube suctioning. Hypercyanotic episodes associated with tetralogy of Fallot and air hunger associated with congestive heart failure are also effectively treated with opioids.

Intermittent dosing of opioids may provide effective analgesia and sedation following surgery, although periods of oversedation and undermedication may occur because of peaks and troughs in drug levels. A continuous infusion is therefore advantageous.

Intermittent morphine 0.05–0.1 mg/kg or as a continuous infusion 50–100 μg/kg per hour, provides excellent postoperative analgesia for most patients. The sedative property of morphine is an advantage over the synthetic opioids; however, histamine release may cause systemic vasodilation and an increase in pulmonary artery pressure. It should therefore be used with caution in patients with limited myocardial reserve and labile pulmonary hypertension.

The synthetic opioids, fentanyl, sufentanil, and alfentanil, have a shorter duration of action than morphine without histamine release, and therefore cause less vasodilation and hypotension. Fentanyl is commonly prescribed following cardiac surgery. It blocks the stress response in a dose-related fashion while maintaining both systemic and pulmonary hemodynamic stability.[134,135] A bolus dose of 10–15 μg/kg effectively ameliorates the hemodynamic response to intubation in neonates.[136] Patients with high endogenous catecholamine levels, e.g. severe cardiac failure or critical aortic stenosis in the neonate, may become hypotensive after a bolus induction dose and fentanyl must be used with caution in these conditions. Chest wall rigidity is an idiosyncratic and dose-related reaction that may occur with a rapid bolus, and can occur in newborns as well as older children.

A continuous infusion of fentanyl 5–10 μg/kg per hour provides analgesia following surgery, although it often needs to be combined with a benzodiazepine to maintain sedation. Large variability between children in fentanyl clearance exists, making titration of an infusion difficult. The experience with ECMO indicates tolerance and dependence to a fentanyl infusion develops rapidly and significant increases in infusion rate may be required.

The development of tolerance is dose- and time-related, and is a particular problem following cardiac surgery in patients who received a high-dose opioid technique to maintain anesthesia. Physical dependence with withdrawal symptoms such as dysphoria, fussiness, crying, agitation, piloerection, tachypnea, tachycardia and diaphoresis may be seen in children and can be managed by gradually tapering the opioid dose or administering a longer acting opioid such as methadone. Methadone has a similar potency to morphine with the advantage of a prolonged elimination half-life between 18 and 24 hours. It can be administered intravenously and is absorbed well orally. It is particularly useful, therefore, to treat patients with opioid withdrawal.

Alternate methods of opioid delivery which are often effective following cardiac surgery include patient controlled analgesia (PCA) and epidural opioids, either as a bolus or continuous infusion. Patients receiving epidural opioids must be closely monitored for potential respiratory depression, and side effects include pruritis, nausea, vomiting, and urinary retention.

Nonsteroidal analgesics

Nonsteroidal anti-inflammatory drugs (NSAIDs) may provide effective analgesia following cardiac surgery, either as a sole analgesic agent or in combination with opioids or local anesthetics. Intravenous ketorolac 0.5 mg/kg eight-hourly is particularly useful as an adjunct to opioids for patients who are weaned and extubated in the early postoperative period. However, there are significant concerns regarding nephrotoxicity and inhibition of platelet aggregation. The incidence of acute renal failure is increased if ketorolac administration is continued for more than three days postoperatively, and in general it should be avoided in patients potentially predisposed to renal failure such as those with hypovolemia, preexisting renal disease, low cardiac output and those receiving medications such as ACE inhibitors. Acute renal failure is more commonly seen after initiation of treatment, or after an increase in dose, and is reversible in most cases.[137]

Inhibition of platelet aggregation and increased bleeding time may occur following a single intravenous dose of ketorolac, although it has not been demonstrated to increase the risk of surgical site bleeding following cardiac surgery.

Anesthetic agents

PROPOFOL

Propofol is an anesthesia induction agent and may be suitable for use in the ICU for short procedures such as transesophageal echocardiography, pericardiocentesis and cardioversion. Its use, however, should be used with caution because of the potential for hypotension from venodilation and direct myocardial depression. Although it has short duration of action and rapid clearance, propofol is currently not approved for longer-term continuous infusion for sedation in pediatric patients. It is a useful agent in some patients who are agitated and difficult to settle during weaning from mechanical ventilation. An infusion of 25–50 μg/kg per minute for four to six hours allows the patient to be sedated comfortably and avoids repeat dosing of benzodiazepines or opioids during this time.

KETAMINE

Ketamine is a 'dissociative' anesthetic agent with a rapid onset and short duration of action. It can be effectively administered intravenously or intramuscularly and provides adequate anesthesia for most ICU procedures including intubation, draining of pleural and pericardial effusions, and sternal wound exploration and closure. It produces a type of catalepsy whereby the eyes remain open, usually with nystagmus and intact corneal reflexes. Occasionally nonpurposeful myoclonic movements may occur. It causes cerebral vasodilation and should be avoided in patients with intracranial hypertension.

Because hemodynamic stability is generally maintained, it is commonly used in ICUs. Heart rate and blood pressure are usually increased through sympathomimetic actions secondary to central stimulation and reduced post-ganglionic catecholamine uptake. However, it is important to remember that this drug does have direct myocardial depressant effects and should be used with caution in patients with limited myocardial reserve, e.g. neonates with critical aortic stenosis.

Dose-related respiratory depression may occur; however, most patients continue to breathe spontaneously after an induction dose of 2–3 mg/kg. Airway secretions are increased, and even though airway reflexes seem intact, aspiration may occur. It is essential that patients be fasted prior to administration of ketamine and complete airway management equipment must be available. An increase in airway secretions may cause laryngospasm during airway manipulation and an antisialagogue such as atropine or glycopyrrolate should be administered concurrently. Side effects of emergence delirium and hallucinations may be ameliorated with the concurrent use of benzodiazepines.

There are conflicting reports about the effect of ketamine on PVR. One small study in children undergoing cardiac catheterization concluded that PVR was increased following ketamine in patients predisposed to pulmonary hypertension.[138] However, another demonstrated minimal effects in young children, either breathing spontaneously or during controlled ventilation.[139] On balance, ketamine has minimal effects on PVR and can be used safely in patients with pulmonary hypertension, provided secondary events such as airway obstruction and hypoventilation are avoided.

Muscle relaxants

Muscle relaxants are more commonly used in pediatric ICUs compared with adult units. Besides being used to facilitate intubation and controlled mechanical ventilation, patients with limited cardiorespiratory reserve also benefit from paralysis because of reduced myocardial work and oxygen demand. However, prolonged paralysis carries the concomitant risks of prolonged ventilatory support and delayed establishment of enteral nutrition, and may result in tolerance and prolonged muscle weakness after discontinuing the muscle relaxant.

Succinylcholine is a depolarizing muscle relaxant with rapid onset and short duration of action. While frequently used in the pediatric ICU to facilitate intubation, the potential for bradycardia and hyperkalemia may be disastrous side effects following cardiac surgery. Its use should therefore be restricted to patients requiring a rapid sequence induction because of the risk for aspiration of gastric contents. The usual intravenous dose of 1 mg/kg should be increased in newborns and infants to 2 mg/kg because of the greater surface area to weight ratio in these patients. It can also be administered intramuscularly in an urgent situation where no vascular access is available, at a dose usual double the intravenous dose (i.e. 3–4 mg/kg). The risk for bradycardia is exaggerated in children, especially after multiple doses, and atropine 20 μg/kg should be administered concurrently.

Rocuronium is an aminosteroid, nondepolarizing muscle relaxant with fast onset and intermediate duration of action. Time to complete neuromuscular blockade for an intubating dose of 0.6 mg/kg ranges from 30 to 180 seconds, although adequate intubating conditions are usually achieved within 60 seconds. It is therefore a suitable alternative to succinylcholine during rapid sequence induction. The duration of action averages 25 minutes although recovery is slower in infants. It is a safe drug to administer to patients with limited hemodynamic reserve and does not cause histamine release.

Vecuronium and cis-atracurium are nondepolarizing muscle relaxants with intermediate durations of actions. They can be administered as a bolus or continuous infusion within the intensive care unit. Both these agents have minimal effect on the circulation and can be administered safely to patients with limited hemodynamic reserve.

Pancuronium is a commonly used, longer duration, nondepolarizing relaxant that may be administered intermittently at a dose 0.1 mg/kg. It may cause a mild tachycardia and increase in blood pressure and is also safe to administer to patients with limited hemodynamic reserve.

CLINICAL PRACTICE GUIDELINES AND FAST TRACK MANAGEMENT

The early tracheal extubation of children following congenital heart surgery is not a new concept, but has received renewed attention with the evolution of 'fast track' management for cardiac surgical patients. Early extubation generally refers to tracheal extubation within a few hours (i.e. four to eight hours) after surgery, although in practice it means the avoidance of routine, overnight mechanical ventilation. Factors to consider when planning early extubation are shown in Table 5.18. For any patient, a thorough review of the preoperative clinical status and surgical procedure is necessary immediately on admission to the ICU, followed by a detailed examination and assessment of monitoring and laboratory data. While this will vary from patient to patient, carefully constructed postoperative order sheets are useful to direct initial management and planning.

Table 5.18 *Considerations for planned early extubation after congenital heart surgery*

Patient factors
- limited cardiorespiratory reserve of the neonate and infant
- pathophysiology of specific congenital heart defects
- timing of surgery and preoperative management

Anesthetic factors
- premedication
- hemodynamic stability and reserve
- drug distribution and maintenance of anesthesia on CPB
- postoperative analgesia

Surgical factors
- extent and complexity of surgery
- residual defects
- risks for bleeding and protection of suture lines

Conduct of CPB
- degree of hypothermia
- level of hemodilution
- myocardial protection
- modulation of the inflammatory response and reperfusion injury

Postoperative management
- myocardial function
- cardiorespiratory interactions
- neurological recovery
- analgesia management

A number of reports have been published describing successful tracheal extubation in neonates and older children following congenital heart surgery, either in the operating room or soon after in the CICU.[140,141] This has been possible without significant compromise of patient care, and a low incidence for reintubation or hemodynamic instability has been reported.

Clinical practice guidelines or critical care pathways are commonly used methods in the ICU to streamline patient management and provide safe as well as cost effective care, although they will vary according to institutional practices. In 1993 we began to establish a program at Children's Hospital Boston for managing selected patients or diagnostic groups after cardiac surgery. The data from commencement of some of our guidelines through to December 2002 are shown in Table 5.19.

The surgical approach and techniques for many cardiac procedures have also substantially changed over recent years, particularly with the development of minimally invasive techniques in both adults and children. While it may be thought that a minimally invasive incision could be associated with a more rapid postoperative recovery because of less pain or analgesic requirements, this has not been demonstrated. In a controlled study of children undergoing ASD repair using either a minimally invasive incision or full sternotomy, we concluded that the primary advantage of the minimally invasive approach was cosmetic, and we were unable to demonstrate any difference in pain scores and other markers of postoperative recovery.[142] The heterogeneity and complexity of congenital cardiac defects means that applying specific management guidelines according to specific diagnoses is difficult. Each patient and his/her circumstances must be viewed individually and managed according to preoperative condition and stability, surgeon preference, any surgical or CPB-related complications and postoperative cardiorespiratory status.

Closed cardiac procedures

Patients undergoing selected nonbypass or closed cardiac surgery and thoracic procedures are suitable for a 'fast track' management plan. Examples include infants and older children undergoing procedures such as patent ductus arteriosus and vascular ring ligation. Infants and older children undergoing repair of coarctation of the aorta may benefit from early extubation and 'fast track' management to avoid the hypertension and tachycardia that often accompanies a slow wean from mechanical ventilation in the ICU following surgery.

In our experience neonates and infants who require surgical modification to pulmonary blood flow, either from placement of a pulmonary artery band or creation of a systemic to pulmonary artery shunt, are not suitable for 'fast track' management protocols; we routinely continue mechanical ventilation and deep sedation for at least the first postoperative night until cardiorespiratory stability is attained.

Open cardiac procedures performed on bypass

Children undergoing relatively short bypass procedures using mild to moderate hypothermia, such as ASD repair, small VSD closure, and right ventricle to pulmonary artery conduit replacement, are often suitable for early extubation either in the operating room or early after ICU admission. These patients generally have a stable preoperative clinical status, demonstrate few complications related to CPB and have an uncomplicated postoperative course. They do not need to be 'weaned' from mechanical ventilation breath by breath, as is frequently the case for longer stay ICU patients who require mechanical ventilation for respiratory support, but rather can be treated as they are emerging from anesthesia and can be quite rapidly converted to a pressure supported mode of ventilation and extubated once awake.

For other postoperative patients, the plan for weaning from mechanical ventilation should be individualized according to age, clinical status, surgical repair and anticipated postoperative management.

NEONATES AND SMALL INFANTS

Two-ventricle repairs

The response to surgery and bypass can vary considerably between neonates and is often unpredictable. Nevertheless, a thorough understanding of the anticipated postoperative

Table 5.19 *Cardiovascular program clinical practice guideline data, Children's Hospital Boston*

CPG diagnosis	Patients (n)	Ventilator time (hours) Median (range)	ICU length of stay (days) Median (range)	Hospital length of stay (days) Median (range)
ASD primum	95	14 (8–45)	3 (2–6)	5 (4–8)
ASD secundum	692	4 (0–68)	1 (0.5–5)	3 (2–11)
Bidirectional Glenn	305	17 (6–432)	2 (0.9–32)	6 (3–77)
Coarctation of the aorta (>1 year)	96	8 (0–36)	2 (0.9–3)	4 (3–5)
RV–PA conduit	167	13 (0–135)	1 (0.8–7)	4 (1–12)
Fenestrated Fontan	421	16 (5–67)	3 (1–76)	9 (4–86)
TGA/IVS	199	40 (25–216)	4 (2–14)	11 (7–29)
TOF/PS (>6 wks)	262	34 (9–120)	4 (1–9)	7 (3–17)
VSD (<6 months)	146	29 (9–144)	3 (0.8–13)	6 (3–13)
VSD (>6 months)	220	15 (0–120)	2 (1–8)	4 (3–15)

course is essential. Early tracheal extubation and 'fast track' management may not be suitable for many neonates and infants undergoing complex two-ventricle or reparative procedures, although such an approach has been reported for selected patients.

In our practice, neonates and infants undergoing two-ventricle repairs are usually managed with sedation and/or paralysis in the immediate postoperative period until hemodynamic and respiratory stability has been attained, although there are clear differences depending on diagnosis and procedure. For example, usually on the first postoperative day following procedures such as an uncomplicated arterial switch operation for d-TGA or repair of an interrupted aortic arch with VSD closure, many of these neonates are sufficiently stable to start to wean from mechanical ventilation and be extubated by the first or second postoperative day.

On the other hand, neonates who have undergone a right ventriculotomy, such as following neonatal repair of tetralogy of Fallot or truncus arteriosus, commonly demonstrate restrictive right ventricle physiology in the immediate postoperative period (see below). Right ventricle compliance usually improves during the first two to three postoperative days, evident by a fall in right sided filling pressures, increased arterial oxygen saturation, and improved cardiac output with warm extremities and an effective diuresis; sedation and/or paralysis can then be discontinued and the patient allowed to wean slowly from mechanical ventilation.

Single ventricle palliation

Neonates undergoing a Norwood-type procedure for hypoplastic left heart syndrome or other forms of single ventricle with aortic arch obstruction, can pose considerable management problems in the immediate postoperative period. Intensive monitoring is essential as the clinical status may change abruptly leading to a rapid deterioration. Deep sedation and paralysis should continue initially following surgery to minimize the stress response and any imbalance between oxygen supply and demand until the patient demonstrates a stable circulation and gas exchange.

INFANTS AND TODDLERS

Infants who are in stable clinical condition prior to surgery and who are undergoing a complete repair using moderate to deep hypothermia on CPB, such as those undergoing closure of a large VSD, complete atrioventricular canal defect or tetralogy of Fallot, are often suitable for early extubation in the first 6–12 hours after surgery, provided they have stable cardiac output, stable gas exchange and no surgical complications such as bleeding.

Infants who have had a large volume load on the ventricle prior to surgery or a labile pulmonary vascular resistance secondary to increased pulmonary blood flow, can be suitable for weaning and extubation in the early postoperative period; however, management should be guided by hemodynamic and respiratory function as patients begin to emerge from sedation. Patients who demonstrate signs consistent with pulmonary hypertension or a low cardiac output state should be managed cautiously; there is no benefit in attempting to advance these patients too early until their clinical course has stabilized with treatment.

CAVOPULMONARY CONNECTION

Following creation of a cavopulmonary connection, whether it be a bidirectional Glenn shunt or a modified Fontan procedure, patients usually benefit from early weaning and tracheal extubation. Effective pulmonary blood flow is enhanced during spontaneous ventilation because of the lower mean intrathoracic pressure. Despite this goal, these patients should only be weaned once hemodynamic stability has been achieved.

In the absence of a pulmonary ventricle, the limitations of the Fontan circulation become readily apparent in the immediate postoperative period if specific complications arise, such as premature fenestration closure, ventricular failure, or loss of atrioventricular synchrony; the subsequent fall in cardiac output will be manifest early as an evolving acidosis, cool extremities, hepatomegaly, ascites, oliguria and often significant chest tube drainage. Once again, intensive monitoring and early intervention and treatment is essential; if there is any doubt or concern for a possible evolving clinical problem, these patients should not be extubated or discharged early from the ICU.

LEFT VENTRICULAR OUTFLOW RECONSTRUCTION

Infants and older children undergoing some types of left ventricular outflow tract repair, including subaortic stenosis repair with the Konno operation or subaortic membrane resection, and aortic valvuloplasty or replacement, usually have well preserved and often hyperdynamic ventricular systolic function. Hypertension and tachycardia are frequently a management concern in these patients in the immediate postoperative period. This is especially a concern during emergence from anesthesia and sedation. Provided ventricular function is stable, hemostasis has been secured, and there are no concerns for ventricular tachyarrhythmias, it is often preferable for these patients to be extubated early after surgery (6–12 hours), rather than undergoing a more prolonged weaning process. Poor recovery of left ventricular function after surgery can also occur secondary to inadequate myocardial protection with cardioplegia in hearts with significant ventricular hypertrophy, and this needs to be thoroughly evaluated prior to considering early extubation. Once extubated, anti-hypertensive management often needs to be continued and titrated according to continuous arterial pressure monitoring, and transfer from the ICU will be delayed until this is achieved.

SPECIFIC MANAGEMENT CONSIDERATIONS

The wide range of surgical procedures undertaken at Children's Hospital Boston over the past five years is demonstrated in Figure 5.8. Despite the heterogeneity, it is possible

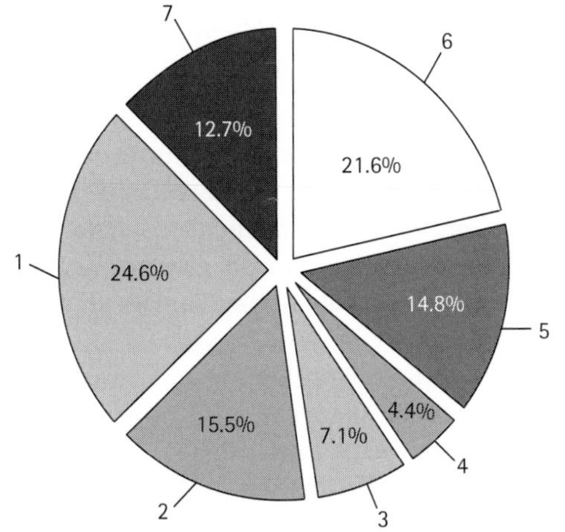

1. Systemic outflow (24.6%)
   - Arterial switch operation 5.0%
   - Coarctation repair 3.1%
   - LVOT obstruction 11.9%
   - Norwood procedure 4.6%
2. Pulmonary outflow (15.5%)
   - Tetralogy of Fallot repair 5.7%
   - Conduit placement/revision 4.8%
   - Other RVOT reconstruction 5.0%
3. Patent ductus arteriosus (7.4%)
4. Permanent pacemaker (4.4%)
5. Other (14.8%)
6. Septal defect (21.6%)
   - ASD repair 7.3%
   - VSD repair 9.8%
   - Complete AV canal repair 4.5%
7. Cavopulmonary connection (12.7%)
   - Fenestrated Fontan 7.1%
   - Bidirectional Glenn shunt 5.6%

Figure 5.8 *Congenital cardiac operations performed at Children's Hospital Boston over a five-year period between 1997 and 2002.*

to apply certain management principles to broad categories of patients, such as those undergoing reconstruction of the systemic ventricular outflow tract, reconstruction of the pulmonary ventricle outflow tract and patients undergoing a pulmonary ventricle exclusion procedure, i.e. a cavopulmonary connection. Specific management issues for these groups are described below.

Transposition physiology with two adequate ventricles

Transposition of the great arteries with an intact ventricular septum or small ventricular septal defect is the most common cardiac cause of cyanosis at birth.

PREOPERATIVE MANAGEMENT

Patients are initially managed with an infusion of prostaglandin E1 at 0.01–0.05 μg/kg per minute to maintain patency of the PDA. There is no dose-response between prostaglandin E1 and size of the PDA; however, complications related to prostaglandin E1 such as apnea and hypotension are more common at the higher dose. A percutaneous balloon atrial septostomy (BAS) should be performed soon after the diagnosis is confirmed to facilitate mixing at the atrial level, thereby increasing cardiac output and SaO_2, and to reduce left atrial pressure. While patients with TGA and a large VSD may have a higher PaO_2 at presentation compared with patients with an intact ventricular septum, a septostomy is often useful to ensure adequate decompression of the LA prior to the arterial switch procedure. If the patient presents in a stable condition with an SaO_2 of more than 65–70%, PaO_2 greater than 25 mmHg and normal pH, the septostomy can be performed semi-electively. Occasionally, an urgent septostomy is indicated for patients who present with severe hypoxemia (PaO_2 less than 20–25 mmHg) and a metabolic acidosis (pH less than 7.20) which indicates very limited mixing of the parallel circulations. On rare occasions when patients present with imminent circulatory collapse, ECMO is life saving.

The septostomy tears the atrial septum and can be performed in the cardiac catheterization laboratory under fluoroscopy or in the ICU using echocardiographic guidance of catheter position. An increase in SaO_2 occurs almost immediately after an adequate septostomy has been created. However, to maintain mixing at the atrial level, volume replacement with colloid or blood products is often necessary. If mechanically ventilated, a low mean airway pressure is essential and occasionally inotrope support with dopamine is necessary to treat hypotension until adequate mixing is achieved. While the prostaglandin E1 infusion can usually be discontinued after an adequate septostomy, it may need to be continued if mixing is inadequate and the PaO_2 remains <25 mmHg.

It is always beneficial to know whether there is a difference between the preductal (right hand) and postductal (lower extremity) SaO_2. A postductal saturation more than 5–10% *higher* than the preductal level, also known as *reverse differential cyanosis*, only occurs in patients with TGA and either pulmonary hypertension or obstruction to systemic outflow (such as coarctation of the aorta or an interrupted aortic arch).

Surgical correction is usually performed in the first week of life after the septostomy, once the patient is hemodynamically stable without signs of end-organ dysfunction. Early surgery is particularly necessary for patients with TGA and an intact ventricular septum because of concerns for involution of the LV muscle mass once PVR decreases after birth. This is less critical for patients with TGA and a large VSD because the RV and LV pressures are equal.

POSTOPERATIVE MANAGEMENT

Following surgery the LA pressure should be closely followed. An increase in LA pressure may be the first indication of myocardial ischemia, but other causes must also be considered at the same time, including an anticipated decrease in ventricular function in response to cardiopulmonary bypass and aortic cross clamp during surgery, residual defects such as an intracardiac shunt or atrioventricular valve regurgitation, and tamponade (see Table 5.3). The sudden onset of heart block or ventricular tachyarrythmia may also herald myocardial ischemia.

Myocardial ischemia is most commonly secondary to mechanical obstruction of the coronary arteries, such as thrombosus, kinking or extrinsic pressure. It is rarely secondary to vasospasm and drugs such as nitroglycerin are ineffective. The sudden onset of ischemia may indicate imminent circulatory collapse and must be treated urgently. For instance, externally pacing a patient who suddenly develops complete heart block after an arterial switch procedure for TGA and intact ventricular septum, may restore the blood pressure temporarily; however, the underlying ischemia is not treated. In this circumstance, it may be preferable to open the sternum and decompress the mediastinum. ECMO should be considered early during resuscitation in a patient who arrests after the arterial switch procedure, because the ischemic myocardium is unlikely to respond to standard resuscitation measures.

Physiologic parallel circulations with a single functional ventricle

For a variety of anatomic lesions, the systemic and pulmonary circulations are in parallel with a single ventricle effectively supplying both systemic and pulmonary blood flow (Table 5.20). The relative proportion of the ventricular output to either pulmonary or systemic vascular bed is determined by the relative resistance to flow in the two circuits. The pulmonary artery and aortic oxygen saturations are equal, with mixing of the systemic and pulmonary venous return within a 'common' atrium. Assuming equal mixing, normal cardiac output and full pulmonary venous saturation, a SaO_2 of 80–85% indicates a Q_p/Q_s of approximately 1.0 and hence a balance between systemic and pulmonary flow.

While there may be specific management issues for certain defects with single ventricle physiology, there are nevertheless common management considerations to balance flow and augment systemic perfusion.

PREOPERATIVE MANAGEMENT

Changes in pulmonary vascular resistance (PVR) have a significant impact on systemic perfusion and circulatory stability (Figure 5.9). In preparation for surgery, it is important that systemic and pulmonary blood flow be as well balanced as possible to prevent excessive volume overload and ventricular dysfunction that reduces systemic and end-organ perfusion. For example, a newborn with HLHS who has an arterial oxygen saturation of more than 90%, and a wide pulse width, oliguria, cool extremities, hepatomegaly and metabolic acidosis, has a severely limited cardiac output and immediate interventions are necessary to prevent imminent circulatory collapse and end-organ injury. In this 'overcirculated' state, manipulation of mechanical ventilation and inotrope support may temporarily stabilize the patient, but surgery should not be delayed or deferred.

Preoperative management should focus on an assessment of the balance between pulmonary (Q_p) and systemic flow (Q_s). This is best achieved by a thorough and continuous re-evaluation of clinical examination for cardiac output state and perfusion, an evaluation of chest radiograph for cardiac size and pulmonary congestion, a review of laboratory data for alterations in gas exchange, acid-base status and end organ function, and imaging with echocardiography to assess ventricular function and A-V valve competence. A central venous line positioned in the proximal SVC may be useful to monitor volume status and sample for mixed venous oxygen saturation as a surrogate of cardiac output and oxygen delivery. Central venous lines are not necessary in all circumstances; they may have significant complications in small newborns and do not substitute for clinical examination.

Initial resuscitation involves maintaining patency of the ductus arteriosus with a prostaglandin E1 infusion at a rate of 0.01–0.05 μg/kg per minute. Intubation and mechanical ventilation is not necessary in all patients. Patients are usually tachypneic, but provided the work of breathing is not excessive and systemic perfusion is maintained without a metabolic acidosis, spontaneous ventilation is often preferable to achieve an adequate systemic perfusion and balance of Q_p and Q_s. A mild metabolic acidosis and low bicarbonate level may be present, but this may not indicate poor perfusion and a

Table 5.20 *Defects amenable to a single ventricle repair*

Atrioventricular valve atresia
- tricuspid atresia
- mitral atresia

Ventricular hypolasia
- hypoplastic left heart syndrome
- double inlet left or right ventricle
- unbalanced atrioventricular canal

Outflow tract obstruction
- Shone's complex
- pulmonary atresia and small right ventricle

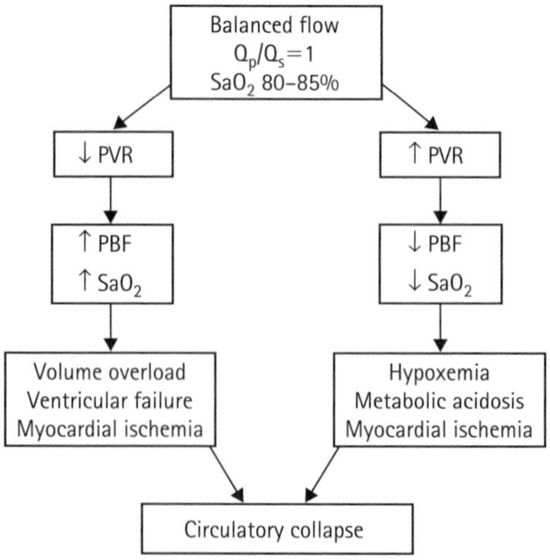

Figure 5.9 *Parallel circulation and hemodynamic stability. PVR = pulmonary vascular resistance; PBF = pulmonary blood flow; SaO_2 = arterial oxygen saturation; Q_p = pulmonary blood flow; Q_s = systemic blood flow.*

lactic acidosis specifically. It is important to evaluate the anion gap at the same time, because a nonanion gap metabolic acidosis may be present secondary to bicarbonate loss from immature renal tubules. Simply assuming that a metabolic acidosis reflects low output in all cases will lead to an unnecessary escalation of circulatory and respiratory support.

Patients require intubation and mechanical ventilation either because of apnea secondary to prostaglandin E1, presence of a low cardiac output state or for manipulation of gas exchange to assist balancing pulmonary and systemic flow. An SaO_2 of more than 90% indicates pulmonary overcirculation, i.e. Q_p/Q_s is greater than 1.0. PVR can be increased with controlled mechanical hypoventilation to induce a respiratory acidosis, often necessitating sedation and neuromuscular blockade, and with a low FiO_2 to induce alveolar hypoxia. Ventilation in room air may suffice, but occasionally a hypoxic gas mixture is necessary. This is achieved by the addition of nitrogen to the inspired gas mixture, reducing the FiO_2 to 0.17–0.19. While these maneuvers are often successful in increasing PVR and reducing pulmonary blood flow, it is important to remember that these patients have limited oxygen reserve and may desaturate suddenly and precipitously. Controlled hypoventilation in effect reduces the FRC and therefore oxygen reserve, which is further reduced by the use of an hypoxic inspired gas mixture. An alternate strategy is to add carbon dioxide to the inspiratory limb of the breathing circuit which will also increase PVR, but because an hypoxic gas mixture is not used, systemic oxygen delivery is maintained.[143,144] Patients who have continued pulmonary overcirculation with high SaO_2 and reduced systemic perfusion despite the above maneuvers require early surgical intervention to control pulmonary blood flow. At the time of surgery, a snare may be placed around either branch pulmonary artery to effectively limit pulmonary blood flow.

Decreased pulmonary blood flow in patients with a parallel circulation is reflected by hypoxemia with an SaO_2 of less than 75%. Preoperatively this may be due to restricted flow across a small ductus arteriosus, increased PVR secondary to parenchymal lung disease, or increased pulmonary venous pressure secondary to obstructed pulmonary venous drainage or a restrictive atrial septal defect. Sedation, paralysis and manipulation of mechanical ventilation to maintain an alkalosis may be effective if PVR is elevated. Systemic oxygen delivery is maintained by improving cardiac output and the hematocrit maintained more than 40%. Interventional cardiac catheterization with balloon septostomy or dilation of a restrictive atrial septal defect may be necessary; however, early surgical intervention and palliation may be indicated.

Systemic perfusion is maintained with the use of volume and vasopressor agents. Inotropic support is often necessary because of ventricular dysfunction secondary to the increased volume load. Systemic afterload reduction with agents such as phosphodiesterase inhibitors may improve systemic perfusion, although they may also decrease PVR and thus not correct the imbalance of pulmonary and systemic flow. It is important to evaluate end organ perfusion and function. Oliguria and a rising serum creatinine level may reflect re-renal insufficiency from a low cardiac output. Necrotizing enterocolitis is a risk secondary to splanchnic hypoperfusion, and we prefer not to enterally feed newborns with a wide pulse width and low diastolic pressure (usually less than 30 mmHg) prior to surgery.

POSTOPERATIVE MANAGEMENT

The management of patients following a Norwood-type operation is complex; intensive monitoring is essential as the clinical status may change abruptly with rapid deterioration. A persistent or progressive metabolic acidosis is a bad prognostic sign and must be aggressively managed. While the balance between Q_p and Q_s is a major focus prior to surgery, in the immediate postoperative period following the Norwood procedure, a low cardiac output state is more likely secondary to ventricular dysfunction. Considerations are shown in Table 5.21.

Deep sedation and paralysis are usually continued following surgery to minimize the stress response until the patient has a stable circulation and gas exchange. Inotrope support with dopamine, and occasionally epinephrine, is usually required, titrated to systemic pressure and perfusion. Afterload

Table 5.21 *Management considerations for patients following a Norwood procedure*

Scenario	Etiology	Management
SaO_2 approx. 85% Normotensive	**Balanced flow** $Q_p = Q_s$	No intervention
$SaO_2 > 90\%$ Hypotension	**Overcirculated** $Q_p > Q_s$ Low PVR Large Blalock-Taussig shunt Residual arch obstruction	*Raise PVR* Controlled Hypoventilation Low FiO_2 (0.17–0.19) *Increase systemic perfusion* Afterload reduction Inotrope support Surgical intervention
$SaO_2 < 75\%$ Hypertension	**Undercirculated** $Q_p < Q_s$ High PVR Small BT shunt	*Lower PVR* Controlled hyperventilation Alkalosis Sedation/paralysis *Increase cardiac output* Inotrope support Hematocrit >40% Surgical intervention
$SaO_2 < 75\%$	**Low cardiac output**	Minimize stress response
Hypotension Low SvO_2	Ventricular failure Myocardial ischemia Residual arch obstruction AV valve regurgitation	Inotrope support Surgical revision ?mechanical support ?transplantation

reduction with milrinone as second-line agents is beneficial to reduce myocardial work and improve systemic perfusion. Monitoring SVC oxygen saturations, as a measure of mixed venous oxygen saturation (SvO_2) and cardiac output is useful in this assessment.[145] Volume replacement to maintain preload is essential, aiming for a common atrial pressure around 10 mmHg.

Closely linked to hemodynamic stability is the tight control of mechanical ventilation and gas exchange. Ideally the pH should be 7.40, $PaCO_2$ 40 mmHg and PaO_2 40 mmHg in room air, reflecting a well balanced circulation. To achieve this, frequent changes in mechanical ventilation settings and FiO_2 may be necessary. Leaving the sternum open after surgery may help facilitate a balanced circulation and stable ventilation pattern.

The type, diameter, length and position of the shunt will also affect the balance of pulmonary and systemic flow. Generally, a 3.5 mm Blalock shunt from the distal innominate artery will provide adequate pulmonary blood flow without excessive steal from the systemic circulation for most full-term neonates. Nevertheless, the shunt results in a low diastolic pressure that in turn effects perfusion to other vascular beds, in particular coronary, cerebral, renal and splanchnic perfusion. This may contribute to a prolonged and difficult postoperative course, and may be obviated by the recently introduced Sano modification of the Norwood procedure in which pulmonary blood flow is provided by a right ventricle to pulmonary artery conduit rather than a shunt directly from the systemic artery.[146] In the immediate postoperative period, mild hypoxemia with an SaO_2 of 65–75% and PaO_2 of 30–35 mmHg is preferable to an overcirculated state with high systemic oxygen saturations. Pulmonary blood flow often increases on the first or second postoperative day as ventricular function improves and PVR falls during recovery from CPB. Pulmonary venous desaturation from parenchymal lung disease such as atelectasis, pleural effusions and pneumothorax requires aggressive management.

Overcirculation in the immediate postoperative period with an SaO_2 of more than 90% may reflect a low PVR, or increased flow across the BT shunt if the shunt size is too large or the perfusion pressure increased from residual aortic arch obstruction distal to the shunt insertion site. The increased volume load on the systemic ventricle results in congestive cardiac failure and progressive systemic hypoperfusion with cool extremities, oliguria, and possibly metabolic acidosis. While manipulation of mechanical ventilation and inspired oxygen concentration may help limit pulmonary blood flow, surgical revision to reduce the shunt size may be necessary.

If there is significant systemic steal through a large shunt, coronary perfusion may be reduced leading to ischemia, low output and dysrhythmias. Rhythm disturbances are uncommon in the immediate postoperative period following a Norwood operation, and a sudden loss of sinus rhythm, and in particular heart block or ventricular fibrillation, should increase the suspicion of myocardial ischemia.

Persistent desaturation and hypotension reflects a low cardiac output from poor ventricular function, thereby decreasing the perfusion pressure across the shunt. The SvO_2 is low (often less than 40%), and treatment directed first at augmenting contractility with inotropes and subsequently reducing afterload with a vasodilator. This is a serious clinical problem with an increased mortality after a Norwood operation. The related myocardial ischemia and acidosis further impair myocardial function and systemic perfusion, leading to circulatory collapse.

Atrioventricular valve regurgitation and residual aortic arch obstruction are important causes of persistent low cardiac output and inability to wean from mechanical ventilation. Echocardiography is useful to assess valve and ventricular function, although less accurate for assessing the degree of residual arch obstruction. Cardiac catheterization is, therefore, preferable and will enable fine tuning of hemodynamic support. Occasionally, surgical revision of the aortic arch or atrioventricular valve is necessary.

More recently a modification to the Norwood procedure has been introduced, which involves placement of conduit from the RV to the PA confluence (ventriculo-pulmonary shunt).[146,147] The primary advantage for this procedure in the immediate postoperative period is improved diastolic perfusion without runoff across an aortopulmonary shunt. Ventricular function is less likely to be compromised after surgery because the volume load to the ventricle is reduced from a lower $Q_p:Q_s$, along with a reduced risk for myocardial ischemia because of improved coronary perfusion. Perfusion to cerebral, renal and splanchnic circulations is also likely to be improved with the lack of diastolic runoff to the pulmonary circulation, and this may also enhance postoperative recovery.

Because pulmonary blood flow occurs only during ventricular systole following an RV–PA conduit procedure, a reduction in ventricular function or restriction to flow across the conduit may result in severe hypoxemia. It is important ventricular preload be maintained and contractility augmented with dopamine if necessary. An increase in pulmonary artery pressure will also limit flow across the conduit, and early extubation is preferable to limit the potential detrimental effects of positive pressure ventilation. Afterload reduction is usually not necessary following this procedure, and may contribute to hypoxemia by lowering the ventricular systolic pressure; the ventricular end-diastolic pressure may also be reduced which could lead to regurgitation of pulmonary arterial blood across the conduit into the ventricle during diastole.

The potential early benefits of this procedure have been described, but longer-term outcome data, particularly related to the ventriculotomy, are to be determined. In our recent experience of patients with hypoplastic left heart syndrome at Children's Hospital Boston, undergoing either an RV–PA conduit or Norwood procedure (based on surgeon preference), we have not observed a reduction in the early mortality or use of ECMO (both $< 10\%$ early mortality); however, the length of stay in the ICU and total hospital stay has been significantly reduced in the RV–PA conduit group (unpublished data).

Cavopulmonary connections

BIDIRECTIONAL CAVOPULMONARY ANASTOMOSIS

In this procedure, the SVC is anastomosed to the right PA, but the pulmonary arteries are left in continuity, and therefore flow from the SVC is bidirectional into both left and right pulmonary arteries. This is the only source of pulmonary blood flow, and inferior vena cava blood returns to the common atrium. Performed between three and six months of age, the bidirectional Glenn shunt has proved to be an important early staging procedure for patients with single ventricle physiology because the volume and pressure load is relieved from the systemic ventricle, yet effective pulmonary blood flow maintained.

The shunt is usually performed on CPB using mild hypothermia with a beating heart. The complications related to CPB and aortic cross clamping are therefore minimal, and patients can be weaned and extubated in the early postoperative period.[148]

Systemic hypertension is common following a shunt. The etiology remains to be determined, but possible factors include improved contractility and stroke volume after the volume load on the ventricle is removed, and brainstem-mediated mechanisms secondary to the increased systemic and cerebral venous pressure. Treatment with vasodilators may be necessary during the immediate postoperative period and during the weaning process.

Following the shunt anastomosis, arterial oxygen saturation should be in the 80–85% range. Persistent hypoxemia is often secondary to a low cardiac output state and low SvO_2. Treatment is directed at improving contractility, reducing afterload and ensuring the patient has a normal rhythm and hematocrit. Increased PVR is an uncommon cause and inhaled nitric oxide is rarely beneficial in these patients. This is not surprising because the pulmonary artery pressure and resistance is simply not high enough following this surgery to see a demonstrable benefit from nitric oxide. Alternatively, ventilation/perfusion mismatch may be a cause for hypoxemia, and nitric oxide may be of benefit in patients with parenchymal lung disease following the shunt because of redistribution of pulmonary blood flow. Persistent hypoxemia should be investigated in the catheterization laboratory to evaluate hemodynamics, look for residual anatomic defects limiting pulmonary flow, such as PA stenosis or a restrictive ASD, and coil any significant venous decompressing collaterals, if present.

FONTAN PROCEDURE

Since the original description in 1971,[149] the Fontan procedure and subsequent modifications have been successfully used to treat a wide range of simple and complex single ventricle congenital heart defects.[150] The repair is 'physiologic' in that the systemic and pulmonary circulations are in series and cyanosis is corrected. However, given the current long-term outcome data, the repair should perhaps be viewed as palliative rather than curative.[151–153] Nevertheless, the mortality and morbidity associated with this surgery has declined substantially over the years and many patients with stable single ventricle physiology are able to lead a normal life.[154]

Ideal physiology immediately following the Fontan procedure

The factors contributing to a successful cavopulmonary connection are shown in Table 5.22 (Figure 5.10). A systemic venous pressure of 10–15 mmHg and a left atrial pressure of 5–10 mmHg, i.e. a transpulmonary gradient of 5–10 mmHg, is ideal.

Intravascular volume must be maintained and hypovolemia treated promptly. Venous capacitance is increased, and as patients rewarm and vasodilate following surgery, a significant volume requirement of around 30–40 ml/kg on the first postoperative night is not unusual.

Table 5.22 *Management considerations following a modified Fontan procedure*

	Aim	Management
• Baffle (pressure 10–15 mmHg)	Unobstructed venous return	Increased preload Low intrathoracic pressure
• Pulmonary circulation	PVR < 2 Wood units/m^2 Mean PA pressure < 15 mmHg Unobstructed pulmonary vessels	Avoid increases in PVR, such as from acidosis, hypo- and hyperinflation of the lung, hypothermia and excess sympathetic stimulation Early resumption of spontaneous respiration
• Left atrium (pressure 5–10 mmHg)	Sinus rhythm Competent AV valve *Ventricle* Normal diastolic function Normal systolic function No outflow obstruction	Maintain sinus rhythm Unchanged or increased rate to increase cardiac output Unchanged or decreased afterload Unchanged or increased contractility PDE inhibitors useful because of vasodilation, inotropic and lusiotropic properties

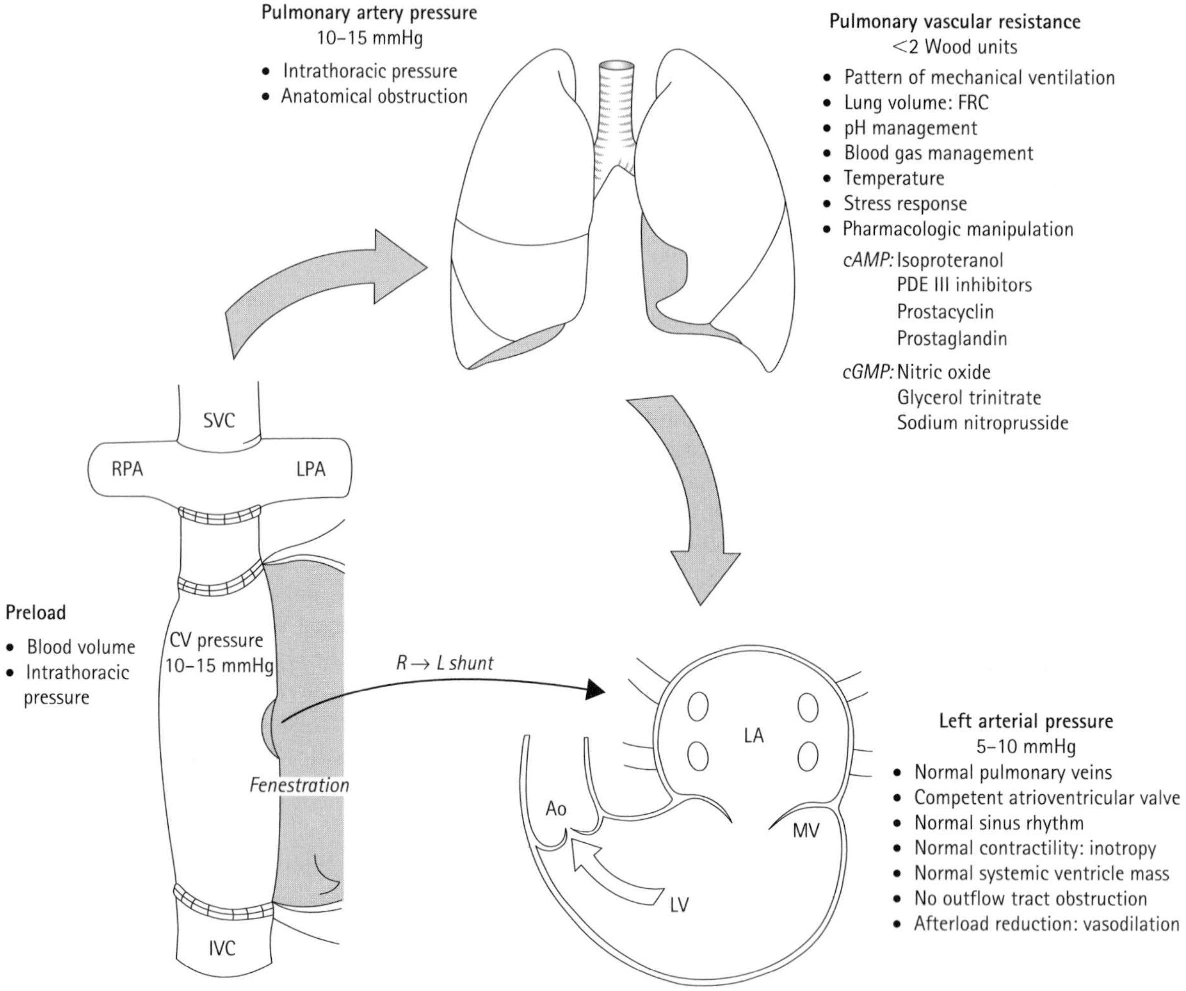

Figure 5.10 *Hemodynamic considerations for optimal pulmonary blood flow and cardiac output in a patient with Fontan physiology.*

Changes in mean intrathoracic pressure and PVR have a significant effect on pulmonary blood flow. Pulmonary blood flow has been shown to be biphasic following the Fontan procedure, and earlier resumption of spontaneous ventilation is recommended to offset the detrimental effects of positive pressure ventilation.[155,156] Using Doppler analysis, it has been demonstrated that pulmonary blood flow predominantly occurs during inspiration in a spontaneously breathing patient, i.e. when the mean intrathoracic pressure is subatmospheric. Therefore, the method of mechanical ventilation following a Fontan procedure requires close observation. A tidal volume of 10–15 ml/kg with the lowest possible mean airway pressure is appropriate. While it is preferable to wean from positive pressure ventilation in the early postoperative period, hemodynamic responses must be closely monitored.

If appropriate selection criteria are followed, patients undergoing a modified Fontan procedure will have a low PVR without labile pulmonary hypertension. Therefore, vigorous hyperventilation and induction of a respiratory and/or metabolic alkalosis is often of little benefit in this group of patients, and the related increase in mechanical ventilation requirements may be detrimental. A normal pH and $PaCO_2$ of 40 mmHg should be the goal, and depending on the amount of right to left shunt across the fenestration, the arterial oxygen saturation is usually in the 80–90% range.

However, PVR may increase following surgery, particularly secondary to an acidosis, hypothermia, atelectasis and hypoventilation, vasoactive drug infusions, and stress response. Any acidosis must be treated promptly. If the cause is respiratory, ventilation must be adjusted. A metabolic acidosis reflects poor cardiac output and treatment directed at the potential causes, including reduced preload to the systemic ventricle, poor contractility, increased afterload and loss of sinus rhythm.

The use of PEEP continues to be debated. The beneficial effects of an increase in FRC, maintenance of lung volume and redistribution of lung water need to be balanced against the possible detrimental effect of an increase in mean intrathoracic pressure. A PEEP of 3–5 cmH_2O, however, rarely has hemodynamic consequence nor substantial effect on effective pulmonary blood flow.

Alternative methods of mechanical ventilation have also been employed for these patients. High frequency ventilation has been used successfully, although the hemodynamic consequences of the raised mean intrathoracic pressure must be continually evaluated.[157] Negative pressure ventilation can be beneficial by augmenting pulmonary blood flow.[158] The development of new negative pressure ventilators and curass and jackets has increased the interest in this mode of ventilation for this group of patients, but experience remains relatively small and indications not defined.

Nonspecific pulmonary vasodilators such as sodium nitroprusside, glycerol trinitrate, prostaglandin E1 and prostacyclin have been used to dilate the pulmonary vasculature in an effort to improve pulmonary blood flow after a Fontan procedure. The results are variable, however. While PVR may fall, pulmonary blood flow could also increase as a result of reduced ventricular end-diastolic pressure following an improvement in ventricular function secondary to the fall in systemic afterload. The response to inhaled nitric oxide is also variable and the improvement may relate to changes in ventilation/perfusion matching rather than a direct fall in PVR.

Afterload stress is poorly tolerated after a modified Fontan procedure because of the increase in myocardial wall tension and end-diastolic pressure. The phosphodiesterase inhibitors, milrinone and amrinone, are particularly beneficial. Besides being weak inotropes with pulmonary and systemic vasodilating properties, their lusitropic action will assist by improving diastolic relaxation and lowering ventricular end-diastolic pressure, thereby improving effective pulmonary blood flow and cardiac output.

Specific complications after the Fontan procedure

Pleuro-pericardial effusions: The incidence of recurrent pleural effusions and ascites has decreased since introduction of the fenestrated baffle technique. Nevertheless, for some patients this remains a major problem with associated respiratory compromise, hypovolemia and possible hypoproteinemia. Usually secondary to persistent elevation of systemic venous pressure, re-evaluation with cardiac catheterization may be indicated.

Rhythm disturbances: Atrial flutter and/or fibrillation, heart block and, less commonly, ventricular dysrhythmia, may have a significant impact on immediate recovery, as well as long-term outcome.[159,160] Sudden loss of sinus rhythm initially causes an increase in left atrial and ventricular end-diastolic pressure, and fall in cardiac output. The SVC or PA pressure must be increased, usually with volume replacement, to maintain the transpulmonary gradient. Prompt treatment with antiarrhythmic drugs, pacing or cardioversion is necessary.

Premature closure of the fenestration: Not all patients require a fenestration for a successful, uncomplicated Fontan operation. Those with ideal preoperative hemodynamics often maintain an adequate pulmonary blood flow and cardiac output without requiring a right to left shunt across the baffle. Similarly, not all Fontan patients who have received a fenestration will use it to shunt right to left in the immediate postoperative period. These patients are fully saturated following surgery, and may have an elevated right sided filling pressure, but nevertheless maintain an adequate cardiac output. The problem is predicting which patients are at risk for low cardiac output after a Fontan procedure, and who will benefit from placement of a fenestration; even patients with ideal preoperative hemodynamics may manifest a significant low output state after surgery. Because of this, essentially all patients having a Fontan procedure are fenestrated at Children's Hospital Boston.

Premature closure of the fenestration may occur in the immediate postoperative period, leading to a low cardiac state output state with progressive metabolic acidosis and large chest drain losses from high right sided venous pressures (Table 5.23). Patients may respond to volume replacement, inotrope support and vasodilation; however, if hypotension and acidosis persists, cardiac catheterization and removal of thrombus or dilation of the fenestration may need to be urgently undertaken.

Persistent hypoxemia: Arterial oxygen saturation levels may vary substantially following a modified Fontan procedure. Common causes of persistent arterial oxygen desaturation less than 75% include a poor cardiac output with a low SvO_2, a large right to left shunt across the fenestration or additional 'leak' in the baffle pathway producing more shunting. An intra-pulmonary shunt, and venous admixture from decompressing vessels draining either from the PA to the systemic venous circulation, or systemic vein to the pulmonary venous system are additional causes. Re-evaluation with echocardiography and cardiac catheterization may be necessary.

Low cardiac output state: An elevated LA pressure after a modified Fontan procedure may reflect poor ventricular function from decreased contractility or increased afterload stress, atrioventricular valve regurgitation and loss of sinus rhythm (Table 5.23). The right sided filling pressure must be increased to maintain the trans-pulmonary gradient, and treatment with inotropes and vasodilators initiated. If a severe low output state with acidosis persists, take down of the Fontan operation and conversion to a bidirectional Glenn shunt anastomosis or other palliative procedure is life saving.

Right ventricular outflow tract reconstruction

Patients undergoing reconstruction of the right ventricular outflow tract are at risk for both systolic and diastolic ventricular dysfunction following surgery. This depends on the age of the patient, the degree of volume or pressure overload imposed on the right ventricle, the duration the RV has been exposed to these loading conditions, and any residual pressure or volume load that remains after surgery. For example, if the right ventricle has been exposed to a significant volume load and is

Table 5.23 *Etiology and treatment strategies for patients with low cardiac output immediately following the Fontan procedure*

Low cardiac output	Etiology	Treatment
Increased TPG		
Baffle > 20 mmHg	*Inadequate pulmonary blood flow*	Volume replacement
LA pressure <10 mmHg	*and preload to left atrium*	Reduce PVR
Clinical state	Increased PVR	Correct acidosis
High SaO_2/low SvO_2	Pulmonary artery stenosis	Inotrope support
Hypotension/tachycardia	Pulmonary vein stenosis	Systemic vasodilation
Poor peripheral perfusion	Premature fenestration closure	Catheter or surgical intervention
SVC syndrome with pleural effusions and increased chest tube drainage		
Ascites/hepatomegaly		
Metabolic acidosis		
Normal TPG		
Baffle >20 mmHg	*Ventricular failure*	Maintain preload
LA pressure >15 mmHg	Systolic dysfunction	Inotrope support
Clinical state	Diastolic dysfunction	Systemic vasodilation if possible
Low SaO_2/low SvO_2	AVV regurgitation and/or stenosis	Establish sinus rhythm or AV synchrony
Hypotension/tachycardia	Loss of sinus rhythm	Correct acidosis
Poor peripheral perfusion	Increased afterload stress	Consider mechanical support
Metabolic acidosis		Surgical intervention, including takedown to BDG or transplantation

TPG = transpulmonary gradient; BDG = bidirectional Glenn anastomosis; AVV = atrioventricular valve.

dilated and contracting poorly prior to surgery, systolic dysfunction is likely to be present in the immediate postoperative period despite correcting the volume overload. Conversely, diastolic dysfunction or restrictive physiology characterized by an elevated RV end-diastolic pressure may be evident after surgery if the RV has been exposed to significant pressure overload and has hypertrophied. The neonate in particular may demonstrate significant restrictive physiology following complete repair of defects including tetralogy of Fallot, pulmonary atresia and truncus arteriosis that require a right ventriculotomy. While there are specific postoperative considerations for each procedure, the considerations for managing restrictive physiology are discussed below.

TETRALOGY OF FALLOT

Complete surgical repair of tetralogy of Fallot has been successfully performed for over forty years with recent studies reporting a 30–35 year actuarial survival of about 85%.[161,162] The anatomical features of tetralogy of Fallot include VSD with anterior malalignment of the infundibular septum, RV outflow tract obstruction which has both fixed and dynamic components, RV hypertrophy and overriding of the aorta. The degree of cyanosis depends upon the amount of outflow obstruction and therefore right to left shunt across the VSD.

Hypercyanotic episodes or 'spells' result from an increase in the amount of right to left shunt secondary to an increase in dynamic outflow obstruction, elevated RV pressure or a fall in SVR. Characteristic features include irritability, profound cyanosis, hyperpnea and syncope. Management is directed at maintaining or increasing SVR, and improving antegrade flow across the RV outflow tract.

Hypercyanotic spells are initially treated with 100% oxygen by face mask, and sedation with opioids or benzodiazepines to treat irritability, hyperpnea, and possibly attenuate dynamic outflow obstruction. If deep cyanosis persists, intravenous crystalloid or colloid (up to 30 ml/kg) should be infused to maintain RV preload. If the patient has a stable blood pressure, a beta-blocker may produce benefit by reducing dynamic outflow obstruction and slowing the heart rate to improve ventricular filling. Attempts at increasing systemic vascular resistance are necessary if the severe cyanosis persists after sedation and volume has been administered. Compression of the femoral arteries or the 'knee-chest' position may be beneficial in the short-term. Occasionally a vasopressor such as phenylephrine 1–2 μg/kg may be necessary to increase SVR if severe hypoxemia persists, and on rare occasions an infusion at 0.01–0.05 μg/kg per minute may be indicated but only as a temporizing measure prior to urgent surgery; ECMO resuscitation is another alternative if an operating room is unavailable.

The risks of cyanosis and complications related to a systemic to pulmonary artery shunt argue for an early complete repair of tetralogy of Fallot. This may be performed in the neonate or young infant depending upon the degree of obstruction and arterial oxygen saturation level. Complete repair in symptomatic neonates and young infants at Children's Hospital Boston often involves a trans-ventricular approach to close the VSD, with pericardial augmentation of the RV outflow tract. A transannular patch is sometimes necessary, and secondary pulmonary regurgitation may compromise ventricular function in the postoperative period (see below). Being smaller and younger, these patients may also be at increased risk for complications associated with CPB and are more likely when very small to require DHCA to facilitate surgical exposure and repair.

Table 5.24 *Factors contributing to RV failure after congenital cardiac surgery*

Surgery and bypass
- ventriculotomy
- myocardial edema
- ischemia

Residual volume load
- pulmonary regurgitation
- residual ventricular septal defect

Residual pressure load
- outflow tract obstruction

Loss of sinus rhythm

RIGHT VENTRICULOTOMY AND RESTRICTIVE PHYSIOLOGY

Right ventricle 'restrictive' physiology in infants and children who have previously undergone congenital cardiac surgery has been described by echocardiography as persistent antegrade diastolic blood flow into the pulmonary circulation following reconstruction of the RV outflow. This occurs in the setting of an elevated RV end-diastolic pressure and RV hypertrophy, and the RV demonstrates diastolic dysfunction with an inability to relax and fill during diastole. The RV is usually not dilated in this circumstance and pulmonary regurgitation limited because of the higher diastolic pressure in the RV.[163–165]

The term 'restrictive' RV physiology is also commonly used in the immediate postoperative period in patients who have a stiff, poorly compliant and sometimes hypertrophied RV. The elevated ventricular end-diastolic pressure restricts filling during diastole and therefore stroke volume and preload to the left ventricle, causes an increase in the right atrial filling pressure and therefore causes systemic venous hypertension, and because of the phenomenon of ventricular-interdependence, changes in RV diastolic function and septal position will in turn affect LV compliance and function. Such a clinical scenario is particularly evident following neonatal right ventricular outflow reconstruction and ventriculotomy, such as following neonatal or newborn truncus arteriosus or tetralogy of Fallot repair. Factors contributing to diastolic dysfunction include lung and myocardial edema following CPB, inadequate myocardial protection of the hypertrophied ventricle during aortic cross clamp, coronary artery injury, residual outflow tract obstruction, volume load on the ventricle from a residual VSD or pulmonary regurgitation and dysrhythmias (Table 5.24).

A low cardiac output state with increased right sided filling pressure (usually more than 10–15 mmHg) is the common feature of neonatal restrictive RV physiology. As a result of the low cardiac output state, patients often have cool extremities, are oliguric and may have a metabolic acidosis. As a result of the elevated right atrial pressure, hepatic congestion, ascites, increased chest tube losses and pleural effusions may be evident.

The patients may be tachycardic and hypotensive with a narrow pulse pressure. Preload must be maintained, despite elevation of the RA pressure. Significant inotrope support is often required (typically dopamine 5–10 μg/kg per minute and/or low dose epinephrine 0.05–0.1 μg/kg per minute), and a phosphodiesterase inhibitor, such as or milrinone, is beneficial because of its lusiotropic properties. Sedation and paralysis are often necessary for the first 24–48 hours to minimize the stress response and associated myocardial work.

While the patent foramen ovale or any ASD is usually closed at the time of surgery in older patients, it is beneficial to leave a small atrial communication following neonatal repair. In the face of diastolic dysfunction and increased RV end-diastolic pressure, a right to left atrial shunt will maintain preload to the left ventricle and therefore cardiac output. Patients may be desaturated initially following surgery (75–85% range typically) because of this shunting. As RV compliance and function improves (usually within two to three postoperative days), the amount of shunt decreases and both antegrade pulmonary blood flow and SaO_2 increase.

Mechanical ventilation may have a significant impact on RV afterload and the amount of pulmonary regurgitation. In addition, an increase in PVR because of hypothermia, acidosis, and either hypo- or hyperinflation of the lung will also increase afterload on the RV and pulmonary regurgitation. Intermittent positive pressure ventilation with the lowest possible mean airway pressure should be the aim, as discussed previously.

Arrhythmias following repair include heart block, ventricular ectopy and junctional ectopic tachycardia. An increase in inotrope or vasoactive support to maintain the blood pressure may also contribute to the tachycardia. It is important to maintain sinus rhythm to avoid additional diastolic dysfunction and an increase in end-diastolic pressure. Atrioventricular pacing may be necessary for heart block. Complete right bundle branch block is typical on the postoperative ECG.

Junctional ectopic tachycardia may cause a significant decrease in cardiac output and be difficult to treat. This is a self-limiting, catechol-sensitive dysrhythmia, usually with an abrupt onset in the first 12–24 hours following surgery. Treatment includes reducing sympathetic stimulation by insuring adequate sedation, optimizing mechanical ventilation and volume status, and reducing vasoactive infusions, if possible.

Inducing hypothermia to 34–35°C may reduce the ectopic rate, thereby enabling capture by external pacing. If these maneuvers are unsuccessful, intravenous procainamide or amiodarone are appropriate antiarrhythmic drugs to reduce the ectopic rate and assist with conversion to sinus rhythm.[166]

Because of the restrictive defect, even a relatively small volume load from a residual VSD or pulmonary regurgitation is often poorly tolerated in the early postoperative period, and it may take two to three days before RV compliance improves following surgery and cardiac output increases. Once RV compliance has improved, as evidenced by a fall in right sided filling pressures, increased arterial saturation and improved cardiac output with warm extremities and an established diuresis, sedation or paralysis is discontinued and the patient allowed to slowly wean from mechanical ventilation.

Left ventricular outflow tract reconstruction

Patients with left ventricular outflow tract obstruction tend to present either as neonates or young infants with significant LV dysfunction and congestive heart failure, or later in childhood with LV hypertrophy but few symptoms. The dramatic presentation of a neonate with circulatory collapse typically occurs with lesions that obstruct systemic blood flow so severely that right to left shunting at the ductus arteriosus is required to perfuse the body. As the ductus significantly narrows or closes, the LV becomes acutely pressure overloaded and begins to fail, leading to pulmonary edema and respiratory distress. When systemic perfusion becomes inadequate, the patient develops hypotension, weak pulses, metabolic acidosis and oliguria. Classic examples include severe (or 'critical') valvar aortic stenosis (AS) and coarctation (CoA).

If the obstruction is less severe, the child can make the transition through ductal closure without notable LV dysfunction and maintain an adequate cardiac output. Over time, however, the pressure overload on the LV stimulates generalized hypertrophy. If untreated and significant, long-term pressure overload can cause LV diastolic dysfunction (compliance falls and end-diastolic pressure rises, causing pulmonary venous hypertension), LV systolic dysfunction, and episodic myocardial ischemia. Clinical manifestations of these changes can include reduced exercise tolerance, exertional chest pain, ventricular dysrhythmias, syncope and sudden death. Significant LV dilation and/or clinical signs of congestive heart failure are ominous findings that are associated with a poor prognosis and increased surgical mortality rate.

AORTIC STENOSIS

The newborn with critical valvar AS who develops hypotension and acidosis as the ductus arteriosus closes requires resuscitation with prostaglandin E1 to restore aortic flow plus mechanical ventilation and inotropic support to achieve stabilization before an intervention is performed. Currently, balloon dilation of the stenotic aortic valve during cardiac catheterization is the preferred intervention at many centers.[167] A surgical valvotomy under direct vision using CPB is the surgical alternative. Despite successful relief of obstruction, significant LV dysfunction and low cardiac output often persist for days after the procedure and require continued treatment with mechanical ventilation and vasoactive drugs. Until LV function recovers and it is able to support the entire cardiac output, a prostaglandin infusion may need to be continued to maintain patency of the ductus arteriosus. Patients should be carefully evaluated after balloon aortic valvuloplasty for residual AS and aortic regurgitation, the chief potential complication of valve dilation, especially if cardiac output does not improve over several days.

Older infants, children, and adolescents with moderate (pressure gradient of 50–70 mmHg at catheterization) or severe (pressure gradient greater than 70 mmHg at catheterization) valvar AS are also generally good candidates for balloon aortic valvuloplasty. If more than mild aortic regurgitation coexists with AS, however, a surgical intervention is preferred to balloon valvuloplasty.

The pathophysiology produced by all types of aortic outflow obstruction is similar, i.e. the pressure-overloaded LV becomes progressively hypertrophied and develops reduced compliance and abnormally elevated end-diastolic pressure.

The initial assessment of obstruction relief can occur when the patient is still in the catheterization laboratory or operating room by either direct pressure measurements or echocardiography. Nevertheless, re-evaluation for residual obstruction by physical examination and/or echocardiography in the ICU as patients recover from anesthesia and baseline physiology returns is important, because outflow gradients can change. A significant residual obstruction should be suspected in any patient with persistent low cardiac output following the intervention. Poor recovery of LV function after surgery can also occur secondary to inadequate myocardial protection with cardioplegia in hearts with significant ventricular hypertrophy. Patients with marked hypertrophy are also at greater risk of developing ventricular tachycardia and ventricular fibrillation early after surgery.

In patients with preserved LV systolic function who undergo an uncomplicated procedure such as aortic valvuloplasty or subvalvar membrane resection, myocardial recovery after CPB is typically rapid and inotropic support is usually not required. Systemic hypertension is more common following relief of LV outflow obstruction, especially during emergence from anesthesia and sedation. Anti-hypertensive therapy in the initial 24–48 hours may be necessary to prevent aortic suture line and reconstructed valve leaflet disruption from excessive stress and to allow adequate hemostasis. Both beta-blockers (e.g. labetalol, propranolol and esmolol) and vasodilators (e.g. nitroprusside), alone or usually in combination, are effective for lowering blood pressure in these patients.

In addition to assessing aortic valve and LV function, an evaluation for complications specific to each procedure is required. For example, if a myectomy is required as part of the resection of fibromuscular subvalvar AS, the possibility of a new VSD, mitral valve injury, and left bundle branch block should all be assessed. Following the Ross procedure, it is important to assess patients for RV as well as LV outflow tract obstruction, because the RV outflow tract is also reconstructed with a valved conduit.

COARCTATION OF THE AORTA

Coarctation of the aorta is a constriction in the descending aorta located at the level of insertion of the ductus arteriosus. Narrowing of the aortic lumen is asymmetric, with the majority of obstruction occurring because of posterior tissue infolding, leading to the common description of a posterior aortic 'shelf.' Depending upon the severity of constriction, patients can present as neonates with severe obstruction (a 'critical' CoA) during ductal closure, as infants with congestive heart failure, or children/adolescents with no symptoms but upper body hypertension (especially with exercise).

Neonates presenting with critical CoA can often be distinguished clinically from patients with critical AS by their clearly discrepant upper versus lower body pulses, perfusion, and blood pressures. Other features at presentation, including evidence of congestive heart failure and inadequate blood flow to tissues, are similar. Because it is common for ductal narrowing or closure to occur after hospital discharge, these patients often become critically ill and suffer end-organ damage before the ductus arteriosus can be reopened and resuscitation accomplished. Intestinal and renal ischemia leading to necrotizing enterocolitis and renal failure, respectively, are well known complications of critical CoA. Echocardiography often reveals additional left sided defects such as bicuspid aortic valve, valvar AS, or aortic arch hypoplasia, and VSD. Preoperative management includes treatment with prostaglandin E1 plus mechanical ventilation, inotropic agents, and diuretic agents, as needed, and adequate time for end-organ recovery before performing an intervention.

CoA also occurs in association with complex defects such as d-TGA, single ventricle, and complete atrioventricular canal defect. If the ductus arteriosus is patent during echocardiographic evaluation of a neonate with suspected congenital heart disease, it is often not possible to predict the severity of CoA with confidence. A patient can have an abnormally narrowed aorta just proximal to the site of ductal insertion (i.e. the aortic isthmus) and a posterior shelf, but still not develop a severe CoA following ductal closure. Therefore, evaluation of the potential severity of CoA in the ICU often involves a strategy of close monitoring for aortic obstruction without prostaglandin E1 to allow the PDA to close, followed by clinical and echocardiographic reassessment. An intervention to reduce aortic obstruction is indicated in any neonate with clinical or echocardiographic evidence of reduced ventricular function or impaired cardiac output. These indications are more important than the systolic blood pressure difference between upper and lower body per se, although differences greater than 30 mmHg are often accompanied by diminished ventricular function.

The postoperative management of patients following surgical repair of CoA can vary depending on age at intervention. However, the key issues for assessment in all patients are adequacy relief of obstruction and preservation of spinal cord function. Upper and lower body blood pressures and pulses should be compared serially and the lower extremities monitored closely for the return of sensation and voluntary movement in the early postoperative period. Equal pulses and a reproducible systolic blood pressure difference less than 10–12 mmHg between upper and lower extremities indicate an excellent repair. Neonates and young infants typically require one or two days of mechanical ventilation after repair, and they are more likely to receive inotropic agents, especially if ventricular function was diminished before surgery. Older children and adolescents can frequently be extubated in the operating room and rarely require inotropic support. In fact, these patients are increasingly likely with older age at repair to have significant hypertension.[168] This should be treated aggressively early after surgery to reduce the risk of aortic suture disruption and bleeding. Beta-blockers and vasodilators along with adequate analgesia and sedation are effective. Patients with longstanding CoA frequently have persistent systemic hypertension despite an adequate repair; continued treatment with ACE inhibitors is advocated to achieve normal blood pressures.

Postcoarctectomy syndrome manifests as abdominal pain and/or distension in older patients and is presumed to be caused by mesenteric ischemia from reflex vasoconstriction after restoration of pulsatile aortic flow. Recurrent laryngeal nerve and phrenic nerve trauma can cause vocal cord paralysis and hemidiaphragm paresis or paralysis, respectively, with neonates and infants at highest risk. Disruption of lymphatic vessels or thoracic duct trauma can produce a chylous effusion and chylothorax which may require treatment by drainage and/or dietary modification.

Catheter directed balloon angioplasty is also used to treat both native and residual CoA.[169–171] The results of native CoA dilation after early follow-up appear similar to published surgical results, but aortic aneurysm formation has been reported.[170] Balloon angioplasty of recurrent CoA after surgery is effective and is now generally preferred to reoperation.

Interrupted aortic arch

Patients with IAA typically present as neonates either with a loud systolic murmur or with circulatory compromise as the ductus arteriosus closes. Patient presentation therefore can be similar to other severe left sided obstructive lesions such as critical AS, critical CoA, and HLHS. Unlike either critical AS or CoA, however, severe pressure overload on the LV does not occur in the presence of an unrestrictive VSD, which functions as a 'pop off' for LV outflow. The approach to resuscitation is similar to that described for the other ductal dependent left sided obstructive lesions, with attention to the possibility of pulmonary overcirculation as for HLHS.

Postoperative management issues specific to patients with IAA include assessment of possible residual left sided obstruction, both in the aortic arch and in the subaortic region, shunting across a residual VSD, hypocalcemia, dysrhythmias and LV dysfunction with low cardiac output secondary to global effects of CPB and DHCA. Left lung hyperinflation on postoperative chest radiographs suggests the possibility of compression of the left mainstem bronchus. This complication tends to occur after difficult arch reconstructions when tension on the aorta causes it to press on the anterior surface of the bronchus, thus producing distal air trapping.

CRITERIA FOR DISCHARGE FROM THE ICU

As patients improve after surgery and require less intensive monitoring and therapy, the timing of discharge from the ICU becomes an important management decision. For the majority of patients who have stable hemodynamics without significant residual defects, and who have been weaned and extubated uneventfully after surgery, the decision to transfer out of the ICU is not difficult. The function of all organ systems should be assessed and considered in this decision, although the focus will be on cardiovascular and respiratory function. Table 5.25 provides a list of cardiovascular and respiratory criteria for consideration prior to patient discharge from the ICU. It is important to emphasize that this decision should be multi-disciplinary, with particular attention paid to nursing availability and experience, and availability of adequate monitoring.

Table 5.25 *General criteria for ICU discharge*

Cardiovascular stability
- stable and appropriate blood pressure without i.v. inotropic or afterload reducing agents
- no requirement for invasive intravascular monitoring
- no requirement for mechanical pacing using temporary wires and an external pacemaker
- stable rhythm (preferably sinus) generating a normal blood pressure and cardiac output

Respiratory status
- no mechanical ventilatory support (possible exception of facial CPAP or BiPAP)
- stable and appropriate ventilation rate, pattern and $PaCO_2$
- stable and adequate oxygenation (PO_2 depends on lesion and physiology after repair or palliation) $\pm$supplemental O_2 via nasal cannula, mask or blow-by
- chest physical therapy or bronchodilator treatments at least three hours apart in frequency
- chest radiograph preferably normal or with focal changes that are stable and improving
- pneumothorax ruled out by chest radiograph after chest drains removed

Organ function
- neurologic status adequate to protect airway from aspiration
- nutrition plan established
- no active or evolving sepsis
- stable or improving renal function and established diuresis

CPAP = continuous positive airway pressure; BiPAP = biphasic positive airway pressure.

ACKNOWLEDGEMENTS

Dr Laussen acknowledges assistance provided by his colleagues and friends of many years, Dr David L Wessel, Children's Hospital Boston, Massachusetts, and Dr Stephen J Roth, Lucile Packard Children's Hospital, Palo Alto, California. Both provided important contributions and advice to the sections relating to pulmonary hypertension, cardiac support and monitoring, and left ventricular outflow tract reconstruction of this chapter. He also acknowledges the expert artwork provided by Emily Flynn-MacIntosh (Figure 5.10).

REFERENCES

1. Kumar RK, Newburger JW, Gauvreau K, Kamenir SA, Hornberger LK. Comparison of outcome when hypoplastic left heart syndrome and transposition of the great arteries are diagnosed prenatally versus when diagnosis of these two conditions is made only postnatally. *Am J Cardiol* 1999; **83**:1649–53.
2. Tworetzky W, McElhinney DB, Reddy VM, Brook MM, Hanley FL, Silverman NH. Improved surgical outcome after fetal diagnosis of hypoplastic left heart syndrome. *Circulation* 2001; **103**:1269–73.
3. Bonnet D, Coltri A, Butera G et al. Detection of transposition of the great arteries in fetuses reduces neonatal morbidity and mortality. *Circulation* 1999; **99**:916–18.
4. Mahle WT, Clancy RR, McGaurn SP, Goin JE, Clark BJ. Impact of prenatal diagnosis on survival and early neurologic morbidity in neonates with the hypoplastic left heart syndrome. *Pediatrics* 2001; **107**:1277–82.
5. American Academy of Pediatrics. Guidelines for Pediatric Cardiovascular Centers. *Pediatrics* 2002; **109**:544–9.
6. du Plessis AJ, Jonas RA, Wypij D et al. Perioperative effects of alpha-stat versus pH-stat strategies for deep hypothermic cardiopulmonary bypass in infants. *J Thorac Cardiovasc Surg* 1997; **114**:991–1000.
7. Anand KJS, Sippell WG, Aynsley-Green A. Randomised trial of fentanyl anaesthesia in preterm babies undergoing surgery: effects on the stress response. *Lancet* 1987; 62–6.
8. Reller MD, Morton MJ, Giraud GD. Severe right ventricular pressure loading in fetal sheep augments global myocardial blood flow to submaximal levels. *Circulation* 1992; **86**:581.
9. Romero TE, Friedman WF. Limited left ventricular response to volume overload in the neonatal period: a comparative study with the adult animal. *Pediatr Res* 1979; **13**:910.
10. Thornburg KL, Morton MJ. Filling and arterial pressure as determinants of RV stroke volume in the sheep fetus. *Am J Physiol* 1983; **244**:H656.
11. Friedman WF. The intrinsic physiologic properties of the developing heart. *Prog Cardiovasc Disease* 1972; **15**:87–111.

12. Baum VC, Palmisano BW. The immature heart and anesthesia. *Anesthesia* 1997; **87**:1529–48.
13. Sagawa K. The end-systolic pressure volume relation of the ventricle: Definition, modifications and clinical use. *Circulation* 1991; **63**:1223–7.
14. Graham TP. Ventricular performance in congenital heart disease. *Circulation* 1991; **84**:2259–74.
15. Howlett G. Lung mechanics in normal infants and infants with congenital heart disease. *Arch Dis Child* 1972; **47**:707–15.
16. Bancalari E, Jesse MJ, Gelband H, Garcia O. Lung mechanics in congenital heart disease with increased and decreased pulmonary blood flow. *J Pediatr* 1977; **90**:192–5.
17. Lees MH, Way RC, Ross BB. Ventilation and respiratory gas transfer of infants with increased pulmonary blood flow. *Pediatrics* 1967; **40**:259–71.
18. Levin AR, Ho E, Auld PA. Alveolar-arterial oxygen gradients in infants and children with left-to-right shunts. *J Pediatr* 1973; **83**:979–87.
19. Rabinovitch M, Haworth SG, Castaneda AR, Nadas AS, Reid LM. Lung biopsy in congenital heart disease: a morphometric approach to pulmonary vascular disease. *Circulation* 1978; **58**:1107–22.
20. Hoffman JIE, Rudolph AM, Heymann MA. Pulmonary vascular disease with congenital heart lesions: pathologic features and causes. *Circulation* 1981; **64**:873–7.
21. Heath D, Edwards JE. The pathology of hypersensitive pulmonary vascular disease: a description of six grades of structural changes in the pulmonary arteries with special reference to congenital cardiac septal defects. *Circulation* 1958; **18**:533–47.
22. Carter BG, Carlin JB, Tibballs J et al. Accuracy of two pulse oximeters at low arterial hemoglobin-oxygen saturation. *Crit Care Med* 1998; **26**:1128–33.
23. Krovetz L, McLoughlin T, Mitchell M et al. Hemodynamic findings in normal children. *Pediatr Res* 1967; **1**:122–30.
24. Lock J. Hemodynamic evaluation of congenital heart disease. In Lock JE, Keane J, Fellows K (eds). *Diagnostic and Interventional Catheterization in Congenital Heart Disease.* Norwell, Martinus Nijhoff, 1987, p 35.
25. Wernovsky G, Wypij D, Jonas RA et al. Postoperative course and hemodynamic profile after the arterial switch operation in neonates and infants. A comparison of low-flow cardiopulmonary bypass and circulatory arrest. *Circulation* 1995; **92**:2226–35.
26. Suga H. Importance of atrial compliance in cardiac performance. *Circ Res* 1974; **35**:39–43.
27. Freed M, Miettinen O, Nadas A. Oximetric detection of intracardiac left-to-right shunts. *Br Heart J* 1979; **42**:690–4.
28. Lang P, Chipman C, Siden H et al. Early assessment of hemodynamic status after repair of tetralogy of Fallot: a comparison of 24 hour (intensive care unit) and 1 year postoperative data in 98 patients. *Am J Cardiol* 1982; **50**:795–9.
29. Vincent R, Lang P, Chipman C et al. Assessment of hemodynamic status in the intensive care unit immediately after closure of ventricular septal defect. *Am J Cardiol* 1985; **55**:526–9.
30. Tabbutt S, Duncan BW, McLaughlin D, Wessel DL, Jonas RA, Laussen PC. Delayed sternal closure after cardiac operations in a pediatric population. *J Thorac Cardiovasc Surg* 1997; **113**:886–93.
31. McElhinney DB, Reddy VM, Parry AJ, Johnson L, Fineman JR, Hanley FL. Management and outcomes of delayed sternal closure after cardiac surgery in neonates and infants. *Crit Care Med* 2000; **28**:1180–4.
32. Verrier EW, Boyle EM. Endothelial cell injury in cardiovascular surgery: an overview. *Ann Thorac Surg* 1997; **64**:S2–8.
33. Hall RI, Smith MS, Rocker G. Systemic inflammatory response to cardiopulmonary bypass: Pathophysiological, therapeutic and pharmacological considerations. *Anesth Analg* 1997; **85**:766–82.
34. Loughead JL, Mimouni F, Tsang RC. Serum ionized calcium concentrations in normal neonates. *Am J Dis Child* 1988; **142**:516–18.
35. Opie LH. Regulation of myocardial contractility. *J Cardiovasc Pharmacol* 1995; **26**:S1–9.
36. Wessel DL. Hemodynamic responses to perioperative pain and stress in infants. *Crit Care Med* 1993; **21**:S361–2.
37. Lawless ST, Zaritsky A, Miles M. The acute pharmacokinetics and pharmacodynamics of amrinone in pediatric patients. *J Clin Pharmacol* 1991; **31**:800–3.
38. Benzing G 3(rd), Helmsworth JA, Schreiber JT et al. Nitroprusside and epinephrine for treatment of low output in children after open heart surgery. *Ann Thorac Surg* 1979; **27**:523–8.
39. Chang AC, Atz AM, Wernovsky G et al. Milrinone: systematic and pulmonary hemodynamic effects in neonates after cardiac surgery. *Crit Care Med* 1995; **23**:1907–14.
40. Hoffman TN, Wernovsky G, Atz AM et al. Prophylactic intravenous use of milrinone after cardiac operation in pediatrics (PRIMACORP) study. Prophylactic intravenous use of milrinone after cardiac operation in pediatrics. *Am Heart J* 2002; **143**:15–21.
41. Hoffman TM, Wernovsky G, Atz AM et al. Efficacy and safety of milrinone in preventing low cardiac output syndrome in infants and children after corrective surgery for congenital heart disease. *Circulation* 2003; **107**:996–1002.
42. Mukharji J, Rehr R, Hastillo A et al. Comparison of atrial contribution to cardiac hemodynamics in patients with normal and severely compromised cardiac function. *Clin Cardiol* 1990; **13**:639–43.
43. Perry JC, Walsh EP. Diagnosis and management of cardiac arrhythmias. In Chang AC, Hanley FL, Wernovsky G, Wessel DL (eds). *Pediatric Cardiac Intensive Care.* Baltimore, Williams & Wilkins, 1998, pp 461–81.
44. Anderson PAW. Physiology of the fetal, neonatal, and adult heart. In Polin RA, Fox WW (eds). *Fetal and Neonatal Physiology.* Philadelphia, WB Saunders, 1992, pp 740–53.
45. Weindling SN, Saul JP, Gamble WJ, Mayer JE, Wessel DL, Walsh EP. Duration of complete atrioventricular block after congenital heart disease surgery. *Am J Cardiol* 1998; **82**:525–7.
46. Munoz R, Laussen PC, Palacio G, Zienko L, Piercey G, Wessel DL. Whole blood ionized magnesium: age-related differences in normal values and clinical implications of ionized hypomagnesemia in patients undergoing surgery for congenital cardiac disease. *J Thorac Cardiovasc Surg* 2000; **119**:891–8.
47. Munoz R, Laussen PC, Palacio G, Zienko L, Piercey G, Wessel DL. Changes in whole blood lactate levels during cardiopulmonary bypass for surgery for congenital cardiac disease: an early indicator of morbidity and mortality. *J Thorac Cardiovasc Surg* 2000; **119**:155–62.
48. Extracorporeal Life Support Organization. *ECLS Registry Report: International Summary*, 2002, Ann Arbor, MI, Extracorporeal Life Support Organization.
49. Ziomek S, Harrell JE Jr, Fasules JW et al. Extracorporeal membrane oxygenation for cardiac failure after congenital heart operation. *Ann Thorac Surg* 1992; **54**:861–7.

50. Walters HL 3rd, Hakimi M, Rice MD, Lyons JM, Whittlesey GC, Klein MD. Pediatric cardiac surgical ECMO. Multivariate analysis of risk factors for hospital death. *Ann Thorac Surg* 1995; **6**:329–36.
51. Aharon AS, Drinkwater DC Jr, Churchwell KB et al. Extracorporeal membrane oxygenation in children after repair of congenital cardiac lesions. *Ann Thorac Surg* 2001; **72**:2095–101.
52. Duncan BW, Hraska V, Jonas RA et al. Mechanical circulatory support in children with cardiac disease. *J Thorac Cardiovasc Surg* 1999; **117**:529–42.
53. Ibrahim AE, Duncan BW, Blume ED, Jonas RA. Long-term follow-up of pediatric cardiac patients requiring mechanical circulatory support. *Ann Thorac Surg* 2000; **69**:186–92.
54. del Nido PJ, Armitage JM, Fricker FJ et al. Extracorporeal membrane oxygenation support as a bridge to pediatric heart transplantation. *Circulation* 1994; **90**(5 Pt 2):II66–9.
55. Slonim AD, Patel KM, Ruttimann UE, Pollack MM. Cardiopulmonary resuscitation in pediatric intensive care units. *Crit Care Med* 1997; **25**:1951–5.
56. Schindler MB, Bohn D, Cox PN et al. Outcome of out-of-hospital cardiac or respiratory arrest in children. *N Engl J Med* 1996; **335**:1473–9.
57. Duncan BW, Ibrahim AE, Hraska V et al. Use of rapid-deployment extracorporeal membrane oxygenation for the resuscitation of pediatric patients with heart disease after cardiac arrest. *J Thorac Cardiovasc Surg* 1998; **116**:305–11.
58. Chen YS, Chao A, Yu HY et al. Analysis and results of prolonged resuscitation in cardiac arrest patients rescued by extracorporeal membrane oxygenation. *J Am Coll Cardiol* 2003; **41**:197–203.
59. del Nido PJ, Dalton HJ, Thompson AE, Siewers RD. Extracorporeal membrane oxygenator rescue in children during cardiac arrest after cardiac surgery. *Circulation* 1992; **86**(5 Suppl):II300–4.
60. Booth KL, Roth SJ, Perry SB, del Nido PJ, Wessel DL, Laussen PC. Cardiac catheterization of patients supported by extracorporeal membrane oxygenation. *J Am Coll Cardiol* 2002; **40**:1681–6.
61. Jaggers JJ, Forbess JM, Shah AS et al. Extracorporeal membrane oxygenation for infant postcardiotomy support: significance of shunt management. *Ann Thorac Surg* 2000; **69**:1476–83.
62. Booth KL, del Nido PJ, Wessel DL, Laussen PC. ECMO support of Fontan and bidirectional Glenn circulation. *Fourth International Symposium on Pediatric Cardiac Intensive Care*, Miami, Florida, Dec 8, 2001.
63. Wessel DL, Almodovar MC, Laussen PC. Intensive care management of cardiac patients on extracorporeal membrane oxygenation. In Duncan BW (ed). *Mechanical Support for Cardiac and Respiratory Failure*. New York, Marcel Dekker, 2000, pp 75–111.
64. Wessel DL, Adatia I, Giglia TM, Thompson JE, Kulik TJ. Use of inhaled nitric oxide and acetylcholine in the evaluation of pulmonary hypertension and endothelial function after cardiopulmonary bypass. *Circulation* 1993; **88**:2128–38.
65. Burch M, Lum L, Elliot M et al. Influence of cardiopulmonary bypass on water balance hormones in children. *Br Heart J* 1992; **68**:309–12.
66. Ationu A, Singer DR, Smith A et al. Studies of cardiopulmonary bypass in children: implications for the regulation of brain natriuretic peptide. *Cardiovasc Res* 1993; **27**:1538–41.
67. Carmichael TB, Walsh EP, Roth SJ. Anticipatory use of venoarterial extracorporeal membrane oxygenation for a high-risk interventional cardiac procedure. *Respir Care* 2002; **47**:1002–6.
68. Karl TR. Extracorporeal circulatory support in infants and children. *Semin Thorac Cardiovasc Surg* 1994; **6**:154–60.
69. Duncan BW. Mechanical circulatory support for infants and children with cardiac disease. *Ann Thorac Surg* 2002; **73**:1670–7.
70. Ishino K, Loebe M, Uhlemann F, Weng Y, Hennig E, Hetzer R. Circulatory support with paracorporeal pneumatic ventricular assist device (VAD) in infants and children. *Eur J Cardiothorac Surg* 1997; **11**:965–72.
71. Akomea-Agyin C, Kejriwal NK, Franks R, Booker PD, Pozzi M. Intraaortic balloon pumping in children. *Ann Thorac Surg* 1999; **67**:1415–20.
72. Wheller J, George BL, Mulder DG, Jarmakani JM. Diagnosis and management of postoperative pulmonary hypertensive crisis. *Circulation* 1979; **70**:1640–4.
73. Heymann MA. Control of the pulmonary circulation in the perinatal period. *J Devel Physiol* 1984; **6**:281–90.
74. Allen K, Haworth SG. Human postnatal pulmonary arterial remodeling: ultrastructural studies of smooth muscle cell and connective tissue maturation. *Lab Invest* 1988; **59**:702–9.
75. Hall SM, Haworth SG. Onset and evolution of pulmonary vascular disease in young children: abnormal postnatal remodeling studied in lung biopsies. *J Pathol* 1992; **166**:183–93.
76. Clapp S, Perry BL, Farooki ZQ et al. Down's syndrome, complete atrioventricular canal, and pulmonary vascular obstructive disease. *J Thorac Cardiovasc Surg* 1990; **100**:115–21.
77. Del Nido PJ, Williams WG, Villamater J et al. Changes in pericardial surface pressure during pulmonary hypertensive crises after cardiac surgery. *Circulation* 1987; **76**(Suppl III):III93–6.
78. Hickey PR, Hansen DD. Pulmonary hypertension in infants: postoperative management. In Yacoub M (ed). *Annual of Cardiac Surgery*. London, Current Science, 1989, pp 16–22.
79. Meyrick B, Reid L. Ultrastructural findings in lung biopsy material from children with congenital heart defects. *Am J Pathol* 1980; **101**:527–42.
80. Koul B, Willen H, Sjöberg T, Wetterberg T, Kugelberg J, Steen S. Pulmonary sequelae of prolonged total venoarterial bypass: Evaluation with a new experimental model. *Ann Thorac Surg* 1991; **51**:794–9.
81. Koul B, Wollmer P, Willen H, Kugelberg J, Steen S. Venoarterial extracorporeal membrane oxygenation – how safe is it? *J Thorac Cardiovasc Surg* 1992; **104**:579–84.
82. Journois D, Pouard P, Mauriat P, Malhère T, Vouhe P, Safran D. Inhaled nitric oxide as a therapy for pulmonary hypertension after operations for congenital heart defects. *J Thorac Cardiovasc Surg* 1994; **107**:1129–35.
83. Kirklin JW, Barratt-Boyes BG. Hypothermia, circulatory arrest, and cardiopulmonary bypass. In *Cardiac Surgery*. New York, Wiley Medical, 1986, pp 29–82.
84. Yndgaard S, Andersen LW, Andersen C, Petterson G, Baek L. The effect of modified ultrafiltration on the amount of circulating endotoxin in children undergoing cardiopulmonary bypass. *J Cardiothorac Vasc Anesth* 2000; **14**:399–401.
85. Journois D, Israel-Biet D, Pouard P, Rolland B et al. High-volume, zero-balanced hemofiltration to reduce delayed inflammatory response to cardiopulmonary bypass in children. *Anesth* 1996; **85**:965–76.
86. Chaturvedi RR, Shore DF, Whilte PA et al. Modified ultrafiltration improves global left ventricular systolic function after open-heart surgery in infants and children. *Eur J Cardiothorac Surg* 1999; **15**:742–6.

87. Elliot M. Modified ultrafiltration and open heart surgery in children. *Paediatr Anaesth* 1999; **9**:1–5.
88. Elliot MJ. Ultrafiltration and modified ultrafiltration in pediatric open heart operations. *Ann Thorac Surg* 1993; **56**:1518–22.
89. Lefer DJ, Flynn DM, Phillips LM, Ratcliffe M, Buda AJ. A novel sialyl Lewis analog attenuates neutrophil accumulation and myocardial necrosis after ischemia and reperfusion. *Circulation* 1994; **90**:2390–401.
90. Gimpel JA, Lahpor JR, van der Mohen AJ, Davien J, Hitchcock JF. Reduction of reperfusion injury of human myocardium by allopurinol: a clinical study. *Free Radic Biol Med* 1995; **19**:251–5.
91. Hopkins RA, Bull C, Haworth SG et al. Pulmonary hypersensitive crises following surgery for congenital heart defects in young children. *Eur J Cardiothorac Surg* 1991; **5**:628–34.
92. Atz A, Adatia I, Wessel DL. Rebound pulmonary hypertension after inhalation of nitric oxide. *Ann Thorac Surg* 1996; **62**:1759–64.
93. Rudolph AM, Yuan S. Response of the pulmonary vasculature to hypoxia and H(+)ion concentration changes. *J Clin Invest* 1966; **45**:399–411.
94. Bergovsky EH, Hass F, Porcelli R. Determination of the sensitive vascular sites from which hypoxia and hypercapnia elicit rises in pulmonary artery pressure. *Fed Proc* 1968; **27**:1420–5.
95. Schreiber MD, Heymann MA, Soifer SJ. Increased arterial pH, not decreased $PaCO_2$, attenuates hypoxia-induced pulmonary vasoconstriction in newborn lambs. *Pediatr Res* 1986; **20**:113–17.
96. Brimioulle S, Lejeune P, Vachiery JL et al. Effects of acidosis and alkalosis on hypoxic pulmonary vasoconstriction in dogs. *Am J Phys* (*Heart Circ Physiol*) 1990; **258**:H347–53.
97. Pepke-Zaba J, Higenbottam TW, Dinh-Xuan A et al. Inhaled nitric oxide as a cause of selective pulmonary vasodilatation in pulmonary hypertension. *Lancet* 1991; **338**:1173–1.
98. Atz A, Wessel DL. Inhaled nitric oxide in the neonate with cardiac disease. *Semin Perinatol* 1997; **21**:441–55.
99. The Neonatal Inhaled Nitric Oxide Study Group: Inhaled nitric oxide in full-term and nearly full-term infants with hypoxic respiratory failure. *N Engl J Med* 1997; **336**:597–604.
100. Roberts JD, Fineman JR, Morin FC et al. Inhaled nitric oxide and persistent pulmonary hypertension of the newborn. *N Engl J Med* 1997; **336**:605–10.
101. Gerlach H, Rossaint D, Pappert D et al. Time-course and dose-response of nitric oxide inhalation for systematic oxygenation and pulmonary hypertension in patients with adult respiratory distress syndrome. *Eur J Clin Invest* 1993; **23**:499–502.
102. Atz A, Wessel DL. Inhaled nitric oxide in sickle cell disease with acute chest syndrome. *Anesth* 1997; **87**:988–90.
103. Goldman AP, Delius RE, Deanfield JE et al. Pharmacologic control of pulmonary blood flow with inhaled nitric oxide after the fenestrated Fontan operation. *Circulation* 1996; **94**(Suppl II): I44–8.
104. Semigran MJ, Cockrill BA, Kacmarek R et al. Hemodynamic effects of inhaled nitric oxide in heart failure. *J Am Coll Cardiol* 1994; **24**:982–8.
105. Loh E, Stamler JS, Hare JM, Loscalzo J, Colucci WS. Cardiovascular effects of inhaled nitric oxide in patients with left ventricular dysfunction. *Circulation* 1994; **90**:2780–5.
106. Bocchi EA, Bacal F, Auler JOC, de Carvalho Carmone MJ, Bellotti G, Pileggi F. Inhaled nitric oxide leading to pulmonary edema in stable severe heart failure. *Am J Cardiol* 1994; **74**:70–4.
107. Lavoie A, Hall JB, Olson DM, Wylam ME. Life-threatening effects of discontinuing inhaled nitric oxide in severe respiratory failure. *Am J Resp Crit Care Med* 1996; **153**:1985–7.
108. Miller OI, Tang SF, Keech A, Celermajer DS. Rebound pulmonary hypertension on withdrawal from inhaled nitric oxide. *Lancet* 1995; **346**:51–2.
109. Atz AM, Wessel DL. Inhaled nitric oxide and heparin for infantile primary pulmonary hypertension. *Lancet* 1998; **351**:1701.
110. Wax D, Garofano R, Barst RJ. Effects of long-term infusion of prostacyclin on exercise performance in patients with primary pulmonary hypertension. *Chest* 1999; **116**:914–20.
111. Atz AM, Wessel DL. Sildenafil ameliorates effects of inhaled nitric oxide withdrawal. *Anesthesiology* 1999; **91**:307–10.
112. Barst RJ, Maislin G, Fishman AP. Vasodilator therapy for primary pulmonary hypertension in children. *Circulation* 1999; **99**:1197–208.
113. Kim NH, Rubin LJ. Endothelin in health and disease: endothelin receptor antagonists in the management of pulmonary artery hypertension. *J Cardiovasc Pharmacol Ther* 2002; **7**:9–19.
114. Rubin LJ, Roux S. Bosentan: a dual endothelin receptor antagonist. *Expert Opin Investig Drugs* 2002; **11**:991–1002.
115. West JB. *Respiratory physiology: The essentials.* Baltimore, Williams and Wilkins, 1995.
116. Hanley FL, Heinemann MK, Jonas RA et al. Repair of truncus arteriosus in the neonate. *J Thorac Cardiovasc Surg* 1993; **105**:1047–56.
117. Watanabe T, Trusler GA, Williams WG et al. Phrenic nerve paralysis after pediatric cardiac surgery. Retrospective study of 125 cases. *J Thorac Cardiovasc Surg* 1987; **94**:383–8.
118. Davies MJ, Njuien K, Gaynor JW. Modified ultrafiltration improves left ventricular systolic function in infants after cardiopulmonary bypass. *J Thorac Cardiovasc Surg* 1998; **115**:361–70.
119. Giuffre RM, Tam KH, Williams WW et al. Acute renal failure complicating pediatric cardiac surgery: A comparison of survivors and non-survivors following acute peritoneal dialysis. *Pediatr Cardiol* 1992; **13**:203–13.
120. Paret G, Cohen AJ, Bohn DJ et al. Continuous arteriovenous hemofiltration after cardiac operations in infants and children. *J Thorac Cardiovasc Surg* 1992; **104**:1222–30.
121. McElhinney DB, Hedrick HL, Bush DM et al. Necrotizing enterocolitis in neonates with congenital heart disease: risk factors and outcomes. *Pediatrics* 2000; **106**:1080–7.
122. Cheng W, Leung MP, Tam PK. Surgical intervention in necrotizing enterocolitis in neonates with symptomatic congenital heart disease. *Pediatr Surg Int* 1999; **15**:492–5.
123. Anand KJS, Hansen DD, Hickey PR. Hormonal-metabolic stress responses in neonates undergoing cardiac surgery. *Anesthesiol* 1990; **73**:661–70.
124. Shew SB, Jaksic T. The metabolic needs of critically ill children and neonates. *Semin Pediatr Surg* 1999; **8**:131–9.
125. Anand KJ, Hickey PR. Halothane-morphine compared with high-dose sufentanil for anesthesia and postoperative analgesia in neonatal cardiac surgery. *N Eng J Med* 1992; **326**:1–9.
126. Gruber EM, Laussen PC, Casta A et al. Stress response in infants undergoing cardiac surgery: a randomized study of fentanyl bolus, fentanyl infusion, and fentanyl-midazolam infusion. *Anesth Analg* 2001; **92**:882–90.
127. Duncan HP, Clotte A, Weir PM et al. Reducing stress responses in the pre-bypass phase of open heart surgery in infants and young

children: a comparison of different fentanyl doses. *Brit J Anaesth* 2000; **84**:556–64.
128. Bichel T, Rouge JC, Schilegel S et al. Epidural sufentanil during paediatric cardiac surgery: effects on metabolic response and postoperative outcome. *Paediatr Anaesth* 2000; **10**:609–17.
129. Kussman BD, Gruber EM, Zurakowski D et al. Bispectral index monitoring during infant cardiac surgery: relationship of BIS to the stress response and plasma fentanyl levels. *Paediatr Anaesth* 2001; **11**:663–9.
130. Lloyd-Thomas AR, Booker PD. Infusion of midazolam in pediatric patients after cardiac surgery. *Brit J Anaesth* 1986; **58**:1109–15.
131. Bergman I, Steeves M, Burckart G et al. Reversible neurologic abnormalities associated with prolonged intravenous midazolam and fentanyl administration. *J Pediatr* 1991; **119**:644–9.
132. Cote CJ. Sedation for the pediatric patient. *Pediatr Clin N Am* 1994; **41**:31–58.
133. American Academy of Pediatrics, Committee on Drugs: Guidelines for monitoring and management of pediatric patients during and after sedation for diagnostic and therapeutic procedures. *Pediatrics* 1992; **89**:1110–15.
134. Hickey PR, Hansen DD, Wessel DL, Lang P, Jonas RA, Elixson EM. Blunting of stress responses in the pulmonary circulation of infants by fentanyl. *Anesth Analg* 1985; **64**:1137–42.
135. Hickey PR, Hansen DD, Wessel DL, Lang P, Jonas RA. Pulmonary and systemic hemodynamic responses to fentanyl in infants. *Anesth Analg* 1985; **64**:483–6.
136. Yaster M. The dose response of fentanyl in neonatal anesthesia. *Anesth* 1987; **66**:433–5.
137. Tarkkila P, Rosenberg PH. Perioperative analgesia with non-steroidal analgesics. *Curr Opin Anaesthesiol* 1998; **11**:407–10.
138. Morray JP, Lynn AM, Stamm SJ. Hemodynamic effects of ketamine in children with congenital heart disease. *Anesth Analg* 1984; **63**:895.
139. Hickey PR, Hansen DD, Cramolini GM. Pulmonary and systemic hemodynamic responses to ketamine in infants with normal and elevated pulmonary vascular resistance. *Anesthesiology* 1985; **62**:287.
140. Barash PJ, Lescovich F, Katz JD et al. Early extubation following pediatric cardiothoracic operations: a viable alternative. *Ann Thorac Surg* 1990; **29**:228–33.
141. Schuller JL, Bovil JG, Nijveld A et al. Early extubation of the trachea after open heart surgery for congenital heart disease. *Brit J Anesth* 1984; **56**:1101–8.
142. Laussen PC, Bichell DP, McGowan FX et al. An evaluation of patient recovery after minimally invasive surgery and full length sternotomy for repair of atrial septal defects in children. *Ann Thorac Surg* 2000; **69**:591–6.
143. Tabbutt S, Ramamoorthy C, Montenegro LM et al. Impact of inspired gas mixtures on preoperative infants with hypoplastic left heart syndrome during controlled ventilation. *Circulation* 2001; **104**:I159–64.
144. Ramamoorthy C, Tabbutt S, Kurth CD et al. Effects of inspired hypoxic and hypercapnic gas mixtures on cerebral oxygen saturation in neonates with univentricular heart defects. *Anesthesiology* 2002; **96**:283–8.
145. Riordan CJ, Randsbaek F, Storey JH. Balancing pulmonary and systemic arterial flows in parallel circulations: The value of monitoring systemic venous oxygen saturations. *Cardiol Young* 1997; **7**:74–9.
146. Sano S, Ishino K, Kawada M et al. Right ventricle–pulmonary artery shunt in first-stage palliation of hypoplastic left heart syndrome. *J Thorac Cardiovasc Surg* 2003; **126**: 504–10.
147. Maher KO, Pizarro C, Gidding S et al. Improved hemodynamic profile following the Norwood procedure with right ventricle to pulmonary artery conduit. *Circulation* 2002; **106**:A2579.
148. Chang AC, Hanley FL, Wernovsky G et al, Castaneda AR. Early bidirectional cavopulmonary shunt in young infants: Postoperative course and early results. *Circulation* 1993; **88**:II149–58.
149. Fontan F, Baudet E. Surgical repair of tricuspid atresia. *Thorax* 1971; **26**:240.
150. Castaneda AR. From Glenn to Fontan: A continuing evolution. *Circulation* 1992; **86**:II80–4.
151. Fontan F, Kirklin JW, Fernandez G et al. The outcome after a 'perfect' Fontan operation. *Circulation* 1990; **81**:1520–36.
152. Driscoll DJ, Offord KP, Feldt RH et al. Five- to fifteen-year follow-up after Fontan operation. *Circulation* 1992; **85**:469–96.
153. Gentles TL, Wernovsky G, Mayer JE et al. Fontan operation in 500 consecutive patients: Factors influencing early and late outcome. *J Thorac Cardiovasc Surg* 1997; **114**:376–91.
154. Gentles TL, Gauvreau K, Mayer JE et al. Functional outcome after the Fontan operation: Factors influencing late morbidity. *J Thorac Cardiovasc Surg* 1997; **114**:392–403.
155. Penny DJ, Redington AN. Doppler echocardiographic evaluation of pulmonary blood flow after the Fontan operation: the role of the lungs. *Br Heart J* 1991; **66**:372–4.
156. Redington AN, Penny DJ, Shinebourne EA. Pulmonary blood flow after total cavopulmonary shunt. *Br Heart J* 1991; **65**:213.
157. Meliones JN, Bove EL, Dekeon MK et al. High frequency jet ventilation improves cardiac function after the Fontan procedure. *Circulation* 1981; **84**:364–8.
158. Shekerdemian LS, Bush A, Shore DF. Cardiopulmonary interactions after Fontan operations: Augmentation of cardiac output using negative pressure ventilation. *Circulation* 1997; **96**:3934–42.
159. Gewillig M, Wyse RK, DeLeval MR. Early and late arrhythmias after the Fontan operation: Predisposing factors and clinical consequences. *Br Heart J* 1992; **67**:72–9.
160. Fishberger SB, Wernovsky G, Gentles TL et al. Factors that influence the development of atrial flutter after the Fontan operation. *J Thorac Cardiovasc Surg* 1997; **113**:80–6.
161. Murphy JG, Gersh BJ, Mair DD. Long term outcome in patients undergoing surgical repair of tetralogy of Fallot. *N Engl J Med* 1993; **329**:593–9.
162. Nollert G, Fischlein T, Bouterwek S et al. Long term survival in patients with repair of tetralogy of Fallot: 36 year-old follow-up of 490 survivors of the first year after surgical repair. *J Am Coll Cardiol* 1997; **30**:1374–83.
163. DiDonato DM, Jonas RA, Lang P et al. Neonatal repair of tetralogy of Fallot with and without pulmonary atresia. *J Thorac Cardiovasc Surg* 1991; **101**:126–37.
164. Cullen S, Shore D, Redington AN. Characterization of right ventricular diastolic performance after complete repair of tetralogy of Fallot. *Circulation* 1995; **91**:1782–9.
165. Redington AN, Penny DJ, Rigby ML. Antegrade diastolic pulmonary arterial flow as a marker of right ventricular restriction after complete repair of pulmonary atresia with intact ventricular

septum and critical pulmonary valve stenosis. *Cardiol Young* 1992; **2**:382–6.

166. Walsh EP, Saul JP, Sholler GF et al. Evaluation of a staged treatment protocol for rapid automatic junctional tachycardia after operation for congenital heart disease. *J Am Coll Cardiol* 1997; **29**:1046–53.
167. Roth SJ, Keane JF. Balloon aortic valvuloplasty. *Progress in Pediatric Cardiology* 1992; **1**:3–16.
168. Anganwu E, Klemm C, Achatzy R et al. Surgery of coarctation of the aorta: a nine-year review of 253 patients. *Thorac Cardiovasc Surg* 1984; **32**:350–7.
169. Lock JE, Bass JL, Amplatz K, Fuhrman BP, Castaneda-Zuniga W. Balloon dilation angioplasty of aortic coarctations in infants and children. *Circulation* 1983; **68**:109–16.
170. Rao PS, Thapar MK, Galal O et al. Follow-up results of balloon angioplasty of native coarctation on neonates and infants. *Am Heart J* 1990; **120**:1310–14.
171. McCrindle BW, Jones TK, Morrow WR et al. Acute results of balloon angioplasty of native coarctation versus recurrent aortic obstruction are equivalent. *J Am Coll Cardiol* 1996; **28**:1810–17.

SECTION 2

Cardiopulmonary bypass

6

The bypass circuit: hardware options

ROBERT HOWE, ROBERT LAPIERRE AND GREGORY MATTE

INTRODUCTION

Some of the most important reasons for the dramatic improvement in outcomes over the past 10–15 years for neonates and infants as well as older children undergoing repair of congenital heart anomalies have been the improvements in cardiopulmonary bypass (CPB) methods and hardware. The subsequent chapters in this section will describe the improvements that have occurred in bypass methods such as pH strategy, degree of hemodilution and flow manipulations. This chapter will focus on the hardware options that are currently available to assemble a bypass circuit that may be applied for repair of a congenital cardiac anomaly.

Oxygenators and other components of the circuit specifically designed for neonatal bypass have only become available over the past decade in spite of the fact that it is more than 50 years since cardiopulmonary bypass was first successfully demonstrated by Gibbon.[1] No doubt this is a reflection of the relatively small size of the commercial pediatric market as well as the large costs that are involved in developing bypass components.

CANNULAS

Introduction

Cannulation is a critically important component of successful cardiopulmonary bypass. While this statement certainly applies to adults with acquired heart disease in whom arterial cannulation may result in dislodgement of atherosclerotic debris, it is even more critically important in the small child with complex arterial and venous anatomy. Many variations of both arterial and venous cannulation are required for congenital cardiac surgery. It is essential that the surgeon should plan carefully the cannulation sites and methods that will be employed in order to allow optimal perfusion of the whole body and particularly the brain throughout the procedure. In addition cannulation must not interfere with an appropriate sequencing of the operative steps. The decision making process for individual anomalies regarding cannulation is covered in the relevant chapter.

Arterial cannulas

The arterial cannula is a highly important component of the extracorporeal circuit. It is a point of narrowing in the pressurized limb of the perfusion circuit. This narrowing causes an increase in flow velocity and can result in turbulence and sheer stress causing damage to the formed elements of blood. In fact the arterial cannula is second only to cardiotomy suction as a source of hemolysis. A properly sized arterial cannula must be of adequate internal diameter to allow blood to pass to the patient with a minimal increase in blood flow velocity, thereby exposing the blood to minimal shear stress and damage. Too small a cannula will also result in an unacceptable increase in the pressure within the arterial side of the bypass circuit. On the other hand the cannula must not be so large as to partially occlude the vessel lumen thereby preventing retrograde flow around the cannula.

Arterial cannulas are sized by internal diameter. A cannula with a thin wall will require a smaller aortotomy and is less likely to partially occlude the lumen than a thicker walled alternative.

Other factors to consider in selecting an arterial cannula are the physical characteristics of the plastic with temperature changes, ability to resist kinking and the ease of insertion.

The extreme temperatures used during pediatric perfusion can cause some arterial cannulas to become rigid thereby applying stress to the aorta during the hypothermic phase of CPB. In general, thin walled wire wound cannulas like the BioMedicus (Medtronic Inc, Minneapolis, MN) (Figure 6.1a) provide the best flow characteristics and are very resistant to kinking. This style of cannula is especially effective for very small aortas, e.g. for interrupted aortic arch, and for minimally invasive procedures. However, they are among the most costly. We use Terumo (formally Bard) arterial cannulas (Figure 6.1b) (Terumo Cardiovascular Systems Corp, Ann Arbor, MI) for most patients. Tables 6.1 and 6.2 display general guidelines for cannula selection based on patient weight used at Children's Hospital Boston.

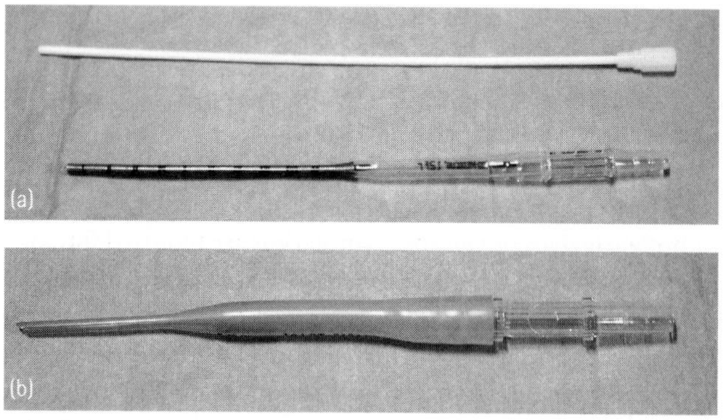

Figure 6.1 *Arterial cannulas used regularly for neonatal and infant bypass. (a) The thin walled, wire wound Biomedicus cannula has excellent flow characteristics and is resistant to kinking including during hypothermic bypass. (b) The Terumo (formerly Bard) arterial cannula is a useful general purpose arterial cannula.*

Table 6.1 *Selection of arterial cannulas based on patient's weight*

	Cannula size (French)	
Weight (kg)	Terumo	BioMedicus pediatric
<5	10	8
5–10	12	10
10–14	14	12
14–28	16	14
28–50	18	NA
>50	20	NA

NA = not applicable.

Table 6.2 *Cannula selection based on patient's weight*

Weight (kg)	Cannula size (French) BioMedicus percutaneous
25–40	15
40–55	17
55–70	19
>70	21

Venous cannulas

Adequate venous return to the bypass circuit is vital to the success of CPB. Unfortunately, having venous cannulas of adequate size and in the proper position does not necessarily guarantee that return to the pump will be adequate. Many additional factors influence the adequacy of venous drainage. One of the most important and often overlooked factors is the size of the vena cava relative to the size of the cannula.[2] If the cannula is so large that there is no space between the caval wall and the cannula then side holes on the cannula will be occluded. Because the cavas, particularly the SVC, vary widely in size in patients with congenital cardiac anomalies, the selection of cannula size will often be a compromise between what might be ideal for the patient with very large cavas versus what is ideal for a patient's specific anatomy. In fact probably the commonest mistake in selecting hardware for the bypass circuit is to select too large a venous cannula.

Other factors that influence venous drainage other than the size of the venous cannula are the flow characteristics of the specific cannula at the flow rate employed, tip style, and the amount of negative pressure applied. There are many factors influencing the amount of negative pressure in the venous line and therefore the cannulas. In the case of vacuum assisted venous drainage, or VAVD, it is simply the amount of suction applied.[3] In the case of conventional gravity drainage the amount of negative pressure is dependent on the venous line diameter and length, the type of reservoir system (i.e. open versus closed) as well as the height difference between the patient and the venous reservoir. Venous reservoirs that allow return to enter the bottom of the reservoir rather than through a straw at the top probably generate less resistance to flow and therefore provide better return. Poiseuille's Law determines the effect of venous line characteristics on flow. Flow is directly related to pressure and the fourth power of radius while inversely proportional to viscosity and length. Considering the factors that can be controlled, optimal venous drainage occurs in a venous line of shortest length and maximal radius for a given patient with an appropriate height difference between the patient and reservoir.

TIP STYLE OF VENOUS CANNULAS

Different venous cannula tip styles may be preferred for right atrial versus caval cannulation. For example, a basket tipped cannula like the Terumo series (Figure 6.2a) works well when cannulating the atrial appendage for right atrial venous drainage. This cannula is used at Children's Hospital Boston (usually as an 18 or 20 French, short) for continuous hypothermic bypass for neonates undergoing procedures like the arterial switch or tetralogy repair. The blunt tip of the cannula is positioned at the SVC/right atrial junction where it is unlikely to entrain air through the tricuspid valve.

Straight lighthouse tipped cannulas like the RMI (Edwards Lifesciences LLC, Irvine, CA) work well when the cavas are cannulated directly and access through the right atrium is not needed by the surgeon, e.g. tetralogy repair in the infant beyond the neonatal period. When right atrial access is needed, thin walled, metal tipped DLP right angled cannulas (Medtronic Inc, Minneapolis, MN) are used (Figure 6.2b). Although they have very good flow characteristics the plastic tubing distal to the metal tip is very thick walled and not ideal for neonatal surgery or minimally invasive surgery. Right angled cannulas can be positioned in the left innominate vein during bidirectional Glenn shunt or Fontan operations allowing the surgeon better access to the SVC. It is particularly important in this setting that the tip of the cannula be sufficiently small to allow flow around the cannula for drainage of the contralateral jugular vein opposite to the tip direction.

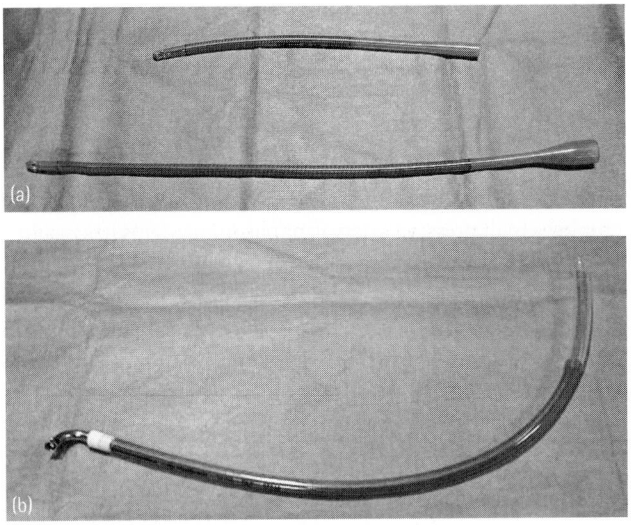

Figure 6.2 *Venous cannulas used for neonatal and infant cardiopulmonary bypass. (a)The basket tipped Terumo venous cannula comes in a shorter infant length as well as in a longer pediatric length. The infant cannula is ideal for continuous hypothermic bypass using a single right atrial cannula. (b) The right angle metal tipped DLP cannula is suitable for continuous bypass with bicaval cannulation.*

One must be cautious when examining the charts of expected flows from venous cannulas because they have been made using a certain set of variables (venous line length and diameter, blood viscosity etc.) and can be misleading depending on local institutional practice for these variables. Each institution should develop a set of charts, as has been done at Children's Hospital Boston (Table 6.3), to determine the optimal cannula sizes for the local patient population and bypass circuit.

BYPASS CIRCUIT

Probably the most important advance that has occurred in cardiopulmonary bypass for neonates and infants over the past 10–15 years has been the reduction in the total volume of priming fluid that has been needed to prime the bypass circuit. The priming volume of current models of neonatal oxygenators is as low as 45–60 ml. Therefore the volume that is sequestered in the PVC tubing that connects the components of the circuit, particularly that which connects the cannulas to the reservoir and oxygenator becomes an important percentage of the total prime volume. Considerable thought has been given by many groups to the positioning of the pump head relative to the patient so as to minimize the tubing length.[4,5] Furthermore modern circuits use considerably smaller tubing diameters than circuits used in the past. Some groups have devised innovative circuits in which the pump head, e.g. a centrifugal pump, is placed close to and at the level of the patient's head which can further decrease tubing length. However, these systems are not in widespread use.

Tubing

For many years there were two standard sizes of tubing used for pediatric perfusion. Quarter-inch tubing was used for neonates and infants and 3/8-inch tubing was used for the

Table 6.3 *Optimal venous cannula sizes at Children's Hospital Boston*

	Cannula size (French)			
	DLP metal tip right angled venous		RMI venous	
Weight (kg)	SVC	IVC	SVC	IVC
<3.5	12	12	16	16
3.5–6	12	14	16	18
6–8	12	16	18	18/20
8–12	14	16	18	20
12–16	14	18	20	20
16–22	16	18	20	22
22–28	16	20	22/24	22/24
28–32	18	20	24/26	24/26
32–40	18	22	26	26/28
>40	20–22	22–28	26/28	26/28

SVC/IVC = superior/inferior vena cava.

toddler and adolescent population. Manufacturers designed connectors for their products to accommodate these tubing sizes based on the flow ratings of the devices. It has now become common for centers including our own to use smaller diameter tubing for the neonatal and infant population, e.g. 3/16 for arterial and venous lines in patients under 2.5 kg. Some centers have even used 1/8 tubing for the arterial side in neonates. However, circuit components such as arterial filters and oxygenators still have 1/4-inch connectors and require adaptors for both 3/16 and 1/8 tubing. It is to be hoped that in the future other manufacturers will introduce connector systems such as seen in the Dideco series of oxygenators which are adaptable to both 3/16 and 1/4-inch tubing. At present the use of 1/8-inch tubing requires multiple adapters. Considering the small saving in prime relative to 3/16 tubing it is presently not recommended that 1/8 tubing be used with present circuit components and connectors.

Cardiotomy suction remains the site where the most damage to the formed elements of blood occurs. Although the cardiotomy pump suckers do not contribute to the initial priming volume, their diameter and length are nevertheless important. Many centers including our own have reduced the length and diameter of suction lines in an attempt to reduce the total surface area of the circuit and the blood to air interface. Additionally minimizing suction head revolutions per minute and thereby reducing the amount of shear stress the blood is exposed to as it travels to the reservoir can reduce the hemolysis associated with pump suction. Reducing the suction line diameter also decreases the impact on venous reservoir volume caused by 'priming' of a suction line during times of high use. We have found that the suction line holdup can be a considerable problem with our smaller patients and circuits, which not uncommonly results in the need for additional blood products to be added to the circuit.

Venous reservoir: 'closed' versus 'open' circuit

Venous reservoirs for cardiopulmonary bypass are termed either open or closed depending on design. More traditional circuits are open in the sense that venous drainage freely flows by gravity into a reservoir which is open to the atmosphere. Any entrained air is naturally vented.

Venous reservoirs are termed closed when the reservoir does not freely communicate with the atmosphere. A collapsible bladder bag collects venous return. This system necessitates a separate open hardshell cardiotomy reservoir to handle both continuous cardiotomy suction flow as well as volume in excess of the capacity of the bladder.

The closed system has the advantage of a limited air to blood interface. Surface tension effects at the air to blood interface have been demonstrated to cause injury to the formed elements of blood.[6] Some systems may also have a smaller priming volume and dynamic volume holdup than an open system but the savings are minimal, if any, when the cardiotomy volume and bladder purge system volume are considered. Furthermore, the closed system does not have multiple screen/depth filters with defoamer and thereby may lead to more microemboli exiting the reservoir.

The primary advantage of open systems for the pediatric population is that volume delineation is clear and that air is automatically purged. Monitoring and actively purging air from a closed system can be distracting to the perfusionist.[7] These factors have led us to practise with open systems at Children's Hospital Boston.

An alternative to the open versus closed system is VAVD. This system utilizes a hard shell reservoir typical of an open system but with no ventilation to the atmosphere. Regulated suction is applied to the reservoir and thereby to the venous line and cannulas to augment venous drainage. The advantages of VAVD are that smaller cannulas and circuit tubing may be used. The principal disadvantage of using a closed hard shell reservoir for vacuum assisted venous drainage is that there is a risk that the reservoir may become pressurized by the air being pumped into the reservoir by the pump suckers. Newer models of hard shell reservoirs for VAVD incorporate a safety vent that prevents excessive pressurization of the reservoir. Failure to employ a high pressure safety vent in some systems has resulted in pressurization of the reservoir followed by massive air embolus.[8] Another disadvantage of VAVD is that there may be an increased microembolic load in the perfusion circuit. With the literature on microembolic load and VAVD conflicting, and our concerns with the additional monitoring and risks, we currently do not employ VAVD for our patient population.

Heparin bonded circuit

There has been considerable interest in recent years in the use of a bypass circuit that is totally heparin bonded. This requires that the cannulas, tubing, oxygenator and filters are all heparin bonded. Studies of inflammatory mediators have confirmed that heparin bonding is effective in reducing complement activation and other markers of the inflammatory response to bypass.[9] Clinical efficacy has also been demonstrated in adults in at least one prospective randomized trial.[10] Further clinical studies need to be undertaken in a pediatric setting to confirm the cost benefit effectiveness of heparin bonded circuits for cardiopulmonary bypass.

PERFUSION PUMPS: THE HEART–LUNG MACHINE

Roller pump

The roller pump, developed by Debakey in 1934, remains the most widely used system for perfusion for congenital cardiac surgery. The principle of operation, i.e. that rollers, usually diametrically opposed, 'milk' a constrained piece of tubing, makes this device both simple and predictable in terms of operation and outcome. This type of pump is capable of generating both positive and negative pressure. It can generate positive pressure to pump blood through the perfusion circuit and to the patient. Roller pumps also generate negative pressure which can be used to pull volume from the venous reservoir and for cardiotomy suction.

It is an important oversimplification to believe that the output from a roller pump can be calculated simply by multiplying the luminal volume of the tubing within the pump head 'raceway' by the number of revolutions per minute. There are several possible sources of error in relying on this calculation alone. Firstly, there is an assumption that the calculation of the luminal volume will be accurate. The most common mistake is to enter the wrong tubing diameter. For example, if 1/4-inch tubing is in the pump head rather than 3/8-inch, the calculated flow rate will actually be considerably less than is believed. Another source of error is the degree of occlusion of the pump head. Many centers believe that the pump head should not be totally occlusive so as to lessen the degree of damage to the formed elements of blood. The rollers are adjusted to allow a minute degree of clearance which is set so as to achieve a measured degree of leakage past the roller head. At Children's Hospital Boston a leak rate of 1 cm per minute is the goal. If this adjustment is not done correctly for both rollers of the pump head or if the equipment is perhaps old and loses this setting during the procedure then once again the calculated flow rate will be greater than the actual flow rate. Another source of error in calculating pump flow rate from a roller pump results from the premise that the elastic recoil of the tubing will be complete irrespective of the revolutions per minute of the pump head. Finally, elastic recoil varies at different temperatures. Due to these limitations, some centers have chosen to incorporate an electromagnetic flow probe to give a more accurate flow reading. Regardless of practice, one needs to be aware of these factors to understand roller pump blood flow measurements during cardiopulmonary bypass.

HEMOLYSIS AND ROLLER PUMPS

In the early years of cardiac surgery there was concern that roller pumps would cause hemolysis. In fact many studies of this question suggest that there is very little hemolysis at the arterial pump head.[11–13] The small amount of hemolysis that does occur can be further reduced by using larger tubing in the raceway of the pump head and by using a minimally non-occlusive pump head setting as described above. In contrast to hemolysis at the arterial pump head there can be considerable hemolysis with high flow suction where blood and air are mixed in the suction line at high velocity. The air–blood interface appears to be the source of hemolysis rather than direct injury to red cells by the roller pump. Minimizing suction head RPM will reduce air entrainment and thereby limit hemolysis.

ROLLER PUMP CONSOLES

There are several consoles currently available that are particularly suitable for pediatric use including the Sorin SC and S3 (Cobe Cardiovascular Inc Division of Sorin Biomedical, Arvada, CO) (Figure 6.3). These consoles have been designed in a compact format with dual mini-pump heads which save space and are especially useful for cardioplegia delivery and left heart venting. Using these newer consoles allows for reduced lengths of tubing, particularly reducing cardiotomy suction tubing. This compact format allows the pediatric perfusionist to connect the various components of the pediatric bypass circuit while reducing the surface area that the patient's blood contacts.

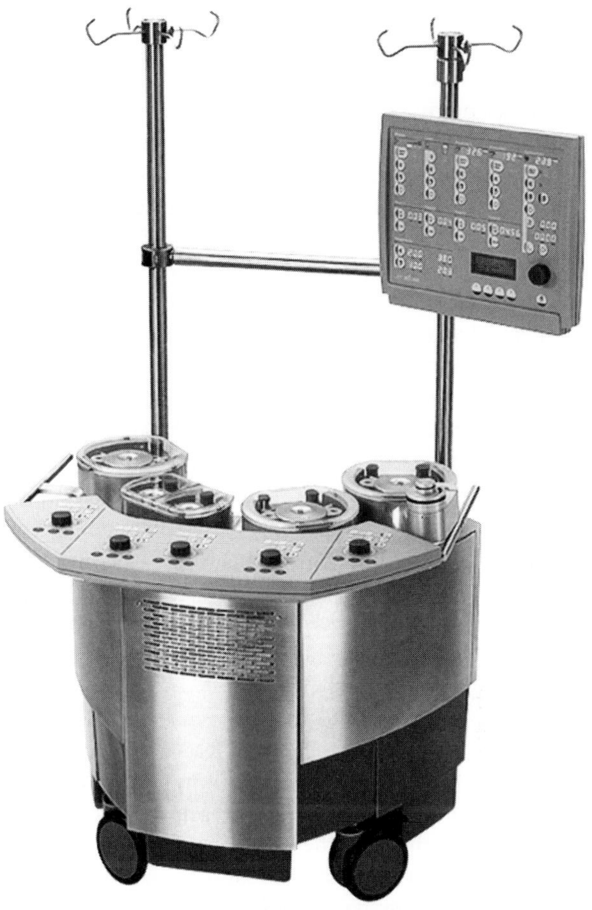

Figure 6.3 *The Sorin SC roller pump console is designed in a compact format that is helpful for pediatric bypass in allowing shorter tubing lengths. This reduces prime volume.*

Centrifugal pumps

Centrifugal pumps have been explored as an alternative to roller pumps for many years but most pediatric institutions have decided to remain with the simplicity and reliability of roller pumps. Centrifugal pumps work on the principle of a high speed rotor with vanes impelling blood to the outlet of the pump head. These pumps all suffer from some degree of after load dependence, i.e. the flow which is generated depends on the afterload resistance.[14] This afterload dependence has been touted as a helpful safety feature in the event of accidental complete occlusion of the arterial line. Under this scenario the pump output will cease and system pressure will not build up causing catastrophic circuit rupture. However, afterload dependence results in constant fluctuations in blood flow. Centrifugal pumps require a separate electromagnetic flow meter, which must be calibrated with each use. The accuracy of these flow probes can be altered by electromagnetic interference and calibration drift. Additional problems associated with centrifugal pumps include local areas of stagnation and vortex zones where high shear stresses may be associated with increased hemolysis. The high speed rotor requires an extremely reliable bearing which must not leak blood. Centrifugal pumps also increase total priming volume. The newer generation heads have a priming volume of approximately 50 ml. Another limitation is that a centrifugal pump cannot be operated in the cardiotomy suction or vent positions. Finally the disposable pump head is a significant additional expense, particularly when contrasted with the disposable component of a roller pump, which is simply a short length of tubing which occupies the arterial head raceway.

Although claims have been made that a centrifugal pump head will not pump gross amounts of air but will simply deprime, careful studies have suggested that considerable volumes of air can indeed be delivered before depriming occurs.[7] And finally since the pump head is not occlusive or even partially occlusive, if the revolutions per minute of the pump head fall below a certain level it is possible for blood to flow retrograde through the pump head and back to the reservoir leading to an undetected loss of blood volume from the patient.[15] Newer systems have incorporated one way valves to attempt to avoid this problem but this adds further complexity and cost.

Pulsatile versus nonpulsatile perfusion

One of the longstanding controversies regarding cardiopulmonary bypass is the importance of pulsatile perfusion. Although many experimental studies have suggested important advantages with pulsatile perfusion it has been difficult to demonstrate a convincing improvement in clinical outcomes with pulsatile systems. However, in the past systems with pulsatile roller pumps were studied. The roller head of such pumps was able to rotate in a discontinuous fashion creating a pulsatile arterial pressure profile. With bubble oxygenators this waveform was more easily achieved because there was only tubing between the roller head and the arterial cannula. Current circuit designs require the pulsatile flow to travel through both a membrane oxygenator and an arterial filter. One needs to realize the effect this has on dampening the pulse. Furthermore in the pediatric setting the very small arterial cannulas that are often employed will further dampen the pressure pulse. Other pulsatile systems that have been examined include pulsatile assist devices in which a balloon placed in the arterial line of the perfusion circuit inflates and deflates. Pulsatile diaphragm pumps analogous to left ventricular assist devices have also been examined but have not come into general usage.[16] We are not currently using pulsatile flow in our perfusion system.

ARTERIAL FILTERS

Arterial filters have only come into widespread use in pediatric cardiac surgery over the last decade. For example, in 1993 Elliott et al[17] reported that at that time only one third of units in the United Kingdom were using arterial filtration routinely. The prospective randomized trial of circulatory arrest versus low flow bypass that was conducted at Children's Hospital Boston between 1988 and 1992 did not include arterial filtration as part of the protocol.[18]

One of the principal objections to the introduction of arterial filtration in children was the relatively large volumes required to prime the filters. In addition to the fact that early filters were thought to increase the total circuit prime volume unreasonably there were also perceived problems related to damage of the cellular components of blood as well as a paradoxical risk of increased particulate embolism from the downstream side of filters.

Arterial filter designs

STANDARD ARTERIAL LINE FILTER

An arterial line filter must remove air and particulate matter while allowing the passage of the cellular elements of blood. In modern practice screen arterial line filters are almost universally used generally with a pore size of 40 μm.[19,20] Arterial filters remove air by causing a sudden decrease in flow velocity as the blood enters the filter. This sudden decrease in velocity causes air bubbles to rise to the top of the filter where they can be purged from the system. The latest generation of filters allows the blood to enter the filter in a tangential pattern thereby increasing the probability that air will be directed to the top of the filter. Screen filters are generally made of polyester woven into a two dimensional screen with a defined pore size between the threads. Most filters are designed with pleats and folds to increase the available surface area for filtration. However, if filtration is required for a prolonged period the efficiency may be reduced by blocking of available pores. Pall Biomedical (Fajardo, PR) offers the AV3SV and AV6SV filters with a microporous hydrophobic membrane integrated into the top of the filter. This membrane allows entrained air to be automatically purged to atmosphere and can handle gross air in the circuit extremely well.

PRE-BYPASS FILTERS

It is helpful to circulate the clear priming solution through the circuit before the blood component has been added. A filter with a pore size ranging from 0.5 to 5 μm is temporarily included in the circuit to remove very small particulate residual debris which may have been created during manufacture of the components of the CPB circuit. The filter is then excluded from the circuit before blood is added.

CRYSTALLOID FILTERS

The most widely used crystalloid filter is the Pall Biomedical CPS02. This filter is a membrane filter with a pore size of 0.2 μm. In addition to filtering out particulate contaminates before entering the CPB circuit this filter is bacteriostatic.

WHITE CELL FILTERS

In recent years there has been increasing recognition of the deleterious effects of circulating activated white cells. These may be either autologous white cells or more importantly homologous white cells from the bank blood added to the circuit. Many centers now choose to use white cell free homologous blood in which the majority of white cells have been removed prior to addition to the bypass circuit. At Children's Hospital Boston this is done by the hospital blood bank service. An alternative method is to pass the bank blood through a white cell filter as it is added to the circuit. Since this can be a prolonged process because of the slow flow rate through white cell filters of this type it is an important logistical advantage to have white cell free homologous blood supplied to the operating room. If autologous white cells as well as homologous white cells are to be removed from the circuit then a white cell filter must be included in the bypass setup which will continuously filter white cells throughout the cardiopulmonary bypass period. Although this is now technically feasible it has the disadvantage of adding further prime volume to the circuit. Furthermore since activated white cells are frequently sequestered in the lungs and spleen and elsewhere during cardiopulmonary bypass to be subsequently released after weaning from bypass it is not clear how effective continuous autologous white cell filtration is.[21,22] This is not a technique that is currently employed at Children's Hospital Boston.

Filtration and gaseous microemboli

Undoubtedly the time period when arterial line filters would have been most helpful was the period when bubble oxygenators were employed. In spite of antifoaming agents bubble oxygenators generated massive numbers of gaseous microemboli. Studies in the animal laboratory at Children's Hospital Boston documented that the number of gaseous microemboli generated by a bubble oxygenator was increased when blood was cooled during the hypothermic period of bypass when gaseous solubility of both oxygen and carbon dioxide was increased.[23] If nitrogen was also added because of use of air rather than 100% oxygen then even more gaseous microemboli were produced. Modern hollow fiber membrane oxygenators generate considerably fewer gaseous microemboli than bubble oxygenators. When an arterial line filter is placed in series with a membrane oxygenator very few gaseous microemboli can be detected under normal circumstances even at hypothermia. However, entrainment of a large amount of air through the venous line, for example using vacuum assisted venous drainage can result in an increased number of gaseous microemboli passing through a membrane oxygenator which can overwhelm an arterial line filter.[24]

Specific arterial filters: brands and models

There are a limited number of pediatric arterial line filters presently available that fulfill reasonable low prime, high flow rating standards.

PALL BIOMEDICAL

The Pall Biomedical LPE 1440 pediatric arterial filter had a low prime volume of 35 ml and a maximum flow rate of 3 liters per minute. It accepted only 1/4-inch tubing. This filter was easy to prime and had a low failure rate but is currently out of production.

TERUMO CAPIOX

The Terumo Capiox CXAFO2 arterial filter (Figure 6.4) has a prime volume of 40 ml but is only rated for 2.5 liters per minute. It is easy to prime and has good flow characteristics. It accepts only 1/4-inch tubing.

DIDECO 736

The Dideco 736 has a flow rating of only 2 liters per minute with a 40 ml prime. The filter is unique in that is has an internal bypass feature. While innovative, we feel that for optimal safety arterial line filters should have an external bypass loop.

HEMOCONCENTRATORS AND ULTRAFILTRATION

In contrast to arterial line filters which are designed to remove particulate debris that is greater than 40 μm in diameter, ultrafilters are designed to hemoconcentrate blood by removing water, dissolved ions and small molecules. The size of the smallest molecules which will be removed by the ultrafilter is dependent on the pore size of the membrane from which the ultrafilter is constructed. For example, albumin, which is relatively small protein molecule with a mass of 65 kDa, must not be removed by an ultrafilter as this would seriously decrease the plasma colloid oncotic pressure. However, many bioactive molecules such as heparin and various inflammatory mediators such as IL-6, C3a and C5a are smaller than albumin and can be removed by the majority of ultrafilters in current clinical usage.

Ultrafiltration can be applied during cardiopulmonary bypass in order to achieve hemoconcentration. This has come

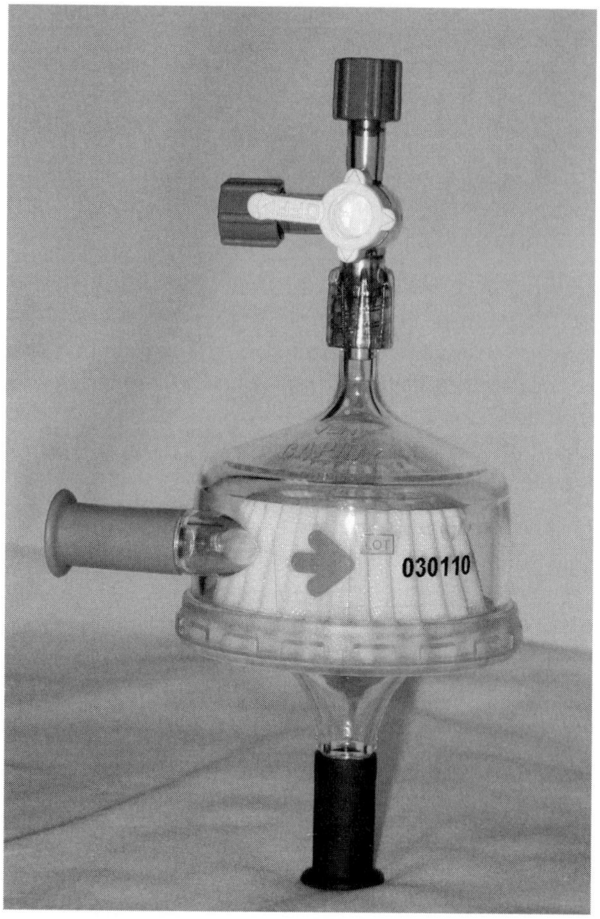

Figure 6.4 *The Terumo Capiox CXAF02 arterial line filter has a prime volume of 40 ml and is rated for a maximal flow of 2.5 liters per minute.*

to be termed 'conventional' ultrafiltration. An alternative technique which is termed 'modified' ultrafiltration was introduced by Elliott a little over 10 years ago and is now widely applied in pediatric cardiac surgery.[25,26]

CONVENTIONAL ULTRAFILTRATION

The ultrafilter is positioned with its inlet connected to the arterial line and its outlet to the venous reservoir. A number of factors will determine the rate of ultrafiltration:

- transmembrane pressure, which is the difference between pressure inside the hollow fibers of the ultrafilter and the pressure on the effluent side of the hollow fibers. Positive pressure from the arterialized blood is applied to the ultrafilter blood inlet. One can increase transmembrane pressure by applying negative pressure to the effluent side of the filter. The greater the transmembrane pressure difference the higher the filtration rate
- blood flow rate to the filter, which is determined by the perfusionist
- characteristics of the specific ultrafilter, including the depth of the pores, i.e. the membrane thickness, the number of pores related to membrane surface area and the size of pores
- the hematocrit of blood – if particularly low because crystalloid has entered the perfusate, then there will be a higher rate of ultrafiltration and therefore a higher rate of hemoconcentration.

MODIFIED ULTRAFILTRATION

This technique allows hemoconcentration of both the patient's circulating blood volume as well as the remaining perfusate in the circuit including the venous reservoir after bypass has been terminated. Blood is drawn retrograde from the arterial cannula as well as from the venous reservoir to the oxygenator and heat exchanger by a roller pump which is connected to the ultrafilter. As with conventional ultrafiltration negative pressure is applied to the ultrafilter to control the rate of filtration. The filtered blood is returned to the patient through the venous line and cannula. Many centers have reported beneficial effects with modified ultrafiltration and it is now widely applied. An improvement in blood pressure and cardiac output has been documented. A number of inflammatory mediators have been documented in the ultrafiltrate.[27] However, not all centers have employed modified ultrafiltration including Children's Hospital Boston. Probably the most important reason why this technique has not been adopted relates to the policy of hemodilution during cardiopulmonary bypass. Centers that find modified ultrafiltration to be particularly effective tend to use lower levels of hematocrit during bypass. Ten years ago when Naik and Elliott described ultrafiltration they suggested that a hematocrit of 20–24% was used by the majority of centers but that levels as low as 10–15% were considered acceptable by some.[28] If the hematocrit is maintained at 30% or perhaps even greater during cardiopulmonary bypass (see Chapter 7), hemoconcentration following bypass is less beneficial. Disadvantages of modified ultrafiltration include the complexity of the circuit, the risk of air entrainment from the arterial cannula, the need to maintain heparinization during the period of ultrafiltration and the additional time required in the operating room. Furthermore the reduced prime volume of modern circuits as well as almost routine application of conventional ultrafiltration have meant that a hematocrit of greater than 30% is often achieved prior to weaning from cardiopulmonary bypass.[29]

Hemoconcentrators; brands and models

The Minntech Hemocor HPH400 hemoconcentrator (Minntech Corp, Minneapolis, MN) has a prime volume of 27 ml and a surface area of 0.3 m^2 (Figure 6.5). It filters to a molecular mass cut off of 65 kDa. Because it is glycerin free it does not need to be flushed with crystalloid before use. As with most hemoconcentrators the Minntech Hemocor comes with only 1/4-inch tubing connections. The arteriovenous shunt flow to the hemofilter can be reduced by stepping down the 1/4-inch connections to pressure tubing on both the inlet and outlet sides of the filters. This minimizes the risk that an

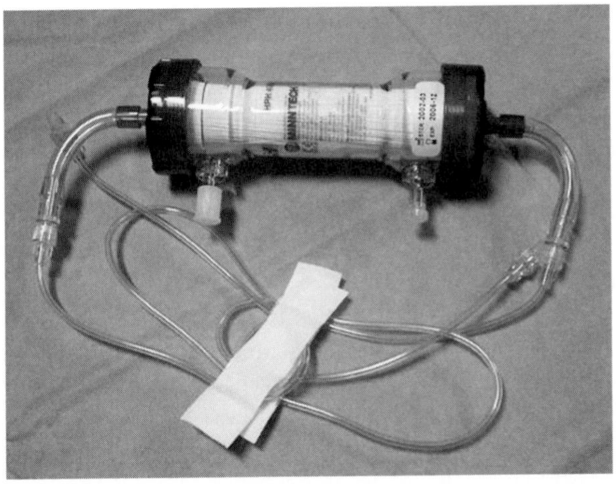

Figure 6.5 *The Minntech Hemocor HPH400 hemoconcentrator has a prime volume of 27 ml.*

excessive steal will be taken from the arterial line thereby reducing blood flow to the patient. The Dideco DHFO.2 (Cobe Cardiovascular Inc, Arvada, CO) hemoconcentrator has a prime volume of 30 ml and a surface area of 0.25 m^2. It also filters molecules less than 65 kDa and is glycerine free.

OXYGENATOR GAS MANAGEMENT: CARBOGEN DELIVERY SYSTEM FOR pH STAT STRATEGY

The advantages of the pH stat strategy relative to the alternative alpha stat strategy are documented in Chapter 8. The pH stat strategy requires the addition of carbon dioxide to the oxygenator gas mixture. This requires that the operating room be equipped with a system capable of safely administering this carbon dioxide.

The use of several different concentrations of oxygen and carbon dioxide or 'carbogen' is used to achieve pH stat. At Children's Hospital Boston concentrations of 97% O_2/3% CO_2, 96/4, 95/5 and 94/6 are used. The decision as to which percentage to use is based on the size of the patient and the level of hypothermia to be used. A system that allows the perfusionist to switch easily from one to another of these concentrations is key to the successful administration of pH stat. The system at Children's Hospital Boston consists of a central bank of tanks that supplies the three cardiac operating rooms. Each carbogen concentration source consists of two cylinders connected to an electronically controlled manifold (Innovator Manifold Control, Western Enterprises, Westlake, OH) (Figure 6.6). The manifold monitors the level of gas in each cylinder. When the tank in use becomes empty the manifold will indicate the tank is empty and switch to a full tank. The gas is piped to the three rooms where it is monitored by a separate panel (MEDAES Area Line Pressure Alarm). This interim panel will generate an audible alarm if both tanks become empty. Each gas then travels to a ball valve where it can be

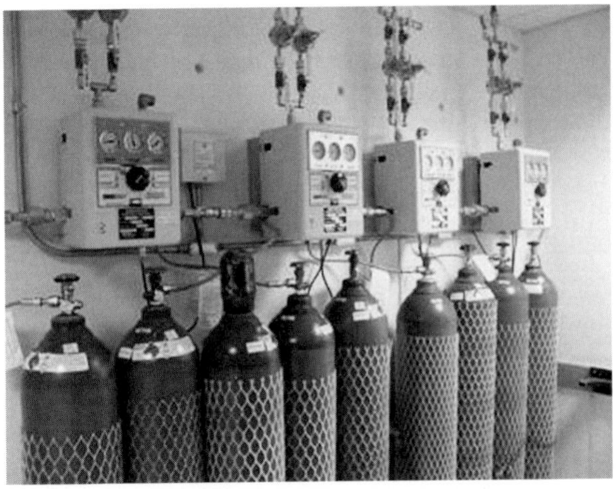

Figure 6.6 *Use of the pH stat strategy requires a reliable source of carbon dioxide in different concentrations to be piped to the cardiac operating rooms. At Children's Hospital Boston there are two cylinders for each of the CO_2 concentrations employed. An electronically controlled manifold switches automatically from empty to full cylinders.*

turned on or off. At this point the gases converge into one pipe which is routed to the back of the perfusionist's gas flow meter during hypothermic bypass. During normothermic bypass the conventional source from the gas blender is employed.

NEONATAL AND PEDIATRIC OXYGENATORS

Introduction

The oxygenator is the most important component of the cardiopulmonary bypass circuit. It is responsible for gas exchange, including oxygen and carbon dioxide as well as volatile anesthetic gases and usually incorporates an integrated heat exchanger that allows cooling and rewarming of the patient. Furthermore, many neonatal and pediatric oxygnators come with integral venous and cardiotomy reservoirs. As a unit, the oxygenator/reservoir holds the greatest proportion of the priming volume and is second only to the cardiotomy suction system as the site where there is the greatest potential for injury to the cellular components of the blood and initiation of inflammatory cascades. It is potentially a major source of microemboli. Important advances in oxygenator design, most notably integration and miniaturization of components, have contributed to the dramatic reduction in the morbidity of cardiopulmonary bypass for the infant and neonate that has been witnessed over the last two decades.

Oxygenator design

SCREEN AND DISC OXYGENATORS

The earliest oxygenators were constructed with mesh screens or solid disks which were coated with a thin film of blood as they rotated through a trough containing blood. It was at this interface that gas exchange occurred. These early oxygenators required a particularly large priming volume and were very injurious to blood. Nevertheless the first successful clinical application of cardiopulmonary bypass by Gibbon in May 1953 employed a disk oxygenator.[1]

BUBBLE OXYGENATORS

Dewall, working with Lillehei in Minnesota, was the first to introduce the concept of a bubble oxygenator into clinical practice.[30] Like screen and disk oxygenators bubble oxygenators were quite injurious to blood. In addition they produced massive amounts of gaseous microemboli. The defoaming agents that were used to remove the macroscopic foaming that occurred when oxygen was bubbled through blood were gradually embolized into the system. Because this was before the years of efficient arterial line filters it is not surprising that many patients in these years suffered from 'post pump lung' or 'post pump delerium'. Bubble oxygenators became obsolete by the late 1980s following the introduction of clinically effective membrane oxygenators.

Membrane oxygenators

There are two basic types of membrane oxygenator. The 'true membrane' oxygenator most closely resembles the human alveolus in that there is an intact membrane separating gas and blood. Other membrane oxygenators do not completely separate blood from gas because of the presence of micropores in the membrane, the so-called 'microporous membrane'. Although membrane oxygenators superficially resemble the human lung, there are in fact important differences. Oxygenators have a much smaller surface area for gas exchange (typically only 10–15%) relative to the natural lungs. In addition the lungs allow red cells to pass through the pulmonary capillaries one at a time, thus markedly decreasing the distance for diffusion. For this reason the 'transit time', i.e. the time during which the red cell is passing along the gas exchanging surface is short, approximately 0.75 s at rest. This translates to a short 'blood path length'. Oxygenators compensate for these disadvantages by creating turbulence along the gas exchange path, thereby increasing exposure of deoxygenated blood to the exchange surface. This increases the potential for blood injury.

TRUE MEMBRANE OXYGENATOR

The material employed in the true membrane oxygenator to separate blood and gas, i.e. the 'membrane' is silicone. Silicone is a 'thermoset plastic'. It has better dimensional stability, heat resistance, chemical resistance and electrical properties than a thermoplastic such as polypropylene, which is employed in microporous membrane oxygenators. Silicone is antithrombogenic because of its physiologic inertness. Its surface charge repels blood components preventing adhesion to the membrane. Silicone is highly permeable to gases. It prevents foaming of blood and denaturization of protein factors.

Gas transfer in a true membrane occurs by molecular diffusion just as in the alveolus. Gas diffuses into the silicone membrane and because of the concentration gradients of carbon dioxide and oxygen, transfer occurs rapidly. The greater the gas pressure differential across the membrane, the more rapid will be the gas transfer. Gas transfer is also directly proportional to the permeability of the membrane which as already noted in the case of silicone, is very high for both carbon dioxide and oxygen.

There is only one true membrane oxygenator series that is commercially available in the United States at present, the Medtronic 600, 800 and 1500 oxygenators (Medtronic World Headquarters, 710 Medtronic Parkway, Minneapolis, MN) previously known as the Sci-Med spiral coil membrane oxygenator. This is the oxygenator series of choice for prolonged pediatric perfusion, particularly for extracorporeal membrane oxygenation.

MICROPOROUS MEMBRANES

These oxygenators represent an intermediate design between the true membrane oxygenator and the bubble oxygenator. The membrane is composed of microporous polypropylene, a thermoplastic which does not allow significant diffusion of gas through the membrane itself. However, at the multiple microporous openings, which are 3–5 μm in diameter there is a transient direct interface between gas and blood. Shortly after the commencement of bypass protein deposits build up at the pores, eliminating direct contact at the pores. In addition, the surface tension of the blood relative to the small size of the pores prevents significant movement of blood through the pores into the gas compartment during bypass. Nevertheless after several hours of use a significant amount of serum may have leaked into the gas compartment which leads to deterioration in gas exchange performance with time.[31] Thus hollow fiber oxygenators are not appropriate for long duration perfusion such as extracorporeal membrane oxygenation. Developments in the method for creating pores in the fibers decreased the risk of serum leakage and increased the duration of efficient function of microporous membrane oxygenators.[32] In the past, the pores in the hollow fibers have been created by extrusion of the polypropylene, that is stretching of the fibers results in minute tears which function as the pores. The new 'microphase separation method' results in more uniform pore size with less tendency for the pores to lengthen under stress and therefore a decreased risk of serum leakage.

Another disadvantage of the microporous membrane oxygenator is that gas embolization can occur if negative pressure develops in the blood side of the membrane. Gas may be entrained into the arterial blood through the micropores and could be pumped into the systemic circulation of the patient if an arterial filter is not in use. Negative pressure can develop, for example, if a blood sample is drawn from the oxygenator when clamps have been applied across the inlet and outlet tubing. In theory turning off water flow through a compliant heat exchanger can also result in a negative pressure in the blood compartment through a 'recoil' phenomenon.

There are two basic designs of the microporous polypropylene membrane oxygenator: hollow fiber and folded membrane.

Hollow fiber

There are two types of hollow fiber membrane oxygenator. Either the gas passes within the fibers surrounded by blood, 'blood outside fiber' or less commonly the blood is within the fibers which are surrounded by the gas, 'blood inside fiber'. Problems which have had to be overcome with the latter style of hollow fiber oxygenator have included the higher resistance to blood flow when blood must pass within the lumen of the polypropylene fibers as well as the risk of thrombosis within the fibers. The Terumo Capiox 300 series are oxygenators which apply the 'blood insider fiber' principle.

Commercially available oxygenators that utilize the 'blood outside fiber' principle include the Sorin/Dideco Lilliput 1 & 2 (Cobe Cardiovascular Inc., Arvada, CO), Polystan Micro (Jostra Corp, The Woodlands, TX) and the Terumo Baby Rx (Terumo Cardiovascular Systems, Ann Arbor, MI). These oxygenators have intrinsically less resistance to blood flow but do potentially suffer from the problem of streaming with resultant decrease in the efficiency of gas exchange. Blood may either flow perpendicular to the fiber pathway or parallel to the fibers. With the latter orientation it is usual for the blood to flow in the opposite direction to the gas flow. The construction of the inlet and outlet manifolds is crucial with the 'blood outside fiber' oxygenator in reducing the probability of streaming and yet at the same time avoiding excessive turbulence.

Folded membrane

In these microporous membrane oxygenators the membrane is a flat sheet which is folded to create plates that separate a blood compartment from the gas compartment. The best known version of the folded plate microporous membrane oxygenator for pediatric use was the Variable Prime Cobe Membrane Lung. This was one of the first membrane oxygenators specifically designed for small infants. It was widely used during the late 1980s and early 1990s prior to the introduction of specific neonatal oxygenators. The folded membrane type microporous oxygenator has been superseded by hollow fiber oxygenators.

Heat exchanger design and principles of function

Cardiopulmonary bypass procedures in neonates and infants are likely to involve much greater extremes in temperature than are used in older children and adults. Thus the risks of gas embolism secondary to the changes in gas solubility which occur with temperature change are greater. Fortunately because of the smaller total mass of infants and neonates the total caloric transfer which must be accomplished with pediatric heat exchanging units is less relative to adult units. Nevertheless because of concerns regarding total prime volume it is important in the pediatric setting that the heat exchanging unit does not increase the prime volume.

In the early years of cardiopulmonary bypass, the heat exchanging units in which the perfusate temperature was changed (as distinct from the 'heater/cooler' units which control the water temperature within the heat exchanger) were separate components from the oxygenator. (Heater/cooler units remain separate units from the heat exchanger.) Many different designs of heat exchanger were used, many of them being custom built in hospital workshops. All functioned on the principle of forced convection, i.e. the perfusate was actively pumped through a coil or series of parallel tubes, usually constructed from stainless steel. Surrounding the coil or tubes was water, the temperature of which was controlled often in relatively crude fashion, such as by the addition of ice or warm water. More sophisticated heater/cooler systems had refrigeration compressors and electrical heating coils whereby the water surrounding the perfusate coils could be thermostatically controlled. Many of the early heat exchanging units were quite inefficient and thus patient temperature could be changed only quite gradually.

There were several disadvantages to the nonintegrated heat exchanger. Most important was the difficulty in cleaning and sterilizing these nondisposable units. In addition they had a large prime volume which made them particularly unsuitable for pediatric perfusion. Because there was a considerable pressure drop across many of these units it was necessary to place them on the arterial side of the oxygenator with a significant risk of gas embolism as cold saturated blood was rewarmed. These important difficulties led to the development of the integrated heat exchanger which was incorporated within the disposable oxygenator. In fact there were several advantages to this type of heat exchanger. It was possible to circulate water through the heat exchanging tubes rather than vice versa so that the pressure drop was much less. This allowed the device to be placed on the venous side of the oxygenator, eliminating the problem of gas embolism with warming of cold blood or at least eliminating the oxygenator as a cause of that gas embolism. (It does not eliminate the risk of gas coming out of solution within the patient's own intravascular space if cold blood is rapidly warmed by a still warm patient during the cooling, rather than the rewarming phase of bypass.) Integrated heat exchanging units in which blood passed around rather than through the elements allowed the additional prime volume of the heat exchanger to be eliminated.

Stainless steel is now widely used for the construction of integrated heat exchanging units. Its advantages included superior corrosive resistance and relative tissue compatibility. These advantages are thought to outweigh the disadvantages of poor heat transfer characteristics and increased cost. To maximize efficiency of heat transfer the total surface area of the heat exchanging coil is increased by the addition of fins to the external surface of the heat exchanging coils. Heat exchange is also improved by allowing the blood and water to flow in opposite directions.

More recent design of heat exchangers have moved away from the traditional convoluted tube and fin design towards a flat sheet design folded in much the same way as for a flat sheet gas exchange unit. Blood is allowed to flow past the folds in very thin layers, thereby increasing the interface surface to mainstream layer ratio. These newer devices have improved heat exchanging efficiency so dramatically that it has been possible to greatly reduce the overall size of the unit and thereby significantly reduce priming requirements.

Apart from the physical limitations to the efficiency of the heat exchanging system, there are physiological reasons to limit the rate of heating and cooling. The most important of these as already alluded to is the risk of gas embolism when fully saturated blood is rapidly warmed. Some studies have suggested that limiting the temperature difference between the water from the heater cooler and the venous temperature of the perfusate to 10°C minimizes this problem, though studies at Children's Hospital Boston have not confirmed this.[23] Most membrane oxygenators place the heat exchanger upstream on the venous side of the gas exchanging unit so that the degree of saturation of the blood adjacent to the heat exchanger will be less. It is important that the blood temperature does not exceed 42°C, the temperature at which protein denaturation occurs. This is the maximum water temperature which should be used. Thus as the patient's temperature approaches normothermia there is a decreasing temperature gradient between the perfusate and patient temperature which limits the efficiency of rewarming. Such constraints do not apply during cooling. It is common practice to lower the water temperature as much as possible during the early phase of cooling, often to as low as 4°C. Thus there will be considerably more than a 10°C gradient between the water and blood temperature during the cooling phase. In larger children because of the large specific heat of the body because of its large water content, the temperature of the venous blood returning to the oxygenator will decrease only slowly so that the arterial temperature will generally not be more than 10–12°C less than esophageal. Thus the risk of microgaseous embolus as the perfusate is rapidly warmed upon entering the vascular space should be small. In neonates and infants however this is not the case; thus very rapid cooling does introduce the risk of producing microgaseous emboli as the cold perfusate enters the warm body. This is an area that requires further investigation both clinically and in the laboratory. Other considerations during cooling relate to the shift to the left of the oxyhemoglobin dissociation curve with cooling. This is further exacerbated by the use of an alkalotic pH strategy such as the alpha stat strategy which is currently in widespread clinical use for adults. Studies at Children's Hospital Boston using near infrared spectroscopy suggest that this combination of factors, i.e. hypothermia and alkalinity may contribute to inefficient function of the cytochrome oxidase chain during the cooling phase of bypass prior to circulatory arrest.[33] These laboratory studies as well as clinical studies argue against very rapid cooling.[34]

Heater/cooler units

Various commercial units are available for controlling the temperature of the water perfusing the heat exchanger, e.g. Cincinatti Sub Zero Hemotherm Model 400 MR (Cincinnati, OH) and Sarns Heater/Cooler TCM2 (Terumo Cardiovascular, Ann Arbor, MI). These modern units have the advantage of separate cooling and rewarming chambers so that it is not necessary to rapidly change the temperature of a large reservoir of water when shifting from cooling to warming. It is this latter difficulty which rendered many older model heater/cooler units very inefficient. The preference at Children's Hospital Boston is to use water from wall outlets which is blended in a manually controlled mixing valve and after passing through the heat exchanger is discarded. Although this may on the surface seem inefficient a cost analysis amortizing the costs of heater/cooler units including back up units as well as electrical costs revealed that wall water was in fact a very cost effective method. In addition it has the advantage of rapid response and accurate control.

Specific oxygenators: brands and models

Table 6.4 summarizes the properties of eight oxygenators.

SORIN/DIDECO D901 LILLIPUT 1 WITH TWIN RESERVOIR

The Lilliput 1 has a priming volume of 60 ml and a membrane surface area of 0.34 m^2 (Figure 6.7). This oxygenator has a reference blood flow of 1200 ml/min with a manufacturer recommended blood flow of 800 ml/min. Considering the oxygenator size, we generally limit its use to patients with an expected maximum blood flow rate of 1150 ml/min. The integrated reservoir has a maximum volume of 675 ml, which is a combination of its 425 ml venous reservoir and 250 ml cardiotomy reservoir. Tubing connections on this unit allow for either 1/4-inch or 3/16-inch tubing.

SORIN/DIDECO D902 LILLIPUT 2

The Lilliput 2 has a priming volume of 105 ml and a membrane surface area of 0.64 m^2 (Figure 6.8). This oxygenator has a reference blood flow of 3300 ml/min with a manufacturer recommended blood flow of 2300 ml/min. Considering the heat exchanger efficiency, we generally limit its use to patients with an expected maximum blood flow rate of 2300 ml/min. The integrated hard shell venous and cardiotomy reservoir has a maximum volume of 1800 ml. Tubing connections on this unit are 1/4-inch for the reservoir outlet and oxygenator and 3/8-inch for the reservoir inlet.

COBE OPTIMIN

At Children's Hospital Boston the Cobe Optimin is used for patients between 23 and 55 kg. It has a priming volume of 170 ml with a surface area of 1.0 m^2 and a maximum flow rate of 5.0 liters per minute. The reservoir has a maximum

Table 6.4 *Oxygenator properties*

Oxygenator	Membrane surface area (m^2)	Membrane material	Structure type	Maximum blood flow (l/min)	Rated blood flow (l/min)	Heat exchanger surface area (m^2)	Blood connectors (inches)	Prime volume (ml)	Maximum reservoir volume (ml)
Sorin/Dideco Lilliput 1 D901	0.34	Microporous polypropylene	Hollow fiber	0.8	1.2	0.02	3/16 and 1/4	60	675
Lilliput 2 D902	0.64	Microporous polypropylene	Hollow fiber	2–3	3.3	0.02	1/4, 3/8 venous	105	1800
Cobe Optimin	1.0	Microporous polypropylene	Hollow fiber	5.0		0.1374	3/8	170	2200
Cobe Optima	1.9	Microporous polypropylene	Hollow fiber	8.0		0.1374	3/8 and 1/2 venous	260	4000
Polystan Micro	0.33	Microporous Polypropylene	Hollow fiber	0.8	1.15	0.05	3/16	52	400
Medtronic perfusion system	0.8, 0.8, 1.5	Silicone rubber	Spiral coil membrane envelope		1.0, 1.2, 1.8	None	Vary by unit	90, 100, 175	Uses a bag system
Capiox Baby RX 05	0.5	Polypropylene	Hollow fiber		1.5	0.035	1/4 and 3/16	43	1000
Terumo Capiox SX 10		Polypropylene	Hollow fiber		3.5	0.13	3/8	135	

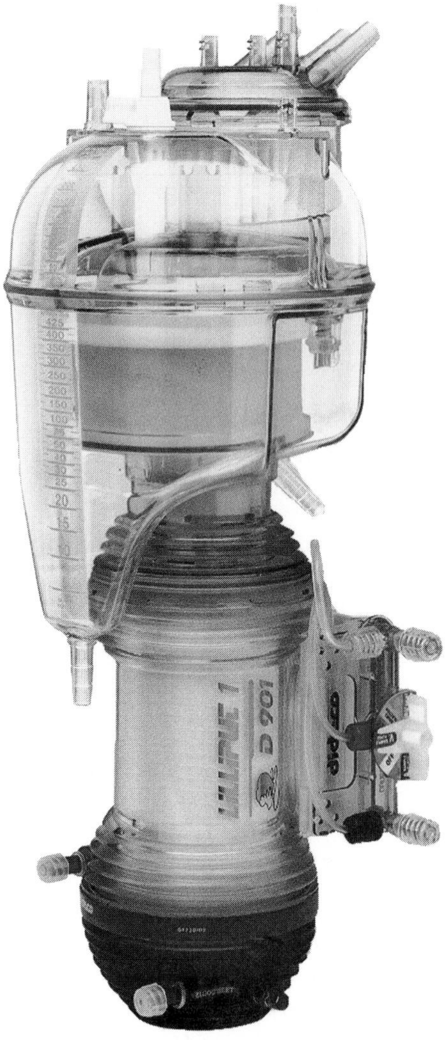

Figure 6.7 *The Sorin/Dideco Lilliput D 901 is an ideal oxygenator for neonates and small infants up to 7.5 kg.*

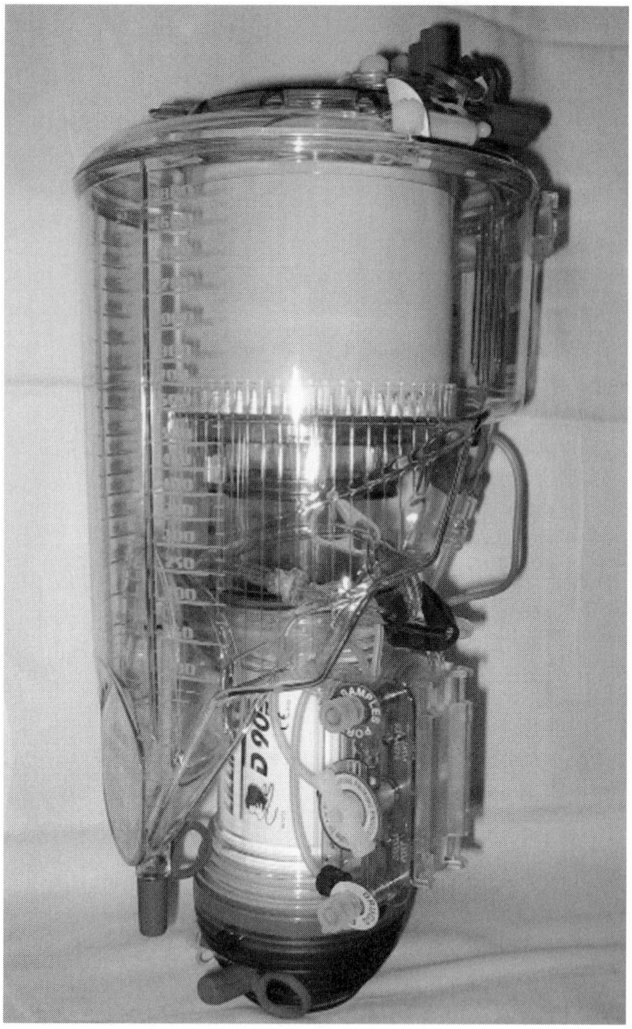

Figure 6.8 *The Lilliput D 902 infant oxygenator can be used for patients up to 23 kg.*

capacity of 2200 ml, a rotating lid and rotating venous inlet for optimum port orientation. The outlet ports on the Optimin are 3/8-inch connections, including the venous connector.

COBE OPTIMA XP WITH HVR/VVR4000i

This is an adult oxygenator that is used at Children's Hospital Boston for all patients that are 55 kg and greater. It has a priming volume of 260 ml, a surface area of 1.9 m^2 and a maximum flow rate of 8.0 liters per minute. The venous reservoir has a capacity of 4000 ml and has a rotating lid for convenient port orientation. It also has a sealed lid and therefore can be used for vacuum assisted drainage.

Other neonatal oxygenators

POLYSTAN MICRO

SAFE MICRO (Jostra Corp, The Woodlands, TX) is a hollow fiber oxygenator with a priming volume of 52 ml and a recommended flow of 800 ml per minute. It incorporates a high efficiency stainless steel heat exchanger with a performance factor of 0.76 at a blood flow of 800 ml per minute. The oxygenator has been specifically designed to provide optimum performance for the neonatal patient with blood inlet and outlet connectors designed to accept either 1/4-inch or 3/16-inch tubing. With top to bottom flow, a totally visible blood flow path and bottom inlet/outlet gas and water connectors, the SAFE MICRO is a convenient and safe oxygenator. We used this oxygenator when it first came to market but discontinued its use when the water pressure ratings for the exchanger were changed. The 400 ml reservoir volume can be a limiting factor for smaller patients who may undergo low flow or circulatory arrest. The dynamics of this reservoir are exceptional. Many centers are currently using the reservoir with the Lilliput 1 oxygenator.

Terumo Baby RX05

This is one of the newest pediatric oxygenators. It has the lowest priming volume at 43 ml. Recommended blood flow is 1500 ml.

The hard shell reservoir has independent venous and cardiotomy filters, a short breakthrough time and a low dynamic priming volume (15 ml). The reservoir is easy to position to allow for shorter tubing lengths for a wide range of setups. It has a storage capacity of 1000 ml.

Infant oxygenator

TERUMO CAPIOX SX10

This pediatric oxygenator has a small dynamic priming volume of 130 ml and a maximum blood flow of 3.5 liters per minute. It has a detachable hard shell reservoir which enhances the versatility of setup with other equipment. The maximum reservoir volume is 1000 ml.

Choosing the best neonatal/infant/pediatric oxygenator

Factors that should influence the final choice of oxygenator include:

- performance specifications including priming volume, heat exchange and gas exchange efficiency
- reliability
- predictability
- ease of setup/use including sufficient number of accessory ports for rapid infusion lines, medication administration, hemoconcentration, additional suckers
- cost.

The final choice as to which oxygenator an institution will use should be made as a joint decision by the perfusion, surgical and anesthesia staff considering the particular needs of their patient population.

REFERENCES

1. Gibbon JH. Application of mechanical heart and lung apparatus to cardiac surgery. *Minn Med* 1954; March:171–85.
2. De Somer F, De Wachter D, Verdonck P, Van Nooten G, Ebels T. Evaluation of different paediatric venous cannulae using gravity drainage and VAVD: An in vitro study. *Perfusion* 2002; **17**:321–6.
3. Humphries K, Sistino JJ. Laboratory evaluation of the pressure flow characteristics of venous cannulas during vacuum-assisted venous drainage. *J Extra Corpor Technol* 2002; **34**:111–14.
4. Darling E, Kaemmer D, Lawson S et al. Experimental use of an ultra-low prime neonatal cardiopulmonary bypass circuit utilizing vacuum-assisted venous drainage. *J Extra Corpor Technol* 1998; **30**:184–9.
5. Horisberger J, Jegger D, Boone Y et al. Impact of a remote pump head on neonatal priming volumes. *Perfusion* 1999; **14**:351–6.
6. Nishida H, Aomi S, Tomizawa Y et al. Comparative study of biocompatibility between the open circuit and closed circuit in cardiopulmonary bypass. *Artif Organs* 1999; **23**:547–51.
7. Morita M, Yozu R, Matayoshi T, Mitsumaru A, Shin H, Kawada S. Closed circuit cardiopulmonary bypass with centrifugal pump for open-heart surgery: new trial for air removal. *Artif Organs* 2000; **24**:442–5.
8. Davila RM, Rawles T, Mack MJ. Venoarterial air embolus: a complication of vacuum-assisted venous drainage. *Ann Thorac Surg* 2001; **71**:1369–71.
9. Jensen E, Andreasson S, Bengtsson A et al. Influence of two different perfusion systems on inflammatory response in pediatric heart surgery. *Ann Thorac Surg* 2003; **75**:919–25.
10. Aldea GS, Soltow LO, Chandler WL et al. Limitation of thrombin generation, platelet activation, and inflammation by elimination of cardiotomy suction in patients undergoing coronary artery bypass grafting treated with heparin-bonded circuits. *J Thorac Cardiovasc Surg* 2002; **123**:742–55.
11. Awad JA, Fortin B, Bernier JP et al. Red blood cell survival after perfusion with a membrane oxygenator. *Am J Surg* 1974; **127**:535–40.
12. Osborn JJ, Cohn K, Hait M et al. Hemolysis during perfusion: sources and means of reduction. *J Thorac Cardiovasc Surg* 1962; **43**:459.
13. Hansbro SD, Sharpe DA, Catchpole R et al. Haemolysis during cardiopulmonary bypass: an in vivo comparison of standard roller pumps, nonocclusive roller pumps and centrifugal pumps. *Perfusion* 1999; **14**:3–10.
14. Leschinsky BM, Itkin GP, Zimin NK. Centrifugal blood pumps – a brief analysis: development of new changes. *Perfusion* 1991; **6**:115–23.
15. Kolff J, Ankney RN, Wurzel D, Devineni R. Centrifugal pump failures. *J Extra Corpor Technol* 1996; **28**:118–22.
16. Gourlay T, Taylor KM. Perfusion pumps. In Jonas RA, Elliott MJ (eds). *Cardiopulmonary Bypass in Neonates, Infants and Young Children.* London, Butterworth-Heinemann, 1994, pp 145–8.
17. Haw MP, Elliott M. Filtration in pediatric cardiac surgery. In Jonas RA, Elliott MJ (eds). *Cardiopulmonary Bypass in Neonates, Infants and Young Children.* London, Butterworth-Heinemann, 1994, p 154.
18. Newburger JW, Jonas RA, Wernovsky G et al. A comparison of the perioperative neurologic effects of hypothermic circulatory arrest versus low flow cardiopulmonary bypass in infant heart surgery. *N Engl J Med* 1993; **329**:1057–64.
19. Gourlay T, Gibbons M, Fleming J, Taylor KM. Evaluation of a range of arterial line filters. Part I. *Perfusion* 1987; **2**:297–302.
20. Gourlay T. The role of arterial line filters in perfusion safety. *Perfusion* 1988; **3**:195–204.
21. Mair P, Hoermann C, Mair J, Margreiter J, Puschendorf B, Balogh D. Effects of a leucocyte depleting arterial line filter on perioperative proteolytic enzyme and oxygen free radical release in patients undergoing aortocoronary bypass surgery. *Acta Anaesthesiol Scand* 1999; **43**:452–7.
22. Baksaas ST, Flom-Halvorsen HI, Ovrum E et al. Leukocyte filtration during cardiopulmonary reperfusion in coronary artery bypass surgery. *Perfusion* 1999; **14**:107–17.
23. Nollert G, Nagashima M, Bucerius J, Shin'oka T, Jonas RA. Oxygenation strategy and neurologic damage after deep hypothermic circulatory arrest. I. Gaseous microemboli. *J Thorac Cardiovasc Surg* 1999; **117**:1166–71.
24. Willcox TW. Vacuum-assisted venous drainage: to air or not to air, that is the question. Has the bubble burst? *J Extra Corpor Technol* 2002; **34**:24–8.
25. Naik SK, Knight A, Elliott MJ. A successful modification of ultrafiltration for cardiopulmonary bypass in children. *Perfusion* 1991; **6**:41–50.

26. Naik SK, Balaji S, Elliott MJ. Modified ultrafiltration improves hemodynamics after cardiopulmonary bypass in children. *J Am Coll Cardiol* 1993; **19**:37.
27. Tassani P, Richter JA, Eising GP et al. Influence of combined zero-balanced and modified ultrafiltration on the systemic inflammatory response during coronary artery bypass grafting. *J Cardiothorac Vasc Anesth* 1999; **13**:285-91.
28. Naik S, Elliott M. Ultrafiltration. In Jonas RA, Elliott MJ (eds) *Cardiopulmonary Bypass in Neonates, Infants and Young Children.* London, Butterworth-Heinemann, 1994, p 160.
29. Wang MJ, Chiu IS, Hsu CM et al. Efficacy of ultrafiltration in removing inflammatory mediators during pediatric cardiac operations. *Ann Thorac Surg* 1996; **61**:651–6.
30. DeWall RA, Bentley DJ, Hirose M, Battung V, Najafi H, Roden T. A temperature controlling (omnithermic) disposable bubble oxygenator for total body perfusion. *Dis Chest* 1966; **49**:207–11.
31. Mottaghy K, Oedekoven H, Starmans H et al. Technical aspects of plasma leakage prevention in microporous membrane oxygenators. *Trans Am Soc Art Organs* 1989; **35**:640–3.
32. Muramato T, Tatebe K, Nogawa A et al. Development of a new microporous hollow fiber membrane for oxygenators. *Jpn J Artif Organs* 1990; **19**:472–5.
33. Sakamoto T, Zurakowski D, Duebener LF et al. Combination of alpha-stat strategy and hemodilution exacerbates neurologic injury in a survival piglet model with deep hypothermic circulatory arrest. *Ann Thorac Surg* 2002; **73**:180–9.
34. Bellinger DC, Wernovsky G, Rappaport LA et al. Cognitive development of children following early repair of transposition of the great arteries using deep hypothermic circulatory arrest. *Pediatrics* 1991; **87**:701–7.

7

Prime constituents and hemodilution

INTRODUCTION

Most cardiac surgeons give little thought to the composition of the prime solution used for the cardiopulmonary bypass circuit. Decisions in this area are usually left to the perfusionists and anesthesiologists who work with the surgeon. Furthermore there has been surprisingly little systematic study of the impact that changes in the prime composition might have on outcomes like fluid accumulation during bypass, subsequent duration of hospitalization or even the risk of death or developmental delay. Not surprisingly the absence of data has resulted in a remarkable variety of approaches being used in different centers. There is no better illustration of this fact than the diversity of approach used for hemodilution.

HEMODILUTION

History of hemodilution

In 1937 John H Gibbon Jr, working in Philadelphia, described the first successful laboratory use of cardiopulmonary bypass to sustain an intact animal.[1] Although considerable thought had been given to the engineering aspects of the pump and oxygenator there was apparently very little deliberation regarding the fluid used to prime the pump.[2] The apparatus was rinsed with two liters of physiological saline after which a 1 : 1000 aqueous solution of the disinfectant metaphen was circulated for 20 minutes before being flushed with a further two liters of saline. The circuit was then primed with heparinized blood obtained from donor animals.[3] By the early 1950s when Gibbon's heart-lung machine was being introduced into clinical practice, the disinfectant was no longer mentioned in papers. However, the circuit was still initially flushed with a physiological saline solution. This aided wetting of the oxygenator screens. The saline was then drained and the entire device was filled with heparinized blood.[4]

Within a short time of Gibbons' report of successful clinical application of the heart-lung machine, Kirklin also described successful clinical application of a pump oxygenator. The prime, like Gibbon's, was whole blood.[5–7] However, as cardiopulmonary bypass became widely applied in the late 1950s many came to recognize the disadvantages of exposing the patient to a large volume of homologous banked blood collected from multiple donors. This problem was particularly apparent in infants and small children whose total blood volume (80 ml × body weight) was very much smaller than the massive priming volumes of early heart-lung machines, which were measured in liters. For example a 10 kg infant was exposed to the equivalent of five total exchange transfusions with the average pump circuit of the late 1950s.

THE HOMOLOGOUS BLOOD SYNDROME

Apart from the risk of blood borne infections such as hepatitis B (more recently including hepatitis C and human immunodeficiency virus), Litwak and Gadboys[8] recognized that the exposure of patients to large volumes of homologous blood was associated with a number of adverse outcomes. It was not uncommon for patients to demonstrate severe pulmonary insufficiency, what was later to be called 'pump lung'. Later this was to be recognized as respiratory distress syndrome, the consequence of multiple factors including exposure to the foreign oxygenator circuit but in addition exposure to a large volume of homologous blood. In some patients multi-organ failure occurred, exacerbated by the presence of sepsis. There is increasing evidence that administration of large volumes of donor blood may alter an organism's immunity, which can increase the risks of systemic sepsis and wound infection. Changes in the immune system may also result in reduced resistance to malignant cell changes and introduce a risk of graft versus host disease, particularly in donor directed transfusion from a parent.

Homologous blood transfusions in the past have also been associated with a 0.2 to 0.5% incidence of anaphylactoid reactions. Improvements in blood banking technology, particularly the removal of white cells as well as the use of reconstituted blood and packed cells has reduced the incidence of these problems. Techniques such as autotransfusion, either by pre-deposited autologous blood or acute preoperative hemodilution have also become widely used in adults.[9] However, pre-deposited blood is not practical for young infants whose small blood volume will not permit removal of an adequate amount of blood. In summary the pressure of multiple factors, most importantly the 'homologous blood syndrome' led to the introduction of hemodilution for cardiopulmonary bypass.

INTRODUCTION OF HEMODILUTION

The first report of successful clinical application of hemodilution for cardiopulmonary bypass was presented by Neptune of Boston at the 1960 meeting of the American Association for Thoracic Surgery.[10] The concept was enthusiastically adopted by many groups, particularly Cooley's group in Texas who soon accumulated a large experience with Jehovah's Witnesses in whom blood transfusion was avoided altogether.[11] By the mid-1960s Kirklin's group at the Mayo Clinic had also stopped using a total blood prime and were using a mixture of 1 liter of 5% glucose with 0.2% sodium chloride in water with concentrated serum albumin plus two liters of blood to make up a total priming volume of approximately three liters.[12] Because there were so many other challenges facing cardiac surgical teams in this era it is perhaps not surprising that much of the experimental work investigating safe limits of hemodilution was not undertaken until well after its widespread clinical application. Furthermore sophisticated methods for assessment of the consequences of hemodilution, for example its influence on cerebral oxygenation, simply were not available.

Physiology of hemodilution

OXYGEN CARRYING CAPACITY

The hemoglobin in red cells allows for remarkably efficient transport of oxygen from the lungs to the cellular mitochondria. It allows transport of very much greater volumes of oxygen by blood than could be carried by dissolved oxygen. In fact the total oxygen content of blood is effectively a linear function of hematocrit.[13,14] Dilution from a normal hematocrit of 40% to a hematocrit of 20% such as is frequently used for cardiopulmonary bypass results in a 50% reduction in total oxygen content. Hemoglobin is not only a remarkable molecule because of the volume of oxygen that it can transport but in addition the oxyhemoglobin dissociation curve allows appropriate pickup or delivery of oxygen according to local conditions. In a more acidotic environment, for example in the capillary bed of a skeletal muscle that is working hard, the oxyhemoglobin dissociation curve is shifted rightward so that oxygen is more freely released. In a more alkaline environment the oxyhemoglobin curve is shifted to the left so that oxygen remains more firmly attached to hemoglobin. Metabolic acidosis, hypercarbia, hyperthermia, and increased 2,3-diphosphoglycerate shift the curve to the right while metabolic alkalosis, hypocarbia, decreased 2,3-diphosphoglycerate and hypothermia shift the curve to the left. Abnormal hemoglobins may have normal, increased or decreased oxygen affinity.[15]

The effect of hemodilution in reducing oxygen delivery to tissues and even limiting oxygen delivery has been studied in mathematical models.[16] Tsai et al[17] developed a model based on the concept that at extreme hemodilution blood is no longer a homogenous continuous source of oxygen at the circulation level, but rather each red cell represents a discrete 'quantum' of oxygen. There is a 'critical cell separation distance' which if exceeded for a given level of oxygen consumption results in cessation of continuous oxygen delivery.[18] Under normal conditions red cell spacing does not affect tissue oxygenation. However, with the decrease in oxygen content accompanying hemodilution the tissue becomes increasingly sensitive to the passage of each quantum of oxygen. Tsai et al[17] demonstrated that nonuniform spacing results in the exposure of red cells to unfavorable gradients for optimal oxygen release. Closely spaced cells experience insufficient gradients while widely spaced cells experience excessive gradients. It is only when cells are perfectly evenly spaced that these deviations are minimized thereby maximizing oxygen release and optimizing tissue oxygenation. In another report, Trouwborst and colleagues[19,20] calculated the 'real arterial oxygen content' defined as the maximum amount of oxygen that can be extracted from hemoglobin before diffusion of oxygen into tissue is compromised and oxygen uptake decreases. This allows for calculation of an 'oxygen extraction ratio' which is the relationship between oxygen consumption and real arterial available oxygen content. Trouwborst also found that another helpful parameter is S35, defined as the saturation of hemoglobin at a PO_2 of 35 mm. He noted that oxygen uptake begins to decline at levels of mixed venous oxygen content of 35 mm or below and that tissue hypoxia may occur when end capillary PO_2 decreases below this level. Trouwborst confirmed that oxyhemoglobin dissociation is influenced by acid-base status, body temperature and red cell 2,3-diphosphoglycerate content. In addition cardiopulmonary bypass per se is accompanied by a leftward shift of oxyhemoglobin dissociation. Although the standard monitoring parameters, i.e. mixed venous oxygen saturation (SvO_2) and oxygen extraction ratio were noted by Trouwborst to be unchanged, nevertheless the S35 was increased as a result of the left shift of oxyhemoglobin dissociation and the consequent decrease in real arterial available oxygen content.

Although the oxygen content of each unit volume of blood is decreased by hemodilution there are a number of compensatory mechanisms that occur in the intact individual not undergoing cardiopulmonary bypass. In fact most laboratory studies of hemodilution have used an anesthetized animal not on bypass. General anesthesia in itself including the muscle relaxation that is employed results in a substantial decrease in oxygen consumption. Even without deliberate cooling to induce hypothermia it is very common for core temperature to decrease somewhat during general anesthesia which further reduces oxygen consumption. Most importantly in the intact animal not on cardiopulmonary bypass there is a compensatory increase in cardiac output which is probably driven in large part by the reduced viscosity which results from hemodilution.

VISCOSITY AND RHEOLOGY

The viscosity of blood is a complex topic. Not only does plasma contain many molecules of various sizes including some with very large molecular weights but in addition it is a suspension of particles including the cellular components of blood as well as chylomicra for lipid transport. Viscosity is defined as shear stress divided by shear rate and is measured in dynes per cm^2 or poise. The shear rate is the velocity gradient which develops between two parallel plates separated by a layer of the fluid under study when a tangential force, defined as *shear stress*, is supplied to one plate. Simple fluids such as water and physiologic saline demonstrate a constant linear increase in viscosity with increasing shear rate. This is even true for plasma despite the complexity of its noncellular elements. These fluids are described as Newtonian. On the other hand blood is nonNewtonian because its viscosity decreases with increasing shear rate. In fact shear rate is the primary determinant of blood viscosity at a given location in the circulation.[21] Thus in the microcirculation where the flow rates are relatively low and therefore shear rate is reduced, blood will be at its most viscous. The complexity of determining the viscosity of blood is complicated by the rheology of the cells which circulate within it. The behavior of a fluid containing a suspension of rigid particles which are nondeformable is more easily predictable. However, deformable nonspherical particles such as red cells change their orientation and shape in response to changes in flow rate. Thus a red cell has a smaller effective particle volume as it aligns with the direction of flow. This contributes to the observation of a decrease in apparent viscosity of blood with increasing shear.[22] On the other hand, aggregation of cells (e.g. rouleaux formation) has an important impact in increasing viscosity. Increased shear per se can result in disaggregation of rouleaux and results in an increase in effective cell concentration.

Shear stress can be transmitted into the interior of red cells causing internal laminar shear and red cell deformation. This property results in a further reduction in the viscous resistance of blood, particularly when passing through a capillary. The associated intracellular flow can supplement oxygen release via intracellular transport of oxyhemoglobin and free oxygen. Any reduction in the ability of red cells to deform can result in changes in flow and oxygen delivery and thus result in cellular damage with spherocytosis being the paradigm. The deformability of red cells is a function of a variety of factors including imposed shear stress, cellular structure and surface area, membrane visco-elastic properties and intracellular viscosity. Despite many statements to the contrary it is interesting that red cell deformability was not demonstrated to be affected by hypothermia in reports from Schmid-Schonbein[23] and Lohrer.[24] In fact Lohrer et al found that red cell deformability and red cell membrane protein composition were unchanged after cardiopulmonary bypass. However, this study was performed at moderate hypothermia so that the findings may not be applicable to deep hypothermia and a long duration of bypass in very young patients. Nevertheless some studies have been done in normal newborns. These studies have demonstrated that the blood of the neonate has the same visco-elastic properties as those observed in adults although mean values for viscosity were higher at all shear rates.[25]

Viscosity in the microcirculation

The architecture of the microcirculation is such that shear rate is highest in capillaries where red cell deformation is needed for cell passage through vessels whose lumina are smaller than the major axis of red cells.[14,26] In vessels smaller than 4 μm in diameter the apparent viscosity of blood increases steeply. This increase in viscosity in small capillaries is especially pronounced if red cell deformability is reduced as is the situation for immature red cells which contain nuclei. In contrast postcapillary venules and veins have the lowest shear rates and thus are the most likely sites of red cell aggregation. Under normal flow conditions the shear rates are relatively high in both pre- and postcapillary segments. However, at low flow rates the lower shear rate in the postcapillary segment (with corresponding higher viscosity) results in an increase in the post- to precapillary resistance ratio with a resulting increase in capillary pressure. This could play a regulatory role in transcapillary fluid exchange and may be relevant to the accumulation of tissue fluid during cardiopulmonary bypass.

Viscosity effects of hemodilution

An exponential relationship exists between hematocrit and the viscosity of blood (Figure 7.1). Variation in imposed shear rate influences this relationship and at lower shear rates more pronounced changes in viscosity result from alterations of hematocrit.[27] Conversely there is a remarkable decrease in the magnitude of change in viscosity with change in shear rate observed at lower hematocrits suggesting that blood becomes more Newtonian in its flow characteristics when dilute.[13,28]

HEMODILUTION, CARDIAC OUTPUT AND PERIPHERAL RESISTANCE

Cardiac output is determined by perfusion pressure and total peripheral resistance. This relationship however is a simplification of the Hagen-Poiseuille equation, i.e.

$$q = \frac{k(p_1 - p_2)r^4}{8\eta l}$$

where q = flow, k is a constant, $p_1 - p_2$ is the pressure drop along a vessel of radius r and length l and η = viscosity.

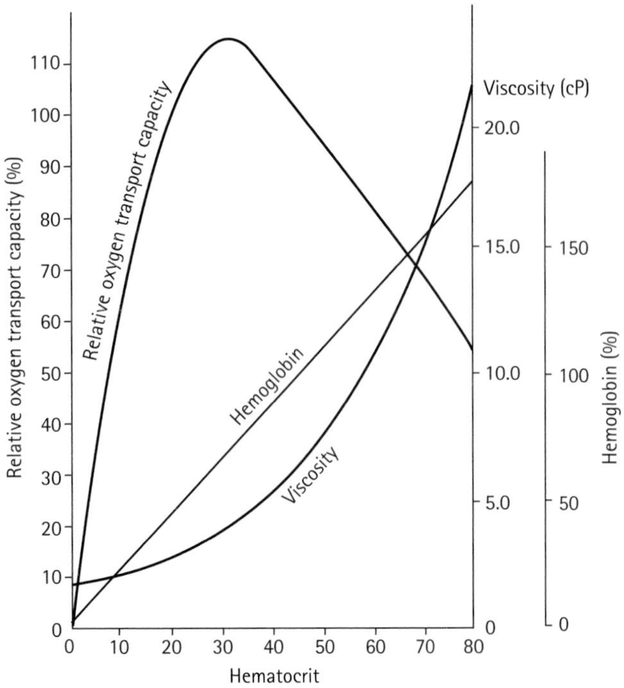

Figure 7.1 *Relationship between hematocrit and apparent viscosity of blood. Because of the exponential relationship between hematocrit and blood viscosity, changes in hematocrit are associated with disproportionate changes in viscosity. This relationship in combination with the linear relationship of oxygen content to hematocrit, results in maximal oxygen carrying capacity at a hematocrit below normal in the intact animal which increases cardiac output in response to hemodilution. This does not apply to the individual on cardiopulmonary bypass. (From Hint H. The pharmacology of dextran and the physiological background for the clinical use of Rheomacrodex and Macrodex.* Acta Anaesthesiol Belg *1968; **19**:119–38, with permission.)*

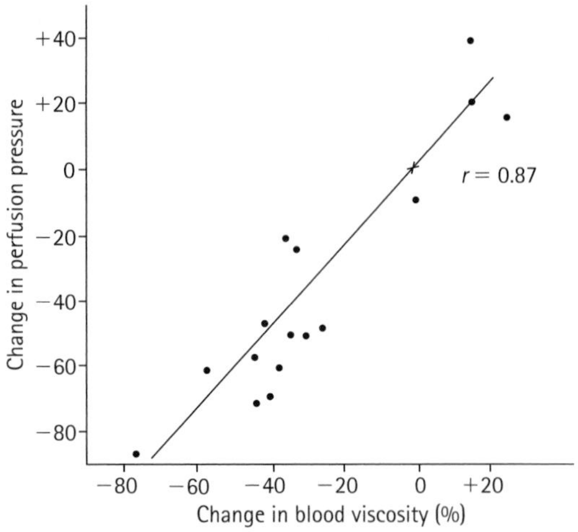

Figure 7.2 *Change in perfusion pressure versus change in viscosity in a series of patients on cardiopulmonary bypass at constant flow rates. (From Gordon et al. Changes in arterial pressure, viscosity and resistance during cardiopulmonary bypass.* J Thorac Cardiovasc Surg *1975; **69**:552–61, with permission.)*

Application of Poiseuille's law to the circulation is limited by the fact that it applies specifically for laminar flow of Newtonian fluids in vessels with rigid walls. However, the relationship draws attention to the important inverse relationship between flow and viscosity. In man the aorta and larger vessels provide little impedance to blood flow while most of the vascular resistance comes from smaller vessels. As vessel diameter decreases shear rate decreases and since blood viscosity is inversely related to shear rate viscosity rises as flow falls. As noted above flow is lowest and viscosity highest in the postcapillary venules.[29]

In the intact individual not on cardiopulmonary bypass hemodilution is associated with an increase in cardiac output. The increase is inversely proportional to hematocrit.[28] as might be predicted from the Hagen-Poiseuille relationship. For example, Bassenge et al[30] demonstrated that an acute decrease in hematocrit from 51% to 13% in conscious dogs was associated with a 93% increase in cardiac output, an 81% increase in heart rate and a 480% increase in coronary blood flow at rest. Under progressive hemodilution when myocardial tissue oxygenation was assessed by measuring coronary sinus effluent PO_2, it was found that myocardial oxygen extraction was virtually complete when the hematocrit reached 25%. This suggested that a further decrease in hematocrit at normothermia would not be fully compensated particularly if a further workload were imposed on the heart. Crystal and Salem[31] reported that although regional blood flow was increased in several organ beds following hemodilution, blood flow was unchanged in the spleen and kidney resulting in a net reduction in oxygen supply in these organs. These results clearly have important implications for the survival of the kidney during cardiopulmonary bypass when there is no compensatory increase in flow rate.

The standard clinical practice of cardiopulmonary bypass does not allow for any increase in perfusion flow rate to compensate for the reduction in total peripheral resistance caused by the reduced viscosity resulting from hemodilution. Thus the most obvious effect of hemodilution is a marked decrease in perfusion pressure at the initiation of bypass. Gordon et al[32] demonstrated that perfusion pressure fell in direct proportion to the change in viscosity resulting from hemodilution (Figure 7.2).

CEREBRAL BLOOD FLOW AND OXYGENATION

There are a number of reports in the stroke literature describing a beneficial effect of hemodilution for the management of cerebral infarcts. For example Hartman et al[33] demonstrated in baboons and subsequently in humans a selective increase in cerebral blood flow to ischemic areas of the brain following hemodilution. The relevance to patients on cardiopulmonary bypass remains unclear because these authors as well as those in many similar reports did not eliminate increased cardiac output as a possible cause for the increased cerebral blood flow seen with hemodilution. Increased cardiac output has been

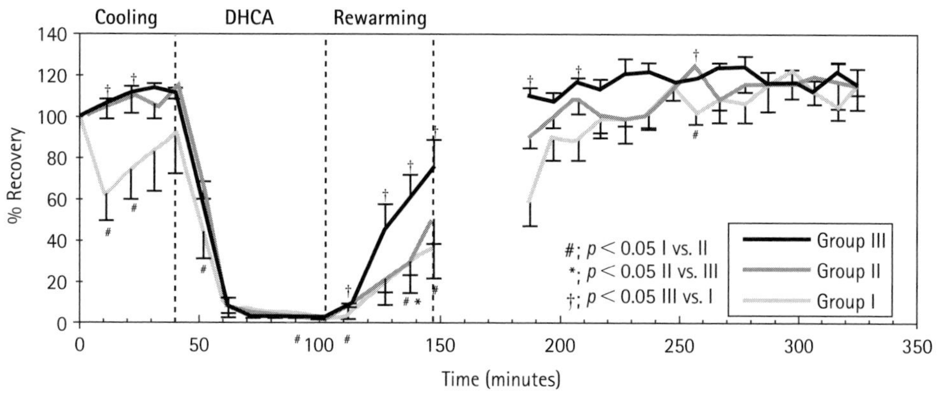

Figure 7.3 *Extreme hemodilution to a hematocrit of 10% (Group I) was associated with a significant decline in cerebral phosphocreatine as measured by magnetic resonance spectroscopy in piglets undergoing cooling to deep hypothermia. Piglets with a hematocrit of 20% (Group II) and 30% (Group III) demonstrated a slight increase in phosphocreatine during cooling. (From Shin'oka et al. Higher hematocrit improves cerebral outcome after deep hypothermic circulatory arrest.* J Thorac Cardiovasc Surg *1996; 112:1610–20, with permission.)*

suggested by others studying a variety of other organs to be of greater importance than rheological changes. The level of hematocrit may affect cerebral vascular reactivity to PCO_2. Using Doppler examinations of the carotid arteries of newborn baboons, Raju and Kim[34] demonstrated that the increase in internal carotid flow velocity in response to increasing PCO_2 was accentuated by a lower hematocrit. The authors postulate three possible explanations for this effect. Firstly the decreased CO_2 buffering capacity associated with a decreased red cell mass resulted in a greater dissolved fraction of CO_2 for a given value of PCO_2. The second explanation is based on Poisseulle's model of steady state flow. Vascular dilation in response to PCO_2 is amplified by the decrease in viscosity associated with hemodilution resulting in a more profound increase in flow. The third possible explanation suggests that endothelial cells may sense varying levels of shear stress. Therefore an increase in viscosity has the effect of increasing sensed shear stress with resulting arterial dilation. Thus decreasing viscosity associated with hemodilution would be expected to lead to arterial constriction.

Piglet study of hemodilution and cerebral oxygenation during circulatory arrest

A study of the cerebral effects of hemodilution was undertaken in 1996 at Children's Hospital Boston[35] using sophisticated techniques for assessment of oxygen delivery to cerebral neurons. Seventeen piglets were randomized into three groups. Group I ($n = 7$) piglets received colloid and crystalloid prime, hematocrit <10%; Group II ($n = 5$) blood and crystalloid prime, hematocrit = 20%; Group III ($n = 5$) blood prime, hematocrit = 30%. All groups underwent 60 minutes of deep hypothermic circulatory arrest at 15°C with continuous magnetic resonance spectroscopy to measure cerebral high energy phosphates and simultaneous near infrared spectroscopy for assessment of cerebral oxygenation. Behavioral recovery was evaluated for four days by a veterinarian who was blinded to treatment assignment. Neurohistological score was assessed after sacrifice on day 4 by an experienced neuropathologist who also was blinded to treatment assignment.

It was found that the extreme hemodilution protocol was associated with evidence of important hypoxic stress during the cooling phase prior to circulatory arrest. There was loss of phosphocreatine (Figure 7.3) and intracellular acidosis. Cytochrome aa3 was more reduced during circulatory arrest in this group relative to the two other groups. The neurological deficit score was best preserved in the high hematocrit group on the first postoperative day although this difference diminished with time. The histological score was worst among the severe hemodilution group. It was concluded that extreme hemodilution during bypass may cause inadequate oxygen delivery during early cooling and that the higher hematocrit achieved with a blood prime is associated with improved cerebral recovery after circulatory arrest.

Hemodilution and plasma proteins

ONCOTIC PRESSURE

Hemodilution results in a decrease in the concentration of circulating plasma proteins and therefore a fall in plasma colloid oncotic pressure. Thus there are many who believe that it is important to add a colloid to the priming solution rather than using a simple crystalloid solution to achieve hemodilution (see below). The fall in plasma colloid oncotic pressure which results from hemodilution plays an important role in the extracellular fluid accumulation that is observed following cardiopulmonary bypass. Tissue edema is in part secondary to the increased capillary permeability which is a manifestation of the systemic inflammatory response caused by cardiopulmonary bypass. However, an accompanying fall in colloid oncotic pressure serves to exacerbate the situation. This appears to be more important in neonates than adults.[36] In an isolated heart model employing immature canine hearts subjected to normovolemic crystalloid hemodilution to a hematocrit of 25% with maintenance of serum osmolarity, differences in response were demonstrated between the immature and mature hearts.[37] The adult group showed no significant change in left ventricular compliance or function after 90 minutes of hemodilution while the puppy group showed a marked decrease in compliance beginning within 30 minutes of the onset of dilution. Electron microscopy demonstrated greater myocardial edema in the puppy group. Although there were no changes in percentage wet weight ratios in either group the authors suggested that there was functionally significant myocardial edema.

COAGULATION FACTORS

Use of any priming solution other than whole blood (including packed cells) results in a reduced concentration of all coagulation factors as well as active platelets. Because cardiopulmonary bypass also activates the fibrinolytic system there is an important risk of increased bleeding because of reduced fibrin formation and increased fibrin breakdown.

IMMUNOGLOBULINS

All of the immunoglobuins including gammaglobulin are reduced by hemodilution which may increase susceptibility to infection. Functional agammaglobulinema, which may persist for over 20 hours, has been described following hemodilution with dextran-60.[28]

In addition to simple hemodilution of immunoglobulins it has been suggested that some of the colloidal agents used in the pump prime can reduce complement activation. For example Bonser et al[38] demonstrated a significant reduction in levels of complement fragments in patients receiving polygeline compared with patients receiving crystalloid or crystalloid with albumin prime.

Clinical application of hemodilution during cardiopulmonary bypass

PRIME VOLUME

The total priming volume is determined by the hardware selected for the circuit to be employed (see Chapter 6). It is important to select a smaller oxygenator that will function at close to its maximal capacity for flow rather than selecting a large oxygenator that will function towards it lower level. One of the most important variables under the control of the surgical and perfusion team is the diameter and length of tubing. With appropriate selection of the venous cannula, height of the table relative to the oxygenator and with appropriate venous drainage characteristics of the oxygenator it is often possible to reduce the diameter of the venous tubing to 3/16-inch in small neonates.

Another important variable in determining the total volume of perfusate is the safety margin with which an individual perfusionist wishes to run the reservoir of the system. Although a more full reservoir allows a longer period of inattention to the level in the reservoir and in that sense provides a greater safety margin for brief periods of inattention by the perfusionist, nevertheless a price is paid in terms of the total perfusate volume to which the patient will be exposed.

HOMOLOGOUS (BANKED) BLOOD REQUIRED FOR PRIMING

A decision must be made initially regarding the desired hematocrit during cardiopulmonary bypass. This is a complex decision that is discussed below (see 'Optimal hematocrit for cardiopulmonary bypass'). When the desired hematocrit has been selected the amount of bank blood that must be added to the prime can be calculated from a simple formula that has been applied for many years:

$$\text{Prime}_{\text{RBC VOL}} = [\text{on-bypass}_{\text{HCT}}] \times [\text{Pt}_{\text{BV}} + \text{Prime}_{\text{BV}}] - [\text{Pt}_{\text{RBC VOL}}]$$

where prime RBC VOL = volume of blood required in prime; on-bypass HCT = desired hematocrit on bypass; Pt BV = patient's calculated blood volume (weight in kg multiplied by 80); prime BV = total priming volume; Pt RBC VOL = Pt BV multiplied by the patient's hematocrit.

If it is necessary to add blood to the prime it should be as fresh as possible. Ideally the blood used for a neonate or infant should be less than 72 hours old though with current testing for viruses this can impose important practical imitations. Therefore the practice at Children's Hospital Boston is to insist upon banked blood that is less than one week old for priming the pump. Fresher units of blood are reserved for transfusion following bypass. There are several reasons for requiring that the blood used for a neonate or infant should be relatively fresh. The level of 2,3-diphosphoglycerate which enhances oxygen availability decreases in stored blood which therefore has a reduced ability to deliver oxygen. The level of various electrolytes and metabolites, particularly potassium, increase outside of the physiological range within 48–72 hours of collection. Fibronectin which is an opsonin of the mononuclear phagocyte system is found in significantly lower levels than normal in blood that is more than 24 hours old.

A number of anticoagulant agents are used for blood storage. Many of these rely on the chelation of calcium by citrate, e.g. citrate phosphate dextrose. It is important to remember that the excess citrate which must be present in banked blood will chelate the patient's own calcium after the onset of bypass. Some groups have 'corrected' this problem by fully heparinizing the unit of blood and then adding calcium to achieve a normal calcium. On the other hand other groups including the group at Children's Hospital Boston believe that there may be advantages in having a lower ionized calcium level during hypothermic bypass (see Chapter 10). Therefore calcium is not corrected until the latter phase of rewarming.

Another approach to avoid citrate is to insist on collection of heparinized blood for neonatal and infant surgery. Some centers in the past have even gone to the extreme of freshly drawn heparinized blood which has never been cooled using a donor who has been pre-screened. However, current medicolegal requirements dictate that all units of blood must be individually tested so that this approach is no longer possible and in any event is of such extreme logistical difficulty that it is difficult to justify. On the other hand some groups continue to use refrigerated (though for less than 48 hours) heparinized blood that has never been exposed to citrate but the logistical challenges for the service's blood bank are immense.

Once again it has been difficult to demonstrate with carefully controlled studies that there are sufficient advantages in this approach and in fact the absence of calcium chelation may be a disadvantage from the point of view of myocardial protection. Many parents of patients undergoing cardiopulmonary bypass focus tremendous attention on the risks of blood transfusion. The current figure that is available from the Red Cross of America regarding the risk of viral transmission from a single unit of blood is 1 in 750 000. This is an exceedingly small risk relative to many of the surgical risks that are faced by the child. Nevertheless it is not uncommon for families to insist upon directed blood donations. Interestingly this has not been shown to reduce the risk of viral transmission. In fact the coercion that may be involved in collecting units of blood from relatives may result in individuals who would not usually volunteer to donate blood doing so in spite of their knowing that they have risk factors which should exclude their donating.

Because the red cells within bank blood are alive and continue to metabolize substrate using the glucose available in the citrate phosphate dextrose solution, there is a progressive development of acidosis within a bank unit of blood. Thus the perfusionist will need to correct the pH of the perfusate using sodium bicarbonate 8.4%.

CRYSTALLOID OR COLLOID

There has been longstanding controversy as to whether the balance of the prime solution other than homologous blood should consist of a crystalloid solution, colloid solution, or a combination of the two. This controversy parallels the controversy that has existed in the trauma literature regarding the management of acute hypovolemia. While colloids theoretically remain within the intravascular space, crystalloid equilibrates rapidly throughout the entire extracellular compartment. Five percent dextrose behaves like free water and equilibrates throughout both intra- and extracellular spaces. There is general agreement that 5% dextrose is inappropriate for volume replacement. However, there is less agreement over a suitable alternative. Proponents of colloid argue that crystalloids fail to maintain an adequate colloid oncotic pressure. The counterargument is that the colloids themselves may leak from capillaries resulting in an increase in interstitial colloid oncotic pressure at the expense of the intravascular pressure. On the other hand supporters of crystalloid reason that in association with reduced intravascular volume the interstitial space is often also depleted and must be replenished. They suggest that the larger volumes required for resuscitation and the concomitant peripheral edema are not harmful.[39] However, there are reports of delayed tissue healing in the presence of edema.[40]

A similar argument over crystalloid versus colloid continues in the setting of the prime solution for cardiopulmonary bypass. The earliest reports of a clear prime describe successful use of 5% dextrose. However, the mortality in these early years of cardiac surgery was extremely high and multiple complications occurred from many sources. Many studies have been done over the years since that time but none has clearly resolved the debate. For example Hoeft et al[41] demonstrated a significant fall in colloid osmotic pressure associated with an increase in extravascular lung water following crystalloid versus colloid prime but this was not reflected in a significant difference in hemodynamic and respiratory states. Hindman et al[42] were unable to demonstrate a difference in brain or renal water content following bypass with an iso-oncotic or hypo-oncotic prime in rabbits. They were, however, able to demonstrate a significant increase in water content of bowel and of smooth muscle.

In adult practice it has been suggested that the increased cost of a colloid prime should result in colloid being reserved for patients with severely compromised ventricular function in whom myocardial edema will be a serious disadvantage. This is substantiated by Foglia et al[43] who showed that a crystalloid prime resulted in marked myocardial edema in adult dogs and was associated with a concomitant reduction in left ventricular compliance and function. The effects were equivalent to one hour of aortic cross clamping with topical hypothermia.

Children appear to derive at least some benefit from a colloid containing prime. Haneda et al[44] studied children undergoing repair of transposition and demonstrated a positive fluid balance during bypass of over 63 ml/kg in infants who had received a crystalloid prime versus 16 ml/kg in those who had a blood/plasma prime. This was associated with a reduction in the length of time in the intensive care unit by 50% as well as a lower mortality.

In general there is a consensus today that crystalloid solutions used for priming the cardiopulmonary bypass circuit for children should not contain dextrose or lactate. The adverse effects of hyperglycemia during bypass pertain not only to the osmotic effects of glucose drawing water from the cells and increasing extracellular fluid but also to the risk of worsening neurological injury. Hyperglycemia should be avoided particularly when hypothermic circulatory arrest is to be used. It is important to remember that the citrate phosphate dextrose storage solution used for homologous banked blood also contains quite high levels of gluose which may importantly elevate the perfusate glucose level.

At Children's Hospital Boston the crystalloid solution which is currently used for priming the circuit is Plasmalyte A (Baxter Healthcare Corp, Deerfield, IL).

Colloids available for prime solutions

Albumin is an important natural colloid. It represents only half of the total plasma protein yet under normal conditions it contributes almost 80% of the intravascular colloid osmotic pressure.[45] Unlike many other colloidal agents, albumin has a uniform molecular size with a molecular mass of 69 kDa. Commercially available human albumin is derived from donated blood by a process of fractionation and/or by plasmapheresis. The albumin solution requires the addition of stabilizing agents before undergoing pasteurization to eliminate the risk of blood-borne infection. Human albumin solution is available as a standard 4.5% concentration with a colloid osmotic pressure similar to plasma or as more concentrated forms which are 10 or 20% solutions and are hyperoncotic.

Gelatin solutions have been widely used in Europe for cardiopulmonary bypass priming. Gelatin is a breakdown product of collagen. The resulting molecules are linked either by succinylation or by urea-linkage, eg. Haemaccel (Beacon Pharmaceuticals, Tunbridge Wells, UK). In common with all the synthetic colloids the gelatins consist of molecules with a wide range of molecular mass averaging around 35 kDa. It is important to note that Haemaccel contains calcium and when given with citrated blood can cause clotting. In common with other synthetic colloids the gelatins have a small risk of anaphylactic reaction.[46]

Hydroxyethyl starches are derived from the maize starch amylopectin. The fundamental structure is similar to glycogen, with D-glucose units linked by $\alpha 1$–4 linkages with $\alpha 1$–6 branch points roughly every 12 glucose units. Amylopectin is readily broken down by hydrolysis by amylase. The product can be stabilized by hydroxyethylation with ethylene oxide. The greater the degree of substitution of hydroxyethyl groups the more resistant is the molecule to degradation and therefore the longer does it survive within the circulation and the body.

Hetastarch (Hespan, Du Pont Pharmaceuticals, Wilmington, DE) has a high degree of substitution with seven hydroxyethyl groups for every ten glucose units. Because of the high degree of substitution Hetastarch persists for a long time, both intravascularly and within the body. This extended survival is due to uptake of the very large molecules by macrophages within the reticuloendothelial system where they do not appear to have any adverse effects on reticuloendothelial cell function.

Pentastarch ((Viastarch) Laevosan-Gesellschaft, Linz, Austria) is also available with five hydroxyethyl groups per 10 of glucose. Although this compound still has a large range of molecular sizes, from less than 50 to 1000 kDa, most are within the range of 100–300 kDa, following elimination of the huge molecules with a mass greater than 1000 kDa. This gives the compound the advantage of a shorter persistence within the body but with a similar efficacy to Hetastarch. By diafiltering Pentastarch a new compound, Pentafraction, has been made. This has no molecules with a molecular weight less than 100 kDa. Preliminary animal work with this fluid suggests that its use is associated with a reduction in capillary leak.

Dextrans, like the hydroxyethyl starches, are also modified polysaccharides. The parent molecule, which is composed of branched glucose residues, is synthesized by the bacterium *Leuconostoc mesenteroides*. Dextrans of different molecular weight distributions are produced by acid hydrolysis of this compound.[47] Similar to the hydroxyethyl starches, their retention within the bloodstream is largely dependent on their molecular weight. The two most commonly encountered dextrans are dextran 40 (molecular mass 40 kDa) and dextran 70 (molecular weight 70 kDa).

Although the dextrans are effective plasma expanders they have fallen out of favor because of a high incidence of unwanted side effects including allergic reactions, red cell aggregation and an interaction with the coagulation system. Like the hydroxyethyl starches the dextrans potentiate von Willebrand's disease and may produce a mild coagulopathy when given in large doses in patients with previously normal clotting.[48]

Fresh frozen plasma and whole blood: It is important to remember that the plasma which is added to the prime when whole blood is used or if red cells are reconstituted with fresh frozen plasma provides an important priming load of colloidal protein. Not only does the plasma contain a considerable quantity of albumin but in addition the coagulation factors will be less diluted relative to using other colloids.

ULTRAFILTRATION

Ultrafiltration is a particularly helpful technique which allows maintenance of a desired hematocrit during cardiopulmonary bypass or in the case of modified ultrafiltration allows hemoconcentration of the patient's blood volume following cardiopulmonary bypass. Negative pressure applied to the ultrafilter results in fluid being drawn through a microporous membrane. The molecules which will be withdrawn in the ultrafiltrate vary according to the pore size of the particular ultrafilter.

Conventional ultrafiltration

Conventional ultrafiltration was first described by Romagnoli et al[49] who described the use of ultrafiltration to concentrate blood in the heart-lung machine. This technique continues to be widely applied in pediatric cardiac surgery. There are numerous sources of fluid that enter the bypass circuit during a cardiac surgical procedure including cardioplegia solution, irrigation solution, iced saline lavage for topical cooling and even the crystalloid used to wet the surgeon's hands during knot tying. Although the patient's own renal function will to some extent eliminate this additional fluid, ultrafiltration allows a specific hematocrit to be achieved. Usually the ultrafilter is placed in a parallel circuit to the patient circuit and a small amount of blood is continuously circulated through the ultrafilter while conventional bypass is ongoing (see Chapter 6). Conventional ultrafiltration can also be applied during a period of circulatory arrest or pre-bypass to concentrate the prime to a desired hematocrit.

Modified ultrafiltration

The technique of modified ultrafiltration was introduced by Elliott at Great Ormond Street and is widely applied at many centers. Figure 7.4 illustrates the setup for modified ultrafiltration. Basically blood is drawn out of the arterial cannula from the patient and is passed through the ultrafilter and returned to the patient through the venous line. Blood is also drawn simultaneously from the oxygenator so that the blood remaining within the reservoir and oxygenator is also hemoconcentrated. Application of modified ultrafiltration for 10–20 minutes after bypass can allow the patient's hematocrit to be increased, for example, from a hematocrit of 25% during bypass to a hematocrit of 40% post-bypass.

Numerous beneficial effects have been reported for modified ultrafiltration including a documented increase in cardiac output, as well as removal of numerous inflammatory products of cardiopulmonary bypass. On the other hand there is a potential risk for technical mishap because of the relative complexity of the procedure including entrainment of air from the aortic cannula. In addition the patient must remain heparinized in the operating room for the additional time that is required. At Children's Hospital Boston modified ultrafiltration is not used. The current technique involves use of a high hematocrit (30–35%) during cardiopulmonary bypass that is maintained by aggressive application of conventional ultrafiltration. During the latter phases of rewarming the hematocrit is increased to even greater than 35%, thereby negating the need for post-bypass modified ultrafiltration.

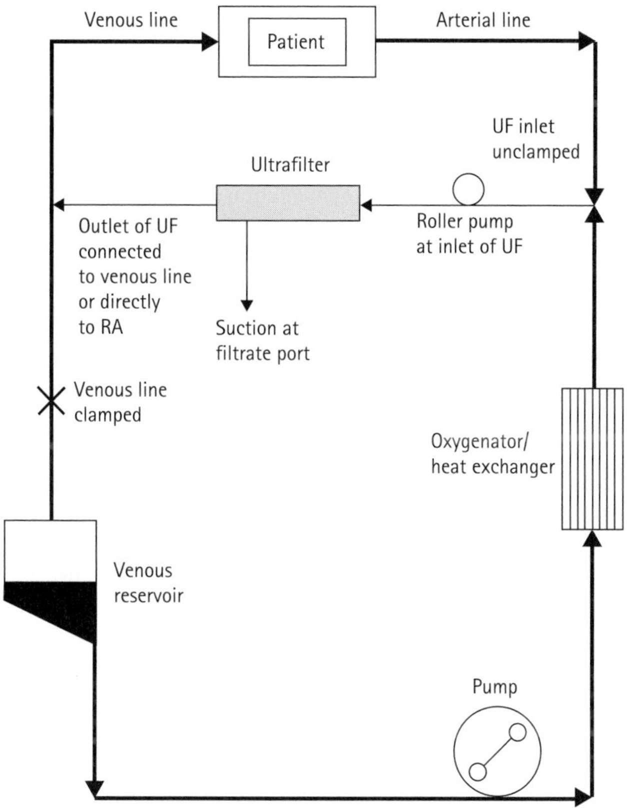

Figure 7.4 *Circuit set up for the technique of 'modified ultrafiltration' as originally described by Elliott. Blood is drawn from the patient through the arterial cannula, is then passed through the ultrafilter (UF) and returns to the patient through the venous cannula. The perfusate within the bypass circuit is also ultrafiltered. (From Jonas RA, Elliott M (eds).* Cardiopulmonary Bypass in Neonates, Infants and Young Children. *London, Butterworth-Heinemann, 1994, with permission.)*

HEMATOCRIT LEVEL DURING CARDIOPULMONARY BYPASS

Optimal hematocrit

The decision regarding selection of an optimal hematocrit during cardiopulmonary bypass is clouded by the large number of reports describing studies which have investigated the optimal hematocrit for nonbypass situations. For example, Hint et al[13] demonstrated an exponential fall in viscosity with a fall in hematocrit while the fall in oxygen transport capacity was almost linear. As viscosity falls, peripheral resistance falls and cardiac output increases. This relationship led Crowell and Smith[50] to suggest that an optimum hematocrit is 27.5%. Messmer et al[28] suggested that oxygen transport peaks at a hematocrit of approximately 30% but noted that there was very little decline in reducing the hematocrit to 25%. As discussed above under 'physiology of hemodilution' the situation during cardiopulmonary bypass is totally different from the nonbypass situation in that it is rare that perfusion flow rate is increased to compensate for the decrease in oxygen transport capacity. The literature in this area is quite vague but implies that the combination of reduction of metabolic rate by anesthesia and hypothermia is more than adequate to compensate for the reduced oxygen carrying capacity of dilute blood and presumably therefore no increase in flow rate is necessary. These statements have usually been predicated on the observation that patients 'appear' to be able to 'tolerate' even very low levels of hematocrit without obvious neurological or other consequences. However, studies from Children's Hospital Boston have suggested that the reduced oxygen carrying capacity of dilute blood may be responsible for cognitive declines that have been observed in children undergoing both atrial septal defect closure as well as repair of more complex anomalies (see below).

A number of texts have recommended and it is common clinical practice that a lower hematocrit is employed when there is a greater degree of hypothermia. It is important to remember, however, that in the early phase of bypass the brain is still warm and has a normal high metabolic rate. Thus although the chosen hematocrit may be acceptable for the target temperature nevertheless injury may occur in the early phase of cooling when the metabolic rate is still high and oxygen delivery is limited. This speculation has been confirmed by numerous laboratory studies at Children's Hospital Boston which have demonstrated by magnetic resonance spectroscopy and near infrared spectroscopy that the early phase of cooling is a period when the brain is particularly at risk for injury.[35,51,52] Although general clinical practice has been to maintain a higher hematocrit for higher temperature bypass (e.g. hematocrit goal equal to the target temperature) an exception to this rule has often been made for simple short procedures such as atrial septal defect closure.

In this setting it has been thought important to avoid any homologous blood transfusion and therefore very low hematocrit levels have been accepted. This has been condoned by laboratory studies by Cook and others,[53–55] which suggest that a hematocrit level even as low as 12% may be safe during cardiopulmonary bypass. This practice may be the explanation for the unexpected finding of a retrospective clinical study of developmental outcome in children who underwent atrial septal defect closure at Children's Hospital Boston either by interventional catheter device closure or surgical closure.[56] The surgical patients were found to have a significantly lower developmental outcome. The only perfusion parameter which approached significance as a predictor of worse developmental outcome was lower hematocrit.

Interaction of hematocrit with pH, temperature and flow rate

It is unlikely that that there is a single optimal hematocrit that suits all patients irrespective of the other conditions of cardiopulmonary bypass. As discussed above under 'Physiology of hemodilution' there are numerous factors other than hematocrit which influence oxygen delivery.[57] Laboratory studies conducted at Children's Hospital Boston have confirmed the important interaction of hematocrit, pH, temperature and flow rate. These studies are discussed in greater depth in Chapter 9. However, in summary the studies have demonstrated that the reduced oxygen carrying capacity of hemodilute blood can be compensated for to some extent by an increased flow rate, reduced temperature or more acidotic pH. However, once again it is important to emphasize that the temperature to be considered should be the maximal temperature experienced at the target hematocrit rather than the minimum temperature.

SUMMARY

Considerable work remains to be done both with clinical studies as well as laboratory studies to define the optimal hematocrit for specific conditions of cardiopulmonary bypass for an individual patient. Until such information is available the current clinical practice at Children's Hospital Boston is to aim for a hematocrit of approximately 30–35% for the majority of patients on bypass.

Minimal acceptable hematocrit

By far the most influential paper that has been widely cited as establishing the minimal acceptable hematocrit on cardiopulmonary bypass was the report by Kawashima et al in 1974.[58] Using a canine model it was found that systemic oxygen consumption was maintained until the hematocrit was diluted below 20%. More recent studies by Cook et al have suggested that so long as the hematocrit is maintained above 9–14%, oxygen delivery is maintained during normothermic bypass.[54,55] It is important to note that these latter studies compensated for the reduced perfusion pressure resulting from hemodilution by an increase in pump flow rate to almost double the normal flow rate. As discussed above under the 'Physiology of hemodilution', a study at Children's Hospital Boston in piglets demonstrates that hemodilution to a hematocrit of 10% during hypothermic bypass caused inadequate oxygen delivery during early cooling and a hematocrit of 30% was associated with improved cerebral recovery after deep hypothermic circulatory arrest both in terms of behavioral recovery as well as histological outcome.[35] A further study from Children's Hospital Boston reported in 1998 by Shin'oka et al studied the relative influence of reduced hematocrit and reduced oncotic pressure in causing the worse outcome noted with a hematocrit of 10%.[51] This study suggests that many of the disadvantages of hemodilution can be overcome by use of a colloidal agent such as pentafraction. Furthermore a higher oncotic pressure on bypass and/or a higher hematocrit produces an improved outcome relative to post-bypass modified ultrafiltration. However, only a higher hematocrit of 30% resulted in optimal cerebral oxygenation before and during one hour of hypothermic circulatory arrest. Many previous reports have suggested that hemodilution is important to counteract the microcirculatory disturbances that occur during deep hypothermia. Bjork and Hultquist[59] were the first to suggest that neurological injury after deep hypothermic circulatory arrest was a result of microcirculatory obstruction. However, until a recent study was conducted at Children's Hospital Boston in which the cerebral microcirculation was directly observed during deep hypothermic bypass there were no reports confirming this speculation.[60] In fact the intravital microscopy study using a piglet model demonstrated not only that higher hematocrit did not impair cerebral microcirculation but hemodilution to a hematocrit of 10% was associated with delayed reperfusion relative to a hematocrit of 30%.

Prospective clinical trial of hematocrit

A single center prospective randomized clinical trial of hematocrit during hypothermic bypass was undertaken at Children's Hospital Boston between 1997 and 2000.[61] There were 147 patients, 74 of whom were assigned to the lower hematocrit strategy (target hematocrit 20%, hematocrit achieved 21.5% ± 2.9%) and 73 were assigned to a higher hematocrit strategy (target hematocrit 30%, hematocrit achieved 27.8 ± 3.2%). It was found that the lower hematocrit group had a lower nadir of cardiac index in the first 24 hours postoperatively ($p = 0.02$) (Figure 7.5a), higher serum lactate 60 minutes after cardiopulmonary bypass ($p = 0.03$), and greater percent increase in total body water on the first postoperative day ($p = 0.006$). Blood product usage and adverse events were similar in the two groups. At one year the lower hematocrit group had worse scores for their psychomotor development index (PDI, a measure of motor skills) (81.9 ± 15.7 versus 89.7 ± 14.7, $p = 0.008$) (Figure 7.5b), as well as more PDI scores at least two standard deviations below population mean (29% versus

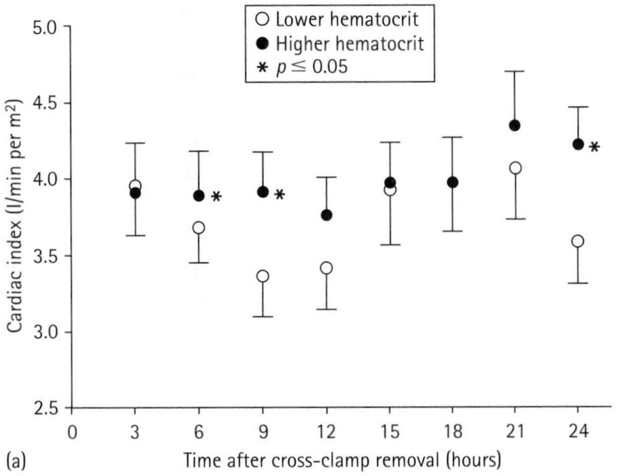

(a)

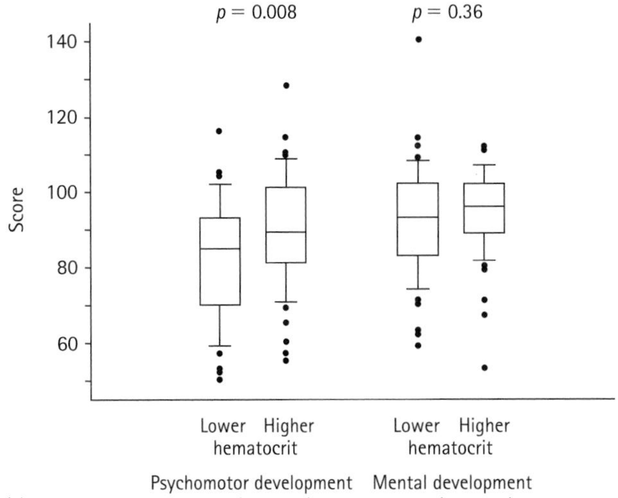

(b)

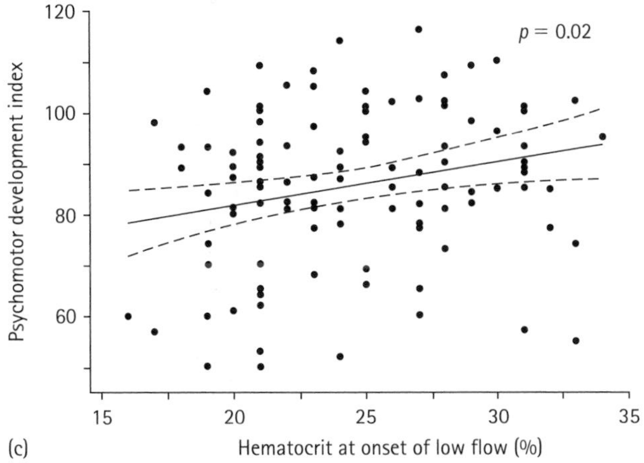

(c)

Figure 7.5 *Results of a randomized prospective clinical trial of lower hematocrit (21.5%) versus higher hematocrit (27.8%) at Children's Hospital Boston. (a) Use of a higher hematocrit (closed circles) was associated with a significantly higher cardiac index at 6 and 9 hours after cross-clamp removal compared with lower hematocrit (open circles). (b) Developmental assessment at one year of age demonstrated a significantly higher psychomotor development index (a measure of motor skills) in patients managed with a higher hematocrit ($p = 0.008$). (c) Analysis using hematocrit as a continuous variable demonstrated a significant association between higher Psychomotor Development Index at one year of age and higher hematocrit during cardiopulmonary bypass.*

9%, $p = 0.01$) which could be classified as developmental delay. Analyses using hematocrit as a continuous variable showed results similar to the intent to treat analyses (Figure 7.5c). This very important study casts considerable doubt on the long held assumption that a hematocrit of 20% is a safe minimal acceptable hematocrit during cardiopulmonary bypass. It is important to note that the pH strategy used during this study was the pH stat strategy. Because of the interaction of hematocrit and pH[57] it is likely that for patients undergoing hypothermic bypass with the alpha stat strategy an even higher minimum hematocrit could result in cognitive decline. It seems reasonable to speculate that the pervasive cognitive deficits observed in adults following cardiopulmonary bypass[62] may at least in part be a consequence of inadequate oxygen delivery secondary to excessive levels of hemodilution. This is not to minimize the important role that microembolization of atheromatous and calcific debris has in causing cognitive deficits in adults which have been widely studied.[63]

In summary and based on the results of the randomized clinical study from Boston it seems reasonable to consider a hematocrit of 25% to be the minimal acceptable hematocrit for any cardiopulmonary bypass conditions. Ongoing studies which include a prospective randomized comparison of hematocrit 25% with hematocrit 35% which is being conducted at Children's Hospital Boston may define an even higher minimal acceptable hematocrit.

ADDITIVES TO THE PRIME OTHER THAN DILUENTS

Anticoagulants

HEPARIN

The discovery in 1916 by Mclean[64] of the anticoagulant heparin from liver extract (hence the name) was an essential prelude to the introduction of cardiopulmonary bypass. Just as important was the discovery by Chargaff and Olson[65] in 1937 that heparin could be neutralized by the peptide protamine. Heparin itself is a polysaccharide that is stored in mast cells. Its role in normal physiology is unclear and should not be confused with the important role of heparan, a related glycose aminoglycan which is attached to endothelial cell membranes and plays an important role in the antithrombogenic property of normal vascular surfaces. The mechanism of action of heparin is to inhibit thrombin by potentiating the activity of the naturally circulating antithrombin factor ATIII. The standard method for monitoring the activity of heparin is to use the activated clotting time (ACT). This is a convenient test that can be performed by the perfusionist. A small quantity of blood is added to a tube containing either diatomaceous earth (celite) or kaolin as the activating agent. A normal ACT before heparin administration is in the region of 130 seconds. Most centers believe that ACT should be maintained at greater than 400 seconds during cardiopulmonary bypass in order to minimize the risk of disseminated intravascular coagulation caused by exposure of coagulation factors to the foreign surfaces of the bypass circuit. (If aprotinin is in use it is important to use kaolin as the activating agent and not the standard celite tubes.) In the case of extracorporeal membrane oxygenation, a lower ACT level can be maintained, generally in the region of 200 seconds. For ventricular assist devices even lower ACT levels are used in clinical practice, e.g. 180 seconds. There are a number of methods for directly assessing heparin concentration in order to allow for a more rational decision regarding the dosage of protamine that should be administered for reversal of heparin at the termination of cardiopulmonary bypass. Nevertheless many centers continue to administer a standard dosage of 4 mg/kg in order to reverse any circulating heparin. It is important to note that heparin is metabolized during cardiopulmonary bypass so that the perfusionist must regularly measure the ACT level to ensure that it is being maintained at greater than 400 seconds. Heparin resistance, i.e. the need for a greater than normal dose of heparin, 4 mg/kg, in order to maintain an ACT level above 400 seconds can be caused by numerous factors as described by Gravelee et al.[66] Another problem with heparin is heparin induced thrombocytopenia, 'HIT'. This syndrome occurs after more than five days of heparin administration and usually does not become apparent for at least nine days. It is most likely immune mediated and results in thrombocytopenia. Somewhat paradoxically this syndrome can result in thrombosis and disseminated intravascular coagulation.

OTHER ANTICOAGULANT AGENTS

A number of other agents have been investigated as possible alternatives to heparin including hirudin and ancrod derived from the Malayan pit viper. Although some studies have reported promise with hirudin in particular neither of these agents has been studied in large clinical trials despite the fact that they have been available for many years. Platelet inhibitors such as prostacyclin have also been studied. Longmore et al[67] added prostacyclin to dogs undergoing cardiopulmonary bypass. The theoretical advantage that prostacyclin would protect platelets was confirmed by this study in that both the platelet count and function were improved. However, Disesa et al found that the severe hypotension secondary to the vasodilation induced by prostacyclin negated any beneficial effect of platelet preservation.[68]

In addition to the systemic use of heparin a number of agents have been studied that are coated on the internal surface of the bypass circuit. Coated circuits allow a lower dose of heparin to be employed. Some studies have suggested that heparin may be completely eliminated if all components of the circuit including the cannulas and oxygenator are coated. Some recent clinical reports have suggested an improved outcome as well as a reduced level of inflammatory mediators when coated circuits are employed.[69]

Procoagulants

APROTININ

Aprotinin is a serine protease inhibitor that has been available for many years. It was traditionally used to reduce the systemic inflammatory response associated with pancreatitis. Its effectiveness in reducing blood loss after cardiopulmonary bypass was noted serendipitously during a trial which was being undertaken to investigate the potential for aprotinin to reduce the inflammatory response to cardiopulmonary bypass.[70] The procoagulant mechanism of aprotinin is not fully understood and is almost certainly complex involving both the coagulation cascade and the fibrinolytic system as well as preservation of platelet activity. Although aprotinin is most effective when administered as a bolus before cardiopulmonary bypass with continuous infusion during bypass as well as post-bypass it is also quite effective when begun postoperatively in the patient who has excessive bleeding post-bypass. There is no question that aprotinin is particularly effective in improving hemostasis in the neonate and young infant following cardiopulmonary bypass. In fact, its effectiveness is so great that there is a significant risk of unwanted thrombosis following its use. For this reason it is wise to avoid aprotinin for procedures that involve placement of small caliber Gortex shunts, e.g. the Norwood procedure or manipulation of the coronary arteries, e.g. the arterial switch procedure or reimplantation of an anomalous coronary artery. Hemostasis can almost always be successfully secured using the methods described in detail in Chapter 2 while acute thrombosis of a shunt or coronary artery is a life threatening problem.

ANTIFIBRINOLYTIC AGENTS

There are a number of antifibrinolytic agents available, most of which have been demonstrated to have similar efficacy. ε-Amino caproic acid (Amicar) is the cheapest of these agents. Like aprotinin it is preferable to commence infusion of an antifibrinolytic agent before cardiopulmonary bypass and to continue infusion through the bypass period as well as for several hours post-bypass. Antifibrinolytic agents are a helpful supplement for hemostasis in complex reoperative patients where bleeding can be expected from large areas of raw surface. However, there is a risk of unwanted thrombosis. It is probably wise for example to avoid an antifibrinolytic agent in a patient undergoing a fenestrated Fontan procedure where there may be an increased risk of thrombosis of the fenestration or even of the entire lateral tunnel or extracardiac conduit though this could not be proven by a study at Children's Hospital Boston.[71]

Anti-inflammatory agents

APROTININ

Aprotinin is effective as an anti-inflammatory agent as well as being procoagulant. The original studies during which aprotinin was discovered to be pro-coagulant did in fact confirm the hypothesis that aprotinin would reduce some markers of inflammation,[72] though in a more recent study there was no effect of aprotinin on complement activiation.[73] There is at least anecdotal evidence that suggests that aprotinin also helps to reduce capillary permeability in neonates and young infants undergoing cardiopulmonary bypass and may therefore accelerate the early postoperative course. Once again, caution should be observed because of the increased risk of unwanted thrombosis in neonates undergoing specific procedures such as a Norwood procedure or arterial switch.

CORTICOSTEROIDS

Corticosteroids have been used in the pump prime at many centers for many years for their anti-inflammatory activities. It is felt that capillary permeability and therefore postoperative edema is reduced. At Children's Hospital Boston, methylprednisolone (Solumedrol) 30 mg/kg is added to the pump prime for all neonatal and infant procedures. Ungerleider's group has extensively studied the timing of steroid administration and has found that administration at least 12 hours preoperatively is beneficial relative to administration in the pump prime.[74] In their preliminary clinical studies, however, this beneficial effect did not translate to earlier extubation or earlier discharge from hospital. Nevertheless more extensive clinical trials are indicated.

Vasoactive agents

VASODILATORS

Many centers believe firmly in the importance of adding a vasodilating agent such as a short acting alpha-blocker, phentolamine, or a longer acting alpha-blocker such as phenoxybenzamine.[75] The scientific basis for this approach has not been well validated for standard cardiopulmonary bypass. Nevertheless when deep hypothermia with circulatory arrest is employed it is clear from clinical experience that intense vasoconstriction can result in delayed warming and large temperature gradients. Laboratory studies at Children's Hospital Boston suggest that endothelial dysfunction may result from the ischemia imposed by circulatory arrest. This was apparent using direct observation of the cerebromicrocirculation by intravital microscopy.[60] In another study infusion of a nitric oxide inhibitor L-NAME which causes intense vasoconstriction resulted in severe cerebral injury following circulatory arrest as determined by magnetic resonance spectroscopy.[76] On the other hand administration of the nitric oxide precursor L-arginine resulted in an improved outcome determined by magnetic resonance spectroscopy. Nitric oxide donors such as nitroglycerin and nitroprusside are also widely employed during cardiopulmonary bypass in order to improve the uniformity of both cooling and rewarming, particularly when deep hypothermia is employed.

VASOCONSTRICTORS

Vasoconstrictors are mentioned only to warn of their disadvantages in the pediatric patient. In the adult patient undergoing cardiopulmonary bypass there are frequently stenoses within the carotid arteries as well as the cerebrovascular tree. The hypotension which results from hemodilution can result in distribution of flow away from downstream watershed areas beyond stenoses. Thus in the adult patient it is reasonable to use a vasoconstricting agent such as phenylephrine to maintain perfusion pressure and to counteract the hypotensive effects of hemodilution.[77] However, in the child who is free of vascular disease and who is more likely to be exposed to deep hypothermia with or without circulatory arrest, a vasoconstrictor will simply exacerbate the problem of vascular spasm that may occur. Therefore vasoconstrictors should be strongly avoided for the pediatric patient on cardiopulmonary bypass and should certainly never be added to the pump prime.

Diuretics

MANNITOL

Mannitol has been a traditional additive to the bypass prime for many years. There are several reasons for this. Mannitol is a potent osmotic diuretic. As early as 1964 Schuster[78] demonstrated that dogs undergoing cardiopulmonary bypass had fewer casts and other cellular debris in their kidneys following introduction of 1.5 g/kg of mannitol. Mannitol is also a free radical scavenger which may play a role in the reduction of reperfusion injury.[79] Finally mannitol has also been shown to be beneficial for ischemic myocardium by improving resting coronary blood flow and subendocardial flow and reducing cell size to normal.[80,81] At Children's Hospital Boston 0.5 g per kg of mannitol is routinely added to the prime.

FUROSEMIDE

At Children's Hospital 0.25 mg per kg of furosemide is added to the pump prime in order to maintain a diuresis during cardiopulmonary bypass. It is felt that the use of the loop diuretic in addition to the osmotic diuretic mannitol is helpful in clearing excess fluid and maintaining renal function during cardiopulmonary bypass though the scientific basis for this practice has not been demonstrated.

Antibiotics

It is important to remember that any drug administered to the patient before bypass will be diluted by the volume of the pump prime. Thus an additional dose of the appropriate prophylactic antibiotic (at Children's Hospital Boston cefazolin 25 mg/kg) is administered into the perfusion circuit before the onset of bypass.

REFERENCES

1. Shumacker HB. *The Evolution of Cardiac Surgery*, Bloomington, IN, Indiana University Press, 1992, pp 242–55.
2. Huskisson L, Elliott M. Prime composition. In Jonas RA, Elliott M (eds). *Cardiopulmonary Bypass in Neonates, Infants and Young Children*. London, Butterworth-Heinemann, 1994, pp 186–97.
3. Gibbon JH. The maintenance of life during experimental occlusion of the pulmonary artery followed by survival. *Surg Gynecol Obstet* 1939; **69**:602–14.
4. Miller BJ, Gibbon Jr JH, Gibbon MH. Recent advances in the development of a mechanical heart and lung apparatus. *Ann Surg* 1951; **134**:694–708.
5. Donald DE, Harshbarger HG, Hetzel PS et al. Experiences with a heart-lung bypass (Gibbon type) in the experimental laboratory. *Proc Staff Meet Mayo Clin* 1955; **30**:113–15.
6. Jones RE, Donald DE, Swan HJC et al. Apparatus of the Gibbon type for mechanical bypass of the heart and lungs. *Proc Staff Meet Mayo Clin* 1955; **30**:105–13.
7. Kirklin JW, DuShane JW, Patrick RT et al. Intracardiac surgery with the aid of a mechanical pump oxygenator system (Gibbon type): report of eight cases. *Proc Staff Meet Mayo Clin* 1955; **30**:201–6.
8. Gadboys HL, Slonim R, Litwak RS. Homologous blood syndrome: I. Preliminary observations on its relationship to clinical cardiopulmonary bypass. *Ann Surg* 1962; **156**:793–804.
9. Boldt J, Bormann BV, Kling D, Scheld H, Hempelmann G. Influence of acute normovolemic hemodilution on extravascular lung water in cardiac surgery. *Crit Care Med* 1988; **16**:336–9.
10. Neptune WB, Bougas JA, Panico FG. Open heart surgery without the need for donor blood priming in the pump oxygenator. *New Engl J Med* 1960; **263**:111–15.
11. Ott DA, Cooley DA. Cardiovascular surgery in Jehovah's Witnesses. Report of 542 operations without blood transfusion. *JAMA* 1977; **238**:1256–8.
12. Cleland J, Pluth JR, Tauxe WN, Kirklin JW. Blood volume and body fluid compartment changes soon after closed and open intracardiac surgery. *J Thorac Cardiovasc Surg* 1966; **52**:698–705.
13. Hint H. The pharmacology of dextran and the physiological background for the clinical use of Rheomacrodex and Macrodex. *Acta Anaesthesiol Belg* 1968; **19**:119–38.
14. Mirhashemi S, Messmer S, Intaglietta M. Tissue perfusion during normovolemic hemodilution investigated by a hydraulic model of the cardiovascular system. *Int J Microcirc Clin Exp* 1987; **6**:123–36.
15. Cooper JR, Slogoff S. Hemodilution and priming solutions for cardiopulmonary bypass. In Gravlee GP, Davis RF, Utley JR (eds). *Cardiopulmonary Bypass Principles and Practice*. Baltimore, Williams & Wilkins, 1993, pp 124–37.
16. Cooper MM, Elliott M. Haemodilution. In Jonas RA, Elliott M (eds). *Cardiopulmonary Bypass in Neonates, Infants and Young Children*. London, Butterworth-Heinemann, 1994, p 86.
17. Tsai AG, Arfors Ke, Intaglietta M. Analysis of oxygen transport to tissue during extreme hemodilution. In Pier J, Goldstrick TK, Meyer M (eds). *Oxygen Transport to Tissue XII. Proceedings of the 17th Annual Meeting of the International Society on Oxygen Transport to Tissue*, New York, Plenum Press, 1991, pp 318–86.
18. Federspiel WJ, Sarelius IH. An examination of the contribution of red cell spacing to the uniformity of oxygen flux at the capillary wall. *Microvasc Res* 1984; **27**:273–85.
19. Trouwborst A, Van Woerkens ECSM, Rating W, Prakash O, Bos E, Wyers-Hille MJ. S35 and derived parameters during extracorporeal circulation together with haemodilution and hypothermia in humans. *Scan J Clin Lab Invest* 1990; **203**:143–7.
20. Trouwborst A, Tenbrinck R, Van Woerkens EC. S35: A new parameter in blood gas analysis for monitoring the systemic oxygenation. *Scan J Clin Lab Invest* 1990; **203**:135–42.
21. Rand PW, Lacombe E, Hunt HE, Austin WH. Viscosity of normal human blood under normothermic and hypothermic conditions. *J Appl Physiol* 1964; **19**:117–22.
22. Cooper MM, Elliott M. Haemodilution. In Jonas RA, Elliott M (eds). *Cardiopulmonary Bypass in Neonates, Infants and Young Children*. London, Butterworth-Heinemann, 1994, p 83.
23. Schmid-Schonbein H. In discussion of Laver and Buckley. In Messmer K, Schmid-Schonbein H (eds). *Hemodilution: Theoretical Basis and Clinical Applications*, New York, Karger, 1972.
24. Lohrer RM, Trammer AR, Dietrich W, Hagl S, Linderkamp O. The influence of extracorporeal circulation and haemoseparation on red cell deformability and membrane proteins in coronary artery disease. *J Thorac Cardiovasc Surg* 1990; **99**:735–40.
25. Walker CHM, Mackintosh TF. The treatment of hyperviscosity syndromes of the newborn with haemodilution. In Messmer K, Schmid-Schonbein H (eds). *Haemodilution: Theoretical Basis and Clinical Application*, New York, Karger, 1972, pp 271–88.
26. Chien S. Present state of blood rheology. In Messmer K, Schmid-Schonbein H (eds). *Haemodilution: Theoretical Basis and Clinical Application*, New York, Karger, pp 1–45.
27. Messmer K, Kessler M, Krumme A et al. Microcirculation changes during normovolemic haemodilution: rheological changes during normovolemic haemodilution. *Arzneim-Forsch (Drug Res)* 1975; **25**:1670.
28. Messmer K, Sunder-Plassman L, Klovekorn WP, Holper K. Circulatory significance of haemodilution: rheological changes and limitations. *Adv Microcirc* 1972; **4**:1–77.
29. Messmer K. Hemodilution. *Surg Clin N Am* 1975; **55**:659–78.
30. Bassenge E, Schmid-Schonbein H, von Restorff W, Volger E. Effect of hemodilution on coronary hemodynamics on conscious dogs. A preliminary report. In Messmer K, Schmid-Schonbein H (eds). *Haemodilution: Theoretical Basis and Clinical Application*, New York, Karger, pp 174–83.
31. Crystal GJ, Salem MR. Myocardial and systemic hemodynamics during isovolemic hemodilution alone and combined with nitroprusside induced controlled hypotension. *Anesth Analg* 1991; **72**:227–37.
32. Gordon RJ, Ravin M, Rawitscher RE, Daicoff GR. Changes in arterial pressure, viscosity and resistance during cardiopulmonary bypass. *J Thorac Cardiovasc Surg* 1975; **69**:552–61.
33. Hartmann A, Rommel T, Dettmers C, Tsuda Y, Lagreze H, Broich K. Hemodilution in cerebral infarcts. *Arzneimittelforschung* 1991; **41**:348–51.

34. Raju TNK, Kim SY. The effect of haematocrit alterations on cerebral vascular CO_2 reactivity in newborn baboons. *Ped Res* 1991; **29**:385–90.
35. Shin'oka T, Shum-Tim D, Jonas RA et al. Higher hematocrit improves cerebral outcome after deep hypothermic circulatory arrest. *J Thorac Cardiovasc Surg* 1996; **112**:1610–20.
36. deLeval M. Perfusion techniques. In Stark J, deLeval M (eds). *Surgery for Congenital Heart Defects*, New York, Grune & Stratton, 1983, p 124.
37. Mavroudis C, Ebert PA. Haemodilution causes decreased compliance in puppies. *Circulation* 1978; **58**:I155–9.
38. Bonser RS, Dave JR, Davies ET et al. Reduction of complement activation during cardiopulmonary bypass by prime manipulation. *Ann Thorac Surg* 1990; **49**:279–83.
39. Ross AD, Angaran DM. Colloids versus crystalloids – a continuing controversy. *Drug Intell Clin Pharm* 1984; **18**:202–12.
40. Chan ST, Kapadia CR, Johnson AW, Radcliffe AG, Dudley HA. Extracellular fluid volume expansion and third space sequestration at the site of small bowel anastomoses. *Br J Surg* 1983; **70**:36–9.
41. Hoeft A, Korb H, Mehlhorn U, Stephan H, Sonntag H. Priming of cardiopulmonary bypass with human albumin or Ringer lactate: effect on colloid osmotic pressure and extravascular lung water. *Br J Anesth* 1991; **66**:73–80.
42. Hindman BJ, Funatsu N, Cheng DC, Bolles R, Todd MM, Tinker JH. Differential effect of oncotic pressure on cerebral and extracerebral water content during cardiopulmonary bypass in rabbits. *Anesthesiol* 1990; **73**:951–7.
43. Foglia RP, Partington MT, Buckberg GD, Leaf J. Iatrogenic myocardial edema with crystalloid primes. Effects on left ventricular compliance, performance and perfusion. *Curr Stud Hematol Blood Transfus* 1986; **5**:53–63.
44. Haneda K, Sato S, Ishizawa E, Horiuchi T. The importance of colloid osmotic pressure during open heart surgery in infants. *Tohoku J Exp Med* 1985; **147**:65–71.
45. Grunert A. Colloid osmotic pressure and albumin metabolism during parenteral nutrition. *Curr Stud Hematol Blood Transfus* 1986; **53**:18–32.
46. Huskisson L, Elliott M. Prime composition. In Jonas RA, Elliott M (eds) *Cardiopulmonary Bypass in Neonates, Infants and Young Children.* London, Butterworth-Heinemann, 1994, p 190.
47. Klotz U, Kroemer H. Clinical pharmacokinetic considerations in the use of plasma expanders. *Clin Pharmacokinet* 1987; **12**:123–35.
48. Strauss RG. Review of the effects of hydroxyethyl starch on blood coagulation system. *Transfusion* 1981; **21**:299–302.
49. Romagnoli A, Hacker J, Keats AS. External hemoconcentration after deliberate haemodilution. *Annual Meeting of the American Society of Anesthesiologists*, extracts of scientific papers, Park Ridge, 1976, p 269.
50. Crowell JW, Smith EE. Determinants of the optimal hematocrit. *J Appl Physiol* 1967; **22**:501–4.
51. Shin'oka T, Shum-Tim D, Laussen PC et al. Effects of oncotic pressure and hematocrit on outcome after hypothermic circulatory arrest. *Ann Thorac Surg* 1998; **65**:155–64.
52. Nomura F, Naruse H, duPlessis A et al. Cerebral oxygenation measured by near infrared spectroscopy during cardiopulmonary bypass and deep hypothermic circulatory arrest in piglets. *Pediatr Res* 1996; **40**:790–6.
53. Cook DJ, Orszulak TA, Daly RC. Minimum hematocrit at differing cardiopulmonary bypass temperatures in dogs. *Circulation* 1998; **98**:II170–4.
54. Liam BL, Plochl W, Cook DJ, Orszulak TA, Daly RC. Hemodilution and whole body oxygen balance during normothermic cardiopulmonary bypass in dogs. *J Thorac Cardiovasc Surg* 1998; **115**:1203–8.
55. Cook DJ, Orszulak TA, Daly RC, MacVeigh I. Minimum hematocrit for normothermic cardiopulmonary bypass in dogs. *Circulation* 1997; **96**(9 Suppl):II200–4.
56. Visconti KJ, Bichell DP, Jonas RA, Newburger JW, Bellinger DC. Developmental outcome after surgical versus interventional closure of secundum atrial septal defect in children. *Circulation* 1999; **100**:II145–50.
57. Sakamoto T, Zurakowski D, Duebener LF et al. Combination of alpha-stat strategy and hemodilution exacerbates neurologic injury in a survival piglet model with deep hypothermic circulatory arrest. *Ann Thorac Surg* 2002; **73**:180–9.
58. Kawashima Y, Yamamoto Z, Manabe H. Safe limits of hemodilution in cardiopulmonary bypass. *Surgery* 1974; **76**:391–7.
59. Bjork VO, Hultquist G. Brain damage in children after deep hypothermia for open heart surgery. *Thorax* 1960; **15**:284–91.
60. Duebener LF, Sakamoto T, Hatsuoka S et al. Effects of hematocrit on cerebral microcirculation and tissue oxygenation during deep hypothermic bypass. *Circulation* 2001; **104**:I260–4.
61. Jonas RA, Wypij D, Roth SJ et al. The influence of hemodilution on outcome after hypothermic cardiopulmonary bypass: Results of a randomized trial in infants. *J Thorac Cardiovasc Surg*, 2003; **126:** 1765–74.
62. Newman MF, Kirchner JL, Phillips-Bute B et al. Longitudinal assessment of neurocognitive function after coronary-artery bypass surgery. *N Engl J Med* 2001; **344**:395–402.
63. Stump DA, Rogers AT, Hammon JW, Newman SP. Cerebral emboli and cognitive outcome after cardiac surgery. *J Cardiothorac Vasc Anesth* 1996; **10**:113–18.
64. McLean J. The discovery of heparin. *Circulation* 1959; **19**:75–8.
65. Chargaff E, Olson KB. Studies on the chemistry of blood coagulation. VI. Studies on the action of heparin and other anticoagulants. The influence of protamine on the anticoagulant effect in vivo. *J Biol Chem* 1938; **125**:671–6.
66. Gravlee GP. Anticoagulation for cardiopulmonary bypass. In Gravlee GP, Davis RF, Utley JR (eds). *Cardiopulmonary Bypass: Principles and Practice.* Baltimore, Williams & Wilkins, 1993, p 363.
67. Longmore DB, Bennett G, Gueirrara D et al. Prostacyclin: a solution to some problems of extracorporeal circulation. Experiments in greyhounds. *Lancet* 1979; **1**:1002–5.
68. DiSesa VJ, Huval W, Lelcuk S et al. Disadvantages of prostacyclin infusion during cardiopulmonary bypass: a double-blind study of 50 patients having coronary revascularization. *Ann Thorac Surg* 1984; **38**:514–19.
69. Aldea GS, Soltow LO, Chandler WL et al. Limitation of thrombin generation, platelet activation, and inflammation by elimination of cardiotomy suction in patients undergoing coronary artery bypass grafting treated with heparin-bonded circuits. *J Thorac Cardiovasc Surg* 2002; **123**:742–55.
70. Royston D, Bidstrup BP, Taylor KM, Sapsford RN. Effect of aprotinin on need for blood transfusion after repeat open-heart surgery. *Lancet* 1987; **2**:1289–91.
71. Gruber EM, Shukla AC, Reid RW, Hickey PR, Hansen DD. Synthetic antifibrinolytics are not associated with an increased incidence of baffle fenestration closure after the modified Fontan procedure. *J Cardiothorac Vasc Anesth* 2000; **14**:257–9.
72. van Oeveren W, Jansen NJ, Bidstrup BP et al. Effects of aprotinin on hemostatic mechanisms during cardiopulmonary bypass. *Ann Thorac Surg* 1987; **44**:640–5.

73. Segal H, Sheikh S, Kallis P et al. Complement activation during major surgery: the effect of extracorporeal circuits and high-dose aprotinin. *J Cardiothorac Vasc Anesth* 1998; **12**:542–7.
74. Lodge AJ, Chai PJ, Daggett CW, Ungerleider RM, Jaggers J. Methylprednisolone reduces the inflammatory response to cardiopulmonary bypass in neonatal piglets: timing of dose is important. *J Thorac Cardiovasc Surg* 1999; **117**:515–22.
75. Poirier NC, Drummond-Webb JJ, Hisamochi K, Imamura M, Harrison AM, Mee RB. Modified Norwood procedure with a high-flow cardiopulmonary bypass strategy results in low mortality without late arch obstruction. *J Thorac Cardiovasc Surg* 2000; **120**:875–84.
76. Hiramatsu T, Jonas RA, Miura T et al. Cerebral metabolic recovery from deep hypothermic circulatory arrest after treatment with arginine and nitro-arginine methyl ester. *J Thorac Cardiovasc Surg* 1996; **112**:698–707.
77. Plestis KA, Gold JP. Importance of blood pressure regulation in maintaining adequate tissue perfusion during cardiopulmonary bypass. *Semin Thorac Cardiovasc Surg* 2001; **13**:170–5.
78. Schuster SR, Kakvan M, Vawter GR et al. An experimental study of the effect of mannitol during cardiopulmonary bypass. *Circulation* 1964; **29**:72–6.
79. Gardner TJ, Stewart JR, Casale AS, Downey JM, Chambers DE. Reduction of myocardial ischemic injury with oxygen derived free radical scavengers. *Surgery* 1983; **94**:423–7.
80. Hottenrott C, McConnell DH, Goldstein SM, Buckberg GD, Nelson RL. Effect of mannitol on coronary flow in ventricles made ischemic by fibrillation or arrest during bypass. *Surg Forum* 1975; **26**:266–8.
81. Willerson JT, Watson JT, Hutton I et al. Reduced myocardial reflow and increased coronary vascular resistance following prolonged myocardial ischemia in the dog. *Circ Res* 1975; **36**:771–81.

8

Carbon dioxide, pH and oxygen management

INTRODUCTION

Despite nearly 50 years experience with cardiopulmonary bypass, the optimal strategies for management of carbon dioxide, pH and oxygen during bypass remain controversial. In the 1950s and 1960s, at a time when oxygenators were inefficient and unreliable, attention was focused on ensuring adequate delivery of oxygen. Thus the strategy for oxygen management was to use pure oxygen and not air. Carbon dioxide was added to the oxygen to maximize cerebral blood flow and to counteract the various effects of hypothermia. However, as the design and reliability of oxygenators improved such that oxygen and carbon dioxide levels could be accurately and consistently set at whatever level was desired, new ideas appeared that questioned whether these were the optimal strategies. By the mid-1980s many centers were no longer adding carbon dioxide and by the mid-1990s many centers were no longer using pure oxygen. However, new information has been emerging that suggests that the original bypass strategies may have been preferable, at least for the management of congenital heart disease. This chapter will examine the physiological background to acid-base and oxygen management during bypass and will review studies that have investigated optimal strategies for blood gas manipulation during clinical application of cardiopulmonary bypass.

CARBON DIOXIDE AND pH

Normal physiology

VASOMOTOR EFFECTS: SYSTEMIC VASODILATION, PULMONARY VASOCONSTRICTION

Carbon dioxide is a powerful systemic vasodilator and conversely alkalosis and a low carbon dioxide level cause systemic vasoconstriction. This includes the cerebral circulation. Evidence of the effects of carbon dioxide and pH on the cerebral circulation are seen regularly by emergency room physicians. Patients suffering an acute anxiety attack can hyperventilate to the point that their carbon dioxide level falls such that a severe degree of cerebral vasoconstriction results. Symptoms of near-syncope or even complete syncope can result. This situation can be remedied by rebreathing in a paper bag to raise the patient's carbon dioxide level thereby restoring adequate cerebral blood flow.

The interpretation of the direct vasomotor effects of carbon dioxide is complicated by the sympathetic response that results from hypercarbia and respiratory acidosis, which may cause sympathetic vasoconstriction. It is also important to remember that the effects of carbon dioxide and pH on the pulmonary circulation are opposite to their effects on the systemic circulation. Thus if there are connections between the systemic and pulmonary circulation such as aortopulmonary collaterals or a systemic to pulmonary arterial shunt (e.g. Blalock shunt), a change in carbon dioxide level and/or pH can cause a marked shift in the distribution of flow between the systemic and pulmonary vascular beds.

ACID-BASE BALANCE

Maintenance of a stable intracellular pH at close to the pH of neutrality of water (pN) is essential for optimal enzyme function.[1,2] At this pH there are an equal number of hydrogen and hydroxyl ions. In humans this corresponds to an intracellular pH of approximately 7.1. In order to maintain intracellular pH at this point extracellular pH is maintained in humans between 7.36 and 7.44. This is achieved through the actions of a number of buffer systems.

Buffers

- *Hemoglobin, proteins:* Proteins provide most of the body's buffering capacity. It is the imidazole moiety, which is found in the amino acid histidine, that is the principal buffer group of proteins.[3] Histidine is widely found in plasma proteins and importantly in hemoglobin. Thus red cells as well as plasma have an essential buffering function that is reduced by hemodilution.

- *Phosphate:* The amount of phosphate present in blood is small and as a result it contributes little to the buffering capacity of blood. It is much more effective intracellularly where it is present in high concentration.
- *Bicarbonate:* The bicarbonate buffer is the principal system available in plasma. However, just as is the case with imidazole, red cells also play an important role in bicarbonate buffering. They achieve this by containing carbonic anhydrase. Carbonic anhydrase facilitates conversion of carbonic acid to carbon dioxide and water thereby preventing accumulation of carbonic acid through subsequent exhalation of carbon dioxide. Because the body can fine tune carbon dioxide levels through respiratory changes and bicarbonate levels through renal excretion, the bicarbonate buffer is a critically important buffer system.

Physiology of carbon dioxide and pH during cardiopulmonary bypass

Cardiopulmonary bypass places the control of acid-base in the hands of the perfusion team and overrides the many homeostatic mechanisms that function during normal physiology. Various manipulations that occur during bypass have an important impact on acid-base balance.

FLOW RATE

Various considerations regarding the perfusion flow rate used for cardiopulmonary bypass are discussed in Chapter 9. In general terms, however, tissue acidosis with a subsequent fall in blood pH will result if the flow rate is inadequate to maintain tissue oxygenation. A flow index of 2.4 l/min per m^2 is usually chosen for full flow normothermic bypass. It is important to remember that this is between a half and two thirds of a normal physiological cardiac output.

Continuous monitoring of venous blood oxygen saturation facilitates the acid-base management of cardiopulmonary bypass and is used to ensure that an adequate perfusion flow rate is being used.[4] There is a strong correlation between lactic acid production and mixed venous oxygen tension. However, the binding of oxygen to hemoglobin is influenced by temperature so that during hypothermia a high oxygen saturation does not as reliably indicate adequate oxygen delivery as it does at normothermia. Furthermore acidosis should be considered in the same way as it is in dealing with hypoperfusion in the intensive care unit: it is a late sign suggesting that tissue damage is imminent or has already occurred. It is a highly insensitive method for monitoring adequacy of tissue perfusion and therefore flow rate.

DILUTION

The contribution to buffering of the nonbicarbonate buffers (the imidazole groups of the proteins contained within plasma and erythrocytes) can be measured and expressed as a buffer strength. Buffer strength is the buffering capacity expressed as the titration of a specific amount of acid or alkali added to a closed system and causing a change of 1 unit of pH. The unit of this measurement is called the *slyke*. Human blood with a normal plasma protein content and hematocrit of 40% contains approximately 30 mmol of imidazole per liter. The nonbicarbonate buffer strength of normal blood is approximately 28 slykes, plasma contributing 8 and erythrocytes 20. If a crystalloid solution is used as the bypass prime, the consequent dilution of the patient's blood will result in a significant reduction in the nonbicarbonate buffer strength. Erythrocyte dilution to a hematocrit of 20%, associated with the same degree of plasma dilution, results in a decrease in buffer strength of approximately 33%, i.e. the buffer strength falls from 28–20 slykes.[2] If the hematocrit is reduced to between 24 and 28% during bypass this will result in a 20% reduction in nonbicarbonate buffering. Hemodilution therefore significantly increases the chance of developing important acidosis.

HYPOTHERMIA

The percentage of water molecules that dissociate into hydrogen ions and hydroxyl ions is temperature dependent. As the temperature increases, more molecules will become dissociated and therefore the number of hydrogen ions increases. At a temperature of 24.52°C the concentration of hydrogen ions in water is 10^{-7} mol/l. Since pH is defined as $-\log[H^+]$ this will mean that the pH is exactly 7.0 at 24.52°C. As water cools the number of hydrogen ions decreases as does the number of hydroxyl ions if neutrality is to be maintained. Thus the pH of water increases as the temperature falls. Another way of expressing this fact is that the pH of neutrality (pN) rises with hypothermia. The relationship between the pH of neutral water and temperature can be described by the equation:

$$\frac{\delta \text{pH}}{°\text{C}} = -0.017.$$

Likewise if the total carbon dioxide content of blood is held constant there is a similar predictable relationship between change in temperature and pH of whole blood. This can be described by the equation:

$$\frac{\delta \text{pH}}{°\text{C}} = -0.0147.$$

Thus a simple nomogram allows calculation of a 'temperature corrected' blood pH. Blood gas analysers measure blood at 37°C by warming the sample to that temperature. The pH which is read from the machine can be temperature corrected to a body temperature of *x*°C by the formula:

$$\text{pH}_{x°\text{C}} = -\text{pH}_{37°\text{C}} + (37 - x)(0.0147).$$

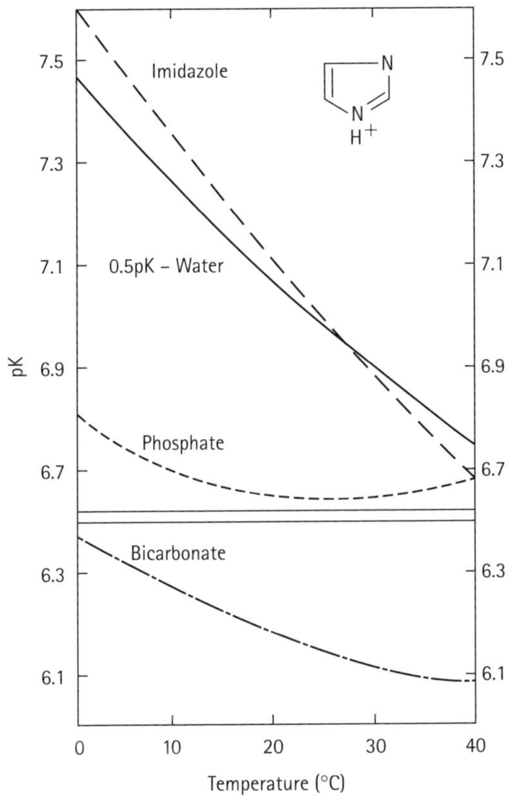

Figure 8.1 *Changes in the dissociation constant (pK) of the major buffering systems in the blood. Because the imidazole moiety of the amino acid histidine in proteins performs the bulk of buffering in blood, the slope of the dissociation constant for blood is similar to the slope of the dissociation constant for water. (From Swan H. The importance of acid-base management for cardiac and cerebral preservation during open heart operations.* Surg Gynecol Obstet *1984;* ***158****:391–414, with permission.)*

It is interesting to note that the fact that the slope of the change in pH with temperature of whole blood is similar to that for neutral water reflects the dominant role of imidazole in the buffering capacity of blood since the dissociation constant (pK) for imidazole is very similar to the dissociation constant for water[5] (Figure 8.1).

Strategies for management of acid-base during cardiopulmonary bypass

Ectothermic ('cold-blooded') animals and hibernating mammals have provided an opportunity for study of the alternative methods whereby different species adjust their physiology in response to the effects of hypothermia. Interestingly different strategies have evolved for species that must remain active while hypothermic versus those that hibernate.

ECTOTHERMS AND THE ALPHA STAT STRATEGY

Ectoterms are animals whose body temperature closely follows ambient temperature. They are faced with the problem of needing to be able to mobilize energy stores efficiently despite their reduced metabolic rate secondary to hypothermia. They achieve optimal energy mobilization by maximizing enzyme efficiency. As their temperature falls these animals allow both intracellular pH and extracellular pH to increase parallel with the rise in the pH of neutrality of water.[6,7] Intracellular pH in fact remains very close to the neutral pH of water. The pH of neutrality of blood retains its usual alkalinity relative to intracellular pH so that there is a constant hydrogen ion concentration gradient between the intracellular and extracellular environments both at normothermia and hypothermia. The pattern of pH change in temperature allows these animals to maintain a constant ratio of hydroxyl to hydrogen ions across a wide range of temperature which they achieve by maintaining a constant carbon dioxide content with reference to an arterial pH of approximately 7.4 at a body temperature of 37°C.[8] This strategy has been termed 'alpha stat' because the ratio (also termed 'alpha') of dissociated to nondissociated imidazole groups remains constant with this strategy.

HIBERNATORS AND THE pH STAT STRATEGY

Hibernating mammals (heterotherms) follow a diametrically opposite strategy to the maintenance of acid-base during hypothermic hibernation relative to ectotherms. Their strategy is to maintain their blood pH constant at 7.4 for all temperatures, i.e. when a blood gas analysis is drawn from a hibernating animal while at a hypothermic body temperature, the pH is always close to 7.4, which, for example at 17°C requires a PCO_2 of 58 mm. If this blood gas sample is read at 37°C the pH will be 7.06 and the $PaCO_2$ will be 156 mm, i.e. a severe respiratory acidosis. This degree of acidosis renders the intracellular environment too acidic for optimal enzymatic activity, thereby depressing metabolism and preserving intracellular substrates.[9,10] This technique of pH management is known as pH stat. Interestingly, it appears that the regulation of intracellular pH in hibernators does not necessarily conform to the pattern of pH stat in all organs. In most tissues of hibernators the intracellular pH during hypothermia does remain constant as does the pH of blood but in contrast in the heart and liver the intracellular pH shifts in an alkaline direction during hypothermia following a pattern similar to the alpha stat system.[11] This suggests that heterotherms may have a mechanism in vital organs enabling their intracellular pH to be regulated independently of blood pH during hypothermia.

ALPHA STAT OR pH STAT FOR CARDIOPULMONARY BYPASS?

Traditional management of acid-base balance during cardiopulmonary bypass in the 1960s and 1970s was to follow the pH stat model. Blood gas analysis performed at 37°C was mathematically temperature corrected using a nomogram to patient temperature and carbon dioxide was added to the oxygen passing through the oxygenator to ensure that the temperature-corrected arterial pH remained at 7.4. As illustrated in Figure 8.2 the blood gas result as read direct from the analyser and as measured at 37°C reveals a considerable respiratory acidosis.

The choice of pH stat management for acid-base control during cardiopulmonary bypass by adding carbon dioxide to the oxygenating gas originated from two suggestions. First, it was suggested that the leftward shift of the oxyhemoglobin dissociation curve which occurs during hypothermia (with the consequent increased affinity of hemoglobin for oxygen), would be reversed by the addition of carbon dioxide which shifts the curve to the right and increases tissue oxygen availability. Secondly, cerebral vasodilation due to carbon dioxide was thought to be beneficial in increasing cerebral blood flow selectively during the stressful period of cardiopulmonary bypass.[12]

During the 1970s, however, a number of reports began to appear describing the alpha stat strategy of pH management utilized by ectotherms as described above.[6,13] The fact that the alpha stat strategy maintained optimal enzyme activity was an appealing rationale to change from the pH strategy to the alpha stat strategy. Interestingly, there were essentially no randomized clinical trials to test the efficacy or even the safety of the alpha stat strategy between the mid-1970s and mid-1980s when the majority of centers including those undertaking congenital heart surgery changed their institutional bypass protocol from the pH stat to the alpha stat strategy. However, laboratory studies were undertaken which demonstrated that the use of pH stat during cardiopulmonary bypass resulted in a loss of cerebral autoregulation and caused cerebral blood flow to be pressure dependent.[14,15] In the setting of full flow bypass this could result in excessive (luxuriant) cerebral blood flow with the potential for an increased number of microemboli.

In contrast the use of alpha stat pH management preserved cerebral autoregulation thereby allowing maintenance of coupling between flow and metabolism down to low temperatures. Moreover, alpha stat pH management appears to extend the lower limit of cerebral autoregulation down to a mean arterial pressure of 30 mm (cerebral perfusion pressure 20 mm).[14,16]

Subsequently at least four randomized prospective clinical trials[17–21] were undertaken in adults comparing outcome after alpha stat management with pH stat management. Although one of the four trials demonstrated no difference in adults undergoing moderately hypothermic relatively high flow bypass, there were three studies which suggested an improved cognitive outcome in adults with the alpha stat strategy. This result has been attributed to a reduced number of microemboli with the alpha stat strategy.

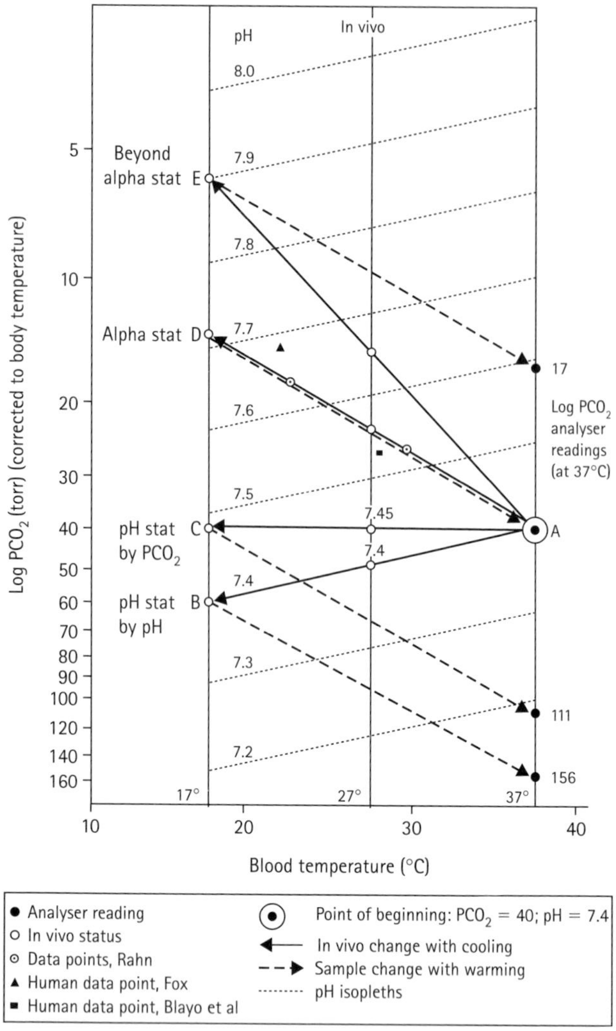

Figure 8.2 *Changes in pH and PCO_2 when the temperature of blood in a closed system is varied between 17°C and 37°C. Four different strategies for management of pH and PCO_2 are illustrated. A–B: pH stat strategy maintaining pH constant at 7.40. It can be seen that rewarming of a blood gas specimen by the blood gas analyser results in a PCO_2 reading of 156 mm. A–C: pH stat strategy maintaining constant PCO_2 at 40 mm. A–D: Alpha stat strategy results in a temperature-corrected pH of 7.7 and PCO_2 of 12. A–E: A very alkaline strategy beyond alpha stat recommended by Swan in an influential review article published in 1984.[8] (Adapted from Swan H. The importance of acid-base management for cardiac and cerebral preservation during open heart operations.* Surg Gynecol Obstet *1984;* **158***:391–414, with permission.)*

IS ALPHA STAT APPROPRIATE FOR BYPASS IN CHILDREN?

In 1985 we changed our pH strategy for hypothermic cardiopulmonary bypass at Children's Hospital Boston to the more alkaline alpha stat strategy. Before 1985 we had used the more acidotic pH stat strategy. Like many other units at that time our rationale for changing our pH management was based solely on comparative physiological studies in cold-blooded vertebrates.[6] Over the next several years we undertook both laboratory and clinical studies to determine the impact of our change in strategy.[22–24] Within a short time considerable evidence accumulated suggesting that our original approach using the pH stat strategy may have been preferable.

Retrospective clinical study of pH strategy

In order to determine the impact of the change in pH strategy on our infant patient population undergoing circulatory arrest

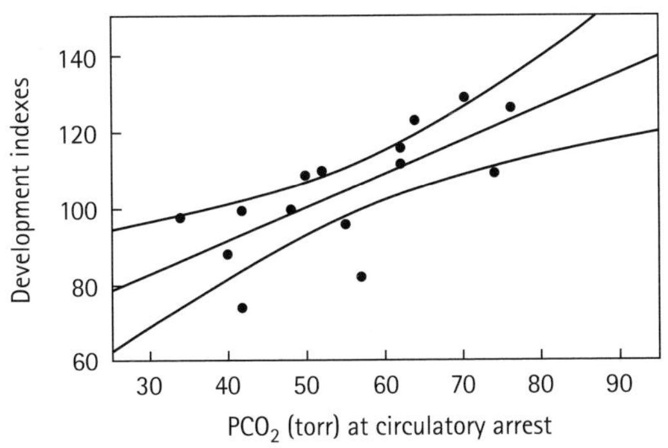

Figure 8.3 *In a retrospective analysis of 16 patients who underwent deep hypothermic circulatory arrest between 1983 and 1988 there was a strong positive correlation between arterial PCO_2 during cooling and developmental score, i.e. children undergoing the alpha stat strategy had a worse developmental outcome. (From Jonas et al. pH strategy and developmental outcome after hypothermic circulatory arrest.* J Thorac Cardiovasc Surg *1993; **106**:362–8, with permission.)*

we undertook a retrospective developmental study with a cohort of patients who had undergone surgery for transposition in a timeframe that straddled our change in pH strategy.[24] Sixteen patients who had undergone Senning procedures between 1983 and 1988 underwent cognitive developmental assessment. Most children scored in the normal range achieving a median developmental score of 109. The mean scores were not associated with any patient related variables. The duration of circulatory arrest was 43 minutes, ranging from 35 to 60 minutes. Duration of circulatory arrest was not associated with cognitive outcome. However, a strong positive correlation was found between arterial PCO_2 during cooling before circulatory arrest and developmental score (Figure 8.3), i.e. children undergoing the alpha stat strategy had a worse developmental outcome. These results had to be interpreted cautiously because of the small sample size and the usual limitations of a retrospective study. For example, there were many changes in perfusion technique during this time such as a change from bubble to membrane oxygenators which may have contributed to this result.

Choreoathetosis and pH strategy

Between 1980 and 1984 there were no cases of choreoathetosis at Children's Hospital Boston. Between 1986 and 1990, following the introduction of the alpha stat strategy in 1985, 19 cases of choreoathetosis occurred.[25] Eleven of these were severe with four of the children dying and six having persistent choreoathetosis. As already noted a number of perfusion protocol changes occurred in the mid-1980s which might have contributed to the virtual epidemic of choreoathetosis. At the same time there was also an increase in the number of children with complex forms of pulmonary atresia with multiple collaterals undergoing surgery. In fact in our review of these cases we found the presence of pulmonary atresia and the use of circulatory arrest to be frequently present factors. We were not able to prove that use of a more alkaline pH strategy was associated with choreoathetosis. Nevertheless it is tempting to speculate that a more alkaline strategy is responsible for a steal of blood from the cerebral to the pulmonary circulation in patients whose pulmonary blood flow is derived from the systemic arterial system because of the opposite effects of alkalosis on cerebral and pulmonary resistance. Decreased cerebral blood flow during cooling may have resulted in inadequate, nonhomogeneous brain cooling before circulatory arrest.

LABORATORY STUDIES OF pH STRATEGY AT CHILDREN'S HOSPITAL BOSTON

In order to better understand the basic mechanisms behind the findings of our clinical studies, we undertook studies using a piglet model of hypothermic circulatory arrest which in many ways replicated the perfusion strategies we used clinically at that time. In the initial acute study,[22] four-week-old miniature piglets weighing approximately 3.5 kg were cooled on cardiopulmonary bypass and underwent circulatory arrest. The animals were rewarmed to normothermia over 45 minutes and were then maintained at normothermia on partial bypass to ensure maintenance of temperature and cardiac output for three more hours. Data collected include cerebral magnetic resonance spectroscopy using a 4.7 tesla horizontal bore magnet, cerebral blood flow by microspheres and electromagnetic flow probe, cerebral metabolism by oxygen and glucose consumption, lactate production and assessment of cerebral edema. A subsequent acute study included near infrared spectroscopy and electroencephalography.[23]

In our first laboratory study of pH strategy all animals underwent one hour of circulatory arrest.[22] Fourteen animals (seven blood flow and metabolism studies, seven magnetic resonance studies) underwent the alpha stat pH strategy during hypothermia and 11 underwent the pH stat strategy (six blood flow and metabolism studies, five magnetic resonance studies). As anticipated we found that the pH stat animals had greater cerebral blood flow during core cooling ($p = 0.001$) because of the cerebral vasodilating effects of the added carbon dioxide.

The intracellular pH determined by magnetic resonance spectroscopy showed an alkaline shift during core cooling in both groups but became more alkaline with alpha stat than pH stat at the end of cooling ($p = 0.013$). Recovery of cerebral ATP ($p = 0.046$) and intracellular pH ($p = 0.014$) in the initial 30 minutes of reperfusion was faster with pH stat. With alpha stat the cerebral intracellular pH became even more acidotic during early reperfusion than it had become during the circulatory arrest period itself, while it showed immediate recovery with reperfusion with pH stat. Brain water content postoperatively was less with pH stat (0.8075) than with alpha stat (0.8124) ($p = 0.05$).

A particularly interesting finding of this study was the redistribution of cerebral blood flow during cooling, which was different between the two groups (Figure 8.4). Animals

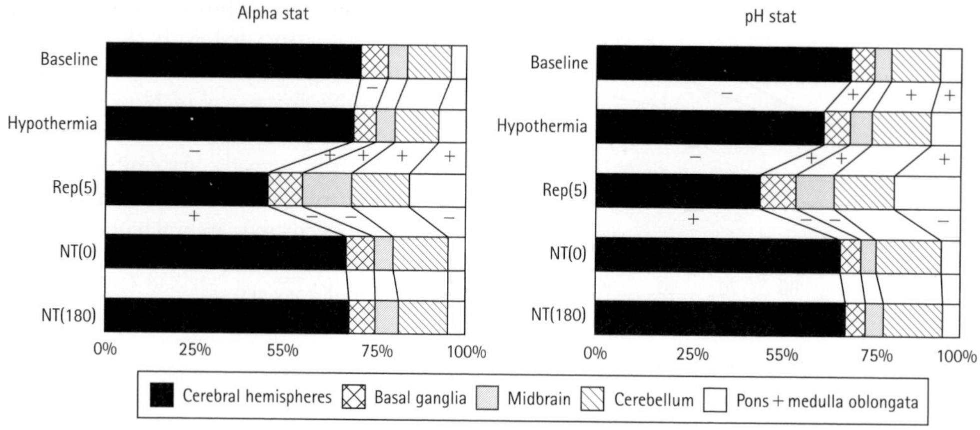

Figure 8.4 *A study of pH strategy in piglets demonstrates that blood flow to the basal ganglia was proportionately decreased during cooling to hypothermia in animals perfused with the alpha stat strategy while the proportion was increased in those perfused with the pH stat strategy. This may be of relevance to the causation of choreoathetosis. NT(0) = after 45 minutes of rewarming, when normothermia was achieved; NT(180) = after 180 minutes of reperfusion at normothermia; Rep(5) = five minutes after initiation of reperfusion and rewarming after one hour of total circulatory arrest. (From Aoki et al. Effects of pH on brain energetics after hypothermic circulatory arrest.* Ann Thorac Surg *1993; 55:1093–103, with permission.)*

undergoing alpha stat had a decrease in the proportion of blood perfusing the basal ganglia in addition to having as expected less total cerebral blood flow than the pH stat animals. Animals undergoing pH stat showed an increase in percentage distribution to the basal ganglia, cerebellum, pons and medulla oblongata with a decrease in percentage distribution to the cerebral hemispheres. But even with the shift in distribution, the absolute regional blood flow to the cerebral hemispheres was not less with pH stat than alpha stat.

Although the findings of our initial study of pH strategy were consistent with our clinical studies of pH strategy, further experiments were required to define whether the mechanism of improved protection with pH stat was operative primarily during the cooling or rewarming phase before or after circulatory arrest respectively. We hypothesized that the apparent improved protection of pH stat might be secondary to greater oxygen availability during the cooling phase before circulatory arrest related to the rightward shift in oxyhemoglobin dissociation (counteracting the leftward shift induced by hypothermia) as well as related to the greater cerebral blood flow secondary to the cerebral vasodilation induced by carbon dioxide with the pH stat strategy. Another explanation might be the greater metabolic suppression caused by pH stat. Alternatively the greater blood flow might be more important in the early reperfusion phase. Furthermore reperfusion after ischemia with a more acidotic reperfusate has been shown in models of both myocardial and cerebral ischemia to be associated with reduced ischemic injury.[26,27] This may be because of competition between calcium and hydrogen ions for intracellular entry with calcium ions causing greater injury than hydrogen ions.

To identify which of these mechanisms was predominant, we studied 49 four-week-old piglets undergoing one hour of deep hypothermic circulatory arrest.[23] Four groups were defined according to cooling/rewarming strategy: alpha stat during cooling/alpha stat during rewarming, alpha/pH, pH/alpha and pH/pH.

As was found in the first study cerebral blood flow was greater with pH stat than alpha stat during cooling ($p < 0.001$). Cytochrome aa3 measured by near infrared spectroscopy (a measure of mitochondrial oxygen availability) became more reduced during cooling with alpha stat than pH stat ($p = 0.049$). Recovery of ATP in the initial 45 minutes of reperfusion was more rapid in the animals in which pH stat was used both during cooling and rewarming compared with the other groups ($p = 0.029$). Recovery of cerebral intracellular pH in the initial 30 minutes was faster in the pH/pH group compared with the alpha/alpha group ($p = 0.026$). Intracellular pH became more acidic during early reperfusion only in the alpha/alpha group whereas it showed continuous recovery in the other groups.

We concluded from this study that there are mechanisms in effect during both the cooling and rewarming phases before and after deep hypothermic circulatory arrest which could contribute to an improved cerebral outcome with pH stat relative to a more alkaline strategy such as alpha stat.

Prospective clinical trial of pH strategy

In light of our epidemic of choreoathetosis in the late 1980s after our change to alpha stat, our retrospective clinical trial suggesting worse developmental outcome with alpha stat and the consistent findings from our laboratory studies suggesting advantages for the pH stat strategy, we planned a clinical study.

In 1992 we began a randomized, prospective single-center trial in which we compared perioperative outcomes and subsequently developmental outcomes in infants undergoing deep hypothermic open heart surgery after use of the alpha stat versus pH stat strategy either with or without circulatory arrest.[28] Admission criteria included reparative and not palliative open heart surgery, age less than nine months, birthweight greater than 2.25 kg, and absence of associated congenital or acquired extracardiac disorders. Among the 182 study infants, diagnoses included dextro transposition of the great arteries ($n = 92$), tetralogy of Fallot ($n = 50$), tetralogy with pulmonary atresia ($n = 6$), ventricular septal defect ($n = 20$), truncus arteriosus ($n = 8$), common arterioventricular canal ($n = 4$), and total anomalous pulmonary venous return ($n = 2$). Ninety patients were assigned to alpha stat and 92 to pH stat. Early mortality occurred in four infants (2%), all in the alpha stat group. Thus even mortality itself was lower with pH stat at close to a 0.05 level of significance ($p = 0.058$). Postoperative seizures determined by continuous EEG monitoring for 48 hours postoperatively occurred in 5 of 57 patients (9%) assigned to alpha stat and 1 of 59 patients (2%) assigned to pH stat ($p = 0.11$).

Clinical seizures occurred in four alpha stat infants (4%) and 2 pH stat infants (2%) ($p = 0.44$). First EEG activity returned sooner among infants randomized to pH stat ($p = 0.03$). Within the homogeneous DTGA subgroup, those assigned to pH stat tended to have a higher cardiac index despite a lower inotrope requirement, less frequent postoperative acidosis ($p = 0.02$) and hypotension ($p = 0.05$); and shorter duration of mechanical ventilation ($p = 0.01$) and intensive care unit stay ($p = 0.01$).

In the majority of patients, i.e. those with transposition and tetralogy, there was a trend towards worse developmental scores at one year of age with alpha stat.[29] In the small subgroup of patients with VSD and complete AV canal there was a significantly higher score for patients with alpha stat. However, this result was strongly influenced by one outlier who was not tested for microdeletion of chromosome 22.

Studies from other centers

A number of both clinical and laboratory studies have been reported from other centers in recent years that have confirmed the advantages of the pH strategy for pediatric bypass.[30,31,32] On the basis of our own studies in conjunction with supporting work from elsewhere we changed our pH strategy to the pH stat strategy in 1996 and use this method for all hypothermic bypass. A review of practice by Groom et al has demonstrated that more than 50% of pediatric centers were using the pH stat strategy by 2000.[33] We have seen no cases of persistent choreoathetosis since we adopted the pH stat strategy.[34]

pH STRATEGY FOR CIRCULATORY ARREST IN ADULTS

The alpha stat strategy is appropriate for normal flow cardiopulmonary bypass in adults because it reduces the microembolic load to the brain by more closely linking cerebral blood flow with cerebral oxygen requirements.[35] However, cerebral blood flow has two functions for any patient undergoing deep hypothermic circulatory arrest, whether that is a child with congenital heart disease or an adult with degenerative aortic arch disease. In addition to supplying oxygen and other substrates, cerebral blood flow is also the principal means by which the brain is cooled. If cerebral blood flow is reduced by use of the alpha stat strategy, the total duration of cooling must increase to compensate. In fact the total volume of blood needed to cool the brain to the desired deep hypothermic temperature will be the same with either alpha stat or pH stat. Thus the total microembolic load will be the same irrespective of the pH strategy used. Thus the pH stat strategy should be preferred not only for the child but also for the adult undergoing deep hypothermic circulatory arrest for all the same reasons:

- pH stat suppresses cerebral metabolism.[9] Recent studies in our laboratory[36,37] have confirmed that pH stat lengthens the safe duration of deep hypothermic circulatory arrest for a given temperature and hematocrit
- pH stat improves oxygen availability by counteracting the leftward shift of oxyhemoglobin induced by hypothermia. This is important in the early cooling phase when the brain is warm but blood is cold
- as described above, the only prospective randomized clinical trial of pH strategy in which many patients underwent deep hypothermic circulatory arrest demonstrated an improved outcome with pH stat.[28] Although this trial was in infants, in view of the facts as noted above we believe the conclusions can be extrapolated to adults undergoing deep hypothermic circulatory arrest.

OXYGENATION STRATEGY FOR CARDIOPULMONARY BYPASS

In the early years of oxygenator technology pure oxygen was used as a safety measure to ensure sufficient blood oxygenation. Recent experimental and clinical data, however, suggest that the hyperoxygenation achieved with modern oxygenators during reperfusion aggravates ischemia–reperfusion injury through generation of oxygen free radicals, particularly in the heart.[38–40] Ihnken and associates,[38] for example, have emphasized the important role of oxygen free radicals in exacerbating myocardial injury during reperfusion after ischemia. They reported higher lipid oxygenation, increased nitric oxide formation and worse cardiac contractility with hyperoxic management of cardiopulmonary bypass after hypoxia and ischemia–reperfusion of immature canine hearts than with normoxic management. Furthermore, recent clinical studies comparing hyperoxic and normoxic management of cardiopulmonary bypass in cyanotic children also revealed higher damage from oxygen free radicals as assessed by products of lipid peroxidation after reperfusion.[41,42]

These data and others have led many pediatric cardiac surgery centers to change from hyperoxic to normoxic management of cardiopulmonary bypass. In order to conduct bypass with a normal arterial oxygen tension it is necessary to replace pure oxygen with a mixture of oxygen and nitrogen (in clinical practice a mixture of air and oxygen). Because the nitrogen in air is less soluble than oxygen there is a risk that normoxic cardiopulmonary bypass might increase gaseous microemboli in the same way that nitrogen bubbles coming out of solution cause 'the bends' in the diver who decompresses too rapidly. Reducing the oxygen content of blood also might reduce the cerebral oxygen supply to a level that could result in hypoxic brain injury during periods of stress such as reduced flow, severe anemia or deep hypothermic circulatory arrest. We therefore undertook two studies at Children's Hospital Boston using laboratory animals to study the net effect of injury from oxygen free radicals versus injury from gaseous microemboli and hypoxia.[43,44]

Risk of gaseous microemboli with normoxic bypass

A laboratory study was undertaken in which 7–10 kg piglets underwent hypothermic cardiopulmonary bypass with either a normoxic gas mixture or with pure oxygen.[43] The animals were cooled to 15°C for 30 minutes on cardiopulmonary bypass and then were rewarmed for 40 minutes to 37°C. In each group three animals underwent bypass with bubble oxygenators without arterial filters while two animals underwent bypass with membrane oxygenators with arterial filters. Cerebral microemboli were monitored continuously by carotid Doppler ultrasonography (8 mHz) and intermittently by fluorescence retinography. The results of this study demonstrated that partially replacing oxygen in the oxygenator gas mixture with 70–80% nitrogen during hypothermia increases the gaseous microembolic load to the brain if bubble oxygenators are used. There was a strong correlation between lower temperature and microembolus count in animals perfused with a normoxic gas mixture confirming the lower solubility of nitrogen in blood relative to oxygen. Use of a membrane oxygenator rather than a bubble oxygenator markedly decreased the number of gaseous microemboli that could be detected. Interestingly with either bubble or membrane oxygenators temperature gradients during both cooling and rewarming had no influence on the number of emboli even though traditional perfusion teaching emphasizes the important role for the temperature gradient in causing gaseous microemboli.

If this conventional wisdom were accurate one would have anticipated that the effect of temperature gradient would be magnified with the addition of nitrogen. However, temperature gradients were not important either with or without nitrogen during either cooling or rewarming. By multivariate analysis embolus count was greater with lower rectal temperature ($p < 0.001$), use of a bubble oxygenator ($p < 0.001$), and lower oxygen concentration ($p = 0.021$) but was not affected by the temperature gradient between blood and body during cooling or rewarming.

Risk of hypoxic injury with normoxic bypass and hypothermic circulatory arrest

A study was undertaken in 10 piglets weighing 8–10 kg to test the hypothesis that normoxic management of cardiopulmonary bypass increases the risk of hypoxic brain injury in the setting of hypothermia and circulatory arrest.[44] In five piglets normoxic bypass was used during cardiopulmonary bypass with PO_2 ranging from 64 to 181 mm. In the other five animals, hyperoxia was employed with PO_2 ranging between 400 and 900 mm. The animals underwent 120 minutes of deep hypothermic circulatory arrest at 15°C, were rewarmed to 37°C and then were weaned from bypass. After six hours of reperfusion the brain was fixed for histological evaluation. Near infrared spectroscopy was used throughout the study to monitor cerebral oxyhemoglobin and oxidized cytochrome aa3 concentration.

The study demonstrated that there was a significant increase in histological evidence of brain injury in the normoxic group, especially in the neocortex and hippocampal regions. Cytochrome aa3 and oxyhemoglobin concentrations tended to be lower during deep hypothermia and circulatory arrest in the normoxic group. There was evidence of increased oxygen free radical activity in both groups. Concentrations of products of lipid peroxidation (malonaldehyde and 4-hydroxy-2e-nonenal) were significantly increased from baseline values after cardiopulmonary bypass and six hours of reperfusion in both groups (55% and 36% respectively, $p < 0.05$). Concentrations of the lipid peroxidation products from the jugular bulb tended to be higher in the hyperoxia group at the end of the experiment.

We concluded from this study that normoxic management of cardiopulmonary bypass results in greater cerebral injury in piglets undergoing 120 minutes of deep hypothermia and circulatory arrest relative to those undergoing hyperoxic management of cardiopulmonary bypass. The difference in injury as determined by histological examination was statistically significant. The trends observed in spectroscopy suggested that the mechanism was hypoxia particularly during the period of extended circulatory arrest.

CONCLUSIONS

Both laboratory and clinical studies support the use of the pH stat strategy for hypothermic cardiopulmonary bypass with or without circulatory arrest in neonates, infants and children. Although the alpha stat strategy is probably appropriate for adults with acquired cardiovascular disease undergoing mildly or moderately hypothermic continuous bypass, the pH stat strategy is more likely appropriate for adults undergoing deep hypothermic circulatory arrest.

Normoxic cardiopulmonary bypass is probably not appropriate for patients of any age undergoing hypothermic circulatory arrest. The only setting in which normoxic bypass is probably as safe as hyperoxic bypass is continuous bypass with a membrane oxygenator and arterial line filter.

REFERENCES

1. Rosenhay FT, Henrod KE. Blood gas studies in the hypothermic dog. *Am J Physiol* 1951; **166**:55–62.
2. White FN, Somero G. Acid base regulation and phospholipids adaptation to temperature; time course and physiological significances of modifying the milieu for protein function. *Phys Rev* 1982; **62**:40–90.
3. Lloyd-Thomas A. Acid base balance. In Jonas RA, Elliott M (eds). *Cardiopulmonary Bypass for Neonates, Infants and Young Children.* London, Butterworth-Heinemann, 1994.
4. Swan H, Sanchez M, Tyndall M, Koch C. Quality control of perfusion: Monitoring venous blood oxygen tension to prevent hypoxic acidosis. *J Thorac Cardiovasc Surg* 1990; **99**:868–72.
5. Severinghaus JW. Blood gas calculator. *J Appl Physiol* 1966; **21**:1108–16.
6. Rahn H, Reeves BR, Howell BJ. Hydrogen ion regulation, temperature and evolution. The 1975 J Burns Amberson Lecture. *Am Rev Resp Dis* 1975; **112**:165–72.
7. Swan H. The hydroxyl-hydrogen ion concentration ratio during hypothermia. *Surg Gynecol Obstet* 1982; **155**:897–912.
8. Swan H. The importance of acid-base management for cardiac and cerebral preservation during open heart operations. *Surg Gynecol Obstet* 1984; **158**:391–414.
9. Wilson E. Theoretical analysis of the effects of two pH regulation patterns on the temperature sensitivities of biological systems in non homeothermic animals. *Arch Biochem Biophys* 1977; **181**:409–19.
10. Sakamoto T, Zurakowski D, Duebener LF et al. Combination of alpha stat strategy and hemodilution exacerbates neurologic injury in a survival piglet model with deep hypothermic circulatory arrest. *Ann Thorac Surg* 2002, **73**:180–90.
11. Swain JA, MacDonald TJ, Robbins RC, Balaban RS. Relationship of cerebral and myocardial intracellular pH to blood pH during hypothermia. *Am J Physiol* 1991; **260**:1640–4.
12. Belsey RHR, Dowlatshahi K, Keen G, Skinner DB. Profound hypothermia in cardiac surgery. *J Thorac Cardiovasc Surg* 1968; **56**:497–509.
13. White FN. A comparative physiological approach to hypothermia. *J Thorac Cardiovasc Surg* 1981; **82**:821–31.
14. Murkin JM, Farrar JK, Tweed WA et al. Cerebral autoregulation and flow metabolism coupling during cardiopulmonary bypass: the influence of $PaCO_2$. *Anesth Analg* 1978; **66**:825–32.
15. Henriksen L. Brain luxury perfusion during cardiopulmonary bypass in humans: A study of cerebral blood flow response to changes in CO_2, O_2 and blood pressure. *J Cereb Blood Flow Metab* 1986; **6**:366–78.
16. Govier AV, Reves JG, MacKay RD et al. Factors and their influence on regional cerebral blood flow during non pulsatile cardiopulmonary bypass. *Ann Thorac Surg* 1984; **38**:592–600.
17. Patel RL, Turtle MR, Chambers DJ, James DN, Newman S, Venn GE. Alpha stat acid base regulation during cardiopulmonary bypass improves neuropsychologic outcome in patients undergoing coronary artery bypass grafting. *J Thorac Cardiovasc Surg* 1996; **111**:1267–79.
18. Stephan H, Weyland A, Kazmaier S, Menck S, Sonntag H. Acid base management during hypothermic cardiopulmonary bypass does not affect cerebral metabolism but does affect blood flow and neurological outcome. *Br J Anaesth* 1992; **69**:51–7.
19. Murkin JM, Martzke JS, Buchan AM, Bentley C, Wong CA. A randomized study of the influence of perfusion technique and pH management strategy in 316 patients undergoing coronary artery bypass surgery. II. Neurologic and cognitive outcomes. *J Thorac Cardiovasc Surg* 1995; **110**:349–62.
20. Bashein G, Townes BD, Nessly ML et al. A randomized study of carbon dioxide management during hypothermic cardiovascular bypass. *Anesthesia* 1995; **110**:1649–57.
21. Murkin JM, Martzke JS, Buchan AM, Bentley C, Wong CJ. A randomized study of the influence of perfusion technique and pH management strategy in 316 patients undergoing coronary artery bypass surgery. I. Mortality and cardiovascular morbidity. *J Thorac Cardiovasc Surg* 1995; **110**:340–8.
22. Aoki M, Nomura F, Stromski ME et al. Effects of pH on brain energetics after hypothermic circulatory arrest. *Ann Thorac Surg* 1993; **55**:1093–1103.
23. Hiramatsu T, Miura T, Forbess JM et al. pH strategies and cerebral energetics before and after circulatory arrest. *J Thorac Cardiovasc Surg* 1995; **109**:948–58.
24. Jonas RA, Bellinger DC, Rappaport LA et al. pH strategy and developmental outcome after hypothermic circulatory arrest. *J Thorac Cardiovasc Surg* 1993; **106**:362–8.
25. Wong PC, Barlow CF, Hickey PR et al. Factors associated with choreoathetosis after cardiopulmonary bypass in children with congenital heart disease. *Circulation* 1992; **86** (Suppl II) II118–26.
26. Bing OH, Brooks WW, Messer JV. Heart muscle viability following hypoxia: protective effect of acidosis. *Science* 1973; **180**:1297–8.
27. Bonventre JV, Cheung JY. Effects of metabolic acidosis on viability of cells exposed to anoxia. *Am J Physiol* 1985; **294**:149–59.
28. du Plessis AJ, Jonas RA, Wypij D et al. Perioperative effects of alpha stat versus pH stat strategies for deep hypothermic cardiopulmonary bypass in infants. *J Thorac Cardiovasc Surg* 1997; **114**:991–1001.
29. Bellinger DC, Wypij D, du Plessis AJ et al. Developmental and neurologic effects of alpha-stat versus pH-stat strategies for deep hypothermic cardiopulmonary bypass in infants. *J Thorac Cardiovasc Surg* 2001; **121**:374–83.
30. Pearl JM, Thomas DW, Grist G, Duffy JY, Manning PB. Hyperoxia for management of acid-base status during deep hypothermia with circulatory arrest. *Ann Thorac Surg* 2000; **70**:751–5.
31. Kurth CD, O'Rourke MM, O'Hara IB. Comparison of pH stat and alpha stat cardiopulmonary bypass on cerebral oxygenation and blood flow in relation to hypothermic circulatory arrest in piglets. *Anesthesiology* 1998; **89**:110–18.
32. Sakamoto T, Kurosawa H, Shin'oka T, Aoki M, Nagatsu M, Isomatsu Y. The influence of pH strategy on cerebral and collateral circulation during hypothermic cardiopulmonary bypass in cyanotic cardiac patients. *J Thorac Cardiovasc Surg* 2004; **127**:12–19.
33. Cecere G, Groom R, Forest R, Quinn R, Morton JA. 10-year review of pediatric perfusion practice in North America. *Perfusion* 2002; **17**:83–9.
34. Menache CC, du Plessis AJ, Wessel DL, Jonas RA, Newburger JW. Current incidence of acute neurologic complications after open-heart operations in children. *Ann Thorac Surg* 2002; **73**:1752–8.
35. Smith P, Taylor K. *Cardiac Surgery and the Brain.* London, Arnold, 1993.
36. Sakamoto T, Hatsuoka S, Stock UA et al. Prediction of safe duration of hypothermic circulatory arrest by near-infrared spectroscopy. *J Thorac Cardiovasc Surg* 2001; **122**:339–50.
37. Sakamoto T, Zurakowski D, Duebener LF et al. Combination of alpha-stat strategy and hemodilution exacerbates neurologic injury

in a survival piglet model with deep hypothermic circulatory arrest. *Ann Thorac Surg* 2002; **73**:180–9.
38. Ihnken K, Morita K, Buckberg GD, Shermann MP, Young HH. Studies of hypoxemic/reoxygenation injury: without aortic clamping. III. Comparison of the magnitude of damage by hypoxemia/reoxygenation versus ischemic reperfusion. *J Thorac Cardiovasc Surg* 1995; **110**:1182–9.
39. Bolling KS, Halldorsson A, Allen BS et al. Prevention of the hypoxic reoxygenation injury with the use of a leukocyte depleting filter. *J Thorac Cardiovasc Surg* 1997; **113**:1081–9.
40. Allen BS, Rahman S, Ilbawi MN et al. Detrimental effects of cardiopulmonary bypass in cyanotic infants: preventing the reoxygenation injury. *Ann Thorac Surg* 1997; **64**:1381–7.
41. Kjellmer I. Mechanisms of perinatal brain damage. *Ann Med* 1991; **23**:675–9.
42. Cazevieille C, Muller A, Meynier F, Bonne C. Superoxide and nitric oxide cooperation in hypoxia/reoxygenation induced neuron injury. *Free Radic Biol Med* 1993; **14**:389–95.
43. Nollert G, Nagashima M, Bucerius J, Shin'oka T, Jonas RA. Oxygenation strategy and neurologic damage after deep hypothermic circulatory arrest. I. Gaseous microemboli. *J Thorac Cardiovasc Surg* 1999; **117**:1166–71.
44. Nollert G, Nagashima M, Bucerius J et al. Oxygenation strategy and neurologic damage after deep hypothermic circulatory arrest. II. Hypoxic versus free radical injury. *J Thorac Cardiovasc Surg* 1999; **117**:1172–9.

9

Hypothermia, reduced flow and circulatory arrest

INTRODUCTION

Predetermined protocols determine many aspects of cardiopulmonary bypass technique such as pH and oxygen strategy as well as prime constituents and the degree of hemodilution. However, the decision regarding the specific minimum temperature to be employed for a given patient during cardiopulmonary bypass as well as the choice of flow rate, including the possibility of hypothermic circulatory arrest, should lie with the surgeon who must balance multiple patient and repair related factors in coming to these decisions. For example, a particularly complex repair requiring deep intracardiac exposure in a small infant who is known to have multiple diffuse collaterals is likely to be managed by most surgeons with quite a different choice of temperature and flow rate from the child who has a simple secundum atrial septal defect. This chapter will examine the many factors that the surgeon needs to consider in coming to such decisions.

HYPOTHERMIA

Advantages of hypothermia

DECREASED INFLAMMATORY RESPONSE OF CARDIOPULMONARY BYPASS

Despite the many improvements in cardiopulmonary bypass hardware and techniques, cardiopulmonary bypass remains far from a physiological state. The deleterious effects of cardiopulmonary bypass are far too numerous and complex to be chronicled in detail in this book. They have been described elsewhere.[1] However, one of the most important general areas is the inflammatory and immune response to bypass, sometimes called 'SIRS' – the systemic inflammatory response.

What is the inflammatory response to cardiopulmonary bypass?

The systemic inflammatory response to bypass consists of activation of multiple humoral cascades as well as activation of cellular components of blood and endothelial cells throughout the body.[2,3]

Humoral cascades: There are multiple humoral cascades which are activated during bypass including the coagulation cascade, the fibrinolytic cascade the complement system and the kallikrein/bradykinin cascade.[4,5] Kirklin and colleagues,[6] for example, have demonstrated that the concentration of the complement degradation product C3a is related to the duration of bypass (Figure 9.1). Previously Chenoweth and colleagues[7] also from the University of Alabama, Birmingham had demonstrated in 1981 that there was a progressive rise in plasma C3a during cardiopulmonary bypass. The amount of C3a generated varied between different oxygenators. Both C3a and C5a are vasoactive anaphylatoxins which increase vascular permeability, release histamine from muscles and cause hypertension and contraction of airway smooth muscle. C5a is rapidly taken up by neutrophils but an increase associated with bypass has been demonstrated. Craddock has shown that complement activated neutrophils sequester within the lung and increase perivascular edema.[8]

Cellular activation by cardiopulmonary bypass: Considerable information has been developed over the last 15 years regarding the complex interaction between white cells and endothelium. The development of monoclonal antibodies has aided the understanding of adhesion molecules such as selectin proteins on endothelial surfaces and carbohydrate ligands which are expressed and are thought to play a major role in attachment of activated leukocytes particularly neutrophils.[9] Early studies suggested that CD62, an endothelial selectin protein was particularly important in bypass related vascular damage because it is an adhesion molecule found in platelets as well as on the endothelium.[10] Blood contact with nonendothelial surfaces leads to CD62 expression on the platelet surface as well as CD18 expression on leukocytes

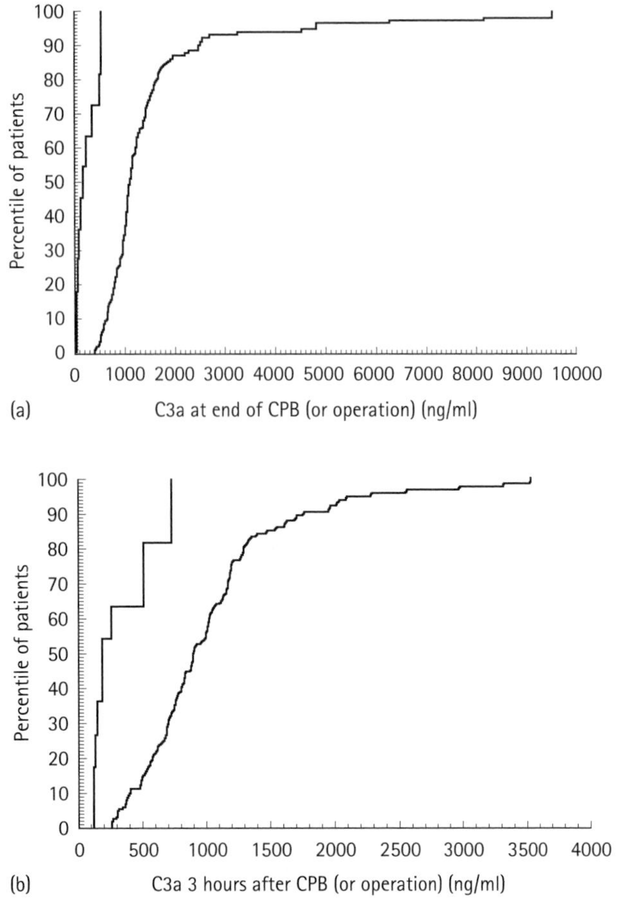

Figure 9.1 *Kirklin and colleagues[6] demonstrated activation of the complement cascade during cardiopulmonary bypass. The figure illustrates percentile distribution of patients according to C3a levels. The steep vertical line on the left represents closed cases and that on the right cases in which cardiopulmonary bypass (CPB) was used. (a) End of cardiopulmonary bypass (or end of operation in closed cases). (b) Three hours after cardiopulmonary bypass (or end of operation in closed cases). (From Kirklin et al. Complement and the damaging effects of cardiopulmonary bypass.* J Thorac Cardiovasc Surg *1983;* ***86****:845–57, with permission.)*

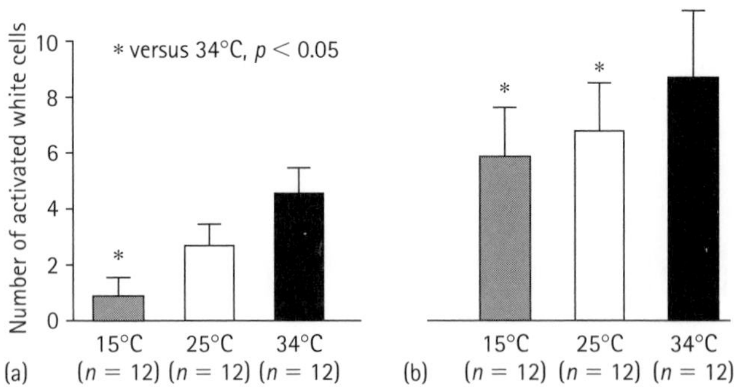

Figure 9.2 *Hypothermic bypass at 15°C was associated with reduced activation of white cells as observed by intravital microscopy of cerebral microvessels in piglets. The number of (a) rolling leukocytes and (b) adherent leuckocytes was significantly less at 15°C relative to 34°C. (From Anttila et al. Higher bypass temperature correlates with increased white cell activation in the cerebral microcirculation.* J Thorac Cardiovasc Surg *2003; in press, with permission.)*

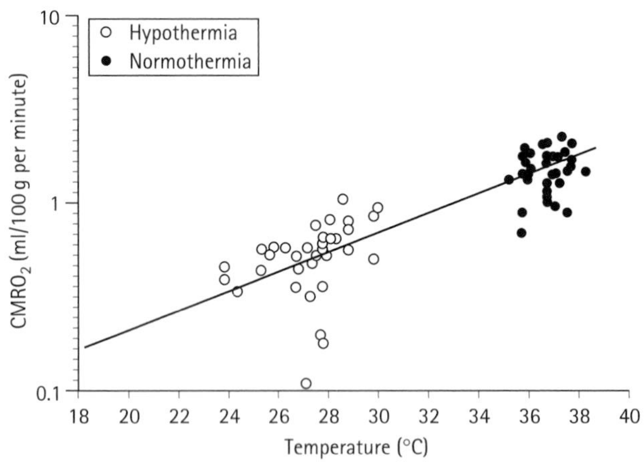

Figure 9.3 *Hypothermia reduces metabolic rate. In a study of 41 adults undergoing hypothermic cardiopulmonary bypass, Croughwell et al[15] found that cerebral metabolic rate determined by oxygen consumption ($CMRO_2$) was reduced by 64% by cooling from 37° to 27°C. (From Croughwell et al. The effect of temperature on cerebral metabolism and blood flow in adults during cardiopulmonary bypass.* J Thorac Cardiovasc Surg *1992;* ***103****:549–54, with permission.)*

leading to platelet aggregation and other neutrophil/platelet amplifying interactions such as leukotriene transcellular synthesis. Synthesis and release of chemoattractants such as leukotrienes promote further neutrophil activation and attraction.[11]

Hypothermia and the inflammatory response to cardiopulmonary bypass

There has been little attention paid to the impact of hypothermia in reducing the inflammatory response to bypass. Not surprisingly the amount of activation of humoral cascades including release of vasoactive substances is reduced by hypothermia.[12] A recent study at Children's Hospital Boston using intravital microscopy in 26 piglets demonstrated that there was reduced activation of white cells with a bypass temperature of 34°C relative to 15°C (Figure 9.2). White cell activation was measured by direct observation of white cell rolling and adhesion in cerebral arterioles.[13]

DECREASED METABOLIC RATE

In contrast to the surprising lack of information regarding the direct effect of hypothermia in reducing the systemic inflammatory response of bypass there is a large body of information regarding the effect of hypothermia in reducing metabolic rate[14,15] (Figure 9.3). Interestingly the observation that hypothermia reduces metabolic rate was not accepted until the very important studies by Bigelow in Canada in 1950.[16,17] Before this time it was thought that hypothermia resulted in an increased metabolic rate. In retrospect this appears to have been related to a failure to abolish shivering because of use of an inadequate level of anesthesia in studies that were undertaken before 1950. Bigelow recognized that the reduction of metabolic rate induced by hypothermia would allow a temporary decrease in perfusion which might allow intracardiac repair of congenital or acquired anomalies. Bigelow's observations were confirmed independently by both Lewis and Swan[18,19] and in 1953 the first open intracardiac repair of a heart malformation was carried out using total body ice water immersion induced hypothermia to allow temporary arrest of the circulation.

Hypothermia was not used in the early years of cardiopulmonary bypass. It was not until Sealy and Brown developed a heat exchanging system which could be combined with cardiopulmonary bypass that hypothermic cardiopulmonary bypass was introduced into clinical cardiac surgery.[20]

The decrease in metabolic rate which occurs with hypothermia has several important consequences for the cardiac surgical team.

Hypothermia allows reduced flow rate: advantages

Although it was recognized early in the history of cardiac surgery that hypothermia would allow complete cessation of bypass, i.e. hypothermic circulatory arrest, the concept that hypothermia allows a safe reduction of perfusion flow rate evolved slowly and somewhat surreptitiously entered into clinical cardiac surgical practice. One of the most important reasons for the slow acceptance of reduced flow rate with hypothermic bypass is a consequence of the fact that there is no good method for directly monitoring the safe lower limit for reduced flow rate. On the other hand it soon came to be realized that there were important advantages, particularly for the congenital surgeon, in working at a reduced flow rate.

Improved intracardiac exposure: Many patients with congenital cardiac anomalies, particularly those which result in cyanosis, will develop multiple profuse collateral vessels which increase the left heart return. This blood flow usually returns to the left atrium through the pulmonary veins but when the pulmonary artery is open it will also result in continuous back bleeding from the pulmonary arteries. When excellent intracardiac exposure is necessary it is often important to reduce the amount of left heart return temporarily. This can be achieved very effectively by reducing the perfusion flow rate. Although left heart venting systems are available it is often difficult in the very small heart to achieve excellent exposure by venting all the left heart return back to the pump circuit.

Low flow decreases the inflammatory response to bypass: As noted above, hypothermia per se reduces the inflammatory effects of bypass including both cellular activation as well as reduced activation of many humoral cascades. Although it has not been well documented it seems probable that an increased perfusion flow rate results in a greater degree of activation of both the cellular components of blood as well as humoral cascades. A higher flow rate results in a larger amount of blood being scavenged by the pump sucker system as well as the left heart vent. The pump suckers and LA vent are particularly powerful activators of the inflammatory response to bypass. It appears that the air blood interface that occurs in the suction system is the primary site of activation. In addition however a greater flow rate results in exposure of a greater volume of blood to the internal tubing surface as well as the surfaces within the oxygenator, heat exchanger, filters and reservoir etc. It is therefore highly probable that the use of a reduced flow rate reduces the inflammatory response in addition to the reduced inflammatory response that results from hypothermia per se.

Decreased emboli and microemboli: Emboli can be either gaseous or particulate. Several studies have demonstrated that the number of *gaseous* emboli emanating from a bubble oxygenator is closely related to the blood flow rate, gas flow rate and the reservoir level within the oxygenator.[21,22] Membrane oxygenators can also produce multiple gaseous microemboli if air is being entrained by the venous cannula and this effect is worse at high flow rates.[23,24]

There is no known relationship between pump flow rate and *particulate* microemboli other than the cardiotomy suction system which is responsible for most of the particles introduced into the bypass circuit.[25,26]

Higher flow rates will generally necessitate greater volumes of cardiotomy return during open extracardiac procedures.

Disadvantages of low flow bypass

The principal disadvantage of low flow bypass is that the safe lower limit for reduced flow remains poorly defined. Kirklin and Barratt-Boyes in their landmark textbook attempted to develop a nomogram which broadly indicates flow rates that may be safe at specific temperatures.[27] This nomogram was developed from a general review of multiple reports which indirectly addressed the topic. However, it should be understood that the principal methods for monitoring safety of cardiopulmonary bypass both in the past and currently remain quite inadequate. Perfusion pressure carries little meaning in a setting of a reduced metabolic rate as well as the reduced viscosity resulting from hemodilution. Many vasoactive mediators are released during bypass which can have a profound effect on systemic vascular resistance. In any event the perfusion pressure is essentially a surrogate marker for perfusion flow rate which should be known directly from the perfusion flow rate being employed. Some allowance must be made for left heart return which can be estimated by the perfusionist based on blood returning from the cardiotomy suckers and the left atrial vent.

The other method for monitoring perfusion adequacy is the systemic venous oxygen saturation.[28] Because hypothermia shifts oxyhemoglobin dissociation to the left it is difficult to be sure that adequate oxygen delivery is being maintained even though the mixed venous oxygen saturation may read greater than 70–80%. Although systemic venous mixed oxygen saturation is very helpful in estimating cardiac output in the normothermic patient not on bypass it is of limited utility in the setting of hypothermia and alkaline pH, particularly with the alpha stat strategy as well as reduced 2,3- diphosphoglycerate resulting from the use of transfused blood in the prime. In the future it will be important that more sophisticated methods for monitoring perfusion adequacy be developed. Techniques such as near infrared spectroscopy hold promise in this area.[29,30] Until more sophisticated monitoring methods are developed however it is likely that cardiac surgeons and perfusion teams will need to select flow rates that carry a significant safety margin relative to minimal acceptable flow rates for the specific bypass conditions of temperature, hematocrit and pH.

Hypothermia enhances safety of cardiopulmonary bypass

In the early years of cardiopulmonary bypass hypothermia provided an important safety element. Cardiopulmonary bypass hardware was not reliable in the early years and there was always a risk of acute failure of an oxygenator or pump system. Because of its effect in reducing metabolic rate, hypothermia allowed a longer safe period of reduced or absent perfusion which would allow time to change out the faulty component of the bypass circuit. Current day bypass hardware is very much more reliable so that the safety factor introduced by hypothermia has become a much less important consideration.

IMPROVED MYOCARDIAL PROTECTION

Hypothermia reduces the metabolic demands of the myocardium as well as the rest of the body. Although local myocardial hypothermia can be attained through infusion of cold cardioplegia solution the temperature of the perfusate has an important effect on the rate of rewarming of the heart, between cardioplegia infusions[31] (Figure 9.4). This is particularly true if partial cardiopulmonary bypass is used, for example with a single venous cannula in the right atrium under which circumstances blood will enter the right ventricle and contribute to rewarming of both the right ventricular myocardium as well as the ventricular septum. Even when there is total cardiopulmonary bypass the temperature of retrocardiac tissues in particular will be determined by perfusate temperature and will affect the rate of myocardial rewarming. Although multiple infusions of cardioplegia solution are well tolerated beyond infancy, in the neonate and younger infant many studies have suggested that multiple reinfusions of cardioplegia result in less good myocardial protection, most likely because of myocardial edema.[32,33] Use of a lower degree of whole body hypothermia allows for more effective maintenance of myocardial hypothermia with a single infusion of cardioplegia (see Chapter 10).

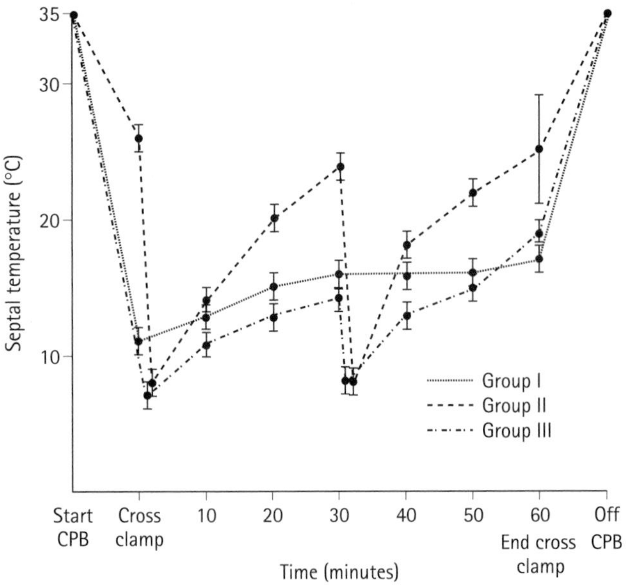

Figure 9.4 *Myocardial rewarming is importantly influenced by systemic temperature during cross-clamp periods. The figure illustrates mean cardiac septal temperature in neonatal pigs. Groups I and III were perfused at deep hypothermia (less than 20°C). Group II was perfused at moderate hypothermia (28°C). Groups II and III had infusions of cardioplegia. Note the rapid rewarming of the interventricular septum in group II relative to the two other groups. (From Ganzel BL, Katzmark SL, Mavroudis C. Myocardial preservation in the neonate.* J Thorac Cardiovasc Surg *1988;* ***96****:414–22, with permission.)*

Disadvantages of hypothermia

PROLONGATION OF CARDIOPULMONARY BYPASS

Use of a more severe degree of hypothermia, i.e. a lower temperature during bypass requires longer periods of cooling and rewarming. The exact duration of cooling and rewarming is determined both by the temperature gradients employed between the water and the heat exchanger, blood temperature and body temperature as well as the mass and specific heat of the individual patient. Because fat has a relatively poor blood supply obese patients require longer periods of cooling and rewarming than patients with a lean body mass. Babies can generally be cooled and rewarmed rapidly probably related to the effectiveness of surface cooling and rewarming as an adjunct to core cooling and rewarming secondary to the higher ratio of surface area to body mass. Babies also tend to be relatively low in total adipose tissue relative to many adult patients.

A longer duration of cardiopulmonary bypass will result in a greater aggregation of the deleterious effects of cardiopulmonary bypass, almost all of which are time related in their degree of severity.

BLEEDING

It is generally considered that use of hypothermic bypass increases the probability of postoperative bleeding.[34] This may be related to the effects of hypothermia on platelet function though bypass per se has a very significant effect on platelet function. The different effects of normothermic and hypothermic bypass on platelet function have not been well documented. Furthermore use of aprotinin and antifibrinolytic agents can be effective in reversing the deleterious effects of bypass and hypothermia on platelet function and coagulation.[35] In general therefore bleeding should not be considered a reason to avoid hypothermic bypass.

INFECTION

Although infection has been documented to be exacerbated by hypothermia in the nonbypass setting it has not been well documented that transient exposure to hypothermic bypass results in a greater incidence of postoperative infection relative to the use of normothermic bypass.

PROLONGED POSTOPERATIVE RECOVERY

Use of moderate hypothermia in adult patients during bypass often results in patients returning to the intensive care unit with a considerable heat debt, i.e. they are likely to remain hypothermic for several hours. It has been well documented that this prolongs the duration of intubation as well as total recovery time in the intensive care unit.[36] In neonates and infants who can be more effectively warmed by surface means than adults and who appear in general to tolerate transient hypothermia better than adults it has not been well documented that early postoperative hypothermia in the intensive care unit significantly prolongs postoperative recovery in the intensive care unit.

DEEP HYPOTHERMIC CIRCULATORY ARREST

Deep hypothermic circulatory arrest involves complete cessation of perfusion at a core body temperature of less than 18°C. Although the technique is now used widely for repair of aortic arch aneurysms in adults, its popularity has declined among congenital surgeons over the last decade. Nevertheless the technique continues to hold important advantages over alternative innovative and unproven methods of continuous though reduced perfusion.

Advantages of deep hypothermic circulatory arrest

DECREASED EXPOSURE TO CARDIOPULMONARY BYPASS

Barratt-Boyes recognized that the technique of deep hypothermic circulatory arrest would allow him to minimize exposure of the infant to cardiopulmonary bypass thereby most likely decreasing the pathological sequelae of the multiple deleterious effects of bypass listed above. The technique of circulatory arrest that Barratt-Boyes popularized was particularly effective in limiting cardiopulmonary bypass time.[37] Most of the cooling is achieved by surface techniques. The child is placed on a cooling blanket and ice bags are applied until the temperature is as low as 23–25°C. Bypass is then established briefly for cooling to a rectal temperature of less than 20°C. This generally requires no more than five minutes of cooling on bypass. The rewarming phase also limits exposure to cardiopulmonary bypass. The child is rewarmed to a rectal temperature of only 32–33°C and the remainder of the warming is achieved by surface means. Thus total exposure of the child to cardiopulmonary bypass may be no more than 20–25 minutes.

IMPROVED EXPOSURE

As described above it is very common for children with congenital heart problems to have greater than usual left heart return. Not only does this increase the risk of global hypoperfusion but in addition the large volume of blood returning to the left atrium through the pulmonary veins can obscure intracardiac exposure. This necessitates placement of an additional cannula, a left heart vent, which frequently is only partially effective in returning blood to the cardiopulmonary bypass circuit.

AVOIDANCE OF MULTIPLE CANNULAS

Although there have been significant advances in cannula design and manufacturing, the need to place at least four cannulas, i.e. one arterial cannula with associated tourniquet, two caval cannulas, each with an associated tourniquet to fix the cannula and a second tourniquet to occlude the cava around the cannula as well as a left heart vent with associated tourniquet means that the operative field becomes crowded. Cannulas also have the potential to distort the heart. This can be of particular importance in procedures that involve valve reconstruction such as repair of complete AV canal. On the other hand procedures that are predominantly extracardiac such as the arterial switch procedure can be comfortably performed on continuous bypass with a single venous cannula in the right atrium. When there is a balloon atrial septal defect present this single cannula drains both right heart and left heart return. A single venous cannula in general does not interfere with accurate performance of a reconstructive procedure.

REDUCED EDEMA

Neonates and young infants have an inherently high capillary permeability. When they develop a systemic inflammatory response to cardiopulmonary bypass this becomes manifest as generalized edema. The degree of edema is further exacerbated by use of a low hematocrit[38] and particularly a low oncotic pressure perfusate.[39] Studies have demonstrated that there is significantly less fluid accumulation in babies undergoing circulatory arrest relative to those undergoing continuous cardiopulmonary bypass.[40]

Declining popularity of deep hypothermic circulatory arrest for congenital cardiac repair in the 1990s

In the 1970s and 1980s there were really only three major centers worldwide that wholeheartedly embraced the concept of primary repair in infancy with application of deep hypothermic circulatory arrest as the support technique. Barratt-Boyes in New Zealand, Castaneda in Boston and Ebert in San Francisco were master technical surgeons who were capable of performing accurate repairs in the limited time available under hypothermic circulatory arrest. The introduction of prostaglandin E1 in the late 1970s[41] opened the door to even greater opportunities for neonatal procedures and led to increasing popularity of procedures such as primary repair of interrupted aortic arch and the development of the stage-1 Norwood procedure by Norwood in Boston. Although there were many centers that continued to oppose both the concept of early primary repair as well as the technique of hypothermic circulatory arrest, nevertheless by the late 1980s many centers worldwide were adopting the concepts of early repair and circulatory arrest.

Improvements in cardiopulmonary bypass for infants and neonates

The 1980s saw the development of membrane oxygenators specifically designed for infants. Not only were the new cardiopulmonary bypass circuits far less injurious but in addition they had a much smaller prime volume so that exposure of the infant to homologous blood was reduced. Improved arterial line filters at last became a reality. More delicate cannulas were introduced (see Chapter 6). The 1980s also saw the introduction of the neonatal arterial switch procedure, a primarily extracardiac procedure that could be performed with equal facility with a single venous cannula on continuous cardiopulmonary bypass or under deep hypothermic circulatory arrest. The stage was now set for a randomized prospective comparison of continuous cardiopulmonary bypass versus deep hypothermic circulatory arrest.

Circulatory arrest trial

Over a four year enrollment period up to March 1992, 171 neonates and young infants under three months of age with transposition with or without a ventricular septal defect were enrolled in a prospective randomized clinical trial at Children's Hospital Boston.[40] Patients were randomized to undergo a arterial switch under either circulatory arrest or continuous low flow bypass at a flow rate of 50 ml/kg per minute. The alpha stat pH strategy and crystalloid hemodilution to a hematocrit of 20% were used for all patients. The mean circulatory arrest duration for those randomized to circulatory arrest was 55 minutes. Perioperative endpoints of the study included the incidence of seizures determined clinically and by continuous EEG. Other endpoints included cumulative release of the brain isoenzyme creatine kinase BB, return of EEG activity, transcranial Doppler assessment of cerebral blood flow velocity, cardiac index, duration of hospitalization as well as complete assessment of fluid and electrolytes, renal and glucose metabolism. A neurological examination was undertaken at regular intervals. At one year of age these same children underwent a brain magnetic resonance imaging scan, neurological examination as well as comprehensive developmental assessment of their motor and cognitive function.[42]

PERIOPERATIVE FINDINGS

The most important finding of the *perioperative* studies was that the use of alpha stat, low hematocrit circulatory arrest is associated with a higher risk of seizures determined both by clinical methods as well as by EEG[40] relative to continuous low flow bypass. Clinical seizures occurred in 12% of infants randomized to circulatory arrest while seizures determined by EEG occurred in 26%. There was a strong correlation between duration of circulatory arrest and the occurrence of seizures ($p = 0.004$) (Figure 9.5). No child who had an arrest time less than 35 minutes had a seizure either clinically or by EEG. Circulatory arrest was also associated with greater release of the brain iso-enzyme creatine kinase BB in the first six hours postoperatively ($p = 0.046$) and longer recovery to first EEG activity ($p < 0.001$). An interesting finding was that

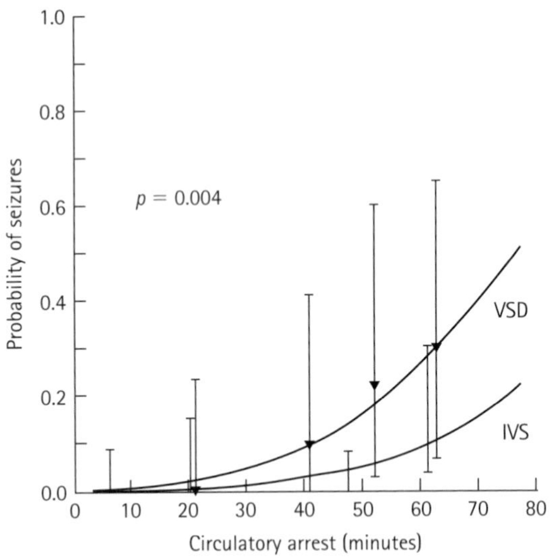

Figure 9.5 *In a randomized prospective trial of low flow bypass versus circulatory arrest (alpha stat, hemodilution to 20%) conducted at Children's Hospital Boston in 1980s using now outmoded bypass equipment, there was a strong correlation between duration of circulatory arrest and the occurrence of seizures. However no child who had an arrest time less than 35 minutes had a seizure either clinically or by encephalography. (From Newburger JW, Jonas RA, Wernovsky G et al. A comparison of the perioperative neurologic effects of hypothermic circulatory arrest versus low flow cardiopulmonary bypass in infant heart surgery.* N Engl J Med *1993;* ***239****: 1057–64, with permission. © 1993 Massachusetts Medical Society. All rights reserved.)*

the presence of an associated ventricular septal defect, which was also associated with older age at the time of surgery, had an important association with risk of seizures. This seemed paradoxical in that the presence of a defect allows improved mixing of the parallel circulations present in transposition, so that these patients are generally less acidotic and less hypoxic than patients with intact ventricular septum and thus are less likely to have suffered a significant preoperative insult. The explanation may lie in the greater cerebral synaptic density of the older patients with a defect (Figure 9.6).

FINDINGS AT ONE YEAR OF AGE

There were 168 survivors of the 171 patients enrolled in the study. Of these 155 returned at one year of age for evaluation.[42]

Developmental testing

The Psychomotor Development Index of the Bayley Scale is a measure of fine and gross *motor ability* in the one year old. Scores were significantly lower among children randomized to circulatory arrest by a mean of 6.5 points ($p = 0.01$). Regression analysis revealed an association between longer duration of circulatory arrest and lower score ($p = 0.02$). The mean score of the two treatment groups combined was 95.1 (predicted 100).

The Mental Development Index does not accurately predict IQ but is a precursor assessment of *cognitive function*. The score of the two treatment groups combined was 105.1 with the current norm being 112. Scores tended to be lower among children assigned to circulatory arrest (mean difference 4.1 points, $p = 0.1$) although the scores did not decrease significantly with an increased duration of circulatory arrest. A diagnosis of associated ventricular septal defect was an independent risk factor for a lower score ($p = 0.004$).

Neurologic examination

A total of 31% of the 154 children who underwent neurologic examination at one year of age had definite abnormalities including hypotonia (18%), hypertonia (8%) and cerebral palsy (3%). All abnormalities were assessed to be mild. Neurologic abnormalities tended to be more common in children randomised to circulatory arrest (41% versus 28%, $p = 0.09$). Possible or definite neurologic abnormalities were associated with a longer duration of circulatory arrest ($p = 0.04$).

Magnetic resonance imaging

Of the 142 children who underwent imaging at one year of age, 15% had definite abnormalities which were mild in 86%. The prevalence of MRI abnormalities was not related to treatment assignment.

Relation between perioperative seizures and one year outcome

As noted above there was a significantly higher incidence of seizures among infants randomized to circulatory arrest compared with those randomized to low flow bypass. In regression analyses with adjustment for the treatment group and the presence or absence of a VSD, the occurrence of EEG

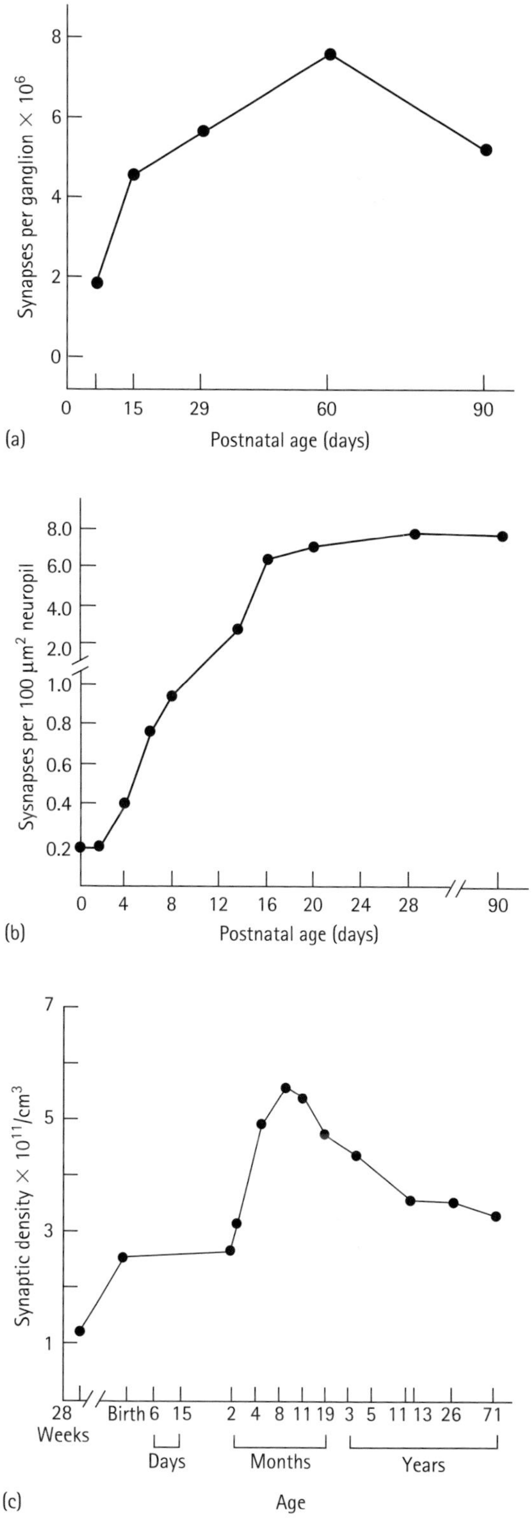

Figure 9.6 *Vulnerability to cerebral insults varies according to age. This is at least in part explained by the rapid increase in synaptic density that occurs in the early months of life. (a) Synapse counts in rat superior cervical ganglion versus postnatal age in days. (b) Synaptic count in rat visual cortex. (c) Synaptic count in human visual cortex. (From Purves D, Lichtman JW.* Principles of Neural Development, *Sunderland, MA, Sinauer Associates, 1985, p 209, with permission.)*

seizures in the early postoperative period was associated with a mean reduction of 11.2 points of the Psychomotor Development Index ($p = 0.002$) and with a significantly higher risk of possible or definite abnormalities on MRI scanning ($p < 0.001$). Infants assigned to circulatory arrest also had an increased risk of clinical seizures in the early postoperative period as noted above. Clinical seizures predicted increased risk of possible or definite neurologic abnormalities at one year of age ($p = 0.05$).

FINDINGS AT FOUR YEARS OF AGE

A total of 158 of the study patients (97%) returned at four years of age for re-evaluation of their neurodevelopmental status.[43] The performance of this cohort as a whole was below population norms on many endpoints. Mean full-scale IQ was 92.6 ± 14.7, verbal IQ was 95.1 ± 15.0 and performance IQ was 91.6 ± 14.5. Treatment groups were similar in terms of IQ, though children in the circulatory arrest group displayed significantly worse motor function and speech. Seizures in the perioperative period, detected either clinically or by EEG, significantly increased the risk of both lower IQ scores and neurologic abnormalities.

FINDINGS AT EIGHT YEARS OF AGE

A total of 155 of the study patients (96%) returned once again at eight years of age for re-evaluation of their neurodevelopmental status.[44,45] As had been seen at four years of age the performance of this cohort as a whole was below expected population means. However, by this time there were no differences in full scale IQ, verbal IQ or performance IQ between the circulatory arrest patients and low flow bypass patients either in the overall scores or on any of the 13 subtests of the Wechsler Intelligence Scale for Children (WISC3) assessment of general intelligence. There were also no differences between circulatory arrest and low flow bypass patients for the overall reading score, overall mathematics score or any Wechsler Individual Achievement Test subscale score which assesses academic achievement. There were also no differences between the groups in the competence scales of the teacher report forms. However, beyond 40 minutes of circulatory arrest time full scale IQ declined in a linear fashion.

Change in attitude towards hypothermic circulatory arrest

There is no question that the early results (i.e. perioperative and four year) of the Boston Circulatory Arrest Study as well as other nonrandomized studies[46] have strongly influenced congenital cardiac surgeons either to avoid completely or at least minimize the use of hypothermic circulatory arrest. Avoidance of hypothermic circulatory arrest has been used almost as a marketing tool by some centers in spite of the fact that few centers have collected or published data to document that their alternative support methods are superior. Interestingly over the same timeframe circulatory arrest has been used more widely for thoracic aortic surgery in adults.

Why circulatory arrest should not be eliminated from use by congenital surgeons

RESULTS OF THE BOSTON CIRCULATORY ARREST STUDY

As described above there are now no differences in IQ between patients who underwent either continuous bypass or circulatory arrest. Furthermore the technique of hypothermic circulatory arrest has been greatly modified and improved in the years since the Boston Circulatory Arrest study was begun.

REFINEMENTS IN THE TECHNIQUE OF DEEP HYPOTHERMIC CIRCULATORY ARREST

A common mistake is to consider deep hypothermic circulatory arrest to be a single immutable factor in potential causation of neurologic injury after cardiac surgery. In fact, circulatory arrest is a technique that has multiple permutations. Over the past 16 years we have undertaken a large number of laboratory and clinical studies that we believe have substantially improved the protection afforded by and safe duration of hypothermic circulatory arrest.

pH strategy

As discussed in detail in Chapter 8, the alkaline alpha stat strategy in which no carbon dioxide is added to the oxygenator gas mixture was applied almost universally between approximately 1985 and 1996. During this period many centers including our own experienced a virtual epidemic of choreoathetosis.[47] Although an association with the change in pH strategy was not proven, the timing was suspicious. Another retrospective study of development showed a strong correlation between a worse developmental outcome with the alpha stat strategy relative to the alternative pH stat strategy in which carbon dioxide is added to the gas mixture.[48] A prospective randomized trial of pH strategy demonstrated that the perioperative outcome was significantly improved with the pH stat strategy.[49] At one year of age there was a strong trend towards an improved outcome in motor skills in patients with transposition and tetralogy.[50] In a very small subgroup of patients with a ventricular septal defect or complete AV canal there was a worse outcome with the pH stat strategy. Subsequent to the completion of the trial of pH strategy the pH stat technique has become our standard strategy not only for deep hypothermic circulatory arrest but for all hypothermic cardiopulmonary bypass.

Hematocrit

The topic of hemodilution during cardiopulmonary bypass is discussed in detail in Chapter 7. In summary hemodilution became a standard practice during the 1960s. By the 1970s a hematocrit of 20% was considered safe and was frequently applied.[51] Some authors suggested that a severe degree of hemodilution was particularly important to avoid microcirculatory disturbances when deep hypothermic circulatory arrest was applied.[52] In the 1980s following the discovery of HIV and hepatitis C viruses as well as the increasing expense of transfused blood there was further pressure to reduce blood usage during cardiopulmonary bypass which led many centers to adopt more severe degrees of hemodilution. Even recent publications have suggested that a hematocrit of 15% can be considered safe.[53] However, laboratory studies conducted at Children's Hospital Boston during the 1990s suggested that hemodilution to a hematocrit of either 10% or 20% resulted in a worse outcome than maintaining a hematocrit of 30% which is the normal hematocrit for a piglet.[38,39] Not only was there an improved behavioral outcome but there was also an improved histological outcome. Magnetic resonance spectroscopy and near infrared spectroscopy suggested that the mechanism was inadequate oxygen delivery with dilute blood, particularly during the cooling phase prior to hypothermic circulatory arrest.

Furthermore a study using intravital microscopy demonstrated that there was no evidence of microcirculatory disturbances with the use of a hematocrit of 30%.[54] In fact it was use of a lower hematocrit of 10% that was associated with delayed reperfusion and areas of 'no reflow'. These laboratory studies led to a prospective randomized clinical trial of hemodilution which was conducted between 1997 and 2000 at Children's Hospital Boston.[55] The trial demonstrated that there was a significantly improved outcome among children randomized to a hematocrit of 30% versus those randomized to a hematocrit of 20%. Not only was there an improved developmental score for motor skills (psychomotor development index) at one year of age but in addition there was reduced edema and an improved cardiac output in the first 24 hours postoperatively with use of a higher hematocrit.

Oxygen

The topic of oxygen strategy during bypass is discussed in detail in Chapter 8. In summary, normoxic cardiopulmonary bypass has been adopted by many centers over the past 10–15 years in the hope that this will reduce the risk of ischemia-reperfusion injury by minimizing generation of oxygen free radicals. However, two laboratory studies undertaken at Children's Hospital Boston demonstrated that the nitrogen which is used to replace oxygen increases the risk of gaseous microemboli, particularly if a bubble oxygenator is employed.[56] In addition brain damage determined by histology was increased with a normoxic technique for hypothermic circulatory arrest relative to circulatory arrest using pure oxygen.[57]

Post-circulatory arrest hyperthermia

A laboratory study at Children's Hospital Boston demonstrated that a fever after circulatory arrest had an extremely powerful effect in exacerbating neurological injury.[58] Piglets whose brain temperature was maintained at 39°C for 24 hours following 100 minutes of deep hypothermic circulatory arrest had very significantly worse behavioral recovery as well as histological outcome relative to animals whose brain temperature was maintained at 34° or 37°C. The mildly hypothermic animals had a slight improvement relative to normothermia but this difference was very much less than the difference between normothermia and hyperthermia (Figure 9.7).

Intermittent reperfusion

Laboratory studies at Children's Hospital Boston have investigated the potential use of a cerebroplegia solution to increase the safe duration of hypothermic circulatory arrest.[59,60] The concept is similar to use of cardioplegia, i.e. cessation of electrical activity induced by chemical means might decrease the metabolic need of cerebral neurons during circulatory arrest.[61,62] Two solutions were studied, namely University of Wisconsin solution as well as an innovative solution developed by the University of Pittsburgh. Neither of these solutions

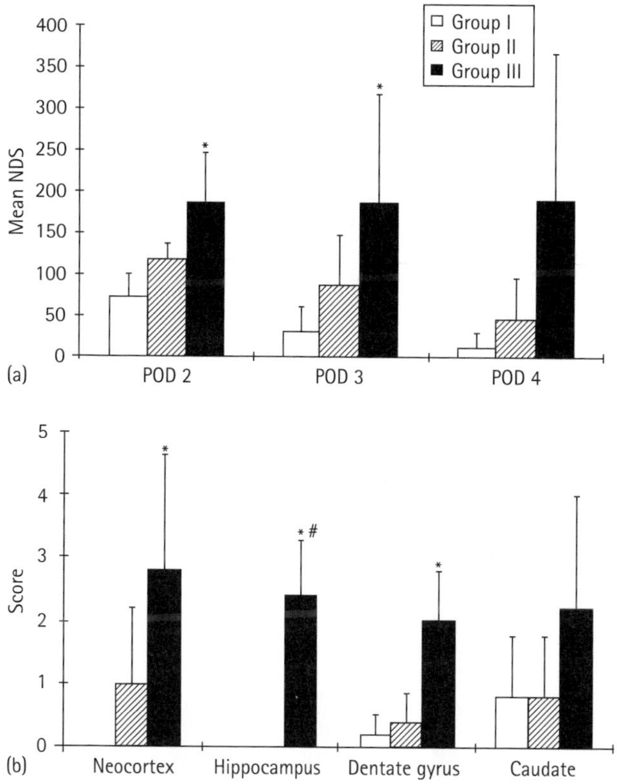

Figure 9.7 *(a) Daily neurologic testing by a blinded observer showed worse neurologic outcome for four days postoperatively in animals maintained at hyperthermia for 24 hours after 100 minutes of deep hypothermia and circulatory arrest (group III) relative to control animals (group II) and animals maintained at a mild degree of hypothermia (group I). NDS = neurological deficit score (higher score is worse). POD = postoperative day; *p < 0.05 group 1 versus group III. (b) Histologic outcome for neocortex, hippocampus, dentate gyrus and caudate nucleus was significantly worse in hyperthermia (group III) animals relative to control (group II) and hypothermic (group I) animals after 100 minutes of circulatory arrest; *p < 0.05 group I versus group III; #p < 0.05 group II versus group III. (From Shum-Tim D, Nagashima M, Shinoka T et al. Postischemic hyperthermia exacerbates neurologic injury after deep hypothermic circulatory arrest.* J Thorac Cardiovasc Surg *1998;* ***116****: 780–92, with permission.)*

extended the safe duration of hypothermic circulatory arrest in our piglet model and in fact both were associated with increased deleterious effects. Interestingly in one study where we used two control groups, i.e. one control group with continuous uninterrupted hypothermic circulatory arrest while the second control group had intermittent periods of reperfusion with the usual perfusate in the pump there was a significantly improved outcome in the intermittent reperfusion group relative to the group receiving the cerebroplegia solution and the group undergoing continuous circulatory arrest[60] (Figure 9.8). This result is similar to the result achieved by the Duke University Group[63] and strongly suggests that intermittent periods of reperfusion for a few minutes perhaps at intervals of 20–30 minutes may be beneficial in increasing the safe duration of hypothermic circulatory arrest.

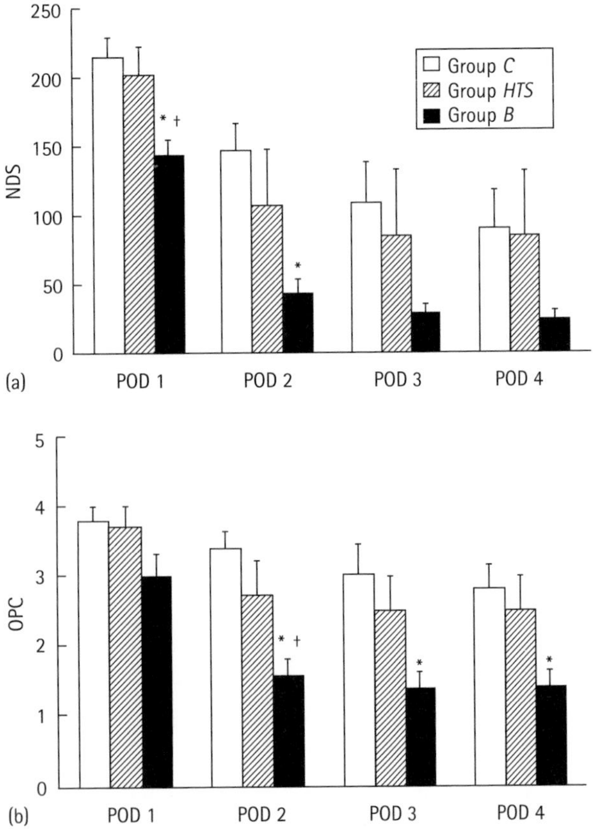

Figure 9.8 *Neurologic and behavioral outcome of piglets exposed to 100 minutes of circulatory arrest at 15°C. There was (a) improved neurologic deficit score (lower neurologic deficit score) and (b) improved overall performance category for group B animals that had intermittent perfusion at 25 minute intervals during circulatory arrest. Control group C underwent 100 minutes of uninterrupted circulatory arrest. Group HTS animals were perfused with preservative solution hypothermosol. POD = postoperative day; NDS = neurologic deficit score; OPC = overall performance category, ⁺$p < 0.05$ versus HTS; *$p < 0.05$ versus C. (From Miura T, Laussen P, Lidov HGW et al. Intermittent whole body perfusion with 'somatoplegia' versus blood perfusate to extend duration of circulatory arrest.* Circulation *1996;* **94**: *II56–62, with permission.)*

Interaction of duration, temperature, pH and hematocrit

Recent laboratory studies at Children's Hospital Boston examined the interaction of pH, hematocrit, temperature and duration of circulatory arrest.[64,65] Studies using near infrared spectroscopy as well as intravital microscopy[54] have confirmed that there is ongoing metabolism and oxygen consumption during hypothermic circulatory arrest (Figure 9.9). While a lower temperature serves to decrease metabolic rate and therefore increase the safe duration of circulatory arrest, the use of the pH stat strategy and a higher hematocrit allow for hyperoxygenation of the brain at the beginning of the circulatory arrest period. By starting at a higher level of oxygenation there is a longer period of declining oxygen level within the brain throughout the early phase of circulatory arrest beyond which there is a plateau with minimal oxygen extraction (Figure 9.10). We have demonstrated that the duration of this latter plateau period termed 'the oxyhemoglobin nadir time' is a useful predictor of behavioral and histological evidence of injury after circulatory arrest.[64] By depressing metabolic rate the pH stat strategy extends the nadir time and particularly the declining oxygenation phase and thereby prolongs the safe duration of circulatory arrest.

Circulatory arrest technique in the 1980s versus current circulatory arrest technique

The technique of hypothermic circulatory arrest that was studied in the Boston Circulatory Arrest study in the 1980s[40] was one that included the alpha stat strategy, crystalloid

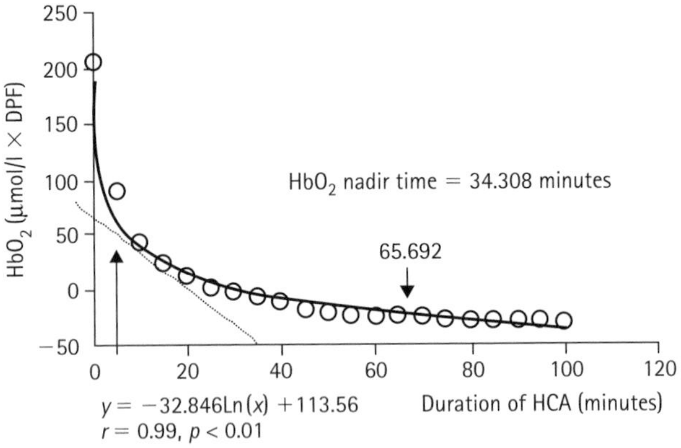

Figure 9.9 *Studies in young piglets have demonstrated ongoing metabolism and oxygen consumption during deep hypothermic circulatory arrest. The nadir value is defined as the point where the HbO_2 signal reaches a plateau state when the slope of the fitting curve, namely the differential coefficient $dHbO_2/dt$ becomes more than −0.5. The duration of arrest beyond the nadir time (oxyhemoglobin nadir time) is a useful predictor of behavioral and histological injury after circulatory arrest. HCA = hypothermic circulatory arrest; DPF = differential pathlength factor. (From Sakamoto T, Hatsuoka S, Stock UA et al. Prediction of safe duration of hypothermic circulatory arrest by near infrared spectroscopy.* J Thorac Cardiovasc Surg *2001; 122: 339–50, with permission.)*

hemodilution to a hematocrit of 20%, use of a relatively high-prime flat sheet membrane oxygenator and no arterial line filter. A relatively long duration of up to 60–75 minutes of circulatory arrest was studied. In spite of what by today's standards is a markedly inferior technique of circulatory arrest, the developmental outcome at eight years of age demonstrates no difference in IQ between patients who underwent continuous hypothermic low flow bypass versus those who underwent the old technique of circulatory arrest. We speculate that with today's technique of circulatory arrest, i.e hematocrit 30%+, pH stat strategy, hyperoxygenation, intermittent reperfusion at 20–30 minute intervals and avoidance of a total duration of greater than one hour it is highly unlikely that any difference could be detected in neurodevelopmental outcome relative to continuous cardiopulmonary bypass. The question that must be answered by those proposing innovative strategies such as retrograde cerebral perfusion,[66] antegrade cerebral perfusion through one arch vessel[67] and other even more innovative procedures[68] is whether such techniques provide homogenous perfusion of the brain and whether they allow equally accurate intracardiac reconstruction. Interestingly, many authors who aggressively promoted the use of retrograde cerebral perfusion for repair of arch aneurysms in adults have now discontinued the use of this technique.

Current indications for deep hypothermic circulatory arrest

The specific situations where an individual surgeon may wish to employ deep hypothermic circulatory arrest will vary according to the speed and accuracy with which he or she can work. Some surgeons may find in spite of the impaired visualization achieved with continuous cardiopulmonary bypass that the absence of the time pressure imposed by the technique of circulatory arrest allows them to achieve a more accurate repair. On the other hand the presence of multiple cannulas can result in distortion of the surgical field which will affect the accuracy of repair in any surgeon's hands. However, situations where it is suggested by the author that circulatory arrest is appropriately applied include neonatal repair of total anomalous pulmonary connection and intracardiac repair in preterm neonates less than 2.5 kg. Although innovative alternatives have been developed the author continues to recommend hypothermic circulatory arrest for the

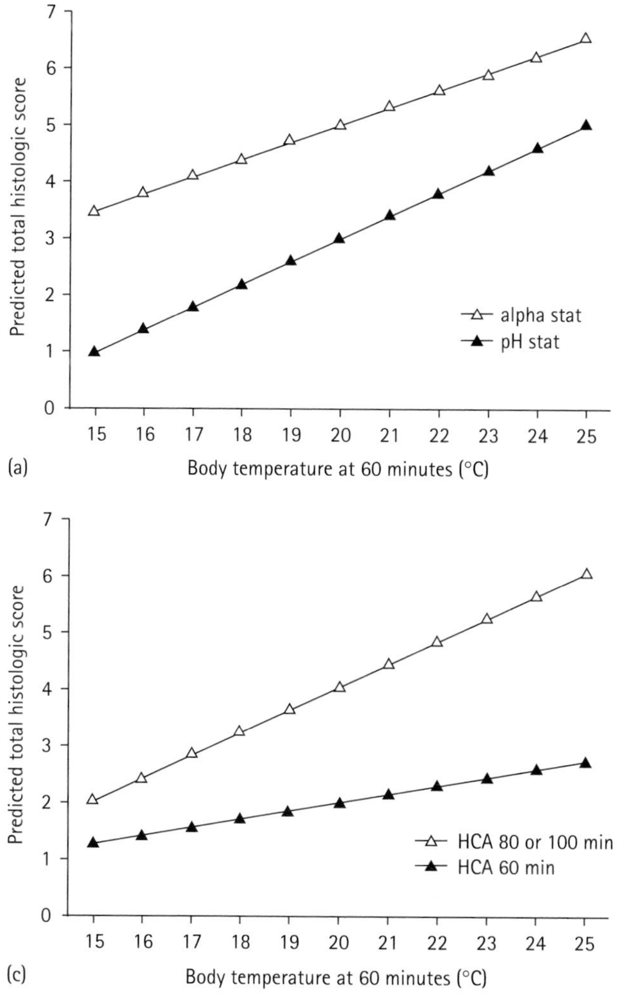

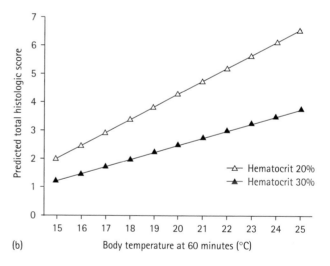

Figure 9.10 *The safe duration of circulatory arrest varies according to the specific conditions including particularly temperature, hematocrit and pH. (a) Interaction of temperature and pH strategy in determining histological injury after circulatory arrest. A higher score represents worse injury. Injury is increased by use of the alpha stat strategy and higher arrest temperature. (b) Interaction of temperature and hematocrit in determining histological injury after circulatory arrest. Injury is increased by use of a lower hematocrit and higher arrest temperature. (c) Interaction of temperature and duration of circulatory arrest in determining histological injury after circulatory arrest. Longer arrest time and higher temperature are associated with worse histologic injury. (From Sakamoto T et al. Interaction of temperature with hematocrit and pH determines safe duration of hypothermic circulatory arrest.* J Thorac Cardiovasc Surg, *in press, with permission from Elsevier.)*

arch reconstruction component of the stage-1 Norwood procedure as well as for repair of interrupted aortic arch. Repair of complete AV canal in the neonate and young infant is unquestionably facilitated by the use of hypothermic circulatory arrest and allows more accurate reconstruction of the AV valves. Small neonates with systemic venous anomalies, e.g. left SVC to coronary sinus also are often best served by the use of hypothermic circulatory arrest.

Summary

Considerable research effort has been expended by a number of groups to define and delineate the limits of hypothermic circulatory arrest. In the future it will be important to focus an equal degree of attention on refining methods of continuous cardiopulmonary bypass including innovative methods that allow avoidance of circulatory arrest. At present there are no clear guidelines available for the congenital surgeon regarding how low flow can be reduced, at what temperature repair should be undertaken and what duration of low flow can be employed for particular circumstances of pH, hematocrit and collateral return. Until such information has been collected, the comprehensive information that has already been gathered regarding circulatory arrest allows this technique to be employed more safely than innovative but unproven methods of continuous cardiopulmonary bypass.

REFERENCES

1. Jonas R. Metabolic response. In Jonas RA, Elliott MJ (eds). *Cardiopulmonary Bypass for Neonates, Infants and Young Children.* London, Butterworth-Heinemann, 1994, pp 205–21.
2. Royston D. Systemic inflammatory responses to surgery with cardiopulmonary bypass. *Perfusion* 1996; **11**:177–89.
3. Utley JR. The history of the concept of inflammatory responses to cardiopulmonary bypass. *Perfusion* 1996; **11**:190–95.
4. Jonas R. Flow reduction and cessation. In Jonas RA, Elliott MJ (eds). *Cardiopulmonary Bypass in Neonates, Infants and Young Children.* Butterworth-Heinemann, London, 1994, p 68.
5. Seghaye MC, Duchateau J, Grabitz RG et al. Complement activation during cardiopulmonary bypass in infants and children. *J Thorac Cardiovasc Surg* 1993; **106**:978–87.
6. Kirklin JW, Westaby S, Blackstone EH et al. Complement and the damaging effects of cardiopulmonary bypass. *J Thorac Cardiovasc Surg* 1983; **86**:845–57.
7. Chenoweth DC, Cooper SW, Hugli TE, Stewart RW, Blackstone EH, Kirklin JW. Complement activation during cardiopulmonary bypass: evidence for generation of C3a and C5a anaphylatoxins. *New Eng J Med* 1981; **304**:497–503.
8. Craddock PR, Fehr J, Brigham KL, Kronenberg RS, Jacob HS. Complement and leukocyte mediated pulmonary dysfunction in hemodialysis. *New Engl J Med* 1977; **296**:769–74.
9. Aoki M, Jonas RA, Nomura F, Kawata H, Hickey PR. Anti-CD18 attenuates deleterious effects of cardiopulmonary bypass and hypothermic circulatory arrest in piglets. *J Card Surg* 1995; **10**:407–17.
10. Rinder CS, Bohnert J, Rinder HM, Mitchell J, Ault K, Hillman R. Platelet activation and aggregation during cardiopulmonary bypass. *Anesthesiology* 1991; **75**:388–93.
11. Seghaye MC, Duchateau J, Grabitz RG et al. Complement, leukocytes, and leukocyte elastase in full-term neonates undergoing cardiac operation. *J Thorac Cardiovasc Surg* 1994; **108**:29–36.
12. Bel A, Elleuch N, Florens E, Menasche P. Temperature and inflammatory response on cardiopulmonary bypass. *Cardiovasc Eng* 2001; **5**:230.
13. Anttila V, Hagino I, Zurakowski D, Lidov HGW, Jonas RA. Higher bypass temperature correlates with increased white cell activation in the cerebral microcirculation. *J Thorac Cardiovasc Surg*, in press.
14. Bering EA. Effect of body temperature change on cerebral oxygen consumption of the intact monkey. *Am J Physiol* 1961; **200**:417–19.
15. Croughwell N, Smith LR, Quill T et al. The effect of temperature on cerebral metabolism and blood flow in adults during cardiopulmonary bypass. *J Thorac Cardiovasc Surg* 1992; **103**:549–54.
16. Bigelow WG, Lindsay WK, Greenwood WF. Hypothermia its possible role in cardiac surgery: An investigation of factors governing survival in dogs at low body temperatures. *Ann Surg* 1950; **132**:849.
17. Bigelow WG, Lindsay WK, Harrison RC, Gordon RA, Greenwood WF. Oxygen transport and utilization in dogs at low body temperatures. *Am J Physiol* 1950; **160**:125.
18. Lewis FJ, Varco RL, Taufic M. Repair of atrial septal defects in man under direct vision with the aid of hypothermia. *Surgery* 1954; **36**:538–56.
19. Swan H, Zeavin I, Blount SG et al. Surgery by direct vision in the open heart during hypothermia. *J Am Med Assoc* 1953; **153**:1081–5.
20. Sealy WC, Brown IW, Young WG et al. Hypothermia and extracorporeal circulation for open heart surgery: Its simplification with a heat exchanger for rapid cooling and rewarming. *Ann Surg* 1959; **150**:627–39.
21. Blauth CI, Smith PL, Arnold JV et al. Influence of oxygenator type on the prevalence and extent of microembolic retinal ischemia during cardiopulmonary bypass. *J Thorac Cardiovasc Surg* 1990; **99**:61–9.
22. Blauth CI, Arnold JV, Schulenberg WE et al. Cerebral microembolism during cardiopulmonary bypass. *J Thorac Cardiovasc Surg* 1988; **95**:668–76.
23. Willcox TW, Mitchell SJ, Gorman DF. Venous air in the bypass circuit: a source of arterial line emboli exacerbated by vacuum-assisted drainage. *Ann Thorac Surg* 1999; **68**:1285–9.
24. Davila RM, Rawles T, Mack MJ. Venoarterial air embolus: a complication of vacuum-assisted venous drainage. *Ann Thorac Surg* 2001; **71**:1369–71.
25. Brooker RF, Brown WR, Moody DM et al. Cardiotomy suction: a major source of brain lipid emboli during cardiopulmonary bypass. *Ann Thorac Surg* 1998; **65**:1651–5.
26. Jewell AE, Akowuah EF, Suvarna SK, Braidley P, Hopkinson D, Cooper G. A prospective randomised comparison of cardiotomy suction and cell saver for recycling shed blood during cardiac surgery. *Eur J Cardiothorac Surg* 2003; **23**:633–6.
27. Kirklin JW, Barratt-Boyes BG. *Cardiac Surgery*, 2nd edn, New York, Churchill Livingstone, 1993, p 91.
28. Harris EA, Seelye ER, Barratt-Boyes BG. On the availability of oxygen to the body during cardiopulmonary bypass in man. *Br J Anesth* 1974; **46**:425.

29. Sakamoto T, Jonas RA, Stock UA et al. Utility and limitations of near-infrared spectroscopy during cardiopulmonary bypass in a piglet model. *Pediatr Res* 2001; **49**:770–6.
30. Nollert G, Jonas RA, Reichart B. Optimizing cerebral oxygenation during cardiac surgery: a review of experimental and clinical investigations with near infrared spectrophotometry. *Thorac Cardiovasc Surg* 2000; **48**:247–53.
31. Doenst T, Schlensak C, Beyersdorf F. Cardioplegia in pediatric cardiac surgery: do we believe in magic? *Ann Thorac Surg* 2003; **75**:1668–77.
32. Bove EL, Stammers AH, Gallagher KP. Protection of the neonatal myocardium during hypothermic ischemia. Effect of cardioplegia on left ventricular function in the rabbit. *J Thorac Cardiovasc Surg* 1987; **94**:115–23.
33. Sawa Y, Matsuda H, Shimazaki Y et al. Comparison of single dose versus multiple dose crystalloid cardioplegia in neonates: Experimental study with neonatal rabbits from birth to 2 days of age. *J Thorac Cardiovasc Surg* 1989; **97**:229–34.
34. Felfernig M, Blaicher A, Kettner SC, Felfernig D, Acimovic S, Kozek-Langenecker SA. Effects of temperature on partial thromboplastin time in heparinized plasma in vitro. *Eur J Anaesthesiol* 2001; **18**:467–70.
35. Bidstrup BP, Royston D, Sapsford RN, Taylor KM. Reduction in blood loss and blood use after cardiopulmonary bypass with high dose aprotinin (Trasylol). *J Thorac Cardiovasc Surg* 1989; **97**:364–72.
36. Christenson JT, Maurice J, Simonet F, Velebit V, Schmuziger M. Normothermic versus hypothermic perfusion during primary coronary artery bypass grafting. *Cardiovasc Surg* 1995; **3**:519–24.
37. Barratt-Boyes BG, Simpson MM, Neutze JM. Intracardiac surgery in neonates and infants using deep hypothermia. *Circulation* 1970; **62**:III73.
38. Shin'oka T, Shum-Tim D, Jonas RA et al. Higher hematocrit improves cerebral outcome after deep hypothermic circulatory arrest. *J Thorac Cardiovasc Surg* 1996; **112**:1610–20.
39. Shin'oka T, Shum-Tim D, Laussen PC et al. Effects of oncotic pressure and hematocrit on outcome after hypothermic circulatory arrest. *Ann Thorac Surg* 1998; **65**:155–64.
40. Newburger JW, Jonas RA, Wernovsky G et al. A comparison of the perioperative neurologic effects of hypothermic circulatory arrest versus low flow cardiopulmonary bypass in infant heart surgery. *N Engl J Med* 1993; **329**:1057–64.
41. Elliott RB, Starling MB, Neutze JM. Medical manipulation of the ductus arteriosus. *Lancet* 1975; **1**:140–2.
42. Bellinger DC, Jonas RA, Rappaport LA et al. Developmental and neurologic status of children after heart surgery with hypothermic circulatory arrest or low flow cardiopulmonary bypass. *N Engl J Med* 1995; **332**:549–55.
43. Bellinger DC, Wypij D, Kuban KCK et al. Developmental and neurological status of children at 4 years of age after heart surgery with hypothermic circulatory arrest or low flow cardiopulmonary bypass. *Circulation* 1999; **100**:526–32.
44. Wypij D, Newburger JW, Rappaport LA et al. The effect of duration of deep hypothermic circulatory arrest in infant heart surgery. *J Thorac Cardiovasc Surg* 2003; **126:**1397–403.
45. Bellinger DC, Wypij D, du Plessis AJ et al. Neurodevelopmental status at eight years in children with D-transposition of the great arteries: The Boston Circulatory Arrest Trial. *J Thorac Cardiovasc Surg*, 2003; **126:**1385–96.
46. Wells FC, Coghill S, Caplan HL, Lincoln C. Duration of circulatory arrest does influence the psychological development of children after cardiac operation in early life. *J Thorac Cardiovasc Surg* 1983; **86**:823–31.
47. Wong PC, Barlow CF, Hickey PR et al. Factors associated with choreoathetosis after cardiopulmonary bypass in children with congenital heart disease. *Circulation* 1992; **86**:II118–26.
48. Jonas RA, Bellinger DC, Rappaport LA et al. Relation of pH strategy and developmental outcome after hypothermic circulatory arrest. *J Thorac Cardiovasc Surg* 1993; **106**:362–8.
49. du Plessis AJ, Jonas RA, Wypij D et al. Perioperative effects of alpha-stat versus pH-stat strategies for deep hypothermic cardiopulmonary bypass in infants. J *Thorac Cardiovasc Surg* 1997; **114**:991–1000.
50. Bellinger DC, Wypij D, du Plessis AJ et al. Developmental and neurologic effects of alpha-stat versus pH-stat strategies for deep hypothermic cardiopulmonary bypass in infants. *J Thorac Cardiovasc Surg* 2001; **121**:374–83.
51. Kawashima Y, Yamamoto Z, Manabe H. Safe limits of hemodilution in cardiopulmonary bypass. *Surgery* 1974; **76**:391–7.
52. Bjork VO, Hultquist G. Brain damage in children after deep hypothermia. *Thorax* 1960; **15**:284.
53. Cook DJ, Orszulak TA, Daly RC. Minimum hematocrit at differing cardiopulmonary bypass temperatures in dogs. *Circulation* 1998; **98**:II170–4.
54. Duebener LF, Sakamoto T, Hatsuoka S et al. Effects of hematocrit on cerebral microcirculation and tissue oxygenation during deep hypothermic bypass. *Circulation* 2001; **104**:I260–4.
55. Jonas RA, Wypij D, Roth SJ et al. The influence of hemodilution on outcome after hypothermic cardiopulmonary bypass: Results of a randomized trial in infants. *J Thorac Cardiovasc Surg* 2003; **126**:1765–74.
56. Nollert G, Nagashima M, Bucerius J, Shin'oka T, Jonas RA. Oxygenation strategy and neurologic damage after deep hypothermic circulatory arrest. I. Gaseous microemboli. *J Thorac Cardiovasc Surg* 1999; **117**:1166–71.
57. Nollert G, Nagashima M, Bucerius J et al. Oxygenation strategy and neurologic damage after deep hypothermic circulatory arrest. II. Hypoxic versus free radical injury. *J Thorac Cardiovasc Surg* 1999; **117**:1172–9.
58. Shum-Tim D, Nagashima M, Shinoka T et al. Postischemic hyperthermia exacerbates neurologic injury after deep hypothermic circulatory arrest. *J Thorac Cardiovasc Surg* 1998; **116**:780–92.
59. Forbess JM, Ibla JC, Lidov HGW et al. University of Wisconsin cerebroplegia in a piglet survival model of circulatory arrest. *Ann Thorac Surg* 1995; **60**:S494–500.
60. Miura T, Laussen P, Lidov HGW et al. Intermittent whole body perfusion with 'somatoplegia' versus blood perfusate to extend duration of circulatory arrest. *Circulation* 1996; **94**:II56–62.
61. Aoki M, Nomura F, Stromski ME et al. Effects of MK-801 and NBQX on acute recovery of piglet cerebral metabolism after hypothermic circulatory arrest. *J Cereb Blood Flow Metab* 1994; **14**:156–65.
62. Hiramatsu T, Jonas RA, Miura T et al. Cerebral metabolic recovery from deep hypothermic circulatory arrest after treatment with arginine and nitro-arginine methyl ester. *J Thorac Cardiovasc Surg* 1996; **112**:698–707.
63. Langley SM, Chai PJ, Miller SE et al. Intermittent perfusion protects the brain during deep hypothermic circulatory arrest. *Ann Thorac Surg* 1999; **68**:4–12.
64. Sakamoto T, Hatsuoka S, Stock UA et al. Prediction of safe duration of hypothermic circulatory arrest by near infrared spectroscopy. *J Thorac Cardiovasc Surg* 2001; **122**:339–50.

65. Sakamoto T, Hatsuoka H, Duebener LF et al. Combination of alpha-stat strategy and hemodilution exacerbates neurological injury in a survival piglet model with deep hypothermic circulatory arrest. *Ann Thorac Surg* 2002; **73**:180–90.
66. Raskin SA, Coselli JS. Retrograde cerebral perfusion overview, techniques and results. *Perfusion* 1995; **10**:51–7.
67. Pigula FA, Siewers RD, Nemoto EM. Regional perfusion of the brain during neonatal aortic arch reconstruction. *J Thorac Cardiovasc* 1999; **117**:1023–4.
68. Reddy VM, Hanley FL, Techniques to avoid circulatory arrest in neonates undergoing repair of complex heart defects. *Sem Thorac Cardiovasc Surg Pediatr Card Surg Annu* 2001; **4**:277–80.

10

Myocardial protection

INTRODUCTION

One of the most important fundamental differences between surgery for congenital heart disease versus surgery for acquired heart disease, is the fact that both the myocardium and the coronary arterial tree are normal in the vast majority of patients with congenital heart disease, particularly in neonates and infants. The congenital cardiac surgeon is not confronted by the difficult problems of uniform delivery of cardioplegia solution, focal areas of scar and global severe impairment of ventricular function. In fact a fundamental premise of this book is that congenital cardiac surgery should be undertaken early in life before the myocardium has been deleteriously affected by the congenital heart problem in question.

The major problem confronting the congenital cardiac surgeon when dealing with myocardial protection during cardiac surgical procedures is the evolving maturity of the myocardium. There are important physiological differences between neonatal and mature myocardium that will be reviewed in this chapter. Almost certainly these physiological differences in function have an impact on the susceptibility of the myocardium to the global ischemia caused by the aortic cross-clamp period. It is probably the evolving maturity of neonatal and infant myocardium that has led surgeons dealing with congenital heart disease to have many different opinions regarding the susceptibility of immature myocardium to ischemia. The bulk of evidence available at present, however, points to the neonatal myocardium being considerably more resistant to ischemia than the mature myocardium. The point of transition remains very poorly defined though it almost certainly occurs in the first year of life and possibly within the first three months of life. The techniques of myocardial protection must be tailored according to the age of the patient in question.

DEVELOPMENTAL DIFFERENCES BETWEEN IMMATURE AND MATURE MYOCARDIUM

Structural differences

As an individual ages myocytes become larger and more oblong, myofibrils become larger and more longitudinally oriented, mitochondria increase in number and sarcoplasmic reticulum becomes more extensive.[1–4]

Substrate metabolism

In the mature heart up to 90% of ATP production is derived from the oxidation of long chain fatty acids.[5] In contrast immature myocardium metabolizes fatty acids, ketones and amino acids, and uses as its principal substrate glucose (Figure 10.1). This is in the spite of the fact that the sensitivity of the neonatal heart to insulin is diminished.[6] For example, the insulin-sensitive glucose transporter (GLUT4) is much less expressed in the immature heart relative to the adult heart whereas the noninsulin-sensitive transporter (GLUT1) is expressed to a higher degree.[7] In general it is accepted that the immature heart has an increased ability to utilize anaerobic metabolism.

Calcium metabolism

The immature myocardium is very much more sensitive to extracellular calcium levels than mature myocardium. In mature hearts most of the calcium required for myocardial contraction is provided by the sarcoplasmic reticulum.[8,9] However, the sarcoplasmic reticulum is underdeveloped in the immature heart and has reduced storage capacity for

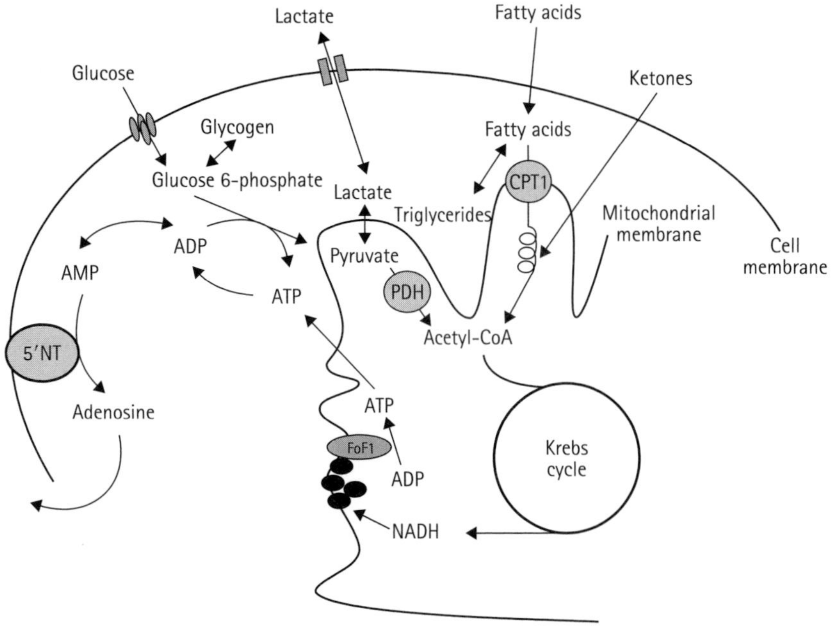

Figure 10.1 *In contrast to mature hearts which derive 90% of their energy supply from long chain fatty acids, immature myocardium metabolizes fatty acids, ketones and amino acids and uses glucose as its principal substrate. CPT1 = carnitine palmitoyl transferase, PDH = pyruvate dehydrogenase, the rate limiting steps for fatty acids and glucose respectively. (From Doenst et al. Cardioplegia in pediatric cardiac surgery: Do we believe in magic?* Ann Thorac Surg *2003; **75**:1668–77, with permission.)*

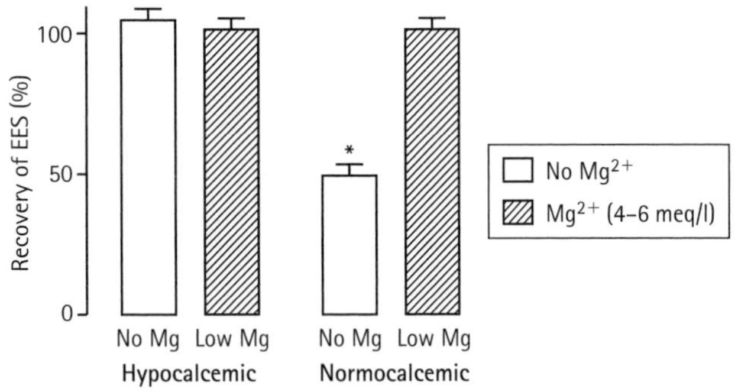

Figure 10.2 *Cardioplegia solutions containing a normal calcium level have poor recovery of end systolic elastance (EES). Addition of magnesium to normocalcemic cardioplegia offsets its detrimental effects in hypoxic neonatal piglet hearts. (From Kronon et al. The relationship between calcium and magnesium in pediatric myocardial protection.* J Thorac Cardiovasc Surg *1997; **114**:1010–19, with permission.)*

calcium.[10] Also the activity of the sarcoplasmic calcium ATPase (SERCA) the enzyme responsible for calcium reuptake into the sarcoplasmic reticulum is reduced relative to mature myocardium. Therefore the ability of the immature heart to release calcium upon stimulation of ryanodine receptors is significantly lower than in mature hearts and reuptake into the sarcoplasmic reticulum is diminished. Therefore immature hearts are much more sensitive to calcium channel blockers than adult hearts. Several reports have described detrimental effects of cardioplegic solutions containing normal or high calcium concentrations and the use of solutions containing subphysiological levels of calcium is recommended[11–13] (Figure 10.2). It has been the experience at Children's Hospital Boston that it is an advantage to have very low levels of ionized calcium during the cooling phase prior to aortic cross clamping and myocardial ischemia.[14] However, some reports have differed from this experience with respect to perfusate calcium levels.[12,15–17]

ENZYME ACTIVITY: ANTIOXIDANTS

Many enzyme systems are less active in immature relative to mature myocardium. For example, oxygen free-radical scavengers such as supraoxide dismutase, catalase and glutathione reductase are less active in immature myocardium.[18] This fact could be important in increasing susceptibility to free radicals generated during reperfusion after ischemia. Clinical studies have demonstrated that in children with tetralogy of Fallot, glutathione reductase activity is significantly reduced.[18–20] Concern regarding free-radical activity has led to the use of leukocyte free blood and leukocyte filters as part of the bypass circuit as a strategy to reduce free-radical generation. However, clinical evidence of efficacy has not been convincingly demonstrated.[21–23]

Another enzyme which is less active in immature myocardium is 5′-nucleotidase (5′NT). This enzyme catalyzes the conversion of ATP to adenosine. Although AMP cannot readily pass out of the cell to the extracellular space, adenosine in contrast is easily lost in the extracellular space through the plasma membrane where 5′NT resides. Loss of adenosine from the mature myocardium itself during ischemia to a level of greater than 50% will inhibit full recovery of contractile function. The fact that the mature heart is less able to convert AMP to adenosine reduces the risk of excessive depletion of the adenine nucleotide pool and may be one explanation as to why immature myocardium is more tolerant to ischemia.[24,25]

Catecholamines

Immature myocardium is less sensitive to catecholamines than mature myocardium. In vitro studies suggest that a decreased coupling of the myocardial β-adrenergic receptors to adenylate cyclase at birth is responsible for this phenomenon.[26] In contrast the kinetics of cyclic AMP hydrolysis and the inhibitory potential of phosphodiesterase inhibitors (e.g. milrinone) are not affected by age. Thus phosphodiesterase inhibitors have come into wide use in the cardiac intensive care unit for managing neonates and infants.

Ischemic preconditioning

There is a marked difference in the effect of ischemic preconditioning on the mature heart relative to the neonatal heart.[27] It has been speculated that the adult heart employs ischemic preconditioning as a mechanism to increase tolerance to ischemia during periods of stress. The lack of a preconditioning effect in the newborn heart may be due to the fact that the mechanisms which are active in preconditioning are already in effect and in part explain the increased tolerance of the neonate to ischemia.

Functional consequences of maturity differences in myocardium

The immature heart has a greater dependence on trans-sarcolemmal calcium movement, has lower intracellular calcium concentration, develops less force, has lower velocity of shortening and has lower velocity of re-extension.

CLINICAL EXPERIENCE: TOLERANCE OF IMMATURE HEART TO ISCHEMIA

A frequently cited report of 200 consecutive pediatric cardiac surgical procedures by one surgeon using St Thomas cardioplegia suggested that myocardial ischemic damage is a common cause of early death in children despite the use of cardioplegia.[28] Rebeyka et al have suggested that the immature myocardium is susceptible to 'rapid cooling contracture'.[14] The proposed mechanism is hypothermia induced calcium accumulation in myocardial cells before the onset of ischemia. However, a number of laboratory studies have suggested that immature myocardium is more resistant to global ischemia than mature myocardium.

The experience at Children's Hospital Boston has been that myocardial failure is a rare primary cause of death after cardiac surgery. A review of the author's experience in one calendar year (1989) with 257 consecutive patients including rapid cooling in all and a high complexity mix (78 neonates, 67 infants) revealed an early mortality of 2%.[29,30] Only two of five patients who died – one with hypoplastic left heart syndrome and one with anomalous left coronary artery from the pulmonary artery – did so in a low output state. Aortic-cross clamp time ranged from 7–191 minutes with total bypass time from 19–272 minutes. There was no relationship between hospital death and myocardial ischemic time. An additional retrospective review of 32 consecutive neonates and infants from the hospital experience who died after cardiac surgery suggests that death could be attributed to a residual anatomical defect in 12 of 18 patients who had a reparative operation and in 4 of 14 patients who had palliative procedures such as first stage palliation of HLHS.

Causes of low output after pediatric cardiac surgery

Although primary myocardial failure is a rare cause of death after pediatric open heart surgery, a fall in cardiac output is seen in most patients between 6 and 18 hours postoperatively (Figure 10.3). In three separate prospective randomized clinical trials performed at Children's Hospital Boston of circulatory arrest,[31] of pH strategy[32] and hematocrit[33] a fall in cardiac output as measured by thermodilution catheters was seen in almost all patients between 9 and 18 hours postoperatively.[34] Thus there is clearly room for improvement in myocardial management techniques.

The most important cause of an excessive fall in cardiac output postoperatively is a residual volume load or pressure load, i.e. an imperfect repair.[29] Other causes include:

- ventricular distention – failure to vent the heart adequately
- retraction/stretch injury to the myocardium
- coronary artery injury
- ventriculotomy
- edema – inappropriate degree of hemodilution of red cells or colloid oncotic pressure
- perfusion factors
- reperfusion conditions, e.g. pressure, calcium, oxygen, additives such as adenosine and free-radical scavengers.

VENTRICULAR DISTENTION: WHY, WHEN AND HOW TO VENT THE LEFT HEART

Although both clinical experience as well as laboratory studies support the notion that immature myocardium is considerably more resistant to ischemia than mature myocardium, there is a definite sense that immature myocardium is considerably more sensitive to stretch injury. The common causes of stretch injury in the operating room are ventricular distention and retraction. Overdistention of the left heart can be caused by a number of mechanisms. Exposure to the full perfusion pressure for even a few seconds appears to have an extremely important impact on subsequent myocardial performance. Furthermore in most situations where distention results there will also be distention of the left atrium and pulmonary veins and a high transcapillary pressure within the

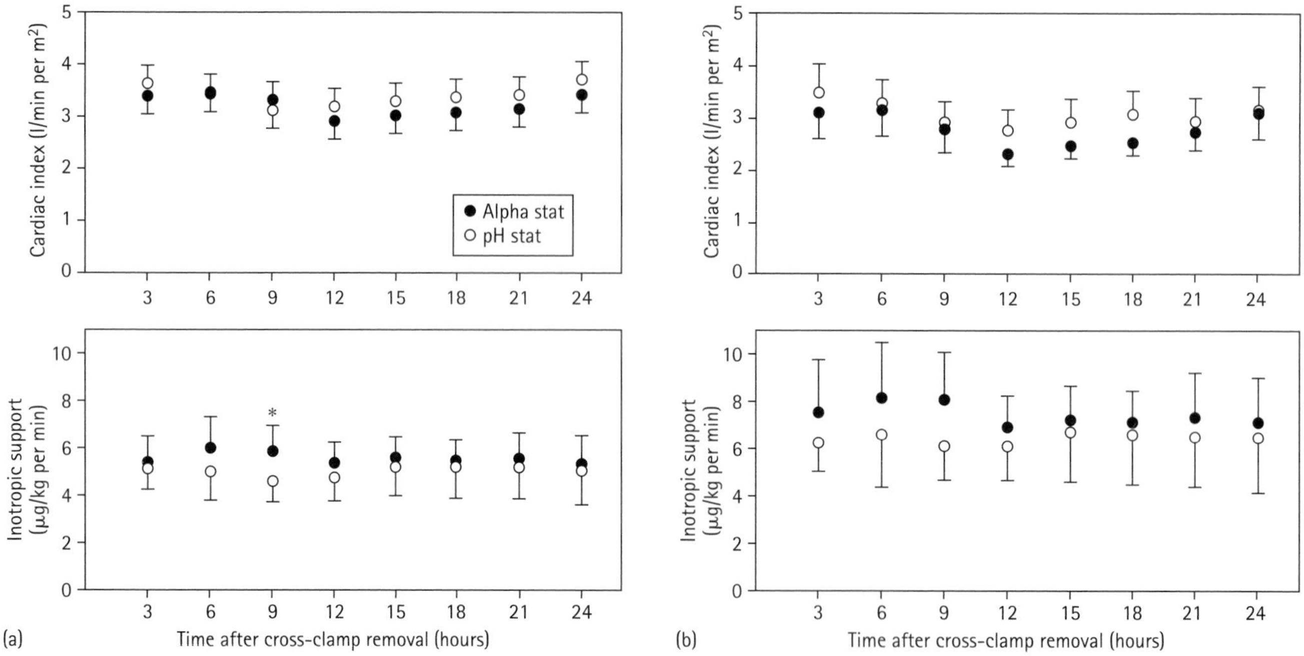

Figure 10.3 *A fall in cardiac output is seen in most pediatric patients between 6 and 18 hours after cross-clamp removal. The figure illustrates serial measurements of cardiac index (top) determined by thermodilution and total inotropic support (bottom) according to treatment group and hours after cross-clamp removal in a prospective randomized trial of pH strategy. (a) Data for all patients. (b) Data for patients with dextro transposition of the great arteries only. Values are depicted as a mean and one side of a 95% confidence interval; *p < 0.05. (From Jonas RA. Myocardial protection for neonates and infants.* Thorac Cardiovasc Surg *1998;* ***46****:288–91, with permission.)*

lungs will result. It is very likely that many cases of so-called 'pump lung' in fact reflect simple mechanical transudation of fluid secondary to left heart distention during cardiopulmonary bypass.

Causes of left heart distention

Virtually all the potential causes of left heart distention are present preoperatively. The fundamental difference that changes these factors from simply an extra volume load for the left heart to a pathological cause of injury is the fact that left heart function is markedly depressed during much of the bypass procedure. For example, systemic to pulmonary artery connections such as a Blalock shunt or multiple aortopulmonary collateral vessels result in increased pulmonary venous return which must be ejected by the left ventricle. Immediately after commencing bypass in the neonate or young infant the rapid fall in ionized calcium level as well as hypothermia result in reduced contractility and a reduced heart rate. The net effect is that the left ventricle is no longer able to accommodate the blood returning to the left atrium. Eventually pressure will equalize between the aorta, the left atrium and the left ventricle unless the left heart is appropriately vented. Another important cause of left ventricular distention other than increased left heart blood return is aortic valve regurgitation. The important difference about aortic regurgitation relative to increased blood return from the lungs is that it can be easily managed by application of the cross clamp. On the other hand it cannot be effectively managed by placement of a vent into the left atrium assuming that the mitral valve is competent. Therefore a vent must be positioned across the mitral valve into the left ventricle in order to adequately decompress the left ventricle in the setting of aortic valve regurgitation.

When to place left heart vent: timing

It is essential that the surgeon constantly monitor the level of left heart distention in order to avoid myocardial and pulmonary injury. This is most easily done by observing the degree of distention of the main pulmonary artery assuming that the cause of left heart distention is increased left heart return. Observation that the left atrial appendage is distended also may be helpful. If the cause of left heart distention is aortic valve regurgitation the surgeon may not be able to observe directly the signs of distention and should have a high level of suspicion that regurgitation is resulting in excessive ventricular distention as the heart rate slows and contractility visibly decreases. LV distention can be monitored by palpation of the left ventricle. The left ventricle can be massaged when it is contracting inadequately or alternatively the aortic cross clamp can be applied. In general it is not wise to place a vent into the left heart while the left heart is beating vigorously, i.e. during the early phase of cooling. An incision into the right superior pulmonary vein may result in air being entrained into the left ventricle which will then be ejected into the systemic circulation. In order to be completely safe it is generally wise to place a left heart vent after the aortic cross clamp has been applied. In urgent situations however the left heart may be decompressed by a stab incision into the left atrium. Above all it is essential to remember that the degree of distention is equal ultimately to aortic perfusion pressure. Therefore an instant method for decreasing left heart distention is to request that the perfusionist immediately drop the flow rate to a very low level until the problem that resulted in left heart distention can be rectified.

Methods for left heart venting

The traditional method for left heart venting is to place a cannula through a purse-string in the right side of the left atrium adjacent to the point of junction of the right pulmonary veins with the left atrium. The cannula should be curved so as to guide it across the mitral valve into the left ventricle. In addition to this traditional method however there are many other steps in the operative strategy and sequence that can allow for adequate left heart decompression. For example in a child with transposition of the great arteries who has had a balloon atrial septostomy a single venous cannula in the right atrium will at all times adequately decompress the left heart. The presence of a large VSD allows a right atrial cannula to temporarily pass across the tricuspid valve for left heart decompression. Very commonly the pulmonary artery is opened during congenital procedures. This too represents a method for decompression of the left atrium from excessive left heart return though it does not decompress the left ventricle if the cause of distention is aortic valve regurgitation.

Danger of left heart venting

It is essential for the surgeon to recognize that placement of a left heart vent places the patient at risk of inadequate systemic perfusion and most importantly of brain injury. If there is a massive amount of left heart return from uncontrolled collateral vessels, the act of decompressing the left heart by returning this blood directly to the pump may avoid injury to the lungs and left ventricle but does not allow the systemic capillary bed to be perfused. Preoperatively this left heart return has been ejected into the systemic circulation. Therefore so long as myocardial contractility is maintained and left heart return is ejected throughout the procedure then there should not be a risk of brain injury. One response by many surgeons when a large amount of left heart return is seen is simply to cool the patient to a lower temperature. However, systemic perfusion of the brain is necessary in order to cool the brain uniformly so that this step in itself is usually not adequate. What should be done is that the perfusion flow rate should be increased or more effectively the source of the excessive left heart return should be controlled, for example by shunt ligation or direct tourniquet control of collaterals. The preoperative diagnostic workup also should include assessment of collateral return so that the surgeon is not placed in an unanticipated situation of excessive left heart return from unknown sources. Frequently coil occlusion of collaterals can be performed in the catheterizaton laboratory, although the decision as to which collaterals to occlude is often complex (see Chapter 25).

When to discontinue venting

During the rewarming phase of bypass, as ventricular contractility is regained, the heart will once again acquire the capacity to eject the volume load resulting from left heart return. When the surgeon judges that there is a reasonable degree of contractility the perfusionist should be asked to reduce the level of vent suction and ultimately to turn the vent off. At this point ejection from the left ventricle should be observed and left atrial pressure should be monitored. The vent must be carefully removed in such a fashion that air is not entrained into the left heart. This can be achieved by insuring that the patient is on partial bypass with partial constriction of the venous line thereby elevating central venous and right atrial pressures. Blood will be returned through the lungs to the left heart ensuring positive left atrial pressure therefore minimizing the risk that air will be entrained.

RETRACTION INJURY TO THE MYOCARDIUM

One of the most challenging aspects of neonatal and infant surgery is to achieve adequate exposure of intracardiac defects such as a VSD using a limited atrial incision and with avoidance of excessive retraction of the myocardium. Neonatal and infant myocardium is extremely soft and easily retracted. It is possible to almost totally evert the right ventricle through the tricuspid valve if one pulls excessively hard on sutures that have already been placed. Excessive force on retractors placed through the tricuspid annulus can damage not only the ventricular myocardium but also the conduction bundle. This may be an explanation for the hyperexcitability of the bundle of His which manifests itself as a His bundle tachycardia or junctional ectopic tachycardia postoperatively. The surgeon must constantly monitor the retraction provided by assistants and at all times avoid excessive force.

CORONARY ARTERY INJURY

Injury to the proximal right coronary or left coronary artery in a neonate or infant is almost certain to be a fatal injury. Fortunately however the proximal main coronary arteries are rarely placed at risk other than in a procedure such as the arterial switch operation. However, smaller branches of the coronary arteries can be damaged during procedures, particularly those which involve either incisions or suture lines in the anterior wall of the right ventricle. For example neonatal repair of tetralogy requires a patch suture line which is frequently no more than 2 or 3 mm from the left anterior descending coronary artery. Excessive tension on the epicardium close to the anterior descending can result in partial ischemia and poor myocardial function. At all times ventriculotomies should be planned in such a fashion as to minimize injury to even very small coronary artery branches.

VENTRICULOTOMY

In addition to avoiding injury to the coronary arteries a ventriculotomy when essential must be minimal in length. Even if the ventriculotomy is an appropriate length it is easy for it to be torn to a greater length through excessive retraction. Once again the surgeon must monitor the retraction force of the assistants in order to reduce this risk.

EDEMA

The neonatal and infant myocardium is particularly susceptible to edema probably secondary to a generalized increase in capillary permeability that is seen in the immature individual.[35,36] However, edema can be exacerbated by an excessive degree of hemodilution, particularly if crystalloid alone is used resulting in a reduction in colloid oncotic pressure. The importance of perfusate hematocrit in optimizing outcome is discussed in detail in Chapter 7.

PERFUSION FACTORS

Hematocrit

Between 1997 and 2000 a prospective randomized trial of hematocrit during cardiopulmonary bypass was performed at Children's Hospital Boston.[33] Seventy four patients under nine months of age undergoing reparative surgery were randomized to a hematocrit of 20% while 73 were randomized to a hematocrit of 30%. Forty percent of patients had transposition of the great arteries, 32% had tetralogy of Fallot and 28% had a VSD. The study groups were comparable at baseline with respect to age at surgery, parental education, gestational age, Apgars and intubation prior to surgery. The total bypass time was similar in both groups at approximately 100 minutes. Median circulatory arrest time was 0. One of the most important findings of the study was that there were developmental differences between the two groups at one year of age with patients in the higher hematocrit group having an improved outcome (see Chapter 7). In addition there were impressive differences in postoperative cardiac index as measured by thermodilution catheter over the first 24 hours postoperatively. The nadir of cardiac index was consistently higher in the patients who had the higher hematocrit. This was associated with a predictable difference in whole body edema as measured by bioimpedance on the first postoperative day ($p = 0.006$). Lowest cardiac index in the higher hematocrit group was 3.1 ± 1.1 l/min per m^2 versus 2.8 ± 1.1 in the lower hematocrit group ($p = 0.02$).

A further point of interest from the hematocrit trial was the fact that two different cardioplegia solutions were employed. There was no difference in cardiac index between patients who received oxygenated crystalloid St Thomas solution (Plegisol, Abbott, Abbott Park, Illinois) versus those who received custom blood cardioplegia solution developed at Children's Hospital Boston. However, an interaction was observed between the cardioplegia solution used and hematocrit such that the effect of hematocrit on cardiac index was exaggerated in patients who received the crystalloid cardioplegia solution. This suggests that the disadvantage of a lower perfusate hematocrit with respect to cardiac output may be secondary to myocardial edema.

pH strategy

A prospective randomized trial of pH strategy during hypothermic bypass was performed at Children's Hospital Boston in 182 patients less than nine months of age undergoing reparative heart surgery.[32] One half of the patients had transposition. Cardiac output was determined by the thermodilution technique beginning three hours after removal of the aortic cross clamp and repeated at three hour intervals over the first 24 hours postoperatively. The pulmonary artery catheter was a 3.5 French double lumen catheter equipped with a radiopaque thermistor. Triplicate measurements of cardiac output were made over one to two minutes using 1 ml injections of iced 5% dextrose into the right atrial line. Cardiac index was calculated by dividing the average output by body surface area. The doses of inotropic, chronotropic and afterload reducing agents were recorded at the time of each set of cardiac output measurements. Total inotrope dose was calculated by adding the doses of dopamine and dobutamine in μg/kg per minute and assigning an arbitrary value of 10 μg/kg per minute inotrope for each 0.1 μg/kg per minute epinephrine.

The pH trial demonstrated that overall infants assigned to the alpha stat group received greater inotropic support nine hours after cross clamp removal ($p = 0.04$); otherwise the two treatment groups did not differ significantly with respect to cardiac index and inotropic support in the first 24 hours postoperatively. However, within the homogeneous D-TGA subgroup, infants in the pH stat group tended to have higher cardiac indices and lower inotropic support at most time points, although these differences did not achieve statistical significance.

Thus there was a consistent trend for patients managed with pH stat to have a higher cardiac output over the first 24 hours postoperatively as determined by thermodilution. This was in spite of higher inotropic support in the alpha stat patients. Consistent with this finding, patients with transposition were extubated significantly sooner and were discharged earlier from the intensive care unit.

The finding of greater cardiac output with the pH stat strategy is consistent with a laboratory study from Children's Hospital which demonstrated that hypercarbic acidotic reperfusion improved recovery of myocardial function after cardioplegic ischemia in neonatal lambs.[37]

REPERFUSION CONDITIONS

The importance of reperfusion conditions, e.g. pressure, calcium, oxygen, additives such as adenosine and free-radical scavengers, in determining the extent of myocardial ischemic injury has been emphasized and extensively explored by Buckberg and colleagues[38–41] However, there is a potential conflict between myocardial and cerebral protection with some of the protective techniques recommended by Buckberg's group which should be recognized.[42]

MYOCARDIAL PROTECTION TECHNIQUES IN CLINICAL PRACTICE

Hypothermia

Hypothermia alone can provide an impressive degree of myocardial protection particularly in the neonate.[43] In fact a

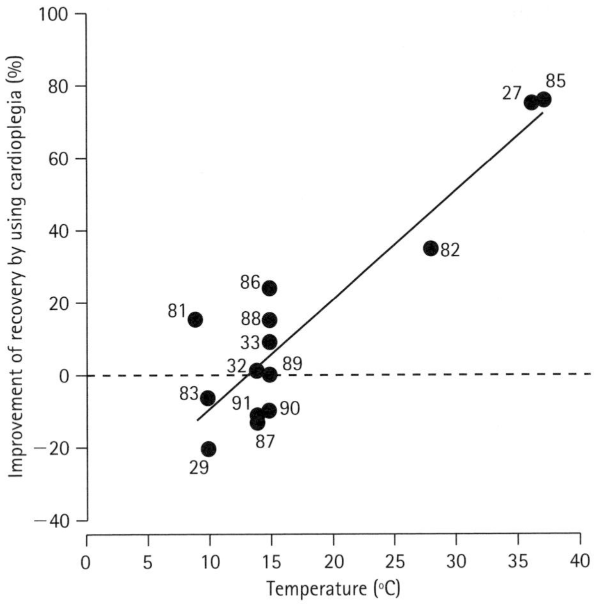

Figure 10.4 *In neonatal hearts various studies (denoted by the closed circles) have failed to demonstrate a consistent important advantage for myocardial protection with hypothermia relative to hypothermia alone at 15°C or less. Studies performed at a higher systemic temperature have tended to show an advantage for the use of cardioplegia. (From Doenst et al. Cardioplegia in pediatric cardiac surgery: Do we believe in magic?* Ann Thorac Surg *2003; 75:1668–77, with permission.)*

considerable number of studies[44–47] suggest that hypothermia alone provides as good or better protection than hypothermia plus cardioplegia. It is important to note however that these studies were performed at a systemic temperature of 15°C or less. Other studies employing temperatures of 15°C or less have suggested that there is some advantage in adding cardioplegia.[48–51] Studies that have been performed at higher systemic temperatures consistently show a benefit for cardioplegia solution for hypothermic use[52–54] (Figure 10.4).

MAINTENANCE OF MYOCARDIAL HYPOTHERMIA

The rate of rewarming of myocardium is strongly associated with the perfusion temperature. Ganzel et al[48] demonstrated in piglets that there was rapid rewarming of the myocardium between cardioplegia infusions of 4°C cardioplegia when a systemic perfusion temperature of 28°C was selected. On the other hand if systemic perfusion was conducted at 15°C the myocardium required less frequent cardioplegia infusion in order to maintain a temperature of less than 15°C. While repeated doses of cardioplegia are well tolerated by mature myocardium there are several reports which suggest that immature myocardium does not tolerate repeated doses of cardioplegia.[53,55–57] Furthermore use of a higher perfusate temperature has been demonstrated to result in an increased level of white cell and endothelial activation.[58] Thus the practice at Children's Hospital Boston for major reconstructive procedures such as the arterial switch operation is deep hypothermia for the systemic perfusion temperature both to improve myocardial protection and to obviate the need for multiple doses of cardioplegia, as well as to reduce the inflammatory effects of bypass both with respect to humoral mediators as well as white cells.

MAINTENANCE OF HYPOTHERMIA: FACTORS OTHER THAN SYSTEMIC TEMPERATURE AND CARDIOPLEGIA INFUSION

There are several factors that are under the control of the surgeon which will influence the rate of myocardial rewarming during the aortic cross-clamp period. It is important to reduce the intensity of overhead lighting directed at the heart during this period. The author's practice is to virtually turn off the overhead lights and to rely on the surgical headlight. Because this is blue halogen-generated light it has a lower level of infrared than more yellow tungsten lights. Nevertheless even the intense headlight spot will result in some degree of rewarming of the neonatal heart. The room temperature should be reduced to approximately 13–14°C. Irrigating solutions which may come in contact with the heart must be very cold, for example, the solution used to study leaflet coaptation during mitral valve repair for complete AV canal. It is not recommended that iced slush be employed as this can result in excessive cooling of the myocardium (the temperature of slush is less than 0°C because of its salt content) and in addition slush has been documented to cause phrenic nerve injury.[59,60] Whenever possible the heart should be kept within the pericardial cavity and in contact with surrounding tissues which are at perfusate temperature.

COLD CONTRACTURE

Some centers have expressed concern that the use of a deeply hypothermic perfusate temperature can result in cold contracture of the neonatal myocardium. For example Rebeyka and co-authors[61] found in immature rabbit hearts that hypothermia before the onset of cardioplegia resulted in worse recovery of function than if the heart was kept warm up to the time of onset of ischemia and the cardioplegia itself was used to both cool and rest the heart. The proposed mechanism of this cold-induced exacerbation of ischemic injury was hypothermia-induced calcium accumulation in the myocardial cells before the onset of ischemia. Also from Toronto Williams and coworkers[62] reported clinical data supporting this hypothesis. Improved patient survival and better myocardial function was reported in patients in whom pre-ischemia hypothermia was avoided. Because other centers have not observed this phenomenon including Children's Hospital Boston we have speculated that the low ionized calcium level used in the perfusate with the Boston perfusion method is a factor which has resulted in the absence of cold contracture being observed.[63]

Cardioplegia

The benefit of cardioplegia in the immature heart as noted above is closely related to myocardial temperature. Early work at Children's Hospital Boston by Fujiwara[64] as well as by others[65,66] all suggest that in the normal heart there is no additional benefit to adding cardioplegia to hypothermia. Nevertheless the practice at Children's Hospital Boston in neonatal procedures is to use a single dose of cardioplegia infusion of 20 ml/kg in combination with systemic deep hypothermia. In patients beyond two to three months of age repeat doses of cardioplegia are employed at approximately 20–30 minute intervals. Beyond the first year of life it is likely that a higher systemic perfusion temperature will be selected and therefore repeat doses of cardioplegia are carefully administered every 20 minutes using an initial dose of 20 ml/kg and subsequent doses of 10 ml/kg.

SPECIFIC CARDIOPLEGIA SOLUTIONS

The author continues to use oxygenated St Thomas crystalloid cardioplegia solution which is marketed in the United States as Plegisol. Other surgeons in the group use custom developed cardioplegia solutions. The lack of firm data regarding optimal cardioplegia recipe is reflected by the fact that more than 150 cardioplegia solutions are clinically used for heart transplantation in the United States.[66] It is surprising that remarkably few clinical studies have been done to compare efficacy of cardioplegia solutions. As noted above one aspect of the prospective randomized trial of hematocrit that was undertaken at Children's Hospital Boston between 1997 and 2000 was that two different cardioplegia solutions were used. No difference was found between oxygenated crystalloid cardioplegia solution (Plegisol) and one of the custom mixes used at Children's Hospital. Hopefully, in future, clinical studies of myocardial protection will be undertaken that will employ measurement of cardiac output during the first 24 hours postoperatively.

CARDIOPLEGIA ADDITIVES FOR THE IMMATURE HEART

The topic of cardioplegia additives for myocardial protection during pediatric cardiac surgery has been addressed in detail in a review article by Allen et al.[11]

Blood

An early study at Children's Hospital Boston by Fujiwara et al[64] found no benefit for blood cardioplegia over crystalloid cardioplegia or hypothermia alone in the normal neonatal lamb. However, Corno et al found that cardioplegia solutions containing blood were associated with improved recovery of function when compared with crystalloid cardioplegia solutions or hypothermia alone.[49] As noted above the hematocrit study at Children's Hospital Boston included a comparison of crystalloid and blood cardioplegia and found no advantage for either solution in a population of patients who were less than nine months of age.

Oxygen

Although studies in mature hearts have suggested improved recovery of function with oxygenation of crystalloid cardioplegia there are no studies in immature myocardium.[67]

Calcium

The ideal calcium level remains unknown and as noted above can be affected by the pre-ischemic perfusate ionized calcium levels.

Magnesium

There is important interaction between calcium and magnesium in that magnesium inhibits cellular entry. The addition of magnesium to a cardioplegia solution may prevent damage from higher cardioplegic calcium concentrations.[11]

CONCLUSION

Many aspects of myocardial protection in the immature heart remain poorly understood. Further improvement in our understanding of the differences between adult and immature myocardium will help to enhance myocardial protection and should lead to elimination of the reduced cardiac output that is so often seen after cardiac surgery in the young.

REFERENCES

1. Olivetti G, Anversa P, Loud AV. Morphometric study of early postnatal development in the left and right ventricular myocardium of the rat. *Circ Res* 1980; **46**:503–12.
2. Sheldon CA, Friedman WF, Sybers HD. Scanning electron microscopy of fetal and neonatal lamb cardiac cells. *J Mol Cell Cardiol* 1976; **8**:853–62.
3. Legato MJ. Cellular mechanisms of normal growth in the mammalian heart. II. A quantitative and qualitative comparision between the right and left ventricular myocytes in the dog from birth to five months of age. *Circ Res* 1979; **44**:263–79.
4. Page E, Early J, Power B. Normal growth of ultrastructures in rat left ventricular myocardial cells. *Circ Res* 1974; **34/35**:II12.
5. Goodwin GW, Ahmad F, Doenst T, Taegtmeyer H. Energy provision for glycogen, glucose and fatty acids upon adrenergic stimulation of isolated working rat heart. *Am J Physiol* 1998; **274**:H1239–47.
6. Clark CMJ. Characterization of glucose metabolism in the isolated rat heart during fetal and early neonatal development. *Diabetes* 1973; **22**:41–9.
7. Depre C, Shipley G, Chen W et al. Unloaded heart in vivo replicates fetal gene expression of cardiac hypertrophy. *Nat Med* 1998; **4**:1269–75.
8. Klitzner TS. Maturational changes in excitation-contraction coupling in mammalian myocardium. *J Am Coll Cardiol* 1991; **17**:218–25.
9. Pieske B, Schlotthauer K, Schattmann J et al. Ca (2+) dependent and Ca (2+) independent regulation of contractility in isolated human myocardium. *Basic Res Cardiol* 1997; **92**:75–86.
10. Boland R, Martonosi A, Tillack TW. Developmental changes in the composition and function of sarcoplasmic reticulum. *J Biol Chem* 1974; **249**:612–23.

11. Allen BS, Barth MJ, Ilbawi MN. Pediatric myocardial protection: An overview. *Sem Thorac Cardiovasc Surg* 2001; **13**:56–72.
12. Bolling K, Kronon M, Allen BS et al. Myocardial protection in normal and hypoxically stressed neonatal hearts: The superiority of hypocalcemic versus normocalcemic blood cardioplegia. *J Thorac Cardiovasc Surg* 1996; **112**:1193–200.
13. Kronon MT, Allen BS, Hernan J et al. Superiority of magnesium cardioplegia in neonatal myocardial protection. *Ann Thorac Surg* 1999; **68**:2285–91.
14. Rebeyka IM, Diaz RJ, Augustine JM et al. Effect of rapid cooling contracture on ischemic tolerance in immature myocardium. *Circulation* 1991; **84**(5 Suppl):III389–93.
15. Pearl JM, Laks H, Drinkwater DC et al. Normocalcemic blood or crystalloid cardioplegia provides better neonatal myocardial protection than does low calcium cardioplegia. *J Thorac Cardiovasc Surg* 1993; **105**:201–6.
16. Kofsky ER, Julia P, Buckberg GD et al. Studies of myocardial protection in the immature heart. V. Safety of prolonged aortic clamping with hypocalcemic glutamate/aspartate blood cardioplegia. *J Thorac Cardiovasc Surg* 1991; **101**:33–43.
17. Baker EJ, Olinger GN, Baker JE. Calcium content of St Thomas' II cardioplegia solution damages ischemic immature myocardium. *Ann Thorac Surg* 1991; **52**:993–9.
18. Teoh KH, Mickle DAG, Weisel RD et al. Effect of oxygen tension and cardiovascular operations on the myocardial antioxidant enzyme activities in patients with tetralogy of Fallot and aorto-coronary bypass. *J Thorac Cardiovasc Surg* 1992; **104**:159–64.
19. del Nido PJ, Mickle DA, Wilson GJ et al. Inadequate myocardial protection with cold cardioplegic arrest during repair of tetralogy of Fallot. *J Thorac Cardiovasc Surg* 1988; **95**:223–9.
20. del Nido PJ, Mickle DA, Wilson GJ et al. Evidence of myocardial free radical injury during elective repair of tetralogy of Fallot. *Circulation* 1987; **76**:174–9.
21. Englander R, Cardarelli MG. Efficacy of leukocyte filters in the bypass circuit for infants undergoing cardiac operations. *Ann Thorac Surg* 1995; **60**:S533–5.
22. Hayashi Y, Sawa Y, Nishimura M et al. Clinical evaluation of leukocyte-depleted blood cardioplegia for pediatric open heart operation. *Ann Thorac Surg* 2000; **69**:1914–49.
23. Kawata H, Sawatari K, Mayer JE. Evidence for the role of neutrophils in reperfusion injury after cold cardioplegic ischemia in neonatal lambs. *J Thorac Cardiovasc Surg* 1992; **103**:908–18.
24. Buckberg G. Update on current techniques of myocardial protection. *Ann Thorac Surg* 1995; **60**:805–14.
25. Bolling SF, Olszanski DA, Bove EL et al. Enhanced myocardial protection during global ischemia with 5'-nucleotidase inhibitors. *J Thorac Cardiovasc Surg* 1992; **103**:73–7.
26. Artman M, Kithas PA, Wike JS et al. Inotropic responses change during postnatal maturation in rabbits. *Am J Physiol* 1988; **255**:H335–42.
27. Awad WI, Shattock MJ, Chambers DJ. Ischemic preconditioning in immature myocardium. *Circulation* 1998; **98**:II206–13.
28. Bull C, Cooper J, Stark J. Cardioplegic protection of the child's heart. *J Thorac Cardiovasc Surg* 1984; **88**:287–93.
29. Jonas RA, Krasna M, Sell JE, Wessel D, Mayer JE, Castaneda AR. Myocardial failure is a rare cause of death after pediatric cardiac surgery. *J Am Coll Cardiol* 1990; **15**:78A.
30. Jonas RA. Myocardial protection for neonates and infants. *Thorac Cardiovasc Surg* 1998; **46**:288–91.
31. Newburger JW, Jonas RA, Wernovsky G et al. A comparison of the perioperative neurologic effects of hypothermic circulatory arrest versus low-flow cardiopulmonary bypass in infant heart surgery. *N Engl J Med* 1993; **329**:1057–64.
32. du Plessis AJ, Jonas RA, Wypij D et al. Perioperative effects of alpha-stat versus pH-stat strategies for deep hypothermic cardiopulmonary bypass in infants. *J Thorac Cardiovasc Surg* 1997; **114**:991–1000.
33. Jonas RA, Wypij D, Roth SJ et al. The influence of hemodilution on outcome after hypothermic cardiopulmonary bypass: Results of a randomized trial in infants. *J Thorac Cardiovasc Surg*, 2003; **126:**1765–74.
34. Wernovsky G, Wypij D, Jonas RA et al. Postoperative course and hemodynamic profile after the arterial switch operation in neonates and infants. A comparison of low-flow cardiopulmonary bypass and circulatory arrest. *Circulation* 1995; **92**:2226–35.
35. Harake B, Power GG. Thoracic duct lymph flow: A comparative study in newborn and adult sheep. *J Dev Physiol* 1986; **8**:87–95.
36. Rosenthal SM, LaJohn LA. Effect of age on transvascular fluid movement. *Am J Physiol* 1975; **228**:134–40.
37. Nomura F, Aoki M, Forbess JM, Mayer JE Jr. Effects of hypercarbic acidotic reperfusion on recovery of myocardial function after cardioplegic ischemia in neonatal lambs. *Circulation* 1994; **90**:II321–7.
38. Ihnken K, Morita K, Buckberg GD, Sherman MP, Ignarro LJ, Young HH. Studies of hypoxemic/reoxygenation injury: with aortic clamping. XIII. Interaction between oxygen tension and cardioplegic composition in limiting nitric oxide production and oxidant damage. *J Thorac Cardiovasc Surg* 1995; **110**:1274–86.
39. Morita K, Ihnken K, Buckberg GD. Studies of hypoxemic/reoxygenation injury: with aortic clamping. XII. Delay of cardiac reoxygenation damage in the presence of cyanosis: a new concept of controlled cardiac reoxygenation. *J Thorac Cardiovasc Surg* 1995; **110**(4 Pt 2):1265–73.
40. Ihnken K, Morita K, Buckberg GD, Young HH. Studies of hypoxemic/reoxygenation injury with aortic clamping: XI. Cardiac advantages of normoxemic versus hyperoxemic management during cardiopulmonary bypass. *J Thorac Cardiovasc Surg* 1995; **110**(4 Pt 2):1255–64.
41. Morita K, Ihnken K, Buckberg GD, Matheis G, Sherman MP, Young HH. Studies of hypoxemic/reoxygenation injury: with aortic clamping. X. Exogenous antioxidants to avoid nullification of the cardioprotective effects of blood cardioplegia. *J Thorac Cardiovasc Surg* 1995; **110**(4 Pt 2):1245–54.
42. Jonas RA. Myocardial protection or cerebral protection: A potential conflict. *J Thorac Cardiovasc Surg* 1992; **104**:533–4.
43. Doenst T, Schlensak C, Beyersdorf F. Cardioplegia in pediatric cardiac surgery: Do we believe in magic? *Ann Thorac Surg* 2003; **75**:1668–77.
44. Magovern JA, Pae WEJ, Waldhausen JA. Protection of the immature myocardium. An experimental evaluation of topical cooling, single-dose and multi-dose administration of St Thomas' cardioplegic solution. *J Thorac Cardiovasc Surg* 1988; **96**:408–13.
45. Baker JE, Boerboom LE, Olinger GN. Cardioplegia induced damage to ischemic immature myocardium is independent of oxygen availability. *Ann Thorac Surg* 1990; **50**:934–9.
46. Hozzeinzadeh T, Tchervenkov CI, Quantz M, Chiu R. Adverse effect of prearrest hypothermia in immature hearts: rate versus duration of cooling. *Ann Thorac Surg* 1992; **53**:464–71.
47. Baker JE, Boerboom LE, Olinger GN. Age and protection of the ischemic myocardium: is alkaline cardioplegia appropriate? *Ann Thorac Surg* 1993; **55**:747–55.
48. Ganzel BL, Katzmark SL, Mavroudis C. Myocardia preservation in the neonate. Beneficial effects of cardioplegia and systemic

hypothermia on piglets undergoing cardiopulmonary bypass and myocardial ischemia. *J Thorac Cardiovasc Surg* 1988; **96**:414–22.
49. Corno AF, Bethencourt DM, Laks H et al. Myocardial protection in the neonatal heart. A comparison of topical hypothermia and crystalloid and blood cardioplegic solutions. *J Thorac Cardiovasc Surg* 1987; **93**:163–72.
50. Konishi T, Apstein CS. Comparison of three cardioplegic solutions during hypothermia ischemic arrest in neonatal blood-perfused rabbit hearts. *J Thorac Cardiovasc Surg* 1989; **98**:1132–7.
51. Diaco M, DiSesa VJ, Sun SC, Laurence R, Cohn LH. Cardioplegia for the immature myocardium. A comparative study in the neonatal rabbit. *J Thorac Cardiovasc Surg* 1990; **100**:910–13.
52. Julia P, Young HH, Buckberg GD et al. Studies of myocardial protection in the immature heart. IV. Improved tolerance of immature myocardium to hypoxia and ischemia by intravenous metabolism support. *J Thorac Cardiovasc Surg* 1991; **101**:23–32.
53. Bove EL, Stammers AH, Gallagher KP. Protection of the neonatal myocardium during hypothermic ischemia. Effect of cardioplegia on left ventricular function in the rabbit. *J Thorac Cardiovasc Surg* 1987; **94**:115–23.
54. Avkiran M, Hearse DJ. Protection of the myocardium during global ischemia. Is crystalloid cardioplegia effective in the immature myocardium? *J Thorac Cardiovasc Surg* 1989; **97**:220–8.
55. Baker JE, Boerboom LE, Olinger GN. Age related changes in the ability of hypothermia and cardioplegia to protect ischemic rabbit myocardium. *J Thorac Cardiovasc Surg* 1988; **96**:717–24.
56. Sawa Y, Matsuda H, Shimazaki Y et al. Comparison of single dose versus multiple dose crystalloid cardioplegia in neonates: Experimental study with neonatal rabbits from birth to 2 days of age. *J Thorac Cardiovasc Surg* 1989; **97**:229–34.
57. Clark BJ, Woodford EJ, Malec EJ, Norwood CR, Pigott JD, Norwood WI. Effects of potassium cardioplegia on high energy phosphate kinetics during circulatory arrest with deep hypothermia in the newborn piglet heart. *J Thorac Cardiovasc Surg* 1991; **101**:342–9.
58. Anttila V, Hagino I, Zurakowski D, Lidov HGW, Jonas RA. Higher bypass temperature correlates with increased white cell activation in the cerebral microcirculation. *J Thorac Cardiovasc Surg*, in press.
59. Mills GH, Khan ZP, Moxham J, Desai J, Forsyth A, Ponte J. Effects of temperature on phrenic nerve and diaphragmatic function during cardiac surgery. *Br J Anaesth* 1997; **79**:726–32.
60. Allen BS, Buckberg GD, Rosenkranz ER et al. Topical cardiac hypothermia in patients with coronary disease. An unnecessary adjunct to cardioplegic protection and cause of pulmonary morbidity. *J Thorac Cardiovasc Surg* 1992; **104**:626–31.
61. Rebeyka IM, Hanan SA, Borges MR et al. Rapid cooling contracture of the myocardium. *J Thorac Cardiovasc Surg* 1990; **100**:240–9.
62. Williams WG, Rebeyka IM, Tibshirani RJ et al. Warm induction blood cardioplegia in the infant. *J Thorac Cardiovasc Surg* 1990; **100**:896–901.
63. Castaneda AR, Jonas RA, Mayer JE, Hanley FL. Myocardial preservation in the immature heart, In *Cardiac Surgery of the Neonate and Infant*, Philadelphia, WB Saunders, 1994, pp 41–53.
64. Fujiwara T, Heinle J, Britton L, Mayer JE. Myocardial preservation in neonatal lambs: Comparison of hypothermia with crystalloid and blood cardioplegia. *J Thorac Cardiovasc Surg* 1991; **101**:703–12.
65. Laks H, Milliken J, Haas G. Myocardial protection in the neonatal heart. In Mancelletti C (ed). *Pediatric Cardiology* 6th edn. Edinburgh, Churchill Livingstone, 1986, pp 13–26.
66. Demmy TL, Biddle JS, Bennet LE, Walls JT, Schmaltz RA, Curtis JJ. Organ preservation solutions in heart transplantation – patterns of usage and related survival. *Ann Thorac Surg* 1997; **63**:262–96.
67. Doherty NE 3rd, Turocy JF, Geffin GA, O'Keefe DD, Titus JS, Daggett WM. Benefits of glucose and oxygen in multidose cold cardioplegia. *J Thorac Cardiovasc Surg* 1992; **103**:219–29.

SECTION 3

Specific congenital cardiac anomalies

11

Patent ductus arteriosus, aortopulmonary window, sinus of Valsalva fistula, aortoventricular tunnel

INTRODUCTION

Patent ductus arteriosus, aortopulmonary window and sinus of Valsalva fistula share common pathophysiology in that each of these lesions usually results in a continuous steal of blood from the systemic circulation during both systole and diastole. Since coronary blood flow occurs during diastole there is a risk that coronary blood flow will be importantly compromised. If the communication is large it can result in a severe degree of congestive heart failure. Aortoventricular tunnel is a closely related anomaly that shares some of the pathophysiologic features of these anomalies.

PATENT DUCTUS ARTERIOSUS

EMBRYOLOGY

A patent ductus arteriosus results from a failure of normal transition from the fetal to the postnatal circulation. Usually ductal closure occurs initially by constriction of smooth muscle within the wall of the ductus.[1] This results in contact between the opposing intimal cushions which leads to thrombosis. There is subsequently fibrosis over several weeks and months and the ductus evolves to become the ligamentum arteriosum.

During fetal life the patency of the ductus is maintained by both local and circulating prostaglandin. After birth increased pulmonary blood flow metabolizes prostaglandin and absence of the placenta removes an important source of prostaglandin. Subsequently there is a marked decrease in the circulating level of prostaglandin. It is also thought that there is an increased level of circulating vasoconstrictive substances.[2,3] In addition to a fall in the level of prostaglandin the increased partial pressure of oxygen in the blood passing through the ductus is another stimulus to ductal constriction. In term infants ductal closure usually occurs within the first 24 hours after birth. In preterm neonates the immature ductal tissue is much less reactive to oxygen and persistent patency of the ductus is therefore much more likely.

Relationship of the ductus to the recurrent laryngeal nerve

Embryologically the ductus represents persistence of the distal component of the left sixth aortic arch.[4] The embryology of the aortic arch is reviewed in detail in Chapter 29. It is important to recall that the left sixth aortic arch originates in the neck (branchial = gill). Therefore the left recurrent laryngeal nerve is carried down into the thoracic cavity as the heart and proximal great vessels migrate from a more cervical to a thoracic position. On the right side there is usually resorption of the right sixth aortic arch as well as the right fifth aortic arch. Thus the right recurrent laryngeal nerve comes to pass around the remnant of the fourth aortic arch which persists as the right subclavian artery.

Atypical ductal anatomy

When there is a right sided aortic arch because of persistence of the right sided embryological arches rather than left sided arches the ductus usually arises from the proximal descending aorta in conjunction with the left subclavian artery.[5] The dilated structure which represents the origin of both the left subclavian artery as well as the ductus is often referred to as the diverticulum of Kommerell. This diverticulum lies posterior to the esophagus. The ductus subsequently passes anteriorly to join the origin of the left pulmonary artery thereby completing a vascular ring. The ductus does not always arise from the diverticulum of Kommerell in cases of right sided aortic arch. When there is mirror image branching, i.e. the first branch of the right sided arch is an innominate artery which branches into a left subclavian artery and left common carotid artery, the ductus often arises more distally from the left subclavian artery or the innominate artery itself.

On occasion the ductus arteriosus may arise from the undersurface of a right sided aortic arch and pass to the right pulmonary artery. Bilateral ducti can also occur but are rare.

ANATOMY

As described above, the location of the ductus is usually left sided arising from the junction of the aortic isthmus with the proximal descending aorta and passing to the origin of the left pulmonary artery. However the ductus may be situated in a number of other locations including origin from the undersurface of a right sided aortic arch and passing to the right pulmonary artery, arising from a diverticulum of Kommerell and passing to the left pulmonary artery or arising from a left sided innominate artery and passing to the left pulmonary artery. Whatever the location of the ductus, the size and shape can be quite variable. The ductus may be extremely wide and short in which case ligation will be dangerous. It may also be long and tortuous. This is seen more frequently with origin from a left innominate artery or left subclavian artery. In general the aortic end of the ductus is larger than the pulmonary artery end. The funnel-like 'ampulla' of the ductus is helpful to the interventional cardiologist who is attempting to close the ductus with a catheter delivered device or coils. It is important for the surgeon to appreciate that the tissue integrity of the ductus varies enormously between the neonate and the older child. The neonatal ductus is an extremely fragile structure particularly if the underlying adventitia is dissected off (which should be avoided). It must always be handled with the greatest respect. It is also not difficult to cut through the ductus in an older child with aggressively firm ligation. Consideration must always be given to division of the short wide ductus between clamps if it is anticipated that there is a chance that tissue integrity is inadequate to allow simple ligation.

ASSOCIATED ANOMALIES

A patent ductus arteriosus may be associated with almost any other congenital cardiac anomaly. Probably the only exception is the absent pulmonary valve syndrome variant of tetralogy of Fallot. In this anomaly absence of the ductus may be a contributing embryological factor in its development.[6]

When a ductus is associated with another cardiac anomaly which causes pulmonary hypertension, e.g. a large VSD, it may be difficult to visualize the ductus by color Doppler mapping because there is minimal pressure differential between the aorta and pulmonary arteries and therefore little flow.

PATHOPHYSIOLOGY AND CLINICAL FEATURES

A patent ductus arteriosus results in a left to right shunt between the aorta and pulmonary arteries. This additional volume work must be handled exclusively by the left ventricle. When the ductus is large pulmonary artery pressure is elevated resulting in increased pressure work for the right ventricle. There is increased pulmonary return to the left atrium resulting in dilation of the left atrium as well as the left ventricle.

As is the case for a ventricular septal defect the degree of left to right shunt will increase in the first weeks and months of life as pulmonary resistance falls from its elevated neonatal level. When the ductus is large it can cause a sufficient degree of elevation of pulmonary artery pressure and flow that pulmonary vascular disease eventually develops.

A large patent ductus arteriosus reduces diastolic pressure and can reduce coronary perfusion which presumably reduces the ability of the left ventricle to manage the increased volume load. In the neonate or preterm infant the patent ductus can result in retrograde flow from the abdominal viscera during diastole.[7–9] This can result in oliguria or even acute renal failure. Even more importantly it is a cause of necrotizing enterocolitis. The preterm infant is at particular risk for this problem if a large ductus is not closed early in life. Patency of the ductus in the preterm infant results in a need for more aggressive ventilation. In the longer term this can result in chronic lung disease in the form of bronchopulmonary dysplasia.

The usual clinical features of a patent ductus arteriosus are the signs and symptoms of left sided heart failure. If the ductus is large there may be tachypnea at rest. The child will be prone to frequent respiratory infections and will fail to thrive. The child's oxygen saturation is normal. The pulse pressure is clearly widened both by palpation and blood pressure measurement when the ductus is large. Auscultation of the chest demonstrates the characteristic systolic murmur extending into diastole or even a continuous machinery murmur which may be best heard posteriorly. All of these same physical findings may be present with aortopulmonary window, sinus of Valsalva fistula and aortoventricular tunnel.

DIAGNOSTIC STUDIES

The plain chest X-ray demonstrates plethoric congested lung fields. The left atrium and left ventricle are enlarged. The pulmonary arteries may appear dilated. The EKG may demonstrate increased left sided forces though if there is important pulmonary hypertension there may also be electrical evidence of right ventricular hypertrophy.

Echocardiography is usually diagnostic. However it is important for the echocardiographer to distinguish a patent ductus arteriosus from an aortopulmonary window which may be distally placed in the ascending aorta. Generally there should be no difficulty distinguishing by echocardiography a patent ductus from a sinus of Valsalva fistula or an aorto left ventricular tunnel.

It should rarely if ever be necessary to confirm the presence of a patent ductus arteriosus by cardiac catheterization in the neonate or infant. However catheterization may be indicated in the older child in whom a particularly large ductus is found. Catheterization is definitely indicated in the older child who is cyanosed because of a right to left shunt at ductal level. Under these circumstances an assessment must be made as to the reactivity of the pulmonary vasculature. If the resistance is markedly elevated, e.g. pulmonary resistance greater than 75% of systemic resistance, and if that resistance is unresponsive to nitric oxide and oxygen then the patient should be considered inoperable because of advanced pulmonary vascular disease.

Magnetic resonance imaging (MRI) is a useful adjunct in situations where there is abnormal aortic arch anatomy and the exact location of the ductus is in doubt. It is important to remember in complex situations that there is always a small possibility of bilateral ducti being present.

MEDICAL AND INTERVENTIONAL THERAPY

Preterm infant ductus

Indomethacin was introduced in 1976 as a pharmacological method for closing the ductus in the preterm infant.[10] Early multi-center studies that attempted to define whether medical therapy was superior to surgical therapy for patent ductus arteriosus in the preterm neonate suggested that treatment arms that included surgery had a higher incidence of pneumothorax and retrolental fibroplasias.[11,12] Therefore the majority of preterm infants with a patent ductus arteriosus today undergo two to three courses of indomethacin usually 12–24 hours apart before being considered for surgical treatment.[13,14] Contraindications to the use of indomethacin include azotemia, evidence of gut ischemia, thrombocytopenia, intracerebral or other hemorrhage and sepsis. Birth weight below 1000 g is generally today not considered to be a contraindication to the use of indomethacin. It is important that the size of the patent ductus be monitored by echocardiography both before and after the administration of indomethacin.[15]

Interventional catheter methods are not available for closure of the ductus in the preterm infant.

The non preterm infant or older child

The medical management of a patent ductus arteriosus in the non preterm infant or older child is standard anticongestive medication with digoxin and diuretics. The situation is somewhat different from the child with a VSD, however, in that spontaneous closure beyond the neonatal period is unlikely. Therefore medical treatment should be seen only as a means to stabilize the child's condition prior to proceeding to closure either in the operating room or catheterization laboratory.

INTERVENTIONAL CATHETER METHODS FOR DUCTUS CLOSURE

This topic is covered in detail elsewhere.[16] In summary a number of different catheter delivered devices have been applied over the years for the management of patent ductus arteriosus. Most recently Dacron covered steel coils have become popular. Multiple coils are introduced if necessary. On occasion the multiple coils can be contained within a synthetic bag (Grifka bag). The advantages of interventional catheterization closure of the ductus include the cosmetic advantage that no incision is required. Relative to a traditional thoracotomy approach there is less discomfort and the child can be discharged from hospital the same day as the procedure.[17] Disadvantages of the technique include the potential complication of embolization of the device or devices, the fact that prosthetic material is left permanently within the endovascular space, the devices frequently project either into the pulmonary artery or aorta, and finally the expense. When one takes into consideration amortization of the expensive catheterization equipment required to undertake this procedure as well as the high cost of the devices themselves some studies suggest a significant cost disadvantage to the catheter approach.[18] In addition there is a significant incidence of persistent patency. Ideally in the future a prospective randomized trial should be conducted comparing catheter techniques for ductal closure with modern techniques of surgical closure such as the video-assisted thoracoscopic approach.

INDICATIONS FOR SURGERY

In the past the diagnosis alone of patent ductus arteriosus has been considered an indication for closure. As the sensitivity of diagnostic modalities such as echocardiography has improved, this approach has required reconsideration. There is no doubt that echocardiography is capable of detecting a hemodynamically insignificant ductus both in the preterm infant as well as in the older infant or child. For example the ductus that is less than 1–1.5 mm in diameter even in a very small preterm infant probably does not warrant surgical intervention when indomethacin therapy has failed.

In the older infant or child a ductus that is as small as 1 or 2 mm is unlikely to cause any measurable hemodynamic impact. Nevertheless there is concern that over the longer term the small patent ductus may be a site for infection in the form of endarteritis. Because there may occasionally be right to left shunting across a small ductus it is thought that bacteria that would normally be filtered by the lungs may enter the systemic circulation or at least become concentrated in the region of the ductus itself. Certainly the ductus which is large enough to be audible to the clinical observer with a stethoscope or the ductus that results in symptoms necessitating medical therapy should be considered in itself to be an indication for closure. However the benefits versus risks of closing an inaudible ductus that is resulting in no hemodynamic impact and which can only be visualized by echocardiography as a very small structure in the region of 1 or 2 mm remain undefined.

SURGICAL MANAGEMENT

History of surgery

The first successful clinical ligation of a patent ductus arteriosus was performed at Children's Hospital Boston in 1938 by Dr Robert Gross.[19] Although Gross performed a ligation for his first successful case he subsequently recommended division and oversewing of the ductus.[20] In 1946 Blalock described the triple ligation technique.[21] In 1963 Decanq reported the closure of a patent ductus in a preterm infant weighing 1400 g.[22] In 1976 Heymann introduced the clinical use of indomethacin to close a patent ductus arteriosus pharmacologically in the preterm infant.[10] In 1971, Portsmann et al described the closure of patent ductus using a catheter delivered device.[23] Another innovator in the area of catheter delivered devices was Rashkind of Philadelphia who was the first to develop an unfolding umbrella device[24] (Rashkind umbrella). Use of catheter delivered coils to close the ductus was described in 1994 by Moore.[25]

Technical considerations

TRADITIONAL THORACOTOMY APPROACH

A traditional thoracotomy approach remains appropriate for the preterm infant undergoing surgical ligation of the ductus or for the older infant or child who has a particularly short and wide ductus that requires division and oversewing.

Ligation of the patent ductus in the preterm infant

Although it is possible to undertake the surgical procedure in the neonatal intensive care unit it is our preference to undertake the procedure in the operating room. However great care must be taken by the team transporting the child to the operating room to avoid overventilation of the child either with an excessively high inspired oxygen level or with excessive pressures which might result in lung injury. It is important to remember that the greater incidence of retrolental fibroplasia that was seen in preterm infants who underwent the surgical arm of clinical trials was attributed to excessive oxygen levels used during transport. Great care must also be taken with temperature maintenance both during transportation as well as when the child is being positioned in the operating room.

The child is positioned with the left side up and with the left arm supported over the head to elevate the left scapula. A left posterior thoracotomy is performed that extends from just below and behind the tip of the scapula to a point between the spine of the scapula and the vertebral column. In a small baby, e.g. 500 g, the length of the incision is likely to be less than 1.5 cm. The muscle layers are divided in the usual fashion. The chest is entered through the third or fourth (not the fifth) intercostal space carefully retracting the intercostal spaces inferiorly to open them out. The cautery is set at an extremely low level and great care is taken to enter the thoracic cavity without injuring the underlying lung. Careful coordination with the anesthesia team is required at this point. The left lung is gently retracted anteriorly. Either one or two small malleable retractors are placed, generally with no underlying gauze sponge as this occupies space within the tiny chest cavity.

Minimal dissection in the region of the ductus is required (Figure 11.1a). Generally the mediastinal pleura is opened above and below the ductus using tenotomy scissors (Figure 11.1b). At this point the left recurrent nerve should be carefully visualized. This is a particularly helpful landmark that not only allows avoidance of recurrent nerve injury but also positively identifies the ductus. The ductus is frequently larger than the aortic arch and the aortic isthmus. It is not difficult to misinterpret the aortic isthmus as the left subclavian artery which can lead to ligation of the left pulmonary artery which is misinterpreted as the ductus. This is probably the commonest error that occurs in undertaking ductal ligation in

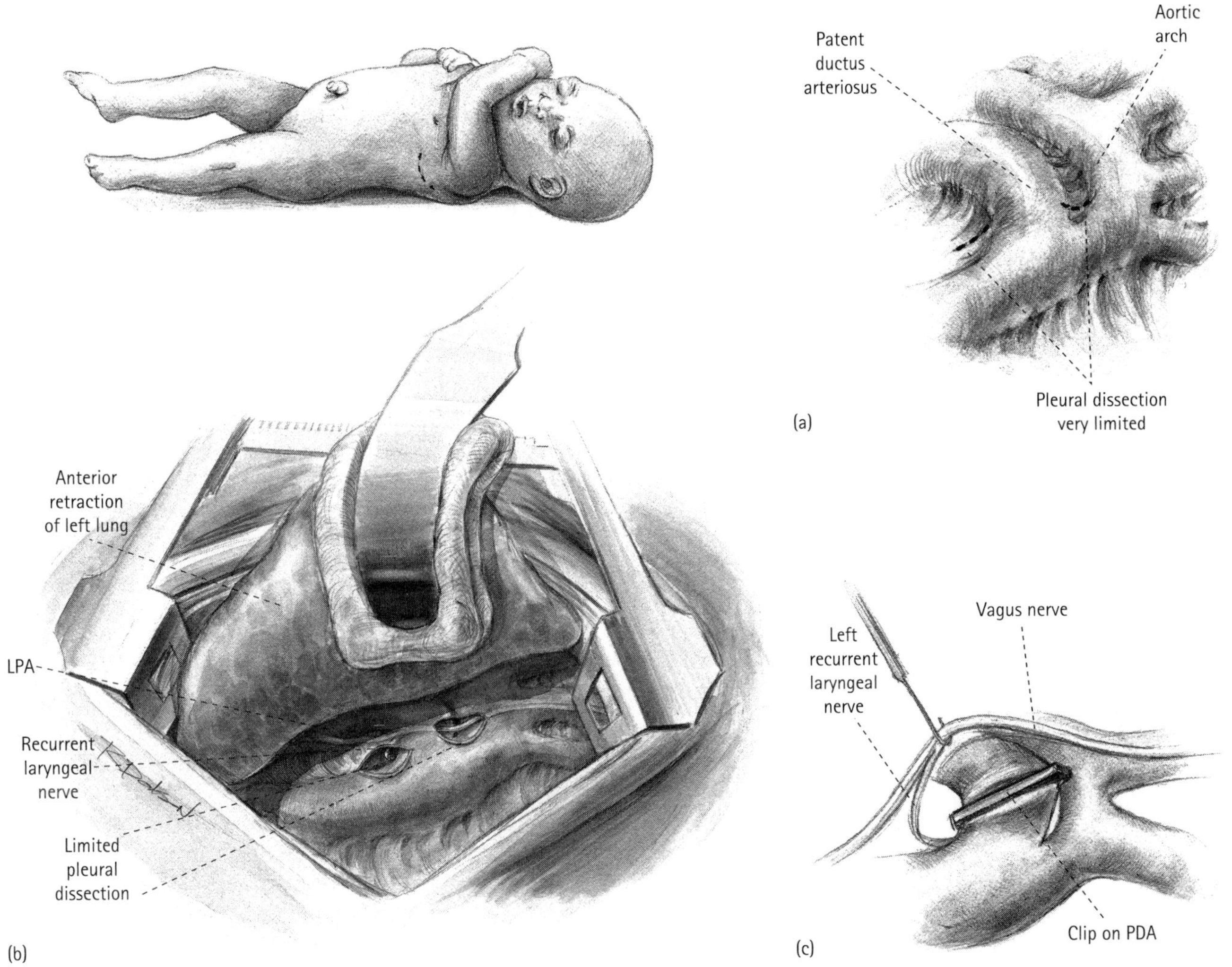

Figure 11.1 *Approach for the ligation of a patent ductus in the preterm neonate is through a limited left posterolateral thoracotomy. (a) Dissection of the mediastinal pleura in the preterm neonate is limited to the tissue above and below the aortic end of the ductus. (b) The left lung is retracted anteriorly. The vagus nerve and left recurrent laryngeal nerve are visualized carefully to aid in positive identification of the ductus. (c) A single surgical clip is used to occlude the ductus.*

the preterm infant. This error must be actively avoided. Having identified the aortic arch and its branches through the mediastinal pleura and having identified the left recurrent laryngeal nerve, a test occlusion of the ductus is performed by gently squeezing it between Debakey forceps. If an arterial line is in place this will result in an increase in diastolic pressure and possibly systolic pressure also. Continuing pulsation should be detectable by pulse oximetry from the distal extremities. An appropriate size vascular clip is selected. Gently lifting the ductus the clip is placed entirely across the duct with careful avoidance of the left recurrent laryngeal nerve which is swept medially by the forceps (Figure 11.1c). The duct is clipped between the forceps and the descending aorta. The malleable retractors are removed, a single small apical chest tube is placed and the chest is closed with absorbable pericostal sutures and absorbable sutures to the muscle layers. If the skin is particularly fragile it is often wise to use interrupted nylon sutures for skin closure.

Division and oversewing of the short, wide ductus in the non preterm infant or child

If preoperative studies have documented that the ductus is particularly short and wide it is preferable to undertake division and oversewing rather than interventional catheter closure or closure by clip ligation using video-assisted thoracoscopy. The surgical approach is through a limited left posterior thoracotomy. The thoracotomy is positioned more posteriorly than laterally. The left lung is retracted using malleable retractors. Generally one retractor serves to hold the left upper lobe while a second retractor retracts the left lower lobe. A single moist gauze sponge placed behind both retractors holds the hilum of the lung out of place without causing excessive direct compression of the hilar structures. The mediastinal pleura is reflected from the aorta in the region of the ductus which is defined by dissection (Figure 11.2a). The left recurrent laryngeal nerve is noted where it arises from the vagus nerve. It is carefully protected at all times. Retraction sutures are used to retract the anterior mediastinal pleural flap. The full length of the ductus is exposed. Generally the pericardium can be kept intact by reflecting it towards the pulmonary artery as part of the dissection. When the ductus has been fully exposed a decision must be made as to whether there is an adequate length of ductus to allow safe division between ductal clamps. Alternatively the juxtaductal aorta should be mobilized over approximately 1 cm. This allows exclusion of the aorta where the ductus arises between two clamps placed across the aorta above and below the ductus. It is important to use the Potts ductus clamps for clamping of the ductus itself (Figure 11.2b). The Potts clamps are designed specifically for this application. They have a single row of relatively sharp teeth which leaves a longer segment of ductus between the clamps for suturing. The relatively sharp teeth are less likely to slip on the ductus relative to Debakey style clamps. A Potts ductus clamp is placed on the pulmonary artery end of the ductus following application of clamps either across the aorta or across the aortic end of the ductus. The ductus is partially divided and a suture is begun on the aortic end. When the suture line has been partially run from anterior to posterior the posterior segment of the ductus is divided and the oversewing suture line is completed. The aortic end of the ductus is now released. The pulmonary artery end of the divided ductus is also oversewn with a continuous running technique using polypropylene (Figure 11.2c). The mediastinal pleura is loosely tacked over the repair area. A single chest tube is inserted. The lungs are re-expanded and the chest is closed in a routine fashion.

Video-assisted thoracoscopic surgery (VATS)

The technique of video-assisted thoracoscopic clip ligation of the patent ductus arteriosus was first published by Laborde in 1993.[26] The technique has rapidly become the standard of care for surgical management of the small to moderate sized ductus that is of adequate length to allow safe ligation. The technique of video-assisted thoracoscopic surgery minimizes the cosmetic disadvantages of surgery in that it results in only three short incisions for introduction of the video camera, a retractor and the electrocautery dissector and subsequently the clip applier (Figure 11.3). Because it is not necessary to spread the ribs there is minimal discomfort. Modern cameras allow excellent visualization and illumination which permits careful identification of the left recurrent laryngeal nerve. As with open ligation of the ductus in the preterm infant dissection is limited to the areas immediately above and below the aortic end of the ductus. The duct is closed with a single vascular clip. Care should be taken to avoid incorporating the left recurrent laryngeal nerve within the medial end of the clip.

Robotically assisted closure of the ductus arteriosus

In 2002 Laborde's group reported successful application of robotic techniques for closure of the patent ductus arteriosus.[27] In the initial series the principal role of the robot was to control camera position using a voice controlled robotic arm (Zeus System, Computermotion, Inc, Goleta, CA). Other robotic systems allow manipulation of more sophisticated instrumentation with complex multidirectional 'wrist' movements. However current instruments are designed for adults and require a large port. They are not useful in small children. Development of instrumentation more specific for pediatrics is under way. However it remains unclear at this point as to what advantages robotic assistance will allow for the relatively simple procedure of ductal ligation. Robotic technology has the potential to allow technically complex manipulations to be performed free of tremor. Robotic technology also allows preprogramming of complex stereotactic measurements derived from noninvasive imaging which is particularly helpful for example in neurosurgery. However since the ductus is readily visualized and complex technical manipulations are not required for its closure it remains unclear whether robotic manipulation will prove to be justifiable when the considerable cost of robotic technology is taken into account.

Results of surgery

TRADITIONAL SURGERY

There have been very few reports in the last decade or so describing the results of traditional surgical management of patent ductus arteriosus. In 1994, Mavroudis et al from Children's Memorial Hospital in Chicago[28] described the results of traditional surgical management for 1108 patients who underwent surgery between 1947 and 1993. A total of 98% of the patients had interruption of the ductus by ligation and division. There were no deaths. The recurrence rate was 0. In recent years the transfusion rate was less than 5% and length of stay was less than three days. The authors suggest that these are the standard against which alternative methods such as video-assisted ligation and catheter occlusion methods should be measured. These results are in many ways similar to the results from the very large report by Panagopoulos et al[29] from more than 30 years ago.

VIDEO-ASSISTED CLIPPING OF THE PATENT DUCTUS

In 1997 Laborde et al[30] from Paris France updated their results with the VATS method for ligation of the patent ductus, the technique which they had pioneered in 1991. Between 1991 and 1996 the authors undertook VATS closure of patent ductus in 332 consecutive patients. Five patients required intraoperative repositioning of the clip to eliminate a residual shunt leaving only one long-term small residual shunt. A total of 1.8% of patients suffered recurrent laryngeal nerve dysfunction which was transient in five patients and persistent in one. The mean operating time was 20 minutes and hospital stay averaged 48 hours for patients who were more than six months of age. The initial experience with the VATS method for ductus closure at Children's Hospital Boston was reported by Burke et al in 1995.[31] The authors described the development of appropriate instruments and procedural training in the animal laboratory. There were no deaths in the first 46 patients who underwent VATS procedures who

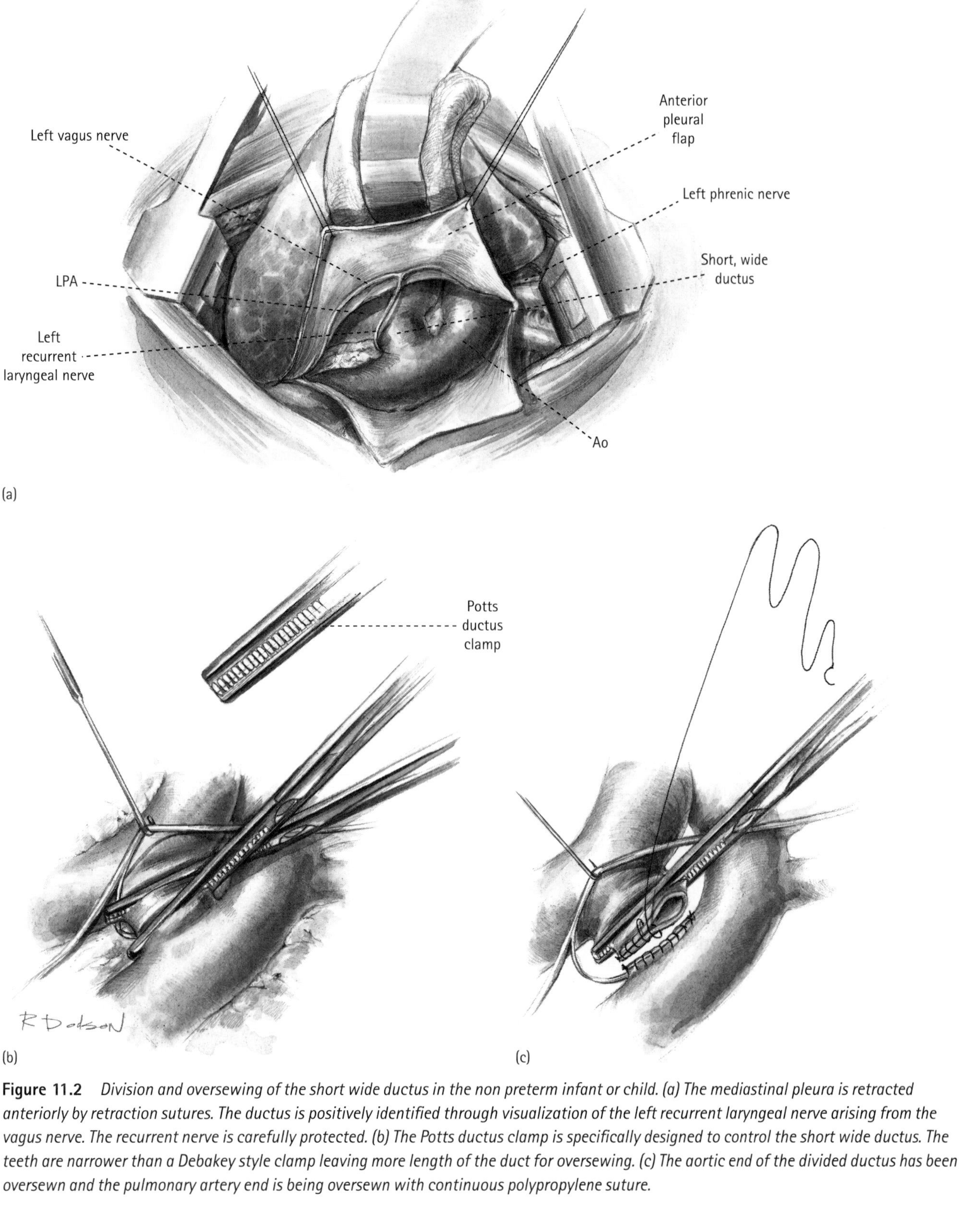

Figure 11.2 *Division and oversewing of the short wide ductus in the non preterm infant or child. (a) The mediastinal pleura is retracted anteriorly by retraction sutures. The ductus is positively identified through visualization of the left recurrent laryngeal nerve arising from the vagus nerve. The recurrent nerve is carefully protected. (b) The Potts ductus clamp is specifically designed to control the short wide ductus. The teeth are narrower than a Debakey style clamp leaving more length of the duct for oversewing. (c) The aortic end of the divided ductus has been oversewn and the pulmonary artery end is being oversewn with continuous polypropylene suture.*

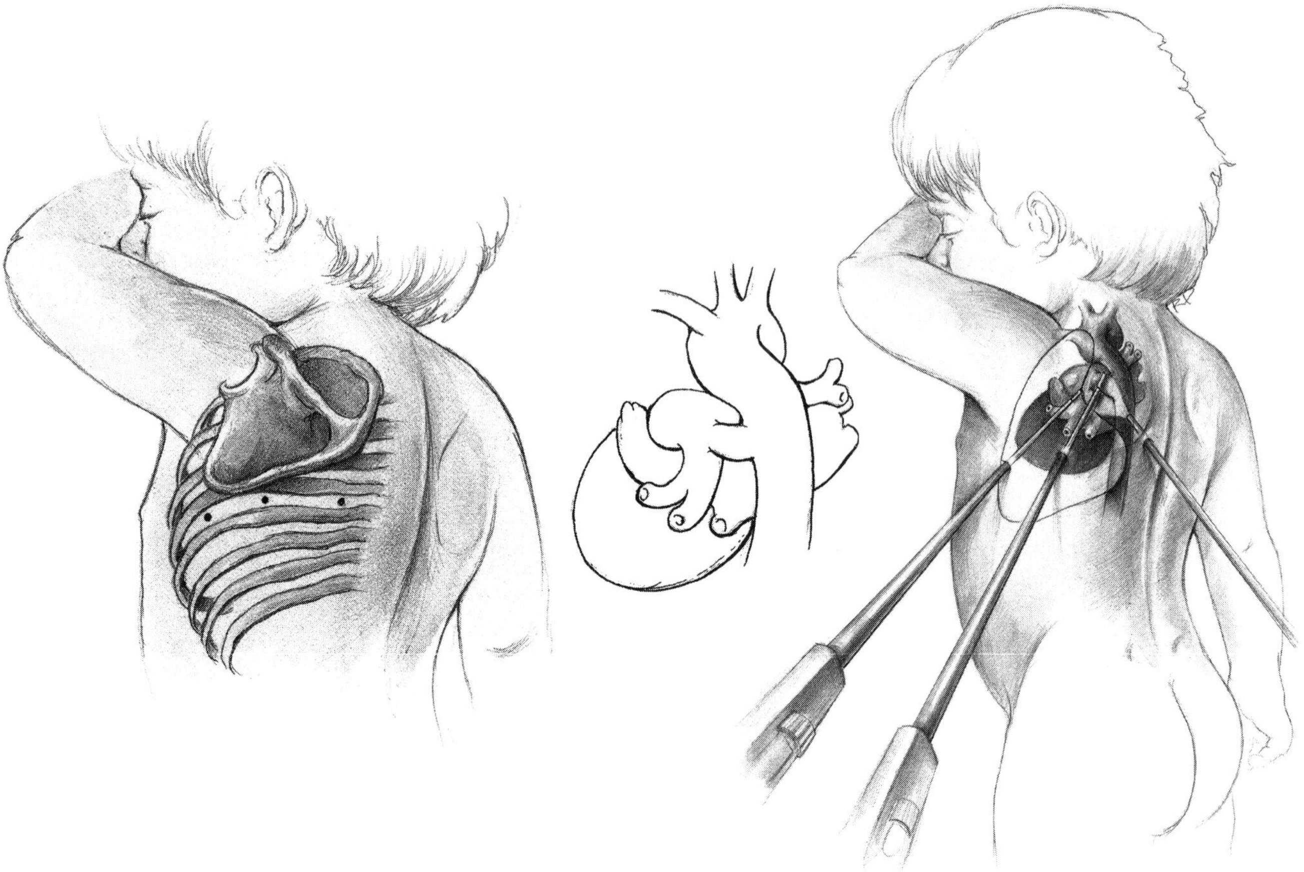

Figure 11.3 *Video-assisted thoracoscopy surgical (VATS) approach to clip ligation of the patent ductus arteriosus. The procedure may be performed through three ports in the fourth interspace.*

included 31 patients with patent ductus as well as other anomalies such as vascular ring. Patients were discharged either on the first or second postoperative day. Residual ductal flow was assessed in the operating room both by intraoperative transesophageal echocardiography which suggested zero residual shunts as well as by Doppler echo at discharge which suggested a 12% incidence of residual shunts. A large experience with VATS closure of patent ductus was reported from Iran by Nezafati et al in 2002.[32] The authors described 300 consecutive patients with a mean age of six years. The authors had no important complications and there were no residual shunts recorded. Three procedures were converted to thoracotomy in adult patients with a dilated ductus. Two patients had transient recurrent laryngeal nerve dysfunction. Similar excellent results were reported by Hines et al[33] from Wake Forest University in North Carolina in 1998. Thirty six of 38 patients who were beyond the neonatal period were discharged from hospital in less than 24 hours. Two of 59 patients suffered a recurrent nerve injury.

SURGICAL CLOSURE OF THE DUCTUS IN THE PRETERM INFANT

Burke et al updated their experience with application of VATS for patent ductus in the preterm infant in 1999.[34] They described 34 preterm infants with a mean weight at surgery of 930 g. Twenty patients weighed less than 1 kg. There was no operative mortality. Echocardiography documented elimination of ductal flow in all patients. Four patients required conversion to open thoracotomy. Two patients died before discharge, one on postoperative day 2 from an intracranial hemorrhage and one on postoperative day 88 because of multiple system organ failure.

In spite of Burke's experience, many centers including Children's Hospital Boston have reverted to a traditional open surgical approach for the premature ductus. In a report by Niinikoski et al from Finland,[35] 101 very low birth weight infants who weighed less than 1500 g at the time of surgery underwent traditional surgical ligation between 1988 and 1998. Operative mortality was 3% and overall mortality was 10%.

EVOLVING CATHETER METHODS

There have been numerous reports over the last decade describing the many different interventional catheter methods which have been tried for occlusion of the patent ductus. Rao has summarized the various devices that are currently available.[36] Because widely different standards have been applied for assessment of these very different methods an advisory panel was convened in order to advise the FDA regarding standards for clinical evaluation of patent ductus occlusion devices.[37] In one of the few very large reports Magee et al[38] described the results of the European registry of catheter occlusion of the ductus. A total of 1291 attempted coil occlusions were undertaken in 1258 patients. The median age at the procedure was four years with a median weight of 29 kg. The immediate occlusion rate was 59% which rose to 95% at one year. In 10% of procedures a suboptimal outcome occurred including coil embolization, abandonment of the procedure, persistent hemolysis, residual leak requiring a further procedure, flow impairment in adjacent structures and duct recanalization. Increasing duct size and the presence of a tubular shaped duct were risk factors for an unfavorable outcome. Residual shunts have been one of the most obvious disadvantages of catheter methods for ductal occlusion relative to surgery. In a report by Pedra et al,[39] 19 patients underwent reocclusion procedures either with Rashkind devices or with coils. Immediate or late complete occlusion was possible in 13 of 19 patients.

Cost of catheter methods versus surgery

A number of reports have attempted to compare the costs of interventional catheter methods with surgery. Although some reports have found that catheter methods are less expensive than surgery, for example reports by Prieto et al[40] and Singh et al,[41] nevertheless others have found that catheter methods are more expensive; for example, Gray et al[42] and Gray and Weinstein.[43]

ROBOTIC VERSUS VATS CLOSURE OF PATENT DUCTUS

In 2002, Labret et al[27] compared 28 patients who underwent VATS closure of a patent ductus with 28 patients who underwent a robotically assisted approach. Operative time was significantly longer in the robotic group. Two patients in the robotic group required reoperation and placement of a second clip while one patient in the VATS group required reoperation. There were no recurrent laryngeal nerve injuries and no important hemorrhage. Mean hospital stay was three days in both groups. The authors conclude that the outcome with robotic closure is similar to the outcome with VATS closure of patent ductus but because of the greater complexity robotic closure requires a longer operative time.

AORTOPULMONARY WINDOW

Aortopulmonary window is a very much rarer anomaly than patent ductus arteriosus. In the past therefore it was not uncommonly misdiagnosed as being a patent ductus. Today with modern diagnostic methods this should rarely if ever happen.

EMBRYOLOGY

An aortopulmonary window results from incomplete development of the conotruncal septum. At the more severe end of the spectrum the anomaly merges with truncus arteriosus while at the less severe end of the spectrum the anomaly is associated with isolated origin of the right pulmonary artery from the aorta.

ANATOMY

There is a wide spectrum of severity of aortopulmonary window. Richardson and coworkers have classified aortopulmonary window as types 1, 2 and 3.[44] Type 1 is a relatively small defect between the ascending aorta and main pulmonary artery immediately above the sinuses of Valsalva (see Figure 11.4a). A type 2 aortopulmonary window is located on the posterior wall of the ascending aorta at the origin of the right pulmonary artery. In type 3 the right pulmonary artery arises from the right side of the ascending aorta and there is complete absence of the aortopulmonary septum. Only the fact that there are separate semilunar valve annuli separated by a thin rim of tissue distinguishes type 3 aortopulmonary window from truncus arteriosus.

ASSOCIATED ANOMALIES

Most series suggest that at least 50% of cases of aortopulmonary window are associated with another anomaly. Table 11.1 illustrates the lesions associated with 18 consecutive cases of aortopulmonary window seen at Children's Hospital Boston. One complex association that has been identified in the literature and that we have seen[45–47] involves a large, confluent aortopulmonary window with separate origin of the right pulmonary artery from the right posterolateral ascending aorta combined with an interrupted aortic arch and patent ductus arteriosus. Interrupted aortic arch, almost exclusively type A, is a common associated lesion in most large series.[48,49]

Table 11.1 *Lesions associated with aortopulmonary window (18 cases)*

Lesion	*n*
Secundum atrial septal defect	5
Patent ductus arteriosus*	4
Ventricular septal defect	4
Interrupted aortic arch	3
Double outlet right ventricle	3
Tetralogy of Fallot	2
Tetralogy of Fallot with pulmonary atresia	2
Hypoplastic left ventricle	2
Right aortic arch	2
Peripheral pulmonary stenosis	2
Partial anomalous pulmonary venous return	1
Coarctation of the aorta	1
Anomalous right subclavian artery	1

*Patent ductus arteriosus occurred only with interrupted aortic arch or coarctation of the aorta.

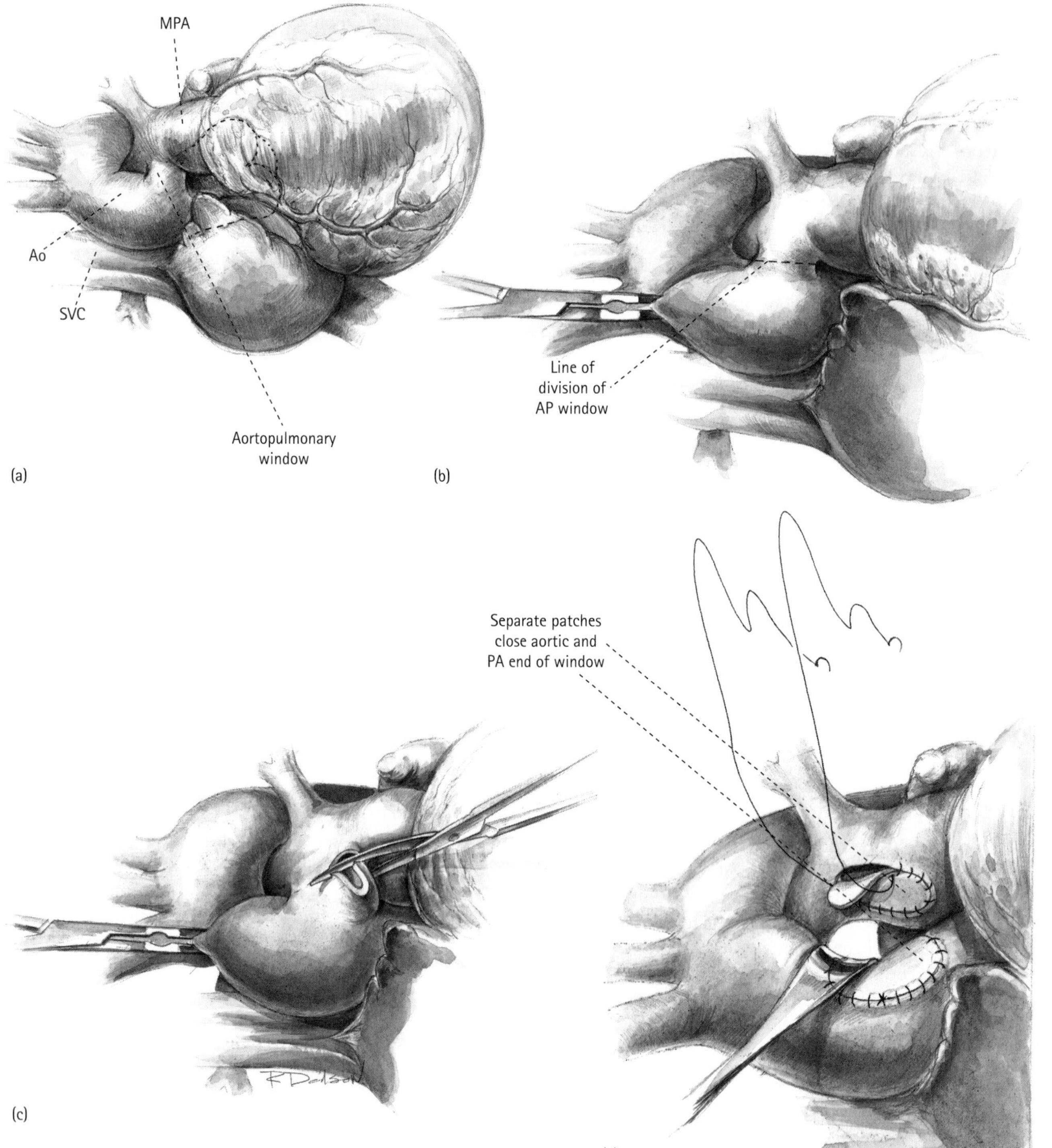

Figure 11.4 *(a) A type 1 aortopulmonary window is a communication between the ascending aorta and main pulmonary artery immediately above the sinuses of Valsalva. (b, c) An isolated aortopulmonary window is best approached by an incision in the aortopulmonary window itself using cardiopulmonary bypass and following application of an aortic cross clamp. (d) The aortic and pulmonary artery end of the divided anteroposterior window should be closed with an autologous pericardial patch.*

PATHOPHYSIOLOGY AND CLINICAL FEATURES

An aortopulmonary window is generally large enough to be nonrestrictive to flow. The hemodynamic consequences are essentially identical to those of a large patent ductus arteriosus. The ausculatory findings are also similar so that it can be extremely difficult on clinical grounds alone to distinguish an aortopulmonary window from a large patent ductus arteriosus. Today echocardiography with color Doppler mapping should allow for accurate diagnosis. As with patent ductus arteriosus, catheterization or other studies are only indicated when there is concern that pulmonary vascular disease might be present or to define associated anomalies.

MEDICAL AND INTERVENTIONAL THERAPY

The medical therapy for aortopulmonary window is the same as for a large patent ductus arteriosus. Because the defect has almost no length and may be closely associated with the semilunar valves it is generally not suitable for closure in the catheterization laboratory either by coils or by device.

INDICATIONS FOR SURGERY

The traditional indication for surgical closure of an aortopulmonary window has been the clinical diagnosis of the anomaly. Unlike patent ductus arteriosus it is exceedingly rare that an aortopulmonary window is so small that it can only be detected by echocardiography and not by clinical means such as auscultation. In the case of a very large lesion where diagnosis has been delayed to the point that pulmonary vascular disease has occurred a careful assessment must be made in the catheterization laboratory. The contraindications for surgery are similar to those described for Eisenmengers syndrome associated with patent ductus arteriosus.

SURGICAL MANAGEMENT

History of surgery

The first successful surgical correction of aortopulmonary window was undertaken by Robert E Gross at Children's Hospital Boston in 1952.[50] Dr Gross performed closed surgical ligation in his initial report. Other closed techniques were subsequently described including closed division with oversewing of the aortic and pulmonary artery defects.[51] The introduction of cardiopulmonary bypass allowed safer and more reliable open techniques to be used. These methods include external division and oversewing and various internal exposures (e.g. transaortic, transpulmonary artery) to either primarily close or patch the defect. In 1978, Johansson et al reported making an incision directly into the anterior wall of the aortopulmonary window itself which provides excellent internal exposure of both the aorta and pulmonary artery adjacent to the defect.[52]

Technical considerations

SIMPLE AORTOPULMONARY WINDOW

Approach is through a median sternotomy with subtotal resection of the thymus. A patch of anterior pericardium is harvested and treated with 6% glutaraldehyde for 20–30 minutes. The aortopulmonary window is inspected externally to confirm the diagnosis. Two semilunar valves should be apparent and the positions of the coronary artery origins noted. Extensive external dissection of the great vessels adds little information concerning the morphologic details of the defect and should be avoided. Following heparinization the ascending aorta is cannulated distally and a single venous cannula is placed in the right atrium. At the institution of cardiopulmonary bypass the pulmonary artery branches are occluded with tourniquets. The procedure can usually be performed using continuous cardiopulmonary bypass at moderately hypothermic temperatures. On occasion in a particularly small child deep hypothermic circulatory arrest may be useful as it allows the surgeon the flexibility of removing the aortic cross clamp to improve exposure by reducing distortion of the great vessels.

Following application of the aortic cross clamp cardioplegia solution is infused into the root of the aorta. At this point the tourniquets may be removed from the branch pulmonary arteries. The isolated defect is best approached directly through an incision in the aortopulmonary window itself (Figures 11.4b, 11.4c). As soon as exposure within the aorta has been obtained the locations of the coronary ostia should be confirmed. After complete division of the window the aortic defect is closed with a small patch of autologous pericardium using continuous 6/0 prolene in the neonate or small infant (Figure 11.4d). Although it is possible to release the aortic cross clamp at this point it is generally preferable to leave the clamp in place to allow accurate closure of the pulmonary artery defect also with an autologous pericardial patch. If the clamp is released the heart will begin to eject blood through the pulmonary artery defect which impairs the accuracy of the suture line. The suture line is usually very close to the pulmonary valve. It is important to carefully avoid picking up the very delicate valve leaflets with the suture. The heart is deaired in routine fashion and the aortic cross clamp is released with the cardioplegia site acting as a further vent for any tiny amounts of residual air.

AORTOPULMONARY WINDOW WITH INTERRUPTED AORTIC ARCH

As mentioned above the aortopulmonary window that is associated with interrupted aortic arch is likely to be more complex than the simple aortopulmonary window. Usually the very large window gives the appearance of complete absence of the septum between the aorta and main pulmonary artery. The right pulmonary artery appears to arise from the right lateral or posterolateral aspect of the ascending aorta (Figure 11.5a). The management of this entity is similar to the management of truncus arteriosus with interrupted aortic arch. The arterial cannulation for cardiopulmonary bypass should be placed distally in the ascending aorta. A single venous cannula is placed in the right atrium. Immediately after commencing bypass tourniquets are tightened around the right and left pulmonary arteries. Blood from the arterial cannula can pass through the aortopulmonary window into the

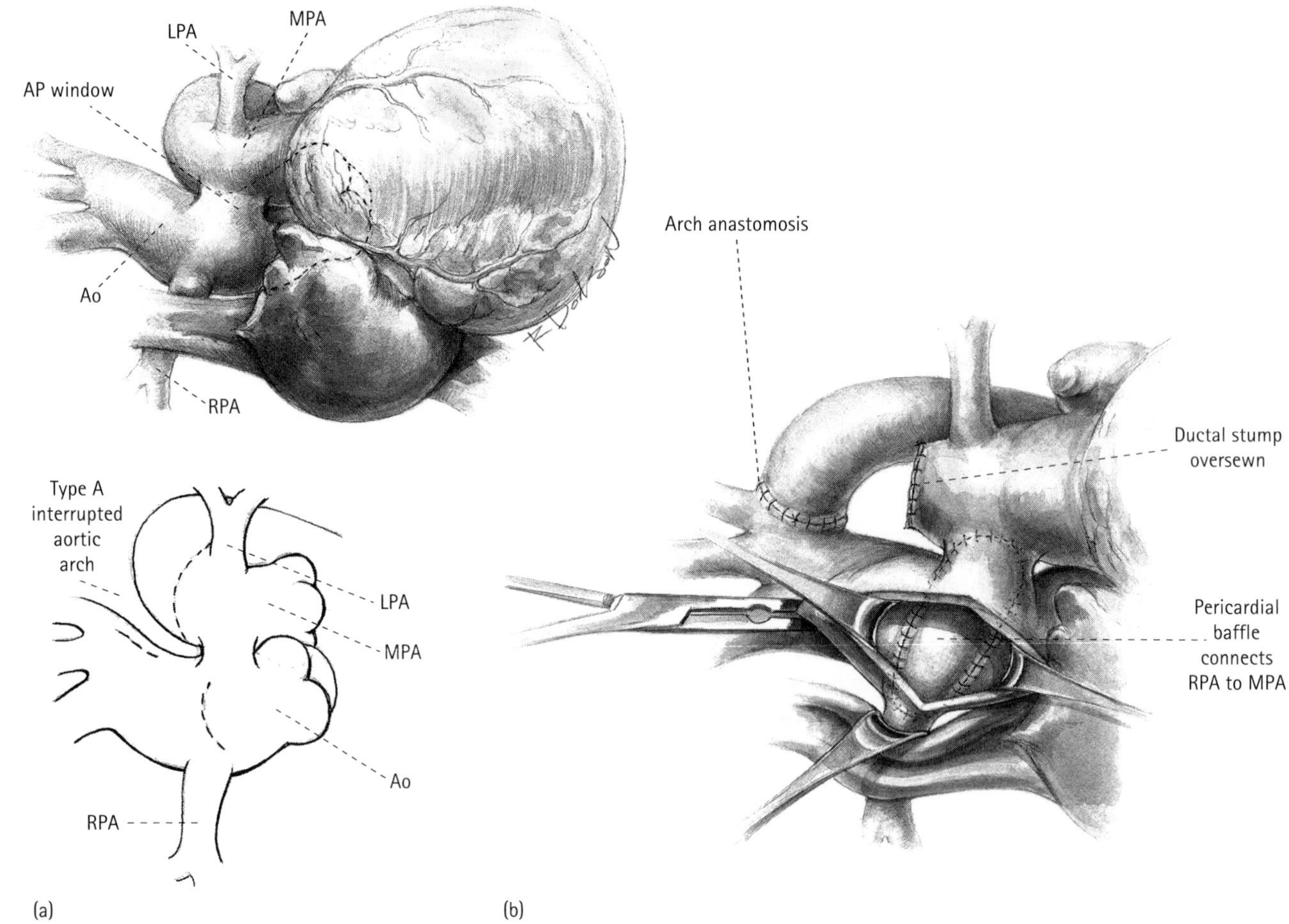

Figure 11.5 *(a) In type 3 aortopulmonary window there is absence of the aortopulmonary septum and the right pulmonary artery arises from the right side of the ascending aorta. Type 3 aortopulmonary window is often associated with interrupted aortic arch. (b) Repair of type 3 anteroposterior window with interrupted aortic arch by direct arch anastomosis and pericardial baffle of the main pulmonary artery to right pulmonary artery across the posterior wall of the ascending aorta.*

pulmonary artery and from there to the ductus arteriosus into the descending aorta to allow cooling of abdominal organs.

When the interruption is type A beyond the left subclavian artery it is often possible to perform the aortic arch anastomosis with bypass continuing. The ductus is controlled with a clamp on its pulmonary artery end. It is divided distally. The pulmonary artery end is oversewn. The distal divided descending aorta is controlled with a C-clamp while it is anastomosed to a longitudinal arteriotomy on the undersurface of the aortic arch (Figure 11.5b). During this time a clamp is applied across the proximal aortic arch and perfusion of the brain continues through the innominate artery. It is recommended that the patient be cooled to deep hypothermia before placing the aortic arch clamp and that flow be reduced to 20 ml/kg/min during the arch anastomosis. When the anastomosis has been completed the clamps can be released from the descending aorta and the aortic arch. The ascending aorta is clamped inferior to the arterial cannula so that the whole body other than the heart is now perfused. Cardioplegia solution is infused into the root of the aorta. Following administration of cardioplegia the tourniquets around the right and left pulmonary artery can be removed. The ascending aorta is opened with a transverse incision at the level of the right pulmonary artery. A pericardial baffle is placed within the aorta to direct blood from the main pulmonary artery to the right pulmonary artery across the posterior wall of the ascending aorta (Figure 11.5b). It is generally preferable to close the ascending aorta anteriorly with a patch also. In the neonate or very small infant it may be preferable to avoid the intraaortic baffling technique described above as this can result in growth related supravalvar aortic stenosis. An alternative procedure that is appropriate for the neonate or small infant is to mobilize the right pulmonary artery widely as is done for an arterial switch procedure. The ascending aorta is transected above and below the level of the right pulmonary artery. The resulting aortic tissue is sutured longitudinally above and below so as to create a tube extension of the right pulmonary artery. This can be anastomosed to the right side of the main pulmonary artery at the level of the aortopulmonary window. The ascending aorta and its arch branches must be well mobilized to allow direct reanastomosis repair of the ascending aorta. It is also necessary to complete closure of the pulmonary artery end of the aortopulmonary window with a patch of autologous pericardium.

Results of surgery

In 2001, Hew et al[53] described the experience at Children's Hospital Boston with surgical management of aortopulmonary window between 1973 and 1999. During this time frame, 38 patients underwent surgery at a median age of five weeks and with a median weight of 3.9 kg. Median follow-up was 6.6 years. A total of 65% of patients had additional defects including interrupted arch, tetralogy of Fallot and VSD. In 45% of patients the defect was approached through an aortotomy, in 31% through the defect itself and in 24% through the pulmonary artery. Closure was achieved using a single patch in 79% of patients. Over this very long time frame there were three hospital deaths and actuarial patient survival at 10 years was 88%. Three patients required reintervention for stenoses of the great arteries. By multivariate analysis approach through a pulmonary arteriotomy had the highest risk of need for reintervention ($p = 0.01$). In 2002, Backer and Mavroudis[54] described a 40 year experience at Children's Memorial Hospital in Chicago with surgical management of aortopulmonary window. Over this time frame 22 patients underwent surgery for aortopulmonary window. Four patients had associated interrupted aortic arch, three had origin of the right pulmonary artery from the aorta and three had an associated VSD. Median follow-up was eight years. There were five early deaths and one late death in the first 16 patients with no deaths in the most recent six patients who underwent transaortic patch closure. Patients who underwent transaortic patch closure demonstrated normal pulmonary artery and aortic growth. In 1993, van Son et al[55] described a 37 year experience with aortopulmonary window at the Mayo Clinic. Over this time frame 19 patients underwent surgery. Associated cardiac anomalies were present in 47%. Early in the experience there were four operative deaths. Risk factors for mortality were early year of operation, division of the aortopulmonary window versus transaortic or transpulmonary closure and a high pulmonary resistance relative to systemic resistance. The authors suggest that patients with a pulmonary to systemic resistance of greater than 40% should be thoroughly assessed to determine operability. Isolated reports have appeared describing transcatheter closure of aortopulmonary window. However in general most defects are either too large or too close to the semilunar valves to allow safe closure with a catheter delivered device.[56]

SINUS OF VALSALVA FISTULA

Like aortopulmonary window, sinus of Valsalva fistula is a very rare entity particularly in Western populations. However unlike aortopulmonary window the anomaly is more acquired than truly congenital. Because the physical findings are usually of recent onset in a young adult, it is generally not difficult to distinguish this entity from the related entities of patent ductus, aortopulmonary window and aortoventricular tunnel which are more truly congenital.

EMBRYOLOGY

Sinus of Valsalva fistula is an acquired lesion that occurs when a sinus of Valsalva aneurysm ruptures. Edwards has suggested that the pathologic basis for a sinus of Valsalva aneurysm is separation between the aortic media and the supporting ventricular fibrous structures.[57] The deficient area protrudes progressively into a low pressure cardiac chamber and progresses in size because of the pressure differential. Thus it is important to remember at the time of surgical repair to not only close the fistula but also to reinforce the deficient wall of the sinus of Valsalva. It is interesting to note that aneurysms and fistulas of the sinus of Valsalva are more common in Oriental than in Western populations, being similar in this respect to subpulmonary VSDs.

ANATOMY

In a review of 154 cases of ruptured aneurysm of the sinus of Valsalva published by Guo Qiang et al,[58] 80% of the aneurysms arose from the right coronary sinus and 20% from the non coronary sinus. This is similar to reports by Chu et al[59] in which 88% of sinuses of Valsalva aneurysms arose from the right coronary sinus. The fistulas communicated with the right ventricle in 75% and with the right atrium in 25% with only one case rupturing into the left ventricle.

ASSOCIATED ANOMALIES

Table 11.2 illustrates the anomalies that were associated with the 154 cases reported by Guo et al. Overall nearly half of the patients (47%) had associated anomalies. Forty-nine percent of patients had an associated VSD. Aortic regurgitation was also common in this relatively older population in which the mean age of the series was 28.8 years.

Table 11.2 *Associated cardiac anomalies*

Cardiac abnormality	*n*	(%)
Ventricular septal defect	62	(49.3)
Aortic regurgitation	36	(23.4)
Tricuspid regurgitation	3	(1.9)
Infundibular pulmonary stenosis	3	(1.9)
Patent arterial duct	2	(1.3)
Patent oval foramen	2	(1.3)
Total	108	(47.4)

PATHOPHYSIOLOGY AND CLINICAL FEATURES

An unruptured aneurysm of the sinus of Valsalva is usually free of symptoms. Clinical examination is also likely to be unremarkable. When there is sufficient distortion of the sinus of Valsalva by the aneurysm to cause aortic regurgitation this is often in the setting of an associated VSD and a diastolic murmur of aortic regurgitation will be audible.

Many patients are able to identify an acute event which was likely to have been associated with rupture. For example, in the series by Guo et al, 70% of patients had a history of a sudden acute episode or acute exacerbation of previous symptoms. In many cases this was associated with strenuous exercise or an abrupt change of posture. The pathophysiology of a ruptured sinus of Valsalva aneurysm is similar to that of a patent ductus arteriosus or aortopulmonary window. There is a left to right shunt which places a volume load on the left ventricle. There is increased pulmonary return to the left atrium. Right ventricular pressure is elevated by the flow returning directly to the right ventricle. Diastolic pressure within the aorta is lowered, resulting in increased pulse pressure. In the report by Guo et al the clinical features of left heart failure were present in most patients. A continuous murmur which is heard maximally over the precordial area, particularly if this is a new finding, should alert the clinician to the possibility of a sinus of Valsalva fistula. The natural history of this lesion is poor with a mean survival time of 3.9 years as reported by Sawyer et al if the lesion is untreated.[60]

DIAGNOSTIC STUDIES

The plain chest X-ray will demonstrate signs of increased pulmonary blood flow and left heart enlargement. If the rupture is into the right atrium there may be considerable dilation of that chamber. The ECG is generally non specific. Two-dimensional echocardiography with color Doppler mapping is usually diagnostic. However in view of the rarity of the lesion as well as the difficulty in distinguishing the lesion from a coronary artery fistula it may be wise to perform cardiac catheterization to delineate the coronary anatomy. Frequently the mouth of the aneurysm within the right coronary sinus is very close to the origin of the right coronary artery.

MEDICAL AND INTERVENTIONAL THERAPY

Medical therapy for a sinus of Valsalva fistula is standard anticongestive therapy. This anomaly is not suitable for management with catheter delivered devices or coils. It is very likely that there will already be some degree of distortion of the aortic valve by the sinus of Valsalva aneurysm which has ruptured to cause the fistula. Furthermore the right coronary ostium is usually very close to the mouth of the sinus of Valsalva aneurysm. Thus devices or coils could easily cause right coronary obstruction or further distortion of a regurgitant aortic valve.

INDICATIONS FOR SURGERY

Because a sinus of Valsalva fistula is an acquired lesion secondary to congenital weakness of the junction between the left ventricle and aortic root it is likely to be progressive. For this reason the diagnosis of sinus of Valsalva fistula in itself should be an indication to proceed to surgery. Although surgery is not indicated on an emergency basis nevertheless it should proceed within a week or two at most of diagnosis. If the patient presents in a compromised state because of untreated congestive heart failure a brief period of intensive medical therapy as an inpatient may be indicated.

SURGICAL MANAGEMENT

History of surgery

One of the earliest reports of surgical treatment of a sinus of Valsalva fistula was by Sawyer et al in 1957.[60] The transaortic approach for repair was described by Shumacker and Waldhausen in 1965.[61] The largest reports have described series of Oriental patients including the reports by Okada et al,[62] Chu et al[59] and Guo et al.[58]

Technical considerations

The aim of surgical repair should not only be to close the fistula between the sinus of Valsalva aneurysm and the affected cardiac chamber (which is usually the right ventricle) but also to reinforce the deficient wall of the sinus of Valsalva. Approach is by a median sternotomy using cardiopulmonary bypass. The arterial cannula is placed distally in the ascending aorta. Bicaval venous cannulation using right angle cannulas should be used. A moderate degree of hypothermia, e.g. 28°C, is appropriate. However the early phase of cooling should be somewhat slower than usual in order to allow time for application of the aortic cross clamp before cardiac action has slowed to the point that distention of the right ventricle will occur because of run off from the fistula. Unless the fistula is particularly large it is reasonable to infuse approximately half of the dose of cardioplegia solution directly into the aortic root aided by massage of the heart. The aorta is then opened with a reverse hockey stick incision extending towards the non coronary sinus (Figure 11.6a). The remainder of the cardioplegia solution is infused directly into the coronary ostia. Caval tourniquets are tightened.

An oblique incision is made in the right atrium. The fistula is easily identified as a parachute like structure with a rupture at its most distal extremity most commonly within the right ventricle and on occasion within the right atrium. It is usually appropriate to oversew the distal end of the fistula (Figure

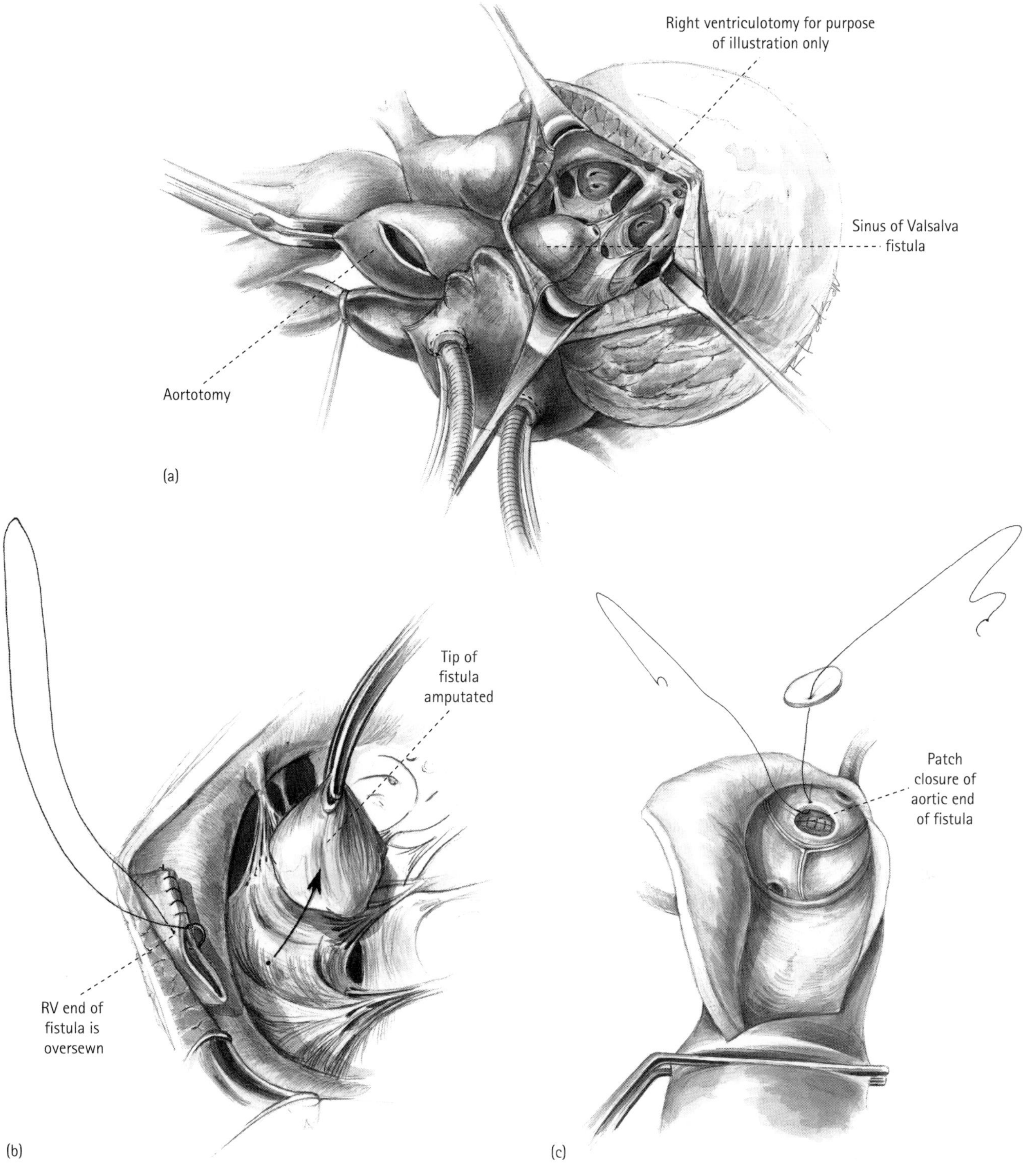

Figure 11.6 *Surgical repair of sinus of Valsalva fistula. (a) Approach should be both at the aortic end of the fistula as well as the distal end of the fistula. A right ventriculotomy such as shown here should rarely be necessary but serves to illustrate the anatomy of the distal end of the fistula. (b) The tip of the fistula has been amputated and the fistula is oversewn on its right ventricular end. (c) A small patch of autologous pericardium is used to close the aortic end of the sinus of Valsalva fistula.*

11.6b). However the principal closure of the fistula should be performed at the aortic end. Generally it is best to use a small patch (Figure 11.6c). In the smaller and younger patient autologous pericardium treated with glutaraldehyde is appropriate. In the larger child or adult a small patch of Gortex is appropriate. The suture line which can be either continuous prolene or interrupted sutures must carefully avoid any distortion of the right coronary ostium or of the aortic valve leaflets.

Yacoub et al[63] have suggested that subpulmonary VSDs also represent a congenital weakness of the junction between the aortic root and the left ventricle. Yacoub recommends direct suture apposition of the aortic root to the crest of the subpulmonary VSD in order to strengthen this area appropriately. However, this technique is generally not applicable in the setting of a ruptured sinus of Valsalva aneurysm as it can result in important distortion of the aortic valve and right coronary artery.

ASSOCIATED AORTIC VALVE REPAIR

Guo et al found that associated aortic regurgitation was a key factor in determining operative results and prognosis. They found a need to perform valvuloplasty or replacement of the aortic valve in 25 of 154 patients. Techniques of aortic valve repair included support of a prolapsed and elongated right coronary leaflet using the technique described by Trusler.[64] Ideally however a sinus of Valsalva fistula should be identified before significant distortion of the aortic valve has occurred.

Results of surgery

In 1994 Professor Guo Qiang et al[58] from Fu Wai Hospital in Beijing, China, described the results of surgical management of 154 patients with sinus of Valsalva fistula. In 79% of cases the fistula originated from the right coronary sinus with the remainder originating from the non coronary sinus. A total of 73% of the fistulas ruptured into the right ventricle and 27% into the right atrium with fewer than 1% rupturing into the left ventricle. Aortic valve regurgitation was present in 23%. Operative mortality was 4.5%. Long-term follow-up was achieved in 80% of patients with a mean duration of nearly six years. The presence of preoperative aortic regurgitation and worse symptoms at the time of surgery were both predictive of a worse long-term outcome. The authors concluded from their analysis that the optimal surgical approach was closure of the distal end of the fistula by direct suture with reinforcement of the aortic sinus with a patch. In 2002 Dong et al[65] updated the experience from Fu Wai Hospital. Between 1996 and 2001, 67 patients underwent repair of sinus of Valsalva fistula. In this more recent experience the majority of fistulas were closed at the distal end of the fistula with an aortotomy being used in only three patients. The aortic valve was replaced in 12 patients. There was one early death and one late death. Late complications included a residual shunt in two patients, paravalvar leak in one and aortic regurgitation in one.

In 1999, Takach et al[66] from the Texas Heart Institute described the results of surgery for 64 patients with sinus of Valsalva fistula. In 61 patients simple plication was used; patch repair was applied in 52 patients with aortic root replacement in 16 patients. Aortic valve replacement or repair was required in 58%. There were five hospital deaths and two patients had strokes during the early postoperative period. Over a mean follow-up of five years the fistula recurred in two patients. The authors recommend early repair to reduce the risk of endocarditis or the need for more extensive surgery.

In a report by Azakie et al[67] from Toronto, 34 patients were reviewed who underwent surgery over a 28-year period. In 10 patients the fistula was closed by direct suture while a patch was employed in 24. Five early fistula recurrences occurred in patients who had primary rather than patch closure. Late aortic valve replacement was necessary in six patients for progressive aortic regurgitation due to bicuspid aortic valve in three, cusp disease of the affected sinus in two patients or aortic root dilation in two. The authors recommend patch closure of the fistula in all cases.

In a review of the Mayo Clinic experience, van Son et al[68] identified 31 patients who underwent surgery between 1956 and 1993. Similar to the first report from Fu Wai the authors found that risk of recurrence and need for operation was lower when an aortotomy, with or without right ventriculotomy, was used during repair versus right ventriculotomy alone. Overall the long-term survival after surgery was excellent.

AORTOVENTRICULAR TUNNEL

INTRODUCTION

An aortoventricular tunnel is an exceedingly rare congenital anomaly. It is indeed as the name suggests a tunnel which connects the lumen of the aorta to the cavity of usually the left ventricle though occasionally aorto right ventricular tunnels have been described. In contrast to a sinus of Valsalva fistula, an aorto left ventricular tunnel is always present at birth and is likely to be symptomatic in the first year of life.[69]

EMBRYOLOGY

Although a detailed explanation of the embryological origin of the aortoventricular tunnel is not available Mackay et al have recently speculated in detail regarding the possible embryological mechanism of formation of such tunnels.[70] The tunnel probably represents abnormal differentiation of the primordial muscle which initially forms both the base of the left ventricle as well as the conotruncus. Abnormal development may involve failure of the outflow cushions to form the sinuses of Valsalva, the valvar leaflets and the fibrous inter leaflet triangles coupled with abnormal separation of the distal outflow tract into the aorta and pulmonary trunk. The association of tunnels with abnormalities of the aortic sinuses, proximal coronary artery and the leaflets themselves is therefore quite predictable.

ANATOMY

The majority of aortoventricular tunnels arise from the right sinus of Valsalva at approximately the level of the sinotubular

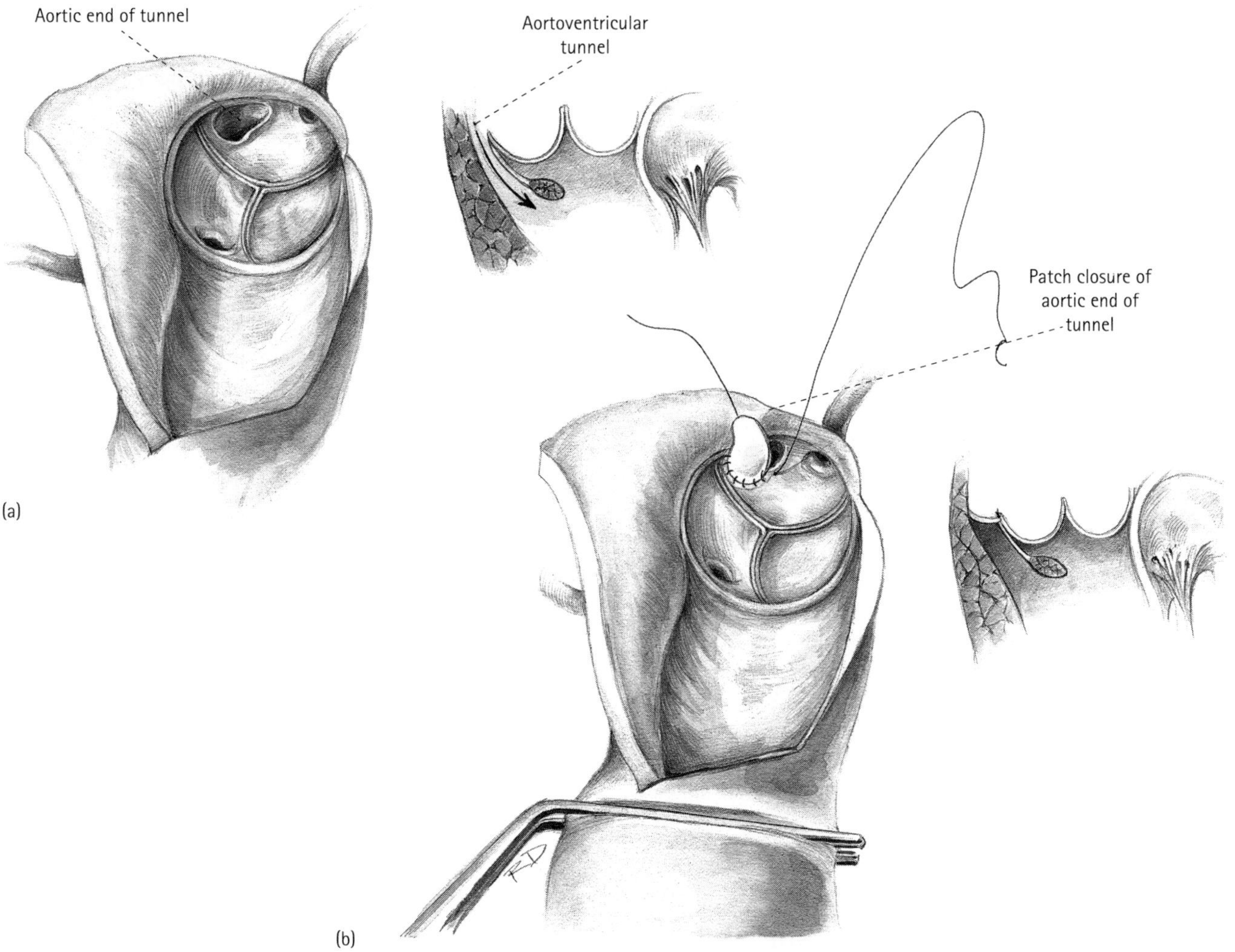

Figure 11.7 *(a) An aortic to left ventricular tunnel usually originates from in the right coronary sinus close to the intercoronary commissure. (b) The aortic to left ventricular tunnel is best managed by autologous pericardial patch closure of the aortic end of the tunnel.*

junction and pass inferiorly through extracardiac tissue before entering the left ventricle immediately below the right coronary leaflet[70] (Figure 11.7a). A typical aorta to left ventricular tunnel produces a large tubular or sacular protuberance that is visible on the anterior aspect of the aortic root. However, not all tunnels pass from the aorta to the left ventricle. There have been at least 10 case reports of tunnel which terminated in the right ventricle.[71,72] There have also been case reports of aorto left ventricular tunnels which have arisen from the left coronary sinus.

Histologically the wall of the tunnel differs at its two ends. The aortic origin consists of fibrous tissue with smooth muscle cells and elastic fibers. At the ventricular opening there is non specific collagen or muscle.

PATHOPHYSIOLOGY

An aorto left ventricular tunnel effectively produces aortic regurgitation. Like patent ductus arteriosus, aortopulmonary window and sinus of Valsalva fistula there is a steal from the systemic circulation during diastole and a widened pulse pressure. However during systole, in contrast to the other lesions, there is no steal and furthermore there is no impact on the pulmonary circulation as there is with the other lesions. In time with distortion of the aortic valve leaflets true aortic valve regurgitation is likely to develop in addition to the regurgitant flow that occurs through the tunnel to the left ventricle.

CLINICAL FEATURES AND DIAGNOSTIC STUDIES

Although there have been occasional reports of patients who were not symptomatic early in life,[73,74] it is thought the majority of patients develop congestive heart failure within the first year of life and in fact many are symptomatic in the neonatal period. Examination reveals bounding peripheral pulses and the blood pressure confirms widening of the pulse pressure. Auscultation reveals a to-and-fro murmur which may be accompanied by systolic and diastolic thrills. Chest X-ray demonstrates cardiac enlargement and in some patients the tunnel itself can be seen as a leftward prominence of the aortic root in the area of the pulmonary trunk.[75] The ECG typically shows left or biventricular hypertrophy with a strain pattern of inverted T waves.

Two-dimensional echocardiography is diagnostic. Color flow imaging documents blood passing through the abnormal channel from the left ventricle to the aorta during systole and in the opposite direction in diastole. The most common diagnostic error is to confuse the ventricular end of the tunnel with a VSD. Cardiac catheterization should only be necessary if the relationship of the tunnel to coronary anatomy is unclear.

MEDICAL AND INTERVENTIONAL MANAGEMENT

Without surgical treatment most patients die early in life from congestive heart failure. Therefore medical management of congestive heart failure should be of limited duration and sufficient only to allow the patient to be in optimal condition at the time of surgery. Although there has been a report of attempted closure of an aorto left ventricular tunnel with an Amplatzer duct occluder,[76] it seems unlikely that the majority of tunnels would be suitable for interventional closure. Since the wall of the tunnel is in part formed by the right coronary leaflet of the aortic valve a device of any type is likely to cause distortion and injury if not perforation of the valve leaflet.

INDICATIONS FOR AND TIMING OF SURGERY

The presence of a tunnel is in itself the indication for surgery. Thus even asymptomatic patients should undergo surgical management. In view of the very poor natural history of this anomaly surgery should be undertaken within a short time, preferably days, of diagnosis.

SURGICAL MANAGEMENT

History of surgery

One of the earliest reports of the aortoventricular tunnel was by Burchell and Edwards in 1957[77] and subsequently by Edwards in 1961.[78] However Levy and colleagues are credited with the first application of the term 'aortico left ventricular tunnel' in 1963.[79]

Technical considerations

CARDIOPULMONARY BYPASS SETUP

The procedure is undertaken on cardiopulmonary bypass generally with a single venous cannula in the right atrium. In the young infant the heart is likely to lose contractility soon after the commencement of bypass so it is advisable to plan for cross clamping of the aorta early. A partial dose of cardioplegia solution can be given directly into the aortic root aided by massage of the left ventricle or by external compression of the tunnel. The remainder of the cardioplegia solution should be infused directly into the coronary ostia after the aorta has been opened.

EXPOSURE OF THE TUNNEL

The aortic end of the tunnel is exposed using a reverse hockey stick incision extending towards the non coronary sinus. The coronary ostia must be carefully identified particularly the right coronary. The right coronary ostium is likely to be within a millimeter or two of the tunnel. Generally the tunnel lies to the left of the right coronary ostium. The aortic end of the tunnel is closed with a small patch of autologous pericardium which can be sutured into position using continuous 6/0 prolene (Figure 11.7b). Although it is possible to visualize the ventricular end of the tunnel through the aortic valve it is generally not advisable to attempt to close the ventricular end of the tunnel. Part of the circumference of the tunnel is formed by the right coronary leaflet so that complete closure of the ventricular end of the tunnel is not possible. Furthermore an attempt to close the ventricular end of the tunnel will leave a dead space between the two patches rather than allowing blood to wash in and out of the residual tunnel. On occasion it is reasonable to reduce the size of the tunnel by external plication of the protuberance that can be seen externally. However great care must be taken if this is done to ensure that the aortic valve is not distorted.

SEPARATION FROM BYPASS

The heart is de-aired in the usual fashion and the aortic cross clamp is released with the cardioplegia site in the ascending aorta bleeding freely. During warming the usual monitoring lines are placed. Separation from bypass should be uneventful and require minimal inotropic support. Because the ventricle has been volume loaded preoperatively there should be excellent ventricular function with the reduced volume load that is present postoperatively.

Results of surgery

Although mortality was high in early series and case reports approaching 20% or more,[80] in recent series mortality has been low.[81] Early reports also suggested a high incidence of late aortic valve regurgitation but these were patients who had been repaired by direct suture of the aortic end of the tunnel often beyond five years of age.[82] More recent series suggest that early repair of the tunnel using a small patch for closure is rarely followed by important aortic valve regurgitation though follow-up is not long.[69,81]

REFERENCES

1. Cassels DE. *The Ductus Arteriosus.* Springfield, IL, Charles C Thomas, 1973, p 75.
2. McMurphy DM, Heymann MA, Rudolph AM, Melmon KL. Developmental change in constriction of the ductus arteriosus. Response to oxygen and vasoactive substances in the isolated ductus arteriosus of the fetal lamb. *Pediatr Res* 1972; **6**:231–238.
3. Oberhansli-Weiss I, Heymann MA, Rudolph AM, Melmon KL. The pattern and mechanisms of response to oxygen by the ductus arteriosus and umbilical artery. *Pediatr Res* 1972; **6**:693–700.
4. Elzenga NJ. *The Ductus Arteriosus and Stenoses of the Adjacent Great Arteries.* Alblassderdam, Grafische Verzorging, 1986.
5. Santos MA, Moll JN, Drummond C, Araujo WB, Romao N, Reis NB. Development of the ductus arteriosus in right ventricular outflow tract obstruction. *Circulation* 1980; **62**:818–822.
6. Zach M, Beitzke A, Singer H, Hofler H, Schellman B. The syndrome of absent pulmonary valve and ventricular septal defect – Anatomical features and embryological implications. *Basic Res Cardiol* 1979; **74**:54–68.
7. Ichihashi K, Shiraishi H, Endou H, Kuramatsu T, Yano S, Yanagisawa M. Cerebral and abdominal arterial hemodynamics in preterm infants with patent ductus arteriosus. *Acta Paediatr Jpn* 1990; **32**:349–356.
8. Meyers RL, Alpan G, Lin E, Clyman RI. Patent ductus arteriosus, indomethacin and intestinal distention: Effects on intestinal blood flow and oxygen consumption. *Pediatr Res* 1991; **29**:569–574.
9. Wong SN, Lo RN, Hui PW. Abnormal renal and splanchnic arterial Doppler pattern in premature babies with symptomatic patent ductus arteriosus. *J Ultrasound Med* 1990; **9**:125–130.
10. Heymann MA, Rudolph AM, Silverman NH. Closure of the ductus arteriosus in premature infants by inhibition of prostaglandin synthesis. *N Engl J Med* 1976; **295**:530–533.
11. Peckham GJ, Miettinen OS, Ellison RC et al. Clinical course to 1 year of age in premature infants with patent ductus arteriosus: Results of a multicenter randomized trial of indomethacin. *J Pediatr* 1984; **105**:285–291.
12. Schmidt B, Davis P, Moddemann D et al. Long-term effects of indomethacin prophylaxis in extremely low birth weight infants. *New Eng J Med* 2001; **344**:1966–1972.
13. De Simone L, Cecchi F, Favilli S et al. Usefulness of pulsed Doppler echocardiography in the diagnosis and medical therapy of patent ductus arteriosus in the newborn with respiratory distress. *G Ital Cardiol* 1991; **21**:409–414.
14. Zanardo V, Milanesi O, Trevisanuto D et al. Early screening and treatment of 'silent' patent ductus arteriosus in premature infants with RDS. *J Perinat Med* 1991; **19**:291–295.
15. McCarthy JS, Zies LG, Gelband H. Age dependent closure of the patent ductus arteriosus by indomethacin. *Pediatrics* 1978; **62**:706–712.
16. Lock JE, Keane JF, Perry SB. *Diagnostic and Interventional Catheterization in Congenital Heart Disease*, 2nd edn. Boston, MA, Kluwer Academic Publishers, 2000.
17. Wessel DL, Keane JF, Parness I, Lock JE. Outpatient closure of the patent ductus arteriosus. *Circulation* 1988; **77**:1068–1071.
18. Hawkins JA, Minich LL, Tani LY, Sturtevant JE, Orsmond GS, McGough EC. Cost and efficacy of surgical ligation versus transcatheter coil occlusion of patent ductus arteriosus. *J Thorac Cardiovasc Surg* 1996; **112**:1635–1639.
19. Gross RE, Hubbard JP. Surgical ligation of a patent ductus arteriosus: report of first successful case. *JAMA* 1939; **112**:729–731.
20. Gross RE. Complete surgical division of the patent ductus arteriosus. *Surg Gynecol Obstet* 1944; **78**:36.
21. Blalock A. Operative closure of the patent ductus arteriosus. *Surg Gynecol Obstet* 1946; **82**:113.
22. Decanq HE Jr. Repair of patent ductus arteriosus in a 1417 g infant. *Am J Dis Child* 1963; **106**:402.
23. Porstmann W, Wierny L, Warnke H, Gerstberger G, Romaniuk PA. Catheter closure of patent ductus arteriosus: 62 cases treated without thoracotomy. *Radiol Clin North Am* 1971; **9**:203–218.
24. Rashkind WJ, Cuaso CC. Transcatheter closure of patent ductus arteriosus. *Pediatr Cardiol* 1979; **1**:3.
25. Moore JW, George L, Kirkpatrick SE et al. Percutaneous closure of small patent ductus arteriosus using occluding spring coils. *J Am Coll Cardiol* 1994; **23**:759–765.
26. Laborde F, Noirhomme P, Karam J, Batisse A, Bourel P, Saint Maurice O. A new video-assisted thoracoscopic surgical technique for interruption of patent ductus arteriosus in infants and children. *J Thorac Cardiovasc Surg* 1993; **105**:278–280.
27. LeBret E, Papadatos S, Folliguet T et al. Interruption of patent ductus arteriosus in children: Robotically assisted versus videothoracosopic surgery. *J Thorac Cardiovasc Surg* 2002; **123**:973–976.
28. Mavroudis C, Backer CL, Gevitz M. Forty-six years of patient ductus arteriosus division at Children's Memorial Hospital of Chicago. Standards for comparison. *Ann Surg* 1994; **220**:402–409.
29. Panagopoulos PG, Tatooles CJ, Aberdeen E, Waterston DJ, Bonham Carter RE. Patent ductus arteriosus in infants and children. *Thorax* 1971; **26**:137–144.
30. Laborde F, Folliguet TA, Etienne PY, Carbognani D, Batisse A, Petrie J. Video-thoracoscopic surgical interruption of patent ductus arteriosus. Routine experience in 332 pediatric cases. *Eur J Cardiothorac Surg* 1997; **11**:1052–1055.
31. Burke RP, Wernovsky G, van der Velde M, Hansen D, Castaneda AR. Video-assisted thoracoscopic surgery for congenital heart disease. *J Thorac Cardiovasc Surg* 1995; **109**:499–507.
32. Nezafati MH, Mahmoodi E, Hashemian SH, Hamedanchi A. Video-assisted thoracoscopic surgical (VATS) closure of patent ductus arteriosus: report of three-hundred cases. *Heart Surg Forum* 2002; **5**:57–59.
33. Hines MH, Bensky AS, Hammon JW Jr, Pennington DG. Video-assisted thoracoscopic ligation of patent ductus arteriosus: safe and outpatient. *Ann Thorac Surg* 1998; **66**:853–858.
34. Burke RP, Jacobs JP, Cheng W, Trento A, Fontana GP. Video-assisted thoracoscopic surgery for patent ductus arteriosus in low birth weight neonates and infants. *Pediatrics* 1999; **104**:227–230.
35. Niinikoski H, Alanen M, Parvinen T, Aantaa R, Ekblad H, Kero P. Surgical closure of patent ductus arteriosus in very-low-birth-weight infants. *Pediatr Surg Int* 2001; **17**:338–341.
36. Rao PS. Summary and comparison of patent ductus arteriosus closure devices. *Curr Interv Cardiol Rep* 2001; **3**:268–274.
37. Proposed standards for clinical evaluation of patent ductus arteriosus occlusion devices. Multiorganization Advisory Panel to FDA for Pediatric Cardiovascular Devices. *Catheter Cardiovasc Interv* 2000; **51**:293–299.
38. Magee AG, Huggon IC, Seed PT, Qureshi SA, Tynan M. Transcatheter coil occlusion of the arterial duct; results of the European Registry. *Eur Heart J* 2001; **22**:1817–1821.
39. Pedra CA, Esteves CA, Pedra SR, Braga SL, Sousa JE, Fontes VF. Indications, technique, results and clinical impact of reocclusion procedures for residual shunts after transcatheter closure of the patent ductus arteriosus. *Arch Inst Cardiol Mex* 1999; **69**:320–329.
40. Prieto LR, DeCamillo DM, Konrad DJ, Scalet-Longworth L, Latson LA. Comparison of cost and clinical outcome between transcatheter coil occlusion and surgical closure of isolated patent ductus arteriosus. *Pediatrics* 1998; **101**:1020–1024.

41. Singh TP, Morrow WR, Walters HL, Vitale NA, Hakimi M. Coil occlusion versus conventional surgical closure of patent ductus arteriosus. *Am J Cardiol* 1997; **79**:1283–1285.
42. Gray DT, Fyler DC, Walker AM, Weinstein MC, Chalmers TC. Clinical outcomes and costs of transcatheter as compared with surgical closure of patent ductus arteriosus. *New Eng J Med* 1993; **329**:1517–1523.
43. Gray DT, Weinstein MC. Decision and cost-utility analyses of surgical versus transcatheter closure of patent ductus arteriosus: should you let a smile be your umbrella? *Med Decis Making* 1998; **18**:187–201.
44. Richardson JV, Doty DB, Rossi NP, Ehrenhaft JL. The spectrum of anomalies of aortopulmonary septation. *J Thorac Cardiovasc Surg* 1979; **78**:21–27.
45. Berry TE, Bharati S, Muster AJ et al. Distal aortopulmonary septal defect, aortic origin of the right pulmonary artery, intact ventricular septum, patent ductus arteriosus and hypoplasia of the aortic isthmus: A newly recognized syndrome. *Am J Cardiol* 1982; **49**:108–116.
46. Ding WX, Su ZK, Cao DF, Jonas RA. One-stage repair of absence of the aortopulmonary septum and interrupted aortic arch. *Ann Thorac Surg* 1990; **49**:664–666.
47. Mendoza DA, Ueda T, Nishioka K et al. Aortopulmonary window, aortic origin of the right pulmonary artery, and interrupted aortic arch: Detection by two-dimensional and color Doppler echocardiography in an infant. *Pediatr Cardiol* 1986; **7**:49.
48. Braunlin E, Peoples WM, Freedom RM et al. Interruption of the aortic arch with aorticopumonary septal defect. An anatomic review. *Pediatr Cardiol* 1982; **2**:329.
49. Kutsche LM, Van Mierop LH. Anatomy and pathogenesis of aorticopulmonary septal defect. *Am J Cardiol* 1987; **59**:443–447.
50. Gross RE. Surgical closure of an aortic septal defect. *Circulation* 1952; **5**:858.
51. Scott HW Jr, Sabiston DC Jr. Surgical treatment for congenital aorticopulmonary fistula. Experimental and clinical aspects. *J Thorac Surg* 1953; **25**:26.
52. Johansson L, Michaelsson M, Westerholm CJ, Aberg T. Aorto-pulmonary window. A new operative approach. *Ann Thorac Surg* 1978; **25**:564–567.
53. Hew CC, Bacha EA, Zurakowski D, del Nido PJ, Jonas RA. Optimal surgical approach for repair of aortopulmonary window. *Cardiol Young* 2001; **11**:385–390.
54. Backer CL, Mavroudis C. Surgical management of aortopulmonary window: a 40-year experience. *Eur J Cardiothorac Surg* 2002; **21**:773–779.
55. van Son JA, Puga FJ, Danielson GK et al. Aortopulmonary window: factors associated with early and late success after surgical treatment. *Mayo Clin Proc* 1993; **68**:128–133.
56. Stamato T, Benson LN, Smallhorn JF, Freedom RM. Transcatheter closure of an aortopulmonary window with a modified double umbrella occluder system. *Cathet Cardiovasc Diagn* 1995; **35**:165–167.
57. Edwards JE, Burchell HB. The pathological anatomy of deficiencies between the aortic root and the heart including aortic sinus aneurysms. *Thorax* 1957; **12**:125–139.
58. Qiang GJ, Dong ZH, Xing XG et al. Surgical treatment of ruptured aneurysm of the sinus of Valsalva. *Cardiol Young* 1994; **4**:347–352.
59. Chu SH, Hung CR, How SS. Ruptured aneurysm of the sinus of Valsalva in Oriental patients. *J Thorac Cardiovasc Surg* 1990; **99**:288–298.
60. Sawyer JT, Adams JE, Scott HW. Surgical treatment for aneurysms of aortic sinus with aorticoarterial fistula. *Surgery* 1957; **41**:26–42.
61. Shumacker HB, King H, Waldhausen JA. Transaortic approach for the repair of ruptured aneurysms of the sinuses of Valsalva. *Ann Surg* 1965; **161**:946–954.
62. Okada M, Muranka S, Mukubo M, Asada S. Surgical correction of the ruptured aneurysm of the sinus of Valsalva. *J Thorac Cardiovasc Surg* 1977; **18**:171–180.
63. Yacoub MH, Khan H, Stavri G, Shinebourne E, Radley-Smith R. Anatomic correction of the syndrome of prolapsing right coronary aortic cusp, dilatation of the sinus of Valsalva, and ventricular septal defect. *J Thorac Cardiovasc Surg* 1997; **113**:253–261.
64. Trusler GA, Moes CAF, Kidd BSL. Repair of ventricular septal defect with aortic insufficiency. *J Thorac Cardiovasc Surg* 1973; **66**:394–403.
65. Dong C, Wu QY, Tang Y. Ruptured sinus of valsalva aneurysm: a Beijing experience. *Ann Thorac Surg* 2002; **74**:1621–1624.
66. Takach TJ, Reul GJ, Duncan JM et al. Sinus of Valsalva aneurysm or fistula: management and outcome. *Ann Thorac Surg* 1999; **68**:1573–1577.
67. Azakie A, David TE, Peniston CM, Rao V, Williams WG. Ruptured sinus of valsalva aneurysm: early recurrence and fate of the aortic valve. *Ann Thorac Surg* 2000; **70**:1466–1470.
68. van Son JA, Danielson GK, Schaff HV, Orszulak TA, Edwards WD, Seward JB. Long-term outcome of surgical repair of ruptured sinus of Valsalva aneurysm. *Circulation* 1994; **90**:II20–II29.
69. Sousa-Uva M, Touchot A, Fermont L et al. Aortico-left ventricular tunnel in fetuses and infants. *Ann Thorac Surg* 1996; **61**:1805–1810.
70. McKay R, Anderson RH, Cook AC. The aorto-ventricular tunnels. *Cardiol Young* 2002; **12**:563–580.
71. van Son JAM, Hambsch J, Schneider P, Mohr FW. Repair of aortico-right ventricular tunnel. *Eur J Cardiothorac Surg* 1998; **14**:214–217.
72. Bharati S, Lev M, Cassels DE. Aortico-right ventricular tunnel. *Chest* 1973; **63**:198–202.
73. Serino W, Andrade FL, Ross D, de Leval M, Somerville J. Aorto-left ventricular communication after closure. Late postoperative problems. *Br Heart J* 1983; **49**:501–506.
74. Ribeiro P, Bun-Tan LB, Oakley CM. Management of aortic left ventricular tunnel. *Br Heart J* 1985; **54**:333–336.
75. Somerville J, English T, Ross DN. Aorto-left ventricular tunnel. Clinical features and surgical management. *Br Heart J* 1974; **36**:321–328.
76. Chessa M, Chaudhari M, De Giovanni JV. Aorto-left ventricular tunnel: transcatheter closure using an amplatzer duct occluder device. *Am J Cardiol* 2000; **86**:253–254.
77. Edwards JE, Burchell HB. The pathological anatomy of deficiencies between the aortic root and the heart, including aortic sinus aneurysms. *Thorax* 1957; **12**:125–139.
78. Edwards JE. *An Atlas of Acquired Disease of the Heart and Great Vessels.* WB Saunders, Philadelphia, PA, 1961.
79. Levy MJ, Lillehei CW, Anderson RC, Amplatz K, Edwards JE. Aortico-left ventricular tunnel. *Circulation* 1963; **27**:841–853.
80. Bjork VO, Hongo T, Aberg B, Bjork B. Surgical repair of aortico-left ventricular tunnel in a 7-day-old child. *Scan J Thorac Cardiovasc Surg* 1983; **17**:185–189.
81. Horvath P, Balaji S, Skovranek S, Hucin B, de Leval MR, Stark J. Surgical treatment of aortico-left ventricular tunnel. *Eur J Cardiothorac Surg* 1991; **5**:113–117.
82. Meldrum-Hanna W, Schroff R, Ross DN. Aortico-left ventricular tunnel: Late follow-up. *Ann Thorac Surg* 1986; **42**:304–306.

12

Coarctation of the aorta

INTRODUCTION

Coarctation of the aorta is a deceptively simple anomaly. While on the surface coarctation might appear to be nothing more than a stenosis of the descending thoracic aorta just beyond the left subclavian artery, the reality is that it is often the tip of the iceberg of a constellation of anatomical and physiological problems related to underdevelopment of the left heart. There are few anomalies that continue to generate more controversy regarding optimal management: whether to balloon dilate the native coarct; which surgical technique to employ, whether resection, subclavian flap or patch plasty; and how and when to deal with associated hypoplasia of the aortic arch. The optimal age at surgery, when to reintervene for recurrent coarctation and the role of balloons and stents for recurrent coarctation are additional controversies.

EMBRYOLOGY

Coarctation of the aorta is associated with a bicuspid aortic valve in at least 50% of patients.[1] Not uncommonly there is also hypoplasia of the mitral valve, left ventricle and/or left ventricular outflow tract. One possible explanation, therefore, for the development of a coarctation is reduction of fetal blood flow through the aortic isthmus with consequent secondary narrowing and kinking at the point of junction with ductal blood flow, which is presumably increased because of the left heart obstruction.[2]

As appealing as the reduced fetal blood flow theory is, there is more evidence supporting an important role for ductal tissue in causing the most common form of juxtaductal coarctation.[3,4] Histologic studies of the aorta at the level of the coarctation have demonstrated infiltration of smooth muscle into the aorta resulting in a noose around the aorta which is often completely circumferential. Contraction of this smooth muscle in the early postnatal period results in constriction of the aorta opposite the ductus. In a sense this represents the opposite of patent ductus arteriosus where there is inadequate smooth muscle constriction leading to persistent patency of the ductus. Interestingly coarctation almost never occurs in the setting of a large intracardiac right to left shunt when there is ductal flow from the aorta to the pulmonary artery as is seen with right heart obstructive anomalies such as tetralogy of Fallot. Perhaps ductal flow from the pulmonary artery to the aorta which is associated with left heart obstruction results in migration of smooth muscle into the proximal descending aorta and hence coarctation formation. A further observation is that the intimal 'coarctation shelf' is similar in appearance to the myxomatous-type tissue seen in the 'intimal cushions' of the ductus. In considering the embryology of coarctation it is important to review the development of the aortic arch and the descending aorta. The aortic arch has branches derived from the embryonic branchial (pharyngeal) arches which develop initially as symmetric structures but undergo a programmed sequence of regression to yield the mature pattern (see Chapter 29). It is suspected that apoptosis is important in achieving this regression and resorption. Interestingly, certain components of the aortic arch such as the distal arch but not the dorsal aorta are populated by cells from the cardiac neural crest.[5] Hypoplasia, interruption or coarctation of the distal arch between the left common carotid and left subclavian artery results from abnormal development of the segment which should have been derived from the left fourth pharyngeal arch. When hypoplasia or coarctation affects the isthmic segment beyond the left subclavian artery, the left embryonic dorsal aorta is involved. Interestingly, interruption of the aorta proximal to the left subclavian artery is frequently associated with microdeletion of chromosome

22 while coarctation beyond the left subclavian artery and type A interruption of the aorta are rarely associated with chromosome 22 microdeletion.[6]

ANATOMY

Simple coarctation

The traditional description of coarctation classifies simple coarctation as either preductal (infantile type) or postductal (adult type). This classification is of little practical value. The majority of coarctations are *juxtaductal* suggesting an important etiological role of ductal smooth muscle extending into the wall of the aorta. In the neonate with *critical coarctation* smooth muscle contraction results in both ductal closure as well as aortic obstruction immediately proximal to the ductus. If the child is able to survive, either because the aortic obstruction is not extremely severe or because of rapid formation of compensatory collaterals, there is a secondary phase of fibrosis that occurs over the first two to three months of life. With further growth of the child and fibrosis of the ligamentum arteriosum a thick fibrous shelf forms within the lumen of the aorta. Frequently the external appearance of the aorta suggests only a mild degree of stenosis while internally the thick intimal shelf opposite the ligamentum arteriosum results in a severe degree of obstruction.

Associated anomalies

BICUSPID AORTIC VALVE

Simple coarctation of the aorta is thought to be associated with a bicuspid aortic valve in approximately 50% of patients.[1] A similar high incidence of bicuspid aortic valve is noted in patients with type B interrupted aortic arch. Type B interrupted aortic arch is very frequently associated with posterior malalignment of the conal septum with resultant subaortic stenosis. In a study of 183 patients with interrupted aortic arch and VSD by the Congenital Heart Surgeons Society[7] the *z* score of the subaortic dimension determined by the long axis view on two-dimensional echocardiography ranged from −4.5 to −9.8. Subaortic stenosis was considerably less common in patients with coarctation of the aorta. In a separate study by the Congenital Heart Surgeons Society[8] the subaortic *z* scores ranged from −2.4 to −8.3 in 326 patients with coarctation. The embryological and genetic relationship between coarctation, bicuspid aortic valve and subaortic stenosis is not understood presently.[6]

AORTIC ARCH HYPOPLASIA

Aortic arch hypoplasia remains poorly defined. Definitions have included qualitative assessment of hypoplasia, functionally important stenosis determined by pressure gradient and echocardiography derived indices. One useful rule of thumb is

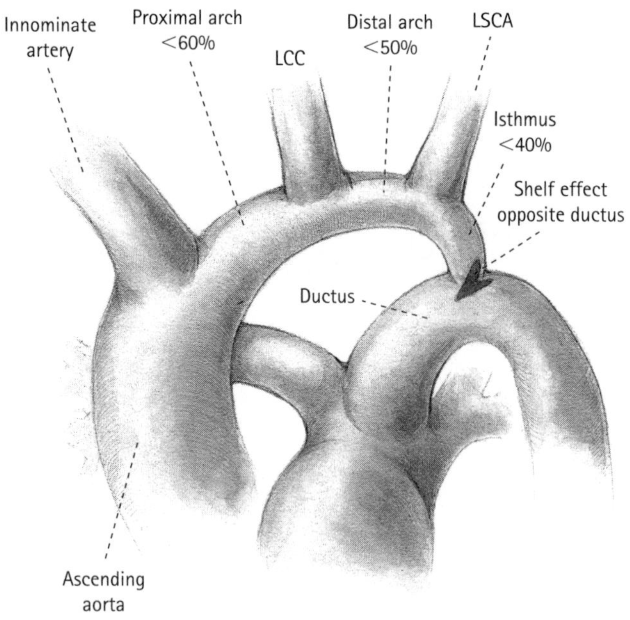

Figure 12.1 *A useful rule of thumb to define aortic arch hypoplasia is that the proximal arch between the innominate artery and left common carotid artery is less than 60% of the diameter of the ascending aorta, the distal aortic arch between the left common carotid (LCC) and left subclavian artery (LSCA) is less than 50% of the diameter of the ascending aorta or the aortic isthmus beyond the left subclavian artery is less than 40% of the diameter of the ascending aorta.*

that the proximal arch should be greater than 60% of the diameter of the ascending aorta, the distal arch greater than 50% and the isthmus greater than 40% (Figure 12.1). Probably most useful is a *z* score for arch diameter of less than −2 calculated by relating the specific segment of the aortic arch in question to normal values. It is important to define the specific segment of the arch under study. The proximal aortic arch between the innominate artery and left common carotid artery is rarely sufficiently hypoplastic in the setting of simple coarctation to warrant surgical intervention. On the other hand, associated hypoplasia of the isthmic segment between the left subclavian artery and the ligamentum arteriosum is very common. In a study by Kaine et al,[9] 37% of patients undergoing balloon angioplasty for native coarctation had a pre-angioplasty aortic isthmus *z* value of less than −2 by echocardiographic assessment. The distal aortic arch between the left common carotid and left subclavian artery appear to have an incidence of hypoplasia intermediate between the proximal arch and the isthmus. In a study by Morrow et al[10] of 14 neonates with isolated coarctation and 14 normal control neonates the mean diameter of the distal aortic arch was 3.5 mm in patients with coarctation versus 5.5 mm for control patients.

BOVINE TRUNK

A not uncommon form of arch hypoplasia is seen in association with a 'bovine trunk' where the innominate artery and left common carotid artery arise as a single trunk from the ascending aorta. The distal arch emerges as a direct leftward

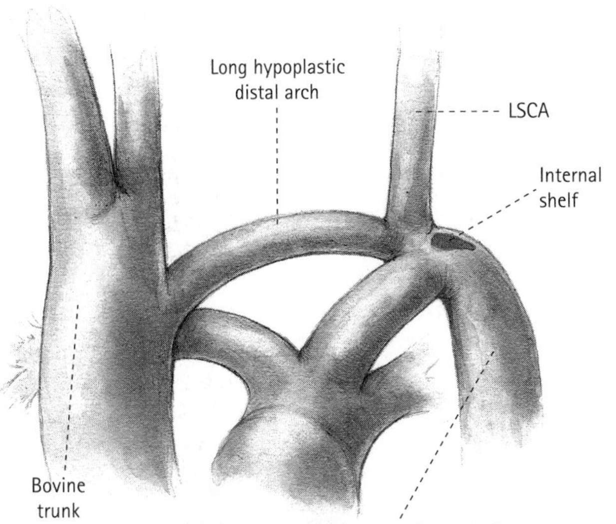

Figure 12.2 *Aortic arch hypoplasia may take the form of a bovine trunk where the innominate artery and left common carotid artery arise as a single trunk from the ascending aorta. The distal arch emerges as a direct leftward branch and may be quite long as well as hypoplastic. In addition there is an internal coarctation shelf opposite the ductus arteriosus. LSCA = left subclavian artery.*

lateral branch and may be quite long as well as hypoplastic (Figure 12.2). If the distal arch is particularly long it may be necessary to modify the choice of surgical technique for dealing with the arch hypoplasia.

VENTRICULAR SEPTAL DEFECT

A review of the literature of coarctation suggests that coarctation with an associated VSD is equally common as simple coarctation. Surgical series which are truly inclusive generally have a distribution of 30% patients with simple coarctation, 30% with an associated VSD and 40% with complex coarctation. A review of 326 patients with coarctation by the Congenital Heart Surgeons Society found that 48% of patients had an associated VSD. Thirty percent of patients had a moderate or large VSD.[8] A total of 64% of isolated VSDs were conoventricular. As noted in Chapter 14, conoventricular VSDs represent a defect between the conal and ventricular septum. The defect is almost always large, approximating the size of the aortic annulus. In addition, there is frequently some degree of malalignment of the conal septum relative to the ventricular septum. Posterior malalignment of the conal septum relative to the ventricular septum is common in VSDs associated with coarctation though not as common as with VSDs associated with interrupted aortic arch. There is often associated hypoplasia of the aortic annulus. Generally in the neonatal period and early infancy there is minimal fibrosis of the left ventricular outflow tract which is rarely tunnel-like at this age. A subaortic membrane is usually an acquired feature. Although perimembranous and posterior malalignment VSDs are most commonly associated with coarctation, VSDs of virtually any location have been reported in association with coarctation as well as multiple VSDs.

ASD, PATENT DUCTUS ARTERIOSUS

A patent ductus arteriosus is rarely associated with a coarctation beyond the neonatal period. As described above under embryology it is closure of the ductus that frequently precipitates presentation of the neonate with critical coarctation. The ductus must be reopened with prostaglandin E1 in order to resuscitate the neonate. A stretched foramen ovale or secundum ASD is quite often associated with a severe coarctation, possibly related to hypoplasia and poor compliance of the left heart. This results in an elevated left atrial pressure which can result in 'stretching' of the foramen ovale and a left to right shunt.

Complex associated heart disease

TAUSSIG-BING DOUBLE OUTLET RIGHT VENTRICLE AND TRANSPOSITION WITH VSD

Patients with Taussig-Bing type double outlet right ventricle have a subpulmonary VSD and transposition physiology. In anomalies of this type as well as true transposition with subpulmonary VSD, the aorta sits atop a long muscular conus. Not uncommonly there is anterior malalignment of the conal septum relative to the ventricular septum, i.e. there is an anterior malalignment VSD. There is often associated hypoplasia of the aortic arch as well as a juxtaductal coarctation.

MALALIGNED COMPLETE ATRIOVENTRICULAR CANAL

When the common atrioventricular valve of complete atrioventricular canal overrides the right ventricle more than the left ventricle, there is often underdevelopment of the left ventricle. In the most severe cases there is also subaortic stenosis and there may be hypoplasia of the aortic arch and coarctation.

SINGLE VENTRICLE WITH SYSTEMIC OUTFLOW OBSTRUCTION

There are many forms of single ventricle with systemic outflow obstruction other than hypoplastic left heart syndrome, for example tricuspid atresia with transposed great arteries, mitral atresia with normally related great arteries and restrictive VSD, and double inlet single left ventricle with restrictive subaortic conus. Hypoplasia of the aortic arch and coarctation are useful markers that intraventricular obstruction to outflow into the aorta is either present or probable in the future.

HYPOPLASTIC LEFT HEART SYNDROME

Coarctation of the aorta is present in at least 80% of patients with hypoplastic left heart syndrome.[11,12] In addition, there is frequently severe underdevelopment of the aortic arch and on occasion interruption of the aorta is associated.

PATHOPHYSIOLOGY AND CLINICAL PRESENTATION

Critical neonatal coarctation

A critical neonatal coarctation is a severe juxtaductal constriction of the aorta which results in profound circulatory collapse in the first month of life. During fetal life flow to the arch vessels is maintained by the left ventricle while circulation to the descending aorta is maintained by the right ventricle through the ductus arteriosus. This latter lower body perfusion is dependent on high pulmonary resistance and continuing patency of the ductus arteriosus. Following birth, however, if a severe coarctation is present, closure of the ductus will restrict blood flow to the lower body. This will result in diminished palpability and ultimate absence of the femoral pulses. The child will appear pale, listless and poorly perfused. There is likely to be tachypnea secondary to increased pulmonary blood flow and perhaps pulmonary edema. Chest X-ray reveals congested lung fields and an enlarged heart. With presentation early in the neonatal period the ECG is likely to show continuing persistence of dominant right heart forces. Arterial blood gas analysis reveals a progressive metabolic acidosis with some attempt at respiratory compensation. Arterial PO_2 is usually normal in spite of the pulmonary edema. If the acidosis is not corrected the child will develop signs of secondary organ damage including renal failure, hepatic failure, necrotizing enterocolitis, seizures and ultimately death.

Infant coarctation

If closure of the ductus has occurred slowly and/or if arterial collateral development has been profuse the infant may present with signs of heart failure which can be managed with appropriate medical therapy. The most common symptoms are tachypnea and failure to thrive. The parents are likely to describe irritability, sweating and difficulty with feedings. There is no cyanosis but these infants can be profoundly ill with obvious wasting and cachexia. Depending on the rapidity of collateral development and aggressiveness of medical therapy it may be possible to manage the child without surgical intervention.

Older child and adult

It is not uncommon for a mild or moderate coarctation to remain undiagnosed beyond infancy. The child or adult may present with a history of exercise intolerance, occasionally with a specific description of fatigue of the lower extremities. When collateral development is excellent it is not at all uncommon for even quite severe coarctation to be completely asymptomatic. Careful physical examination, however, will reveal elevation of blood pressure in the upper extremities beyond two standard deviations above mean for the child's age. In addition there will be a diminished pulse pressure and delay of the femoral pulses. Measurement of blood pressure in the arms and legs will usually reveal an important blood pressure gradient though this alone is not sufficient to determine the severity of the coarctation because of variable collateral development. Chest X-ray in the older child and adult frequently reveals a radiographic image of the coarctation itself in the form of the classic 'reverse three' sign. Enlarged intercostal vessels which bypass the coarctation segment cause erosion of the ribs. This results in the other classical radiological sign of coarctation, namely 'rib notching'.

DIAGNOSTIC STUDIES

A fundamental problem in assessing the severity of coarctation is the variable development of an arterial collateral circulation. Enlargement of the internal mammary arteries and peri-scapular arteries can produce almost normal pulsation in the femoral arteries despite the presence of a very severe coarctation. Thus, assessment of coarctation severity by either blood pressure cuff measurement or even direct measurement by catheter is inadequate per se to determine whether surgery is indicated. It is essential to image the coarctation area to determine the anatomical degree of narrowing. When there is greater than 50% diameter loss, surgery is indicated even though there may be only a mild blood pressure gradient of perhaps less than 20 mm.

Methods of imaging

ECHOCARDIOGRAPHY

Two-dimensional echocardiography provides excellent images during the neonatal period and infancy. The thymus is usually large and invests the aortic arch resulting in high quality images of the arch and juxtaductal area. Beyond infancy as the thymus involutes and as the proximal descending aorta becomes invested more by the lung than thymus, it becomes increasingly difficult to assess the degree of severity of coarctation. Doppler echocardiography provides additional useful information in that it should confirm absence of a normal upstroke during systolic flow. Blunting of the pressure wave in the descending aorta is characteristic of an important coarctation.

ANGIOGRAPHY

Although cardiac catheterization with a pressure pullback and aortography are the traditional gold standards for assessment of a coarctation, it should rarely be necessary to assess a coarctation by this invasive technique today. There is no advantage in collecting directly measured hemodynamic information because of the inability to assess the hemodynamic impact of collaterals.

MAGNETIC RESONANCE IMAGING

The aortic arch and proximal descending aorta are assessed very well by MRI. In fact this has been one of the first important anomalies in which MRI has produced better images in the older child and adult than any other noninvasive technique. MRI also provides excellent images for assessment of collateral development.

MEDICAL AND INTERVENTIONAL THERAPY

Critical neonatal coarctation

The medical management for critical neonatal aortic coarctation follows similar lines to those applied for hypoplastic left heart syndrome and interrupted aortic arch. It is essential to achieve secure intravenous access and delivery of prostaglandin E1. It is important to optimize the ratio of pulmonary to systemic resistance. This is usually achieved by reducing FiO_2 to 21% and maintaining PCO_2 above 45 mm. Generally intubation of the child is advisable because of possible apneic episodes precipitated by prostaglandin E1. Intubation and controlled ventilation also facilitate achieving the desired level of hypercarbia. It is often useful to optimize cardiac output with dopamine at 5 μg/kg per minute. Medical therapy should be maintained until the child has achieved normal acid base status and a normal creatinine. Enteral feeding should be avoided and a careful watch should be kept for signs of necrotizing enterocolitis such as abdominal distention or heme-positive stools.

Congestive heart failure beyond the neonatal period

Congestive heart failure beyond the neonatal period can be managed medically with standard anticongestive therapy including digoxin and diuretics.

Balloon angioplasty

There is ongoing controversy regarding the advisability of balloon angioplasty for native coarctation. However, balloon angioplasty remains the standard of care for *recurrent* coarctation following previous surgical repair.

BALLOON ANGIOPLASTY FOR NATIVE COARCTATION

It is generally accepted that the risk of recurrence is extremely high after balloon angioplasty in the setting of neonatal coarctation. Even when there is an associated medical problem such as intraventricular hemorrhage it is doubtful that balloon angioplasty is indicated. It is probably preferable to palliate the child medically including an ongoing prostaglandin infusion rather than subjecting the neonate to the risks of the invasive procedure of balloon angioplasty.

In the infant or older child there are a number of reports[13,14] that suggest that the risk of coarctation recurrence after balloon angioplasty is acceptable and perhaps equivalent to the risk of recurrence following surgery. The technique is not completely free of the risk of paraplegia.[15] Furthermore there is concern that abnormal ductal tissue is not removed with this technique.[16] In fact the technique is dependent on tearing of the media and intima. In the setting of abnormal ductal tissue this may result in a high incidence of late aneurysm formation. Certainly aneurysm formation has been described already in at least 5% of patients with relatively short long-term follow-up.[14,17,18] One of the serious consequences of aneurysm formation is that subsequent surgical intervention carries a higher risk of paraplegia because there has been no ongoing stimulus for collateral formation though this risk appears to be very small.[19] Furthermore it has generally proved necessary to replace the aneurysm segment with a prosthetic graft. Perhaps in the future it will be possible to predict patients who are at risk of aneurysm formation.

INDICATIONS FOR AND TIMING OF SURGERY

Symptoms and signs indicating need for surgery

Many children with coarctation are asymptomatic and the decision regarding whether to undertake surgery and optimal timing may be controversial. However, the presence of symptoms which are unresponsive to medical therapy is an absolute indication for surgery for coarctation. As described above under clinical presentation the neonate with a critical coarctation will present with the signs of shock while beyond the neonatal period there may be the usual signs and symptoms of congestive heart failure.

Indications for surgery in the asymptomatic child

HYPERTENSION

Profuse collateral development may result in a child being free of symptoms and having a relatively mild blood pressure gradient between arms and legs (less than 20–30 mm). However, if upper body blood pressure is greater than two standard deviations above normal and if imaging studies confirm a diameter loss of 50% or greater at the level of the coarctation, then surgery is indicated.

BLOOD PRESSURE GRADIENT

The gradient across the coarctation whether measured by blood pressure cuff between the arms and legs, by Doppler echocardiography or by direct pullback of a catheter is unreliable as a method for determining whether surgery is indicated. Certainly a gradient of greater than 20–30 mm in the setting of a coarctation that can be imaged to have a diameter loss of 50% or greater should be considered an absolute indication for surgery. However, a lower gradient may be present in spite of important evidence of stenosis by imaging because of the presence of profuse collateral development.

Imaging studies

If there is greater than 50% stenosis at the level of the coarctation surgery is indicated. Beyond infancy if echocardiography is unable to provide a clear assessment of the diameter loss, it may be necessary to perform MRI.

DESCENDING AORTIC FLOW

Doppler echocardiographic assessment of flow in the ascending aorta may provide additional information when imaging studies are equivocal in their assessment as to the degree of anatomical severity of a coarctation. However, this information alone should be used rarely to decide appropriateness of surgery.

Timing of surgery in the asymptomatic patient

Early in the history of coarctation surgery there was concern that it was likely in the young child that there would be inadequate growth of a circumferential aortic anastomosis.[20] However, experience in the 1980s and 1990s with the arterial switch procedure has demonstrated that in the absence of ductal tissue and excessive tension, an aortic anastomosis will almost always grow normally. Because there is continuing fibrosis and maturation of a coarctation in the first one to two months of life it is probably not advisable to undertake elective coarctation surgery in the asymptomatic infant during this period. However, there appears to be no important advantage in deferring surgery beyond the first two to three months of life. Deferring surgery beyond 5–10 years of age almost certainly increases the risk of essential hypertension appearing relatively early in adult life despite successful coarctation repair with no residual gradient.[21,22]

SURGICAL MANAGEMENT

History of surgery for coarctation

Following his success in achieving the first successful closure of a patent ductus arteriosus in 1938, Robert E Gross took up the challenge of pioneering the surgical correction of coarctation of the aorta. Gross was particularly concerned that there might be patients in whom end to end anastomosis would not be feasible. Accordingly he investigated the use of tubes of aortic homograft tissue as interposition grafts. He studied different methods for sterilization such as irradiation and antibiotic treatment, different methods of homograft storage such as CO_2 freezing, simple freezing, freeze drying and storage at 4°C. Gross published the results of these studies in a landmark article in the *New England Journal of Medicine* in 1945.[23] While correcting the proofs of that paper he appended a statement that he had performed his first clinical correction of coarctation. However, the first successful repair of coarctation had already been performed by Craaford in Sweden several months earlier.[24] Craaford had visited Gross' laboratory and had observed his work with homografts. In 1962, Schuster and Gross[20] reported the results of their first 500 repairs of coarctation by resection and end to end anastomosis or by interposition graft. In that paper they described concern regarding the growth of the circumferential anastomosis. They recommended that the optimal age for surgery should be about 10 years of age since by this time the child's aorta would have achieved 50% of adult size. In 1961, von Reuden[11] proposed an isthmus plasty procedure as well as synthetic patch aortoplasty with the goal being to avoid a circumferential anastomosis. Concern regarding growth of a circumferential anastomosis also led Waldhausen in 1966[25] to propose the ingenious left subclavian patch aortoplasty procedure. This procedure eliminated a circumferential anastomosis but failed to eliminate the abnormal ductal tissue.[16]

In 1987 Elliott et al[26] proposed management of the hypoplastic arch associated with coarctation by extended end to end anastomosis and radically extended end to end anastomosis. Other innovative techniques that have been described include the subclavian flap procedure with maintenance of left subclavian artery continuity by Meier et al[27] and De Mendonca et al[28] as well as the reverse subclavian flap procedure.[29]

Technical considerations

RESECTION AND END TO END ANASTOMOSIS

Resection and end to end anastomosis is currently the preferred technique for management of coarctation at Children's Hospital Boston. An arterial monitoring catheter should be placed in the *right* radial artery. A urinary catheter is usually inserted. With the patient in the right lateral decubitus position approach is via a left third or fourth but not fifth interspace thoracotomy incision which is predominantly posterior. The left lung is retracted anteriorly. The mediastinal pleural is reflected from the area of coarctation and stay sutures are placed in the anterior edge of the pleura to retract this anteriorly. Care is taken to identify the vagus nerve and the left recurrent laryngeal nerve (Figure 12.3a). Initially mobilization is carried out of the proximal vessels starting with the left subclavian artery. It is important to identify the large lymphatic vessel which frequently passes over the proximal left subclavian artery. Injury to this lymphatic which is passing to the thoracic duct can result in a postoperative chylothorax. The lymphatic vessels should be either ligated or cauterized. Great care should be taken in mobilizing behind the proximal left subclavian artery or the adjacent distal aortic arch to avoid injury to Abbott's artery which frequently arises from this area. The distal aortic arch is mobilized up to the level of

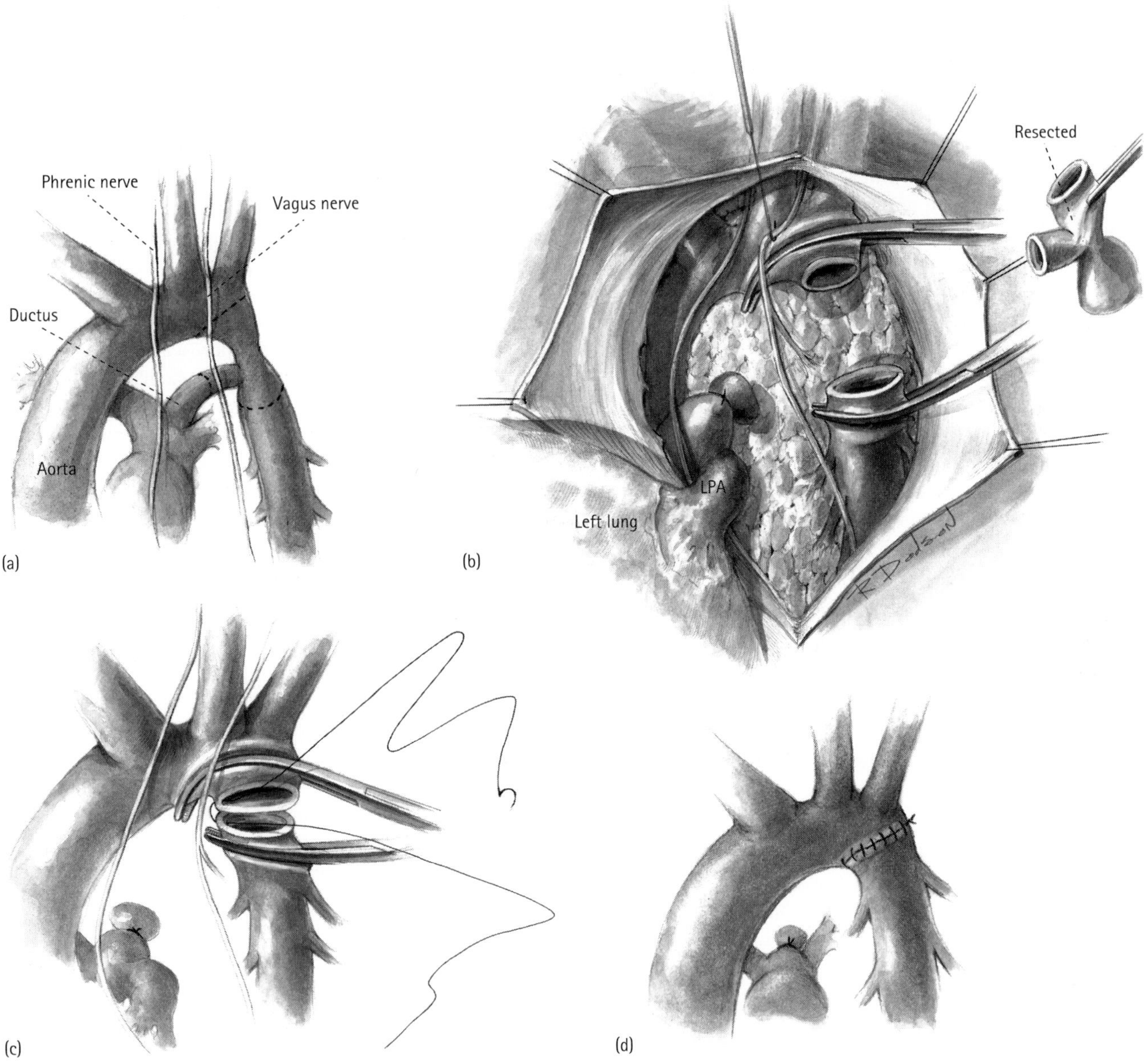

Figure 12.3 *(a) The vagus and phrenic nerves lie in close proximity to the area of coarctation surgery and must be carefully preserved. The lines of coarctation resection are indicated. (b) The ductus arteriosus has been ligated. The area of coarctation has been resected. (c) Following resection an end to end anastomosis is constructed using a continuous suture technique. The posterior wall is sutured first working inside the lumen (inverting suture line) followed by an everting external suture line across the anterior wall. (d) The completed end to end anastomosis following resection of coarctation.*

the left common carotid artery. When proximal control has been achieved such that it would be possible to place a controlling clamp if injury occurred at the time of dissection of the descending aorta and its attendant collateral vessels, the next area for dissection is the lateral side of the descending aorta and its collateral vessels (enlarged intercostals). The ligamentum arteriosum is dissected free with careful visualization and preservation of the left recurrent laryngeal nerve. The final area for dissection is the medial proximal descending thoracic aorta. This area is left until last since injury to a collateral vessel here can result in difficult bleeding. If necessary one can now place clamps, transect the aorta and pursue the retracted bleeding collateral vessel. Collateral vessels must be dissected with the utmost respect since in the older child or adult in particular they can be very thin-walled and fragile.

Mobilization of the descending aorta and proximal vessels is continued until it is clear that approximation of the vessels will be possible without undue tension following resection of the coarctation. The ligamentum arteriosum is ligated medially. Clamps are applied after communication with the anesthesia staff that they should anticipate a rise in blood pressure. Often for proximal control it is useful to apply a C-clamp which will include both the distal aortic arch as well as the left subclavian artery. A straight or angled Debakey clamp is often appropriate for the descending thoracic aorta. Heparin is usually not given and is thought to be unnecessary because the vessels of young children are free of atherosclerotic disease. Thus, this is not analogous to vascular surgery in an atherosclerotic adult population. However, some centers choose to infuse 1 mg/kg of heparin prior to clamp application.

The coarctation area is excised (Figure 12.3b). It is not necessary to excise the isthmic segment which should be filleted open along its lesser curve. The resultant aortotomy almost always is extended into the distal arch. Elliott has termed this an 'extended end to end anastomosis'. An end to end anastomosis is fashioned using either absorbable Maxon or PDS or a continuous prolene suture (Figure 12.3c). Great care is taken at the toe of the anastomosis to avoid purse-stringing. As described in Chapter 2, narrow bites are taken in the distal arch while wider bites are taken in the proximal descending thoracic aorta. Several bites should be run before the clamps are pulled together so as to minimize the tension on each suture before it is pulled up. Following removal of the distal clamp first to allow de-airing and subsequently the proximal clamp, the mediastinal pleura is approximated over the repair site. The anesthesia team should be warned before clamp release because there may be transient hypotension with lactic acid 'washout'. This can usually be managed with intravenous fluid replacement only. The pulse oximeter on a lower extremity should now easily detect pulsatile flow. Initially there may be a gradient by blood pressure cuff between arms and legs, perhaps because of lower extremity vasoconstriction in the setting of systemic hypothermia. Within 15–30 minutes, however there should be less than a 10 mm gradient unless there is arch hypoplasia. In the setting of a simple coarctation a residual arch gradient of up to 20 mm may be acceptable. Residual arch hypoplasia should be more aggressively addressed if an intracardiac left to right shunt is present, e.g. with an associated VSD for which spontaneous closure is anticipated. In the infant and small child a single chest tube is adequate. The incision is closed with interrupted pericostal absorbable suture with careful closure of the muscle layers with absorbable continuous suture technique and subcutaneous and subcuticular absorbable suture completing wound closure.

RADICALLY EXTENDED END TO END ANASTOMOSIS

One technique for dealing with the hypoplastic aortic arch is radically extended end to end anastomosis as proposed by Elliott (Figure 12.4). The approach is as for simple anastomosis or extended end to end anastomosis. However, dissection is carried along the proximal aortic arch and up to the distal ascending aorta. The proximal innominate artery is also defined. A particularly important step in this procedure is to ensure that there is a method for monitoring perfusion of the innominate artery during the period that clamps will be applied. Ideally a right radial arterial line is placed though care should be taken to ensure that there is not an aberrant right subclavian artery. In addition, it is useful to have a pulse oximeter on the right hand and right ear. A C-clamp is applied which partially occludes the distal ascending aorta and proximal innominate artery (Figure 12.4b). The aortotomy is extended across the entire surface of the aortic arch into the distal ascending aorta. By wide mobilization of the head vessels as well as the descending aorta it is possible to bring the toe of the descending aorta up to the ascending aorta in the same way that a direct anastomosis to the ascending aorta is fashioned for type B interrupted aortic arch. Great care must be taken with the toe of the anastomosis to ensure that this area is not stenosed since there will be at least moderate tension on the anastomosis (Figure 12.4c,d). In addition it is important to ensure that retraction on the proximal C-clamp does not importantly interfere with perfusion of the innominate artery. Cerebral perfusion during the clamp period is dependent on flow through the circle of Willis from the right vertebral artery and the right common carotid artery. Both the left common carotid artery and left subclavian arteries must be occluded during the clamp period.

LEFT SUBCLAVIAN PATCH AORTOPLASTY

Approach is as for resection and end to end anastomosis (Figure 12.5). The left subclavian artery is mobilized to the level of the first rib. In theory the left vertebral artery should be ligated in order to prevent a subsequent left subclavian steal phenomenon. However, it is almost certainly important not to ligate multiple branches of the distal subclavian artery as this can increase the risk of left limb ischemia. Cases of arm gangrene and amputation have been described. The left subclavian artery is ligated distally. Clamps are applied across the distal aortic arch and proximal descending aorta following ligation of the ductus or ligamentum. The left subclavian artery is divided proximal to its ligature. It is opened longitudinally with the incision being carried along the isthmus of the aorta and several millimeters beyond the coarctation shelf (Figure 12.5a). The subclavian artery is turned down as a flap. The toe of the flap is sutured into the most distal extent of the descending aortotomy (Figure 12.5b). Although some authors have recommended excision of the coarctation shelf, there is concern that this increases the risk of subsequent aneurysm formation.

REVERSE LEFT SUBCLAVIAN PATCH AORTOPLASTY (Figure 12.6a)

This is a very useful technique for dealing with hypoplasia of the distal aortic arch. It is usually performed in conjunction with resection and end to end anastomosis. In the neonate with a patent ductus arteriosus receiving a prostaglandin infusion it is possible to perform the subclavian flap component of the combined procedure without interrupting flow to the descending aorta. Approach is as for resection and end to end anastomosis. The left subclavian artery is mobilized as described for the antegrade subclavian flap procedure. In addition the

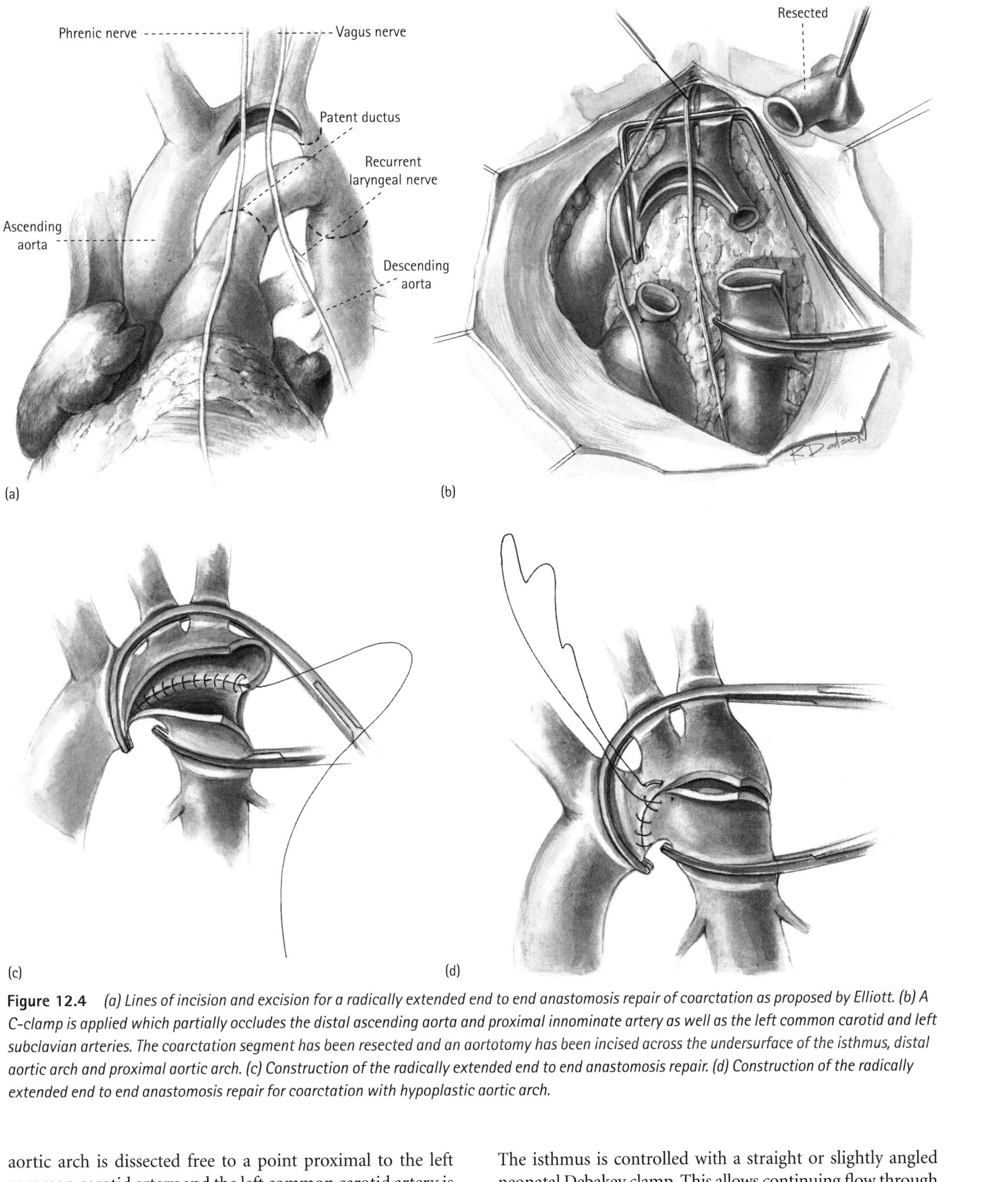

Figure 12.4 *(a) Lines of incision and excision for a radically extended end to end anastomosis repair of coarctation as proposed by Elliott. (b) A C-clamp is applied which partially occludes the distal ascending aorta and proximal innominate artery as well as the left common carotid and left subclavian arteries. The coarctation segment has been resected and an aortotomy has been incised across the undersurface of the isthmus, distal aortic arch and proximal aortic arch. (c) Construction of the radically extended end to end anastomosis repair. (d) Construction of the radically extended end to end anastomosis repair for coarctation with hypoplastic aortic arch.*

aortic arch is dissected free to a point proximal to the left common carotid artery and the left common carotid artery is also dissected free over at least 5–6 mm. Proximal control is obtained with a C-clamp which incorporates the proximal aortic arch as well as the distal left common carotid artery. The isthmus is controlled with a straight or slightly angled neonatal Debakey clamp. This allows continuing flow through the ductus to perfuse the lower body in the neonate with a patent ductus (Figure 12.6b). Following ligation of the distal subclavian artery, it is transected. The subclavian artery is

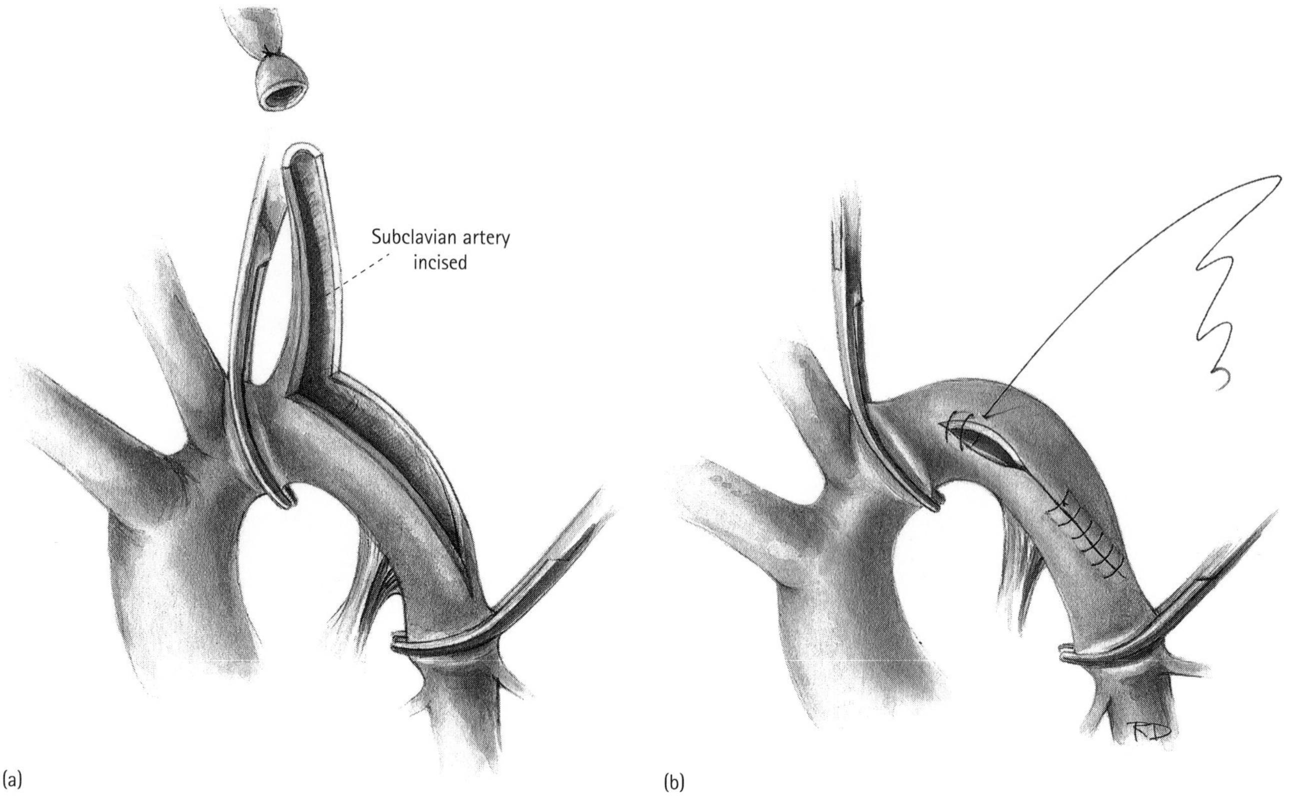

(a)

(b)

Figure 12.5 *(a) The left subclavian patch aortoplasty is performed by first ligating the left subclavian artery distally. The aorta is controlled between clamps and the left subclavian artery is transected. A longitudinal incision is extended along the full length of the left subclavian artery and across the area of coarctation opposite the ductus. (b) The left subclavian patch is turned down and is sutured into the aortotomy using a running suture technique.*

opened longitudinally along its rightward aspect with the incision extended across the superior surface of the distal aortic arch and then distally along the left common carotid artery opposite to the left subclavian incision. The flap is turned back retrograde towards the left common carotid artery with the toe being sutured into the common carotid incision. The body of the left subclavian patch is sutured across the incision in the distal aortic arch thereby supplementing the circumference of the distal arch. Generally continuous 6/0 prolene or an absorbable 6/0 suture such as Maxon or PDS is employed. Following release of the clamps and having secured hemostasis, attention can now be directed to the coarctation area itself. A resection and end to end anastomosis is performed as described above with the proximal incision being carried to a point under the retrograde left subclavian flap (Figure 12.6c). This procedure has the advantage that less tension on the anastomosis results because it is not necessary to pull the toe of the descending aorta as far proximally on the aortic arch. In addition suturing is achieved with better exposure and there is little risk that there will be compromise of flow in the innominate artery. The cross clamp time during which descending aortic flow is interrupted should be considerably shorter than that required for a radically extended end to end anastomosis because half the procedure is performed with perfusion to the lower body continuing through the ductus.

MODIFICATIONS OF LEFT SUBCLAVIAN PATCH AORTOPLASTY

The technique described by Meier[27] avoids a circumferential aortic anastomosis but provides ongoing continuity of the left subclavian artery (Figure 12.7). Approach is once again as for resection and end to end anastomosis. The left subclavian artery is widely mobilized but ligation of the vessel itself and the vertebral artery are not required. The distal subclavian artery is controlled with a small bulldog clamp or with a fine tourniquet during the cross clamp period. The left subclavian artery is divided at its origin from the aorta. It is filleted open on its rightward face. The aortotomy is extended from the point of left subclavian origin across the coarctation and beyond for several millimeters (Figure 12.7b). The mobilized left subclavian artery is now advanced and is sutured into the aortotomy as a flap (Figure 12.7c). Although this procedure has the advantage of maintaining flow to the left arm it suffers from the same disadvantage as the standard subclavian flap procedure in that it does not include excision of the abnormal ductal tissue resulting in a risk of late aneurysm formation at this site.

SYNTHETIC PATCH AORTOPLASTY (Figure 12.8)

Although this approach was popular in the 1970s and was particularly championed by Ebert and Mavroudis,[30] it is now

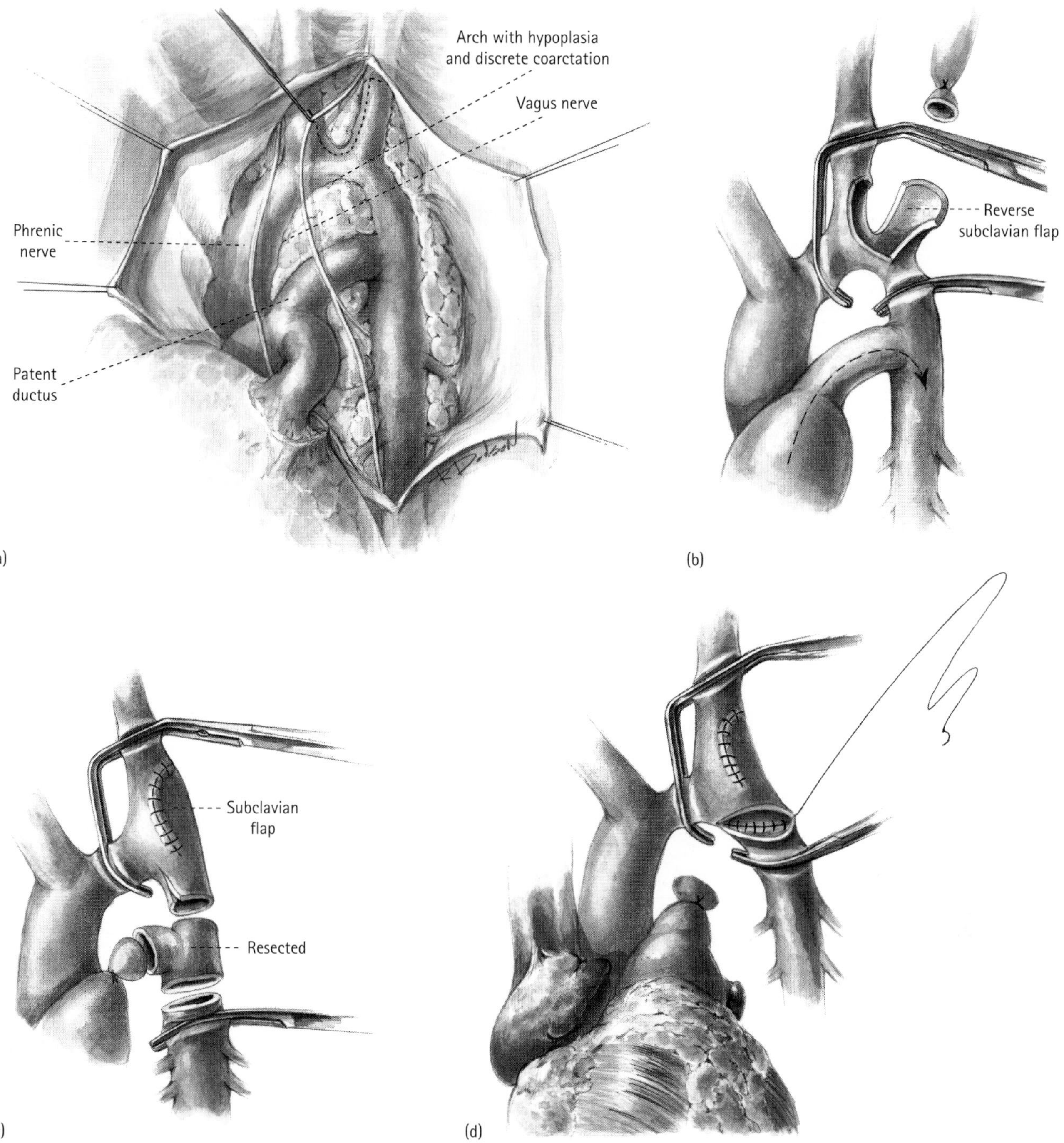

Figure 12.6 *(a) The reverse subclavian patch aortoplasty is a useful technique for dealing with distal aortic arch hypoplasia associated with coarctation. The dashed line indicates the incision along the right side of the subclavian artery, the superior surface of the distal aortic arch and the left side of the origin of the left common carotid artery. (b) The left common carotid artery and proximal aortic arch are controlled with a C-clamp while the isthmic segment is controlled with a straight or slightly angled neonatal Debakey clamp. This allows continuing perfusion of the lower body through the patent ductus (dashed arrow). The left subclavian artery is turned back in a reverse direction as a flap to complement the hypoplastic distal arch. (c) The reverse subclavian flap has been completed. Following a period of reperfusion, clamps are applied as indicated and the area of coarctation is resected. (d) An end to end anastomosis which extends under the arch segment supplemented by the reverse subclavian flap is performed.*

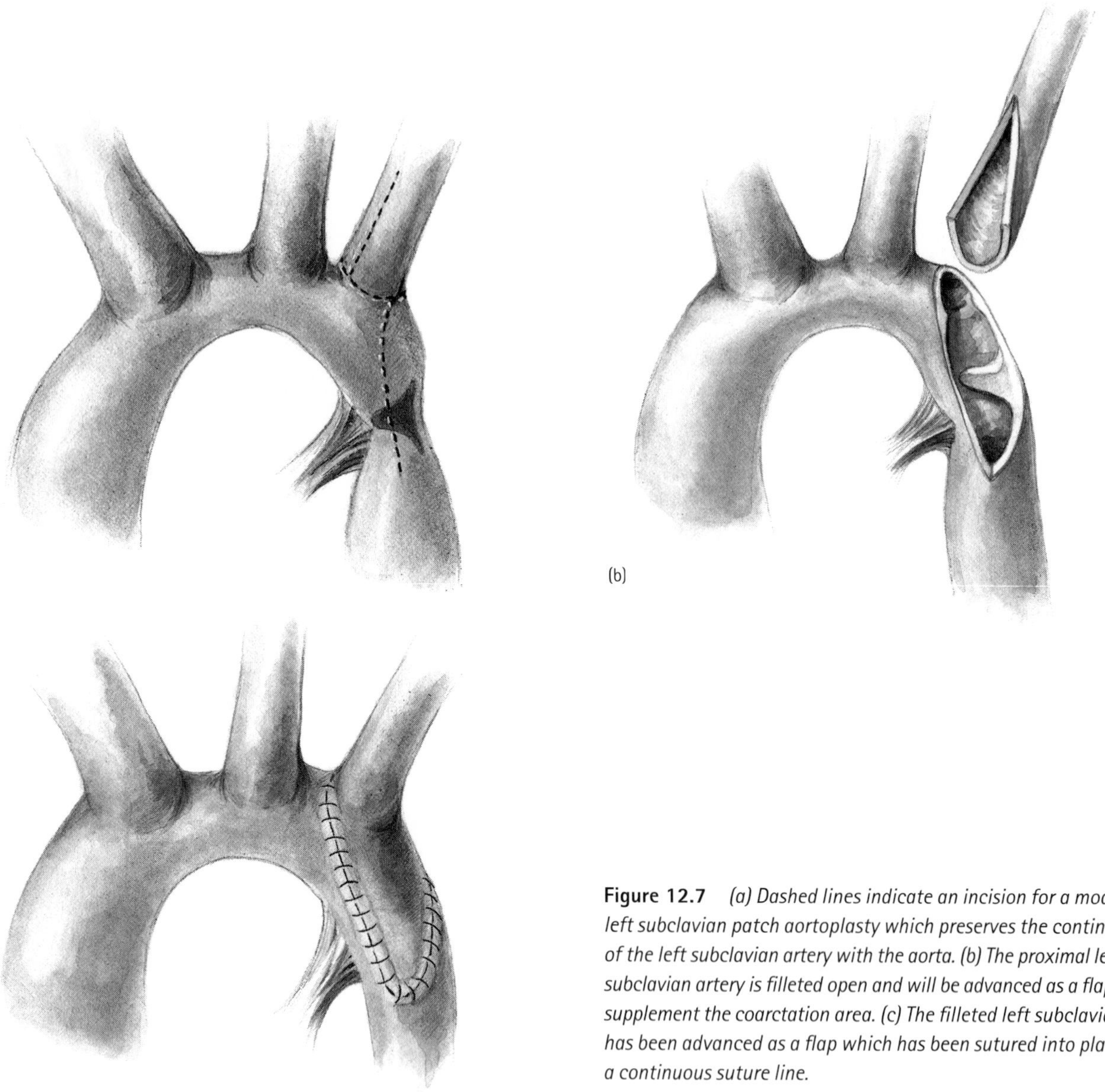

(a) (b) (c)

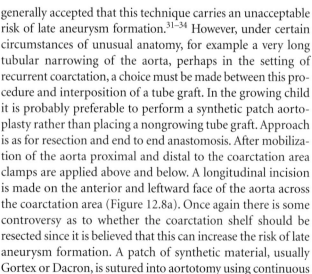

Figure 12.7 *(a) Dashed lines indicate an incision for a modified left subclavian patch aortoplasty which preserves the continuity of the left subclavian artery with the aorta. (b) The proximal left subclavian artery is filleted open and will be advanced as a flap to supplement the coarctation area. (c) The filleted left subclavian artery has been advanced as a flap which has been sutured into place using a continuous suture line.*

generally accepted that this technique carries an unacceptable risk of late aneurysm formation.[31–34] However, under certain circumstances of unusual anatomy, for example a very long tubular narrowing of the aorta, perhaps in the setting of recurrent coarctation, a choice must be made between this procedure and interposition of a tube graft. In the growing child it is probably preferable to perform a synthetic patch aortoplasty rather than placing a nongrowing tube graft. Approach is as for resection and end to end anastomosis. After mobilization of the aorta proximal and distal to the coarctation area clamps are applied above and below. A longitudinal incision is made on the anterior and leftward face of the aorta across the coarctation area (Figure 12.8a). Once again there is some controversy as to whether the coarctation shelf should be resected since it is believed that this can increase the risk of late aneurysm formation. A patch of synthetic material, usually Gortex or Dacron, is sutured into aortotomy using continuous nonabsorbable suture (Figure 12.8b). If a Gortex patch is employed it is generally wise to use Gortex suture since bleeding through needle holes at aortic pressure can be persistent.

ONE STAGE REPAIR OF VSD AND COARCTATION

There is considerable controversy regarding the optimal approach to repair of a coarctation associated with a VSD which is judged unlikely to close spontaneously. For example, a large conoventricular VSD, often with some degree of posterior malalignment and close to the size of the aortic annulus or larger has a small probability of spontaneous closure. One approach is to use a left thoracotomy incision and to place a pulmonary artery band at the time of coarctation repair. The VSD is then closed at a later time through a median sternotomy after perhaps as short an interval period as two weeks. During this time the child's symptoms of congestive heart failure will

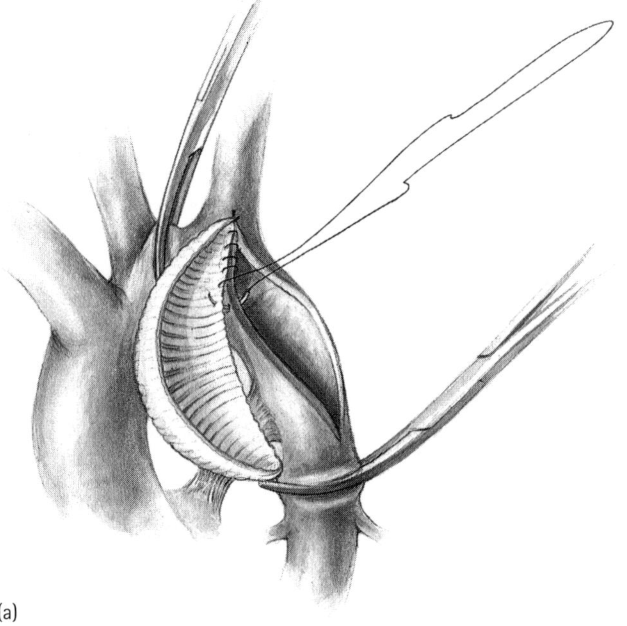

(a)

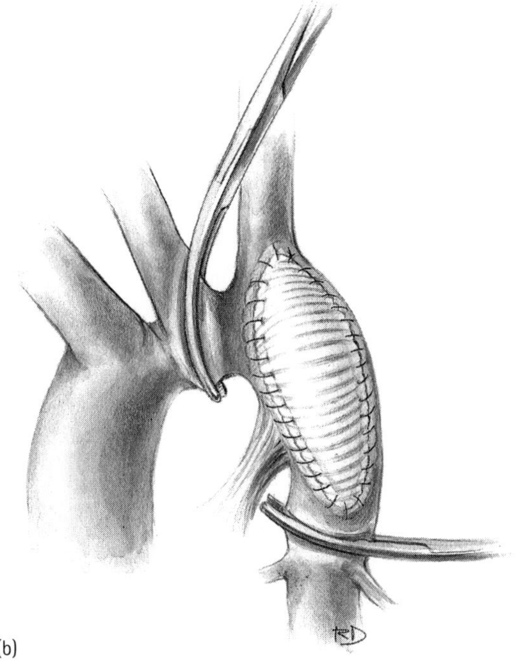

(b)

Figure 12.8 *(a) Synthetic patch aortoplasty. A longitudinal incision has been made in the aorta opposite the coarctation area. A patch of crimped Dacron has been sutured into the aortotomy using a continuous suture technique. (b) The completed synthetic patch aortoplasty.*

have improved. This approach also might reduce the probability of requiring a period of circulatory arrest. The disadvantage of this approach includes the need for an extended hospitalization, the risks of two operations rather than one, the expense of two operations rather than one, additional psychological stress for the family and the cosmetic disadvantage of two incisions rather than one. Therefore it is our preference to undertake a one stage approach.

MEDIAN STERNOTOMY FOR ONE STAGE REPAIR OF VSD AND COARCTATION

A routine median sternotomy incision is performed. Cannulation of the ascending aorta is modified in that a flexible thin walled narrow gauge (e.g. eight French Biomedicus cannula) is inserted into the right lateral side of the mid ascending aorta. Venous cannulation can be performed with either two caval cannulas or a single venous cannula depending on the child's size and the surgeon's preference as to the method of VSD closure. Immediately after commencing bypass the ductus arteriosus is suture ligated. During cooling to deep hypothermia, the arch vessels are thoroughly mobilized as well as the proximal descending aorta. Considerable care is taken to preserve the left recurrent laryngeal and vagus nerves as well as the phrenic nerves. When the rectal temperature is less than 18°C a fine neonatal vascular clamp is placed across the proximal aortic arch and a C-clamp is placed on the descending aorta. The left common carotid and left subclavian arteries are controlled with fine tourniquets. The coarctation area can be excised and an extended end to end anastomosis performed. Alternatively if there is extensive hypoplasia of the aortic arch either a radical extended end to end anastomosis can be fashioned or a patch plasty can be performed using glutaraldehyde treated autologous pericardium. These procedures will necessitate the use of a period of hypothermic circulatory arrest which should not exceed 15 minutes. The patient is then reperfused for a period of at least five minutes if another period of circulatory arrest is to be used for VSD closure. Generally VSD closure should not require use of more than 20 minutes of hypothermic circulatory arrest so that the cumulative arrest time can be kept to less than 35–40 minutes. The details of VSD closure are described in Chapter 14.

Complications of coarctation surgery and how to minimize them

EARLY COMPLICATIONS

Paraplegia

By far the most devastating complication reported with coarctation surgery is paraplegia. Brewer et al[35] undertook a survey of 12 000 cases of coarctation in 1972 and found a 0.5% incidence of paraplegia following coarctation surgery in that era. In the current era, however, the risk of paraplegia is almost certainly much less. This may be because the risk of paraplegia is less in younger patients perhaps because there is less likely to be major hemorrhage secondary to injury of the fragile collateral vessels which develop with age. In addition the smaller aorta of the smaller child necessitates a very much shorter suture line and therefore quicker cross-clamp time. Drawing on the adult experience with paraplegia with aneurysm surgery, it is very likely that an extended cross-clamp time, for example, more than 30 minutes, as well as hypotension, are important predisposing factors for the development of paraplegia. Brewer's landmark article reviews the blood supply of the spinal cord. It is important to remember that the anterior spinal artery is supplied by branches from the right and left vertebral artery which arise from the subclavian arteries. Thus presence of an aberrant right subclavian artery increases the risk of compromise of blood flow to the anterior spinal artery. Brewer's article emphasizes the possibility of discontinuity of the anterior spinal artery as a cause of spinal cord ischemia. If multiple intercostals vessels are occluded during the cross clamp and most particularly the artery of Adamkiewicz then the risk of paraplegia will be increased. Accordingly it is important to preserve flow through as many collateral vessels as possible and to avoid division of collateral vessels unless absolutely necessary.

One factor which is not discussed in Brewer's article is the use of hypothermia. It is a common practice in the pediatric operating room to aggressively maintain temperature with heating lamps and warming blankets. This almost certainly increases the risk of neuronal injury in the spinal cord. It is our practice to use a mild degree of systemic hypothermia to 34°C or 35°C by use of a cooling blanket during the cross-clamp period. Direct cooling of the spinal cord with iced saline lavage in the thoracic cavity introduces a risk of ventricular fibrillation and should be avoided. Some reports[36] have described direct cooling of the spinal cord through placement of an epidural catheter but this is probably not necessary in the setting of a pediatric coarctation repair where the cross-clamp period rarely should exceed 15–20 minutes. The importance of careful temperature control continues in the postoperative period where it is equally important in at least the first 24 hours to avoid hyperthermia. If the cross-clamp period has been long, e.g. greater than 30 minutes, a mild degree of ongoing hypothermia, for example 34.5–35°C for the first 18–24 hours is almost certainly protective against paraplegia.

As described by Brewer, hypotension increases the risk of paraplegia. Generally the cause of hypotension is hemorrhage but it is important also to avoid iatrogenic hypotension. Application of the clamps will result in upper body hypertension but the anesthesia team should not respond to this with aggressive antihypertensive therapy. A moderate to severe degree of hypertension should be tolerated through the cross-clamp period to encourage collateral perfusion of the lower body. Generally techniques that are applied for aneurysm surgery to maintain lower body perfusion such as left atrial to femoral bypass or femoro-femoral bypass are not necessary and introduce unnecessary risks. However, it is important for the individual surgeon to be able to estimate an approximate cross-clamp duration and if this seems likely to exceed 20–30 minutes because of complicating factors, then serious consideration should be given to measurement of distal aortic pressure following application of clamps. If this pressure is less than a mean pressure of approximately 50 mm in the older child or 40 mm in the younger child, consideration should be given to supporting lower body perfusion by one of the techniques mentioned.

Hemorrhage

The most common cause of important hemorrhage is the tearing of sutures related to excessive tension on individual sutures. For this reason a running suture technique, particularly across the posterior wall is preferred. By placing multiple suture loops the tension on each individual suture is reduced before the anastomosis is pulled together. The tension should be supported during the anastomosis by the assistant holding the clamps (with careful compression of the clamps' ratchets). Attempting to tie individual sutures placed posteriorly undoubtedly increases the risk of suture tears, subsequent hemorrhage and subsequent need for multiple hemostatic sutures thereby negating any possible advantage of interrupted sutures in allowing a wider anastomosis.

Chylothorax

There is very frequently an important lymphatic vessel crossing the left subclavian artery, usually quite close to its origin. It is important to identify this vessel and to ligate it with a fine ligature or cauterize it. Careful closure of the mediastinal pleura probably also decreases the risk of persistent chylothorax postoperatively.

Left recurrent laryngeal nerve palsy

The left recurrent laryngeal nerve should be visualized during mobilization of the ligamentum arteriosum. In addition great care should be taken when mobilizing the medial pleural flap to avoid injury to the vagus nerve. Excessive tension on the pleural flap by retraction sutures also should be avoided to minimize the risk of a postoperative recurrent laryngeal nerve palsy. Fortunately surgery is rarely required today for recurrent coarctation because of the success of balloon angioplasty. In the setting of recurrent coarctation with dense scarring in the region of the recurrent laryngeal nerve, particular care must be taken in dissecting this area.

Paradoxical hypertension

It is extremely common for the patient to have at least a moderate increase in blood pressure in the first days to weeks postoperatively. In the early phase over the first 24–48 hours this is probably related to elevated catecholamine levels secondary to the stress of surgery in the setting of a patient with hyper-reactive systemic vasculature. During this phase management with an agent such as labetalol,[37] which blocks both α- and β-receptors, is useful. Alternatively a continuous infusion of a short acting beta-blocker agent such as esmolol is useful.[38] The latter phase of the elevated blood pressure that is seen following coarctation surgery is most likely secondary to increased angiotensin levels.[39,40] Elevated renin/angiotensin levels are usually observed in patients with coarctation presumably secondary to the diminished and less pulsatile blood pressure that the kidneys are exposed to. Over the first few days to weeks postoperatively this hormonal hypertension will usually resolve in the younger child (teenager or less), though in the older teenager or adult it may be persistent. The most appropriate therapy is an ACE inhibitor such as enalapril.

LATE COMPLICATIONS

Hypertension

Early onset of essential hypertension is common in patients who have not had their coarctation repaired until 5–10 years of age. It is important to exclude a recurrent coarctation as the cause of the elevated blood pressure. This problem should be prevented by early diagnosis and management in early childhood.[21]

Recurrent coarctation

The definition of recurrent coarctation remains controversial. Different reports[41] have applied varying levels of severity to define this problem. Some centers believe that even an exercise induced gradient of greater than 15–20 mm with no gradient at rest justifies the term. In general, however, a resting blood pressure gradient of 20–30 mm with a diagnosis by imaging modality of a diameter loss of 50% or greater is accepted as coarctation recurrence. Recurrence of coarctation can be minimized by excision of all ductal tissue, minimization of tension on the anastomosis by wide mobilization of the arch and head vessels as well as the descending thoracic aorta and meticulous suture technique. The details of suture technique are covered in Chapter 2. In summary purse-stringing of the anastomosis should be minimized by avoiding wide spacing of continuous suture bites and careful focus on alignment of the descending aorta with the arch, even if this results in some degree of stenosis of the takeoff of the left subclavian artery.

The management of recurrent coarctation is by balloon angioplasty with or without stent placement.[42,43]

The long-term risks of stent placement in this setting are at present unknown.

Aneurysm formation

Many studies have now documented the risk of late aneurysm formation following synthetic patch aortoplasty.[31–34] Initially this appeared to be more likely when the procedure was performed in older children and teenagers although with longer follow-up it appears that even with repair earlier in life this complication can occur. Most likely the problem is secondary to residual ductal tissue as well as a mismatch in the compliance of the synthetic patch with the native aortic wall. However, aneurysms have also been reported in a number of patients following subclavian patch aortoplasty[44,45] so it would appear that the abnormal ductal tissue is the more important factor. Aneurysm formation is also an important complication following balloon angioplasty. It may be an immediate consequence of angioplasty and require relatively urgent surgery. Dilation of the aorta to beyond 150% of its normal diameter is the most common definition that is currently applied for an aneurysm at the coarctation site. Continuing growth of an aneurysm beyond this size is an indication for surgery. Surgical management should involve particular care to minimize the risk of paraplegia using the techniques described above. It should be anticipated that there will be poor collateral development and therefore measurement of distal aortic pressure following application of clamps should be undertaken. Support of the lower body perfusion may be necessary. Interposition of a synthetic tube graft is generally required.

RESULTS OF SURGERY

The literature describing the results of management of coarctation is extremely extensive, no doubt reflecting the many controversies that persist as outlined in the introduction to this chapter. More recently much of the literature has focused on the risks and benefits as well as the intermediate results of balloon angioplasty and stent placement. This is an evolving area and one that is beyond the scope of this book.

Neonatal coarctation

The most extensive report describing the outcome of surgical management of coarctation in neonates is the multi-institutional report of the Congenital Heart Surgeons Society published in 1994.[8] Quaegebeur et al reviewed 326 severely symptomatic neonates who had either isolated coarctation or coarctation with an associated VSD. Some of these patients had associated underdevelopment of left heart structures, for example 5% had important mitral valve anomalies, 5% had underdevelopment of the left ventricle and 9% had left ventricular outflow tract obstruction. Overall the survival at 24 months was 84% (Figure12.9a). The most frequently used technique for repair was resection and end to end anastomosis. However, multi-variate analysis did not demonstrate any particular advantage for this technique versus the subclavian flap technique. However, repairs which included augmentation of the proximal aortic arch were associated with an increased risk of mortality (Figure 12.9b). Recurrent coarctation was seen most commonly following patch graft repair. The results of the Congenital Heart Surgeons Society study are similar to the results of the study undertaken by Ziemer et al from Children's Hospital Boston.[46] One hundred consecutive neonates who underwent repair between 1972 and 1984 were reviewed. This included patients with both simple coarctation (29%), patients with an associated VSD (32%) as well as patients with additional complex heart disease. In this early timeframe, predating the introduction of prostaglandin, early mortality was relatively high with actuarial survival at four years being 86% for patients with simple coarctation and 80% for patients with an associated VSD. This study did not

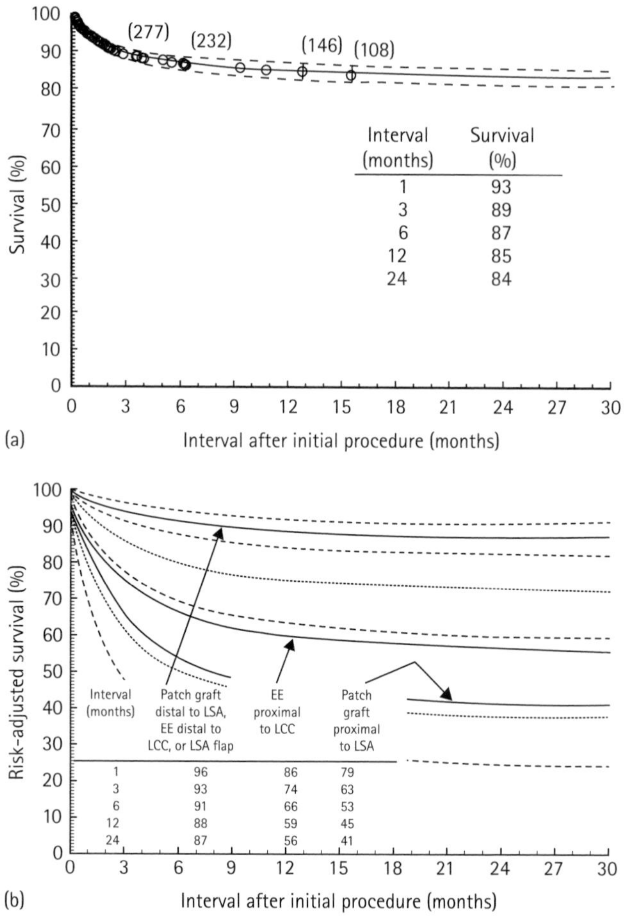

Figure 12.9 *(a) Survival after the initial intervention (at time zero) in 322 neonates with coarctation with and without ventricular septal defect studied by the Congenital Heart Surgeons Society between 1990 and 1992. Survival at 24 months was 84%. (b) Survival after coarctation repair according to technique of repair. Repairs which included augmentation of the proximal aortic arch were associated with an increased risk of mortality. (Modified from Quaegebeur JM et al. Outcomes in seriously ill neonates with coarctation of the aorta. A multiinstitutional study.* J Thorac Cardiovasc Surg *1994; 108:845, 847, with permission from Elsevier.)*

demonstrate any advantage with respect to recurrence rate for the subclavian flap technique relative to resection and end to end anastomosis. In fact, freedom from reintervention for recoarctation after five years was 92.9% for patients who underwent end to end anastomosis and 75.2% for those who underwent a subclavian flap aortoplasty. Following this study the technique of resection and end to end anastomosis was adopted as the standard technique for management of coarctation at all ages at Children's Hospital Boston. In another, more recent report from Children's Hospital Boston,[47] Bacha et al reviewed the results of surgery in 18 neonates who were all less than 2 kg at the time of coarctation repair. Surgery was undertaken between 1990 and 1999. Median weight was 1330 g. A VSD was present in five patients and Shones complex in four. Sixteen patients had resection and end to end anastomosis and two had resection combined with a subclavian flap. There was one early death and two late deaths. Eight patients had a residual or recurrent coarctation which was managed by balloon dilation in five patients. Shones complex and a hypoplastic aortic arch were independent risk factors for decreased survival ($p < 0.001$). The authors concluded that coarctation repair can be undertaken with a relatively low risk even in very low birth weight preterm infants but there should be a high expectation of recurrent coarctation.

Long-term follow-up after coarctation surgery

A landmark paper describing very long-term results following coarctation surgery was published by Clarkson et al from Green Lane Hospital in New Zealand in 1983.[21] The late survival was remarkably satisfactory. The probability of survival at 20 years of patients discharged from hospital after surgery between the ages of 1 and 19 years was only slightly less than that of the general population (95% versus 97%). However, patients who underwent surgery at an older age had a significantly less good late survival than the general population and those who were more than 40 years of age at the time of surgery had a markedly decreased late survival. One of the most important findings of the Clarkson study was that the age of operation influenced the risk of late hypertension. Patients who were more than 20 years of age at the time of surgery were more likely to have late hypertension than those operated on between 5 and 19 years of age ($p = 0.007$). In a more recent study of long-term follow-up after coarctation repair, Salazar et al[48] described the late results of surgery for 274 patients who underwent coarctation surgery at the University of Minnesota between 1948 and 1976. The authors found, like Clarkson, that systemic hypertension was predicted by older age at operation. Other predictors of late systemic hypertension were the blood pressure at the first postoperative visit as well as the occurrence of paradoxical hypertension following surgery. Another recent report, which suggests that early repair reduces the risk of late hypertension, was published in 1998 by Serafi et al[49] from New England Medical Center. The authors reviewed surgical outcomes of 176 consecutive patients who underwent repair of coarctation over a 25-year period. There was no mortality in the 113 patients with isolated coarctation. Persistent or late hypertension was identified in 18 of the 107 patients who were followed for more than five years. Late hypertension was rare in patients operated on during infancy (4.2%) versus 27.1% of patients operated on beyond one year of age. The authors conclude that elective repair of coarctation should be performed in the first year of life to minimize the risk of persistent hypertension.

ANEURYSM FORMATION AFTER COARCTATION SURGERY

Although considerable attention has been focused on the risk of aneurysm development following balloon dilation of coarctation, it is important to remember that aneurysms have also been reported following surgical repair. Von Kodolitsch et al[50] described 25 patients who required corrective surgery of aortic aneurysms following previous coarctation surgery. Eight of these aneurysms were located in the ascending aorta while 17 were at the site of the coarctation repair. The authors found that advanced age at coarctation repair and use of a patch plasty technique independently predicted local aneurysm formation. Ascending aortic aneurysm was associated with the presence of a bicuspid aortic valve, advanced age at coarctation repair and a high preoperative peak systolic pressure gradient.

The problem of aneurysm formation after coarctation surgery has been reviewed in detail by Serfontein and Kron in the 2002 Pediatric Cardiac Surgery Annual.[41]

Arch hypoplasia and coarctation

Arch hypoplasia associated with aortic coarctation remains an important problem particularly in young infants. In 1994 van Heurn et al[51] described the results of the extended end to end arch aortoplasty which was introduced by Elliott in 1987.[26] A total of 151 infants under three months of age underwent repair of coarctation at Great Ormond Street Hospital between 1985 and 1990. Hypoplasia of the isthmus was present in 25% and 33% had hypoplasia of the arch. A number of different techniques were applied for repair. Actuarial freedom from recoarctation at four years was 57% after subclavian flap angioplasty, 77% after standard end to end anastomosis, 83% after extended end to end anastomosis and 96% after radically extended end to end anastomosis. The alternative technique of reverse subclavian flap repair of hypoplastic aortic arch has been less widely used than extended end to end anastomosis. This is in spite of the fact that it has the important advantage of minimizing tension on the repair. Kanter et al[52] described 162 infants less than three months of age who underwent repair at Emory University after 1988. A total of 46 had a reverse subclavian flap aortoplasty at a median age of 11 days and mean weight of 3.2 kg. There were two hospital deaths, one in a patient who had subsequently undergone a Norwood procedure and the other from sepsis. At a mean follow-up of 38 months five patients had recurrent obstruction of which three were at the coarctation site rather than at the arch repair. The authors concluded that reverse subclavian flap aortoplasty is an excellent technique for relief of arch hypoplasia with a low recurrence rate and acceptable operative and intermediate term survival.

REFERENCES

1. Becker AE, Becker MJ, Edwards JE. Anomalies associated with coarctation of the aorta. Particular references to infancy. *Circulation* 1970; **41**:1067–1075.
2. Rudolph AM, Heymann MA, Spitznas U. Hemodynamic considerations in the development of narrowing of the aorta. *Am J Cardiol* 1972; **30**:514–525.
3. Elzenga NJ, Gittenberger-deGroot AC, Oppenheimer-Dekker A. Coarctation and other obstructive aortic arch anomalies. Their relationship to the ductus arteriosus. *Int J Cardiol* 1986; **13**:289–308.
4. van Son JA, Lacquet LK, Smedts F. Patterns of ductal tissue in coarctation of the aorta in early infancy. *J Thorac Cardiovasc Surg* 1993; **105**:368–369.
5. Kappetein AP, Gittenberger-deGroot AC, Zwinderman AH, Rohmer J, Poelmann RE, Huysmans HA. The neural crest as a possible pathogenetic factor in coarctation of the aorta and bicuspid aortic valve. *J Thorac Cardiovasc Surg* 1991; **102**:830–836.
6. McElhinney DB, Anderson RH. Developmental anomalies of the outflow tracts and aortic arch: towards an understanding of the role of deletions within the 22nd chromosome. *Cardiol Young* 1999; **9**:451–457.
7. Jonas RA, Quaegebeur JM, Kirklin JW, Blackstone EH, Daicoff GO. Outcomes in patients with interrupted aortic arch and ventricular septal defect. A multiinstitutional study. Congenital Heart Surgeons Society. *J Thorac Cardiovasc Surg* 1994; **107**:1099–1109.
8. Quaegebeur JM, Jonas RA, Weinberg AD, Blackstone EH, Kirklin JW. Outcomes in seriously ill neonates with coarctation of the aorta. A multiinstitutional study. *J Thorac Cardiovasc Surg* 1994; **108**:841–851.
9. Kaine SF, Smith EO, Mott AR, Mullins CE, Geva T. Quantitative echocardiographic analysis of the aortic arch predicts outcome of balloon angioplasty of native coarctation of the aorta. *Circulation* 1996; **94**:1056–1062.
10. Morrow WR, Huhta JC, Murphy DJ, McNamara DG. Quantitative morphology of the aortic arch in neonatal coarctation. *J Am Coll Cardiol* 1986; **8**:616–620.
11. von Rueden TJ, Knight L, Moller JH, Edwards JE. Coarctation of the aorta associated with aortic valvular atresia. *Circulation* 1975; **52**:951–954.
12. Elzenga NJ, Gittenberger de Groot AC. Coarctation and related aortic arch anomalies in hypoplastic left heart syndrome. *Int J Cardiol* 1985; **8**:379–389.
13. Hijazi ZM, Geggel RL, Marx GR, Rhodes J, Fulton DR. Balloon angioplasty for native coarctation of the aorta: acute and mid-term results. *J Invasive Cardiol* 1997; **9**:344–348.
14. Rao PS, Najjar HN, Mardini MK, Solymar L, Thapar MK. Balloon angioplasty for coarctation of the aorta: immediate and long-term results. *Am Heart J* 1988; **115**:657–665.
15. Ussia GP, Marasini M, Pongiglione G. Paraplegia following percutaneous balloon angioplasty of aortic coarctation: a case report. *Catheter Cardiovasc Interv* 2001; **54**:510–513.
16. Jonas RA. Coarctation: Do we need to resect ductal tissue? *Ann Thorac Surg* 1991; **52**:504–607.
17. Ovaert C, McCrindle BW, Nykanen D, MacDonald C, Freedom RM, Benson LN. Balloon angioplasty of native coarctation: clinical outcomes and predictors of success. *J Am Coll Cardiol* 2000; **35**:988–996.
18. Fawzy ME, Sivanandam V, Galal O et al. One- to ten-year follow-up results of balloon angioplasty of native coarctation of the aorta in adolescents and adults. *J Am Coll Cardiol* 1997; **30**:1542–1546.
19. Minich LL, Beekman RH 3rd, Rocchini AP, Heidelberger K, Bove EL. Surgical repair is safe and effective after unsuccessful balloon angioplasty of native coarctation of the aorta. *J Am Coll Cardiol* 1992; **19**:389–393.
20. Schuster SR, Gross RE. Surgery for coarctation of the aorta: A review of 500 cases. *J Thorac Cardiovasc Surg* 1962; **43**:54–70.

21. Clarkson PM, Nicholson MR, Barratt-Boyes BG, Neutze JM, Whitlock RM. Results after repair of coarctation of the aorta beyond infancy. *Am J Cardiol* 1983; **51**:1481–1488.
22. Brouwer RMHJ, Erasmus ME, Ebels T, Eijgelaar A. Influence of age on survival, late hypertension and recoarctation in elective aortic coarctation repair. *J Thorac Cardiovasc Surg* 1994; **108**:525-531.
23. Gross RE, Hufnagel CA. Coarctation of the aorta: Experimental studies regarding its surgical correction. *New Eng J Med* 1945; **233**:287–293.
24. Crafoord C, Nylin G. Congenital coarctation of the aorta and its surgical treatment. *J Thorac Surg* 1945; **14**:347–361.
25. Waldhausen JA, Nahrwold DL. Repair of coarctation of the aorta with a subclavian flap. *J Thorac Cardiovasc Surg* 1966; **51**:532–533.
26. Elliott MJ. Coarctation of the aorta with arch hypoplasia: improvements on a new technique. *Ann Thorac Surg* 1987; **44**:321–323.
27. Meier MA, Lucchese FA, Jazbik W, Nesralla IA, Mendonca JT. A new technique for repair of aortic coarctation. Subclavian flap aortoplasty with preservation of arterial blood flow to the left arm. *J Thorac Cardiovasc Surg* 1986; **92**:1005–1012.
28. de Mendonca JT, Carvalho MR, Costa RK, Franco Filho E. Coarctation of the aorta: a new surgical technique. *J Thorac Cardiovasc Surg* 1985; **90**:445–447.
29. Hart JC, Waldhausen JA. Reversed subclavian flap angioplasty for arch coarctation of the aorta. *Ann Thorac Surg* 1983; **36**:715–717.
30. Backer CL, Paape K, Zales VR, Weigel TJ, Mavroudis C. Coarctation of the aorta. Repair with polytetrafluoroethylene patch aortoplasty. *Circulation* 1995; **92**:II132–136.
31. Bergdahl L, Jungqvist A. Long-term results after repair of coarctation of the aorta by patch grafting. *J Thorac Cardiovasc Surg* 1980; **80**:177–181.
32. Bromberg BI, Beekman RH, Rocchini AP et al. Aortic aneurysm after patch aortoplasty repair of coarctation: A prospective analysis of prevalence, screening tests and risks. *J Am Coll Cardiol* 1989; **14**:734–741.
33. Hehrlein FW, Mulch J, Rautenburg HW, Schlepper M, Scheld HH. Incidence and pathogenesis of late aneurysms after patch graft aortoplasty for coarctation. *J Thorac Cardiovasc Surg* 1986; **92**:226–230.
34. Heikkinen L, Sariola H, Salo J, Ala-Kulju K. Morphological and histopathological aspects of aneurysms after patch aortoplasty for coarctation. *Ann Thorac Surg* 1990; **50**:946–948.
35. Brewer LA, Fosburg RG, Mulder GA, Verska JJ. Spinal cord complications following surgery for coarctation of the aorta. *J Thorac Cardiovasc Surg* 1972; **64**:368–378.
36. Cambria RP, Davison JK. Regional hypothermia with epidural cooling for spinal cord protection during thoracoabdominal aneurysm repair. *Semin Vasc Surg* 2000; **13**:315–324.
37. Bojar RM, Weiner B, Cleveland RJ. Intravenous labetalol for the control of hypertension following repair of coarctation of the aorta. *Clin Cardiol* 1988; **11**:639–641.
38. Gidding SS, Rocchini AP, Beekman R et al. Therapeutic effect of propranolol on paradoxical hypertension after repair of coarctation of the aorta. *New Engl J Med* 1985; **312**:1224–1228.
39. Parker FB, Farrell B, Streeten DH, Blackman MS, Sondheimer HM, Anderson GH. Hypertensive mechanisms in coarctation of the aorta: Further studies of the renin-angiotensin system. *J Thorac Cardiovasc Surg* 1980; **80**:568–573.
40. Parker FB, Streeten DH, Farrell B, Blackman MS, Sondheimer HM, Anderson GH. Preoperative and postoperative renin levels in coarctation of the aorta. *Circulation* 1982; **66**:513–514.
41. Serfontein SJ, Kron IL. Complications of coarctation repair. *Semin Thorac Cardiovasc Surg Pediatr Card Surg Annu* 2002; **5**:206–211.
42. Castaneda-Zuniga WR, Lock JE, Vlodaver Z et al. Transluminal dilatation of coarctation of the abdominal aorta. An experimental study in dogs. *Radiology* 1982; **143**:693–697.
43. Mann C, Goebel G, Eicken A et al. Balloon dilation for aortic recoarctation: morphology at the site of dilation and long-term efficacy. *Cardiol Young* 2001; **11**:30–35.
44. Kino K, Sano S, Sugawara E, Kohmoto T, Kamada M. Late aneurysm after subclavian flap aortoplasty for coarctation of the aorta. *Ann Thorac Surg* 1996; **61**:1262–1264.
45. Martin MM, Beekman RH, Rocchini AP, Crowley DC, Rosenthal A. Aortic aneurysms after subclavian angioplasty repair of coarctation of the aorta. *Am J Cardiol* 1988; **61**:951–953.
46. Ziemer G, Jonas RA, Mayer JE, Perry S, Castaneda AR. Surgery for coarctation of the aorta in the neonate. *Circulation* 1986; (suppl I): I25–31.
47. Bacha EA, Almodovar M, Wessel DL et al. Surgery for coarctation of the aorta in infants weighing less than 2 kg. *Ann Thorac Surg* 2001; **71**:1260–1264.
48. Toro-Salazar OH, Steinberger J, Thomas W, Rocchini AP, Carpenter B, Moller JH. Long-term follow-up of patients after coarctation of the aorta repair. *Am J Cardiol* 2002; **89**:541–547.
49. Seirafi PA, Warner KG, Geggel RL, Payne DD, Cleveland RJ. Repair of coarctation of the aorta during infancy minimizes the risk of late hypertension.*Ann Thorac Surg* 1998; **66**:1378–1382.
50. von Kodolitsch Y, Aydin MA, Koschyk DH et al. Predictors of aneurysmal formation after surgical correction of aortic coarctation. *J Am Coll Cardiol* 2002; **39**:617–624.
51. van Heurn LW, Wong CM, Spiegelhalter DJ et al. Surgical treatment of aortic coarctation in infants younger than three months: 1985 to 1990. Success of extended end-to-end arch aortoplasty. *J Thorac Cardiovasc* Surg 1994; **107**:74–85.
52. Kanter KR, Vincent RN, Fyfe DA. Reverse subclavian flap repair of hypoplastic transverse aorta in infancy. *Ann Thorac Surg* 2001; **71**:1530–1536.

13

Atrial septal defect

INTRODUCTION

An atrial septal defect is the simplest intracardiac anomaly. It was the first congenital cardiac anomaly to be repaired using cardiopulmonary bypass. More recently it has been the first intracardiac anomaly that has been successfully managed by a catheter delivered device. At present the roles of traditional surgical closure on cardiopulmonary bypass, closure using minimally invasive surgery, catheter delivered device closure and robotic surgery are in a state of flux and not yet fully defined.

EMBRYOLOGY

Like patent ductus arteriosus, a *secundum* atrial septal defect represents a failure in the transition from the fetal circulation to the postnatal circulation. Before birth oxygen rich blood from the inferior vena cava carrying blood from the placenta via the ductus venosus is directed into the left atrium by the foramen ovale. The foramen ovale consists of the fibromuscular crescent called the limbus of the fossa ovalis (Figure 13.1). The septum primum is a thin membranous flap of tissue which opens into the left atrium so long as the pressure in the right atrium is higher than the pressure in the left atrium. Following birth when there is increased blood return to the left atrium because the lungs have expanded, the septum primum should normally close against the left side of the limbus of the fossa ovalis. For several weeks to months it is possible to reopen the foramen ovale if the pressure in the right atrium is higher than the pressure in the left atrium. Thus a newborn infant with no congenital cardiac anomaly can temporarily appear quite blue when straining with a Valsalva movement thereby forcing systemic venous flow into the left atrium. In approximately 25% of individuals the foramen ovale remains 'probe patent' for life.[1] In these individuals there is the potential for paradoxical embolism of thrombotic material into the left atrium with subsequent risk of stroke. If the septum primum is either absent or heavily fenestrated a secundum atrial septal defect results. In contrast to a secundum ASD a *primum* ASD represents a failure of development of the component of the atrial septum adjacent to the atrioventricular valves which is formed by endocardial cushion tissue.[2] Primum atrial septal defects are covered in Chapter 21. Less common forms of atrial septal defect include the *sinus venosus* ASD and the *coronary sinus septal* defect. The sinus venosus septal defect represents a failure in the formation of the sinus venosus component of the atrial septum. This component of the atrial septum is adjacent to the orifices of the cavas and the pulmonary veins. Not surprisingly it is often associated with anomalous connection of the pulmonary veins, particularly the right upper lobe pulmonary vein. The right upper lobe may be drained by several small veins rather than the usual single vein. Frequently these anomalous veins will join the superior vena cava thereby creating a true form of partial anomalous pulmonary venous connection. Even when the right upper lobe vein enters normally, absence of the sinus venosus component of the atrial septum adjacent to the superior vena cava/right atrial junction results in what is effectively anomalous pulmonary venous connection of the right upper lobe to the right atrium. A *coronary sinus* septal defect represents a failure of formation of the common wall separating the left atrium from the coronary sinus as it passes in the left atrioventricular groove towards the coronary sinus ostium.

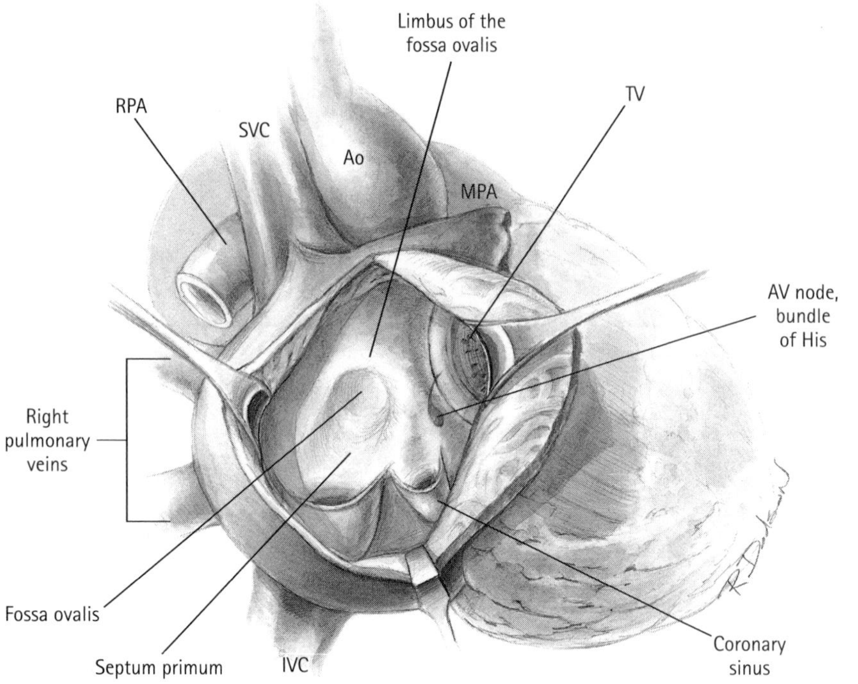

Figure 13.1 *Normally the foramen ovale closes during the transition from the prenatal to postnatal circulation by apposition of the thin septum primum against the limbus of the fossa ovalis. RPA = right pulmonary artery; SVC = superior vena cava; Ao = aorta; MPA = main pulmonary artery; TV = tricuspid valve; AV = atrioventricular; IVC = inferior vena cava.*

ANATOMY

Secundum ASD

A secundum ASD is always situated within the fossa ovalis. It may vary in size from a miniscule perforation of the septum primum to a small defect representing stretching of the septum primum ('stretched foramen ovale' – Figure 13.2a1) to complete absence of the septum primum (Figure 13.2b1). The limbus of the fossa ovalis are almost always present to some degree. When there is complete absence of the atrial septum including the limbus of the fossa ovalis, the anomaly is more correctly termed 'common atrium'. Generally this is seen as part of heterotaxy (see Chapter 20).

Primum atrial septal defect

The anatomy of the primum ASD with its associated maldevelopment of the atrioventricular valves is covered in Chapter 21.

Sinus venosus ASD

A sinus venosus ASD is most commonly situated immediately inferior to the junction of the superior vena cava and the right atrium (Figure 13.3a). It is relatively uniform in size being usually similar in diameter to that of the superior vena cava. Anomalous pulmonary venous drainage of the right upper lobe to the SVC is very common (Figure 13.4). Although the majority of sinus venosus ASDs are close to the SVC/right atrial junction there are occasional sinus venosus ASDs that are situated at the inferior vena caval/right atrial junction or directly posteriorly, i.e. midway between the SVC and IVC junctions with the right atrium. When a sinus venosus ASD is situated at the IVC/right atrial junction there is more likely to be anomalous drainage of the right lung to the inferior vena cava, e.g. 'scimitar' syndrome rather than anomalies of the right upper lobe pulmonary veins.

Coronary sinus septal defect

A hemodynamically important coronary sinus septal defect is almost always associated with enlargement of the coronary sinus ostium. The actual defect itself can vary in size from a few millimeters to complete absence of the wall of the coronary sinus within the left atrium. In this latter situation the coronary sinus ostium is itself the atrial septal defect (Figure 13.5a).

Associated anomalies

PARTIAL ANOMALOUS PULMONARY VENOUS CONNECTION

Partial anomalous pulmonary venous connection is most commonly associated with a sinus venosus ASD. It usually takes the form of one or several small veins from the right upper lobe draining directly to the superior vena cava (Figure 13.4). *Scimitar syndrome* (Figure 13.6) is a rare anomaly in which the right pulmonary veins join to form a single vertical trunk which descends in a curve (scimitar) to enter the inferior vena cava, generally close to the IVC/right atrial junction. If an ASD is present it is usually a low sinus venosus

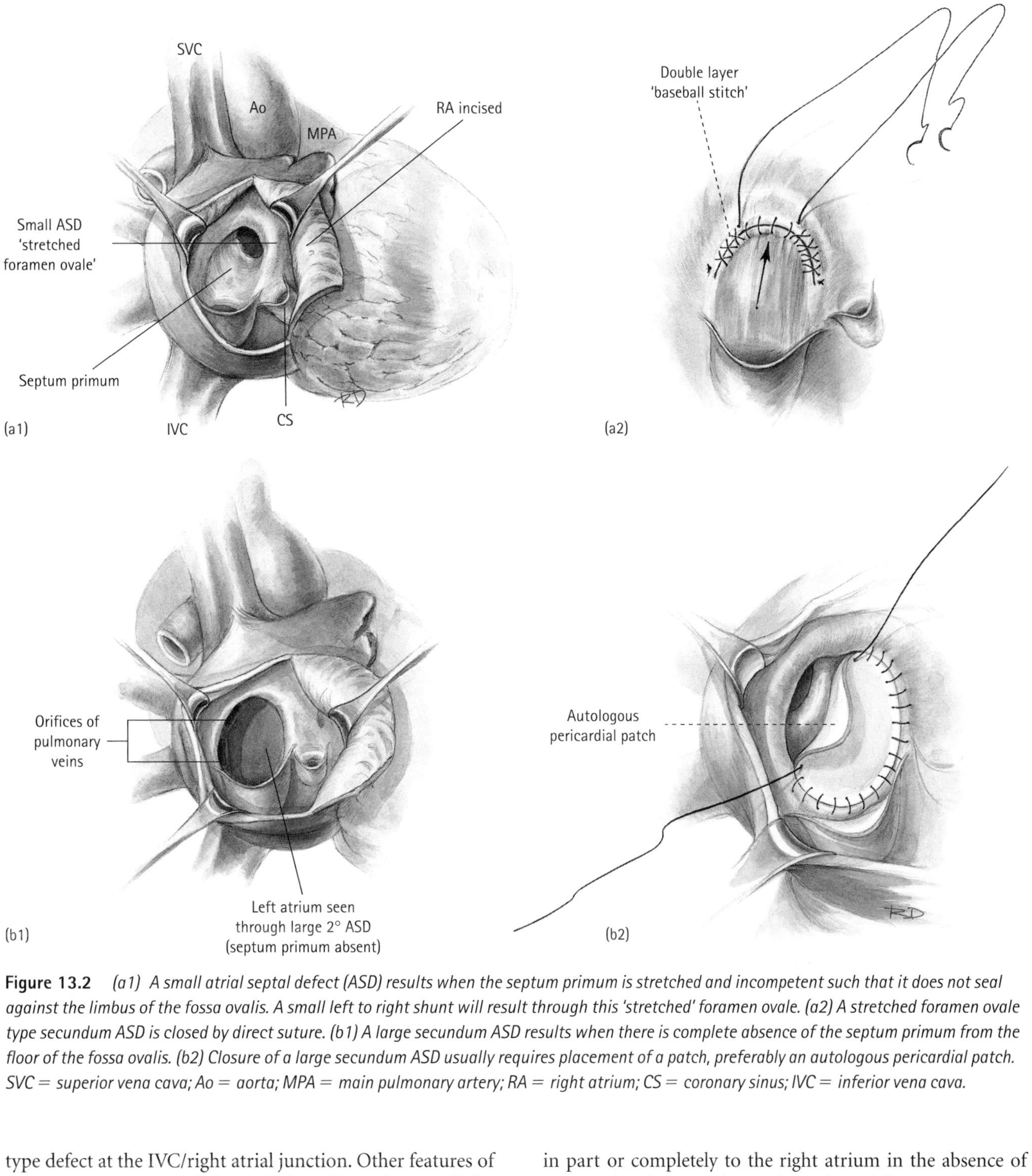

Figure 13.2 *(a1) A small atrial septal defect (ASD) results when the septum primum is stretched and incompetent such that it does not seal against the limbus of the fossa ovalis. A small left to right shunt will result through this 'stretched' foramen ovale. (a2) A stretched foramen ovale type secundum ASD is closed by direct suture. (b1) A large secundum ASD results when there is complete absence of the septum primum from the floor of the fossa ovalis. (b2) Closure of a large secundum ASD usually requires placement of a patch, preferably an autologous pericardial patch. SVC = superior vena cava; Ao = aorta; MPA = main pulmonary artery; RA = right atrium; CS = coronary sinus; IVC = inferior vena cava.*

type defect at the IVC/right atrial junction. Other features of scimitar syndrome include right lung hypoplasia and the presence of aortopulmonary collateral vessels supplying either the right lower lobe or the entire right lung rather than supply from the true pulmonary artery. Partial anomalous pulmonary venous connection can occur in the absence of an ASD. Most commonly the left upper pulmonary vein drains to an ascending vertical vein which is similar to a left sided superior vena cava and usually connects to the left innominate vein. Less commonly the right pulmonary veins drain in part or completely to the right atrium in the absence of an associated ASD. Obstruction of partial anomalous pulmonary veins is extremely rare. The hemodynamics therefore are similar to those of a left to right shunt at the atrial level.

LEFT SUPERIOR VENA CAVA TO LEFT ATRIUM

Persistence of a left sided superior vena cava can occur in association with almost any congenital cardiac anomaly including atrial septal defect. It is particularly commonly associated

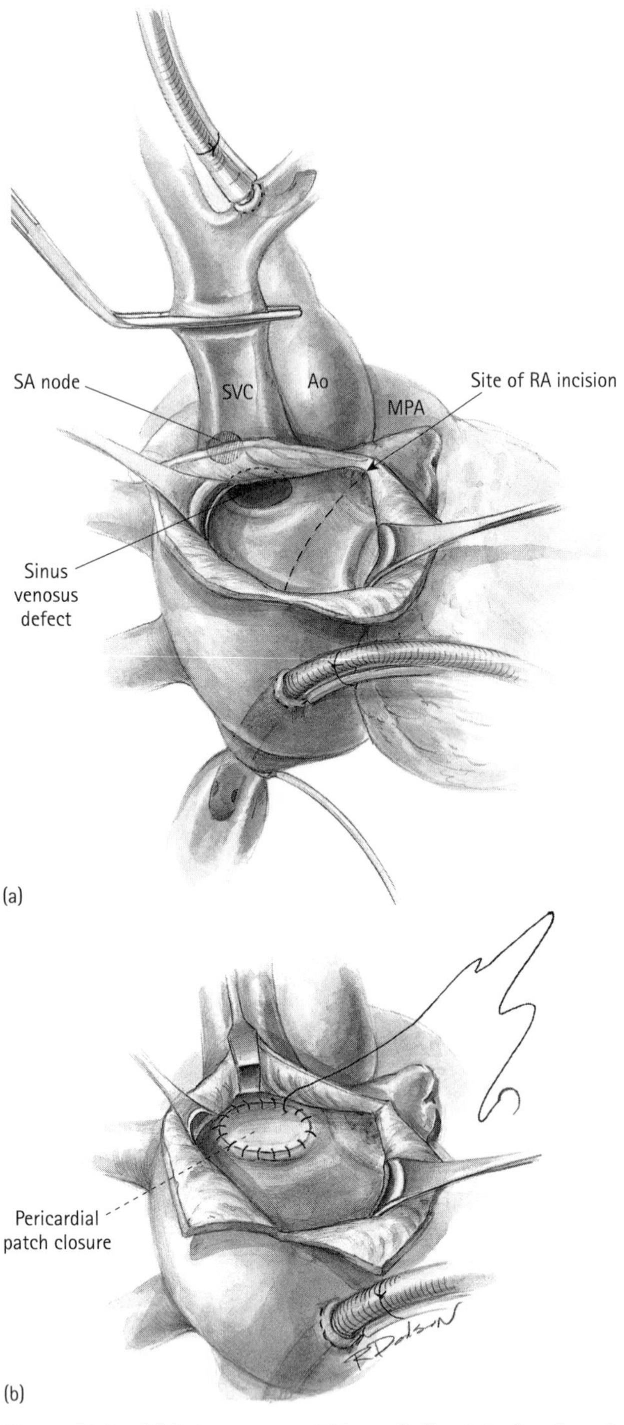

Figure 13.3 *(a) A sinus venosus ASD usually lies at the junction of the superior vena cava and right atrium. It is often similar in diameter to the diameter of the superior vena cava.*
(b) A sinus venosus ASD which is not associated with partial anomalous pulmonary venous connection into the superior vena cava is closed using an autologous pericardial patch. SA node = sinoatrial node.

with common atrium as part of heterotaxy. However, it may also occur in association with a coronary sinus septal defect or any of the other ASDs. The size of the left SVC relative to the right SVC is variable. There may be a communicating left innominate vein though this too can be of variable size or completely absent.

PATHOPHYSIOLOGY AND CLINICAL FEATURES

Normally left atrial pressure is higher than right atrial pressure reflecting the greater compliance of the right heart relative to the left heart. The greater compliance of the right heart results at least in part from the fact that pulmonary artery pressure is much less than systemic pressure and therefore the right ventricle is very much less hypertrophied than the left ventricle. When there is a defect in the atrial septum blood will flow from the left atrium to the right atrium, through the pulmonary circulation returning once again to the left atrium. The amount of blood which will pass left to right though the ASD depends on the size of the defect and the relative compliance of the right and left heart. As an individual ages the compliance of the left heart gradually deteriorates at least in part related to an increase in systemic blood pressure as individuals approach middle age. Thus the degree of left to right shunt, which is quantitated as the $Q_p : Q_s$, tends to increase with time. In some individuals, however, perhaps 5–10%, who are susceptible to the development of pulmonary vascular disease, there may be a decrease in left to right shunt with age and by late teenage years or the third decade of life there may be shunt reversal, i.e. the patient has developed Eisenmenger's syndrome.[3] This is much less common than occurs in the setting of a ventricular septal defect which will commonly raise not only the pulmonary blood flow but also the pulmonary artery pressure. An atrial septal defect without associated anomalies is unlikely to be associated in the first decade or two of life with an increase in pulmonary artery pressure. Why some individuals nevertheless remain susceptible to the development of pulmonary vascular disease remains unclear. The exact percentage of individuals who are at risk of pulmonary vascular disease if an ASD is untreated also remains unclear and is unlikely to be answered with any degree of accuracy because of the widespread early management of ASDs today.

Because the young child has excellent compliance of both the right heart and the left heart there are likely to be no symptoms from an ASD in the first decade or two of life. By the fourth or fifth decade as left ventricular compliance begins to decrease symptoms such as exertional dyspnea may appear. Occasionally a large atrial septal defect is accompanied by important symptoms of congestive heart failure in infancy.[4] There is also some evidence to suggest that an ASD may be associated with growth retardation in many children based on the observation that they tend to shift to an accelerated growth curve following ASD closure.[5]

Cyanosis is not a feature of an atrial septal defect unless Eisenmenger's syndrome has developed. However, cyanosis may be seen if there is a left SVC draining to the left atrium associated with the ASD.

The physical examination is often unremarkable apart from reasonably subtle auscultatory findings. Because the

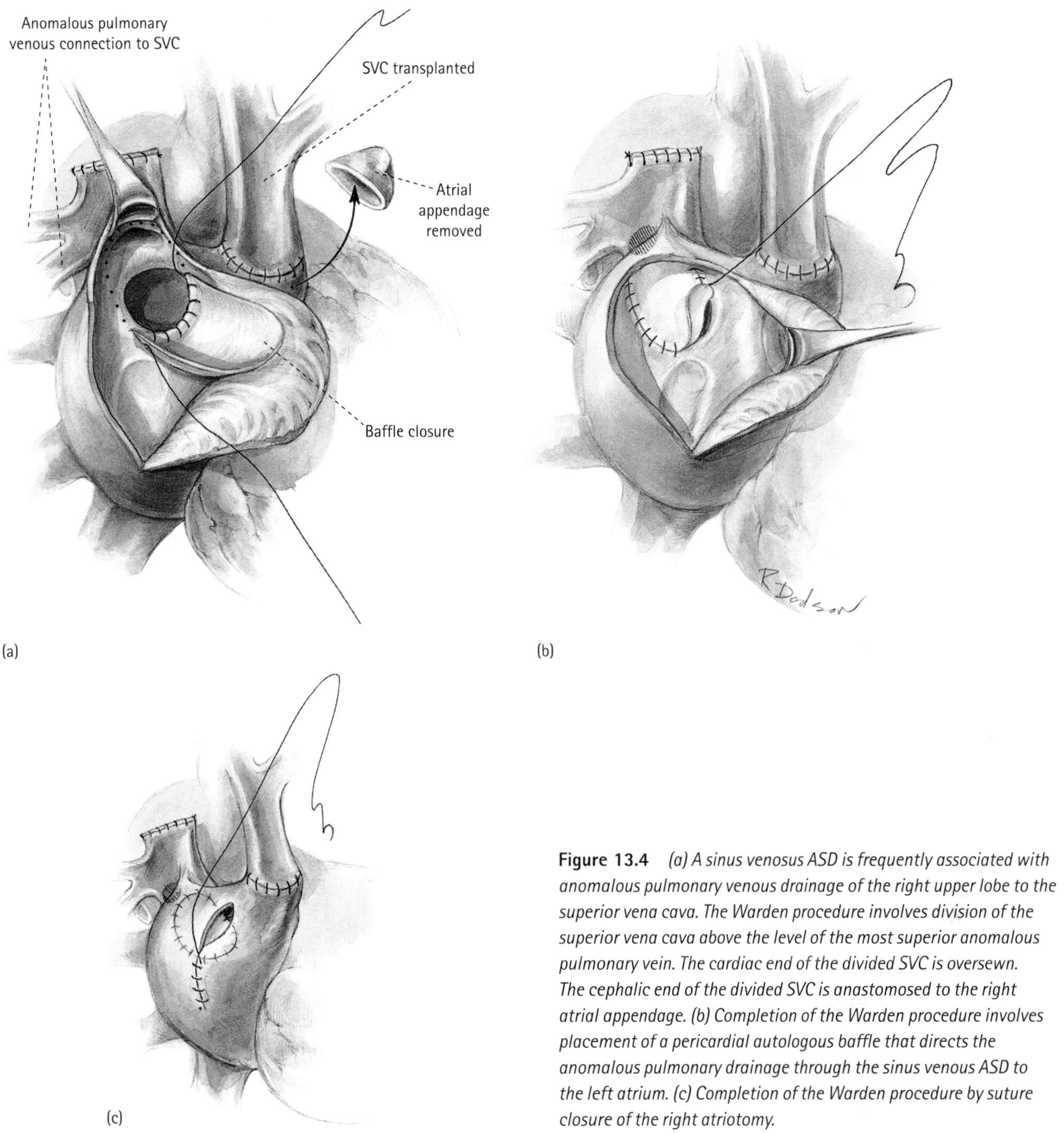

Figure 13.4 *(a) A sinus venosus ASD is frequently associated with anomalous pulmonary venous drainage of the right upper lobe to the superior vena cava. The Warden procedure involves division of the superior vena cava above the level of the most superior anomalous pulmonary vein. The cardiac end of the divided SVC is oversewn. The cephalic end of the divided SVC is anastomosed to the right atrial appendage. (b) Completion of the Warden procedure involves placement of a pericardial autologous baffle that directs the anomalous pulmonary drainage through the sinus venous ASD to the left atrium. (c) Completion of the Warden procedure by suture closure of the right atriotomy.*

pressure difference between the right and left atrium is only a few millimeters of mercury and the size of the ASD is usually relatively large, there is no murmur generated by the left to right flow within the atrium. There may be a subtle systolic ejection murmur audible over the pulmonary artery reflecting the increased flow passing through the pulmonary valve. Even though the pulmonary valve is usually structurally normal it becomes functionally stenotic because of the large amount of flow passing through it. The most important finding is 'fixed splitting' of the second heart sound. Because pulmonary closure is delayed because of the large amount of flow passing through it, there is no longer the usual variability of splitting between the aortic and pulmonary valve closures which occurs with respiration.

DIAGNOSTIC STUDIES

A plain chest X-ray is helpful because it will demonstrate the enlarged main pulmonary artery at the left border of the heart. The right and left pulmonary artery will also be prominent at the hilum of each lung and the lung fields are

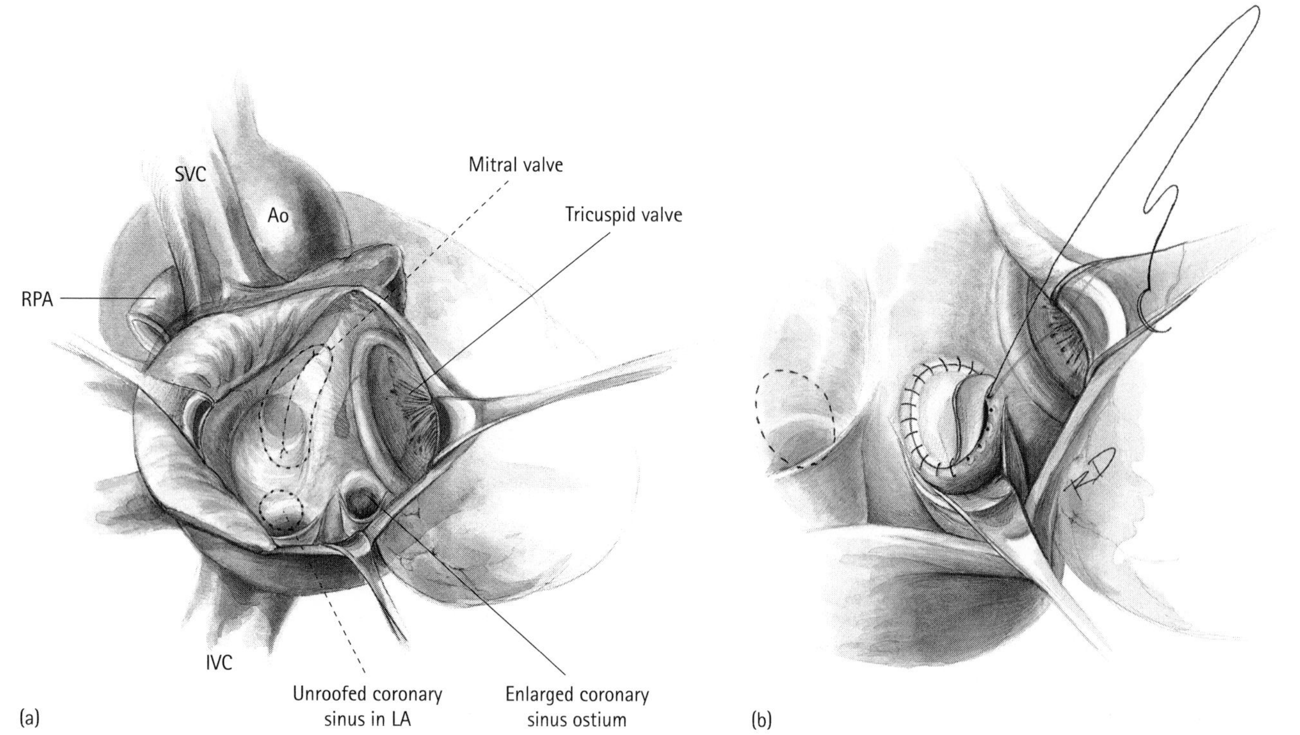

Figure 13.5 *(a) A coronary sinus septal defect results when there is partial or complete unroofing of the coronary sinus in the left atrium. The coronary sinus ostium is usually dilated. (b) Closure of a coronary sinus septal defect by placing an autologous pericardial patch. The patch should be sutured within the mouth of the coronary sinus if possible to reduce the risk of injury to the AV node thereby avoiding complete heart block. Coronary sinus venous return now enters the left atrium resulting in a trivial right to left shunt.*

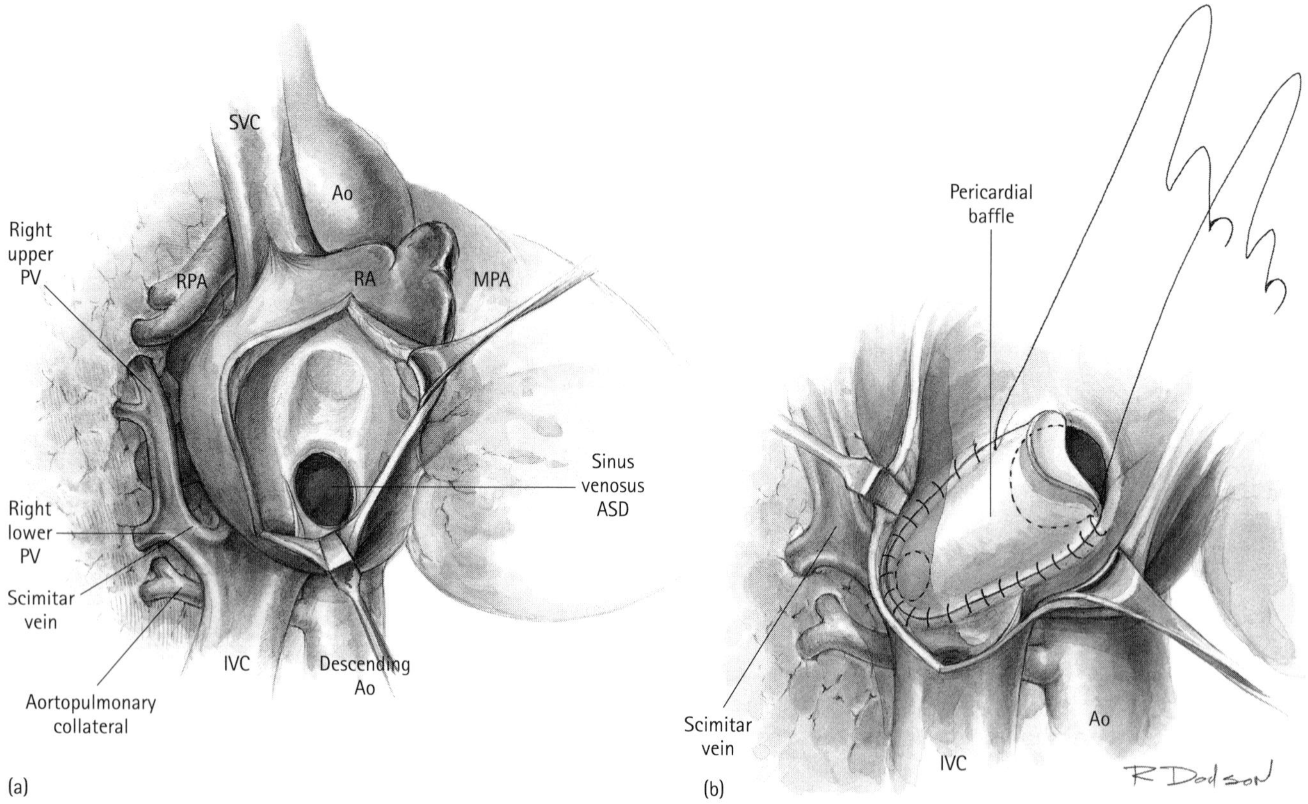

Figure 13.6 *(a) Scimitar syndrome is a constellation of anomalies including a sinus venosus ASD usually close to the junction of the inferior vena cava with the right atrium, anomalous pulmonary venous (PV) drainage of most of the right lung connecting to the IVC/right atrial junction, aortopulmonary collateral blood supply to the right lower lobe and hypoplasia of the right lung. (b) Scimitar syndrome is usually best managed by placement of an autologous pericardial baffle directing the anomalous pulmonary venous return through the sinus venosus ASD to the left atrium. The baffle also closes the ASD eliminating any left to right shunt.*

plethoric. The ECG may be relatively normal though the axis can be helpful in differentiating a primum ASD from the other forms of ASD. Because the triangle of Koch where the AV node and bundle of His are usually located is absent in the setting of a primum ASD, the bundle must pass in a more inferior direction to gain access to the ventricular septum. This is associated with left axis deviation and a counterclockwise loop. It is extremely rare for there to be left axis deviation with a secundum ASD where the axis is more likely to be rightward than leftward depending on the degree of right ventricular hypertrophy. It is not uncommon to see a partial right bundle branch block reflecting right ventricular intraventricular conduction delay. A two-dimensional echocardiogram is usually diagnostic of an atrial septal defect. In the years before color Doppler mapping was available it was not uncommon for 'false dropout' to result in an incorrect false positive diagnosis of a secundum ASD. However, color flow mapping has essentially eliminated this problem. The echocardiogram, however, is not accurate in diagnosing associated anomalies of pulmonary venous connection. This is particularly true when there are small anomalous pulmonary veins draining to the superior vena cava. Because the lung wraps over the superior vena cava it is particularly difficult for ultrasound to define this area clearly. Two-dimensional echocardiography is helpful in quantitating the hemodynamic impact of an ASD. An assessment is made of the degree of right ventricular volume overload by observing the size of the right atrium and right ventricle relative to the left heart. In addition diastolic flattening of the ventricular septum suggests an important volume overload of the right heart. An absolute measurement of the width of color flow through the atrial septum is also helpful. Cardiac magnetic resonance imaging is emerging as a useful modality in defining pulmonary venous drainage when a sinus venous ASD has been diagnosed by initial echocardiography. There is little or no role today for diagnostic cardiac catheterization though catheterization has emerged as an important therapeutic modality for atrial septal defect.

MEDICAL AND INTERVENTIONAL THERAPY

Because atrial septal defects are usually asymptomatic it is rarely necessary to use anticongestive therapy. However, occasionally a large ASD can cause symptoms in infancy. Under these circumstances standard anticongestive therapy with digoxin and diuretics may be indicated. Over the years many devices have been developed for the purpose of closing a secundum ASD in the catheterization laboratory. The topic has been reviewed extensively elsewhere.[6] No device is suitable for closure of a primum ASD or is designed to be applicable for a coronary sinus septal defect or sinus venosus ASD.

The Amplatzer device consists of two mushroom shaped wire meshes containing thrombus inducing fabric connected by a central stalk. By positioning each end of the device on either side of the atrial septum and then screwing the two halves together the 'mushrooms' become flattened and the central stalk expands to fill the ASD. The device has the advantage that it 'centers' itself on the ASD because the central stalk itself plays a role in the septal defect closure. On the other hand the 'mushroom' ends of the device are bulky and tend to partially fill both the right atrium and left atrium. Over time the metal mesh becomes incorporated into the ASD though the long-term effect of a relatively rigid metal structure within the constantly moving heart remains unclear. Late perforation and cardiac tamponade have been seen (J Gold, personal communication). The long term risk of thromboembolism appears to be relatively low but over the very long term remains unknown.[7] Likewise the long-term risk of bacterial endocarditis remains unknown. There have been cases of serious early infection reported. The current alternative to the Amplatzer device is a variation on a device originally designed by Rashkind.[8,9] This device consisted of fine stainless steel arms supporting polyurethane foam. The device was modified by Dr James Lock to become a 'clamshell' in which the spring loaded stainless steel arms clamp down on each other sandwiching the atrial septum between two layers of Dacron fabric.[10] The Dacron fabric becomes incorporated into the atrial septum. This device has a much lower profile than the Amplatzer device. It has the disadvantage that in its original form it was not self-centering so that the device must be very much larger than the ASD. The long thin arms of the clamshell device have a risk of entanglement in other cardiac structures such as the atrioventricular valves. There is also a risk of perforation of the atrial wall and aorta. Fractures of the metal arms have been observed. As with the Amplatzer device the risk of thromboembolism from the device has been quite low as has the risk of infection. Nevertheless the very long term risk of these problems remains unclear. The advantages of a catheter delivered device include a complete avoidance of cardiopulmonary bypass with its attendant risks as well as the avoidance of the pain and cosmetic disadvantage of a surgical incision. These latter problems have been reduced somewhat by the introduction of the minimally invasive approach to ASD closure (see below). In addition the future holds out the promise for even less invasive surgical techniques including the application of robotic technology.

INDICATIONS FOR AND TIMING OF SURGERY

ASDs occur in a wide spectrum of size ranging from tiny fenestrations of the septum primum to complete absence of the atrial septum. Clearly at the more severe end of the septum surgical closure is indicated because of the risk of pulmonary vascular obstructive disease as well as the almost certain development of right heart failure in middle age following many years of right ventricular volume loading. The problem as to where to draw the line defining when surgical closure is not indicated for the very small ASD has been complicated in recent years by the introduction of echocardiography. This has meant that many small ASDs are now detected even though there may be no symptoms and indeed no physical findings. In the years before echocardiography an atrial septal effect was generally only detected because of the presence of physical findings such as a pulmonary outflow murmur and fixed splitting of the second sound. These physical findings usually could not be detected unless there was a left to right shunt ($Q_p:Q_s$) of 1.5 : 1 or greater.[11] A shunt of this size was generally considered to be sufficiently large to warrant surgical closure. Today a judgment must be made in the child who is free of symptoms and who has no findings on physical examination as to whether an ASD is causing sufficient hemodynamic load to warrant closure. This judgment must be made by the echocardiographer who will determine the degree of right ventricular volume overload. In general this will correspond to an ASD that is at least 5–6 mm in diameter. However, it is important to understand that the shape of the color flow jet can be quite irregular so that measurement in at least two planes is necessary. The recommended age for ASD closure has changed over the last decade or so. Traditionally elective closure of a secundum ASD was recommended in the year prior to a child beginning school, i.e. four or five years of age. Today the second year of life is considered the optimal time for ASD closure. Spontaneous closure of a small secundum ASD has been documented in the first year of life so in general elective closure should not be undertaken in infancy.[12] On the other hand, if important symptoms are present such as congestive heart failure and failure to thrive then ASD closure should definitely be undertaken during infancy. If an ASD is still present beyond 12 months of age and there is evidence of right ventricular volume overload usually associated with a color flow jet that is at least 5–6 mm in diameter then surgery should be arranged for a convenient time during the next year. There are important psychological advantages for the family who will otherwise remain anxious for several years awaiting surgery at a later time. They are likely to be overprotective towards the child which can interfere with psychological development. Furthermore in the second or third year of life the child will be quite free of any anxiety related to surgery while a school age child may become quite anxious. The introduction of minimally invasive surgery has further increased the advantages of repair early in life. In the second or third year of life the thoracic cage is more flexible and can easily be retracted to allow excellent exposure of the heart even through a very tiny incision. Very small cannulas are adequate for drainage. In an older child exposure of the aorta through a short and low cosmetic incision becomes increasingly difficult.

SURGICAL MANAGEMENT

History of surgery

Because of their anatomic simplicity, atrial septal defects were the subject of some of the earliest attempts at surgical repair of intracardiac defects. Several ingenious closed methods for closure, such as the atrioseptopexy method of Bailey et al[13] and the closed suture technique of Sondergaard,[14] were applied in the late 1940s and early 1950s. Open repair, using the atrial well technique, was performed at Children's Hospital Boston by Gross and coworkers in 1952[15] and repair under direct vision using moderate hypothermia and inflow occlusion was performed in 1953 by Lewis and Taufic.[16] In 1954, Gibbons introduced cardiopulmonary bypass for closing an atrial septal defect.[17] In the present era cardiopulmonary bypass is used almost exclusively for surgical closure of atrial septal defects. Various minimally invasive surgical approaches have become popular since the mid-1990s.[18,19]

Minimally invasive surgical closure of secundum ASDs

Minimally invasive partial lower sternotomy approach has become the standard surgical management for the secundum ASD over the last decade. Although alternative approaches are available they have important disadvantages.

LIMITED ANTEROLATERAL THORACOTOMY

The principal disadvantage of the anterolateral thoracotomy is that it is impossible to define subsequent breast development in the prepubertal girl.[20] Significant distortion of breast development frequently occurs following the use of this approach. In addition there can be denervation of skin over the breast. A high incidence of phrenic nerve weakness has been reported using this approach. Exposure of the aorta can be difficult particularly in the older child.

POSTEROLATERAL THORACOTOMY

Planche has championed the use of the posterolateral thoracotomy which avoids the problem of breast distortion and results in a transverse scar on the back.[21] Exposure of the aorta is improved relative to the anterolateral approach. However, scoliosis has been described in association with posterolateral thoracotomy, particularly when performed very early in life. Although some have suggested that this is primarily related to an association of vertebral anomalies with congenital cardiac anomalies requiring a thoracotomy, nevertheless careful follow-up will be required of these patients to demonstrate that scoliosis does not become a problem in the teenage growth years.

LIMITED LOWER STERNOTOMY

It is possible to limit the skin incision for secundum ASD closure, particularly in the smaller child less than two to three years of age to between 3.5 and 4 cm.[18,19] This incision still allows passage of all cannulas through the incision itself. Although various modifications are possible in which cannulas are passed through chest tube incisions or femoral bypass is used, today we do not apply such modifications. It is

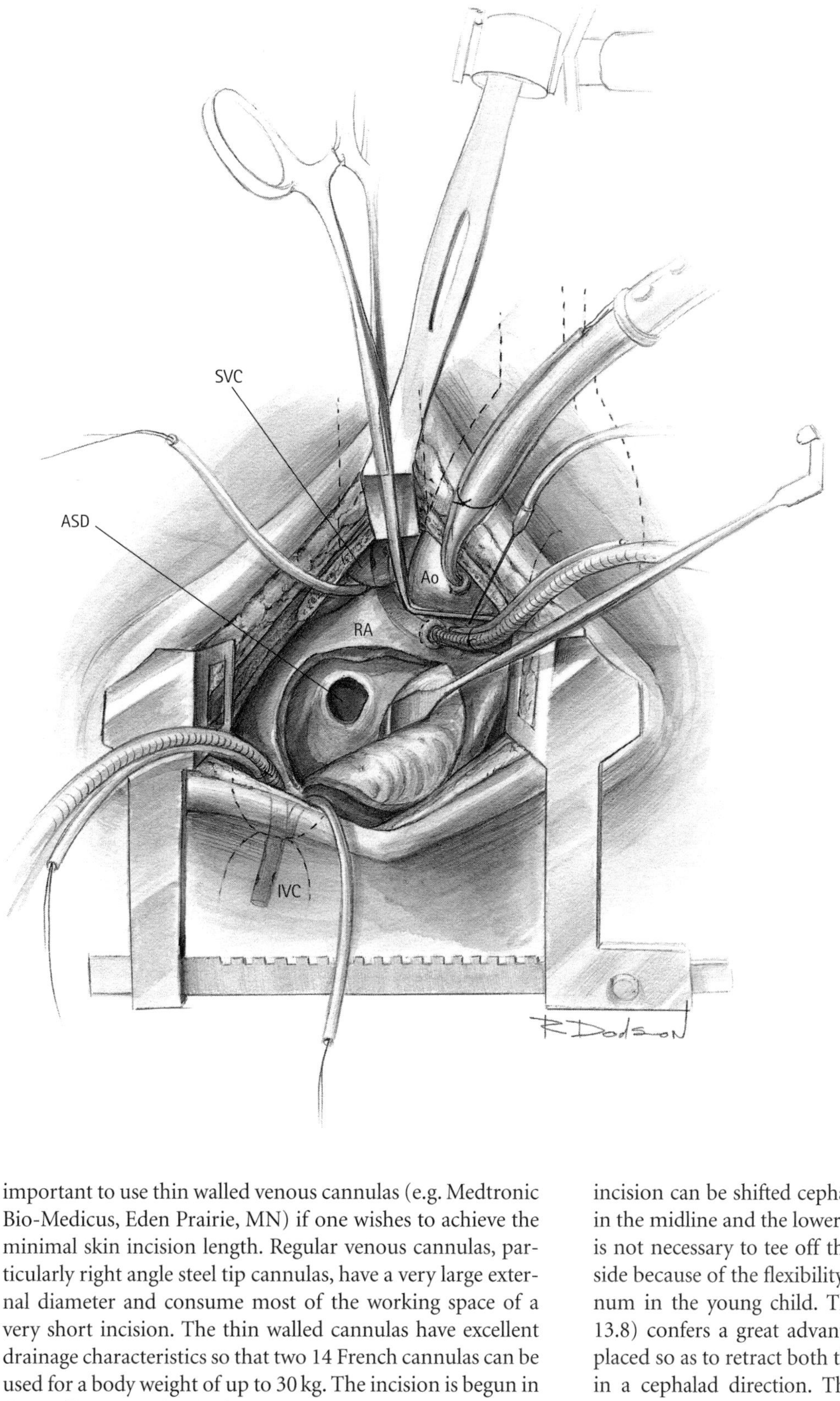

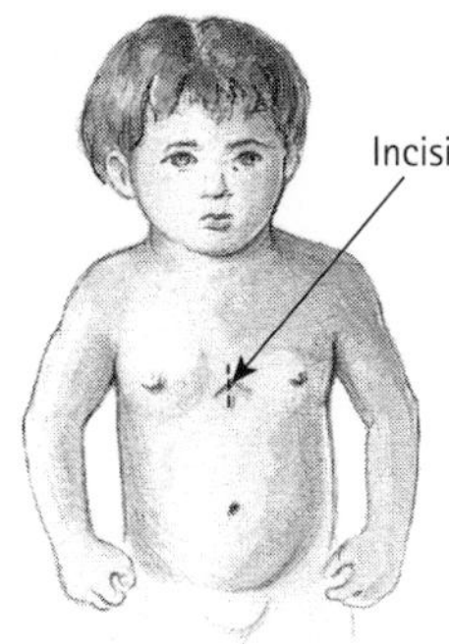

Figure 13.7 *A limited lower partial median sternotomy is the preferred approach for minimally invasive surgical closure of a secundum ASD. The inset illustrates that the incision is begun at about the level of the nipples and is carried down for 3.5 to 6 cm. Thin walled venous cannulas are particularly helpful in allowing standard cannulation and yet leaving adequate room to manipulate instruments for the ASD closure. The aorta is cross clamped in the standard fashion and cardioplegia solution is infused into the root of the aorta.*

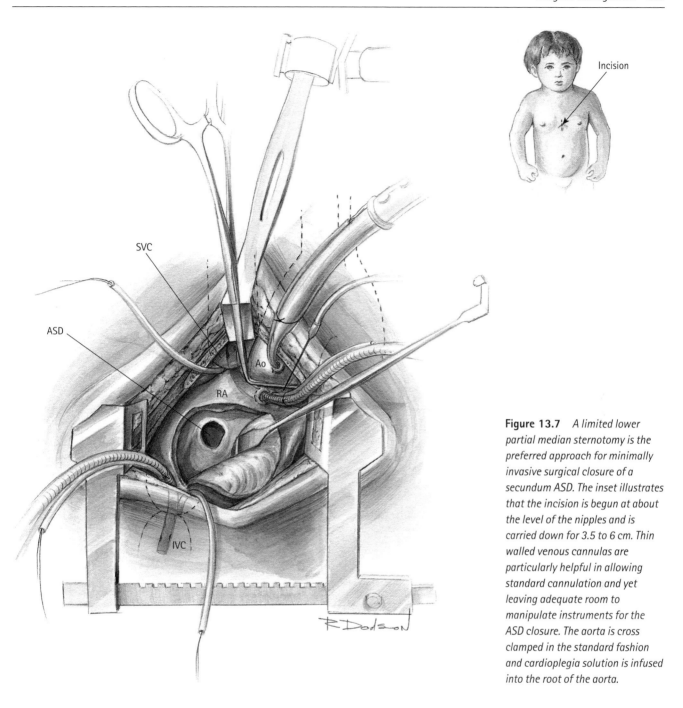

important to use thin walled venous cannulas (e.g. Medtronic Bio-Medicus, Eden Prairie, MN) if one wishes to achieve the minimal skin incision length. Regular venous cannulas, particularly right angle steel tip cannulas, have a very large external diameter and consume most of the working space of a very short incision. The thin walled cannulas have excellent drainage characteristics so that two 14 French cannulas can be used for a body weight of up to 30 kg. The incision is begun in the midline at the level of the nipples and is carried down for 3.5–4 cm (Figure 13.7). If the operator is less experienced a slightly longer incision of up to 5–6 cm increases the ease of the procedure considerably. A plane is developed between the subcutaneous fat and the prepectoral fascia so that the skin incision can be shifted cephalad. The xiphoid process is split in the midline and the lower half of the sternum is divided. It is not necessary to tee off the sternal bone incision to either side because of the flexibility of the costal cartilages and sternum in the young child. The Bookwalter retractor (Figure 13.8) confers a great advantage. This fixed arm retractor is placed so as to retract both the sternum and the skin incision in a cephalad direction. This allows excellent exposure of the aorta while maintaining the original incision in a very low cosmetic location. It is not necessary to remove any thymus. The two lobes of the thymus are partially separated at their lower poles. A patch of the anterior and inferior pericardium is harvested and treated with 0.6% glutaraldehyde

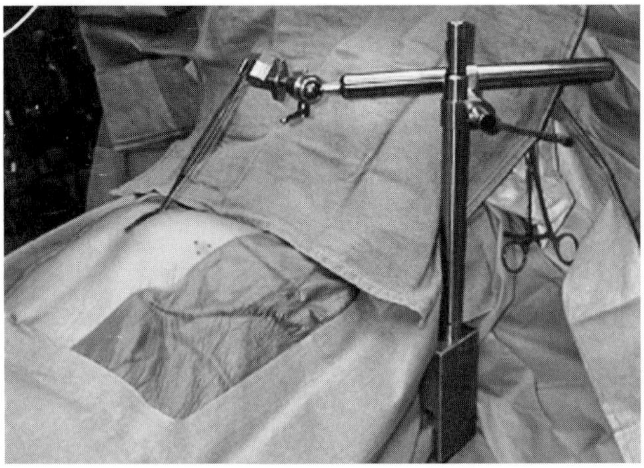

Figure 13.8 *The Bookwalter fixed arm retractor is helpful when performing minimally invasive ASD closure. The entire thoracic cavity is retracted cephalad improving exposure for aortic cannulation in particular.*

for 20 minutes. The pericardium is not split behind the thymus. The retractor blade of the Bookwalter retractor system is inserted within the pericardium and aids in the creation of a pericardial cradle as well as retracting the thymus, sternum and skin. Pericardial suspension sutures are placed in the usual fashion.

Cannulation site

It is not necessary to cannulate the cavas directly. The venous cannulation sutures can be placed approximately 2 cm apart in the right atrial appendage and the right atrial free wall. The aortic cannulation suture is placed on the anterior surface of the aorta at approximately its midpoint. Following heparinization the cannulas are introduced. Arterial cannulation can be performed in the standard fashion using a side biting clamp which draws the aorta down into better view. Alternatively a Seldinger type technique can be used introducing a guide wire into the lumen of the aorta and then threading an introducer and Biomedicus cannula. The Biomedicus venous cannulas are inserted with the plastic introducer in place so that a curve can be used to angle each cannula directly into the superior vena cava and inferior vena cava.

Cardiopulmonary bypass and cardioplegia

Standard cardiopulmonary bypass is begun and the patient is cooled to a mild degree of hypothermia such as 32°C. During this time tourniquets are placed around the superior vena cava and inferior vena cava and a cardioplegia stitch is inserted into the aortic root. The aortic cross clamp is applied, cardioplegia is infused in the usual fashion and the caval tourniquets are tightened.

ASD exposure

The right atrium is opened through a limited oblique incision between the cannulas. Care should be taken to avoid dividing any arteries visible in the atrial free wall which may in part supply the sinus node. In addition the crista terminalis should not be divided. With appropriate retraction of cannulas excellent exposure of the secundum ASD is usually possible despite the skin incision being 4 cm or less in length.

ASD closure

Direct suture closure: Small to moderate sized ASDs can be closed by direct suture (see Figure 13.2a2). It is generally an advantage to use a Castro Viejo type needle holder which is more ergonomically appropriate for a limited incision. The defect is closed with two layers of continuous 5/0 polypropylene using a single double-ended polypropylene suture. By placing several throws after the initial stitch, two independent suture lines are created. Thus recurrence of the ASD related to suture fracture is highly unlikely. Furthermore the knot that is tied when completing two suture lines is very much more secure than the knot that is tied when a single suture is tied to itself at the end of the suture line. The suture line should be begun at the lower, most dependent end of the incision, generally adjacent to the inferior vena caval right atrial junction. Not only does this follow the general principle of working from the more difficult end of a suture line to the easier end but in addition it is important in minimizing the introduction of air into the left atrium.

Patch closure of secundum atrial septal defect: If the secundum ASD is too large to allow direct suture closure, an autologous pericardial patch should be employed (Figure 13.2b2). Use of an autologous pericardial patch eliminates essentially any prosthetic material from ASD closure and should thereby minimize the risk of thromboembolism and late endocarditis. These a re important advantages of the surgical closure of a secundum ASD relative to device closure that involves placement of large amounts of potentially thrombogenic fabric and metal which must be left permanently within the right atrium and left atrium.

Autologous pericardium is treated with 0.6% glutaraldehyde (Poly Scientific, Bay Shore, NY) for approximately 20 minutes. The patch is sutured to the margins of the ASD using continuous polypropylene suture. As with the direct suture closure the suture line should begin at the most dependent inferior part of the ASD. This allows air to be eliminated from within the left atrium. Care should be taken to avoid suctioning within the left atrium which should remain almost full throughout the procedure.

De-airing

It is not recommended that the blood level be lowered in the left atrium in order to observe the internal orifices of the pulmonary veins. The left atrium should remain full of blood at all times and no air should be introduced. Partial anomalous pulmonary venous connection is rare in association with a secundum ASD. The echocardiographer should have made a note in their report regarding the usual connection of a superior and inferior right pulmonary vein entering the left atrium. This can be confirmed by external and not internal observation at the time of surgery.

The suture line should proceed from inferior to superior so that if a tiny amount of air has been introduced into the left atrium it should spill out into the right atrium as closure is completed. As a further precaution the cardioplegia needle should now be removed and the left ventricle gently massaged from apex towards base. The aortic cross clamp is released with the cardioplegia site bleeding freely.

Right atrial closure and weaning from bypass

During warming the right atriotomy is closed with two layers of fine prolene suture. There is a tendency for sutures to be spaced far too closely in the atrial wall. Wide spacing of sutures results in the suture line purse-stringing itself together and results in a shorter ultimate scar than is seen if multiple fine sutures are placed in the atrium. It is just as important to de-air the right heart as right atrial closure is completed as it is to de-air the left heart. When the child has been rewarmed to a rectal temperature of 35°C weaning bypass is discontinued. It is generally not necessary to monitor central venous pressure with a right atrial catheter and no pacing wires are placed. The cannulas are removed and protamine is given.

Creation of a pleuro-pericardial window

In order to reduce the risk of late pericardial tamponade a pleuro-pericardial window should be created. The right sided pleura is opened and the pericardium is opened posteriorly to within approximately 1 cm of the phrenic nerve. A single chest tube is inserted through a short vertical incision approximately 2 cm below the inferior end of the main incision. A single straight chest tube, perhaps with additional side holes cut to allow adequate mediastinal drainage is inserted with the tip in the right pleural cavity and the additional side holes lying close to the atrial incision.

Incision closure

Although a heavy absorbable suture such as polydioxanone can be used for sternal closure the large knots which result can be palpable for many weeks or even months and can be bothersome to parents and children. We therefore use light gauge stainless steel wire to approximate the lower end of the sternum. Two wire sutures are generally needed. The remainder of the closure is routine with continuous Vicryl to the presternal fascia and linea alba with continuous Vicryl to the subcutaneous fat and subcuticular Vicryl completing wound closure. It is important that a light gauge Vicryl be employed to minimize the risk of a reaction to the suture material.

Surgical management of the primum ASD

The surgical management of the primum ASD is covered in Chapter 21.

Surgical management of the sinus venosus ASD

Although it is possible to manage the sinus venosus ASD through a minimally invasive approach, we generally use a full sternotomy to allow complete inspection of the superior vena cava for partial anomalous pulmonary venous connection. The upper end of the skin incision can be somewhat limited to improve cosmesis though if a Warden procedure (see below) is to be used then the skin incision cannot be very limited at its upper end. However, the lower end of the skin incision can be limited under these circumstances.

DISSECTION OF THE SUPERIOR VENA CAVA

Unless a cardiac MRI has been obtained and has excluded the possibility of anomalous pulmonary venous connection to the superior vena cava, it is generally advisable to dissect out the superior vena cava to exclude the possibility of anomalous pulmonary veins draining to the superior vena cava. Even if the right upper lobe pulmonary vein draining to the right atrium appears relatively normal this does not eliminate the possibility of additional small veins draining directly to the superior vena cava. Dissection of the superior vena cava before bypass facilitates recognition of the pulmonary veins as distinct from the azygous vein by the color of the blood within the veins. Dissection of the superior vena cava should be undertaken with great care to avoid disturbing the right phrenic nerve.

CANNULATION FOR THE SINUS VENOSUS ASD

Whichever surgical technique is used for management of a sinus venous ASD it is helpful to have the superior vena cava cannula remote from the ASD. If a Warden procedure is to be performed then a right angle metal tip cannula should be placed in the left innominate vein. The cannula should have a sufficiently small tip that blood can pass around the cannula from the contralateral internal jugular vein as is done for venous cannulation for the bidirectional Glenn shunt (see Figure 13.3a). A regular straight cannula can be inserted through the right atrial free wall into the inferior vena cava.

CARDIOPULMONARY BYPASS AND CARDIOPLEGIA

Mildly hypothermic bypass with cooling to 30–32°C is generally appropriate. Standard cardioplegic arrest is employed.

STANDARD SINUS VENOSUS ASD PATCH CLOSURE

If there are no anomalous pulmonary veins connecting to the superior vena cava the sinus venosus ASD can be closed with an autologous pericardial patch (Figure 13.3b). A standard oblique incision in the right atrium is made with careful preservation of coronary arteries passing across the atrial free wall and care taken not to divide the crista terminalis. A retractor is placed in the internal orifice of the superior vena cava with gentle retraction to avoid injury to the sinus node. An autologous pericardial patch is sutured into place. Care should be taken to avoid purse-stringing the caval orifice or the orifice of the right upper lobe pulmonary vein. Relatively wide bites should be taken on the patch with much closer bites being taken on the patient. A continuous polypropylene suture is employed. The usual measures for de-airing are employed and the clamp is then released. The atriotomy is closed during warming.

WARDEN PROCEDURE

If there are anomalous pulmonary veins entering the superior vena cava it is often advisable to perform a Warden procedure (see Figure 13.4). A clamp is applied across the superior vena cava just below the junction of the left innominate vein and right innominate vein. The azygous vein is doubly ligated and divided. After application of the aortic cross clamp and infusion of cardioplegia solution as well as tightening of the IVC tourniquet, an oblique incision is made in the right atrium in a standard fashion. The superior vena cava is divided above the most cephalad anomalous vein. The cardiac end of the divided SVC is oversewn with continuous 5/0 prolene with care to avoid stenosing the uppermost pulmonary vein (see Figure 13.4a). A pericardial patch is sutured into the right atrium so as to baffle the superior vena caval orifice through the sinus venosus ASD (see Figure 13.4b). In this way pulmonary venous return is now baffled through the superior vena cava into the left atrium and the ASD has been closed. All that remains to do is to anastomose the amputated tip of the right atrial appendage at the cephalad end of the divided SVC. Generally a continuous absorbable Maxon suture is employed. Care should be taken to avoid purse-stringing this anastomosis. Generally the SVC/appendage anastomosis is not under tension because of the dilated nature of the right atrium including the right atrial appendage.

Coronary sinus septal defect

The usual approach for closure of a coronary sinus septal defect is a minimally invasive partial sternotomy. Cannulation is as for a standard minimally invasive approach. Usually the coronary sinus ostium is closed with a patch of autologous pericardium (see Figure 13.5b). Care is taken to suture within the ostium so as to avoid placing sutures within the triangle of Koch which would risk the AV node and potentially cause complete heart block. Coronary sinus effluent will drain through the unroofed segment of coronary sinus into the left atrium but this results in an acceptable small right to left shunt. If there is a left sided superior vena in continuity with the coronary sinus it may be necessary to take an alternative approach.

Persistent left sided superior vena cava

A persistent left sided superior vena cava can be found in association with a number of anomalies including ASD. It is important for the echocardiographer to determine if there is a left innominate 'communicating' vein connecting the left SVC to the right SVC. If an adequate sized vein is present then it is reasonable to simply ligate the left SVC if it is not draining to the right atrium through a totally roofed coronary sinus. If there is no communicating vein a number of options are available for dealing with a persistent left SVC. A judgment must be made as to the relative size of the left SVC relative to the right SVC. If it is extremely small then it can be safely tied off. If it is similar in size to the right SVC or larger then consideration should be given to internal baffling of the left SVC to the right atrium. In the setting of a common atrium for example the pericardial patch which is constructed to septate the common atrium is diverted leftward so as to incorporate the left SVC orifice on the right side of the pericardial patch. If there were a coronary sinus septal defect then consideration would need to be given to closing the actual coronary sinus septal defect itself rather than the ostium of the coronary sinus which is the more usual surgical technique for dealing with a coronary sinus septal defect. Occasionally circumstances arise where the left SVC can be divided close to its junction with the left atrium. The left atrial end is oversewn and the cephalad end is anastomosed to the tip of the right atrial appendage. Another option is to ligate the left SVC below the point of entry of the hemi-azygous vein. In very rare circumstances a Gortex conduit can be sutured between the left SVC and the right atrial appendage. It is generally not advisable to attempt to suture such a conduit directly to the right SVC as this risks occlusion of both cavas which is poorly tolerated.

CANNULATION TECHNIQUES FOR LEFT SIDED SVC

It is usually not necessary to place a third venous cannula within a left sided superior vena cava. If an ASD is to be closed it is generally possible to perform cannulation of the right sided SVC and inferior vena cava and to handle drainage from the left SVC with a coronary sinus sucker. A flexible sucker, for example, can be advanced through the coronary sinus ostium into the left SVC. If bilateral cannulation is attempted and both SVCs are relatively small there is a risk of injury to the cavas which can result in occlusion. Dissection around the left SVC to enable cannulation also increases the risk of a phrenic nerve injury on the left.

Partial anomalous pulmonary venous connection

The management of partial anomalous pulmonary venous connection from the right upper lobe to the superior vena cava in association with a sinus venous ASD has been described above with the description of the Warden procedure. Alternative strategies may be applied for other forms of partial anomalous pulmonary venous connection.

SCIMITAR SYNDROME

The arterial blood supply to the right lung must be carefully defined preoperatively. This will generally necessitate cardiac catheterization. If there is duplicate aortopulmonary collateral supply, usually to the right lower lobe, it should be closed by coil embolization at the time of catheterization. The point of junction of the scimitar vein with the inferior vena cava should also be clearly defined though this is usually well seen by echocardiography. It is generally helpful to apply deep hypothermic circulatory arrest for placement of an autologous pericardial baffle which re-directs the anomalous venous return. It is advisable to place a straight caval cannula during the cooling phase rather than directly cannulating the IVC as this could result in some narrowing close to the baffle when the purse-string for the cannula is tied. When deep hypothermia has been achieved, the aortic cross clamp has been applied and cardioplegia infused then circulatory arrest is begun. The caval cannula is removed. An autologous pericardial patch is sutured around the internal orifice of the Scimitar vein with care taken to avoid purse stringing the orifice (see Figure 13.6b). The baffle is then sutured around the orifice of the low sinus venosus ASD. Care should be taken to avoid making the baffle excessively redundant which might narrow the IVC. The left atrium and baffle are carefully de-aired before tying the suture line. In rare circumstances the scimitar vein enters the IVC so low that placement of an internal baffle is inadvisable. Under these circumstances the vein can be divided and reimplanted directly into the left atrium. However, this approach is accompanied by a significant risk of anastomotic stenosis and should be avoided if possible.

PARTIAL ANOMALOUS PULMONARY VENOUS CONNECTION WITH ASSOCIATED ASD

Left upper lobe pulmonary venous connection to an ascending left sided vertical vein

This is the most common form of partial anomalous pulmonary venous connection. It can be found in association with a number of other anomalies or occasionally be isolated. Surgical management is indicated if the left to right shunt is calculated to be greater than 1.5 : 1. It may be necessary to undertake catheterization to quantitate the degree of shunting. The ascending vertical vein is divided just below its junction with the left innominate vein. It is partially filleted open and is anastomosed to the base of the left atrial appendage which is opened longitudinally. It is important to avoid torsion of the anomalous vein. Therefore the anterior surface of the vein should be marked before it is divided. The anastomosis is rarely under any degree of tension since the ascending vertical vein supplies plenty of length to allow for the anastomosis.

Right sided pulmonary veins draining to right atrium

If there is no ASD in association with partial anomalous pulmonary venous connection of the right pulmonary veins to the right atrium it is necessary to create one. This can usually be done in the base of the fossa ovalis. An autologous pericardial patch is sutured around the orifices of the right pulmonary veins and the surgically created secundum ASD. It is important to place wide bites on the pericardial patch and close bites around the orifices of the pulmonary veins and the ASD in order to avoid purse-stringing either end of the baffle pathway. Purse-stringing can result in subsequent problems with growth related narrowing of the pulmonary venous pathway.

RESULTS OF SURGERY

There is a remarkably extensive body of literature regarding management of atrial septal defects. In recent years much of this information has focused on the development of interventional catheter delivered devices and various approaches for minimally invasive surgical repair of ASDs. There are few recent reports describing traditional surgical management of the secundum ASD.

Traditional surgical management

In 1996, Mavroudis[22] in an editorial briefly described the results of traditional surgical management of secundum ASD over a 10-year period between 1985 and 1995 at Children's Memorial Hospital in Chicago. A total of 212 patients had an isolated secundum ASD closed. A total of 47% had pericardial patch closure and 53% had primary suture closure. There were no deaths, no reoperations for bleeding, no neurologic complications and no residual ASDs. In 2001 Jones et al[23] described a retrospective review of 87 children who underwent standard surgical closure of secundum ASD in Brisbane, Australia. There were no deaths. However, there was a relatively high incidence of postoperative pericardial effusions and post pericardiotomy syndrome. The authors did not employ the technique of creating a pleuro pericardial window at the time of surgery in order to minimize the risk of need for postoperative pericardiocentesis.

Minimally invasive surgical closure of ASD

In 2001, Bichell et al[24] described the results of surgery for the first 135 patients who underwent a minimally invasive approach for repair of ASD at Children's Hospital Boston. The median age at the time of surgery was five years. A 3.5–5 cm midline incision centered over the xiphoid with division of the xiphoid or of the lower sternum (mini-sternotomy) was performed. There were no early or late deaths and no bleeding or wound complications. No patient suffered a clinically detectable neurological complication. No procedure required conversion to a full sternotomy and no cannulation attempt was abandoned for an alternative site. Cross clamp and cardiopulmonary bypass times were equivalent to a concurrent group of patients who underwent a full sternotomy. The length of hospital stay in the mini-sternotomy group was 2.7 days. We concluded from this study that the mini-sternotomy approach results in a satisfactory cosmetic result without compromising the safety or accuracy of ASD repair.

Further details regarding the postoperative recovery of patients after mini-sternotomy were documented in a paper by Laussen et al from Children's Hospital Boston.[25] The authors compared 17 patients who underwent a mini-sternotomy with 18 patients who underwent a full length sternotomy. A comprehensive prospective assessment of both intraoperative course and postoperative course was undertaken. Postoperative comparisons included pain scores at 6, 12 and 24 hours, frequency of emesis, analgesic requirements, respiratory rate and gas exchange and length of intensive care unit and total hospital stay. No significant differences were identified between the mini and full sternotomy approaches. No adverse outcomes were detected. Only improved cosmesis was identified as an advantage for the mini-sternotomy approach. In 1999, Khan et al[26] described an experience with minimally invasive surgical repair of ASD at UCSF California. Over a five-year period 115 consecutive patients underwent minimally invasive surgical closure of secundum ASD using a partial sternotomy. There were no deaths and no major complications. Patients were discharged a median of four days postoperatively. The authors also concluded that the mini-sternotomy approach results in a cosmetically superior result for the patient without compromising safety.

Minimally invasive repair – right thoracotomy approach

A number of reports, particularly in the Asian literature, have described the use of a right anterolateral or posterolateral thoracotomy approach. For example Yoshimura et al[27] reviewed the long-term results of 126 patients in whom an ASD was closed through a right posterolateral thoracotomy. There was no operative or late mortality. The majority of patients were pleased with the cosmetic result.

Daebritz et al[28] described the use of a right anterolateral thoracotomy for ASD closure in 87 female patients. The mean age of the patients at the time of surgery was 20 years reflecting the fact that many of these patients were postpubertal. The problem of predicting the submammary fold in prepubertal patients is an important one. Breast deformity with this approach can be important.[20] Daebritz et al also mention the increased incidence of phrenic nerve damage as was previously identified by Helps et al.[29]

Comparison of interventional catheter and surgical closure of ASD

Numerous reports have appeared in recent years comparing interventional catheter and surgical methods for ASD closure. Very few of these reports describe a randomized or even a prospective comparison of these alternative methods for ASD closure.

In 2002, Hughes et al[30] reported a prospective observational study in which they compared standard surgical closure and catheter delivered device closure in 62 children. Nineteen of the patients had surgical repair and 43 had closure with an Amplatzer device. There were no differences in complications. None of the patients receiving devices required management in the intensive care unit or transfusion with blood products. The median values for postoperative pain score, analgesia use and convalescence time were greater for surgical patients. The median cost of the procedure was similar. Also in 2002, Du et al[31] described a multicenter, nonrandomized comparison of catheter delivered devices and surgery. A total of 442 patients were assigned to device closure and 154 patients to surgery. There were differences between the groups including the age at the time of the procedure and the size of the defect. The procedure was unsuccessful in 4% of the catheter assigned group and none of the surgical group. The authors concluded that there were no statistical differences in the success rates of patients in whom the procedure could be completed though the complication rate was lower and length of hospital stay was shorter for device closure. In a report from the United Kingdom, Thomson et al[32] compared 27 patients assigned for catheter delivered device closure with 19 patients who had surgical closure. In 11% of patients the attempt to close the defect with a device was unsuccessful. The authors concluded that there is a higher probability of requiring a second procedure if a patient is assigned to device closure. There were more complications in the surgical group but these were minor and did not require any change in management. Resolution of right ventricular dilation was similar for both techniques. However, the time spent in hospital and away from work or school was shorter for the device group. The cost of both techniques was similar.

In 2001 Cowley et al[33] compared the results of closure of secundum ASDs by surgery with device closure. Of 45 patients who were assigned to the catheter group, 36 had successful ASD closure with no residual shunts detectable by oximetry. All 44 patients assigned to surgery had successful ASD closure with no residual shunts. The authors conclude that there are advantages to both approaches for the treatment of secundum ASD. Transcatheter closure using the Amplatzer device has fewer short term complications, avoidance of cardioplegia and cardiopulmonary bypass, shorter hospitalization, reduced need for blood products and less patient discomfort. However, the surgeon's ability to close any ASD regardless of anatomy remains an important advantage of surgery. In 1999, Visconti et al[34] described a retrospective study in which developmental outcome was compared after surgical versus device closure of secundum ASD. There were important differences between the two groups including the age at the time of assessment. Patients in the device group were smaller at the time of closure and had smaller defects. Families of device patients tended to have a higher parent IQ, higher level of maternal education and higher level of maternal occupation. In regression analyses with adjustment for age at testing and parent IQ surgical repair was associated with a 9.5 point deficit in full scale IQ and a 9.7 point deficit in performance IQ. However, there were some tests in which surgical patients performed better than the device patients. Also scores of achievement were not different between the two groups. The only bypass related variable that had any trend towards significance was lowest hematocrit. These surgical patients were operated on in a timeframe when hematocrits as low as 13% were tolerated and not infrequently occurred because of larger priming volumes and less sophisticated circuits than are available currently.

Late complications of ASD devices

It is beyond the scope of this book to discuss the results of placement of catheter delivered devices in detail. However, surgical reports are beginning to appear regarding surgical management of late complications of ASD devices including hemopericardium and endocarditis. For example, Mellert et al[35] described five patients who required surgical procedures to deal with late complications of ASD devices. Three patients required emergency surgery, including one patient for hemopericardium with tamponade due to late cardiac perforation.

Late results of surgical closure of ASDs

A number of reports have described very long-term follow-up following ASD closure. For example, Murphy et al[36] studied 123 patients who had undergone closure of a secundum or sinus venosus ASD at the Mayo Clinic 27–32 years prior to review. The overall 30-year actuarial survival was 74% compared with 85% among matched controls. However, among patients in the younger two quartiles there were no differences in survival relative to controls, namely 97% and 93%. When repair was performed in older patients, late cardiac failure, stroke and atrial fibrillation were significantly more frequent. The authors conclude that it is important to close ASDs before the age of 25. Another long-term follow-up from the Cleveland Clinic by Moodie et al[37] reviewed 25-year outcome after ASD closure. The authors found excellent survival with low morbidity.

There has been concern that electrophysiological abnormalities have been seen late after ASD surgery. However, some studies have suggested that electrophysiological anomalies may be an inherent part of the ASD complex. For example, Karpawich et al[38] found that ASD closure improved nodal and atrial muscle electrophysiological function presumably by relieving stress on atrial impulse propagation. However, preoperatively sinus node recovery time was already prolonged and there was an abnormal AV nodal response to rapid atrial pacing in several patients. These anomalies persisted late postoperatively. A study by Gatzoulis[39] suggests that the risk of atrial flutter or fibrillation in adults with atrial septal defects is related to the age at the time of surgical repair and the pulmonary artery pressure. The authors recommend early closure of ASD to minimize the risk of late atrial flutter or fibrillation.

ASD repair in adults

A number of reports have reviewed the question regarding advisability of ASD closure in adults. For example Attie et al[40] reviewed 521 patients in Mexico City who were more than 40 years of age at the time they were referred for ASD treatment. The authors concluded that surgical closure was superior to medical treatment in reducing overall mortality and cardiovascular events. They recommend surgical closure for ASDs in adults more than 40 years of age so long as the pulmonary artery pressure is less than 70 mm and the pulmonary to systemic flow ratio is greater than 1.7 : 1. In a report by Jemielity et al[41] which reviewed 76 patients retrospectively in Poland who underwent surgical closure of ASDs at more than 40 years of age a similar conclusion was derived, namely that clinical status and right ventricular dilation can be improved by ASD closure.

The important problem of ASDs associated with pulmonary vascular obstructive disease was reviewed in 1987 by Steel et al from the Mayo Clinic.[42] Of 702 patients with an isolated ASD seen between 1953 and 1978, 6% had pulmonary vascular disease defined as a total pulmonary resistance greater than 7 units/m^2. Out of these 40 patients, 26 underwent surgical closure and 14 received medical treatment. All four surgically treated patients with a total pulmonary resistance of greater than 15 units/m^2 died. The authors concluded in this early study that high pulmonary resistance is uncommon in association with an ASD and that surgery should be undertaken if total pulmonary resistance is less than 15 units/m^2. Fortunately the problem of undiagnosed ASD has become exceedingly rare with more thorough screening of the general population. Echocardiography has also been important in differentiating an ASD from a benign murmur. Furthermore reactivity to nitric oxide as well as oxygen is now a helpful adjunct in the catheterization laboratory in deciding whether there is any reasonable chance that a patient may benefit from ASD closure.

Sinus venosus ASD

The innovative 'Warden' procedure for sinus venous ASD with partial anomalous pulmonary venous connection was initially described by Warden et al in 1984.[43] In 1989, Gustafson et al[44] updated the results of surgery for this procedure. A total of 27 patients with partial anomalous pulmonary connection underwent the Warden procedure between 1964 and 1987. One 31-year-old woman with severe pulmonary hypertension died early. In one patient a technical error resulted in SVC obstruction. One patient developed sick sinus syndrome. No patient other than the one mentioned developed SVC obstruction and there were no cases of pulmonary venous obstruction. Walker et al, from Children's Hospital Boston,[45] reviewed sinus node function following repair of sinus venosus defects. Even with traditional repair the incidence of sinus node dysfunction was rare.

Scimitar syndrome

Scimitar syndrome is a very rare anomaly. In a paper by Gao et al,[46] 13 consecutive infants with scimitar syndrome who underwent cardiac catheterization in the first six months of life at the Hospital for Sick Children in Toronto were reviewed. Twelve of the 13 patients had pulmonary hypertension at the time of diagnosis. Six patients died despite specific treatment. However, 11 of 13 infants had associated cardiac malformations and nine had large systemic arterial collateral vessels to the right lung. Seven patients had anomalies involving the left side of the heart, particularly hypoplasia of the left heart or aorta and six of these patients died. The authors concluded that the severe symptoms and pulmonary hypertension found in infants with scimitar syndrome can be caused by a number of associated anomalies. In many patients the important associated anomalies significantly increased the risk of death or serious complications.

REFERENCES

1. Edwards JE. Congenital malformations of the heart and great vessels. A. Malformations of the atrial septal complex. In Gould SE (ed). *Pathology of the Heart*, 2nd edn. CC Thomas, Springfield, IL, pp 260–293.
2. Van Mierop LHS. Embryology of the atrioventricular canal region and pathogenesis of endocardial cushion defects. In Feldt RH, McGoon DC, Ongley PA et al (eds). *Atrioventricular Canal Defects*. Philadelphia, WB Saunders, 1976.
3. Besterman E. Atrial septal defect with pulmonary hypertension. *Br Heart J* 1961; **23**:587–598.
4. Fyler DC, Buckley LP, Hellenbrand WE et al. Report of the New England Regional Infant Cardiac Program. *Pediatrics* 1980; **65**:376–460.
5. Rhee EK, Evangelista JK, Nigrin DJ, Erickson LC. Impact of anatomic closure on somatic growth among small, asymptomatic children with secundum atrial septal defect. *Am J Cardiol* 2000; **85**:1472–1475.
6. Lock JE, Keane JF, Perry SB (eds). *Diagnostic and Interventional Catheterization in Congenital Heart Disease*, 2nd edn. Boston, Kluwer Academic, 2000.
7. Chessa M, Carminati M, Cao QL et al. Transcatheter closure of congenital and acquired muscular ventricular septal defects using the Amplatzer device. *J Invasive Cardiol* 2002; **14**:322–327.
8. Rashkind W. Transcatheter treatment of congenital heart disease. *Circulation* 1983; **67**:711–716.
9. Beekman R, Rocchini A, Snider A, Rosenthal A. Transcatheter atrial septal defect closure: preliminary experience with the Rashkind occluder device. *J Intervent Cardiol* 1989; **2**:35–41.
10. Rocchini AP, Lock JE. Defect closure: umbrella devices (technology, methodology in atrial septal defect, ventricular septal defect, fenestrated Fontan, PDA, others. In Lock JE, Keane JF, Perry SB (eds). *Diagnostic and Interventional Catheterization in Congenital Heart Disease*, 2nd edn. Boston, Kluwer Academic, 2000, pp 179–198.
11. Fyler DC. Atrial septal defect secundum. In Fyler DC (ed). *Nadas' Pediatric Cardiology*. Philadelphia, Hanley & Belfus, 1992, pp 513–524.
12. Cockerham JT, Martin TC, Gutierrez FR, Hartmann AF Jr, Goldring D, Strauss AW. Spontaneous closure of secundum atrial septal defect in infants and young children. *Am J Cardiol* 1983; **52**:1267–1271.
13. Bailey CP, Nichols HT, Bolton HE et al. Surgical treatment of forty-six interatrial septal defects by atrio-septo-pexy. *Ann Surg* 1954; **140**:805–815.
14. Sondergaard T. Closure of atrial septal defects: Report of three cases. *Acta Chir Scan* 1954; **107**:492–496.
15. Gross RE, Pomeranz AA, Watkis E Jr et al. Surgical closure of defects of the interauricular septum by use of an atrial well. *N Engl J Med* 1952; **247**:455–461.
16. Lewis FJ, Taufic M. Closure of atrial septal defects with the aid of hypothermia. Experimental accomplishments and the report of one successful case. *Surgery* 1953; **33**:52–59.
17. Gibbons JH. Application of a mechanical heart-lung apparatus to cardiac surgery. *Minn Med* 1954; **March**:171–175.
18. del Nido PJ, Bichell DP. Minimal-access surgery for congenital heart defects. *Semin Thorac Cardiovasc Surg* 1998; **10**:75–80.
19. Gundry SR, Shattuck OH, Razzouk AJ, del Rio MJ, Sardari FF, Bailey LL. Facile minimally invasive cardiac surgery via ministernotomy. *Ann Thorac Surg* 1998; **65**:1100–1104.
20. Cherup LL, Siewers RD, Futrell JW. Breast and pectoral muscle maldevelopment after anterolateral and posterolateral thoracotomies in children. *Ann Thorac Surg* 1996; **41**:492–497.
21. Houyel L, Petit J, Planche C et al. [Right postero-lateral thoracotomy for open heart surgery in infants and children. Indications and results.] *Arch Mal Coeur Vaiss* 1999; **92**:641–646.
22. Mavroudis C. VATS ASD closure: a time not yet come. *Ann Thorac Surg* 1996; **62**:638–639.
23. Jones DA, Radford DJ, Pohlner PG. Outcome following surgical closure of secundum atrial septal defect. *J Paediatr Child Health* 2001; **37**:274–277.
24. Bichell DP, Geva T, Bacha EA, Mayer JE, Jonas RA, del Nido PJ. Minimal access approach for the repair of atrial septal defect: the initial 135 patients. *Ann Thorac Surg* 2000; **70**:115–118.
25. Laussen PC, Bichell DP, McGowan FX, Zurakowski D, DeMaso DR, del Nido PJ. Postoperative recovery in children after minimum versus full-length sternotomy. *Ann Thorac Surg* 2000; **69**:591–596.
26. Khan JH, McElhinney DB, Reddy VM, Hanley FL. A 5-year experience with surgical repair of atrial septal defect employing limited exposure. *Cardiol Young* 1999; **9**:572–576.
27. Yoshimura N, Yamaguchi M, Oshima Y, Oka S, Ootaki Y, Yoshida M. Repair of atrial septal defect through a right posterolateral thoracotomy: a cosmetic approach for female patients. *Ann Thorac Surg* 2001; **72**:2103–2105.
28. Daebritz S, Sachweh J, Walter M, Messmer BJ. Closure of atrial septal defects via limited right anterolateral thoracotomy as a minimal invasive approach in female patients. *Eur J Cardiothorac Surg* 1999; **15**:18–23.
29. Helps BA, Ross-Russell RI, Dicks-Mireaux C, Elliott MJ. Phrenic nerve damage via a right thoracotomy in older children with secundum ASD. *Ann Thorac Surg* 1993; **56**:328–330.
30. Hughes ML, Maskell G, Goh TH, Wilkinson JL. Prospective comparison of costs and short term health outcomes of surgical versus device closure of atrial septal defect in children. *Heart* 2002; **88**:67–70.
31. Du ZD, Hijazi ZM, Kleinman CS, Silverman NH, Larntz K. Comparison between transcatheter and surgical closure of

secundum atrial septal defect in children and adults: results of a multicenter nonrandomized trial. *J Am Coll Cardiol* 2002; **39**:1836–1844.

32. Thomson JD, Aburawi EH, Watterson KG, Van Doorn C, Gibbs JL. Surgical and transcatheter (Amplatzer) closure of atrial septal defects: a prospective comparison of results and cost. *Heart* 2002; **87**:466–469.
33. Cowley CG, Lloyd TR, Bove EL, Gaffney D, Dietrich M, Rocchini AP. Comparison of results of closure of secundum atrial septal defect by surgery versus Amplatzer septal occluder. *Am J Cardiol* 2001; **88**:589–591.
34. Visconti KJ, Bichell DP, Jonas RA, Newburger JW, Bellinger DC. Developmental outcome after surgical versus interventional closure of secundum atrial septal defect in children. *Circulation* 1999; **100**:II145–150.
35. Mellert F, Preusse CJ, Haushofer M et al. Surgical management of complications caused by transcatheter ASD closure. *Thorac Cardiovasc Surg* 2001; **49**:338–342.
36. Murphy JG, Gersh BJ, McGoon MD et al. Long-term outcome after surgical repair of isolated atrial septal defect. *New Eng J Med* 1990; **323**:1645–1650.
37. Moodie DS, Sterba R. Long-term outcomes excellent for atrial septal defect repair in adults. *Cleve Clin J Med* 2000; **67**:591–597.
38. Karpawich PP, Antillon JR, Cappola PR, Agarwal KC. Pre- and postoperative electrophysiologic assessment of children with secundum atrial septal defect. *Am J Cardiol* 1985; **55**:519–521.
39. Gatzoulis MA, Freeman MA, Siu SC, Webb GD, Harris L. Atrial arrhythmia after surgical closure of atrial septal defects in adults. *N Engl J Med* 1999; **340**:839–846.
40. Attie F, Rosas M, Granados N, Zabal C, Buendia A, Calderon J. Surgical treatment for secundum atrial septal defects in patients >40 years old. *J Am Coll Cardiol* 2001; **38**:2035–2042.
41. Jemielity M, Dyszkiewicz W, Paluszkiewicz L, Perek B, Buczkowski P, Ponizynski A. Do patients over 40 years of age benefit from surgical closure of atrial septal defects? *Heart* 2001; **85**:300–303.
42. Steele PM, Fuster V, Cohen M, Ritter DG, McGoon DC. Isolated atrial septal defect with pulmonary vascular obstructive disease – long term follow-up and prediction of outcome after surgical correction. *Circulation* 1987; **76**:1037–1042.
43. Warden HE, Gustafson RA, Tarnay TJ, Neal WA. An alternative method for repair of partial anomalous pulmonary venous connection to the superior vena cava. *Ann Thorac Surg* 1984; **38**:601–605.
44. Gustafson RA, Warden HE, Murray GF, Hill RC, Rozar GE. Partial anomalous pulmonary venous connection to the right side of the heart. *J Thorac Cardiovasc Surg* 1989; **98**:861–868.
45. Walker RE, Mayer JE, Alexander ME, Walsh EP, Berul CI. Paucity of sinus node dysfunction following repair of sinus venosus defects in children. *Am J Cardiol* 2001; **87**:1223–1226.
46. Gao YA, Burrows PE, Benson LN, Rabinovitch M, Freedom RM. Scimitar syndrome in infancy. *J Am Coll Cardiol* 1993; **22**:873–882.

14

Ventricular septal defect

INTRODUCTION

Although a bicuspid aortic valve is the most common congenital cardiac anomaly, ventricular septal defects are the commonest anomalies managed by pediatric cardiologists and cardiac surgeons.[1] There are a number of anatomical variants. Because many VSDs have the potential to close spontaneously while others have the potential to cause pulmonary vascular disease, they present a challenge to the pediatric cardiologist and cardiac surgeon most particularly in the area of indications and timing of surgery. Unlike surgical closure of an ASD, surgical closure of a VSD can present a number of technical challenges to the congenital cardiac surgeon.

EMBRYOLOGY

After the primitive cardiac tube has looped either in a dextro (d-loop) or levo (l-loop) direction during the fourth week of gestation, septation of the ventricular component of the cardiac tube begins from what will ultimately be the diaphragmatic or inferior surface of the heart.[2] The muscular intraventricular septum forms by an infolding of ventricular muscle. It will usually align with the conal septum which separates the right ventricular outflow tract from the left ventricular outflow tract. Van Praagh has described the way in which the muscular intraventricular septum from below interdigitates with the conal septum in the Y formed by the bifurcation of the septal band.[3] The final area of closure of the ventricular septum is the membranous area adjacent to the anteroseptal commissure of the tricuspid valve. The membranous septum lies below the anterior half of the non coronary leaflet of the aortic valve and under the commissure between the non and right coronary leaflets. Septation is usually complete between 38 and 45 days of gestation.

ANATOMY

It is important at all times to remember that the ventricular septum is not a straight wall between the right ventricle and left ventricle, as it is often represented in two-dimensional diagrams. It is a curved structure because of the circular shape of the normal left ventricle and the crescent shape of the right ventricle which wraps around the anterior and rightward aspects of the left ventricle (Figure 14.1). It is also important to remember that the structure of the ventricular septum varies according to location. For example, as viewed from the left ventricular aspect the septum is smooth walled with fine trabeculations as is seen in the remainder of the left ventricle. At the apex of the right ventricle the septum is heavily trabeculated. In the region of the right ventricular outflow the septum is much less heavily trabeculated particularly in the region of the conal septum itself. The septal band extends inferiorly from the conal septum and continues as the moderator band which connects to the anterior papillary muscle of the tricuspid valve which arises from the parietal, i.e. free wall of the right ventricle. The septal band separates what is classified as the anterior muscular septum and what is predominantly the outflow component of the septum from the sinus or inflow component of the ventricular septum. The mid-muscular septum is a poorly defined area that is approximately in the middle of the ventricular septum between the apex of the right ventricle and the pulmonary valve as well as being in the middle of the axis connecting the diaphragmatic surface of the heart to the anterior free wall.

Perimembranous (paramembranous, membranous, subaortic, infracristal) VSD

When the membranous area of the ventricular septum fails to form completely, a ventricular septal defect results adjacent to the commissure between the anterior and septal

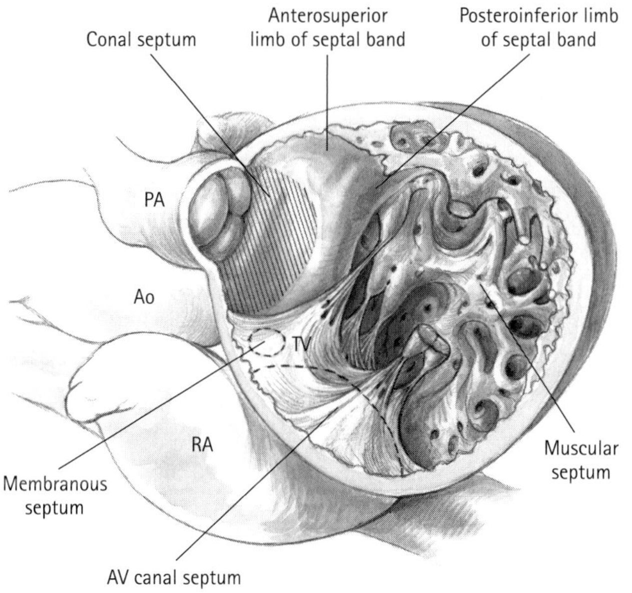

Figure 14.1 *A view of the right ventricular aspect of the ventricular septum showing the components of the ventricular septum, i.e. the muscular interventricular septum, AV canal septum, membranous septum and conal septum.*

leaflets of the tricuspid valve. Not only is this type of defect in the *membranous* area but in addition it is likely to be surrounded by fibrous, *membranous* tissue (Figure 14.2). It is this fibrous tissue which can gradually result in spontaneous closure of the perimembranous VSD. This fibrous tissue has also been termed 'accessory tricuspid valve tissue'. On occasion it forms a 'windsock' type structure. Van Praagh has distinguished the true membranous VSD, which is a small defect limited exclusively to the area of the membranous septum, from a larger 'paramembranous' VSD which is a more accurate term than perimembranous VSD, a literal interpretation of which would imply that the membranous area is intact and that there is a defect surrounding the membranous area.[4] Nevertheless the term perimembranous is in common usage. The perimembranous VSD is intimately associated with the bundle of His which in a d-loop heart passes through the tricuspid annulus at the posterior and inferior corner of the VSD. The bundle soon branches into the right and left bundle branch (Figure 14.3).

Conoventricular (subaortic, infracristal) VSD

The conoventricular VSD, a term developed by the Van Praaghs, describes a VSD which lies between the conal and muscular interventricular septa[4,5] (see Figure 14.2). It is frequently associated with at least some degree of malalignment of the conal septum relative to the muscular septum, for example, the anterior malalignment VSD of tetralogy or the posterior malalignment VSD of interrupted aortic arch. Unlike a perimembranous VSD the conoventricular VSD is almost always large and unrestrictive to pressure. It does not have fibrous margins but is muscular other than in the region where there may be fibrous continuity between the tricuspid and aortic valve. The defect usually extends more superiorly

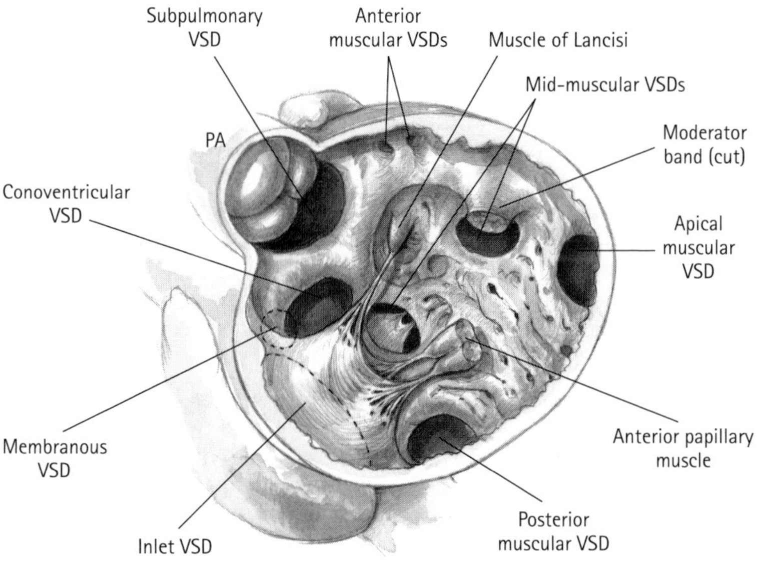

Figure 14.2 *There are many synonyms for the different morphological subtypes of ventricular septal defect. The nomenclature system used at Children's Hospital Boston classifies a VSD as membranous, conoventricular, inlet, subpulmonary or muscular.*

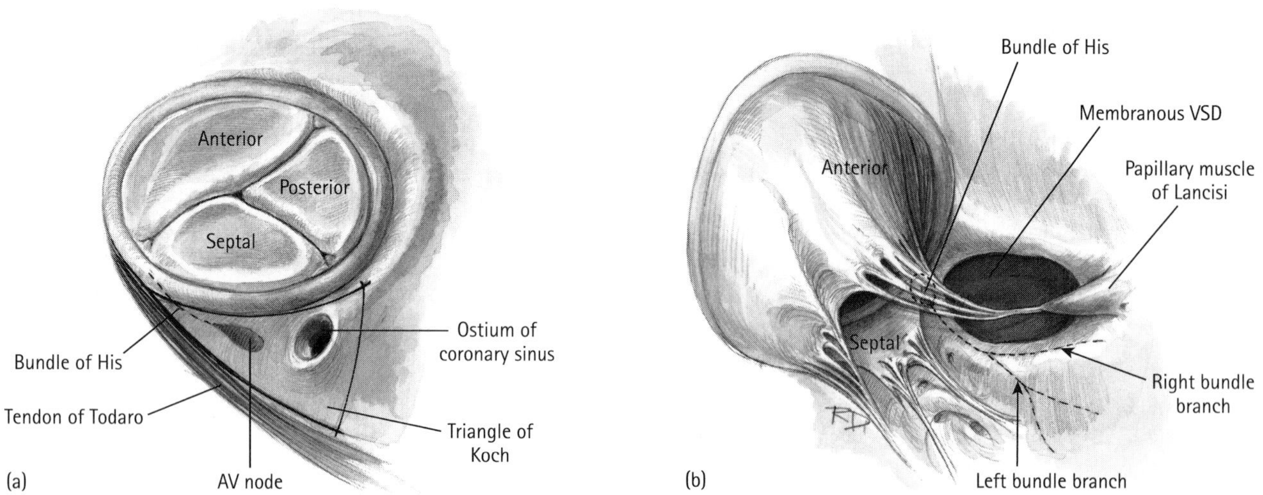

Figure 14.3 *(a) Atrial view – the bundle of His originates from the AV node in the triangle of Koch, which is bounded by the tendon of Todaro, the tricuspid annulus and the coronary sinus. The bundle penetrates the fibrous skeleton of the heart close to the anteroseptal commissure of the tricuspid valve. (b) Ventricular view of a membranous VSD which is intimately associated with the bundle of His. The papillary muscle of Lancisi is a useful landmark which indicates the point beyond which the bundle has bifurcated into the right bundle branch and left bundle branch.*

and anteriorly than a perimembranous VSD. Like the perimembranous VSD it is close to the bundle of His which penetrates the fibrous skeleton of the heart, i.e. the tricuspid annulus at its posterior and inferior margin.

Subpulmonary (supracristal, conal, intraconal) VSD

The subpulmonary VSD is very much more common in oriental populations than it is in Western countries.[6] As the name suggests, this defect lies closely adjacent and immediately below the pulmonary valve (see Figure 14.2). It is usually a defect within the conal septum and can therefore also be termed an intraconal VSD. Because this defect lies immediately below the belly of the right coronary cusp of the aortic valve, there is an important risk of aortic valve prolapse and subsequent aortic valve regurgitation developing. This defect is quite distant from the bundle of His so that the risk of complete heart block during surgical closure should be extremely small.

Inlet (atrioventricular canal type) VSD

The inlet septum or AV canal septum is formed from endocardial cushion tissue. When deficient there is a defect immediately below the septal leaflet of the tricuspid valve (see Figure 14.2). There is no muscle between the tricuspid annulus and an inlet defect. An inlet VSD is the most likely type of defect to be associated with straddling atrioventricular valve chordae (see below).

An inlet 'extension' is not uncommonly associated with a conoventricular type VSD. An inlet VSD may coexist with a perimembranous VSD, with a bar of muscle running between the two defects. This bar of muscle presumably also carries the bundle of His.

Muscular VSD

VSDs can occur anywhere in the muscular intraventricular septum and are termed 'muscular VSDs' (see Figure 14.2). Probably the most common location is in the mid-muscular septum. These defects are closely related to the point where the moderator band arises from the septal band. It is usually possible to pass an instrument both below and above the origin of the moderator band through the ventricular septum when there is a mid-muscular VSD. Another common location for muscular VSDs is in the anterior muscular septum immediately anterior to the point where the septal band bifurcates to encompass the conal septum. Apical muscular VSDs can be particularly difficult for the surgeon to identify since they occur in the heavy trabeculated apical component of the right ventricle. The Van Praaghs have described an apical recess in the right ventricle into which many apical muscular VSDs open.[7,8]

ASSOCIATED ANOMALIES

A VSD is one component of many anomalies including tetralogy of Fallot, double outlet right ventricle, complete AV canal, and interrupted aortic arch. It is seen in about one third of patients who have transposition of the great arteries. In any anomaly where there is a large left to right shunt, including an isolated VSD, there is likely to be hypoplasia of the ascending aorta and aortic arch. There may also be an associated coarctation. Because of the large volume of blood returning to the left atrium the foramen ovale may become 'stretched' and allow a left to right shunt at atrial level as well as ventricular level. There may also be a true associated secundum ASD or patent ductus arteriosus.

Double chambered right ventricle, aortic valve prolapse and regurgitation

Over time, some patients with a VSD will develop muscular obstruction within the mid-body of the right ventricle creating a 'double chambered right ventricle'. Children whose moderator band is situated a little more towards the outflow region of the right ventricle may be at greater risk of developing this problem.[9] Another acquired anomaly, which can occur as early as three or four years of age but usually later, is prolapse of the aortic valve resulting in associated aortic regurgitation.[10]

Straddling tricuspid or mitral chordae

Chordae are described as 'straddling' when they pass from their ventricle of origin through a VSD and attach to the contralateral AV valve. This is most commonly seen when the VSD is of the inlet type. The term straddling should be distinguished from 'overriding' which describes the relationship of an AV valve to the underlying ventricle, e.g. a tricuspid valve may partially override the left ventricle but there may or may not be straddling of tricuspid chords into the left ventricle. Nevertheless straddling of chords is more likely in the setting of an overriding AV valve.

PATHOPHYSIOLOGY AND CLINICAL FEATURES

An isolated VSD results in a left to right shunt at ventricular level. This causes an increase in pulmonary blood flow, i.e. $Q_p : Q_s > 1$. It may also result in an increase in pulmonary artery pressure depending on both the magnitude of the left to right shunt as well as the pulmonary resistance.

In the newborn pulmonary resistance is relatively high. It usually decreases substantially in the first days of life with a continuing important decline over the next four to six weeks and a slow gradual decline beyond that for several months. However, because of the high resistance at birth it is not uncommon for a VSD to be undetected initially since there may be insufficient left to right shunt to result in a clearly audible murmur. Over the first four to six weeks of life an increasingly loud murmur may develop and is often accompanied by the onset of symptoms of congestive heart failure. Thus the child will become increasingly tachypneic, particularly related to feeding. There may be sweating, also usually associated with feeding. Most importantly the child will fail to gain weight. Physical examination usually demonstrates hepatomegaly. It is usually possible to manage the symptoms of congestive heart failure with appropriate medical therapy including digoxin and lasix. However, if the pulmonary resistance falls to a very low level and if the ventricles are not capable of generating an extremely elevated cardiac output without a substantial increase in filling pressures, then the child is likely to fail to thrive and will progressively fall off the growth curve.

However, this does not happen to all children. In some patients, most commonly those who start with a relatively smaller VSD, there can be quite rapid accumulation of fibrous tissue around the margins of the VSD, particularly a perimembranous VSD. This tissue will decrease the size of the defect and may ultimately result in its complete closure. Muscular VSDs also appear to have an increased propensity to spontaneous closure. Perhaps the muscular hypertrophy that results from increased ventricular pressure contributes to closure of the muscular VSD. Gradual spontaneous closure of a VSD results in the interesting change in physical examination whereby the murmur becomes increasingly prominent because the velocity of the jet passing through the defect increases. This can be documented by echocardiography as an increasing Doppler gradient across the VSD, i.e. paradoxically the smaller the VSD the louder the murmur. Eventually when the defect closes completely the murmur disappears.

Unfortunately a gradual improvement in symptoms during the first year of life does not necessarily mean that the VSD has become smaller. As a result of the increased flow and pressure in the pulmonary resistance vessels there is likely to be both intimal proliferation as well as smooth muscle hypertrophy of the media of pulmonary arterioles. This is the beginning of pulmonary vascular disease. In fact in some patients there is a complete failure of transition from the normal fetal pulmonary vasculature to the more mature state in which smooth muscle extends less distally into the pulmonary artery tree. With further progression of vascular disease pulmonary arterioles become fibrosed and even occluded with thrombus. There may be formation of arteriovenous malformations and fibrinoid necrosis.[11–13] The exact sequence of histopathological changes of pulmonary vascular disease is poorly understood since pulmonary vascular disease today is exceedingly rare. It is difficult to predict which children will develop an early and accelerated form of pulmonary vascular disease. There is almost certainly an individual predisposition which at present cannot be predicted. Although in general it is unlikely that a child will develop fixed and irreversible pulmonary vascular disease from a simple VSD earlier than about two years of age, nevertheless there are many exceptions to this rule. Accordingly the child who initially starts with congestive heart failure early in life and who is known to have a relatively large VSD and who subsequently appears to have a reduction in symptoms should be very carefully assessed.

DIAGNOSTIC STUDIES

The plain chest X-ray demonstrates that the child with a VSD and important left to right shunt has enlargement of both ventricles as well as the left atrium. The pulmonary arteries are prominent and the lung fields are congested and plethoric. The ECG will demonstrate right ventricular hypertrophy if right ventricular pressure is elevated either because of a relatively unrestrictive VSD or an elevation in pulmonary resistance. Echocardiography is diagnostic. Doppler color flow mapping now allows extremely sensitive detection of even tiny VSDs.[14] Echocardiography is also very helpful in localizing a VSD since the defect can be viewed in many different planes. This is in contrast to the situation with cineangiography in the catheterization laboratory where generally a limited number of dye injections are made. If there are multiple defects there may be overlap such that the multiple nature of the VSDs is not detected. Magnetic resonance imaging is emerging as a new modality that will be helpful in localizing VSDs in the future, although it is unlikely to exceed the sensitivity of echocardiography with color flow mapping.

MEDICAL AND INTERVENTIONAL THERAPY

The medical treatment of a VSD resulting in congestive heart failure is the standard medical treatment for congestive heart failure. The child's status must be very carefully monitored by the pediatric cardiologist since there can be important failure to thrive which is probably associated with developmental delay. A large left to right shunt also is associated with an important risk of serious viral respiratory infection, particularly respiratory syncitial virus (RSV) during the winter months. An RSV pneumonia in a child with a large VSD can be fatal. The cardiologist will need to adjust the child's medical therapy dosage as the child grows. There must be regular assessment of pulmonary artery pressure and the size of the VSD so as to assess the ongoing risk of pulmonary vascular disease.

Catheter delivered device closure of VSDs

The majority of VSDs are intimately associated with either inlet or outlet valves and/or chordal support apparatus of the tricuspid valve. For this reason it seems unlikely that catheter delivered devices will ever be able to achieve accurate and complete closure for the majority of VSDs without endangering valve function. On the other hand muscular VSDs are ideally suited to device closure. Because the left ventricular aspect of any of the muscular VSDs is smooth walled and finely trabeculated, a device can fit flush against the left ventricular aspect of the ventricular septum. The higher pressure in the left ventricle serves to seal the device against the ventricular septum. Catheter delivered devices have indeed proven to be particularly successful in muscular VSD closure and are at present our method of choice for muscular VSD closure.[15] The only limitation relates to the large sheath size that is required which necessitates the child being at least 8–10 kg in weight. Therefore it may be necessary to place a pulmonary artery band to protect the pulmonary vasculature as well as to reduce symptoms of congestive heart failure. Regrettably this subsequently requires the child to undergo a surgical procedure for removal of the pulmonary artery band and reconstruction of the main pulmonary artery.

INDICATIONS FOR SURGERY

The decision regarding timing of surgery and indications for surgery for an isolated VSD is a complex one. Fortunately the risks of surgery are now so low with a mortality rate of well under 1% that it should not be necessary to accept even a relatively small risk that a child will develop pulmonary vascular disease.

Symptoms

If a child has persistent symptoms in spite of medical therapy, surgical closure of the VSD is definitely indicated. Symptoms not uncommonly include failure to thrive with the child falling progressively off the growth curve as well as frequent respiratory infections.

PULMONARY ARTERY PRESSURE GREATER THAN HALF SYSTEMIC

If the pulmonary artery pressure is assessed to be greater than about 50% of systemic pressure, then it is advisable to undertake surgical closure by the end of the first year of life at the latest. Often a defect that results in greater than 50% systemic pressure in the pulmonary arteries is clearly a large defect which probably has a low probability of spontaneous closure. This is definitely the case if the defect is situated in the inlet septum or is a true conoventricular or subpulmonary type VSD. If imaging demonstrates accumulation of fibrous tissue particularly as a windsock or aneurysm in the membranous area then there may be a higher probability of spontaneous closure. If echocardiography has documented a large VSD with pulmonary artery pressure greater than 50% of systemic pressure it is probably advisable to proceed with VSD closure early in infancy.

PULMONARY ARTERY PRESSURE LESS THAN HALF SYSTEMIC

The child whose pulmonary artery pressure is less than half systemic is unlikely to develop pulmonary vascular disease and can in general be safely followed for several years. However, it is important to remember that a VSD, particularly in the subpulmonary as well as membranous area, can be associated with aortic valve prolapse. Therefore the child needs to be closely monitored with regular examinations including echocardiography to observe the competence and anatomy of the aortic valve. Hopefully there will be evidence of progressive closure of the defect which will encourage an approach of ongoing conservative therapy rather than proceeding to surgery. There is, however, an ongoing risk of bacterial endocarditis so the parents need to receive frequent reinforcement regarding the importance of antibiotic prophylaxis in association with dental work or other invasive procedures.

Very small VSD in the teenager or young adult

There is ongoing controversy regarding the need to close very small defects. Many argue that VSDs are rarely found in middle aged or elderly adults at routine autopsy suggesting that spontaneous closure of VSDs can occur in later life. On the other hand others argue that the ongoing risk of bacterial endocarditis as well as the need for regular surveillance for monitoring of the aortic valve argue in favor of surgical closure of the very small defect by the time a child reaches mid-teenage years.[16] A counter argument that has been postulated is that VSD closure may not change the risk of bacterial endocarditis.[17,18] The usual recommendation is that antibiotic prophylaxis should be continued even when VSD closure has been successfully achieved.

SURGICAL MANAGEMENT

History of surgery

The concept of banding the main pulmonary artery to reduce pulmonary artery pressure and thereby palliate the child with a VSD was introduced by Muller and Dammann in 1952.[19] In 1954 Lillehei et al[20] described VSD closure using cross circulation in which one parent functioned as the oxygenator for the child during the procedure. Rather remarkably for the time, five of the first eight patients were infants and three of these survived. VSD closure employing cardiopulmonary bypass with the heart lung machine was first described by Kirklin et al in 1955.[21] Lillehei and Kirklin used a ventriculotomy to approach the VSD. The concept of transatrial closure was introduced by Stirling et al in 1958.[22] Despite initial attempts to perform primary repair of VSDs in the 1950s the mortality was so high in these days that a two stage approach evolved with initial pulmonary artery banding and later repair for patients who were importantly symptomatic in infancy. It was not until 1969 that Barratt-Boyes et al popularized the concept of early primary repair of infants with a large VSD.[23] Barratt-Boyes was able to demonstrate that the combination of surface cooling, brief cooling on cardiopulmonary bypass, a period of circulatory arrest with subsequent rewarming using a combination of cardiopulmonary bypass and surface warming could be undertaken with a remarkably low mortality.

Cardiopulmonary bypass setup

Most VSDs are closed today using continuous mildly or moderately hypothermic cardiopulmonary bypass. The ascending aorta is cannulated in a routine fashion. Caval cannulation with metal tipped right angle cannulas is often convenient though straight cannulas inserted through the atrium can also be used. The pH stat strategy should be employed and the hematocrit should be maintained at at least 30%. When bypass flow has been stabilized the ascending aorta is cross clamped and cardioplegic solution is infused into the root of the aorta. Caval tourniquets are then tightened. Deep hypothermic circulatory arrest is useful in very small children, i.e. babies less than 3–3.5 kg. In a small baby who has pulmonary hypertension and in whom circulatory arrest will be used it is advisable to ligate the ductus arteriosus even if patency has not been demonstrated. In fact there may be little flow across a patent ductus in the setting of pulmonary hypertension caused by the VSD. Furthermore during the circulatory arrest period there is a potential for air to enter the aortic arch when blood is drained from the pulmonary artery and right ventricle.

Technical considerations

The incision for all procedures is a median sternotomy. A minimally invasive partial sternotomy can be used but is not routine. When the usual right atrial approach is employed as it is for most VSDs it is helpful to lift the right side of the pericardium but to avoid pericardial suspension sutures on the left side. The operating table is positioned away from the surgeon. Often some degree of Trendelenberg tilt is also helpful.

RIGHT ATRIAL APPROACH

The majority of VSDs are closed working through a right atriotomy and through the tricuspid valve. The exceptions to this are the anterior malalignment VSD of tetralogy where there is important ventricular obstruction and a ventriculotomy will be used to relieve right ventricular outflow tract obstruction. The same infundibular incision is employed for VSD closure. A subpulmonary VSD is generally best approached through an incision in the pulmonary artery and an apical VSD may occasionally be best approached through an apical right ventricular incision.

The right atrial free wall should be studied before an incision is made in order to determine the blood supply of the sinus node. Quite often a large vessel will run from the middle of the right AV groove across the right atrial free wall to the sinus node. It is helpful to plan the atrial incision to avoid division of this vessel (Figure 14.4a). It is also best to avoid division of the crista terminalis. An appropriate retractor is placed in the atrial incision and passes though the tricuspid annulus. Care should be taken to avoid excessive retraction of the tricuspid annulus as this can not only result in complete heart block but can also damage the ventricular muscle of the neonate and young infant. The VSD is identified at the commissure between the septal and anterior leaflets of the tricuspid valve if it is either a perimembranous VSD or a conoventricular type VSD.

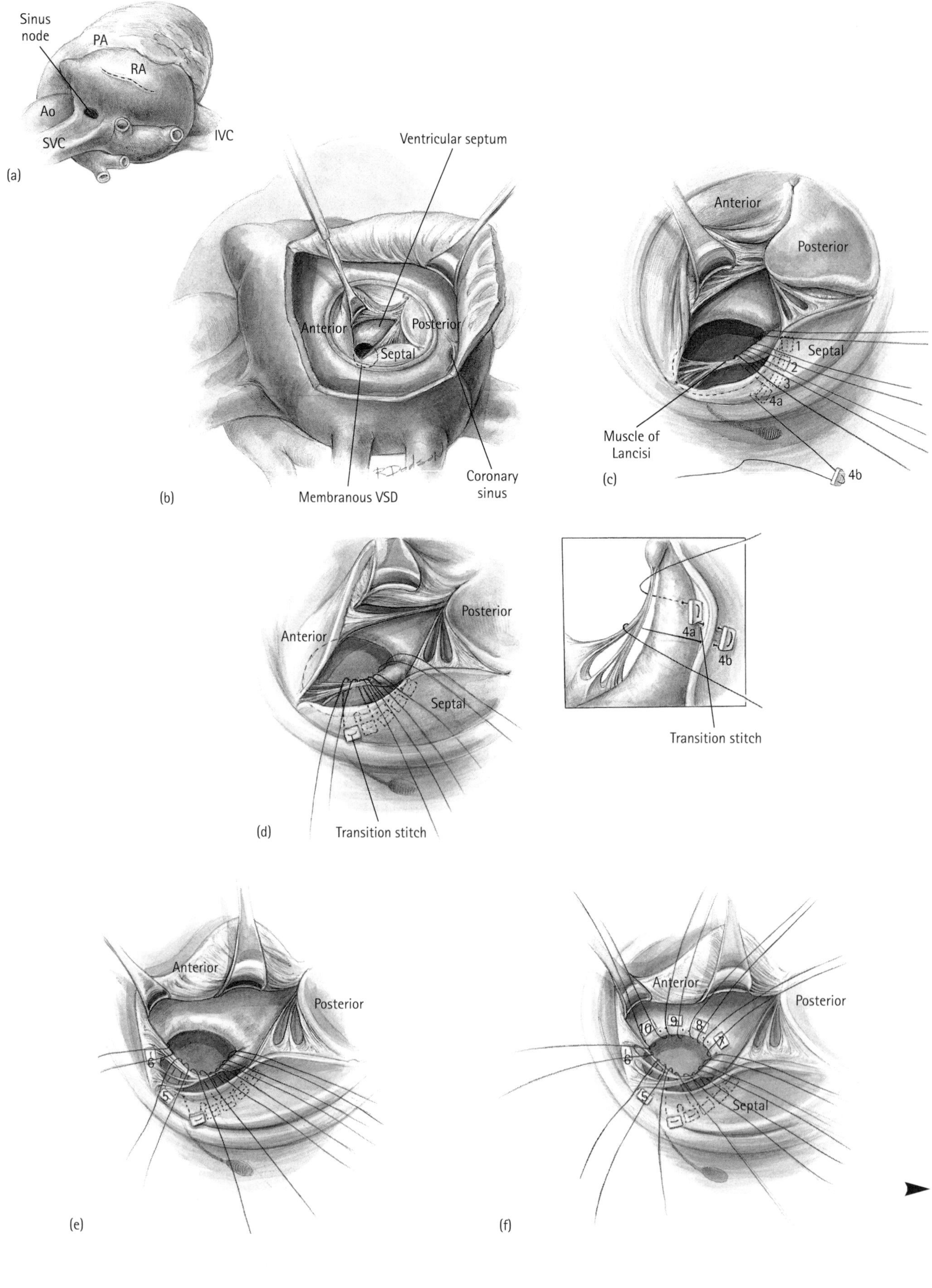
Sinus node
PA
RA
Ao
SVC
IVC
(a)
Ventricular septum
Anterior
Posterior
Septal
Membranous VSD
Coronary sinus
(b)
Anterior
Posterior
Septal
1
2
3
4a
4b
Muscle of Lancisi
(c)
Anterior
Posterior
Septal
Transition stitch
(d)
4a
4b
Transition stitch
Anterior
Posterior
6
5
(e)
Anterior
Posterior
Septal
10
9
8
7
6
5
(f)

SUTURE PLACEMENT FOR THE PERIMEMBRANOUS OR CONOVENTRICULAR VSD

Although it is possible to close VSDs in neonates and infants with a continuous technique, use of an interrupted pledgetted technique, using braided polyester sutures with very small Teflon pledgets allows more consistent and secure closure of VSDs in very small infants and neonates. The initial suture is placed at 3–4 o'clock as indicated in Figure 14.4c. Sutures are placed sequentially working in a clockwise direction with great care in the region of the conduction bundle at the posterior and inferior angle of the defect. It is particularly important that the needle should not only enter the right ventricular aspect of the septum but should also exit the right ventricular aspect of the septum. As sutures approach the tricuspid annulus they should be placed at least 2 or 3 mm inferior to the inferior margin of the defect (Figure 14.4c). In fact it is usually advisable to use a 'transition' stitch as demonstrated in Figures 14.4c,d. Two pledgets are used for the transition stitch, one lies against the muscle of the ventricular septum while the second lies on the right atrial aspect of the septal leaflet of the tricuspid valve. An additional two or three sutures are placed backhand through the septal leaflet close to but not in the annulus of the tricuspid valve with the pledgets also lying on the right atrial aspect of the tricuspid valve (Figure 14.4e). The most superior of these atrial sutures will pass through the leaflet very close to the annulus and emerge in conal septal muscle. With this suture also it is important that the tip of the needle remain on the right ventricular aspect of the septum. If the suture were to be passed through into the left ventricular aspect of the septum there would be a risk of injuring the aortic valve. If there is any doubt as to the exact location of the aortic valve it is helpful to infuse cardioplegia solution briefly. This often demonstrates that the aortic valve is immediately adjacent to this most cephalad suture. Occasionally it is helpful to place a transition suture at the superior and posterior corner analogous to the transition suture placed at the inferior and posterior corner.

Suturing is now begun again from the start point at 3–4 o'clock (Figure 14.4f) and is taken in a counterclockwise direction. Each previous suture is used for retraction to expose the superior margin of the VSD. Exposure in this area can be particularly difficult when there is a large conoventricular VSD and particularly when the conal septum is anteriorly malaligned. Often a combination of traction on the suture that was placed at the superior and posterior corner as well as traction on the most recently placed suture aids in the exposure of the final difficult superior-most aspect of the VSD.

PATCH MATERIAL

Generally a choice is made between one of three different materials for VSD closure. As discussed in Chapter 3, knitted Dacron velour is an excellent material to use for the majority of VSDs. It is reasonably flexible and will mold to the irregular contours of most VSDs. It excites a fibrous reaction that is probably helpful in sealing off tiny residual VSDs that are often seen by echocardiography in the early postoperative period. On the other hand, if the VSD patch is more of a baffle as for VSD closure for double outlet right ventricle or transposition of the great arteries with a Rastelli procedure, then the fibrosis that is stimulated can be a disadvantage since it may increase the risk of left ventricular outflow tract obstruction. Under these circumstances autologous pericardium treated with glutaraldehyde is often preferred, particularly when the material must adopt a complex three-dimensional shape. Under these circumstances Dacron may buckle or kink inwards in spite of the higher pressure on its left ventricular aspect. Pericardium or stretch PTFE is probably also preferable when the VSD patch will lie against a valve leaflet as is often the case, for example, with a subpulmonary VSD.

CUTTING THE PATCH

It is important to remember that the patch should be cut slightly larger than the suture line which is quite a bit larger than the VSD itself. There should be a margin of at least 1.5 mm from the edge of the patch to be sure that each of the mattress sutures will lie entirely on the surface of the patch itself. The sutures are passed carefully through the patch when it is has been cut and it is then threaded down into position. It should not be necessary for these sutures as they are tied to bring the patch down into contact with the ventricular septum; the patch should already be lying in the appropriate location before these sutures are tied.

SUTURE TYING

Tying of VSD sutures must be done with great delicacy since the muscle is very soft in the neonate and young infant in particular. It is very easy to overtie these sutures and to cause the muscle to tear. Even the tearing out of one suture can result in an unacceptable residual VSD. Each suture should

Figure 14.4 *(a) The incision in the right atrial free wall used to approach a membranous VSD should be planned to avoid injury to coronary vessels which sometimes run from the right AV groove to the sinus node. (b) A membranous VSD is exposed at the anteroseptal commissure of the tricuspid valve. Retraction of the anterior leaflet improves exposure of the defect. (c) Interrupted pledgetted sutures are placed several millimeters below the inferior margin of a membranous VSD in order to avoid injury to the bundle of His. A transition stitch (pledgets 4a and 4b) is helpful in laying the patch directly over the bundle. (d – inset) The transition stitch is completed by passing the suture back through the septal leaflet of the tricuspid valve so that one pledget lies under the leaflet while one lies on the atrial aspect of the septal leaflet. (e) Additional sutures (pledgets 5 and 6) are placed through the septal leaflet (not the tricuspid annulus). (f) Remaining sutures (pledgets 7–10) are placed working in a counterclockwise direction. Traction on suture 6 as well as the most recently placed suture aids exposure of the superior margin of the defect.*

be carefully visualized as it is tied down and the pledgets should be seen to be lying appropriately. The sutures are laid down in such a fashion that each bite lies flat against the patch and does not bunch the patch up. This can be achieved by tensioning the suture away from the most recently tied suture. A suture tying technique that uses a 'slip knot' technique is most appropriate. This allows tensioning of the knot. The 'noose' is then tightened to set the appropriate tension and then the suture is locked by throwing throws in opposite directions. Teflon coated polyester sutures require at least five or six throws to be securely locked into position.

DE-AIRING

Left heart return is often minimal in the child who has had a large left to right shunt. For this reason it may be necessary to fill the left heart with saline and to simultaneously vent air through the cardioplegia infusion site. Often it is helpful to place a blunt needle through the foramen ovale and to inject saline through the left atrium. Air should be gently massaged and milked from the apex towards the base of the heart and then out through the ascending aorta at the cardioplegia site. When this maneuver has been repeated several times and it is clear that no more air is being milked out of the ventricle, the flow rate of the pump is reduced and the aortic cross clamp is released while the cardioplegia site bleeds freely.

PLACEMENT OF MONITORING CATHETERS AND PACING WIRES

During the rewarming period a left atrial monitoring line is inserted through the right superior pulmonary vein. It is also helpful to place a pulmonary artery monitoring line particularly if the child is likely to have some degree of pulmonary hypertension postoperatively. A pulmonary artery monitoring line also allows for measurement of a residual oxygen stepup between the right atrial line and the pulmonary artery line. Although the sample drawn from the right atrial line is not a true mixed venous sample nevertheless it is reassuring when the right atrial and pulmonary artery saturations are within 2 or 3%. A stepup of more than 5–10% should stimulate the search for a residual VSD. This search should be even more carefully conducted by intraoperative transesophageal echocardiography if pulmonary artery pressure is also elevated. The absolute value of the pulmonary artery saturation is also helpful. If this exceeds 80% then this is often an indication that the child is likely to have a shunt of greater than 2:1 one year postoperatively.[24] Since sutures have been placed in the region of the conduction bundle it is advisable to place two atrial and one ventricular pacing wire. Atrial pacing wires allow cardiac output to be optimized and are particularly helpful if the child should develop junctional tachycardia. This is most commonly seen when an anterior malalignment VSD has been closed, particularly when this has been done transatrially. Presumably this results from the greater degree of retraction of the tricuspid annulus that is required for this approach.

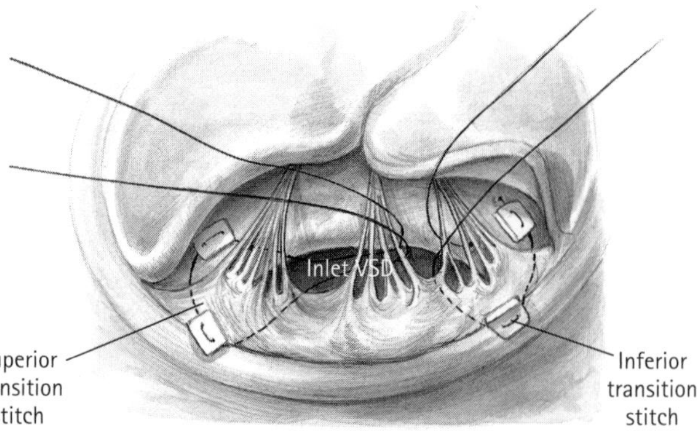

Figure 14.5 *It is often wise to place a superior transition suture for an inlet VSD in addition to an inferior transition suture as there can be no certainty whether the bundle of His passes immediately above or immediately below a large inlet VSD.*

SUTURE PLACEMENT FOR INLET VSDs

Usually when the entire inlet septum is absent as with complete AV canal the conduction bundle is displaced inferiorly. Under these circumstances there is counterclockwise rotation of the electrical axis of the heart as noted on the ECG preoperatively. However, under some circumstances the membranous area may be left relatively intact which allows the conduction bundle to penetrate in the usual location so that the bundle lies superior to the VSD. Since there is no way of knowing for sure whether the bundle in the case of an inlet VSD is passing superior or inferior to the defect it is generally wise to take appropriate precautions in both locations. This can easily be achieved by use of appropriate transition sutures (Figure 14.5).

DIRECT SUTURE CLOSURE OF THE MID-MUSCULAR VSD ASSOCIATED WITH MODERATOR BAND

The commonest location for a large mid-muscular VSD is immediately under the septal band at the point of origin of the moderator band. It is usually possible to pass a right angle instrument through the defect both from above and below the moderator band. Although our practice in the past was to excise the overlying moderator band and septal band and to attempt to place a patch to close a defect of this type, our more recent approach has been to use the overlying muscle. Figure 14.6b illustrates the placement of several doubly pledgetted VSD sutures which wedge the septal band and moderator band into the septal defect. Muscular VSDs in other areas of the ventricular septum also can be decreased in size or even obliterated by compressing the adjoining muscle between doubly pledgetted sutures taking very large bites of muscle. The sutures should not be tied unduly tightly.

TRANSPULMONARY ARTERY APPROACH

The transpulmonary artery approach is helpful and indeed may be essential when there is underdevelopment of the conal septum. This is often the case with an isolated subpulmonary

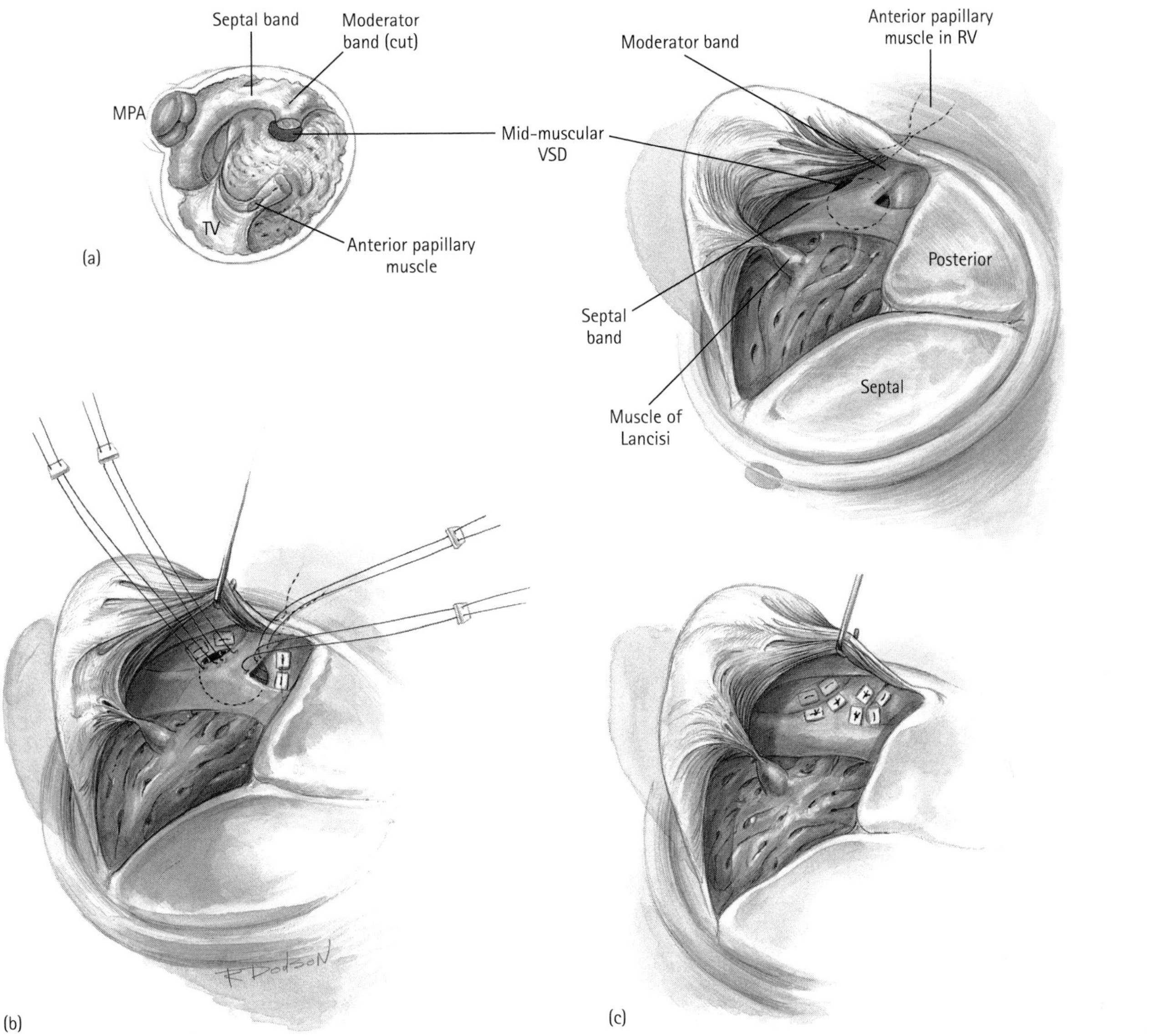

Figure 14.6 *(a) The most common location for a large mid-muscular VSD is under the septal band at the site of origin of the moderator band from the septal band. (b) Several interrupted doubly pledgetted sutures are placed so as to wedge the origin of the moderator band together with the adjoining septal band into the right ventricular aspect of the large mid-muscular VSD. (c) The mid-muscular VSD has been successfully obliterated by direct suture closure using the moderator band and septal band.*

VSD where the pulmonary valve essentially forms the superior margin of the VSD. This situation is also seen not uncommonly with the posterior malalignment VSD that occurs with interrupted aortic arch. Careful study of the preoperative echocardiogram will help to determine whether a transpulmonary artery or transatrial approach is more appropriate for the child with interrupted aortic arch and VSD.

PULMONARY ARTERY INCISION AND EXPOSURE

A transverse incision is made a few millimeters above the tops of the commissures of the pulmonary valve (Figure 14.7a). A retractor is placed through the pulmonary valve and retraction is directed inferiorly. Generally this provides excellent exposure of the subpulmonary or posterior malalignment VSD since the pulmonary artery and pulmonary annulus are usually quite enlarged under these circumstances (Figure 14.7b).

SUTURE PLACEMENT

Interrupted pledgetted horizontal mattress sutures are placed around the circumference of the defect. Because this defect is some distance above the conduction tissue no particular precautions need to be taken across the inferior margin of the defect. Nevertheless as a general principle it is best to keep both the entrance and exit points of each suture on the right ventricular aspect of the septum. The crest of the ventricular septum should under no circumstances ever be encircled by the sutures.

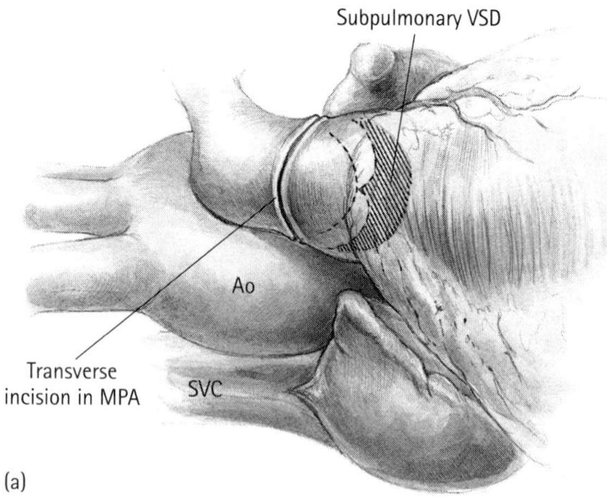

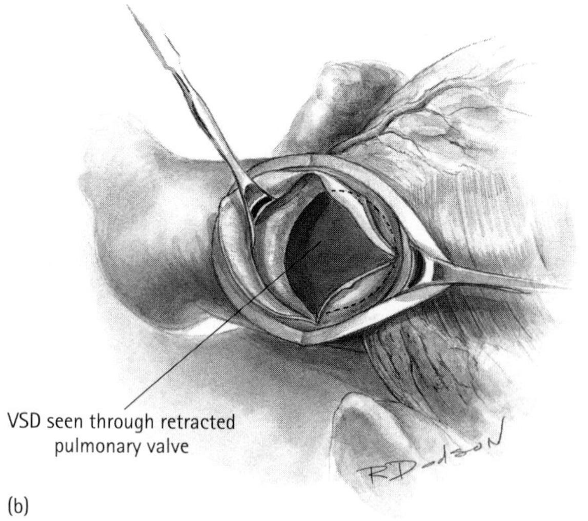

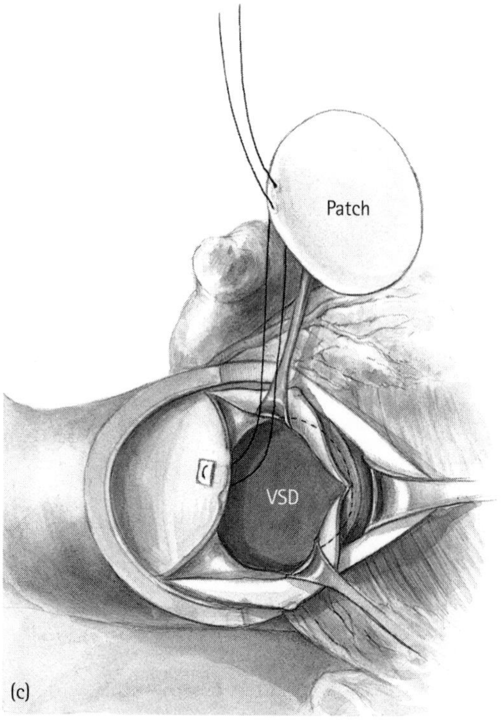

Figure 14.7 *(a) A subpulmonary VSD is usually best approached by a transverse incision in the main pulmonary artery immediately above the pulmonary valve. (b) Exposure of a subpulmonary VSD through the pulmonary valve is usually excellent because the main pulmonary artery and pulmonary annulus are quite dilated. (c) If the conal septum is absent immediately below the pulmonary valve it is helpful to place at least one suture through the base of the appropriate leaflet (s) of the pulmonary valve. The pledgets will lie above the pulmonary valve.*

Where there is virtual absence of the conal septum sutures should be placed through the pulmonary annulus with the pledgets lying within the sinuses of Valsalva of the pulmonary valve (Figure 14.7c).

PATCH MATERIAL

As noted above it is probably advisable in the setting of the VSD patch abutting directly against the valve leaflet tissue of the pulmonary valve that Dacron should be avoided. Generally under these circumstances it is appropriate to use autologous pericardium.

RESULTS OF SURGERY

There are very few reports describing large series of patients who have undergone standard surgical management of an isolated VSD during the last decade or so. Almost certainly this is because the results of surgery for VSD closure have been excellent for many years. Recent reports have tended to focus on new developments such as device management of muscular VSDs, surgical management of apical muscular VSD and the potential role for less invasive surgical techniques including video-assisted methods.

Surgical closure of isolated VSD

In 1995 van den Heuvel[25] described 263 consecutive patients with isolated VSDs who were managed in Rotterdam, The Netherlands. Forty three of the patients underwent surgical closure of the VSD while 220 patients were managed conservatively. Spontaneous closure of the VSD occurred in 30% of the patients. There were no deaths in either group. The patients who were managed surgically had non restrictive defects and were operated on during the first year of life. The morphology of the VSD significantly influenced the probability of spontaneous closure. Patients who were managed conservatively were more likely to have growth delay relative to surgical patients. In 1994 the same group from Rotterdam[26] described the long-term results after surgical closure of a VSD between 1968 and 1980. There were 176 infants and children. Mean follow-up was 14.5 years. At physical examination all patients who were followed were in good health. The mean exercise capacity was 100 ± 17% of predicted values. The authors concluded that the long-term results of surgical closure of VSD in infancy and childhood are good with a low risk of pulmonary hypertension. Personal health assessment is comparable to that of the normal population as is exercise capacity.

In another report Kuribayashi et al[27] from Japan described more than 10 years of follow-up for 49 infants who underwent primary closure of VSD between 1971 and 1982. Even though these patients had a right ventriculotomy as part of the procedure all survivors were growing normally and maintaining a good quality of life with no late deaths. Mean cardiac index was 3.4 L/minute per m^2 and left ventricular ejection fraction was 64%. In 1993, the second report of the major multi-institutional study known as the Natural History Study described the outcome for patients treated with a VSD in the early years of cardiac surgery. A total of 1280 patients were admitted to the study between 1958 and 1969.[18] Patients with small defects and pulmonary vascular disease were managed medically while patients with large VSDs in general were managed surgically. Overall probability of 25-year survival was 87%. Of the patients who were managed surgically, 5.5% required a second operation. At late follow-up there was an extremely low incidence of bacterial endocarditis but a higher than normal prevalence of serious arrhythmias. Apart from patients who had pulmonary vascular disease most patients had an excellent or good final clinical status.

It is difficult to know how to interpret information from this large natural history study because of the relatively primitive state that cardiac surgery was in at the time these patients were enrolled.

Another report of very long-term follow-up after surgery for VSD closure[28] described the results 30–35 years after surgery in 296 consecutive patients from the University of Minnesota. Only 2% of patients were lost to follow-up. There was a surprisingly high late mortality of 20% but these were patients who in general were more than five years of age at the time of surgery or with a pulmonary vascular resistance of greater than 7 units or with complete heart block. Eight of 37 patients with transient heart block after surgery died. There were 20 other patients who had other arrhythmias after surgery but none of these died. During the follow-up period nine episodes of endocarditis occurred. Once again, it is difficult to interpret this report because of the very early years in which surgery was undertaken, namely 1954–1960. In 1994, Castaneda et al[29] described the outcome of surgery for 427 infants who underwent surgical repair of VSD between 1973 and 1990 at Children's Hospital Boston. The early mortality for isolated VSDs was 2.3% with no deaths after 1984. Hospital mortality tended to be highest among infants with pre-existing respiratory problems or with hemodynamically significant residual lesions postoperatively.[30] Three patients died after discharge from the hospital. Two of the deaths were sudden suggesting an arrhythmic event. Lung biopsy specimens were obtained from 49 patients. Even though pulmonary vascular abnormalities were identified in all biopsies they were not predictive of hemodynamic findings at catheterization one year after surgery. We concluded in this previous report that primary surgical closure of VSDs during the first year of life is a low risk and effective option for most symptomatic infants. After successful VSD closure the majority of infants demonstrate prompt reduction in pulmonary artery pressure and relief of symptoms. Early VSD closure in infancy prevents the development of irreversible pulmonary vascular obstructive disease.

In 1991, Weintraub et al[31] reviewed the postoperative growth of 52 infants who underwent surgical closure of a large VSD before seven months of age. The authors found at a mean age of 5.7 years that the weight, length and head circumference had normalized for 35 patients who were of a normal birth weight. In general the catchup growth occurred within 6–12 months of surgery. However, among 11 infants with a low birth weight all three variables remained abnormal at long-term follow-up.

VSDs with associated pulmonary vascular disease

There is little useful recent information regarding management of the older patient with a large VSD and established pulmonary vascular disease. The guidance for management of such patients must be derived from early reports such as the report by Dushane and Kirklin in 1973.[32] In one more recent report, Neutze[33] described catheterization findings in 87 patients with VSD, 58 of whom had moderate or severe elevation of pulmonary arteriolar resistance. The authors found that the response to isoprenaline infusion was a helpful guide as to the subsequent course after surgery. They suggest that if preoperative resistance is less than 7 units/m^2 and there is a good response to a vasodilator the patient is likely to do well postoperatively. If the preoperative resistance remains greater than 7 units/m^2, despite infusion of isoprenaline, then a good postoperative course is unlikely.

Surgical closure of apical muscular VSDs

In 2000 Stellin et al described a new approach to surgical closure of the apical muscular VSD. The authors describe an 'apical recess' into which an apical muscular VSD often enters. The authors suggest that an incision into the apical recess allows safe patch closure.[7] In 2002, the same authors followed up with a report which included 14 postmortem cases, two explanted hearts and nine patients who had undergone successful surgery.[8] Another report describing successful surgical approach to the apical muscular VSD was described by Tsang et al, also in 2002.[34] These authors felt that it was unlikely that the now more conventional approach of multiple device placement within the apical recess would have been feasible in the three patients reported.

Management of multiple VSDs

Multiple VSDs almost always appear in multivariate analyses of early mortality risk as a predictor of increased risk. Various approaches have been described. The traditional surgical approach through a left ventricular incision is now not recommended based on unsatisfactory late left ventricular function.[35] One report has suggested that biologic glue may be useful for closure of multiple VSDs. Leca et al[36] used fibrin glue in 15 children with multiple VSDs between 1986 and 1991. The authors suggested that there were at most trivial residual shunts by color flow mapping in the 13 long-term survivors. Patients did not experience neurological complications though comprehensive neurological examinations were not undertaken.

In 1998, Kitagawa et al[37] described the management of 33 patients with multiple VSDs who underwent repair at Ann Arbor, Michigan, between 1988 and 1996. In most patients a right atriotomy procedure alone was used though an apical left ventriculotomy was used for apical defects. Among patients who had pulmonary hypertension preoperatively there were no early or late deaths and no episodes of complete heart block or significant residual VSDs. However, in patients who had protected pulmonary vasculature preoperatively secondary to right ventricular outflow tract obstruction of some form there was one early death and complete heart block occurred in two patients. This report highlights the important concept that a residual VSD will be better tolerated in the patient who had been exposed to high pulmonary flow and pressure preoperatively. On the other hand in the patient with a protected pulmonary circulation such as the patient with tetralogy of Fallot failure to close multiple VSDs adequately may result in a large postoperative shunt which may result in serious symptoms. Multiple muscular VSDs may be dealt with either intraoperatively or preoperatively using catheter delivered devices. In 1997 Murzi et al[38] described intraoperative use of double umbrella devices. Five patients had multiple muscular VSDs closed by Rashkind devices. In four of these patients there was minimal residual shunt while there was a moderate residual shunt in one. In an earlier report Fishberger et al[39] described intraoperative placement of umbrella devices in nine patients. There were three early deaths, two in patients who were moribund preoperatively. One other patient died due to severe ventricular dysfunction which may have resulted from the considerable retraction that was required in order to manipulate the large delivery device. This experience emphasizes the importance of specific devices being developed for intraoperative delivery. The approach of preoperatively closing multiple muscular VSDs by transcatheter device delivery has in general proved to be more practical than intraoperative closure. Bridges et al in 1991[15] described successful delivery of umbrella devices to close 21 muscular defects in 12 patients.

Device closure of VSDs

A complete review of the results of catheter delivered devices for VSD closure is beyond the scope of this book. However, it is interesting to note that some recent reports have explored the possibility of closure of membranous VSDs by catheter delivered devices. For example, in 2002 Hijazi et al[40] described placement of a new Amplatzer device in six patients with membranous VSDs. The median age of patients was 10.5 years and median weight was 29 kg. One patient developed trivial aortic regurgitation following device placement. The authors concluded that transcatheter occlusion of membranous VSDs is safe and effective. However, additional challenges will be faced in closing VSDs in infancy which is when the majority of patients require intervention. In an earlier report, Rigby and Reddington[41] had described successful placement of a Rashkind double umbrella device in 10 of 13 patients with membranous VSDs in which the procedure was attempted. The authors, however, acknowledge that the procedure is difficult and the mean procedure time was greater than 120 minutes. They suggest that this may be an alternative to surgery in some patients but overall did not recommend its routine use even with the introduction of large devices.

Surgical closure of VSDs with adjunctive procedures such as VATS

In 2002, Yu et al described the application of video-assisted thoracoscopic surgery (VATS) in nine patients undergoing septal defect closure.[42] Three of the patients aged 10–22 years had a VSD. A mini-thoracotomy with a length of 2–3 cm was made. A thoracoscope was used to assist primary closure of the defect. Patients were placed on femoro-femoral bypass during defect closure and the aorta was cross clamped. In an earlier report Miyaji et al in 2001[43] described the use of video-assisted cardioscopy for management of 12 patients with either an ASD or VSD. However, the skin incision was still relatively long at 5.4 cm and mean hospital stay was eight days.

REFERENCES

1. Fyler DC. Trends. In Fyler DC (ed). *Nadas' Pediatric Cardiology.* Philadelphia, Hanley & Belfus, 1992, pp 273–280.
2. Van Praagh R, Van Praagh S. Embryology and anatomy: Keys to the understanding of complex congenital heart disease. *Coeur* 1982; **13**:315.
3. Van Praagh R, Geva T, Kreutzer J. Ventricular septal defects: How shall we describe, name and classify them? *J Am Coll Cardiol* 1989; **14**:1298–1299.
4. Smolinsky A, Castaneda AR, Van Praagh R. Infundibular septal resection: Surgical anatomy of the superior approach. *J Thorac Cardiovasc Surg* 1988; **95**:486–494.

5. Soto B, Ceballos R, Kirklin JW. Ventricular septal defects: A surgical viewpoint. *J Am Coll Cardiol* 1989; **14**:1291–1297.
6. Tatsuno K, Ando M, Takao A, Hatsune K, Konno S. Diagnostic importance of aortography in conal ventricular septal defect. *Am Heart J* 1975; **89**:171–177.
7. Stellin G, Padalino M, Milanesi O et al. Surgical closure of apical ventricular septal defects through a right ventricular apical infundibulotomy. *Ann Thorac Surg* 2000; **69**:597–601.
8. Van Praagh S, Mayer JE, Berman NB, Flanagan MF, Geva T, Van Praagh R. Apical ventricular septal defects; Follow-up concerning anatomic and surgical considerations. *Ann Thorac Surg* 2002; **73**:48–57.
9. Wong PC, Sanders SP, Jonas RA et al. Pulmonary valve moderator band distance and association with development of double chambered right ventricle. *Am J Cardiol* 1991; **68**:1681–1686.
10. Van Praagh R, McNamara JJ. Anatomic types of ventricular septal defect with aortic insufficiency. *Am Heart J* 1968; **75**:604–619.
11. Heath D, Edwards JE. The pathology of hypertensive pulmonary vascular disease. *Circulation* 1958; **18**:533–547.
12. Rabinovitch M, Castaneda AR, Reid L. Lung biopsy with frozen section as a diagnostic aid for inpatients with congenital heart disease. *Am J Cardiol* 1981; **47**:77–84.
13. Rabinovitch M, Keane JF, Norwood WI, Castaneda AR, Reid L. Vascular structure in lung tissue obtained at biopsy correlated with pulmonary hemodynamic findings after repair. *Circulation* 1984; **69**:655–667.
14. Spevak PJ, Mandell VS, Colan SD et al. Reliability of color flow mapping in the identification and localization of multiple ventricular septal defects. *Echocardiography* 1993; **10**:573–581.
15. Bridges ND, Perry SB, Keane JF et al. Preoperative transcatheter closure of congenital muscular ventricular septal defects. *New Eng J Med* 1991; **324**:1312–1317.
16. Backer CL, Winters RC, Zales VR et al. Restrictive ventricular septal defect: How small is too small to close? *Ann Thorac Surg* 1993; **56**:1014–1019.
17. Waldman JD. Why not close a small ventricular septal defect? *Ann Thorac Surg* 1993; **56**:1011–1012.
18. Kidd L, Driscoll DJ, Gersony WM et al. Second natural history study of congenital heart defects. Results of treatment of patients with ventricular septal defects. *Circulation* 1993; **87**:I38–51.
19. Muller WH, Dammann JF. The treatment of certain congenital malformations of the heart by the creation of pulmonic stenosis to reduce pulmonary hypertension and excessive pulmonary blood flow: A preliminary report. *Surg Gynecol Obstet* 1952; **95**:213.
20. Lillehei CW, Cohen M, Warden HE et al. The results of direct vision closure of ventricular septal defects in eight patients by means of controlled cross circulation. *Surg Gynecol Obstet* 1955; **101**:446.
21. Kirklin JW, Harshbarger HG, Donald DE et al. Surgical correction of ventricular septal defect: Anatomic and technical considerations. *J Thorac Surg* 1957; **33**:45.
22. Stirling GR, Stanley PH, Lillehei CW. The effects of cardiac bypass and ventriculotomy upon right ventricular function with report of successful closure of ventricular septal defect by use of atriotomy. *Surg Forum* 1958; **8**:433.
23. Barratt-Boyes BG, Neutze JM, Harris EA (eds). *Heart Disease in Infancy: Diagnosis and Surgical Treatment.* Edinburgh, Churchill Livingstone, 1973.
24. Lang P, Chipman CW, Siden H, Williams RG, Norwood WI, Castaneda AR. Early assessment of hemodynamic status after repair of TOF. A comparison of 24 hour and 1 year postoperative data in 98 patients. *Am J Cardiol* 1982; **50**:795–799.
25. van den Heuvel F, Timmers T, Hess J. Morphological, haemodynamic, and clinical variables as predictors for management of isolated ventricular septal defect. *Br Heart J* 1995; **73**:49–52.
26. Meijboom F, Szatmari A, Utens E et al. Long-term follow-up after surgical closure of ventricular septal defect in infancy and childhood. *J Am Coll Cardiol* 1994; **24**:1358–1364.
27. Kuribayashi R, Sekine S, Aida H et al. Long-term results of primary closure for ventricular septal defects in the first year of life. *Surg Today* 1994; **24**:389–392.
28. Moller JH, Patton C, Varco RL, Lillehei CW. Late results (30 to 35 years) after operative closure of isolated VSD from 1954 to 1960. *Am J Cardiol* 1991; **68**:1491–1497.
29. Castaneda AR, Jonas RA, Mayer JE, Hanley FL. *Cardiac Surgery of the Neonate and Infant.* Philadelphia, W.B. Saunders, 1994, p 198.
30. Yeager SB, Freed MD, Keane JF, Norwood WI, Castaneda AR. Primary surgical closure of ventricular septal defect in the first year of life: Results in 128 infants. *J Am Coll Cardiol* 1984; **3**:1269–1276.
31. Weintraub RG, Menahem S. Early surgical closure of a large ventricular septal defect: Influence on long term growth. *J Am Coll Cardiol* 1991; **18**:552–558.
32. DuShane JW, Kirklin JW. Late results of the repair of ventricular septal defect with pulmonary vascular disease. In Kirklin JW (ed). *Advances with Cardiovascular Surgery.* Orlando, Grune & Stratton, 1973, p 9.
33. Neutze JM, Ishikawa T, Clarkson PM, Calder AL, Barratt-Boyes BG, Kerr AR. Assessment and follow-up of patients with ventricular septal defect and elevated pulmonary vascular resistance. *Am J Cardiol* 1989; **63**:327–331.
34. Tsang VT, Hsia TY, Yates RW, Anderson RH. Surgical repair of supposedly multiple defects within the apical part of the muscular ventricular septum. *Ann Thorac Surg* 2002; **73**:58–63.
35. Hanna B, Colan SD, Bridges ND, Mayer JE, Castaneda AR. Clinical and myocardial status after left ventriculotomy for ventricular septal defect closure. *J Am Coll Cardiol* 1991; **17**:110A.
36. Leca F, Karam J, Vouhe PR et al. Surgical treatment of multiple ventricular septal defects using a biologic glue. *J Thorac Cardiovasc Surg* 1994; **107**:96–102.
37. Kitagawa T, Durham LA 3rd, Mosca RS, Bove EL. Techniques and results in the management of multiple ventricular septal defects. *J Thorac Cardiovasc Surg* 1998; **115**:848–856.
38. Murzi B, Bonanomi GL, Giusti S et al. Surgical closure of muscular ventricular septal defects using double umbrella devices (intraoperative VSD device closure). *Eur J Cardiothorac Surg* 1997; **12**:450–454.
39. Fishberger SB, Bridges ND, Keane JF et al. Intraoperative device closure of ventricular septal defects. *Circulation* 1993; **88**:II205–209.
40. Hijazi ZM, Hakim F, Haweleh AA et al. Catheter closure of perimembranous ventricular septal defects using the new Amplatzer membranous VSD occluder: initial clinical experience. *Catheter Cardiovasc Interv* 2002; **56**:508–515.
41. Rigby ML, Redington AN. Primary transcatheter umbrella closure of perimembranous ventricular septal defect. *Br Heart J* 1994; **72**:368–371.
42. Yu SQ, Cai ZJ, Cheng YG et al. Video-assisted thoracoscopic surgery for congenital heart disease. *Asian Cardiovasc Thorac Ann* 2002; **10**:228–230.
43. Miyaji K, Murakami A, Kobayashi J, Suematsu Y, Takamoto S. Transxiphoid approach for intracardiac repair using video-assisted cardioscopy. *Ann Thorac Surg* 2001; **71**:1716–1718.

15

Transposition of the great arteries

INTRODUCTION

Transposition of the great arteries is one of the commonest congenital cardiac anomalies resulting in cyanosis. In untreated patients with transposition and intact ventricular septum, death occurs early in infancy, generally following ductal closure at a few days of age. In patients with an associated VSD or ASD, pulmonary vascular disease occurs rapidly and aggressively and can be fatal by the end of the first year of life. Not surprisingly therefore there were many attempts in the early years of open heart surgery in the 1950s to undertake surgical correction for these unfortunate blue babies. However, it was not until the late 1980s that anatomical correction in the form of the arterial switch procedure became the standard of care.

Transposition of the great arteries has been important for the development of both interventional catheter techniques and congenital heart surgery. Balloon atrial septostomy, introduced by Rashkind in Philadelphia[1] was one of the first widely applied interventional catheter techniques. The neonatal arterial switch procedure introduced by Norwood and Castaneda at Children's Hospital Boston[2] was critically important in demonstrating that corrective neonatal surgery could be performed with remarkably low mortality. And finally these children who have few associated extracardiac anomalies or genetic associations have demonstrated that it is possible to take a child with a critical, life threatening heart anomaly to the operating room shortly after birth and to perform a major corrective open heart procedure with every expectation of an excellent outcome both in the short and longer term.

EMBRYOLOGY

Transposition, like double outlet right ventricle and tetralogy, is an anomaly of the conotruncus. The embryology of the conotruncal malformations is described in greater detail in Chapter 23. In summary the classic theory of conotruncal malseptation suggests that failure of the septum to spiral in the usual fashion results in ventricular/great vessel discordance, i.e. transposition.[3] The alternative theory of van Praagh[4] suggests that the primary problem is underdevelopment of the subpulmonary conus. This results in fibrous continuity between the pulmonary and mitral valves, a hallmark of transposition.

The common, dextro form of transposition is referred to using van Praagh's segmental approach as 'd' or 'd-loop' transposition, in reference to the direction of looping of the primitive cardiac tube in the early stage of cardiac development (S,D,D). With a d-loop the ventricles lie in their usual relationship with the morphological left ventricle on the left and the morphological right ventricle anterior and on the right. d-Loop transposition should not be confused with d-malposition of the aorta relative to the pulmonary artery which is of little functional importance (S,D,D). In contrast levo or l-loop transposition has entirely different pathophysiology relative to d-loop transposition (see Chapter 28).

Embryology of the coronary arteries in d-transposition

The coronary circulation develops in similar fashion to the pulmonary arterial and pulmonary venous circulation. For example, the distal pulmonary venous system is derived from the original systemic venous system and invests the primitive foregut as it buds to form the primitive bronchi and subsequently the lungs. The original communications of the pulmonary veins with the systemic veins resorb through a system of programmed cell death similar to apoptosis. This resorption occurs when communication has been established with the primordial pulmonary vein which buds from the posterior surface of the left atrium. Failure of the pulmonary bud to link with the venous complex results in persistence of the systemic venous connection and hence total anomalous pulmonary venous connection. In a similar fashion the proximal main coronary arteries arise as buds in the sinuses of Valsalva (usually the aortic but sometimes the pulmonary). These buds must fuse with a primitive vascular plexus that forms from angioblasts in the mesoderm of the developing heart tube. The major coronary vessels, i.e. the right and left coronary artery, originate from angioblasts in the atrioventricular sulcus. As Van Praagh has pointed out,[5] the very name coronary artery reflects their circular course at the atrioventricular septum (*corona* = crown (Latin)). Each ventricle, right and left, has its own distinct and different coronary arterial pattern. When there are variations in the positions of the great vessels and/or the ventricles relative to the usual location there is interference with the normal connection of the main trunks of the coronary arteries with the sinus of Valsalva buds. Perhaps not surprisingly the commonest coronary 'anomaly' with transposition in fact represents the most efficient connection of the main coronary trunks to the aorta and therefore should be termed 'usual' distribution for a given anomaly such as transposition. Although this distribution is not 'normal' in the sense that with normally related great arteries and normally positioned ventricles (d-loop) the left main coronary artery passes behind the pulmonary artery, nevertheless for d-loop transposition of the great arteries the usual distribution is for the left main coronary artery to pass anterior to the pulmonary artery and from there to the left sided atrioventricular groove. Similarly the right main coronary artery passes directly from the closest sinus to the right sided atrioventricular groove. In addition to the many variations in the connections of the main coronary trunk into the sinuses of Valsalva, there can be anomalies of the coronary buds themselves. This can result in coronary ostial atresia, coronary ostial stenoses, oblique origin of the coronary ostium and intramural coronary arteries.[6]

ANATOMY

Transposition is part of an anatomical spectrum of conotruncal anomalies extending from tetralogy, in which the aorta is primarily connected to the left ventricle and the pulmonary artery is connected to the right ventricle, through double outlet right ventricle in which both great vessels primarily arise from the right ventricle, and finally transposition, in which the aorta arises from the right ventricle and the pulmonary artery from the left ventricle. The complexity of distinguishing the border zones between these classifications is described in Chapter 23.

One of the most important distinguishing features of transposition is that the aortic valve is lifted away from the other three valves of the heart by an infundibulum or conus. In hearts with d-loop transposition the pulmonary valve is in fibrous continuity with the mitral valve in the same way that the aortic valve should be in fibrous continuity with the mitral valve when the great vessels are normally related. An important effect of the subaortic conus is that the aortic valve lies at a higher level than the pulmonary valve. Thus when the coronary arteries are transferred as part of the arterial switch they will lie above the level of the sinuses of Valsalva if the coronaries are kept at the same level.

The ascending aorta often lies directly anterior to the main pulmonary artery or slightly to the right (S, D, D). When there is an intact ventricular septum, the great vessels are likely to be of a similar size.

Associated anomalies

It is not uncommon for the ductus to remain patent or to be kept patent by infusion of prostaglandin E1. The foramen ovale may be stretched or there may be a true secundum ASD.

VENTRICULAR SEPTAL DEFECT

Approximately 20% of children with transposition have an associated VSD.[7] When a VSD is present the aorta is usually between half and two thirds the diameter of the main pulmonary artery. The aorta is also smaller than the main pulmonary artery when there is underdevelopment of the aortic annulus or subaortic conus as is likely to be the case if the VSD is of the anterior malalignment type, i.e. the conal septum projects anteriorly into the right ventricular outflow tract relative to the muscular interventricular septum. There may be associated underdevelopment of the right ventricle, tricuspid valve, aortic arch hypoplasia and coarctation or interrupted aortic arch.

If the VSD is of the posterior malalignment type, i.e. the conal septum projects into the left ventricular outflow tract, there is likely to be hypoplasia of the pulmonary annulus. There may be pulmonary valve stenosis or at least a bicuspid pulmonary valve. In this setting the main pulmonary artery may be smaller than the aorta. Approximately 20% of patients with transposition and VSD have left ventricular outflow obstruction at birth. However, obstruction may not become apparent until later so that the incidence is often cited as 30–35% among patients with transposition with VSD.[8]

Isolated left ventricular outflow obstruction

Left ventricular outflow tract obstruction occurs occasionally with transposition in the absence of an associated VSD.

It may be functional where it is usually caused by the septum bulging to the left because of the pressure differential in favor of the right ventricle when pulmonary resistance has fallen. In time the obstruction can progress from a dynamic state to more of a fixed and fibrous, tunnel-like left ventricular outflow obstruction.

ANATOMICAL VARIANTS OF THE CORONARY ARTERIES

Coronary ostial abnormalities

Coronary ostial atresia and coronary ostial stenosis are self explanatory. As described in the section above they result embryologically from a failure of the normal fusion of the main coronary trunks with the sinus of Valsalva bud emerging from the aorta. Less well understood are the intramural coronary arteries and the oblique ostium resulting in a potentially stenotic coronary artery.

Intramural coronary artery

From a surgeon's perspective the ideal coronary artery for surgical transfer during the arterial switch procedure should be positioned relatively high in the appropriate sinus of Valsalva as well as centrally located between the two commissures of that sinus. In fact there are a tremendous number of variations that can increase the difficulty of transfer. For example, the ostium may be situated very low in the sinus of Valsalva close to the hinge point of the valve cusp associated with the sinus. This will reduce the amount of button that can be harvested from the sinus below the coronary ostium and necessitates more careful and finer suturing with a higher risk of subsequent hemorrhage. In addition to variation in the height within a given sinus it is not at all uncommon for the ostium to be placed closer to one or other commissure, more commonly the more posterior commissure. When an ostium is placed eccentrically within a sinus it is not uncommon for its appearance to be somewhat slit like when viewed from within the aorta. A centrally placed ostium will usually have a circular appearance such that a probe can be passed directly into the ostium at right angles to the wall of the sinus. In contrast, the oblique ostium necessitates the probe being placed at an acute angle relative to the sinus. There is some evidence to suggest that even with normally related great arteries and an oblique ostial origin of this nature there is an increased risk of acute coronary ischemia, generally associated with exercise, and increased risk of sudden death.[9] In the case of coronary transfer for an arterial switch procedure it is the author's opinion that these variants of coronary arterial anatomy also increase the risk of post-transfer ischemia. In a more extreme example of the eccentrically placed ostium the coronary arises not from the immediately adjacent sinus of Valsalva but from the same sinus. This usually results in two ostia that are relatively close together: one ostium arises in a normal location centrally in the sinus while the other, usually the left ostium, arises between the right ostium and the posterior commissure. Rather than emerging at right angles to the sinus the anomalous coronary passes very obliquely and in fact remains within the wall of the aorta, i.e. 'intramurally'.[10,11] It does not emerge until it is adjacent to the appropriate sinus of Valsalva. Thus when viewed externally the coronary artery may appear to have 'usual' distribution but when viewed internally the distribution is clearly not usual because both ostia arise from the same sinus. It is important to understand that the intramural coronary artery frequently passes behind the posterior commissure of the aortic valve. This commissure of the neopulmonary valve will need to be detached in order to harvest a button that contains the full length of the intramural coronary artery.

Single coronary ostium

A single coronary ostium frequently represents an extreme example of the intramural coronary artery. Because of a longer intramural course the anomalous ostium comes to lie immediately adjacent to the other coronary ostium or indeed may completely fuse with that ostium so that there is truly a single coronary ostium.[12]

Coronary artery branching patterns in d-transposition

A number of different conventions have been developed to describe the many coronary artery branching patterns that are seen in association with transposition.

LEIDEN CONVENTION

The Leiden convention is a widely used method of classification of the coronary artery branching patterns seen with d-transposition. It was initially proposed by the anatomists Gittenberger-DeGroot and Sauer who were working with Quaegebeur's group in Leiden, Holland.[10] As depicted in Figure 15.1 and described in Table 15.1, the classification defines the sinus of origin for each of the three main coronary arteries. The sinuses are numbered by a convention in which the perspective of an individual looking from the aorta to the pulmonary artery labels the sinus adjacent to the pulmonary artery on the right hand side of the observer as sinus 1, whereas sinus 2 is the sinus adjacent to the pulmonary artery on the left hand side of the observer. Thus for the commonest type of coronary distribution, sinus 1, i.e. usually the anatomically leftward and posterior sinus, gives rise to the anterior descending and circumflex coronary arteries, whereas sinus 2, the anatomically rightward and posterior sinus, gives rise to the right coronary artery. This can be abbreviated as (1AD, CX; 2R) (Figure 15.1). Yamaguchi and others[13] have proposed a further level of classification to distinguish the epicardial course of the coronary arteries, for example, anterior or posterior to the main pulmonary artery. Using the Leiden

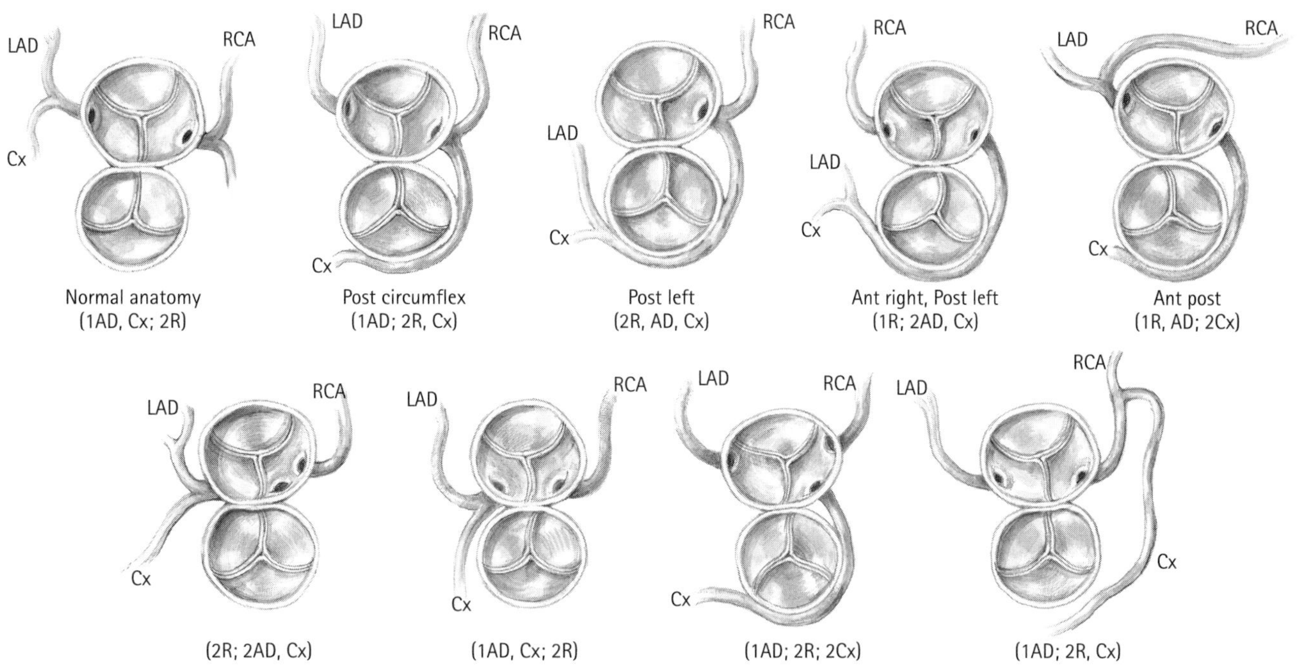

Figure 15.1 *The Leiden classification for coronary artery anatomy in d-transposition of the great arteries. The facing sinuses in the aorta are labeled from the perspective of an individual standing within the aorta and facing the pulmonary artery. Sinus 1 is on the observer's right side and sinus 2 is on the observer's left side. Usual coronary artery for transposition becomes (1AD, CX; 2R), i.e. the anterior descending and circumflex coronary arteries arises from sinus 1 and the right coronary artery arises from sinus 2.*

Table 15.1 *Classification of the coronary anatomy in d-transposition of the great arteries*

*Leiden classification of coronary origin**

SINUS

Using the perspective of an individual looking from the aorta to the pulmonary artery:

- sinus 1 – adjacent to the pulmonary artery on the right-hand side of the observer
- sinus 2 – adjacent to the pulmonary artery on the left hand side of the observer

CORONARY ARTERIES

- right coronary artery
- anterior descending artery
- circumflex artery

Supplemental descriptive classification

- epicardial course of major coronary branches:
  - anterior – passing anterior to the aorta
  - posterior – passing posterior to the pulmonary artery
  - between – passing between the great arteries (usually intramural)
- unusual origins
- commissural – a coronary origin near an aortic commissure
- separate – separate origin of two coronary branches from the same aortic sinus
- remote or distal – origin of the circumflex artery and the posterior descending artery as a distal bifurcation of the right coronary artery
- aortic position relative to the pulmonary artery
- right or anterior, left, side by side or posterior

*A comma is used to indicate that major branches arise from a common vessel, whereas a semicolon denotes separate origins.

convention, a single coronary artery arising from the rightward and posterior facing sinus with the left coronary artery passing posterior to the pulmonary artery would be designated (2R, AD, CX) posterior left course.

YACOUB AND RADLEY-SMITH CLASSIFICATION

Another popular method for classifying coronary artery branching patterns with transposition was originally described by Yacoub and Radley-Smith in 1978.[14] Figure 15.2 depicts the Yacoub classification. It can be seen that the usual distribution is classified in this scheme as type A. In Type B there is a single coronary ostium with the right coronary artery passing between the aorta and pulmonary artery.

DESCRIPTIVE CLASSIFICATION OF CORONARY ARTERY BRANCHING PATTERNS

At Children's Hospital Boston we have not adopted either the Leiden classification or the Yacoub classification. There are so many potential variations of coronary anatomy that in general we have used a descriptive method that specifies an individual child's anatomy. For example, the relative positions of the aorta and pulmonary artery must first be described, e.g. aorta directly anterior to pulmonary artery, aorta 45° to right and anterior of pulmonary artery. When the aorta lies more than 45° anterior to the pulmonary artery, the coronaries are usually described as arising from a rightward and posterior facing sinus and a leftward and posterior facing sinus. For example, with the usual distribution of the coronary arteries, the left

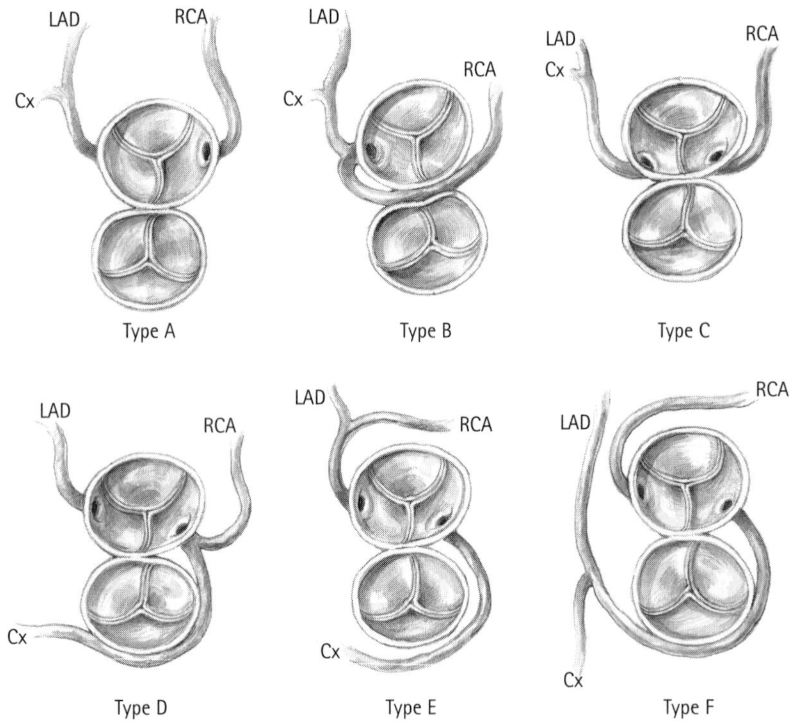

Figure 15.2 *The Yacoub and Radley-Smith classification for coronary artery anatomy in d-transposition.*

main coronary artery is described as arising from the leftward and posterior facing sinus while the right main coronary artery is described as arising from the rightward and posterior facing sinus. Although this system provides a full description of the patient's anatomy for those managing the individual child, it is not adequate when computer coding of coronary artery anatomy is necessary. A system that we have used for analysis of surgical outcomes has been reported previously.[15] This system has been applied in several reports from Children's Hospital Boston and was also used in reports compiled by the Congenital Heart Surgeons Society. Table 15.2[16] illustrates the coronary anatomy in 470 patients who underwent arterial switch procedures at Children's Hospital Boston between 1983 and 1992. In addition to analysing outcome relative to individual coronary artery branching patterns a group analysis was undertaken using the following groupings:

- all coronary arteries arising from a single sinus
- all variations of intramural coronary arteries
- patterns with a retropulmonary course of the entire left coronary system
- patterns with a retropulmonary course of the circumflex only
- any left coronary supply from the posterior facing sinus.

Anatomical variations of single coronary artery

Figure 15.3 illustrates the ostial origin and course in the atrioventricular (AV) groove of 53 patients with single coronary artery associated with transposition managed at Children's Hospital Boston between January 1, 1983 and June 30, 2000.[17] In 27 patients there was a single ostium in the rightward and posterior facing sinus. The left main coronary artery branched from the single coronary trunk and passed posterior to the pulmonary artery before branching into the circumflex and left anterior descending while the right coronary artery ran a usual course in the right AV groove. In 16 of the 53 patients there was a single ostium in the leftward and posterior facing sinus. The right coronary passed anterior to the aorta to enter the right AV groove while the left coronary artery ran a usual course. In 5 of 53 patients the single ostium arose from the rightward posterior facing sinus and the left main coronary artery passed anteriorly to enter the left AV

Table 15.2 *Coronary anatomy in 470 patients who underwent arterial switch procedures at Children's Hospital Boston between 1983 and 1992*

Nomenclature	Sinus 1**	Sinus 2**	n	%
Usual	LAD, Cx	R	289	61
Circumflex from RCA	LAD	CxR	103	22
Single RCA		LADCxR	21	4
With additional small LAD from sinus 1			2	0.4
Single LCA	RLADCx		10	2
Inverted origins	R	LADCx	13	3
Inverted RCA/Cx	RLAD	Cx	19	4
Intramural LCA		LADCxR	9	2
Intramural LAD		LADCxR	3	0.6
Intramural RCA	LADCxR		1	0.2

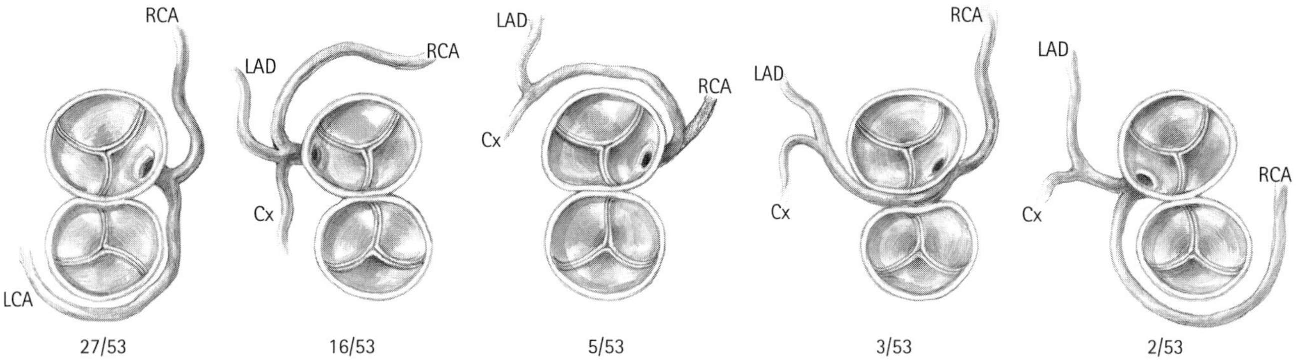

Figure 15.3 *Anatomical variations of single coronary arteries with d-transposition of the great arteries seen at Children's Hospital Boston between 1983 and 2000.*

groove. The right coronary artery pursued a normal course in the right AV groove. In 3 of 53 patients there was a single ostium in the right posterior facing sinus with the left main coronary artery passing between the aorta and pulmonary artery in order to enter the left AV groove. The right coronary artery pursued a normal course. In the least common pattern, two patients had a single ostium in the left posterior facing sinus. The right coronary artery passed posterior to the pulmonary artery to enter the right AV groove. The left coronary artery pursued a normal course in the left AV groove.

PATHOPHYSIOLOGY

The hallmark of 'transposition physiology' is that the oxygen saturation in the main pulmonary artery is higher than the saturation in the aorta. This results from the presence of two parallel circulations, i.e. the systemic venous return coming back to the right ventricle is pumped back to the systemic arterial circulation and likewise the pulmonary venous circulation returns to the lungs. There must be a point of mixing between the parallel circulations for the child to survive. In the first days of life this is likely to be the ductus. After the ductus has closed the child will not survive unless there is an associated VSD or ASD.

During fetal life the pressure is the same in the right and left ventricle irrespective of the presence of transposition. This results from the presence of an unrestrictive ductus arteriosus. Because the pressure in the right ventricle is the same as the pressure in the left ventricle, the muscle of the right ventricle at birth is similar in thickness to the muscle of the left ventricle. After birth the pulmonary resistance soon begins to fall with a corresponding fall in left ventricular pressure if the ventricular septum is intact. By 4–6 weeks of age the left ventricle will be unprepared to acutely take over the pressure load required for the systemic circulation.[18] Another consequence of the fall in pulmonary resistance is that there is an increase in pulmonary blood flow which may become three or four times greater than systemic flow. This is accomplished by dilation of the left ventricle. Thus transposition is a cyanotic anomaly in which pulmonary blood flow is not decreased but is actually increased relative to normal.

If a VSD is present the pressure in the left ventricle will be maintained at a level that is determined by the degree of restriction of the VSD. However, as is the case for patients with normally related great arteries, a membranous VSD has a tendency to close spontaneously so that within weeks left ventricular pressure may have decreased from close to systemic to less than two thirds. At this level left ventricular muscle mass is not likely to be maintained adequately to allow an arterial switch without preliminary preparation of the ventricle.

Pulmonary vascular disease

Pulmonary vascular disease occurs rapidly and aggressively in untreated patients with transposition, particularly if a VSD is present.[19–21] Presumably the combination of high flow, high pressure and the presence of a high oxygen saturation in pulmonary arterial blood results in the rapid development of fixed and irreversible vascular disease. It is not uncommon for patients with transposition and VSD to become inoperable by as early as six months. Even if the ventricular septum is intact the child may be inoperable by 12 months of age.

Left ventricular outflow tract obstruction

When there is important LV outflow obstruction, pulmonary blood flow is reduced. The combination of transposition physiology and reduced pulmonary blood flow results in a profound degree of cyanosis.

Reverse differential cyanosis

When there is a coarctation or interruption of the aortic arch, blood flow to the lower body must be maintained by patency of the ductus. However, the blood flowing to the lower body from the left ventricle through the ductus is fully saturated while that flowing to the upper body is desaturated. This results in pink toes and blue fingers, a diagnostic feature of transposition with aortic arch obstruction termed 'reverse differential cyanosis'.

CLINICAL FEATURES AND PREOPERATIVE DIAGNOSIS

The diagnosis of d-transposition of the great arteries is usually made in the first 24 hours of life. As the ductus closes the child becomes profoundly hypoxic and acidotic. The chest X-ray demonstrates increased pulmonary blood flow despite the cyanosis. The great vessel appearance in the mediastinum is also characteristic. Because the aorta lies anterior to the pulmonary artery the superior mediastinum appears narrow. The heart is usually egg-shaped so that the appearance has been described as an 'egg-on-a-string'.

Echocardiography

The two-dimensional echocardiogram is diagnostic of transposition. In the neonatal period the thymus invests the great vessels and the base of the ventricles producing an excellent medium for ultrasound conduction. Thus very clear images are obtained which are almost always sufficiently precise to allow accurate diagnosis of coronary as well as great vessel anatomy. The echocardiographer should also define the relative positions of the aortic root and pulmonary root, i.e. whether the aorta is directly anterior to the pulmonary artery or for example 45° anterior and rightward. The relative sizes of the pulmonary and aortic valve and ascending aorta versus main pulmonary trunk should be defined both in absolute terms in millimeters as well as normalized by z score. The coronary ostia should be defined as well as the location of the right and left main coronary artery. It is also necessary to define the venous drainage, e.g. is there a left SVC, if so, is there a communicating left innominate vein and what are the relative sizes of the right SVC and left SVC? In addition the size and site of septal defects should be defined. It is important to define the size of the aortic arch, isthmus and juxtaductal area as these can be hypoplastic and there can be an associated coarctation. Arch hypoplasia and/or the presence of a coarctation should alert the echocardiographer to carefully review the subaortic area which may be hypoplastic. Often this is because of malalignment of the conal septum anterior to the ventricular septum associated with an anterior malalignment VSD. Arch hypoplasia or coarctation should also alert the echocardiographer to measure carefully the size of the tricuspid annulus and to assess the adequacy of the right ventricle.

Limited role for cardiac catheterization and angiography

Although performance of a balloon atrial septostomy is useful in the stabilization and subsequent intraoperative management of the child with transposition this does not necessitate a full catheterization including collection of hemodynamic and angiographic data.

In the early years of the arterial switch procedure, particularly when it was felt that certain coronary patterns might contraindicate an arterial switch procedure, and in the years before there was a large experience in diagnosing coronary artery anatomy by echocardiography, it was a common practice at Children's Hospital Boston to undertake coronary angiography in the newly diagnosed neonate with transposition. This was generally performed in a steep laid back position, with balloon occlusion of the distal ascending aorta and injection in the aortic root.[22] Coronary angiography in this fashion, however, can be equally difficult to perform and interpret as echocardiography. The balloon catheter may not achieve complete occlusion of the ascending aorta. There may be overlap of other structures but more importantly it is particularly difficult to derive information regarding the location of the coronary ostia so that an intramural coronary artery for example may not be diagnosed as easily with angiography as echocardiography. For all these reasons it is exceedingly rare for coronary angiography to be undertaken preoperatively in the infant with transposition in the current era.

MEDICAL AND INTERVENTIONAL THERAPY

Balloon atrial septostomy should be performed on a semi-urgent basis within hours of the diagnosis of d-transposition of the great arteries with no associated ASD or VSD. Although it is possible to manage the child with a prostaglandin infusion to maintain ductal patency, this often results in a steal away from the systemic circulation, particularly the abdominal organs, which predisposes the neonate to necrotizing enterocolitis. Since there are two parallel circulations, any flow that passes from the ductus into the pulmonary circulation unless it subsequently returns to the systemic circulation with bidirectional ductal shunting will return to the left atrium and can result in left atrial hypertension. Ideally this is decompressed back to the systemic circulation at atrial level through a balloon septostomy defect.

It is our preference to stabilize the neonate in the intensive care unit for a day or two in general before proceeding to surgery. This allows the child to recover from the trauma associated with birth as well as the possible additional insult of ductal closure, hypoxia and resulting acidosis. The child should be assessed for renal, hepatic, mesenteric and cerebral function by the usual methods. Ideally all organ systems should be functioning normally by the time of surgery. It is not necessary that the child be intubated during this period though if there is inadequate mixing at the atrial level following the balloon septostomy it may be necessary to reintroduce prostaglandin, and under these circumstances intubation is sometimes preferred to guard against possible apneic episodes. It is also not necessary to have an indwelling arterial catheter as the child's oxygen saturation can be monitored adequately by pulse oximeter. However, in preparation for an expeditious setup time in the operating room it is generally advisable to place an arterial catheter in a radial artery as well as establishing secure intravenous access prior to going to the operating room. We avoid placement of a central venous line either in the internal jugular or subclavian vein. Neonates are susceptible to SVC thrombosis and this risk is increased if a central venous line is placed. The risk is further increased with a larger gauge double lumen or multi-lumen catheter through which parenteral nutrition or other hyperosmolar solutions are subsequently infused. Thrombosis of the superior vena cava can be a particularly debilitating problem in the neonate and in many cases is ultimately fatal. On the other hand there is little benefit to be gained in placement of a central venous line. There should be no risk of excessive blood loss in a primary sternotomy and since single venous cannulation in the right atrium is to be applied it is not necessary for monitoring of central venous pressure intraoperatively. Postoperatively a right atrial line should be brought transcutaneously through the chest wall for monitoring of right atrial pressure.

INDICATIONS FOR AND TIMING OF SURGERY

The diagnosis of transposition is in itself an indication for surgery. As discussed in the history of the development of surgery for transposition (see below), the arterial switch procedure is now firmly established as the procedure of choice. There are almost no situations which would justify the performance of a Senning or Mustard procedure for d-transposition. For this reason these procedures are described in Chapter 28.

With the advent of fetal echocardiography and accurate diagnosis at birth for almost all children with important heart disease, the question as to how late a primary arterial switch procedure can be safely performed rarely arises. However, the situation can arise in countries without comprehensive screening of neonates and in the occasional situation in which a child is too ill from sepsis or intracranial hemorrhage, for example, to allow surgery in the newborn period.

The left ventricle remains prepared for a one stage arterial switch procedure so long as there is a VSD or patent ductus that is large enough to maintain left ventricular pressure greater than two thirds systemic pressure. However, if the ventricular septum is intact the left ventricle becomes measurably thinner within a few weeks of birth.[18] Early in the neonatal switch experience we believed empirically that at approximately four weeks of age the majority of children with an intact septum and no ductus were at too great a risk to allow a one stage switch. Subsequent data from the multi-institutional Congenital Heart Surgeons Society study suggested that the time limit should be drawn at three weeks of age.[23] However, this was very early in the arterial switch experience for many surgeons. Subsequent reports from deLeval and Mee suggested that with greater experience and with liberal use of mechanical ventricular support an upper limit of eight weeks of age was reasonable.[24,25] Beyond eight weeks it is probably wise to prepare the ventricle by a preliminary procedure designed to raise LV pressure (see 'Two stage arterial switch' below).

SURGICAL MANAGEMENT

History

Among the earliest attempts at surgical correction in the mid-1950s were procedures designed to correct transposition anatomically, i.e. division and reanastomosis of the great vessels as well as transfer of the coronary arteries. These initial attempts were uniformly unsuccessful for a number of reasons. Firstly the majority of babies had an intact ventricular septum and an intact atrial septum and therefore became profoundly sick at the time of ductal closure. Although Blalock and Hanlon had introduced an ingenious palliative procedure to create an atrial septectomy surgically[26] this resulted in intrapericardial adhesions and increased the difficulty and risks of subsequent repair. Furthermore, there was no appreciation in the early years of cardiac surgery that in patients with intact ventricular septum the left ventricular pressure decreases to such a low pressure within a few days of birth that within a month or two of birth the left ventricle is unprepared to take over acutely the workload of the systemic circulation. Early heart-lung machines were particularly deleterious to the very small patient so that the requirement that all patients with transposition undergo surgery very early in life resulted in their being exposed to the many deleterious effects of cardiopulmonary bypass. Finally in the 1950s and even the early 1960s surgeons simply had not yet developed the microvascular instrumentation and techniques required to successfully undertake transfer of the coronary arteries, an essential component of the arterial switch procedure. In the late 1960s following the development of coronary artery bypass grafting for acquired coronary artery disease, there was a rapid acceleration in learning by surgeons of techniques that would allow microvascular anastomosis.

By the late 1960s and early 1970s Barratt Boyes in New Zealand and Castaneda in Boston were beginning to demonstrate that primary repair in infancy for a wide range of congenital anomalies could be undertaken with an acceptably low mortality risk so long as one minimized exposure to cardiopulmonary bypass. Barratt-Boyes popularized the use of deep hypothermic circulatory arrest to achieve this.[27] By this time, i.e. the early 1970s, Rashkind had introduced his balloon septostomy procedure,[1] a tremendous advance in allowing palliation of neonates with an intact atrial and ventricular septum and closing ductus arteriosus. In addition Senning[28] and subsequently Mustard[29] introduced their atrial level repairs. In the late 1970s Brom repopularized the Senning procedure and reported with Quaegebeur extremely low mortality rates for the Senning procedure.[30] In Toronto where Mustard had pioneered his atrial level procedure, Trusler and Williams were also reporting an extremely low surgical mortality risk for the Mustard procedure.[31] However, by this time, Jatene in Brazil had demonstrated the technical feasibility of anatomical correction.[32] He did this in a child who was well beyond the neonatal period and who had a VSD which maintained left ventricular pressure and therefore the preparedness of the left ventricle.

Yacoub in the United Kingdom began to adopt the arterial switch procedure for patients with transposition.[33] He chose to perform a two stage procedure in which the child's left ventricle was prepared for the arterial switch procedure by initial application of a pulmonary artery band. The arterial switch procedure was then performed approximately one year later. In Boston, Castaneda and Norwood took the bold approach for that time of performing a primary neonatal arterial switch procedure in children who had an intact ventricular septum, i.e. the majority of patients with transposition.[2] The success of this procedure was based on the premise that the left ventricle was exposed to systemic pressure prenatally in patients with transposition because of patency of the ductus arteriosus (in the same way that the right ventricle is exposed to systemic pressure prenatally in the child with normally related great arteries). It is important to remember at this time, i.e. the early 1980s, there was only a rudimentary understanding by surgeons of the many potential variations in coronary artery anatomy that could occur in association with transposition of the great arteries. Initially Castaneda and Norwood believed that there were several rare coronary branching patterns that were unsuitable for translocation and recommended that these children should have a Senning procedure. However, Yacoub argued at this time that all coronary types could be transferred and time has indeed proven him to be correct.[14] Nevertheless it is true to say that some of the rarer coronary branching patterns, particularly origin of both main coronary arteries from a single ostium, represent a considerably greater technical challenge to the congenital cardiac surgeon.

Technical considerations

ARTERIAL SWITCH PROCEDURE

Working through a standard median sternotomy, the thymus is subtotally resected. Marking sutures are placed on the proximal pulmonary artery to indicate the points where the coronaries will be translocated. The sites selected are simply the points at which the artery will most comfortably rotate after mobilization of the first 3 or 4 mm. The arterial cannulation purse-string sutures is placed immediately proximal to the innominate artery. The venous cannulation stitch is placed in the tip of the right atrial appendage. The ductus arteriosus is dissected free and will be doubly suture ligated with 5/0 Prolene immediately after commencing bypass with subsequent division (Figure 15.4a).

The patient is placed on cardiopulmonary bypass and is cooled to a rectal temperature of less than 18°C using a single venous cannula placed in the right atrium. The tip of the cannula rests in the orifice of the superior vena cava. During cooling the branch pulmonary arteries are mobilized into their hilar branches. The aorta is cross clamped and a single dose of cardioplegia solution is infused into the root of the aorta. The aorta is divided at approximately its midpoint opposite the pulmonary bifurcation (Figure 15.4b). The coronary arteries are excised with a button composed of the majority of the adjoining sinus of Valsalva (Figure 15.4b inset). The first 2–4 mm of the coronary arteries are mobilized with careful preservation of all branches (Figure 15.4c). If necessary, small epicardial branches are mobilized from under the epicardium.

The main pulmonary artery is divided just proximal to its bifurcation (Figure 15.4d). A Lecompte maneuver[34] is performed, bringing the pulmonary bifurcation anterior to the ascending aorta. Appropriate U-shaped areas of tissue are excised from the proximal neoaorta. The bottoms of the U-shaped areas are generally at the level of the tops of the commissures of the neoaortic valve. It is important that the original marking sutures be used as a guide to the area of neoaorta that is excised.

The coronary buttons are sutured into the neoaorta using continuous 7/0 Prolene (Figure 15.4e). The sutures are tied at each end. The suture line is very carefully examined for any very minor imperfections and any suspicious areas are reinforced with interrupted sutures. The areas under the coronary arteries themselves, particularly on the left, are very difficult to expose at the completion of the procedure; therefore, it is critically important that there be no bleeding here.

An alternative to excising U-shaped areas from the neoaorta is to make a J-shaped incision as indicated in the inset and to rotate a medially based trapdoor flap (Figure 15.4f). This allows for less rotation of the coronary artery but increases the circumference of the proximal neoaorta, which is generally already somewhat larger than the distal divided ascending aorta. We very rarely find it useful to perform this maneuver. Once again, it can be seen that the coronaries are inserted above the level of the neoaortic valve and, thus, should not interfere long-term with the function of the valve.

If an intramural coronary artery is present, it is usually dealt with by excising a longer button including detachment of the posterior neopulmonary valve commissure if necessary (Figure 15.4g). This commissure can be resuspended when the pulmonary artery has been reconstructed with pericardium.

The aortic anastomosis is fashioned using continuous 6/0 Prolene (Figure 15.4h). A continuous suture technique is employed. The points of junction with the coronary suture lines are reinforced with mattress sutures.

The proximal neopulmonary artery is reconstructed with a patch of autologous pericardium treated with 0.6% glutaraldehyde for at least 20 minutes. Continuous 6/0 Prolene is employed (Figure 15.4i). The circulation is now briefly arrested, though the cannulas are not removed.

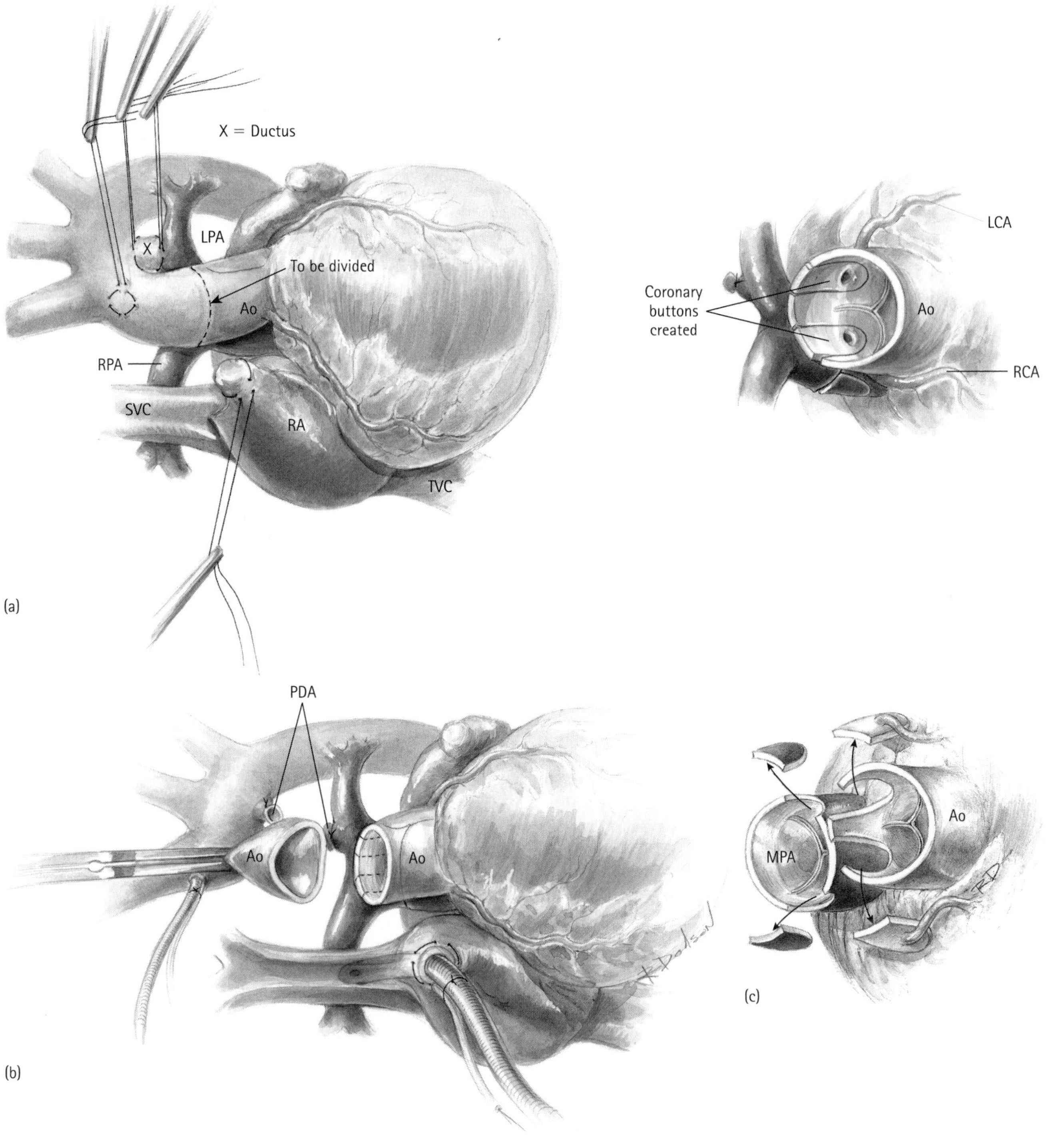

Figure 15.4a–c *Preliminary steps for the arterial switch procedure. (a) The aortic cannulation suture is placed distally in the ascending aorta. A single venous cannula is placed through the right atrial appendage. The ductus will be suture ligated as indicated. The ascending aorta will be divided at approximately its midpoint as indicated by the dashed line. (b) The ductus has been suture ligated and divided. The ascending aorta has been cross clamped and has been divided at its midpoint. The coronary arteries will be excised as indicated. Inset: details of excision of the coronary buttons. (c) The first 2–4 mm of the coronary arteries have been mobilized. Appropriate U-shaped areas of tissue are excised from the proximal neoaorta guided by marking sutures which were placed before bypass was commenced.*

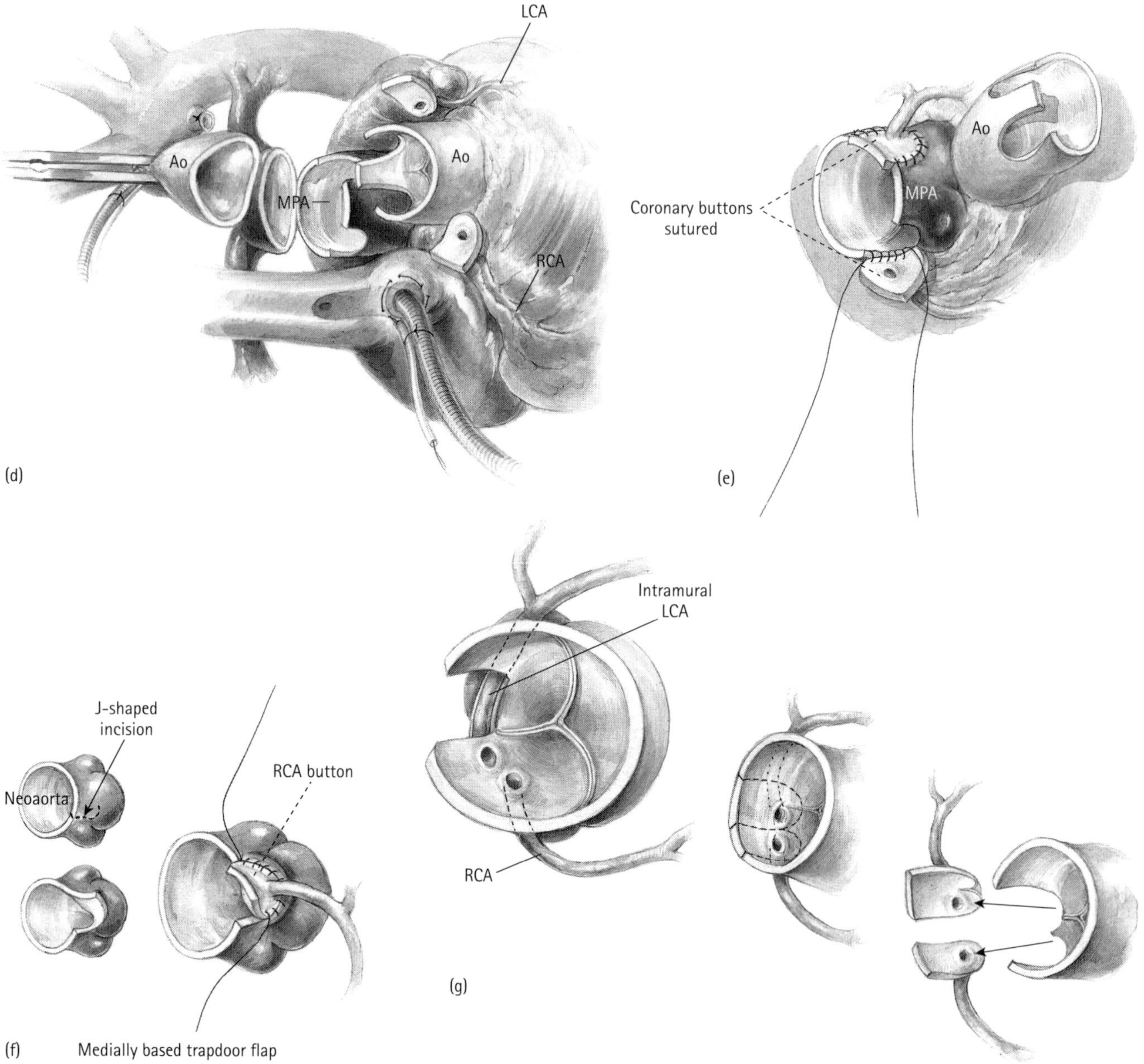

Figure 15.4d–g *(d) The main pulmonary artery has been divided just proximal to its bifurcation. A Lecompte maneuver will subsequently be performed bringing the pulmonary bifurcation anterior to the ascending aorta. (e) The coronary buttons are sutured into the neoaorta using continuous 7/0 Prolene. It is important to reinforce any points of transition of suture technique, e.g. from an inverting to an everting technique. (f) The medially based trapdoor flap is an alternative to excision of a U-shaped area of tissue. The flap is achieved by creation of a J-shaped incision. The trapdoor flap requires less rotation of the coronary buttons but adds to the circumference of the proximal neoaorta. (g) The most common form of intramural coronary artery is a left main coronary artery which has its ostium in the right posterior facing sinus with the coronary vessel itself emerging externally from the left posterior facing sinus. The intramural segment of the artery frequently passes behind the top of the posterior commissure of the original aortic valve. The inset demonstrates that the intramural coronary artery is usually best dealt with by separating the two closely spaced coronary ostia and excising a larger than usual left coronary button often with detachment of the posterior commissure of the neopulmonary valve.*

A short oblique incision is made low in the right atrial free wall. The ASD is closed by direct suture with continuous 5/0 Prolene.

The aortic cross clamp is released. Satisfactory perfusion of all areas should be observed. The pulmonary anastomosis is fashioned using continuous 6/0 Prolene (Figure 15.4j). When the posterior layer has been completed rewarming is begun.

During rewarming a left atrial monitoring line is inserted through the right superior pulmonary vein. Two atrial and one ventricular pacing wire are inserted. With rewarming completed, the child should wean from bypass with dopamine sup-

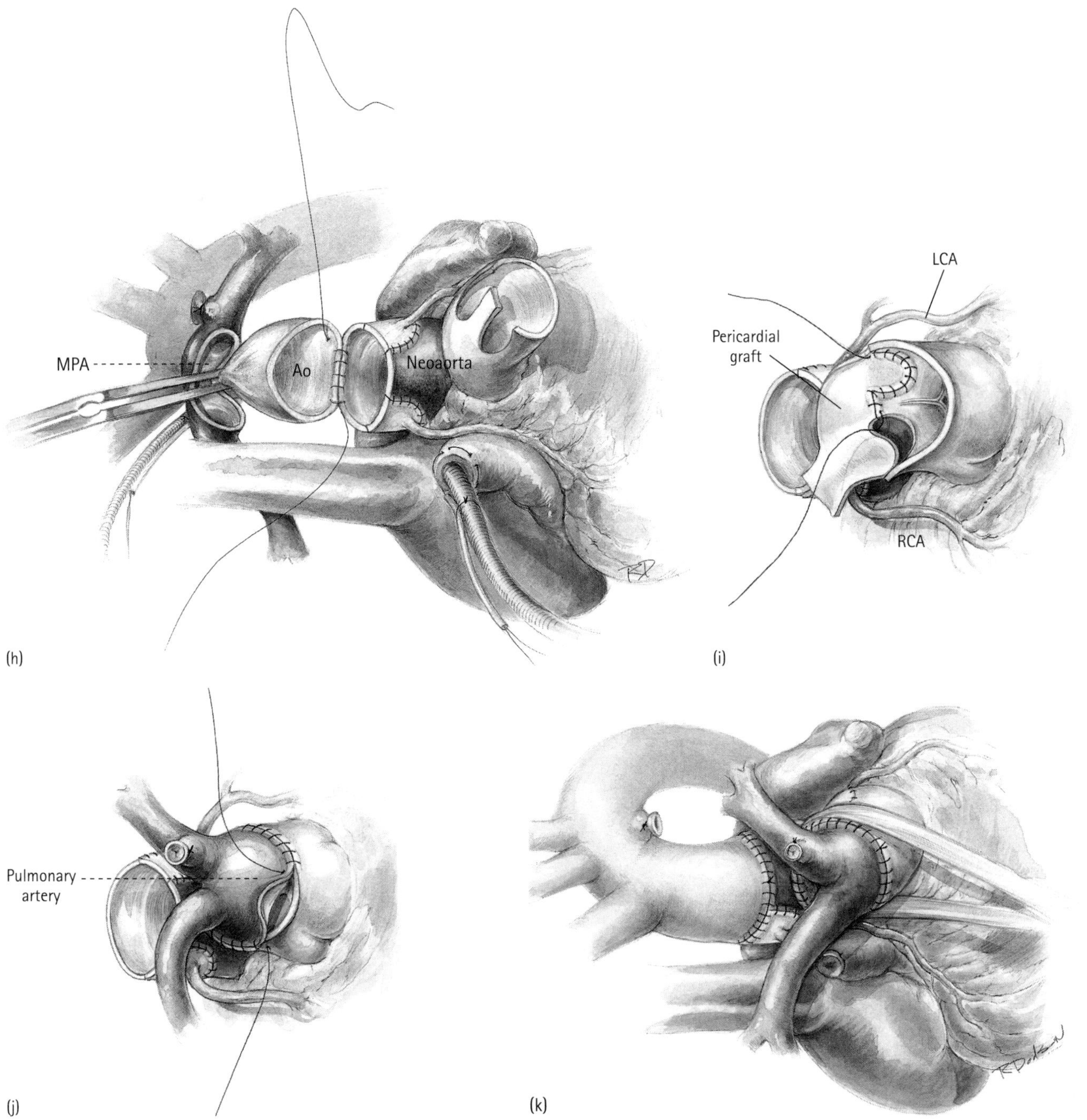

Figure 15.4h–k *(h) After completion of the coronary suture line the aortic anastomosis is fashioned using continuous 6/0 Prolene. The points of junction with the coronary suture lines are reinforced with mattress sutures. (i) The coronary donor areas are filled with a single bifurcated patch of autologous pericardium lightly treated with glutaraldehyde. (j) The pulmonary anastomosis is fashioned following release of the aortic cross clamp. A continuous suture technique is employed. (k) The completed arterial switch procedure.*

port at 5 μg/kg per minute. After removal of the cannulas, protamine is given. Hemostasis is assisted with thrombin soaked gelfoam. A right atrial line is inserted through the right atrial appendage. Chest tubes are inserted. The chest is closed with interrupted stainless steel wires to the sternum with continuous Vicryl to the presternal fascia and subcutaneous and subcuticular Vicryl completing wound closure.

Management of high risk coronary arteries

Single coronary artery from right posterior facing sinus with posterior left main: a positive feedback loop: coronary ischemia and left ventricular dilation: Relatively early in the arterial switch experience it was appreciated that there was a greater degree of difficulty in transferring the second most common coronary branching pattern where the circumflex coronary artery arises from the right coronary artery which itself arose from the rightward and posterior facing sinus. The circumflex then commonly takes a course posterior to the pulmonary artery before entering the left AV groove and supplying much of the obtuse margin of the left ventricle as well as frequently the posterior aspect of the septum. It was thought that this problem was primarily related to the tendency of the circumflex to kink on itself because of the acute angle resulting from transfer to the neopulmonary artery. One method for minimizing this kinking is to create a medially based trapdoor flap as described above.

In addition to the kinking problem, further experience with the arterial switch elucidated another important mechanism resulting in left ventricular ischemia.[35] In the commonest type of single coronary artery the ostium is placed in the rightward and posterior facing sinus. The left main coronary artery arises from the single coronary trunk and passes posterior to the main pulmonary artery before entering the left AV groove. From this point it branches into the anterior descending and circumflex coronary arteries and supplies essentially all of the left ventricle other than perhaps a small amount of the posterior wall if there is a very dominant right coronary system. Several factors can result in a mild degree of left ventricular ischemia. These include the kinking effect noted above. In addition if there has been inadequate mobilization of the left main coronary artery it may be under some degree of tension. There also may be a tendency to hinge or kink on the epicardium if the coronary artery has not been mobilized out of its epicardial fat. The initial mild degree of left ventricular global ischemia will result in left ventricular distention. In the neonate the apex of the heart begins to point out of the chest and in fact may completely emerge from the chest cavity. This results in additional stress being placed on the left main coronary artery which further exacerbates either the tension or the kinking problem. A positive feedback loop is setup which can be very difficult to break. Secondary myocardial edema will ensue as a consequence of the myocardial ischemia as well as the additional transfusion and higher filling pressures that are necessitated in order to maintain an adequate arterial pressure.

How to break a positive feedback loop causing left ventricular ischemia: The most important point is to avoid developing this feedback loop. The problem can be extremely difficult to fix once established. It may be possible to mobilize an additional length of the left main coronary artery so that it is able to loop more freely rather than angling at the point where dissection from epicardial fat was stopped. Reimplantation of the coronary with repositioning using small autologous pericardial patches can be attempted but this can be a difficult undertaking since this usually necessitates taking down the pulmonary anastomosis in order to achieve satisfactory exposure. The cross clamp must be reapplied and cardioplegia must be reinfused. All of these procedures add considerably to bypass time which is likely to further increase myocardial swelling so that the feedback loop once again is set in motion. By far the most important treatment is prevention. There are several points that should be carefully followed in order to prevent this problem from developing.

The very first maneuver in transfer of the coronary arteries is critically important. While the heart is beating normally and the great vessels are under normal pressure, marking sutures of fine Prolene should be placed at the point to which the coronary arteries will be transferred. The site that is selected is simply the point at the same level as the original coronary ostium with a minimal degree of rotation of the coronary. Although initially it was thought to be an advantage to replace the coronary artery more distally in this setting we no longer believe this to be the case.

It is exceedingly important to avoid rotation at the ascending aortic anastomosis. If the proximal neoaortic root is rotated by the anastomosis then the coronaries will come to lie in an incorrect location. Some surgeons find it useful to place marking traction sutures directly anteriorly and at 120° to the left and the right before division of the pulmonary trunk is completed. Great care should be taken to avoid rotation of the ascending aorta when it is cross clamped.

The 'U' that is excised from the proximal neoaorta should lie entirely above the sinotubular junction of the neoaortic valve. It is important to remember that because the original aortic valve lies on a subaortic conus it is more distally placed than the neoaortic valve. When tissue is excised for reimplantation of the coronary arteries this height differential will usually result in the bottom of the 'U' being at the level of the tops of the commissures of the neoaortic valve. It is rare that the 'U' is placed over the midpoint of a sinus of Valsalva. More commonly it is close to or even immediately distal to the top of a commissure of the neoaortic valve.

The suturing of the button into the U-shaped defect is critically important. The surgeon should think of the sutures as small guy ropes that are being placed so as to pull the ostium open as a uniform circle. It is easy to distort the ostium by uneven placement of sutures. Even a slight flattening of the ostium can result in coronary ischemia thereby setting up the highly undesirable feedback loop.

It is important to mobilize adequate lengths of the proximal single main coronary artery as well as the proximal right main and left main coronary artery. In the early years we often divided small branches including the sinus node artery. Today it is exceedingly rare that any branches should be divided. The branches can be mobilized from the epicardium over several millimeters, even up to a centimeter in length if necessary. Using a low level setting of electrocautery the vessels are mobilized from their epicardial location by incision of the adjacent epicardium in much the same way that an internal mammary artery pedicle is raised. The coronary vessels themselves are extremely elastic once mobilized from their epicardial location and will accommodate a surprising amount of stretch that is not possible when they are still tethered by the epicardium and surrounding epicardial fat.

In constructing the overlying pulmonary artery anastomosis it is important to avoid a tightly draped main or right pulmonary artery which can compress the coronaries at their origin. It is rare that this is a problem with this form of coronary artery though it is a not uncommon problem with the second most common form.

Management of cardiopulmonary bypass

It is important to avoid myocardial and whole body edema as this in itself can begin to initiate the positive feedback loop. Several bypass related factors as noted below have been modified over the past 10–15 years which have dramatically decreased the amount of whole body edema that is seen postoperatively.

Cardiopulmonary bypass and edema – venous cannulation: Although many centers prefer direct caval cannulation with two right angle venous cannulas it is our preference to use a single venous cannula placed through the atrial appendage into the right atrium. In the presence of a balloon atrial septal defect the single atrial cannula also functions as a left atrial vent and drains left heart return which can otherwise be profuse. Direct cannulation of the cavae introduces a significant risk of an imbalance in venous drainage between the upper and lower body which can result in an imbalance of perfusion and possible edema of the obstructed area.

Hematocrit: It was previously believed that hemodilution was a necessary component of deep hypothermic bypass and circulatory arrest. There was concern that the increased viscosity of blood at deep hypothermia would result in obstructed microvascular circulation. In fact, multiple studies from our laboratory have suggested that hemodilution can result in inadequate oxygen delivery. In addition the reduced oncotic pressure results in edema. The reduced level of coagulation factors can exacerbate bleeding postoperatively leading to a need for increased homologous blood transfusion which also can exacerbate edema (see Chapter 7).

pH strategy: Both laboratory and a prospective randomized clinical study have revealed a lower incidence of intraoperative and postoperative complications when the pH stat strategy (addition of carbon dioxide) is applied relative to the alpha stat strategy (see Chapter 8). A laboratory study which specifically examined brain edema demonstrated greater cerebral edema with the alpha stat strategy after hypothermic circulatory arrest relative to the pH stat strategy.[36]

Flow rate: It remains unclear as to the optimal flow rate to use during the arterial switch procedure. Although there are proponents of full flow deep hypothermic bypass, full flow moderate hypothermic bypass and even full flow normothermic bypass, our own preference is to use reduced flow deeply hypothermic bypass (see Chapter 9). Deep hypothermia in the neonate probably contributes importantly to myocardial protection and allows one dose only of cardioplegia to be infused even for myocardial ischemic times as long as 2.5 hours. Repeated doses of cardioplegia in the neonate have previously been demonstrated to result in myocardial edema (see Chapter 10).

Management of calcium: We use homologous blood stored in citrate in order to increase the hematocrit to at least 25–30%. The citrate chelates calcium and results in an extremely low ionized calcium level during the cooling phase of cardiopulmonary bypass. This may be helpful in improving myocardial protection which may reduce the amount of postoperative myocardial edema.

Vasodilating agents: It is common to observe vasoconstriction following periods of circulatory arrest or markedly reduced perfusion. This may be secondary to endothelial injury resulting in reduced nitric oxide synthase activity. Vasodilator agents such as phentolamine, phenoxybenzamine, milronone and nitroglycerin are almost certainly useful in reversing this post insult vasospasm.

Single coronary artery from the left anterior facing sinus

The second most common form of single coronary artery associated with transposition does not present a risk of inducing the ischemic positive feedback loop described above. This coronary pattern is most commonly seen when the great vessels are close to being side by side (Figure 15.5). The single coronary ostium lies in the more anterior of the two facing sinuses. The single main trunk gives rise to a right coronary artery which passes anterior to the aorta to reach the right AV groove. The challenge in transferring this coronary artery is that the button must be moved in a direction that is 180° opposite to the right main coronary artery. This is in contrast to the usual transfer which is a simple rotation of the button to an adjacent great vessel. In general it is possible to mobilize the right main coronary artery from its epicardial bed and this will provide enough mobility to allow the right coronary to stretch and the button can be implanted into the neoaorta without undue tension. On occasion, however, even extensive mobilization of the right coronary artery will still result in excessive tension. Under these circumstances it is necessary to extend the button by creating a small tube of autologous pericardium which can be sutured to the usual site of excision in the neoascending aorta (Figure 15.5b). The autologous pericardial tube should be approximately 4 mm in diameter so that even with no growth it will be of adequate size as an adult coronary ostium. The button is sutured to the top of this pericardial tube extension in the usual fashion. The length of the extension should generally be no more than 4 or 5 mm. Figure 15.5b2 illustrates that it is often important in this setting to move the pulmonary artery anastomosis rightward to prevent compression of the single coronary artery by the main pulmonary artery.

Single coronary artery between aorta and pulmonary artery

In the rare case of a single coronary artery running between the pulmonary artery and aorta, it is not possible to rotate the coronary button through 180° (Figure 15.6). The button is rotated through approximately 90° and is then roofed with pericardium.

Management of d-transposition with mild and/or dynamic left ventricular outflow tract obstruction

If a child presents at a time when pulmonary resistance has already fallen and left ventricular pressure is quite a bit lower

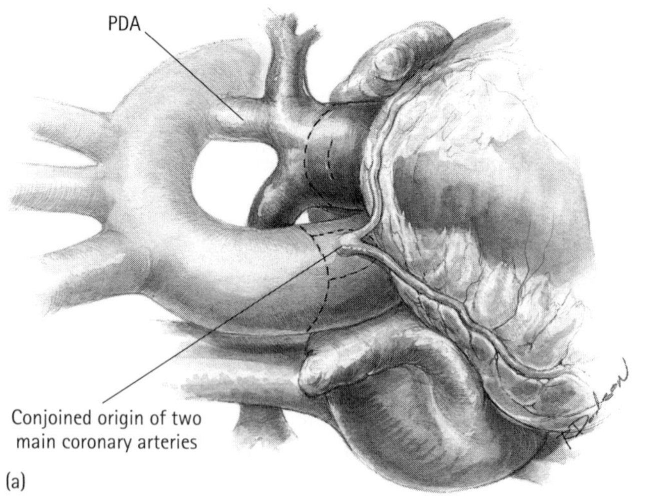

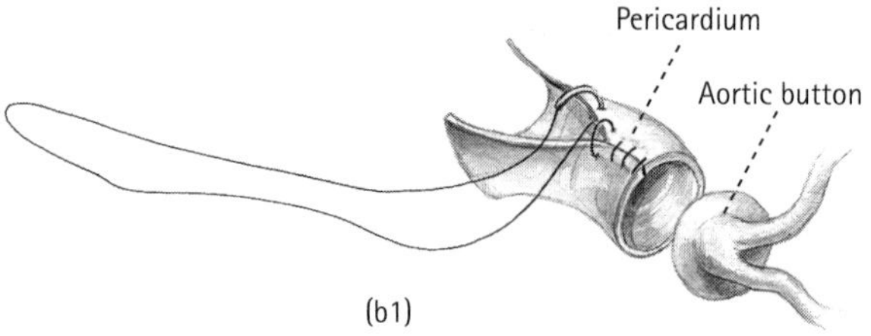

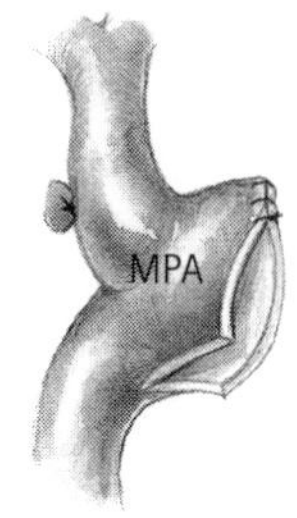

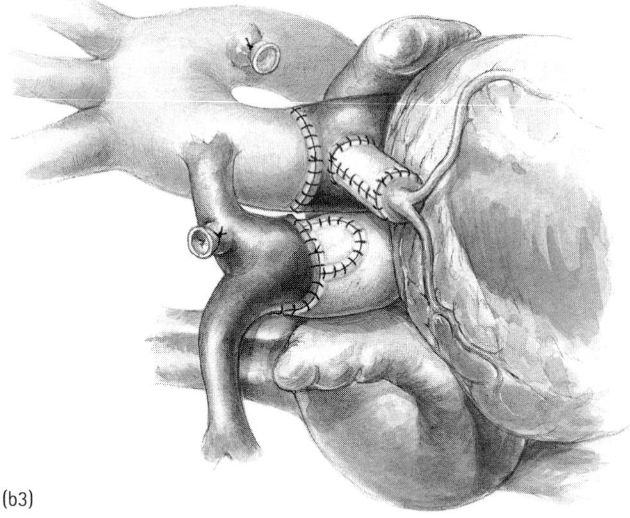

Figure 15.5 *Single coronary artery from the left anterior facing sinus. (a) This single coronary pattern is usually found with side by side great arteries. The dashed lines indicate incisions for division of the main pulmonary artery and aorta as well as excision of the single coronary button. (b) If direct coronary implantation results in excessive tension on the right coronary artery despite extensive mobilization, a tube of autologous pericardium should be created and used for extension of the single coronary artery. The inset above (b1) demonstrates creation of an autologous pericardial tube. The inset below (b2) demonstrates that it is often helpful to shift the pulmonary anastomosis rightward in order to prevent compression of the transferred single coronary artery by the main pulmonary artery.*

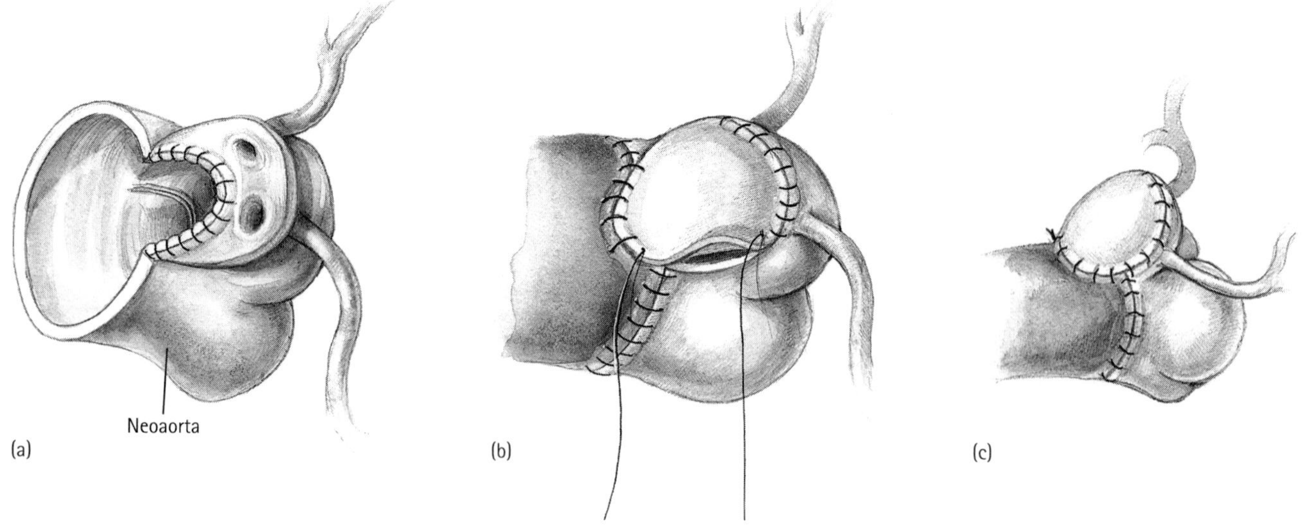

Figure 15.6 *In the extremely rare instance of a single coronary artery running between the pulmonary artery and aorta the button is rotated though 90° and roofed with pericardium.*

than right ventricular pressure, the echocardiogram will demonstrate that the ventricular septum bulges to the left. The septum may contribute to dynamic left ventricular outflow tract obstruction. This can usually be determined preoperatively and is very obvious intraoperatively. After division of the main pulmonary artery passage of an instrument through the neoaortic valve shows that the muscular septum can readily be moved out of the way.

The presence of a bicuspid pulmonary (neoaortic) valve is not an absolute contraindication to an arterial switch procedure.[37] The z score for the size of the valve should be determined and, if it is at least -2.5 to -2, it is probably reasonable to proceed. If there is also severe fixed LV outflow tract obstruction, e.g. a fibrous tunnel or important septal attachments of the mitral valve, it may be necessary to consider a Rastelli or Nikaidoh procedure (see below). However, in general it is preferable to have a less than ideal result with an arterial switch rather than a perfect initial result with a Rastelli procedure.

RASTELLI AND NIKAIDOH PROCEDURES

These procedures are performed for d-transposition with VSD and severe left ventricular outflow tract obstruction. They are described in Chapter 23.

D-TRANSPOSITION WITH INTERRUPTED ARCH OR COARCTATION

The presence of arch hypoplasia, interruption or coarctation should alert the echocardiographer to examine carefully the right ventricular outflow tract, right ventricular volume and tricuspid valve. If the right ventricle is very small and/or if the tricuspid valve is smaller than $z = -2.5$ to -3, a two ventricle repair may be contraindicated. If the neopulmonary annulus is smaller than -2.5 to -3 it may be necessary to place a transannular patch. If a coronary artery crosses the infundibulum it may even be necessary to place a right ventricle to pulmonary artery conduit.

The aortic arch is best dealt with at the time of the arterial switch procedure while working through a median sternotomy. Because the ascending aorta is shifted posteriorly as part of the arterial switch it is generally possible to perform a direct anastomosis for interrupted arch or coarctation with very little tension on the anastomosis. If there is hypoplasia of the arch it is best dealt with by a longitudinal pericardial patch plasty using autologous pericardium treated with glutaraldehyde (Figure 15.7b). This has the advantage also of increasing the size of the ascending aorta so that it will better match the size of the proximal original pulmonary artery, thereby facilitating the neoaortic anastomosis. The plasty or arch anastomosis is best performed under a brief period of hypothermic circulatory arrest which should be sequenced after the coronary transfer. This allows for a long period of cooling of the brain before the circulatory arrest. It is usually not necessary to place an arterial cannula in the main pulmonary artery for descending aortic perfusion as adequate flow is achieved through the circle of Willis even when there is interruption of the aorta. The lower body will readily tolerate an arrest period of 15–20 minutes even if a profound degree of hypothermia is not achieved though this is usually not a problem.

Because the right ventricular infundibulum is often hypoplastic it may be necessary to make an infundibular incision for division of muscle bundles. A pericardial outflow patch is used to close the incision (Figure 15.7d).

POSTOPERATIVE MANAGEMENT IN THE INTENSIVE CARE UNIT FOLLOWING THE ARTERIAL SWITCH

Monitoring catheters should have been placed in the right and left atrium. In addition, two atrial pacing wires and one ventricular pacing wire also should be available. Intensive care management should be routine (see Chapter 5).

Results of surgery

THE CONGENITAL HEART SURGEONS SOCIETY STUDY OF TRANSPOSITION

The most extensive multi-institutional study of the results of surgery for transposition of the great arteries has been conducted by the Congenital Heart Surgeons Society.[38] A total of 829 neonates from 24 institutions were entered into the study between 1985 and 1989. This covered the period when many institutions were transitioning from an atrial level repair to an arterial repair. Of these, 516 patients had an arterial switch procedure, 285 had an atrial repair and 28 had a Rastelli procedure. This study drew attention to the importance of deaths that occur before repair. In this particular study this accounted for a 2.5% mortality. Follow-up of these patients has confirmed that the ongoing late risk of death is significantly higher for an atrial level repair relative to an arterial repair. Thus in the current era where early mortality is similar for the two procedures there is no question that an arterial switch procedure is to be preferred over an atrial level repair.

Another important report from the Congenital Heart Surgeons Society study was published in 1997.[39] The focus of the report was outflow obstruction after the arterial switch procedure. The late incidence of right ventricular outflow tract obstruction in this early cohort of patients is 0.5% per year which is very much higher than the risk of obstruction in the reconstructed aortic root, which appears to be 0.1% per year. Risk factors for infundibular obstruction or obstruction at the level of the pulmonary valve were a side by side position of the great vessels, presence of coexisting coarctation, use of prosthetic material in sinus reconstruction, earlier era of surgery and institution. Obstruction in the pulmonary root or pulmonary artery was associated with lower birth weight, left coronary artery arising from the rightward and posterior sinus (sinus 2), coronary explantation using a circular button separate from the transection of the aorta, earlier date of surgery and institutional factors.

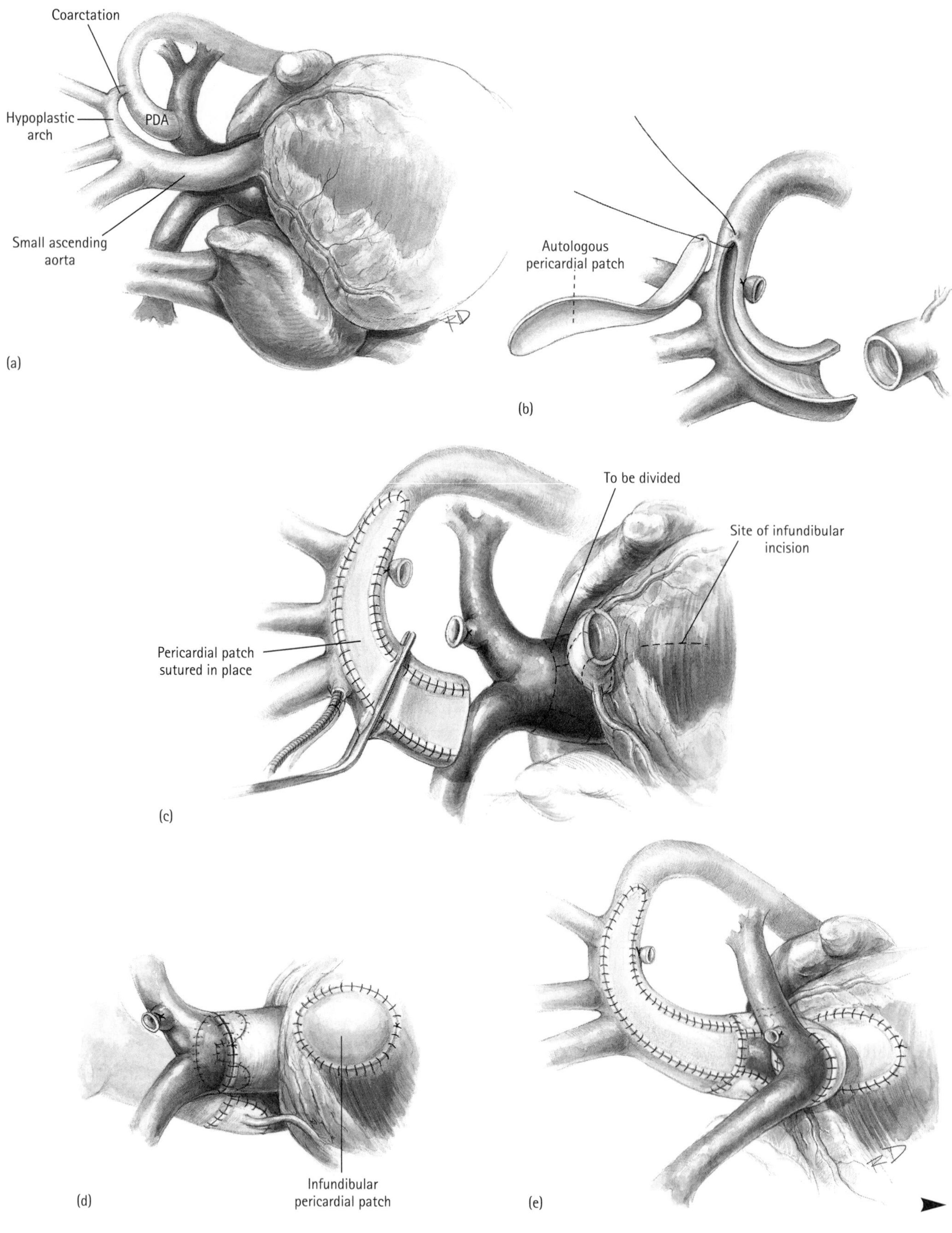

Coarctation
Hypoplastic arch
PDA
Small ascending aorta
(a)
Autologous pericardial patch
(b)
To be divided
Site of infundibular incision
Pericardial patch sutured in place
(c)
Infundibular pericardial patch
(d)
(e)

RESULTS OF THE ARTERIAL SWITCH PROCEDURE AT CHILDREN'S HOSPITAL BOSTON

A number of reports have been published from Children's Hospital Boston regarding the neonatal arterial switch procedure which now encompasses a 20 year time span following the first procedure in January 1983. A number of these papers have been summarized in a review in the 1998 Pediatric Cardiac Surgery Annual by Blume and Wernovsky.[40] An important collection of three articles appeared contiguously in the *Journal of Thoracic and Cardiovascular Surgery* in 1995. Colan et al[41] reviewed the status of the left ventricle after the arterial switch procedure. In patients who underwent a primary arterial switch procedure echo indices of left ventricular size, shape and function were normal. In contrast, patients who underwent a rapid two stage arterial switch procedure had mildly reduced echo indices of left ventricular function and contractility both compared with normal as well as with patients undergoing a primary arterial switch procedure. Rhodes et al[42] examined arrhythmias and intracardiac conduction after the arterial switch procedure. In contrast to the experience with the Senning and Mustard procedures sinus rhythm was present in 99% of patients during 24 hour Holter monitor studies at a mean of 2.1 years after the operation. The incidence of supraventricular tachycardia was very low as was the incidence of other important arrhythmias. Wernovksy et al[16] examined factors influencing early and late outcome of the arterial switch procedure. This study identified specific features of coronary anatomy as being a risk factor for both mortality as well as a risk factor for reintervention for pulmonary arterial stenosis. A more detailed analysis of the influence of coronary artery anatomy on outcome after the arterial switch procedure follows.

THE INFLUENCE OF CORONARY ARTERY ANATOMY ON THE RESULTS OF SURGERY FOR THE ARTERIAL SWITCH PROCEDURE

One of the first papers to review the influence of coronary artery anatomy on outcome was published by Yacoub and Radley Smith in 1978,[14] five years before the first primary neonatal arterial switch procedure was performed and nearly 10 years before the arterial switch was to become the standard of care for transposition of the great arteries. In their seminal article entitled 'Anatomy of the coronary arteries in transposition of the great arteries and methods for their transfer in anatomical correction' Yacoub and Radley Smith stated that all types of coronary artery pattern are amenable to transfer. However, in that very early report Yacoub did not describe experience with a single right, single left or the 'inverted coronary patterns', i.e. the right coronary artery arising from the left facing sinus and passing anterior to the aorta into the right AV groove with the left coronary artery arising from the right posterior facing sinus and passing behind the pulmonary artery. The other 'inverted coronary pattern' is that in which the circumflex coronary artery arises from the right facing sinus while the right coronary artery arises with the anterior descending coronary artery from the left posterior facing sinus. In these two situations much of the left ventricle (all in the case of inverted main coronary arteries) is supplied by a coronary vessel passing behind the pulmonary artery which places the patient at risk of the ischemic positive feedback loop described above.

In a subsequent early report, Quaegebeur et al[30] described an eight year experience with 66 patients undergoing the arterial switch procedure. They stated that there was no impact of coronary artery patterns on outcome when analysed by multivariate analysis. There were five patients in this series who had either a single right or inverted coronary patterns, although there was one late death in this series of unknown cause in a patient with a single right coronary artery.

The potential challenge of coronary artery transfer was highlighted by a 1988 paper published by Brawn and Mee.[43] The authors described 50 patients of whom 11 had had serious coronary artery transfer problems. The authors were successful in correcting all of these problems except one by either relocating the coronary ostia, inserting pericardial patches at the coronary to neoaortic anastomosis or placing tacking sutures to adjust the position of the pulmonary artery to relieve coronary compression. The one patient who clearly died from coronary problems had an inverted coronary pattern. Also a second patient with unstated coronary anatomy died of 'sudden myocardial failure' within 24 hours of surgery.

In a report by Serraf et al in 1993[44] an analysis was undertaken of 432 consecutive neonates who underwent an arterial switch procedure in Paris between 1984 and 1992. The authors found that the risk of surgical mortality was increased in any coronary pattern in which either one or both of the great vessels passed between the great vessels. In this setting the coronary relocation requires turning the ostial patch through 180° which creates a risk of torsion obstruction of the main coronary arteries. A technique similar to that described in the surgical techniques section above must be applied to avoid this

Figure 15.7 *(a) d-Transposition with aortic arch hypoplasia and coarctation of the aorta. The ascending aorta is often approximately half the diameter of the main pulmonary artery. (b) Aortic arch hypoplasia is often best managed by a longitudinal autologous pericardial patch which extends along the full length of the small ascending aorta. The patch serves to bring the ascending aortic diameter closer to the diameter of the proximal neoaorta. (c) The pericardial plasty of the aortic arch is performed under a brief period of hypothermic circulatory arrest. The aortic cross clamp is then applied and perfusion is recommenced while the remainder of the patch is sutured into the ascending aorta. (d) There is often infundibular hypoplasia associated with aortic arch hypoplasia. It may be necessary to perform an infundibular incision, divide infundibular muscle bundles and place an infundibular pericardial outflow patch. (e) Completed arterial switch procedure and arch augmentation together with right ventricular infundibular outflow patch.*

risk. In another report from Paris in 1988, Planche et al[45] had previously reported a similar finding to the 1993 report from Paris, namely that passage of the coronary arteries between the great vessels was associated with a higher mortality. In many cases this was in the setting of an intramural coronary artery.

As noted above the largest series reported of patients undergoing the neonatal arterial switch procedure is the multi-institutional report from the Congenital Heart Surgeons Society.[46] In the first report of this series in which Castaneda was the first author, 187 patients were described in 1988. At this time the overall mortality rate was high with only 81% of patients surviving at one year. There was no difference in mortality risk whether patients entered a protocol for neonatal arterial switch or later atrial switch. In this initial report coronary artery anatomy did not emerge as a risk factor. However, it is likely that during the early learning phase of this new operation that there were many factors contributing to mortality which almost certainly masked the influence of coronary anatomy. In the next report from the Congenital Heart Surgeons Society also published in 1988[7] in which Norwood was the first author, a total of 466 neonates had now been entered into the 20 institution study. The type of coronary anatomy was once again not identified as a risk factor for death either in the overall group or in low risk institutions. However, the authors point out that at this time there was still a tendency for surgeons to select out patients who had complex coronary anatomy and this too might have masked a potential effect of coronary anatomy on outcome. In the 1992 paper describing the ongoing results of the Congenital Heart Surgeons Society study of transposition, Kirklin et al[47] described 513 neonates who had now been entered into the same study and who had undergone an arterial switch procedure. In this report coronary artery anatomy emerges for the first time as a risk factor. In fact this was the only risk factor specifically related to patient morphology that influenced early survival. Origin of the left main coronary artery or only the left anterior descending or circumflex coronary artery from the rightward posterior facing sinus (sinus 2) was a risk factor for death. An intramural course of the left main or left anterior descending coronary artery also increased risk. Arteries with an intramural course nearly always arose from an ostium near the commissure between the two posterior facing sinuses.

Thus the Congenital Heart Surgeons Society study confirms the importance of the feedback loop mechanism as described above in that each of these patterns places either all or an important segment of the left ventricle at risk of ischemia if there is dilation of the left ventricle resulting in tension on a coronary artery passing posterior to the pulmonary artery.

Another report which describes coronary branching pattern as influencing survival was the 2000 report by Daebritz et al[48] from Aachen, Germany. In this series describing 312 patients operated on between 1982 and 1997, single coronary artery origin either from the right posterior facing sinus with the left main coronary passing behind the pulmonary artery (B1) or single coronary artery arising from the left posterior facing sinus with the right coronary artery passing anterior to the aorta (A2) were associated with reduced operative survival. A single coronary ostium was also associated with reduced late survival.

Experience with mortality risk for the arterial switch procedure according to coronary anatomy at Children's Hospital Boston

In 1990, Mayer et al[35] undertook an analysis of 314 patients who had undergone the arterial switch procedure at Children's Hospital Boston between 1983 and 1989. The analysis reveals that to that time there was a moderately increased risk for an arterial switch operation when two of the less common coronary artery patterns were encountered, i.e. either single right coronary artery or either of the inverted coronary artery patterns. This report did not find that an intramural course of either coronary artery was a risk factor. The increased risk of the intramural coronary had previously been suggested by Quaegebeur et al though they had been unable to demonstrate this fact statistically. However, in a report by Day et al from UCLA,[49] of 70 patients having the arterial switch procedure patients with an intramural coronary artery had significantly greater morbidity and mortality secondary to coronary ischemia relative to patients with the most common coronary patterns. In a 1999 report from Children's Hospital Boston, Blume et al[50] reviewed the 'evolution of risk factors influencing the early mortality of the arterial switch operation'. They reviewed 223 patients who underwent an arterial switch procedure between January 1, 1992 and December 31, 1996. This included patients who had aortic arch obstruction or interruption, multiple VSDs and prematurity. Overall there were 16 early deaths (7%) with three deaths in the 109 patients considered low risk (2.7%). In this analysis coronary artery pattern was not associated with an increased risk of death. However, compared with usual coronary artery pattern inverted coronary patterns with single right coronary patterns were associated with morbidity as indicated by increased incidence of delayed sternal closure and longer duration of mechanical ventilation. Blume et al concluded that the arterial switch procedure can be performed in the current era without excess early mortality related to an uncommon coronary artery pattern.

Results of surgery for single coronary artery at Children's Hospital Boston

Between 1983 and 2000, 844 patients underwent the arterial switch procedure at Children's Hospital, Boston. Of these patients, 53 (6.3%) had a single coronary pattern. Seven (13%) with a single coronary pattern died. Since July of 1991 no patient with a single coronary pattern has died. Revision of the coronary anastomosis at the time of the arterial switch was required in seven patients (13%) intraoperatively due to myocardial ischemia. Patients with a single right ostium with the circumflex or left main coronary artery passing behind the pulmonary artery were estimated to have an approximately eightfold increased risk of early death compared with other single coronary patterns. In addition, patients with a side by side position of the great arteries were estimated to have a significantly higher risk of mortality (approximately sixfold) compared with other positions.

A similar experience has been described by the group from Toronto in a report published in 2000 by Shukla et al.[51] Although the mortality was 38% in patients with transposition/intact ventricular septum and a single coronary artery and 41% with patients with transposition with associated VSD nevertheless in the 3.5 years immediately preceding the close of the series, the mortality of six consecutive neonates with single coronary artery was zero. The authors describe in this article a number of technical maneuvers similar to those described in this review.

Late coronary problems following the arterial switch procedure

In 1996 Bonhoeffer et al from Paris[52] described 'long term fate of the coronary arteries after the arterial switch operation in newborns with transposition of the arteries'. A total of 12 coronary occlusions were identified in 165 children who underwent selective coronary angiography at an average age of approximately six years. In a report by Tanel et al[53] from Children's Hospital Boston, 13 patients (3%) were identified as having previously unsuspected coronary abnormalities among 366 patients who underwent postoperative catheterization after the arterial switch procedure. Of these 13 patients, one patient died suddenly three years after surgery, one patient was lost to follow-up and the remaining 10 patients were alive and asymptomatic up to 11 years after surgery.

DEVELOPMENTAL OUTCOME AFTER THE ARTERIAL SWITCH

A not unexpected finding in the most recent report from the Congenital Heart Surgeons Society[38] is the high prevalence of psychosocial deficits as reported by parents, especially learning difficulties. This finding is not surprising when one considers the era in which this cohort of patients underwent surgery. At that time (the late 1980s) the use of long periods of hypothermic circulatory arrest was common. More importantly patients were managed with severe degrees of hemodilution and an alkaline pH strategy that frequently was more alkaline than the alpha stat strategy. As discussed in Chapter 9, this combination of factors has been clearly demonstrated to be associated with a higher incidence of perioperative neurological complications[54] as well as evidence of developmental impairment in subsequent follow-up studies.[55–57]

In a prospective randomized trial of pH strategy in the mid-1990s[58] patients with transposition had significantly higher mental (109.4 $\pm$ 14.7) and psychomotor (99.0 $\pm$ 16.8) development index scores than had either the tetralogy or VSD subgroups. This probably in part reflects the fact that microdeletion of chromosome 22 rarely if ever occurs in patients with transposition. However, in addition it also demonstrates the improved developmental outcome that had occurred consequent to cardiopulmonary bypass hardware and methodologic changes that had occurred between the late 1980s when the first developmental outcomes cohort was enrolled versus the latter study. Further improvements in developmental outcome have occurred subsequent to changes in hematocrit management.[59] Thus it seems highly probable that in the current era with use of the pH stat strategy, a hematocrit of greater than 25–30 and limited use of hypothermic circulatory arrest, children with transposition are likely to score within the normal range for developmental outcome.

Two stage arterial switch

The concept of a two stage arterial switch was introduced by Yacoub in 1976.[60] Many of Yacoub's patients presented to him beyond the neonatal period and therefore did not have a prepared left ventricle for a one stage switch. Yacoub placed a pulmonary artery band to increase left ventricular pressure which caused left ventricular hypertrophy thereby 'preparing' the ventricle. He empirically waited an interval period of several months to a year or so before undertaking the arterial switch. This work predated description of the Lecompte maneuver.[34] Yacoub used a conduit to connect the right ventricle to the distal divided pulmonary arteries.

The long interval two stage switch described by Yacoub had a number of disadvantages. The band caused scarring that complicated pulmonary artery reconstruction. Scarring also could distort the neoaortic valve and did lead to an important incidence of neoaortic valve incompetence. Adhesions caused by the band obscured coronary artery anatomy and made the coronary transfer more difficult. Finally for the family there were the logistical difficulties imposed by two hospitalizations separated by an interval period of medical management.

In the early 1980s the Chief of Cardiology at Children's Hospital Boston, Dr Bernardo Nadal-Ginard, was undertaking cutting edge research into the molecular biology of cardiac hypertrophy.[61] His work demonstrated not only that there were important shifts in the isoforms of heavy chain myosin in response to a pressure load, but in addition those changes were apparent within hours of the stress being imposed. Measurement of the rate of muscle protein synthesis demonstrated that maximal synthesis was occurring by 48 hours from the onset of the pressure load. Dr Nadal and the Chief of cardiac surgery at the time, Dr Aldo Castaneda, reasoned that preparation of a left ventricle for an arterial switch in a human should be possible in days rather than months. This concept was supported by data that had already been collected from athletes engaging in training programs in whom monitoring of cardiac muscle mass had been done with echocardiography. Thus a program of 'rapid two stage arterial switching' was begun at Children's Hospital Boston in 1986.[62]

INDICATIONS FOR A TWO STAGE ARTERIAL SWITCH

A two stage arterial switch is indicated in the child presenting beyond four to eight weeks of age whose left ventricular pressure is less than approximately 66% of systemic pressure. If left ventricular pressure has been maintained by a patent ductus or VSD beyond the immediate neonatal period it may be possible to exceed four to eight weeks. However, even within a timeframe of four to eight weeks it is possible that a child will have inadequate left ventricular muscle mass to survive an arterial switch unless a period of ventricular support with extracorporeal membrane oxygenation or a ventricular assist device is provided following the arterial switch.[63]

A two stage arterial switch may also be indicated in a child who has a failing atrial level repair of transposition, i.e. a Senning or Mustard procedure. Although anecdotal successes have been described beyond early teenage years we and others[64] have generally been disappointed with the results of this approach in young adults and suggest a heart transplant when there is late right ventricular dysfunction.

TECHNICAL ASPECTS OF RAPID TWO STAGE ARTERIAL SWITCH

Stage one

Approach is through a midline sternotomy. The thymus is subtotally resected. A 3.5 mm modified right Blalock shunt is constructed in all patients from the distal innominate artery and proximal subclavian artery to the right pulmonary artery using longitudinal arteriotomies and continuous 6/0 Prolene for both anastomoses. Although it may seem that some patients will tolerate banding alone, a safer approach which avoids dangerous desaturation in the interval period is to place a relatively small shunt in all patients. When the clamps on the shunt have been released a silastic Dacron impregnated band approximately 3 mm in width is passed through the transverse sinus and then between the aorta and main pulmonary artery to encircle the main pulmonary artery. A pressure monitoring catheter is placed in the proximal main pulmonary artery. Usually it is found that the shunt alone has resulted in an increase in pressure to at least 50% of systemic pressure. The band should be tightened so that the proximal pulmonary artery pressure is at least 66% of systemic pressure. Although our practice in the past was to tighten the band to greater than 75% more recent information suggests that this may result in late ventricular dysfunction.[65]

Interval period

It is important to understand that the stage one preparatory procedure imposes a large volume load on the systemic right ventricle which may require considerable support in the first few days following the procedure.[66] Approximately one third of babies will need to remain intubated and receiving inotropic support throughout an interval period of five to seven days, one third can be extubated but must remain in the intensive care unit and one third have very little difficulty during the preparatory period. Daily echo studies should be undertaken to track ventricular function and ventricular mass. By 5–7 days the left ventricle should have recovered normal function after an initial period of importantly depressed function.

Second stage arterial switch

The second stage is no different than a primary arterial switch other than the need to remove the band and to clip and divide the shunt. At 5–7 days there are usually only fibrinous adhesions that are easily broken down and do not obscure coronary anatomy. Postoperative management is also routine.

Two stage arterial switch following a previous Mustard or Senning

Because the child who has had a Mustard or Senning has a normal arterial oxygen saturation it is not necessary to place a shunt to maintain the arterial oxygen saturation. Nevertheless these individuals can be quite unstable, particularly following the arterial switch when there is a real risk of sudden ventricular fibrillation unheralded by ventricular ectopy or ST changes.[64]

RESULTS OF TWO STAGE ARTERIAL SWITCH PROCEDURE

Between 1986 and 1988, 11 patients at Children's Hospital Boston underwent first stage preparation for a two stage arterial switch procedure at a mean age of 4.5 months. The median interval period was nine days before the arterial switch procedure. Serial echocardiography documented that left ventricular mass increased by a mean of 85% during this short interval. Mean left ventricular to right ventricular pressure ratio was increased by the preparatory first stage from 0.5 to 1.04. There were no deaths following the first stage procedure and no early deaths in the 10 patients who had an arterial switch procedure. One patient underwent a Senning procedure because of an intramural coronary artery. Late studies of ventricular function[65] have documented that echo indices of left ventricular function and contractility are slightly reduced relative to normal and relative to patients who have undergone a primary arterial switch procedure.

REFERENCES

1. Rashkind WJ, Miller WW. Creation of an atrial septal defect without thoracotomy: A palliative approach to complete transposition of the great arteries. *JAMA* 1966; **196**:991–992.
2. Castaneda AR, Norwood WI, Jonas RA, Colan SD, Sanders SP, Lang P. Transposition of the great arteries and intact ventricular septum: anatomical repair in the neonate. *Ann Thorac Surg* 1984; **38**:438–443.
3. Pexieder T. Conotruncus and its septation at the advent of the molecular biology era. In Clark EB, Markwald RR, Takao A (eds). *Developmental Mechanisms of Heart Disease.* Armonk, NY, Futura Publishing Company, 1995, pp 227–248.
4. Van Praagh R, Van Praagh S, Nebesar RA, Muster AJ, Sinha SN, Paul MH. Tetralogy of Fallot: Underdevelopment of the pulmonary infundibulum and its sequelae. *Am J Cardiol* 1970; **26**:25–33.
5. Van Praagh S, Davidoff A, Chin A et al. Double outlet right ventricle: Anatomic types and developmental implications based on a study of 101 autopsied cases. *J Cardiol* 1982; **12**:389–483.

6. Sim EK, van Son JA, Edwards WD, Puga FJ. Congenital ostial membrane of right coronary artery in complete transposition of the great arteries. *J Thorac Cardiovasc Surg* 1994; **107**:1538–1539.
7. Norwood WI, Dobell AR, Freed MD, Kirklin JW, Blackstone EH and the Congenital Heart Surgeons Society. Intermediate results of the arterial switch repair. *J Thorac Cardiovasc Surg* 1988; **96**:854–862.
8. Shrivastava S, Tadavarthy SM, Fukuda T, Edwards JE. Anatomic causes of pulmonary stenosis in complete transposition. *Circulation* 1976; **54**:154–159.
9. Kimbris D. Anomalous origin of the left main coronary artery from the right sinus of Valsalva. *Am J Cardiol* 1985; **55**:765–769.
10. Gittenberger-deGroot AC, Sauer U, Quaegebeur J. Aortic intramural coronary artery in three hearts with transposition of the great arteries. *J Thorac Cardiovasc Surg* 1986; **91**:566–571.
11. Sachweh JS, Tiete AR, Jockenhoevel S et al. Fate of intramural coronary arteries after arterial switch operation. *Thorac Cardiovasc Surg* 2002; **50**:40–44.
12. Scheule AM, Jonas RA. Management of transposition of the great arteries with single coronary artery. *Semin Thorac Cardiovasc Surg Pediatr Card Surg Annu* 2001; **4**:34–57.
13. Yamaguchi M, Hosokawa Y, Imai Y et al. Early and midterm results of the arterial switch operation for transposition of the great arteries in Japan. *J Thorac Cardiovasc Surg* 1990; **100**:261–269.
14. Yacoub MH, Radley-Smith R. Anatomy of the coronary arteries in transposition of the great arteries and methods for their transfer in anatomical correction. *Thorax* 1978; **33**:418–424.
15. Wernovsky G, Sanders SP. Coronary artery anatomy and transposition of the great arteries. *Coron Artery Dis* 1993; **4**:148–157.
16. Wernovsky G, Mayer JE, Jonas RA et al. Factors influencing early and late outcome of the arterial switch operation for transposition of the great arteries. *J Thorac Cardiovasc Surg* 1995; **109**:289–301.
17. Scheule AM, Zurakowski D, Blume ED et al. Arterial switch operation with a single coronary artery. *J Thorac Cardiovasc Surg* 2002; **123**:1164–1172.
18. Bano-Rodrigo A, Quero-Jimenez M, Moreno-Granado F, Gamallo-Amat C. Wall thickness of ventricular chambers in transposition of the great arteries: Surgical implications. *J Thorac Cardiovasc Surg* 1980; **79**:592–597.
19. Clarkson PM, Neutze JM, Wardill JC, Barratt-Boyes BG. The pulmonary vascular bed in patients with complete transposition of the great arteries. *Circulation* 1976; **53**:539–543.
20. Newfeld EA, Paul MM, Muster AJ, Idriss FS. Pulmonary vascular disease in complete transposition of the great arteries. A study of 200 patients. *Am J Cardiol* 1974; **34**:75–82.
21. Viles PH, Ongley PA, Titus JL. The spectrum of pulmonary vascular disease in transposition of the great arteries. *Circulation* 1969; **40**:31–41.
22. Mandell VS, Lock JE, Mayer JE, Parness IA, Kulik TJ. The 'laid-back' aortogram: An improved angiographic view for demonstration of coronary arteries in TGA. *Am J Cardiol* 1990; **65**:1379–1383.
23. Kirklin JW, Blackstone EH, Tchervenkov CI, Castaneda AR. Clinical outcomes after the arterial switch operation for transposition. Patient, support, procedural, and institutional risk factors. Congenital Heart Surgeons Society. *Circulation* 1992; **86**:1501–1515.
24. Foran JP, Sullivan ID, Elliott MJ, de Leval MR. Primary arterial switch operation for transposition of the great arteries with intact ventricular septum in infants older than 21 days. *J Am Coll Cardiol* 1998; **31**:883–889.
25. Davis AM, Wilkinson JL, Karl TR, Mee RB. Transposition of the great arteries with intact ventricular septum. Arterial switch repair in patients 21 days of age or older. *J Thorac Cardiovasc Surg* 1993; **106**:111–115.
26. Blalock A, Hanlon CR. The surgical treatment of complete transposition of the aorta and the pulmonary artery. *Surg Gynecol Obstet* 1950; **90**:1.
27. Barrratt-Boyes BG, Neutze JM, Harris EA (eds). *Heart Disease in Infancy*. Edinburgh, Churchill Livingstone, 1973.
28. Senning A. Surgical correction of transposition of the great vessels. *Surgery* 1959; **45**:966.
29. Mustard WT. Successful two stage correction of transposition of the great vessels. *Surgery* 1964; **55**:469.
30. Quaegebeur JM, Rohmer J, Brom AG. Revival of the Senning operation in the treatment of transposition of the great arteries. Preliminary report on recent experience. *Thorax* 1977; **32**:517–524.
31. Trusler GA, Williams WG, Izukawa T, Olley PM. Current results with the Mustard operation in isolated transposition of the great arteries. *J Thorac Cardiovasc Surg* 1980; **80**:381–389.
32. Jatene AD, Fontes VF, Paulista PP et al. Anatomic correction of transposition of the great vessels. *J Thorac Cardiovasc Surg* 1976; **72**:364–370.
33. Yacoub MH, Radley-Smith R, Maclaurin R. Two stage operation for anatomical correction of transposition of the great arteries with intact interventricular septum. *Lancet* 1977; **1**:1275–1278.
34. Lecompte Y, Neveux JY, Leca F et al. Reconstruction of the pulmonary outflow tract without prosthetic conduit. *J Thorac Cardiovasc Surg* 1982; **84**:727–733.
35. Mayer JE Jr, Sanders SP, Jonas RA, Castaneda AR, Wernovsky G. Coronary artery pattern and outcome of arterial switch operation for transposition of the great arteries. *Circulation* 1990; **82**(5 Suppl):IV139–145.
36. Aoki M, Nomura F, Stromski ME et al. Effects of pH on brain energetics after hypothermic circulatory arrest. *Ann Thorac Surg* 1993; **55**:1093–1103.
37. Wernovsky G, Jonas RA, Colan SD et al. Results of the arterial switch operation in patients with transposition of the great arteries and abnormalities of the mitral valve or left ventricular outflow tract. *J Am Coll Cardiol* 1990; **16**:1446–1454.
38. Williams WG, McCrindle BW, Ashburn DA, Jonas RA, Mavroudis C, Blackstone EH. Outcomes of 829 neonates with complete transposition of the great arteries 12–17 years after repair. *Eur J Cardiothorac Surg* 2003; **24**:1–9.
39. Williams WG, Quaegebeur JM, Kirklin JW, Blackstone EH and the Congenital Heart Surgeons Society. Outflow obstruction after the arterial switch operation: A multiinstitutional study. *J Thorac Cardiovasc Surg* 1997; **114**:975–990.
40. Blume ED, Wernovsky G. Long-term results of arterial switch repair of transposition of the great vessels. *Semin Thorac Cardiovasc Surg Pediatr Card Surg Annu* 1998; **1**:129–113.
41. Colan SD, Boutin C, Castaneda AR, Wernovsky G. Status of the left ventricle after arterial switch operation for transposition of the great arteries. Hemodynamic and echocardiographic evaluation. *J Thorac Cardiovasc Surg* 1995; **109**:311–321.
42. Rhodes LA, Wernovsky G, Keane JF et al. Arrhythmias and intracardiac conduction after the arterial switch operation. *J Thorac Cardiovasc Surg* 1995; **109**:303–310.
43. Brawn WJ, Mee RB. Early results for anatomic correction of transposition of the great arteries and for double outlet right ventricle with subpulmonary ventricular septal defect. *J Thorac Cardiovasc Surg* 1988; **95**:230–238.

44. Serraf A, Lacour-Gayet F, Bruniaux J et al. Anatomic correction of transposition of the great arteries in neonates. *J Am Coll Cardiol* 1993; **22**:193–200.
45. Planche C, Bruniaux J, Lacour-Gayet F et al. Switch operation for transposition of the great arteries in neonates. A study of 120 patients. *J Thorac Cardiovasc Surg* 1988; **96**:354–363.
46. Castaneda AR, Trusler GA, Paul MH, Blackstone EH, Kirklin JW. The early results of treatment with simple transposition in the current era. *J Thorac Cardiovasc Surg* 1988; **95**:14–27.
47. Kirklin JW, Blackstone EH, Tchervenkov CI, Castaneda AR. Clinical outcomes after the arterial switch operation for transposition. Patient, support, procedural and institutional risk factors. *Circulation* 1992; **86**:1501–1515.
48. Daebritz SH, Nollert G, Sachweh JS, Engelhardt W, von Bernuth G, Messmer BJ. Anatomical risk factors for mortality and cardiac morbidity after arterial switch operation. *Ann Thorac Surg* 2000; **69**:1880–1886.
49. Day RW, Laks H, Drinkwater DC. The influence of coronary anatomy on the arterial switch operation in neonates. *J Thorac Cardiovasc Surg* 1992; **104**:706–712.
50. Blume ED, Altmann K, Mayer JE et al. Evolution of risk factors influencing early mortality of the arterial switch operation. *J Am Coll Cardiol* 1999; **33**:1702–1709.
51. Shukla V, Freedom RM, Black MD. Single coronary artery and complete transposition of the great arteries: A technical challenge resolved? *Ann Thorac Surg* 2000; **69**:568–571.
52. Bonhoeffer P, Bonnet D, Piechaud JF et al. Coronary artery obstruction after the arterial switch operation for transposition of the great arteries in newborns. *J Am Coll Cardiol* 1997; **29**:202–206.
53. Tanel RW, Wernovsky G, Landzberg MJ et al. Coronary artery abnormalities detected at cardiac catheterization following the arterial switch operation for transposition of the great arteries. *Am J Cardiol* 1995; **76**:153–157.
54. Newburger JW, Jonas RA, Wernovsky G et al. A comparison of the perioperative neurologic effects of hypothermic circulatory arrest versus low-flow cardiopulmonary bypass in infant heart surgery. *N Engl J Med* 1993; **329**:1057–1064.
55. Bellinger DC, Rappaport LA, Wypij D, Wernovsky G, Newburger JW. Patterns of developmental dysfunction after surgery during infancy to correct transposition of the great arteries. *J Dev Behav Pediatr* 1997; **18**:75–83.
56. Bellinger DC, Wypij D, Kuban KC et al. Developmental and neurological status of children at 4 years of age after heart surgery with hypothermic circulatory arrest or low flow cardiopulmonary bypass. *Circulation* 1999; **100**:526–532.
57. Newburger JW, Wypij D, Bellinger DC et al. Length of stay after infant heart surgery is related to cognitive outcome at age 8 years. *J Pediatr* 2003; **143**:67–73.
58. Bellinger DC, Wypij D, du Plessis AJ et al. Developmental and neurologic effects of alpha-stat versus pH-stat strategies for deep hypothermic cardiopulmonary bypass in infants. *J Thorac Cardiovasc Surg* 2001; **121**:374–383.
59. Jonas RA, Wypij D, Roth SJ et al. The influence of hemodilution on outcome after hypothermic cardiopulmonary bypass: Results of a randomized trial in infants. *J Thorac Cardiovasc Surg* 2003; **126**:1765–1774.
60. Yacoub MH, Radley-Smith R, Hilton CJ. Anatomical correction of complete transposition of the great arteries and ventricular septal defect in infancy. *Br Med J* 1976; **1**:1112–1114.
61. Izumo S, Nadal-Ginard B, Mahdavi V. Protooncogene induction and reprogramming of cardiac gene expression produced by pressure overload. *Proc Natl Acad Sci* 1988; **85**:339.
62. Jonas RA, Giglia TM, Sanders SP et al. Rapid, two-stage arterial switch for transposition of the great arteries and intact ventricular septum beyond the neonatal period. *Circulation* 1989; **80**(3 Pt 1):I203–208.
63. Mee RB, Harada Y. Retraining of the left ventricle with a left ventricular assist device (Bio-Medicus) after the arterial switch operation. *J Thorac Cardiovasc Surg* 1991; **101**:171–173.
64. Poirier NC, Mee RB. Left ventricular reconditioning and anatomical correction for systemic right ventricular dysfunction. *Semin Thorac Cardiovasc Surg Pediatr Card Surg Annu* 2000; **3**:198–215.
65. Boutin C, Wernovsky G, Sanders SP, Jonas RA, Castaneda AR, Colan SD. Rapid two-stage arterial switch operation. Evaluation of left ventricular systolic mechanics late after an acute pressure overload stimulus in infancy. *Circulation* 1994; **90**:1294–1303.
66. Wernovsky G, Giglia TM, Jonas RA, Mone SM, Colan SD, Wessel DL. Course in the intensive care unit after 'preparatory' pulmonary artery banding and aortopulmonary shunt placement for transposition of the great arteries with low left ventricular pressure. *Circulation* 1992; **86**(5 Suppl):II133–139.

16

Tetralogy of Fallot with pulmonary stenosis

INTRODUCTION

Tetralogy of Fallot is slightly more common than transposition of the great arteries and therefore is the commonest congenital cardiac anomaly producing cyanosis.[1] It lies somewhere close to the middle of the spectrum of complexity of congenital heart disease. Lesions such as complete AV canal, truncus arteriosus and hypoplastic left heart syndrome that are more complex than tetralogy can be considered complex congenital heart disease, while those lesions less complex than tetralogy, such as atrial and ventricular septal defects and patent ductus arteriosus can reasonably be considered simple congenital heart disease. Results of surgery for tetralogy with pulmonary stenosis have been and continue to be a useful benchmark to assess the capabilities of a congenital cardiac surgical program. In the current era the risk of mortality for a patient undergoing repair of tetralogy of Fallot with pulmonary stenosis, without complicating additional anomalies such as absent pulmonary valve syndrome or complete AV canal, should be less than 2%.[2]

In the past it was customary to consider tetralogy of Fallot with pulmonary stenosis and tetralogy of Fallot with pulmonary atresia as a single entity and part of a continuous spectrum. While this may be true from an embryological and morphological perspective, it is not useful when one considers surgical management. In tetralogy of Fallot with pulmonary atresia it is common for much of the pulmonary blood flow to be derived from aortopulmonary collateral vessels, i.e. vessels other than the true pulmonary arteries. This is exceedingly rare in the patient with tetralogy of Fallot with pulmonary stenosis. Therefore a reasonable inference can be made for the patient with tetralogy of Fallot and pulmonary stenosis that since the child has been able to achieve adequate oxygenation through the true pulmonary arteries to remain alive preoperatively, the true pulmonary arteries and the pulmonary vascular bed are sufficiently well developed to allow one stage complete repair. Thus, for patients with tetralogy of Fallot with pulmonary stenosis much of the complex decision making associated with staged repair in tetralogy of Fallot with pulmonary atresia is unnecessary. There are a number of ongoing controversies regarding the management of tetralogy of Fallot with pulmonary stenosis which will be examined in this chapter. Despite its advantages elective one stage repair in early infancy is not universally accepted.[3]

The optimal management of symptomatic patients in early infancy also remains controversial. Some centers prefer a two stage approach involving placement of an initial systemic to pulmonary artery shunt while others prefer one stage repair. The optimal surgical approach whether transatrial or transventricular remains controversial.[4] Finally, the management of the stenotic, hypoplastic pulmonary valve remains unclear. Some centers advocate placement of a monocusp valve at the time of initial repair[5] while others advocate pulmonary valve replacements in many of their patients late postoperatively.[6,7] Even percutaneous transcatheter insertion of a pulmonary valve has been described.[8]

EMBRYOLOGY

To understand the embryology of tetralogy of Fallot, it is important to review the embryology of the development of the pulmonary arteries. The lung buds as they arise from the primitive foregut carry the arteries and veins which invest the foregut and which are derived from the systemic arterial and systemic venous circulations. The proximal mediastinal pulmonary arteries, on the other hand, are derived from the sixth dorsal aortic arches which coalesce with the more distal vasculature. The proximal main pulmonary artery is formed by division of the original conotruncus.

Classic theory of development of tetralogy of Fallot

The conotruncus ('bulbus' or 'bulbus cordis') is usually subdivided by a process of spiral septation into relatively equally sized great vessels, namely the aorta and the main pulmonary artery.[9] If the process of septation is unequal the main pulmonary artery may be hypoplastic relative to the aorta. The conotruncus is in continuity with the dorsal aorta. The transition points between the main pulmonary artery and the branch pulmonary arteries (right and left pulmonary artery) can be points of stenosis. There may also be multiple points of stenosis more distally, perhaps representing points of junction of the sixth dorsal aorta with the peripheral pulmonary vasculature.

Van Praagh's theory of the embryology of tetralogy of Fallot

Van Praagh has postulated that tetralogy of Fallot is a consequence of a single problem, namely underdevelopment of the subpulmonary conus.[10] The consequence of underdevelopment of the subpulmonary infundibulum is that the aortic valve comes to lie more anteriorly, superiorly and rightwards relative to the pulmonary valve than usual. In addition, the underdevelopment of the subpulmonary infundibulum results in less blood flow through the pulmonary valve and main pulmonary artery so that these structures are usually hypoplastic.

ANATOMY

Although Fallot initially described four anatomical features, there are only two anatomical features that are of particular relevance to the surgeon approaching the surgical repair of the child with tetralogy of Fallot.

Ventricular septal defect

The VSD in tetralogy of Fallot with pulmonary stenosis is almost always large and unrestrictive and of the anterior malalignment type (Figure 16.1a). This means that the defect is between the conal septum and ventricular septum and therefore can also be termed 'conoventricular'. It also extends to the membranous area and therefore is labeled by some as a perimembranous VSD though this is not accurate. In fact there is often a remnant of the membranous septum which can be useful for VSD closure.[11] There is a variable degree of anterior malalignment of the conal septum relative to the ventricular septum. It is the anteriorly protruding conal septum that is at least in part responsible for the right ventricular outflow tract obstruction which is the other essential component of tetralogy of Fallot (Figure 16.1b). The VSD is remarkably uniform in size across the majority of the spectrum of tetralogy of Fallot. It is almost always large enough to be unrestrictive from a pressure perspective so that right ventricular pressure is equal to left ventricular pressure and is therefore systemic. Very occasionally the VSD can be restrictive. This may be because it is simply small though more likely it is in part obstructed by adjacent tricuspid valve tissue. If there is associated severe right ventricular outflow tract obstruction the pressure in the right ventricle can be suprasystemic which can result in severe right ventricular hypertrophy and increase the risk of surgery importantly if correction is not undertaken early in infancy.

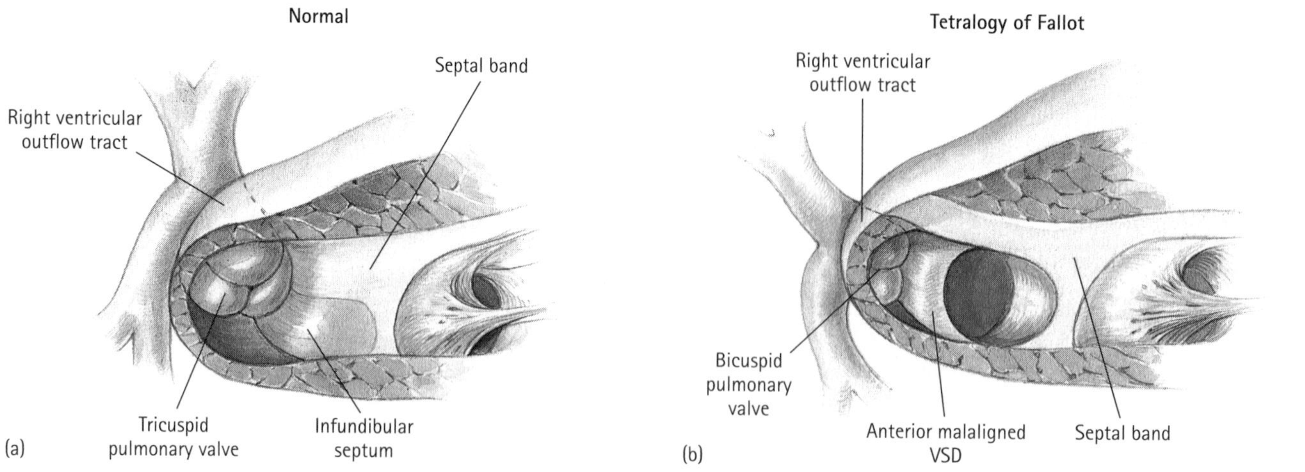

Figure 16.1 *(a) Normally the infundibular septum lies between the limbs of the septal band which bifurcates into two divisions. The pulmonary valve is tri-leaflet. (b) In tetralogy of Fallot anterior malalignment of the infundibular septum relative to the ventricular septum results in an anterior malalignment type of conoventricular VSD between the limbs of the septal band and the anteriorly displaced infundibular septum. The infundibular septum crowds the right ventricular outflow tract because of its anterior displacement. The pulmonary valve is usually bicuspid.*

Right ventricular outflow tract obstruction

As noted above, the VSD of tetralogy is an anterior malalignment VSD so that the conal septum projects into the right ventricular outflow tract and usually contributes to some degree of crowding of the infundibulum of the right ventricle. In addition the pulmonary valve is frequently bicuspid. Just as is the case with a bicuspid aortic valve, there is often commissural fusion, thickening of the valve leaflets and hypoplasia of the pulmonary annulus. There may be tethering of the free edges of the valve cusps to the pulmonary artery wall resulting in an hourglass like narrowing at the sinotubular junction, i.e. supravalvar pulmonary stenosis. The features described to this point are those that are likely to be encountered during repair in the neonatal period or early infancy. In time, however, there will be progression of right ventricular hypertrophy which can lead to a positive feedback loop in which hypertrophied muscle bundles within the infundibulum of the right ventricle including the moderator band and other muscle bundles towards the mid-body of the right ventricle exacerbate obstruction and thereby increase right ventricular pressure which further exacerbates muscular hypertrophy. Although this does not result in a progressive increase in right ventricular pressure which remains at systemic level because of the unrestrictive nature of the VSD, it will result in a progressive worsening of the child's degree of cyanosis. As the obstruction becomes increasingly muscular rather than fixed, i.e. secondary to valvar pulmonary stenosis and pulmonary annular hypoplasia, there is an increasing risk of cyanotic spells during which the child temporarily can become profoundly hypoxic.

Other anatomical features of tetralogy of Fallot with pulmonary stenosis

RIGHT VENTRICULAR HYPERTROPHY

It is normal for the right ventricle to be exposed to systemic pressure during in-utero development so that the right ventricle is similar in wall thickness to the left ventricle until birth, even in children who do not have congenital heart disease. Following birth when pulmonary resistance decreases there is a decrease in the thickness of the right ventricle relative to the left ventricle. In patients with tetralogy of Fallot who by definition have an unrestrictive VSD and right ventricular outflow tract obstruction, right ventricular pressure remains at systemic pressure and therefore there is no involution of the right ventricle relative to the left ventricle. Beyond the early years of childhood the muscular hypertrophy will acquire an increasing component of fibrosis which is accompanied by worsening diastolic dysfunction.[12]

DEXTROPOSITION OF THE AORTA

As discussed above, tetralogy of Fallot can be thought of as an underdevelopment of the infundibulum of the right ventricle.[10] In the normal heart the right ventricular infundibulum carries the pulmonary valve anteriorly and superiorly away from the other three valves which are in fibrous continuity with each other. As the infundibulum becomes progressively less well developed the pulmonary valve moves posteriorly and inferiorly relative to its usual position with respect to the aorta. Relative to the pulmonary valve therefore the aorta comes to lie more anteriorly which was described originally by Fallot as 'dextroposition' of the aorta. As one moves further into the spectrum of tetralogy of Fallot one approaches double outlet right ventricle, where a conus is beginning to form under the aortic valve which will lift the aortic valve even further anteriorly and superiorly relative to the pulmonary valve. As one passes through the spectrum of double outlet right ventricle and reaches transposition, there is now fibrous continuity between the pulmonary valve and the mitral valve; the aortic valve is separate from the other three valves with its own subaortic conus or infundibulum.

Associated cardiac anomalies

CORONARY ARTERY DISTRIBUTION

As the aorta moves forward relative to the pulmonary artery the distance that the left main coronary artery must traverse in order to pass posteriorly behind the pulmonary artery before bifurcating into the anterior descending and circumflex coronary arteries increases. Not surprisingly, therefore, a small number of patients (about 5%) have anomalous coronary distribution where the anterior descending coronary artery arises from the right coronary artery and passes leftward across the infundibulum of the right ventricle before turning inferiorly in the anterior intraventricular groove.[13,14] The circumflex coronary artery continues to arise from the usual location and passes posterior to the main pulmonary artery before entering the left atrioventricular groove. Very occasionally the right coronary artery arises from the left coronary artery and passes rightward across the infundibulum of the right ventricle.

OTHER CORONARY 'ANOMALIES'

It is very common to see a particularly large branch of the right coronary artery passing obliquely across the anterior wall of the right ventricle towards the apex of the heart. Branches of this coronary artery run leftward, usually overlying the hypertrophied muscle bundles which lie within the infundibulum of the right ventricle. It is our impression that a large conal coronary artery and anterior right ventricular branch are so common that they should be considered a standard feature of tetralogy of Fallot.

MULTIPLE VSDs

Multiple VSDs can occur in the usual locations, particularly the mid-muscular septum and anterior and apical muscular septum. The incidence of multiple VSDs has been reported to lie between 3 and 15%.[15] As will be discussed below this is of particular importance in the surgical management of tetralogy of Fallot.

DISCONTINUOUS PULMONARY ARTERIES

As stated in the Introduction above, in the absence of large collateral vessels it can be assumed that the pulmonary arteries are of adequate size to carry a full cardiac output in virtually all patients with tetralogy and pulmonary stenosis. In fact a careful radiographic study of 200 patients from the University of Alabama and Children's Hospital Boston demonstrated that important hypoplasia of the right and left pulmonary artery was exceedingly rare although it is usual for the main pulmonary artery to be underdeveloped.[16] However, it is common for ductal tissue to extend into the origin of the left pulmonary artery and to cause an origin stenosis.[15] At the severe end of the spectrum the pulmonary arteries become discontinuous, usually between the main pulmonary artery and left pulmonary artery. Early in life the LPA is supplied by the ductus but following ductal closure it is unlikely to grow. If not identified and repaired early in life, the LPA and left lung will become severely hypoplastic.

PATENT FORAMEN OVALE

There is almost always a patent foramen ovale associated with tetralogy of Fallot. Occasionally this can be larger and allow a left to right shunt postoperatively if it is not partially closed at the time of surgery.

RIGHT AORTIC ARCH

About 25% of patients with tetralogy of Fallot have a right aortic arch.

PATHOPHYSIOLOGY AND CLINICAL PRESENTATION

The functional consequences of abnormal anatomy in tetralogy of Fallot depend primarily on the amount of fixed obstruction to right ventricular outflow as well as the dynamic, muscular component of right ventricular outflow tract obstruction. As noted above, the VSD is usually unrestrictive. Therefore as the degree of fixed valvar pulmonary stenosis and hypoplasia worsens an increasing percentage of right ventricular blood will pass right to left through the VSD and into the aorta and the level of resting cyanosis will worsen. A systolic ejection murmur is audible and is maximal over the pulmonary area. Beyond early infancy the progression of secondary right ventricular hypertrophy will lead to an increase in the dynamic component of right ventricular outflow tract obstruction. In the setting of increased catecholamines there is likely to be dynamic infundibular obstruction of the right ventricle which can result in an exacerbation of cyanosis. Cyanosis is also exacerbated by a fall in systemic vascular resistance. Stimulation of β-adrenergic receptors which occurs in the setting of high intrinsic catecholamine levels will result in a combination of infundibular spasm and a decrease in peripheral resistance secondary to dilation of resistance vessels in skeletal muscle. Thus it is readily understandable why treatment with a beta-blocking agent such as propranolol can be effective in temporarily palliating infants who have reached the point of having 'cyanotic spells'. During a cyanotic spell the typical systolic murmur is either reduced in intensity or absent because of reduced flow across the obstruction. When cyanosis is chronic because of a severe degree of fixed obstruction, the usual consequences of long-term cyanosis will ensue including polycythemia with all of its attendant complications including cerebral thrombosis and cerebral abscess. Clubbing of the extremities and nose is prominent.

DIAGNOSTIC STUDIES

Pulse oximetry

Pulse oximetry confirms cyanosis at rest with exacerbation during cyanotic spells. A resting saturation of less than 80–85% should be an indication for surgery. Intermittent falls of saturation to less than 65–70% should be an indication for urgent surgery.

Chest X-ray and electrocardiography

If pulmonary blood flow is importantly reduced this may be apparent on the chest X-ray in that the lung fields will be oligemic (dark). The hypoplasia of the main pulmonary artery also may be visible so that the cardiac contour is boot shaped (*coeur en sabot*). The ECG, while normal at birth, will demonstrate an abnormal degree of right ventricular hypertrophy beyond the neonatal period.

Two-dimensional echocardiography

The two-dimensional echocardiogram is usually adequate to define all relevant anatomical features required for surgical repair. So long as there is patency of the pulmonary valve and major aortopulmonary collateral vessels cannot be identified arising from the descending aorta by color Doppler mapping, then it is not necessary to define the specific arborization and size of the distal pulmonary vasculature by cardiac catheterization.[16] A very careful assessment should be made of the ventricular septum to exclude additional VSDs since even relatively small additional muscular VSDs can cause important hemodynamic consequences in the early postoperative period.[17]

Although it is useful to know about the presence of an anomalous anterior descending from the right coronary artery across the infundibulum of the right ventricle preoperatively, this is not essential information. At a first-time operation the anatomy of the coronary arteries should be very obvious to the surgeon. Any corrective operation for tetralogy should take into account very carefully the coronary anatomy in the planning of the ventriculotomy. It is important for the echocardiographer to define the anatomy of the interatrial septum. A patent foramen ovale or small secundum ASD is useful in the early postoperative period to allow right to left decompression. On the other hand a large secundum ASD will have to be reduced in size. If the interatrial septum is intact a small ASD should be created. It is not important to define the size of the right and left branch pulmonary arteries in the setting of tetralogy with pulmonary stenosis versus atresia, despite suggestions to the contrary by many centers. Measurement preoperatively gives little indication of the potential postoperative size of the pulmonary arteries since the distending pressure is likely to be quite different pre- and post and postoperatively. The compliance of the pulmonary arteries in patients with tetralogy who have not had previous surgery is usually excellent so that the postoperative diameter is likely to be considerably greater than the preoperative diameter at low pressure. Furthermore in the child whose resting arterial oxygen saturation is greater than 70–80% preoperatively it can be assumed that close to one cardiac output is already passing through the true pulmonary arteries (this assumption is not valid if there are major aortopulmonary collateral vessels but this is very rarely the case with tetralogy of Fallot with pulmonary stenosis). If the pulmonary arteries are able to carry close to a full cardiac output preoperatively there is no reason to suspect that they will not be able to maintain a full cardiac output in the postoperative period when the pressure in the pulmonary arteries is increased.

Because many centers observe low cardiac output following repair of tetralogy (for reasons which will be discussed below) there has been a long-held assumption that the left ventricle is frequently underdeveloped in patients with tetralogy and may be of inadequate volume to sustain a normal cardiac output once the VSD is closed. While it is true that both the right and left ventricle contribute to systemic cardiac output preoperatively, it is exceedingly rare that the left ventricle is of inadequate volume to sustain normal systemic cardiac output following VSD closure. The dimensions of the mitral valve should be measured and a z score (number of standard deviations above or below the normal mean dimension for age) calculated. The length of the left ventricle should be determined relative to the apex of the heart. In our experience so long as the length of the left ventricle is at least 80% of the distance from the AV valve to the apex of the heart, and so long as the mitral valve dimensions are not more than 2–2.5 z scores below normal it can be confidently assumed that the left ventricle will be able to manage a full cardiac output postoperatively.[18]

Cardiac catheterization

It should be exceedingly rare that cardiac catheterization is undertaken in the child who has not previously undergone surgery for tetralogy of Fallot with pulmonary stenosis. This is important because catheterization carries a real risk of catecholamine and direct catheter induced spasm of the infundibular outflow of the right ventricle, precipitating emergency surgery which without question carries an increased risk relative to elective surgery. Cardiac catheterization is indicated if there is doubt regarding the presence of important aortopulmonary collateral vessels or multiple muscular VSDs. It is not necessary to define coronary artery anatomy for primary surgery and is also not necessary to define the size and arborization of the true pulmonary arteries in contradistinction to the situation with tetralogy of Fallot with pulmonary atresia.

Magnetic resonance imaging

Magnetic resonance imaging is presently in a state of rapid evolution and can now provide an enormous amount of both structural and functional information. However, the need for general anesthesia in order to obtain the controlled apnea and immobility necessary for a good quality study at present is an important limitation. The additional cost of an MRI scan relative to echocardiography is another consideration.

MEDICAL AND INTERVENTIONAL THERAPY

Although it is possible to palliate the child with tetralogy medically who is having cyanotic spells using a beta-blocking agent such as propranolol, this approach is not reliable and should rarely be used. α-Adrenergic agents such as phenylephrine, which elevate systemic vascular resistance, are effective in temporarily reversing right to left shunting and relieving cyanosis but they do nothing to treat the underlying pathophysiology and have no role in longer term management.

It is a particular disadvantage to use a vasoconstricting agent immediately prior to the onset of cardiopulmonary bypass and even more so if hypothermic circulatory arrest is to be employed.[19] It is probably preferable to tolerate relatively low arterial oxygen saturations transiently before bypass rather than vasoconstricting the child with phenylephrine immediately before bypass. Recently there has been some enthusiasm for balloon dilation and even stenting of the right ventricular outflow tract for palliation prior to repair of tetralogy.[20–22] There has been speculation that this might reduce the need for a transannular patch, though to date there is no evidence to support this contention. Furthermore, there appear to be fewer long term deleterious effects of a transannular patch relative to leaving a hypoplastic and stenotic pulmonary valve in place.[23,24]

Another important disadvantage of balloon dilation of the outflow tract is that it can produce excessive pulmonary blood flow if the right ventricular outflow tract obstruction is primarily valvar. Following acute effective relief of severe pulmonary valve stenosis there is likely to be a massive left to right shunt through the anterior malalignment VSD which can result in pulmonary edema and even death. An important complication of attempted dilation of the right ventricular outflow tract has been perforation of the infundibulum which has on occasion required emergency surgery including institution of extracorporeal membrane oxygenation in the catheterization laboratory.

INDICATIONS FOR AND TIMING OF SURGERY

Considerable controversy persists regarding the optimal timing for repair of tetralogy of Fallot. Although primary repair was attempted in the early years of open heart surgery[25] the morbidity of early heart-lung machines led to a high mortality and acceptance of a routine two stage approach with an initial palliative shunt.[26] However, it subsequently became apparent that shunts also carried significant mortality and morbidity. In particular early shunts such as the Potts shunts[27] and Waterston shunts[28] were very damaging to patients with tetralogy because they resulted in severe distortion of the left or right branch pulmonary artery and often an elevation in pulmonary resistance. The classical Blalock shunt often thrombosed when performed in the neonatal period or early infancy. It was not until the introduction of the modified Blalock shunt with a PTFE interposition graft by de Leval in the early 1980s that the Blalock shunt became more consistently successful.[29]

However, even the modified Blalock shunt usually results in scarring and distortion at the level of the distal anastomosis which is an important consideration in the child who requires a highly compliant pulmonary arterial tree to ameliorate the deleterious effects of the pulmonary regurgitation which accompanies a transannular patch.

Advantages of early primary repair

As discussed in Chapter 1, there are multiple advantages for all developing organ systems of the body to have a normal circulation as early in life as possible. In children with tetralogy of Fallot the developing pulmonary vasculature is exposed to abnormally low pressure as well as reduced flow. There is evidence to indicate that this results in a reduced ratio of gas exchanging capillaries relative to alveoli.[30]

Lung development continues for the first several years of life but deferring surgery beyond this time may result in a reduced cross sectional area for gas exchange.

Development of the heart is also abnormal in the child with unrepaired tetralogy. The right ventricle is exposed to systemic pressure in the child with the usual unrestrictive anterior malalignment VSD. Persistence of systemic pressure in the right ventricle results in abnormal right ventricular hypertrophy with subsequent fibrosis and decreased compliance. In the normal heart the right ventricle is highly compliant allowing an enormous increase in pulmonary blood flow with little or no change in systemic venous pressure. Failure to repair tetralogy early in life is likely to lead to a lifetime decrease in right ventricular compliance. There is also evidence that left ventricular function is less good when repair of tetralogy is delayed.[31] Arrhythmias are also more common late after repair if repair is performed beyond infancy.[32]

The organ which undergoes the most rapid development in the first year of life is the brain. It seems highly probable that chronic cyanosis in the first year of life will be accompanied by a reduced developmental outcome relative to what might otherwise have been achieved.[33]

In addition to the multiple developmental advantages for the child there are additional important economic and psychosocial advantages of early primary repair for the young family with a child born with tetralogy of Fallot. It is not difficult to empathize with young inexperienced parents who are told by their physician that their child has a potentially fatal cardiac condition which can result in sudden cyanotic spells and death if the child is allowed to become agitated. One can only imagine the fear that a single cry at night from this child will cause. One option adopted by many centers is to defer reparative surgery beyond 6–12 months and to undertake a preliminary shunt if the child becomes symptomatic within that timeframe.[2,3] The family must then endure a second hospitalization with its attendant stresses and costs. It seems infinitely preferable from the perspective of the family as well as the cost to society to undertake single stage elective repair early in infancy before the development of symptoms.

Specific indications for surgery

SYMPTOMS

Prostaglandin dependent neonate

Occasionally a child will be born with a sufficiently severe degree of fixed right ventricular outflow tract obstruction that the child is prostaglandin dependent from birth. In this setting it is particularly important to exclude the presence of important aortopulmonary collateral vessels as the child is likely to be close to having tetralogy of Fallot with pulmonary atresia. Mediastinal continuity of the true pulmonary arteries should also be carefully confirmed.

Worsening cyanosis

Right ventricular outflow tract obstruction almost always progressively worsens in the first weeks and months of life usually due to increasing muscular outflow tract obstruction but on occasion because of worsening valvar stenosis. This may result in the resting oxygen saturation gradually decreasing from a level of greater than 90% at birth to less than 75–80%. This should be an indication to move ahead relatively urgently with surgery.

Cyanotic spells

Cyanotic spells are usually observed in a child who is initially agitated. This is followed by a period of profound cyanosis with an arterial oxygen saturation of less than 20–30%. In a classic cyanotic spell the child subsequently becomes gray, pale and comatose, presumably related to a fall in cardiac output secondary to hypoxia. Cyanotic spells can result in brain injury and death and should be an indication for immediate hospitalization and surgical repair. In the past both parents and hospital staff were taught maneuvers to reverse cyanotic spells though today it should be rare that a child progresses to the point of having recurrent cyanotic spells. The child's agitation should be treated with morphine. Systemic vascular resistance can be increased by placing the child in a knee to chest position. (This is equivalent to the 'squatting' position often adopted by the older, untreated child.) Oxygen should also be given. If necessary the child should be anesthetized, intubated, paralysed and ventilated. Systemic resistance can be further increased pharmacologically with α-adrenergic agents such as phenylephrine (Neosynephrine) and the catecholamine drive exacerbating the spell can be diminished by administration of a beta-blocking agent such as propranalol.

ELECTIVE REPAIR

At present it is our practice to schedule elective repair following diagnosis which is usually made within a few days of birth. This allows the parents and caregivers time to plan the necessary logistics and for the financial aspects of the procedure to be put in place usually over a four to six week period. Over this timeframe, ductal tissue which may extend into the origin of the left pulmonary artery will declare itself as a possible stenosis at the origin of the left pulmonary artery. Although there was concern that repair in early infancy resulted in a higher probability of transannular patch placement, this in fact seems to not be borne out by experience with elective repair.[18]

Analysis of early reports of tetralogy repair in early infancy reveals that almost all patients in early reports were symptomatic and therefore had a more severe degree of right ventricular outflow tract obstruction with a correspondingly higher probability of transannular patch placement. In a comparison of primary repair in infancy versus a two stage approach contrasting the experience at Children's Hospital Boston with that at the University of Alabama at Birmingham, Kirklin et al found that the incidence of transannular patching in the two institutions was very similar.[18]

CONTRAINDICATIONS TO EARLY PRIMARY REPAIR

In the current era there should be essentially no contraindications to early primary repair. In the past the following associated anomalies have been considered contraindications but we would dispute that they should remain so.

Anomalous coronary artery

It has been stated that an anomalous anterior descending coronary artery arising from the right coronary artery and passing across the infundibulum of the right ventricle should be considered a contraindication to a primary repair, because it may necessitate placement of a conduit from the right ventricle to the pulmonary arteries. In fact, it is frequently possible with a transatrial approach and placement of outflow patches either above or below or both relative to the coronary artery to avoid conduit placement.[34]

In the very occasional child in whom it is necessary to place a small conduit, every attempt should also be made to enlarge the native outflow tract. With a double outlet right ventricle thereby created, it is probable that the conduit will last several years and will not increase the total number of procedures required relative to initial elective placement of a modified Blalock shunt.

Multiple muscular VSDs

Although it is true that additional VSDs are an important additional risk factor for mortality and morbidity in the early postoperative period after tetralogy repair, it is frequently possible to reduce the size of the additional muscular VSDs by appropriate suture placement as discussed below. Only in the very rare setting of a Swiss cheese like septum would we consider deferring surgery until the child has reached the size where catheter delivered device placement of associated muscular VSDs is possible.

Discontinuous central pulmonary arteries

It is important to establish continuity between the main, and right and left pulmonary arteries as early in life as possible to promote development of normal pulmonary architecture. This is best accomplished as part of an early repair. Although the anastomosis between the discontinuous and main pulmonary artery may require subsequent balloon angioplasty this is a relatively simple, low risk procedure. An alternative to early, direct anastomosis is delayed repair following placement of a systemic arterial shunt to the discontinuous pulmonary artery. However, this is likely to result in excessive pressure within the single pulmonary artery with a risk of development of pulmonary vascular occlusive disease. In addition, placement of a shunt will result in fibrosis surrounding the vessel and will reduce the probability that direct anastomosis will be possible at the time of subsequent repair. In this case placement of a conduit connection from the main pulmonary artery to the discontinuous pulmonary artery will be necessary at the time of complete repair.

SURGICAL MANAGEMENT

History of surgery

Surgical treatment of tetralogy of Fallot was initiated by Blalock and Taussig in 1945 with the establishment of the subclavian artery to pulmonary artery anastomosis.[35] Klinner et al in 1962 were the first to interpose a prosthetic conduit between the subclavian artery and the pulmonary artery,[36] a technique that was further refined by de Leval and colleagues.[29] Laks and Castaneda added a helpful modification of the Blalock-Taussig shunt, using the subclavian artery ipsilateral to the aortic arch.[37]

In 1946, Potts et al[38] introduced the descending aorta to left pulmonary artery anastomosis, in 1955 Davidson reported the first central aortopulmonary shunt by direct suture[39] and in 1962 Waterston[40] performed the ascending aorta to right pulmonary artery anastomosis, an important alternative to the Blalock-Taussig and Potts operations. In 1948, both Sellors and Brock expanded the scope of palliative operations by adding closed pulmonary valvotomy and infundibulotomy.[41,42]

In an imaginative and daring effort, on April 31, 1954, Lillehei and collaborators[43] using controlled cross circulation in a 10-month-old boy, carried out the first intracardiac repair of tetralogy of Fallot; this included closure of the VSD and relief of the right ventricular outflow tract obstruction under direct vision. In Lillehei's original cross circulation series of 11 repairs of tetralogy of Fallot, six patients were less than two years old. The first successful repair using a heart-lung machine was accomplished by Kirklin and associates in 1955.[44] Lillehei recognized the need for enlarging the right ventricular infundibulum with a patch and extended the patch across a stenotic pulmonary valve annulus as early as 1956.[45] The use of a nonvalved prosthetic conduit from the right ventricle to the pulmonary artery for the treatment of tetralogy of Fallot with pulmonary atresia was first reported by Klinner.[46] Ross and Somerville first reported the interposition of a valved aortic homograft for repair of tetralogy of Fallot with pulmonary atresia in 1966.[47] However, after the initial success with repair of tetralogy of Fallot in infancy, subsequent attempts at early repair carried a high mortality rate and the two stage repair became universally favored. In 1969, Barratt-Boyes and Neutze[48] successfully reinitiated primary repair of symptomatic infants with tetralogy of Fallot with pulmonary stenosis applying the technique of hypothermic circulatory arrest. In 1972, Castaneda[49] introduced early repair of symptomatic infants with tetralogy of Fallot, including infants within the first three months of life at Children's Hospital Boston.

Technical considerations

METHOD OF CARDIOPULMONARY BYPASS

Elective repair of tetralogy of Fallot is generally carried out when the child is between one and three months of age. At this age these babies usually weigh in the range of 4–6 kg. In this weight range repair can comfortably be undertaken on continuous cardiopulmonary bypass with double caval cannulation. The ascending aorta is cannulated with an arterial cannula in the standard fashion. Venous cannulation can be undertaken with either straight or right angle caval cannulas. In general moderate to deep hypothermia is employed to aid myocardial protection and alleviate the need for multiple doses of cardioplegia.

In the child who is larger than 5–6 kg and older than three months, moderate hypothermia at 25°C or above and multiple doses of cardioplegia are employed.

In children less than 3.5–4 kg in weight it is our preference to use a single venous cannula in the right atrium and to rely on tricuspid valve competence to prevent air being entrained into the cannula. Depending on the chordal attachments of the tricuspid valve as well as the proximity of the edge of the VSD to the tricuspid valve, it may be necessary to discontinue bypass for a period of approximately 10 minutes during placement of sutures around the posterior and inferior corner of the VSD. Deep hypothermia is employed when a single venous cannula is utilized so that circulatory arrest can be employed without delay when necessary.

In children less than 2–2.5 kg in weight it is usually preferable to employ elective hypothermic circulatory arrest. Much of the initial phase of the surgery can be undertaken on continuous cardiopulmonary bypass with a single venous cannula. The ventriculotomy, division of infundibular muscle and placement of initial sutures can be undertaken on bypass. In general it is advisable to complete VSD closure as well as to begin placement of the outflow patch under hypothermic circulatory arrest. Generally no more than 30–40 minutes of circulatory arrest time is necessary.

VENTRICULAR APPROACH TO REPAIR OF TETRALOGY OF FALLOT WITH PULMONARY STENOSIS

The ventricular approach remains our preferred technique for the majority of patients with tetralogy of Fallot with pulmonary stenosis. This approach offers several advantages over the atrial approach. It allows the infundibulum to be enlarged without aggressive resection of muscle which can lead to extensive endocardial scar formation. It also allows VSD exposure without undue traction on the tricuspid annulus thereby avoiding traction injury to the tricuspid valve and conduction bundle. Several technical considerations need to be carefully observed if the ventricular approach is to be used correctly.

Decision regarding a transannular patch

During the cooling phase of cardiopulmonary bypass the pulmonary bifurcation area including the origin of the left pulmonary artery as well as the main pulmonary artery are dissected free. Usually there is only a very small ligamentum arteriosum but if there is a patent ductus arteriosus it should be ligated immediately after commencing bypass. The size of the main pulmonary artery and the diameter of the pulmonary annulus should be directly measured and compared with the preoperative echo determinations. If the pulmonary annulus and main pulmonary artery are more than two to three standard deviations below normal a transannular patch will be indicated (Figure 16.2a).

Location of the ventriculotomy

During cooling the anatomy of the coronary artery distribution needs to be carefully studied. An incision should be planned which will avoid division of the large right ventricular coronary artery that extends towards the apex of the heart. It is usually necessary to divide the branch of this artery which runs transversely at the narrowest area of muscular obstruction in the infundibulum. There is frequently a dimpling seen in the infundibulum at this level. This coronary artery branch presumably supplies the hypertrophied muscle which is contributing to obstruction so that division of this branch

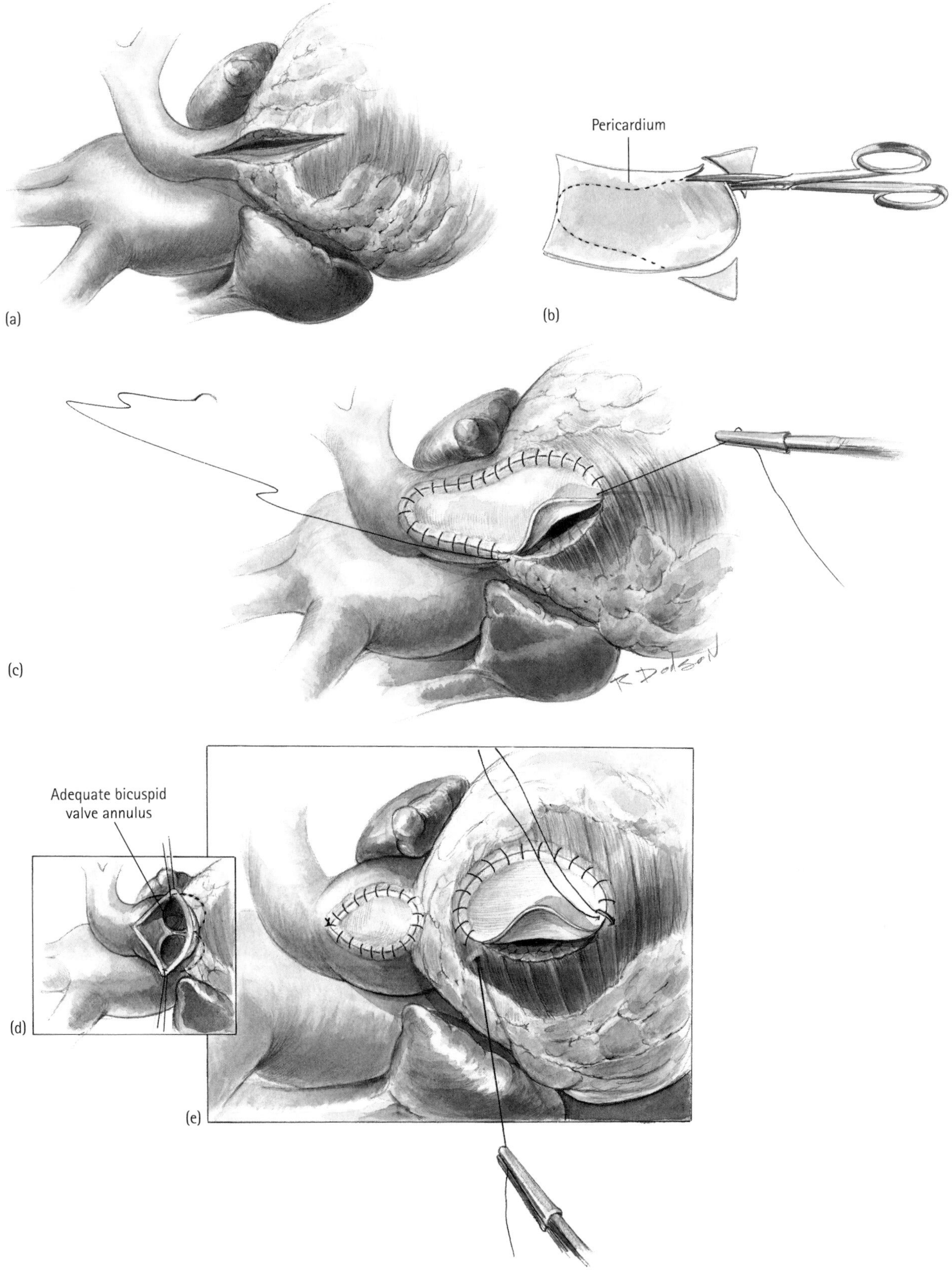

Figure 16.2 *(a) A ventriculotomy approach is preferred for repair of tetralogy of Fallot when there is moderate or severe infundibular obstruction. The incision should be extended across the annulus (transannular incision) when the z score of the pulmonary annulus is smaller than 2–3 standard deviations below normal. (b) Autologous pericardium lightly tanned with glutaraldehyde is ideal for use as a right ventricular outflow tract patch. The patch should usually be pear shaped as indicated. (c) Placement of a transannular pericardial right ventricular outflow tract patch. (d) On occasion there may be an adequate pulmonary annulus but moderate or severe hypoplasia of the supravalvar main pulmonary artery. (e) Two separate patches are placed, one in the main pulmonary artery for management of supravalvar pulmonary stenosis and one in the infundibulum of the right ventricle for infundibular obstruction.*

should not compromise right ventricular function. It is, however, extremely important to preserve the major branch of the right coronary artery which extends towards the apex. This will often require a slightly oblique incision in the infundibulum. If the incision is to be extended across the annulus it should curve superiorly along the full length of the main pulmonary artery beyond the takeoff of the right pulmonary artery (Figure 16.2b, 2c, 2d, 2e). If there is anything more than mild stenosis at the origin of the left pulmonary artery the incision should be extended across this origin stenosis for at least 3 or 4 mm.

Length of the ventriculotomy

It is important to limit the length of the ventriculotomy to the length of the infundibulum. (Note that the figures in this chapter have an expanded ventriculotomy to allow visualization of intracardiac structures.) The length of the incision will be dependent on the length of the conal septum which is quite variable in patients with tetralogy. If the conal septum is hypoplastic or absent the incision can be limited to no more than 5–6 mm. In all cases the incision should finish several millimeters cephalad to the connection of the moderator band to the free wall of the right ventricle which is also the origin of the anterior papillary muscle of the tricuspid valve.

DIVISION OF INFUNDIBULAR MUSCLE BUNDLES

Van Praagh describes an anterior malalignment VSD as a defect which lies between the parietal and septal extensions of the septal band. These two muscle bundles usually fuse with the conal septum and in a sense fix it in its anterior location. By dividing both the parietal (free wall) and septal connections of the conal septum, the conal septum is able to be brought posteriorly by the VSD patch. In practical terms this means that the surgeon simply incises the left and right ends of the conal septum (Figure 16.3a, 3b, 3c). It is important to do this at a sufficient distance from the point where the VSD sutures will be placed as sutures placed in cut muscle hold poorly. It is the endocardium which provides the support for VSD sutures so that its integrity should not be disrupted at any point where VSD sutures will be placed.

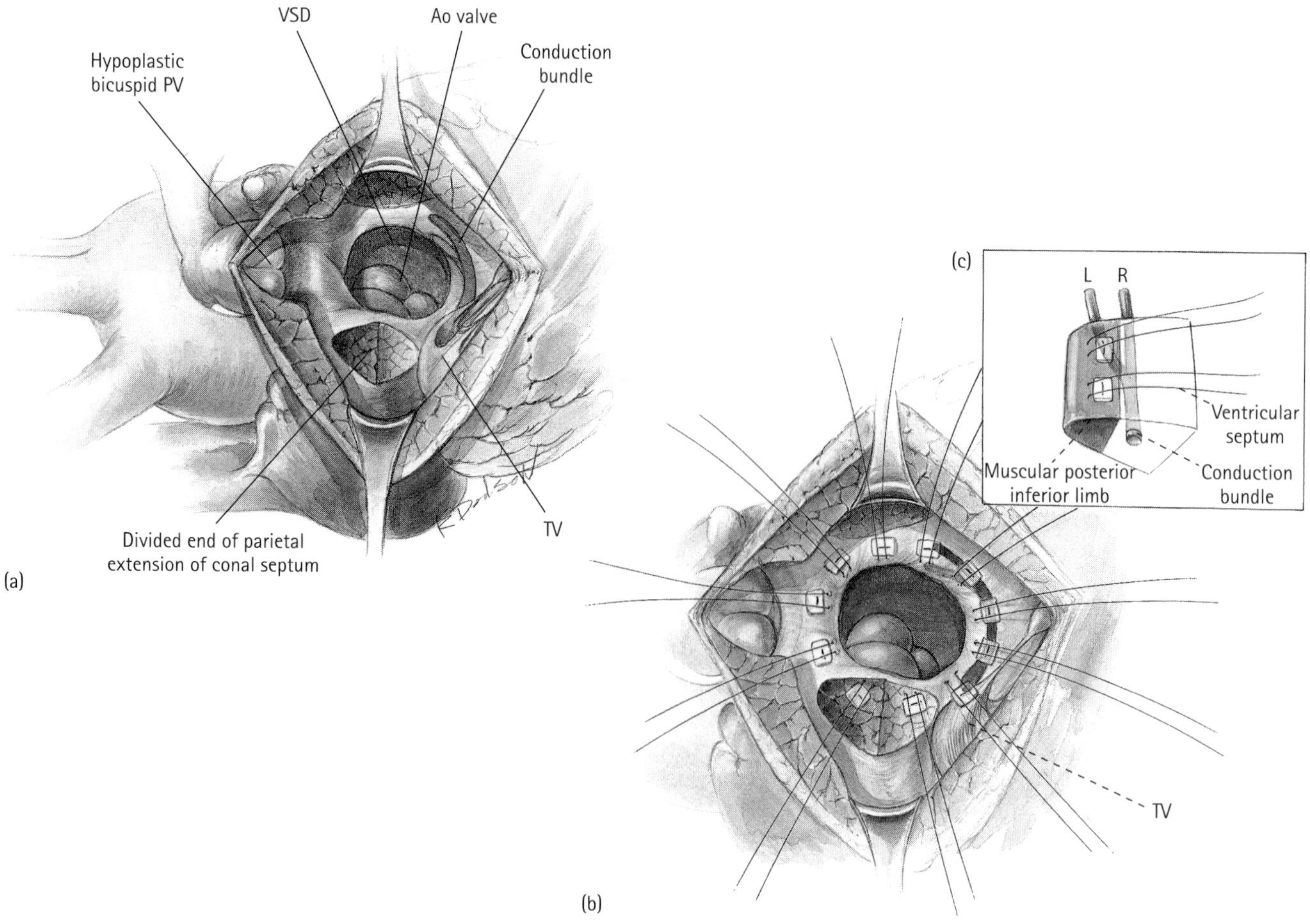

Figure 16.3 *(a) Division of the parietal (free wall) and septal extensions of the conal septum will allow the conal septum to move posteriorly when the VSD patch is anchored to it. (b) Placement of multiple interrupted pledgetted 5/0 sutures for closure of the anterior malalignment VSD. In this patient there is considerable muscular separation between the tricuspid and aortic valves so that sutures can be placed into the muscle ridge in this area. Sutures would usually not be separated from each other as depicted here. The inset (c) demonstrates that sutures are placed on the right ventricular aspect of the septum. The muscle bar separates the edge of the VSD from the conduction bundle.*

PRESERVATION OF MODERATOR BAND

It is particularly important to identify the moderator band specifically and to preserve this structure. It functions as a central pillar of the right ventricle and as such tethers the anterior free wall to the posterior septal wall. In older children the moderator band may be quite hypertrophied and can contribute to right ventricular outflow tract obstruction. In this setting it should be partially but not completely divided. There are likely to be additional muscle bundles on the septal surface associated with the septal band which should also be divided in the older child. In the neonate and young infant it is rarely necessary to actually excise muscle. Simple division of muscle bundles is quite effective in relieving obstruction.

TRANSVENTRICULOTOMY VSD CLOSURE

Although some surgeons prefer a continuous suture technique it is our preference to use interrupted pledgetted horizontal mattress sutures using a 5/0 coated polyester suture and small Teflon pledgets. A very small half circle custom needle is employed. After placement each suture is useful for retraction to expose the site for the next suture. The initial suture is placed at approximately 3:00 with the middle of the conal septum representing 12:00 and the posterior and inferior corner of the VSD representing 6:00. The initial sutures are placed quite deeply to allow the traction necessary for exposure of the more difficult superior margin of the VSD. When the papillary muscle of the conus has been passed working in a clockwise direction, sutures are placed so as to emerge approximately 2 mm below the inferior edge of the VSD. The conduction bundle is close to the posterior and inferior margin of the VSD though it is not as exposed as in the patient with a membranous VSD or inlet VSD. Nevertheless, care should be taken at the posterior and inferior corner. It is often useful to employ the fibrous remnant of the membranous septum which is frequently present (Figure 16.4a, 4b, 4c, 4d). If there is fibrous

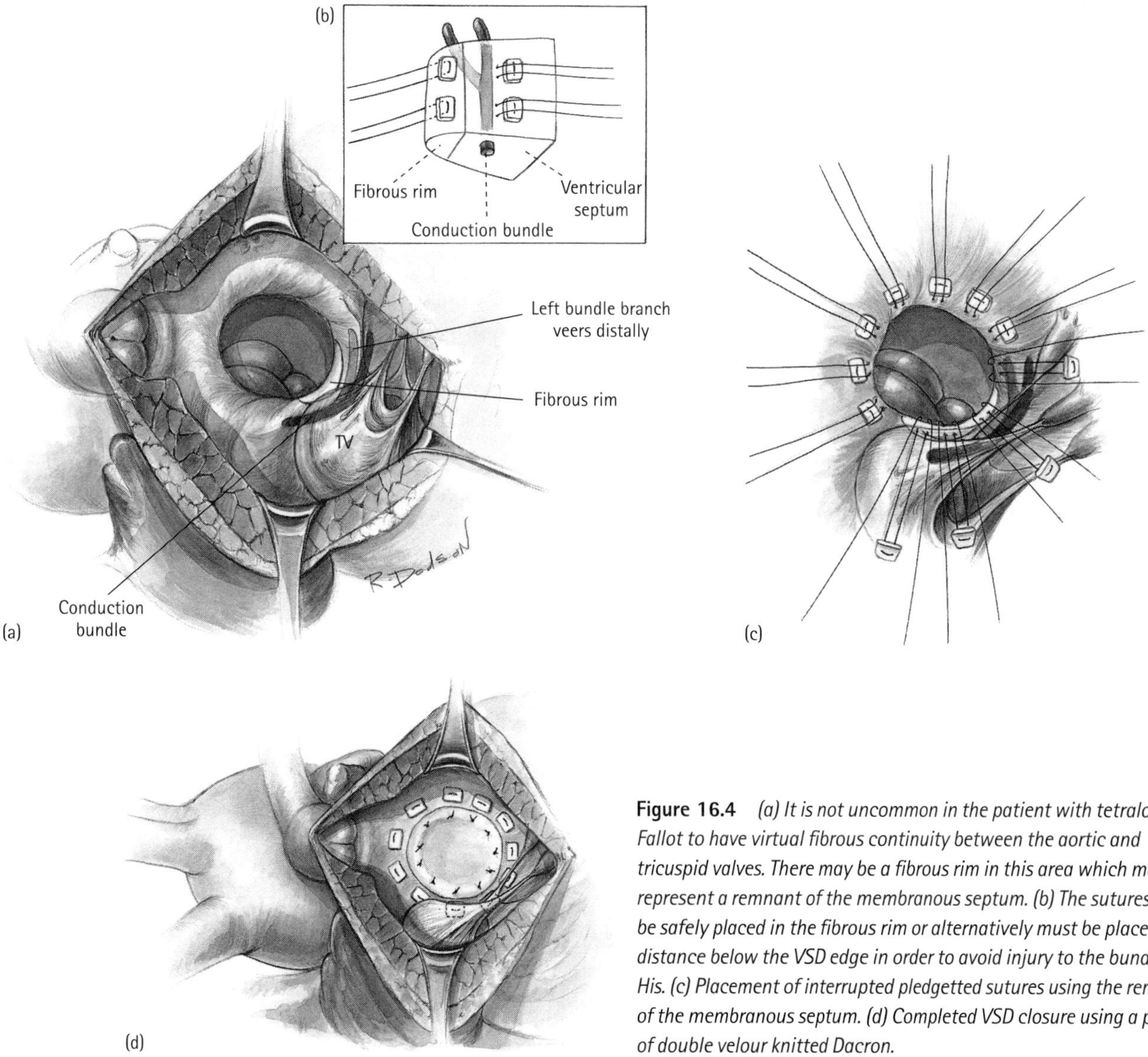

Figure 16.4 *(a) It is not uncommon in the patient with tetralogy of Fallot to have virtual fibrous continuity between the aortic and tricuspid valves. There may be a fibrous rim in this area which may represent a remnant of the membranous septum. (b) The sutures may be safely placed in the fibrous rim or alternatively must be placed some distance below the VSD edge in order to avoid injury to the bundle of His. (c) Placement of interrupted pledgetted sutures using the remnant of the membranous septum. (d) Completed VSD closure using a patch of double velour knitted Dacron.*

continuity between the tricuspid and aortic valves as is often the case, an alternative approach is to open the tricuspid valve and place sutures through from the right atrial side of the septal leaflets with the pledgets coming to lie in the right atrium. It is critically important for the surgeon to avoid even the slightest entanglement with tricuspid chords which can be extremely fine and delicate. It is also important to avoid taking large bites of folded tricuspid valve leaflet tissue as this will compromise subsequent tricuspid valve function.

Having passed in a clockwise direction across the tricuspid valve the surgeon must now ascend the aortic valve annulus. Frequently there are ridges and valleys of muscle bundles that extend right up to the level of the aortic annulus. It is crucial to avoid placing the patch in such a fashion that it straddles one of these valleys as a residual intramyocardial VSD will result.[50]

Although the suture entrance points can be some distance from the aortic annulus and not precisely radial in their orientation, the exit points should be within the fibrous aortic annulus so that the patch lies right up to the level of the aortic annulus. Anchoring the sutures through the fibrous annulus ensures that the sutures can be tied firmly and will not cut through the very soft muscular tissue of the young infant. Once the conal septum has been reached anteriorly there are no longer ridges and valleys as the conal septum is smooth and featureless up to the aortic valve. Sutures can be passed through the full thickness of the conal septum. In the particularly small child it is important to consider subsequent growth of this area. The Teflon pledgets are quite large relative to the outflow area in a child who is less than 2 kg in weight. In this setting it is useful to custom cut small pericardial pledgets. This will decrease the risk of subsequent right ventricular outflow tract obstruction. The final sutures are placed between 12:00 and 3:00 usually without difficulty. A knitted velour Dacron patch is threaded onto the sutures. Dacron offers the advantage that it excites a fibrous reaction which helps to seal the irregularities around the margin of the VSD. Although autologous pericardium will tie down somewhat more easily than Dacron it is our impression that small residual VSDs are more persistent with autologous pericardial patches relative to Dacron. Presumably the catheter delivered devices that utilize Dacron make use of the same fibrous reaction. The patch should be tied into place with great care beginning at about 4:00 or 5:00. The sutures have been deeply anchored and the patch can be firmly tied at this point. In the region of the conduction bundle across the posterior and inferior angle the sutures need to be tied with particular care. The pledgets should be visualized to ensure they are appropriately seated and not caught in tricuspid chordae.

RIGHT VENTRICULAR OUTFLOW TRACT PATCH

An autologous pericardial patch which has been soaked in 0.6% glutaraldehyde for 20–30 minutes is cut to shape (Figure 16.2b). As noted in Chapter 2, it is particularly important that the ends of the patch be blunt and not the 'diamond shape' that is often described. This permits augmentation of the left pulmonary artery or main pulmonary artery diameter with the toe of the patch and augmentation of the inferior end of the ventriculotomy with the heel of the patch. The placement of sutures is begun at the toe of the patch using continuous 6/0 or 5/0 prolene on a small needle such as a BV1 or RB2. Sutures should be more widely spaced on the patch relative to the artery so that the artery diameter is augmented. The patch should be sufficiently wide that the main pulmonary artery has a normal appearance when subsequently distended with blood. It may be useful to place a Hegar dilator that is of normal diameter for the child's size in order to check that the patch is of appropriate width. This is particularly critical at the level of the annulus. The patch should widen somewhat as it extends on to the ventricle so that it is pear shaped. At the apex of the ventriculotomy particularly wide bites should be taken on the patch while bites should be very closely spaced in the ventricular muscle.

AVOIDANCE OF CORONARY INJURY BY SUTURES

In the neonate and small infant it is usually preferable to leave the aortic cross clamp in place until the patch suture line is well beyond coronary arteries because they are at risk of being caught up in the suture line. The suture line will usually be within 3–4 mm of the left anterior descending coronary artery and within 2–3 mm of the long anterior right ventricular branch extending from the right coronary to the apex of the heart. The suture line can be all but completed prior to cross-clamp removal. Leaving a small portion of the suture line open at the time the aortic cross clamp is removed will allow decompression of both the right and left heart until ejection commences. When the heart is beating effectively the suture line can be closed.

MONITORING LINES AND PACING WIRES

Following de-airing of the heart and release of the cross clamp a left atrial line is inserted through a mattress suture in the right superior pulmonary vein as described previously. Two atrial pacing wires are routinely placed as a means to diagnose and treat junctional ectopic tachycardia (JET). JET is a relatively common occurrence following neonatal and infant repair of tetralogy particularly when an atrial approach is utilized. We continue to place a pulmonary artery pressure line through a mattress suture in the infundibulum of the right ventricle. This allows for assessment of residual VSD by oxygen saturation data. In addition, pullback of the line into the right ventricle on the first postoperative day quantitates any residual right ventricular outflow tract gradient. A single ventricular pacing wire is also placed.

MANAGEMENT OF THE FORAMEN OVALE

It is important to leave the foramen ovale patent. In the early postoperative period the right ventricle is likely to be the limiting factor for total cardiac output. This is in part because of the acute volume load imposed by pulmonary regurgitation secondary to a transannular patch. There has also been considerable retraction of the right ventricle during the period of myocardial ischemia. The hypertrophied right ventricle which has adapted for the pressure load of pulmonary stenosis and an unrestrictive VSD is not well suited to accommodate a sudden increase in volume work and right atrial pressure may increase importantly. A high right atrial pressure, e.g. more than 10–12 mm, is poorly tolerated by the neonate and young infant and will result in a 'leaky capillary syndrome'. On the other hand a mild degree of cyanosis which will result from a right to left shunt at atrial level is well tolerated by the neonate who is adapted to the low oxygen environment of the prenatal circulation. Cardiac output is maintained, urine output is maintained and the vicious cycle of tissue edema, pleural effusions and ascites is avoided.

WEANING FROM BYPASS

Weaning from bypass should be uncomplicated. A low dose dopamine infusion at 5 μg/kg/minute is often useful. If the child does not wean easily from bypass there is almost certainly a residual anatomical problem.

Residual right ventricular outflow tract obstruction

Residual right ventricular outflow tract obstruction is easily detected with simultaneous monitoring of the previously placed pulmonary artery pressure line and exploratory needle pressure measurement within the body of the right ventricle. Right ventricular outflow tract obstruction severe enough to produce suprasystemic right ventricular pressure is the most likely reason for failure to wean from bypass. A right ventricular pressure that is less than 80–90% of systemic pressure is rarely sufficient cause alone for failure to wean from bypass. Dynamic obstruction of the right ventricular outflow tract can be seen in the immediate postbypass period particularly in the setting of relative hypovolemia and inotrope induced hypercontractility. Intraoperative transesophageal echocardiography (TEE) may be useful in instances where the level of the obstruction is uncertain despite simultaneous pressure measurements. Complete assessment requires use of both two-dimensional imaging and Doppler analysis. Echocardiographic imaging can provide visualization of the extent and severity of the obstruction while spectral Doppler can be used to quantitate the pressure gradient. However, TEE assessment of residual right ventricular outflow tract obstruction is not without limitations. Echocardiographic images can lead to an overestimation of the severity of right ventricular outflow tract obstruction if the image plane is through a particularly narrow portion of an otherwise widely patent outflow tract. Underestimation of the true pressure gradient will occur if the Doppler beam can not be aligned parallel to the area of peak velocity within the outflow tract. Nonetheless, a persistently high pressure gradient across an intact annulus detected either directly or by TEE is an indication for a return on bypass to extend the outflow patch across the annulus.

Residual VSD

Despite care visualizing all margins of the VSD patch as it is tied down and reinforcing sutures in areas of soft muscle residual VSDs may occur. A residual VSD will be characterized by an elevated left atrial pressure and systemic hypotension. Normally, right atrial pressure would be expected to be higher than left atrial pressure in the immediate postoperative period following tetralogy repair. In the presence of a residual VSD left atrial pressure will be disproportionately elevated. The diagnosis can be confirmed by demonstrating a marked stepup in the oxygen saturation of blood taken from the right atrium (e.g. 65%) relative to that taken from the pulmonary artery (e.g. 87%). TEE can be useful in localizing and sizing the VSD as well. The TEE exam must be conducted so as to differentiate a peripatch leak from a muscular VSD. Muscular VSDs which were undetected may become detectable once the repair is completed and right ventricular pressure is subsystemic. Similarly, previously detected small muscular VSDs may appear more prominent following repair.

A residual VSD is very poorly tolerated in the patient with tetralogy for several reasons. The peripheral pulmonary arteries are thin walled and distensible and pulmonary vascular resistance is generally not elevated. As a result there is potential for a very large left to right shunt with attendant left and right ventricular volume overload and dilation. Pulmonary regurgitation from a transannular patch and tricuspid regurgitation from right ventricular dilation will exacerbate right ventricular volume overload. An acute volume load is particularly poorly tolerated in the setting of diastolic dysfunction. Restrictive right ventricular diastolic physiology may occur in older patients as the result of the concentric hypertrophy which accompanies chronic exposure to systemic pressure or to the combined effects of myocardial edema, cardiopulmonary bypass and a ventriculotomy in neonates. Finally, the ventricles have been adapted to a state of relative pressure and not volume overload prior to repair. Thus, the child with a residual VSD after effective relief of right ventricular outflow tract obstruction can rapidly develop a profound low cardiac output state.

Coronary obstruction

If the outflow tract patch suture line has passed extremely close to a coronary artery, particularly the left anterior descending, tension within the epicardium can cause partial obstruction of the coronary artery. This should be apparent by both ECG ST segment changes and discoloration of the affected area of myocardium. TEE evidence of regional wall motion abnormalities (hypokinesis, akinesis) will further confirm this suspicion. It may become necessary to return on bypass, take down the suture line where it is closest to the coronary artery and pass sutures from within the ventricle. When this is undertaken, it is useful to use interrupted pledgetted sutures with the pledgets lying on the endocardial surface of the free wall to minimize tension in the region of the coronary artery.

RESULTS OF SURGERY

Early mortality

Pigula et al[51] undertook a retrospective review of 99 children with both tetralogy of Fallot with pulmonary stenosis as well as tetralogy of Fallot with pulmonary atresia who underwent early complete repair at Children's Hospital Boston between 1988 and 1996. All patients were less than 90 days of age with a median age of 27 days. Of the 99 patients, 59 were prostaglandin dependent. Overall 91% of patients were considered symptomatic because of cyanosis with or without cyanotic spells. The early mortality was 3% with the mortality for patients with tetralogy of Fallot with pulmonary stenosis in this timeframe being 2.7%. The results from Children's Hospital Boston are similar to those from several other reports during the 1990s. Sousa-Uva et al described an overall mortality of 3.6% among 56 patients undergoing repair of tetralogy in the first six months of life.[52] Hennein et al described no hospital deaths among 30 neonates with symptomatic tetralogy of Fallot.[53] Karl et al described a review of 366 patients with a median age of 15.3 months. There were two hospital deaths for a hospital mortality of 0.5%.[2] In an important study described by Kirklin et al the results of an approach of primary repair were compared with a two stage approach.[18] One hundred consecutive patients from the University of Alabama were compared with 100 consecutive patients from Children's Hospital Boston undergoing correction of tetralogy of Fallot between 1984 and 1989. The authors concluded that there was a possible disadvantage for the two stage approach employing preliminary shunting and later repair.

Long-term results after early primary repair

Bacha et al reported in 2001[23] the late results of early primary repair of tetralogy performed at Children's Hospital Boston between 1972 and 1977 in 57 patients who were less than 24 months of age at the time of surgery. Recent follow-up was obtained for 45 of the 49 long-term survivors. Median follow-up was 23.5 years. Although there were eight early deaths in this early timeframe there was only one late death 24 years after the initial repair. The overwhelming majority of patients (41 of 45 traced patients) were completely free of symptoms. There was no influence of a transannular patch on late survival (Figure 16.5a). In fact lack of a transannular patch tended to be associated with a higher risk for reintervention (Figure 16.5b). The majority of reintervention procedures which 10 patients underwent were for recurrent right ventricular outflow tract obstruction which was necessary in eight patients. Six of these patients had not had a transannular patch although the majority of patients (65%) had undergone placement of a transannular patch at the initial procedure. Other reinterventions included one patient who had a homograft pulmonary valve replacement 20 years postoperatively performed at another institution and one patient who required a defibrillator for inducible ventricular tachycardia.

Long-term follow-up studies from other centers have suggested that residual or recurrent right ventricular outflow tract obstruction is a more serious late problem and a more common cause of need for reoperation than pulmonary regurgitation. Chen and Moller[54] followed 144 patients for 10 years. They found that patients with right ventricular outflow tract obstruction had the worst late results. A large right ventricular to pulmonary artery pressure gradient was noted in three

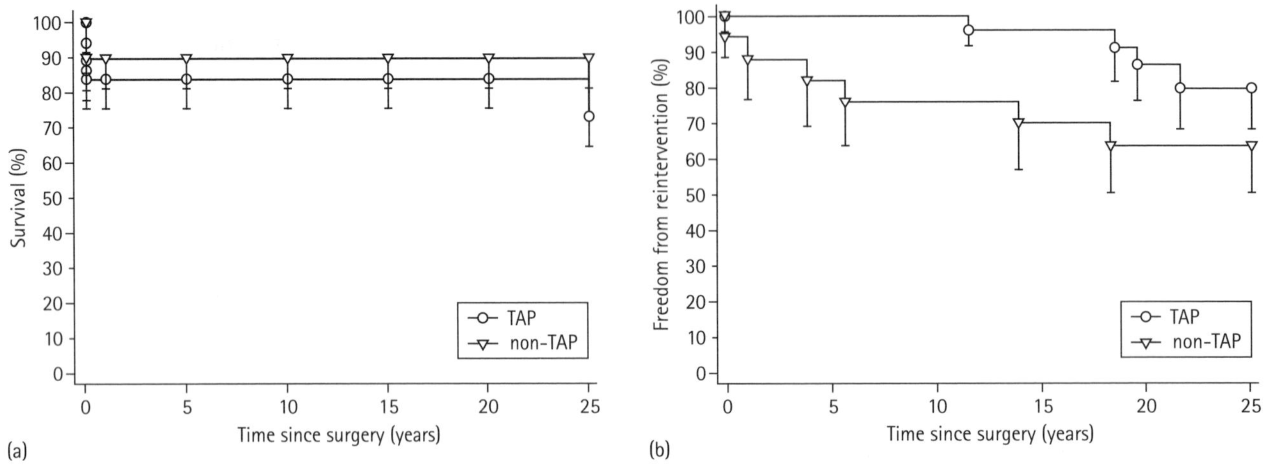

Figure 16.5 *(a) The impact of a transannular patch (TAP) on late survival among 57 patients who underwent repair of tetralogy of Fallot with pulmonary stenosis in the first two years of life between 1972 and 1977. (b) The impact of a transannular patch on freedom from reintervention among 57 patients who underwent repair of tetralogy of Fallot with pulmonary stenosis in the first two years of life between 1972 and 1977. There is a trend towards a higher rate of reintervention for patients who did not have a transannular patch. (From Bacha et al. Long-term results after early primary repair of tetralogy of Fallot.* J Thorac Cardiovasc Surg *2001; 122:157,158, with permission from Elsevier.)*

of four patients who died late suddenly. Lillehei et al[24] reviewed 106 patients who underwent repair of tetralogy at the University of Minnesota between 1954 and 1960. Similar to the experience from Boston the commonest cause for reoperation was recurrent right ventricular outflow tract obstruction. No patient required late pulmonary valve replacement.

TRANSANNULAR PATCH NO LONGER A RISK FACTOR

Although placement of a transannular patch was demonstrated as a risk factor for early mortality in the first decades of surgery for tetralogy of Fallot, in the current era most studies do not identify the use of a transannular patch as a risk factor. For example, this was true in the two institutional study reported by Kirklin et al[18] comparing the results of surgery with a two stage approach as practiced at that time at the University of Alabama with an approach of early primary repair as practiced at Children's Hospital Boston. In fact a high post repair pressure ratio, i.e. residual obstruction, was a risk factor for death after repair.

Primary versus two stage repair

A small number of centers continue to support an approach of initial palliation with a modified Blalock shunt in the first 6–12 months of life followed by subsequent repair.[2,3] However, the majority of centers have accepted the fact that early primary repair can be performed with excellent low mortality and an acceptable low rate of reintervention, particularly when the rate of reintervention is compared with the mandatory reintervention required with a two stage approach. Furthermore although some centers have described a low mortality for shunt procedures a number of excellent centers have described significant risk. For example in a 1997 report by Gladman et al[55] overall survival for patients who had a two stage approach at the Hospital for Sick Children in Toronto was 90% while in patients who had primary repair the survival was 97%.

Transatrial versus transventricular repair

A number of studies over the last decade have presented excellent results using a primarily transatrial approach to repair of tetralogy of Fallot. For example Karl et al[2] and Hirsch et al[56] have described excellent results using the transatrial approach with a limited ventriculotomy. These authors have focused attention on the length of the ventriculotomy as an important determinant of late right ventricular function. However, it is important to remember that centers which mainly use a ventriculotomy approach to the repair of tetralogy focus attention on a number of other factors which determine late right ventricular function. These factors include

- the width of the outflow tract patch
- preservation of the moderator band
- avoidance of excessive division of right ventricular muscle
- careful preservation of tricuspid valve function by avoidance of sutures snaring tricuspid chords or leaflet tissue
- careful planning of the ventriculotomy to minimize damage to coronary artery branches
- careful avoidance of distal pulmonary artery obstruction.

Late pulmonary valve replacement

The majority of centers have found that pulmonary valve replacement is rarely indicated even decades after repair of tetralogy of Fallot.[24] However, some centers have described a relatively high incidence of late pulmonary valve replacement. For example Ilbawi et al[57] described 49 patients who required pulmonary valve replacement 2–20 years after repair of tetralogy of Fallot. The primary indications for valve implantation were progressive cardiomegaly and evidence of right ventricular dilation or dysfunction. Other reports of beneficial effects of late pulmonary valve replacement include those by Warner et al[6] from New England Medical Center and by Finck et al[7] from the Mayo Clinic. In the future percutaneous transcatheter insertion of a pulmonary valve as described by Bonhoeffer[8] may become an attractive alternative to surgical reintervention.

The role of the monocusp valve

Although some centers have expressed enthusiasm for placement of a monocusp valve at the time of initial tetralogy repair follow-up studies have suggested that the function of such 'valves' is transient at best. For example Bigras et al[58] compared postoperative echocardiographic findings of 24 patients who had undergone transannular patch repair with a monocusp valve with 17 patients who had undergone patch repair without a monocusp valve and 20 patients who had undergone repair without a transannular patch. The authors found no significant differences in the degree of early postoperative pulmonary regurgitation or in clinical outcomes such as mortality, number of reoperations or hospital stay. Gundry et al[5] described 19 patients who had monocusp valves placed and were assessed up to 24 months postoperatively. Although 16 of 19 patients had competent monocusp valves immediately postoperatively by 24 months only one of seven patients had a competent valve. No patient had monocusp stenosis though this is likely to be an important late consequence of monocusp valve insertion.

TETRALOGY OF FALLOT WITH ABSENT PULMONARY VALVE SYNDROME

Tetralogy of Fallot with complete AV canal is considered in Chapter 21.

Introduction

Tetralogy of Fallot with absent pulmonary valve syndrome is a variant of tetralogy of Fallot with pulmonary stenosis in which respiratory symptoms are usually more problematic than cardiac symptoms. The distinguishing feature of this lesion is the potential for enormous dilation of the mediastinal, i.e. main, right and left pulmonary arteries. This can result in severe compression of the trachea, mainstem and peripheral bronchi. In addition, the small pulmonary arteries can be affected.[59] The normal pattern of single segmental arteries is replaced by a network of intertwining arteries which compress intrapulmonary bronchi.

As with many other anomalies there is an extremely wide spectrum of severity. At the severe end of the spectrum the outlook is dismal. The pulmonary arteries are dilated along their entire length to the periphery of the lung, and airway compression is severe occurring along the length of the bronchial tree and into the small airways. On the other hand at the mild end of the spectrum there is minimal or no tracheal/bronchial involvement, the small airways are not involved and the management is comparable to that of tetralogy of Fallot with pulmonary stenosis.

Embryology

Presumably the basic cardiac malformations which occur with the absent pulmonary valve syndrome are of the same embryological origin as tetralogy of Fallot with pulmonary stenosis. There is an anterior malalignment VSD and usually a mild degree of right ventricular outflow tract obstruction including pulmonary annular hypoplasia. One of the intriguing observations about the absent pulmonary valve syndrome is that the ductus arteriosus is never present when the pulmonary arteries are in continuity. It is felt that in the presence of a ductus arteriosus this lesion is incompatible with fetal survival to birth.[60] In the setting of a VSD and an absent pulmonary valve the presence of a ductus will create the physiologic equivalent of severe aortic insufficiency. The majority of left ventricular output flows retrograde through the ductus into the right ventricle and across the VSD back into the left ventricle. This has led to speculation that the absence of a pulmonary valve promotes premature closure and subsequent obliteration of the ductus[61] or that only those fetuses without a ductus survive to birth. The dilated central pulmonary arteries are thought to enlarge secondary to the to-and-fro flow between the pulmonary artery and the right ventricle in utero. Histological study of the central pulmonary arteries has failed to define the presence of a connective tissue disorder though there is usually fracture of elastin fibers.[59]

Anatomy

There is an anterior malalignment VSD similar in size and location to that found in tetralogy of Fallot with pulmonary stenosis. The conal septum is often underdeveloped. The pulmonary annulus is mildly to moderately hypoplastic. There are vestigial nubbins of primitive myxomatous tissue at the level of the valve annulus but no true formation of valve leaflets. Immediately beyond the pulmonary annulus the main pulmonary artery is usually dilated to at least 2–3 times its usual diameter. The right and left branch pulmonary arteries which are normally 4–5 mm in diameter are commonly 2–3 times that diameter. At the hilar level the lobar branches are often of a normal size although they may be dilated as well. The origin of the right main bronchus may be compressed at the point where it lies just posterior to the dilated right pulmonary artery. Similarly, the left main bronchus may be compressed at the point where the dilated left pulmonary artery passes over the bronchus. The carina itself may be compressed by the distal main pulmonary artery and the origin of the right pulmonary artery.

Pathophysiology and clinical presentation

Hypoxemia in this syndrome is the result of both intrapulmonary and intracardiac pathology. Pulmonary venous desaturation can result from ventilation–perfusion mismatch and intrapulmonary shunting. Right to left shunting at the ventricular level will also contribute to hypoxemia though it is rare for there to be sufficiently severe right ventricular outflow tract obstruction to cause a large right to left shunt. In fact, in the absence of pulmonary venous desaturation pulmonary blood flow is often balanced such that the child does not have congestive heart failure and is not hypoxemic. While cardiac symptoms are usually mild, pulmonary problems can be severe. Many neonates present with respiratory distress from the time of birth. Air trapping is encountered leading to overinflated lungs. Ventilation is inefficient and the work of breathing is high. Hypercarbia commonly ensues with a resultant respiratory acidosis which can be severe enough to reduce pH below 7.10. In instances where airway compression is less severe the child may present later in infancy with frequent respiratory infections and a history of wheezing. In the least severe forms of this syndrome, respiratory symptoms will be minimal and the diagnosis will be established on the basis of a murmur and cyanosis.

Diagnostic studies

CHEST X-RAY

The chest X-ray will reveal hyper-expansion of the lung. Individual lobes or the entire lung may be involved depending on the site of bronchial obstruction (Figure 16.6).

Unilateral obstruction commonly leads to a considerable mediastinal shift to the contralateral side.

ECHOCARDIOGRAPHY

Two-dimensional echocardiography is diagnostic. In addition to the usual cardiac features of tetralogy of Fallot the

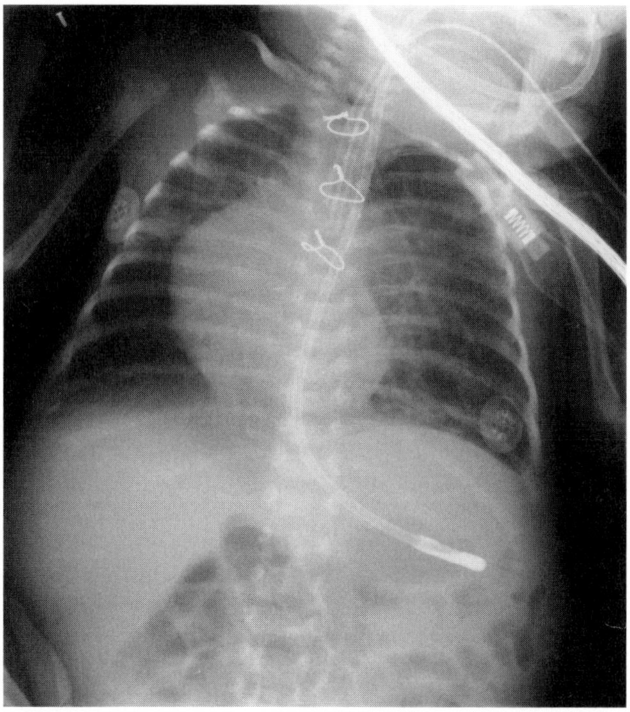

Figure 16.6 *Chest X-ray of a four-month-old child with absent pulmonary valve syndrome demonstrates segmental collapse in the right lung with patchy hyperinflation of both lungs, particularly in the right lower zone.*

location and extent of pulmonary artery dilation can be delineated.

COMPUTED TOMOGRAPHY AND MAGNETIC RESONANCE IMAGING

If there is any doubt that respiratory symptoms are related to dilation of the central pulmonary arteries, either a CT or MRI scan can define the specific relationship between sites of airway compression and dilation of the central pulmonary arteries. Sedation or general anesthesia may be necessary to obtain a diagnostic quality scan. When the airway is compromised anesthesia or ICU personnel experienced in the management of these patients should be available.

BRONCHOSCOPY

Bronchoscopy can provide a baseline measure of the degree of airway compression. In addition, when pulmonary artery dilation is mild bronchoscopy can be used to rule out tracheal and bronchial compression as a source of respiratory symptoms. As with the CT and MRI scan, bronchoscopy carries some risk if the airway is tenuous and carbon dioxide retention is problematic.

CARDIAC CATHETERIZATION

Angiography at the time of cardiac catheterization provides better delineation of peripheral pulmonary artery dilation beyond the hilum than echocardiography. However, because such dilation is not medically or surgically treatable and because children with such dilation are likely to have severe respiratory compromise, cardiac catheterization is rarely indicated for absent pulmonary valve syndrome.

Medical and interventional therapy

If the child has respiratory distress when breathing spontaneously, intubation and positive pressure ventilation are indicated. Paralysis may be helpful but is not always. One of the most important maneuvers in the medical palliation of this condition is to place the child in the prone position. Presumably this allows the pulmonary arteries to fall forwards and takes some pressure off the airway. Even though it is possible to palliate the child in this position for some time nevertheless surgery should not be deferred but should proceed shortly after diagnosis has been established. At present there are no effective nonsurgical interventional procedures for managing absent pulmonary valve syndrome. Stenting of the airways should not be employed except under the most extreme circumstances.

Indications for surgery

The diagnosis of absent pulmonary valve syndrome is in itself an indication for surgical management as there is no probability of spontaneous resolution and there are no alternatives to surgical management. Decision making then hinges on determining the optimal timing of surgery.

SYMPTOMS

Profound respiratory compromise in the neonate

Severe respiratory compromise shortly after birth is an indication for emergent or urgent surgical correction.

Wheezing, frequent respiratory infections in infancy

In this circumstance surgical correction should be undertaken shortly after the diagnosis has been established.

ELECTIVE REPAIR

In the child who is free of symptoms surgery should be scheduled electively in the first months of life or shortly after diagnosis has been established.

Surgical management

COMPLETE REPLACEMENT OF THE CENTRAL PULMONARY ARTERIES INCLUDING INSERTION OF HOMOGRAFT PULMONARY VALVE

The child who presents with severe respiratory compromise shortly after birth or in early infancy should be managed aggressively. Use of a pulmonary homograft to replace the dilated main and branch pulmonary arteries and the dysplastic pulmonary valve following their resection is almost always indicated.[62]

ANESTHESIA AND GENERAL SETUP

Method of cardiopulmonary bypass

In the small, sick neonate who is difficult to ventilate, surface cooling is a useful adjunct prior to the onset of cardiopulmonary bypass. The room temperature should be lowered and the cooling blanket on which the child lies should be activated during the placement of monitoring and intravenous lines.

Cardiopulmonary bypass should be established with standard ascending aortic cannulation and a single venous cannula inserted through the right atrial appendage. There will be severe mediastinal crowding by the hyperinflated lung fields making it unwise to attempt bicaval cannulation. Deep hypothermia is achieved by cooling to a rectal temperature less than 18°C and the procedure is undertaken at a reduced flow rate of 50 ml/kg per minute.

PRELIMINARY DISSECTION

During cooling the branch pulmonary arteries are mobilized out to the hilar branches (Figure 16.7a). Following application of the aortic cross clamp the main pulmonary artery is transected at the level of the pulmonary annulus and the right and left pulmonary artery are transected leaving a sufficient cuff of tissue proximal to the hilar branches to allow subsequent suturing without stenosing the hilar branches (Figure 16.7b). At this point a decision is made regarding selection of a pulmonary homograft. A homograft with both the appropriate pulmonary annulus and branch pulmonary

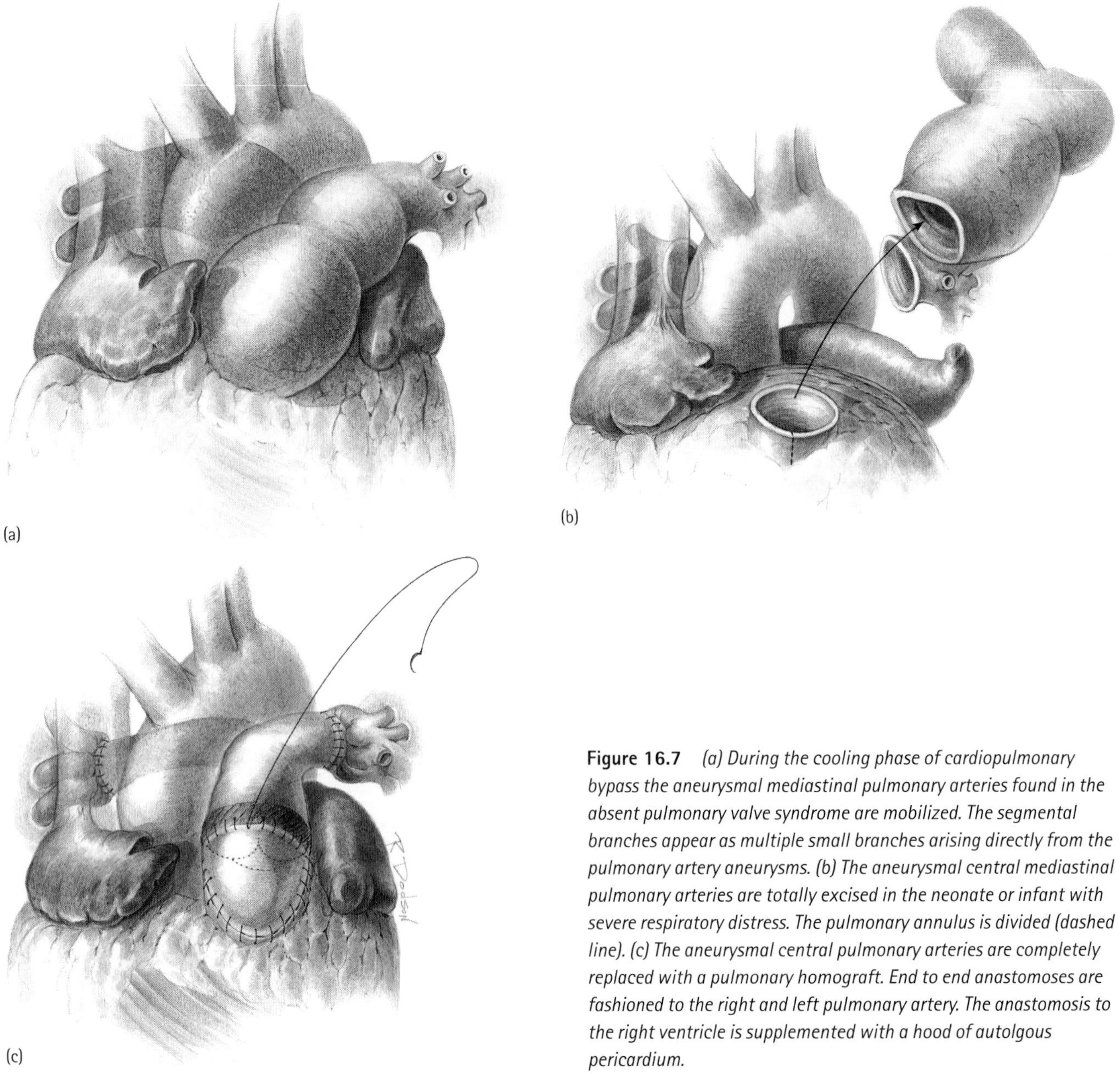

Figure 16.7 *(a) During the cooling phase of cardiopulmonary bypass the aneurysmal mediastinal pulmonary arteries found in the absent pulmonary valve syndrome are mobilized. The segmental branches appear as multiple small branches arising directly from the pulmonary artery aneurysms. (b) The aneurysmal central mediastinal pulmonary arteries are totally excised in the neonate or infant with severe respiratory distress. The pulmonary annulus is divided (dashed line). (c) The aneurysmal central pulmonary arteries are completely replaced with a pulmonary homograft. End to end anastomoses are fashioned to the right and left pulmonary artery. The anastomosis to the right ventricle is supplemented with a hood of autolgous pericardium.*

artery dimensions should be chosen. The homograft should be thawed and rinsed during VSD closure.

VSD CLOSURE AND INFUNDIBULAR MUSCLE BUNDLE DIVISION

The infundibular incision is made across the pulmonary annulus and infundibular muscle bundles are divided as indicated. The VSD is closed with a knitted velour Dacron patch using interrupted pledgetted horizontal mattress 5/0 coated polyester sutures in the usual fashion. It may be necessary to discontinue bypass briefly during placement of sutures across the posterior and inferior angle of the VSD. However, bypass can be recommenced for the remainder of the procedure.

PULMONARY HOMOGRAFT INSERTION

The pulmonary homograft is trimmed so that the right and left homograft branches are of an appropriate length. A simple end to end anastomosis is fashioned to the patient's right and left pulmonary artery with particular attention paid to avoiding stenosis of the hilar branches (Figure 16.7c). It is better to err on the side of leaving a greater margin from the hilar branches than might be thought to be necessary. Continuous 6/0 polypropylene suture is usually appropriate.

The pulmonary homograft annulus is now sutured to the patient's pulmonary annulus posteriorly. In some instances it may be possible to use the homograft annulus to primarily close the infundibular incision. In all likelihood, however, use of a small pericardial patch will be necessary to close the infundibular incision with the cephalad end of the pericardial patch sutured to the pulmonary homograft annulus anteriorly (Figure 16.7c). Continuous 5/0 polypropylene with a slightly larger needle than is used for the branch pulmonary artery anastomoses (RB2 rather than BV1) is usually appropriate. Prior to completion of the homograft anastomosis the heart is allowed to fill with blood and air is vented through the cardioplegia site. The aortic cross clamp is released with the cardioplegia site bleeding freely.

MONITORING LINES

The usual monitoring lines for tetralogy of Fallot with pulmonary stenosis should be placed, i.e. a left atrial line, pulmonary artery line and right atrial line. Two atrial pacing wires and a single ventricular pacing wire should be placed as well.

MANAGEMENT OF THE FORAMEN OVALE

The foramen ovale should be left patent in order to allow right to left decompression in the early postoperative period as is standard practice for tetralogy of Fallot with pulmonary stenosis.

WEANING FROM BYPASS

The principal challenge will be management of ventilation. There should be a marked improvement in the tendency for air trapping but complete resolution of this problem is unlikely due to persistence of tracheo- and bronchomalacia and distal small airway obstruction. Tracheo- and bronchomalacia may persist for several weeks to months and will continue to compromise ventilation. It may be useful to delay sternal closure to avoid cardiovascular compromise from persistent lung hyperinflation in the early postoperative period.

ELECTIVE SURGICAL MANAGEMENT WITH MODERATE DILATION OF THE CENTRAL PULMONARY ARTERIES

In the child who has little or no respiratory compromise replacement of the central pulmonary arteries and/or pulmonary valve with homograft material is usually not necessary. Avoidance of unnecessary homograft placement obviates the need for mandatory reoperations.

REDUCTION PULMONARY ARTERIOPLASTY

In addition to the usual management of tetralogy of Fallot with pulmonary stenosis, i.e. Dacron patch closure of the anterior malalignment VSD, division of infundibular muscle bundles and appropriate patch enlargement of the infundibulum and pulmonary annulus, it is necessary to reduce the main and branch pulmonary arteries in size by an appropriate plasty.[63] It may also be appropriate to perform a plasty with a running suture line across the posterior wall of the branch pulmonary arteries internally without resection. Care should be taken to avoid excessively narrowing the central pulmonary arteries if the child's symptoms are mild. On occasion the child with absent pulmonary valve syndrome will have such a mild degree of enlargement of the central pulmonary arteries and complete absence of respiratory symptoms such that neither plasty of the pulmonary arteries nor insertion of an orthotopic pulmonary valve is indicated.

WHEN SHOULD AN ORTHOTOPIC PULMONARY VALVE BE PLACED?

Because absent pulmonary valve syndrome is a rare anomaly it is difficult to answer this question with certainty. The child who has severe respiratory symptoms and documented severe compression of the airways should at a minimum have an extensive plasty of the central pulmonary arteries as well as insertion of a pulmonary valve.[62] In the older child who has chronic respiratory symptoms orthotopic pulmonary valve replacement may also be indicated. However, an alternative more conservative approach would be to perform a repair including VSD closure, relief of infundibular obstruction, a limited plasty of the central pulmonary arteries and subsequent observation. If the child continues to have respiratory symptoms and if there is redilation of the central pulmonary arteries at reoperation an orthotopic pulmonary valve can be placed.

Results of surgery

Because absent pulmonary valve syndrome is a particularly rare anomaly and in addition it exists in a wide spectrum of severity, it is difficult to know what the risks are for the surgical management of an individual child. The fact that numerous surgical approaches were described in the first decades of cardiac surgery suggests that results until the last decade have been unsatisfactory. In 1969 Waldhausen and colleagues described the use of the Glenn shunt to alleviate bronchial obstruction.[64] Osmon and colleagues described aneurysmoraphy.[65] Bove et al[66] described suspension of the pulmonary arteries to the retrosternal fascia in addition to aneurysmorrhaphy. Litwin and colleagues[67] described an innovative procedure in which the left pulmonary artery was removed from the mediastinum and replaced anterior to the ascending aorta using a tubular prosthetic interposition graft.

Layton and associates[68] reported successful use of a valved homograft in two teenage patients in 1972. Snir et al[69] described use of a valved homograft in 22 patients in 1991. Danilowicz[70] was the first to describe successful use of a homograft in one neonate and one infant in 1993. In 2002 Hraska et al[71] described an innovative procedure similar in principle to the procedure described by Litwin but with elimination of the conduit placed between the main pulmonary artery and right pulmonary artery. Effectively a Lecompte maneuver is performed to bring the right pulmonary artery anterior to the ascending aorta.

Not all centers agree that homograft replacement of the central pulmonary arteries is necessary even for symptomatic infants. In 1997 Godard et al reported a series of 37 consecutive patients who underwent surgery for absent pulmonary valve syndrome in Paris between 1977 and 1995.[72] The hospital mortality was 8%. The late mortality was 5%. The authors conclude that pulmonary arterioplasty is required to reduce bronchial obstruction but there is no need for pulmonary valve insertion.

In 2002 Hew et al described a retrospective review of 59 consecutive patients with absent pulmonary valve syndrome who were admitted to Children's Hospital Boston for surgical management between 1960 and 1998.[62] Fifteen patients underwent VSD closure, total resection of dilated central pulmonary arteries and reconstruction of the right ventricular outflow tract and pulmonary arteries with a homograft. A total of 21 patients had VSD closure, reconstruction of the right ventricular outflow tract with a transannular patch and aneurysmorrhaphy. Twelve patients had miscellaneous procedures. The operative survival rates at 1, 5 and 10 years were 83%, 80%, 78% and 78% respectively. Risk factors for operative mortality by multivariate analysis were the presence of respiratory distress ($p = 0.04$), surgery in the neonatal period ($p = 0.02$), weight less than 3 kg ($p = 0.02$), palliative surgery leaving an open VSD ($p = 0.02$) and surgery before 1990 ($p = 0.04$). After 1990 the operative mortality decreased to 11%. In patients with respiratory distress survival with homograft replacement of the central pulmonary arteries was 73% versus 41% with other techniques ($p = 0.2$). The patients were followed for 72 ± 50 months. There were no significant differences in freedom from reintervention rates among the surgical groups ($p = 0.08$). Hew et al concluded from this review that aggressive homograft replacement of the pulmonary arteries has been associated with improved survival in patients with absent pulmonary valve syndrome, particularly in neonates with severe respiratory distress.

REFERENCES

1. Fyler DC. Report of the New England Regional Infant Cardiac Program. *Pediatrics* 1980; **65**:375–461.
2. Karl TR, Sano S, Pornviliwan S, Mee RB. Tetralogy of Fallot: favorable outcome of nonneonatal transatrial, transpulmonary repair. *Ann Thorac Surg* 1992; **54**:903–907.
3. Fraser CD, McKenzie ED, Cooley DA. Tetralogy of Fallot: surgical management individualized to the patient. *Ann Thorac Surg* 2001; **71**:1556–1561.
4. Coles JG. Transatrial repair of tetralogy of Fallot. *Ann Thorac Surg* 1995; **59**:1363.
5. Gundry SR, Razzouk AJ, Boskind JF, Bansal R, Bailey LL. Fate of the pericardial monocusp pulmonary valve for right ventricular outflow tract reconstruction. *J Thorac Cardiovasc Surg* 1994; **107**:908–912.
6. Warner KG, Anderson JE, Fulton DR, Payne DD, Geggel FL, Marx GR. Restoration of the pulmonary valve reduces right ventricular volume overload after previous repair of tetralogy of Fallot. *Circulation* 1993; **88**:II189–197.
7. Finck SJ, Puga FJ, Danielson GK. Pulmonary valve insertion during reoperation for tetralogy of Fallot. *Ann Thorac Surg* 1988; **45**:610–613.
8. Bonhoeffer P, Boudjemline V, Qureshi SA et al. Percutaneous insertion of the pulmonary valve. *J Am Coll Cardiol* 2002; **39**:1664–1669.
9. Pexieder T. Conotruncus and its septation at the advent of the molecular biology era. In Clark EB, Markwald RR, Takao A (eds). *Developmental Mechanisms of Heart Disease.* Armonk, NY, Futura Publishing Company, 1995, pp 227–248.
10. Van Praagh R, Van Praagh S, Nebesar RA, Muster AJ, Sinha SN, Paul MH. Tetralogy of Fallot: Underdevelopment of the pulmonary infundibulum and its sequelae. *Am J Cardiol* 1970; **26**:25–33.
11. Kurosawa H, Morita K, Yamagishi M, Shimizu S, Becker AE, Anderson RH. Conotruncal repair for tetralogy of Fallot: midterm results. *J Thorac Cardiovasc Surg* 1998; **115**:351–360.
12. Munkhammar P, Cullen S, Jogi P, deLeval MR, Elliott M, Norgard G. Early age at repair prevents restrictive right ventricular physiology after surgery for tetralogy of Fallot. *J Am Coll Cardiol* 1998; **32**:1083–1087.
13. Dabizzi RP, Caprioli G, Aiazzi L et al. Distribution and anomalies of coronary arteries in tetralogy of Fallot. *Circulation* 1980; **61**:95–102.
14. Fellows KE, Freed MD, Keane JF, Van Praagh R, Bernhard WF, Castaneda AR. Results of routine preoperative coronary angiography in tetralogy of Fallot. *Circulation* 1975; **51**:561–566.
15. Fellows KE, Smith J, Keane JF. Preoperative angiocardiography in infants with tetrad of Fallot. Review of 36 cases. *Am J Cardiol* 1981; **47**:1279–1285.
16. Shimazaki Y, Blackstone EH, Kirklin JW, Jonas RA, Mandell V, Colvin EV. The dimensions of the right ventricular outflow tract and pulmonary arteries in tetralogy of Fallot and pulmonary stenosis. *J Thorac Cardiovasc Surg* 1992; **103**:692–705.
17. Spevak PJ, Mandell VS, Colan SD et al. Reliability of Doppler color flow mapping in the identification and localization of multiple ventricular septal defects. *Echocardiography* 1993; **10**:573–581.
18. Kirklin JK, Blackstone EH, Jonas RA et al. Morphologic and surgical determinants of outcome events after repair of tetralogy of Fallot

with pulmonary stenosis: A two institution study. *J Thorac Cardiovasc Surg* 1992; **103**:706–723.

19. Hiramatsu T, Jonas RA, Miura T et al. Cerebral metabolic recovery from deep hypothermic circulatory arrest after treatment with arginine and nitro-arginine methyl ester. *J Thorac Cardiovasc Surg* 1996; **112**:698–707.
20. Sluysmans T, Neven B, Rubay J et al. Early balloon dilation of the pulmonary valve in infants with tetralogy of Fallot. Risks and benefits. *Circulation* 1995; **91**:1506–1511.
21. Sreeram N, Saleem M, Jackson M et al. Results of balloon pulmonary valvuloplasty as a palliative procedure in tetralogy of Fallot. *J Am Coll Cardiol* 1991; **18**:159–165.
22. Arab SM, Kholeif AF, Zaher SR, Abdel Mohsen AM, Kassem AS, Qureshi SA. Balloon dilation of the right ventricular outflow tract in tetralogy of Fallot: A palliative procedure. *Cardiol Young* 1999; **9**:11–16.
23. Bacha EA, Scheule AM, Zurakowski D et al. Long-term results after early primary repair of tetralogy of Fallot. *J Thorac Cardiovasc Surg* 2001; **122**:154–161.
24. Lillehei CW, Varco RL, Cohen M et al. The first open heart corrections of tetralogy of Fallot. A 26–31 year follow-up of 106 patients. *Ann Surg* 1986; **204**:490–502.
25. Lillehei CW, Varco RL, Cohen M, Warden HE, Patton C, Moller JH. The first open-heart repairs of ventricular septal defect, atrioventricular communis, and tetralogy of Fallot using extracorporeal circulation by cross-circulation: a 30-year follow-up. *Ann Thorac Surg* 1986; **41**:4–21.
26. Kirklin JW, Blackstone EH, Pacifico AD, Brown RN, Bargeron LM. Routine primary vs two stage repair of tetralogy of Fallot. *Circulation* 1979; **60**:373–386.
27. Lansing AM, Haiderer O. Transaortic closure of the Potts anastomosis in the complete repair of tetralogy of Fallot. *J Thorac Cardiovasc Surg* 1973; **66**:279–282.
28. Alfieri O, Locatelli G, Bianchi T, Vanini V, Parenzan L. Repair of tetralogy of Fallot after Waterston anastomosis. *J Thorac Cardiovasc Surg* 1979; **77**:826–830.
29. de Leval MR, McKay R, Jones M, Stark J, Macartney FJ. Modified Blalock-Taussig shunt. Use of subclavian artery orifice as flow regulator in prosthetic systemic-pulmonary artery shunts. *J Thorac Cardiovasc Surg* 1981; **81**:112–119.
30. Rabinovitch M, Herrera-deLeon V, Castaneda AR, Reid L. Growth and development of the pulmonary vascular bed in patients with tetralogy of Fallot with or without pulmonary atresia. *Circulation* 1981; **64**:1234–1249.
31. Borow KM, Green LH, Castaneda AR et al. Left ventricular function after repair of tetralogy of Fallot and its relationship to age at surgery. *Circulation* 1980; **61**:1150–1158.
32. Walsh EP, Rockenmacher S, Keane JF, Hougen TJ, Lock JE, Castaneda AR. Late results in patients with tetralogy of Fallot repaired during infancy. *Circulation* 1988; **77**:1062–1067.
33. Newburger JW, Silbert AR, Buckley LP, Fyler DC. Cognitive function and age at repair of transposition of the great arteries in children. *N Engl J Med* 1984; **310**:1495–1499.
34. Tchervenkov CI, Pelletier MP, Shum-Tim D, Beland MJ, Rohlicek C. Primary repair minimizing the use of conduits in neonates and infants with tetralogy or double-outlet right ventricle and anomalous coronary arteries. *J Thorac Cardiovasc Surg* 2000; **119**:314–323.
35. Blalock A, Taussig HB. The surgical treatment of malformations of the heart in which there is pulmonary stenosis or pulmonary atresia. *JAMA* 1945; **128**:189–202.
36. Klinner VW, Pasini M, Schaudig A. Anastomose zwischen System- und Lungenarterie mit hilfe von Kunststoffprothesen bei Cyanotischen Herzvitien. *Thoraxchirugie* 1962; **10**:68.
37. Laks H, Castaneda AR. Subclavian arterioplasty for the ipsilateral Blalock-Taussig shunt. *Ann Thorac Surg* 1975; **19**:319.
38. Potts WJ, Smith S, Gibson S. Anastomosis of the aorta to a pulmonary artery. *JAMA* 1946; **132**:627–631.
39. Davidson JS. Anastomosis between the ascending aorta and the main pulmonary artery in the tetralogy of Fallot. *Thorax* 1955; **10**:348.
40. Waterston DJ. Treatment of Fallot's tetralogy in children under one year of age. *Rozhl Chir* 1962; **41**:181.
41. Brock RC. Pulmonary valvulotomy for relief of congenital pulmonary stenosis. Report of 3 cases. *Br Med J* 1948; I1121–1126.
42. Sellors TH. Surgery of pulmonary stenosis (a case in which pulmonary valve was successfully divided). *Lancet* 1948; **1**:98.
43. Lillehei CW, Cohen M, Warden HE et al. Direct vision intracardiac surgical correction of the tetralogy of Fallot, pentalogy of Fallot and pulmonary atresia defects: Report of the first 10 cases. *Ann Surg* 1955; **142**:418.
44. Kirklin JW, DuShane JW, Patrick RT et al. Intracardiac surgery with the aid of a mechanical pump-oxygenator system (Gibbon type): Report of eight cases. *Proc Staff Meet Mayo Clin* 1955; **30**:201.
45. Gott VL. C. Walton Lillehei and total correction of tetralogy of Fallot. *Ann Thorac Surg* 1990; **49**:328–332.
46. Klinner W. Indikationsstellung und operative technik fur die korrektur der Fallotschen tetralogy. *Langenbecks Archiv fur Klinische Chirurgie* 1964; **308**:40.
47. Ross D, Somerville J. Correction of pulmonary atresia with a homograft aortic valve. *Lancet* 1966; **2**:1446–1447.
48. Barratt Boyes BG, Neutze JM. Primary repair of tetralogy of Fallot in infancy using profound hypothermia with circulatory arrest and limited cardiopulmonary bypass. A comparison with conventional two-stage management. *Ann Surg* 1973; **178**:406–411.
49. Castaneda AR, Lamberti J, Sade RM, Williams RG, Nadas AS. Open-heart surgery during the first three months of life. *J Thorac Cardiovasc Surg* 1974; **68**:719–731.
50. Preminger TJ, Sanders SP, van der Velde ME, Castaneda AR, Lock JE. Intramural residual interventricular defects after repair of conotruncal malformations. *Circulation* 1994; **89**:236–224.
51. Pigula FA, Khalil PN, Mayer JE, del Nido PJ, Jonas RA. Repair of tetralogy of Fallot in neonates and young infants. *Circulation* 1999; **100**(Suppl II): II157–161.
52. Sousa-Uva M, Lacour-Gayet F, Komiya T et al. Surgery for tetralogy of Fallot at less than six months of age. *J Thorac Cardiovasc Surg* 1994; **107**:1291–1300.
53. Hennein HA, Mosca RS, Urcelay G, Crowley DC, Bove EL. Intermediate results after complete repair of tetralogy of Fallot in neonates. *J Thorac Cardiovasc Surg* 1995; **109**:332–344.
54. Chen D, Moller JH. Comparison of late clinical status between patients with different hemodynamic findings after repair of tetralogy of Fallot. *Am Heart J* 1987; **113**:767–772.
55. Gladman G, McCrindle BW, Williams WG, Freedom RM, Benson LM. The modified Blalock-Taussig shunt: Clinical impact and morbidity in Fallot's tetralogy in the current era. *J Thorac Cardiovasc Surg* 1997; **115**:25–30.
56. Hirsch JC, Mosca RS, Bove EL. Complete repair of tetralogy of Fallot in the neonate: results in the modern era. *Ann Surg* 2000; **232**:508–514.
57. Ilbawi MN, Idriss FS, DeLeon SY, Muster AJ, Berry TE, Paul MH. Long-term results of porcine valve insertion for pulmonary

regurgitation following repair of tetralogy of Fallot. *Ann Thorac Surg* 1986; **41**:478–482.
58. Bigras JL, Boutin C, McCrindle BW, Rebeyka IM. Short-term effect of monocuspid valves of pulmonary insufficiency and clinical outcome after surgical repair of tetralogy of Fallot. *J Thorac Cardiovasc Surg* 1996; **112**:33–37.
59. Rabinovitch M, Grady S, David I et al. Compression of intrapulmonary bronchi by abnormally branching pulmonary arteries associated with absent pulmonary valves. *Am J Cardiol* 1982; **50**:804–813.
60. Yeager SB, van der Velde ME, Waters BL, Sanders SP. Prenatal role of the ductus arteriosus in absent pulmonary valve syndrome. *Echocardiography* 2002; **19**:489–493.
61. Zach M, Beitzke A, Singer H, Hofler H, Schellman B. The syndrome of absent pulmonary valve and ventricular septal defects – anatomical features and embryological indications. *Basic Res Cardiol* 1979; **74**:54–68.
62. Hew CC, Daebritz SH, Zurakowski D, del Nido PJ, Mayer JE, Jonas RA. Valved homograft replacement of aneurysmal pulmonary arteries for severely symptomatic absent pulmonary valve syndrome. *Ann Thorac Surg* 2002; **73**:1778–1785.
63. Stellin G, Jonas RA, Goh TH, Brawn WJ, Venables AW, Mee RBB. Surgical treatment of absent pulmonary valve syndrome in infants: Relief of bronchial obstruction. *Ann Thorac Surg* 1983; **36**:468–475.
64. Waldhausen JA, Friedman S, Nicodemus SH, Miller WW, Rashkind W, Johnson J. Absence of the pulmonary valve in patients with tetralogy of Fallot. Surgical management. *J Thorac Cardiovasc Surg* 1969; **57**:669–674.
65. Osmon MZ, Meng CCL, Girdany BR. Congenital absence of the pulmonary valve: report of eight cases with review of the literature. *Am J Roentgenol* 1969; **106**:58–69.
66. Bove EL, Shaher RM, Alley R, McKneally M. Tetralogy of Fallot with absent pulmonary valve and aneurysm of the pulmonary artery: report of two cases presenting as obstructive lung disease. *J Pediatr* 1972; **81**:339.
67. Litwin SB, Rosenthal A, Fellows K. Surgical management of young infants with tetralogy of Fallot, absence of the pulmonary valve and respiratory distress. *J Thorac Cardiovasc Surg* 1973; **65**:552–558.
68. Layton CA, McDonald A, McDonald L, Towers M, Weaver J, Yacoub M. The syndrome of absent pulmonary valve. Total correction with aortic valvular homografts. *J Thorac Cardiovasc Surg* 1972; **63**:800–808.
69. Snir E, de Leval MR, Elliott MJ, Stark J. Current surgical technique to repair Fallot's tetralogy with absent pulmonary valve syndrome. *Ann Thorac Surg* 1991; **51**:979–982.
70. Danilowicz D, Presti S, Colvin SB, Doyle EF. Repair in infancy of tetralogy of Fallot with absence of leaflets of the pulmonary valve (absent pulmonary valve syndrome) using a valved pulmonary artery homograft. *Cardiol Young* 1992; **2**:25–29.
71. Hraska V, Kantorova A, Kunovsky P, Haviar D. Intermediate results with correction of tetralogy of Fallot with absent pulmonary v alve using a new approach. *Eur J Cardiothorac Surg* 2002; **21**:711–714.
72. Godart F, Houyel L, Lacour-Gayet F et al. Absent pulmonary valve syndrome: surgical treatment and considerations. *Ann Thorac Surg* 1996; **62**:136–142.

17

Valve surgery

INTRODUCTION

In Chapter 3 the many options available for valve replacement are described. Chapter 3 also emphasizes that all presently available valve replacement options have important disadvantages. Most importantly all replacement options including the Ross procedure do not incorporate growth potential. For this reason emphasis has shifted to developing valve repair options for essentially all congenital valve anomalies. Although repair does not create a perfect valve it does allow the child to live a good quality life free of the risk of thromboembolism and free of the need to take anticoagulant medication. Eventually valve replacement will be required for the majority of children. However, there is hope that with development of tissue engineered valves,[1] improved options will be available in the future.

AORTIC VALVE DISEASE

The topic of aortic valve stenosis is covered in Chapter 18. The management of pure congenital aortic valve stenosis at any age is balloon dilation.

AORTIC VALVE REGURGITATION

Aortic valve regurgitation is often secondary to one of a number of congenital cardiac problems. Pure primary congenital aortic regurgitation (AR) where the valve itself is congenitally structurally abnormal is a relatively rare entity, certainly much less common than congenital aortic valve stenosis.

Anatomy

PRIMARY CONGENITAL AORTIC VALVE REGURGITATION

Congenital aortic valve regurgitation is often the result of incomplete formation of a bicuspid valve.[2,3] The right coronary leaflet is frequently affected. It may be very hypoplastic and incompletely fused with either the non or left leaflet. The resulting fused leaflet may have poor commissural support and tend to prolapse. With time the aortic annulus enlarges secondary to the large volume load passing through the valve. This results in even more regurgitation and sets up a deteriorating spiral. The regurgitant jet also damages the free edges of the valve leaflets which become thickened and rolled. A quadricuspid aortic valve may be importantly incompetent.[4]

AORTIC REGURGITATION FOLLOWING BALLOON DILATION

In an early series of balloon dilations of the aortic valve at Children's Hospital Boston, aortic regurgitation was seen in approximately 13% of patients immediately following balloon dilation, increasing to 38% during follow-up.[5] The most common anatomical problem that has been seen is detachment of the right coronary leaflet at the anterior commissure (Figure 17.1). This probably results from the tendency of the balloon to straighten out relative to the posterior curve of the arch of the aorta as the balloon is inflated. In an analysis of 21 valves by Bacha et al[5] the following problems were seen: the

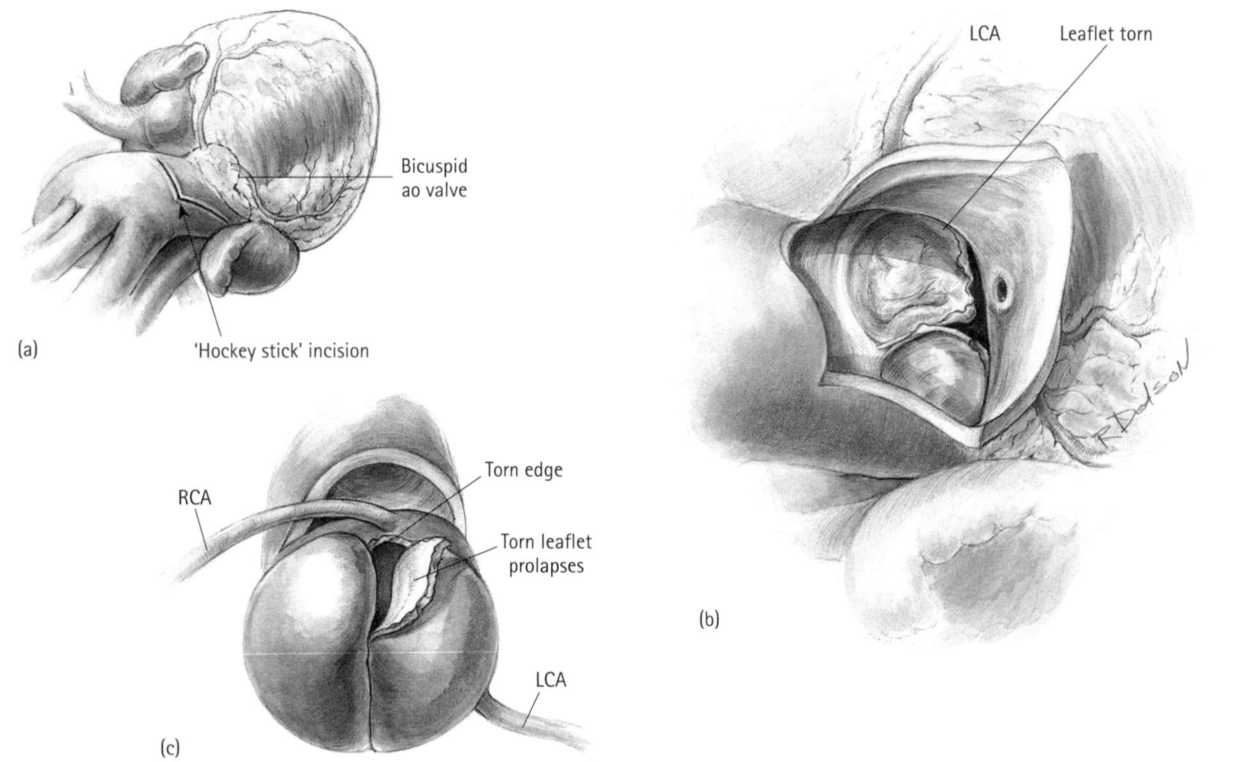

Figure 17.1 *Aortic valve regurgitation following balloon dilation. (a) The aortic valve is approached through a traditional reverse hockey stick incision extending into the noncoronary sinus. The stenotic aortic valve is frequently bicuspid. (b) Balloon dilation often results in detachment of the anterior commissure, particularly the anterior part of the right coronary leaflet. (c) View from below of the detached and prolapsing right coronary leaflet following balloon dilation of the stenotic bicuspid aortic valve.*

valve was bicuspid in 19 patients, tricuspid in one and unicuspid in one. Fusion of left coronary cusp (LCC) and right coronary cusp (RCC) was predominant in 15 (71%) patients, of the RCC-noncoronary cusp (NCC) in four, and fusion of both LCC-RCC and RCC-NCC in one. Predominant factors contributing to AR were a combination of anterior commissural avulsion in 10, cusp dehiscence with retraction (presumably secondary to longstanding balloon dilation-induced tear) in nine, simple cusp tear in five (anterior in four, posterior in one), central incompetence in two (from calcified cusps in one, from sinus of Valsalva dilation in one), perforated cusp in one, and free cuspal edge adhesion to aortic wall in one patient. The RCC was the most frequently involved cusp (20/21 patients).

AORTIC REGURGITATION ASSOCIATED WITH VSD

A subpulmonary VSD lies immediately below the belly of the right coronary cusp of the aortic valve. A longstanding jet can result in prolapse of this valve leaflet secondary to the Venturi effect of the jet (Figure 17.2).[6] Valve leaflet prolapse is less likely with a membranous VSD which lies below the right/non commissure where the valve is better supported. However, because membranous VSDs are much more common than subpulmonary VSDs, it is more common in Western populations to find aortic regurgitation associated with a membranous VSD. Prolapse is particularly likely in the setting of a membranous VSD if the valve is bicuspid.[7]

AORTIC REGURGITATION SECONDARY TO SUBAORTIC STENOSIS

A subaortic membrane or tunnel subaortic stenosis sets up turbulence that eventually damages the aortic valve and causes aortic regurgitation. The valve leaflets may adhere to the membrane which contracts and draws the affected leaflet into the left ventricular outflow tract. The leaflets may become thickened and rolled along their free edges resulting in poor coaptation.[8]

AORTIC REGURGITATION ASSOCIATED WITH AORTIC ROOT DILATION

Connective tissue disorders such as Marfan's syndrome and Ehlers-Danlos syndrome are associated with aortic root dilation which can result in aortic valve regurgitation if sufficiently severe.[9] The tops of the commissural posts are distracted resulting in central regurgitation (Figure 17.3). The valve leaflets themselves may be affected by the disease process resulting in stretching and prolapse. Occasionally aortic root dilation is seen late after tetralogy repair (particularly if this has been delayed and performed at an older age in a child with pulmonary atresia).

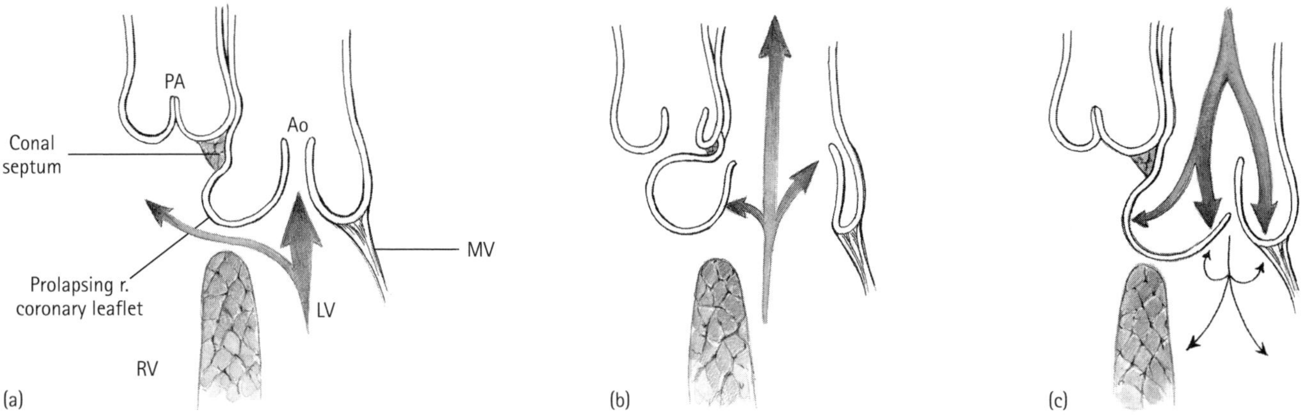

Figure 17.2 *Mechanism of aortic valve regurgitation associated with a ventricular septal defect. (a) The jet passing through a VSD can cause a Venturi effect which results in prolapse of the right coronary leaflet. This is more likely if the VSD is subpulmonary in location. (b) With time, systolic pressure directly exacerbates prolapse of the aortic valve leaflet. (c) The prolapsing right coronary leaflet may result in almost complete closure of the VSD. However, by this time aortic regurgitation is apparent.*

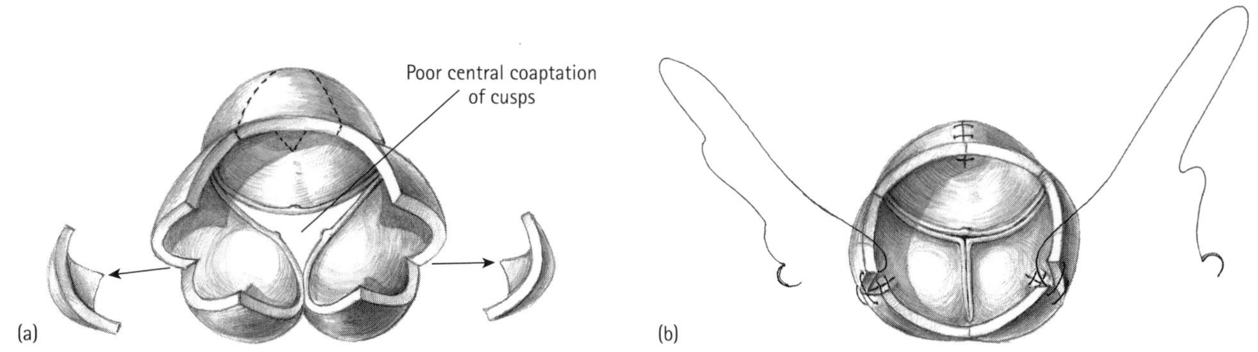

Figure 17.3 *(a) Dilation of the aortic root such as is seen in a connective tissue disorder like Marfan's syndrome results in central regurgitation because of distraction of the tops of the commissures of the aortic valve. (b) Wedge excision of the sinuses of Valsalva is helpful in reducing central regurgitation secondary to aortic root dilation.*

MISCELLANEOUS CAUSES OF AORTIC REGURGITATION

Aortic regurgitation is seen in association with a number of anomalies such as aorto left ventricular tunnel and sinus of Valsalva aneurysm and fistula (see Chapter 11). It also may occur secondary to injury or scarring of the aortic valve caused by bacterial endocarditis. Although the single semilunar valve in patients with truncus arteriosus is not strictly an aortic valve, it has the functional role of such.

Pathophysiology and clinical features

A detailed analysis of the pathophysiology of aortic valve regurgitation can be found in textbooks of acquired heart disease. The fundamental problem for the child is that the 'regurgitant fraction' of blood refluxes back through the valve into the left ventricle and must be re-ejected with the next cycle. Thus the ventricle is volume-loaded and must dilate to cope with this increased work-load. The wall thickness of the left ventricle must increase to maintain a stable wall stress. The aortic diastolic pressure will be low and this reduces coronary perfusion. However, flow in many vascular beds will be affected. With severe regurgitation it is possible to see retrograde flow in the descending aorta which compromises mesenteric flow in particular which can be dangerous for example in the neonate with truncus and associated truncal regurgitation. The left ventricular end diastolic pressure is increased and transmits this pressure back to the pulmonary circulation perhaps elevating pulmonary artery and right ventricular pressure.

Mild or moderate aortic regurgitation is tolerated very well for many years by children as it is by adults. Severe regurgitation will result in the usual signs of congestive heart failure, particularly failure to thrive. Pulses are water hammer like to palpation. The diastolic blood pressure may be very low or unobtainable.

Diagnostic studies

The chest X-ray demonstrates cardiomegaly. The ECG shows predominant left ventricular forces reflecting the compensatory hypertrophy. Echocardiography is essential in both grading the severity as well as demonstrating the mechanism of regurgitation. Three dimensional echo reconstruction of the valve can be very helpful in planning surgical reconstruction.[10]

Medical and interventional therapy

There are no interventional catheter techniques that are useful for aortic valve regurgitation. Medical therapy is standard drug treatment of congestive heart failure.

Indications for surgery

The presence of symptoms that are not controlled by medical therapy is certainly an indication to move ahead with surgery. Serial echocardiography is very helpful in defining the ventricular volume, wall thickness and contractility of the left ventricle. A decline in preload independent contractility indices or dilation beyond two standard deviations are reasonable indications to proceed.[11]

It is important to understand that the goal in treating aortic regurgitation in the young child is to avoid valve replacement. Thus the traditional indications for aortic valve replacement are not applicable in the pediatric setting. Furthermore experience with valve repair surgery suggests that earlier surgery is associated with a higher probability of a successful result. Longstanding regurgitation is associated with damage to the free edges of aortic valve leaflets as well as aortic annular dilation. Both these factors increase the difficulty of reconstruction. If a valve appears particularly suitable for repair, e.g. a circumscribed perforation secondary to healed endocarditis then the indications to proceed should be quite a bit less stringent relative to the valve that appears quite unsuitable for repair and which may require replacement.

Surgical management

TECHNICAL CONSIDERATIONS

The operation is performed on cardiopulmonary bypass with moderate systemic hypothermia. Cooling should be slower than usual to minimize the risk of early ventricular fibrillation. A pericardial patch is harvested and fixed in 0.6% glutaraldehyde for 20–30 minutes. The aortic cross clamp is applied before the heart is at risk of distention because of bradycardia and reduced contractility. Often it is helpful to infuse part of the first dose of cardioplegia while gently massaging the left ventricle to prevent distention and before making the aortotomy or placing the vent. A left ventricular vent is placed through the right superior pulmonary vein. An aortotomy is made transversely and is extended towards the noncoronary sinus of Valsalva. The remainder of the first dose of cardioplegia is infused selectively into both coronary ostia.

A decision to perform valve reconstruction is at the surgeon's discretion, and is a judgment based on preoperative echocardiography, intraoperative TEE and direct inspection of the valve. Anatomic elements necessary for valve repair include a sufficient annular diameter to not require left ventricular outflow tract enlargement, mobile cusps or cusps that can be made mobile by resection or shaving of excess fibrous tissue, as well as an ability to achieve coaptation without inducing stenosis.

A variety of valvuloplasty techniques are available and have been described by us[5] and others.[12–16] The valve is studied using fine forceps to approximate the length, depth and mobility of the cusps. The diameter of the central opening of the valve as well as the location and mobility of the commissures and raphes is noted.

Primary repair

Excess fibrous tissue, which has a tendency to build up around raphes (rudimentary fused commissures), is aggressively removed (so-called 'shaving'), giving the cusp more mobility. Fused commissures with adequate suspension to the aortic wall are opened with a scalpel. Simple tears involving otherwise competent cusps are repaired primarily, usually with a 5/0 Prolene running suture. If the native cusps are deemed adequate, tears involving the anterior commissure (right coronary (RCC)-noncoronary cusp (NCC) commissure) in bicuspid valves are repaired by resuspending the commissure with sutures passed through the aortic wall. Otherwise, the commissure is resected and reconstructed (see below). Prolapsed but otherwise competent and pliable cusps are shortened by resuspension of the cusps to the commissures with pledget-supported sutures. In cases of central cusp incompetence with dilation of the sinuses of Valsalva, a sinus of Valsalva reduction plasty is performed to reduce commissural splaying. This is done by resecting a wedge of noncoronary sinus, followed by primary closure of the aortotomy (Figure 17.3b).

Treated autologous pericardial patch repair

Perforated cusps are repaired with a pericardial patch sutured into the perforation. Deficient cusps, usually resulting from a longstanding balloon-induced tear with retraction of the free cusp edge (see Figure 17.1), are augmented by suturing a half-moon-shaped autologous pericardial patch to the free edge of the retracted cusp (Figure 17.4). The patch is deliberately tailored so that it overlaps the opposite free cusp edge by a few millimeters. However, if the opposite cusp is too far or deficient as well, the patch is not extended; rather, the opposite cusp edges are supplemented with strips of fixed pericardium. The free edge of the patch should be slightly longer and redundant so that most patches are further anchored to at least one commissure (usually anteriorly), thereby resuspending the leaflet. If the native cusp is very stiff or calcified, the cusp is partially or completely resected and reconstructed with a pericardial patch. Generally however, as much as possible of the native valve is left intact because large patches in young children have a risk of accelerated calcification. If the two cusps are deficient at a commissure,

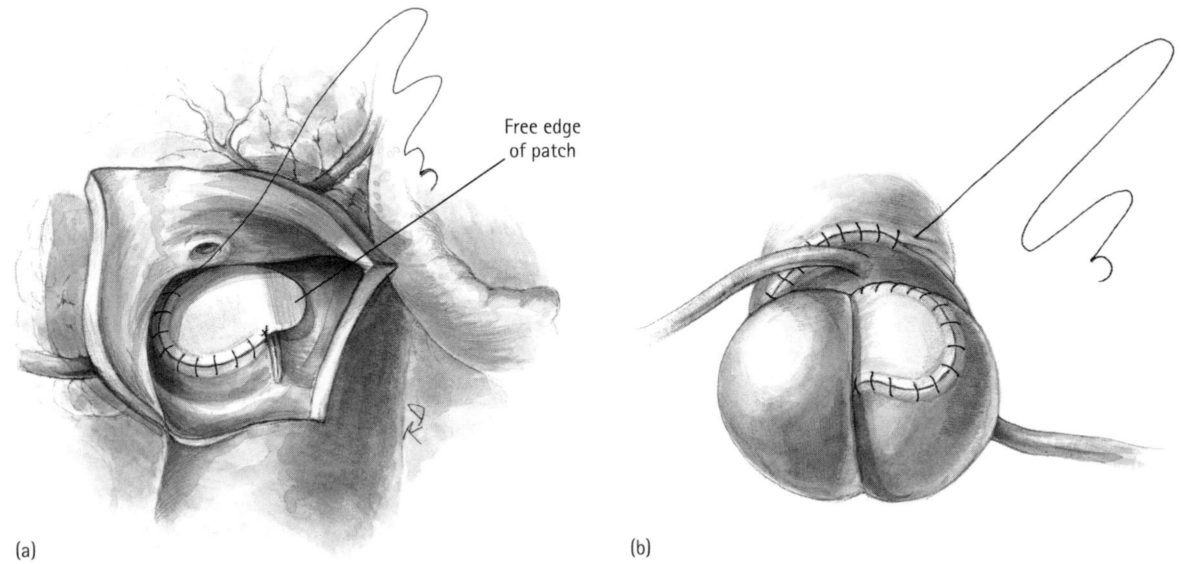

Figure 17.4 *Autologous pericardial patch repair of the regurgitant aortic valve. (a) A small autologous pericardial patch, lightly tanned with glutaraldehyde, is used to resuspend the prolapsing right coronary leaflet, which has been detached at the anterior commissure by balloon dilation. (b) View from below of anterior repair of the right coronary leaflet with an autologous pericardial patch.*

two pericardial patches are used to augment the deficient cusps and reconstruct the commissure.

Results of surgery

Bacha[5] reported the results of 21 patients who underwent aortic valve reconstruction at Children's Hospital Boston between 1988 and 1999. There were no early or late deaths. Mean hospital stay was 5 ± 2 days. Mean follow-up was 31 ± 27 months. A pericardial effusion necessitating percutaneous drainage occurred in one. In another, severe recurrent AR occurred prior to discharge following pericardial patch reconstruction with anterior commissural reconstruction of a partially resected cusp. At reoperation, a patch suture line had dehisced and was repaired with marked reduction in aortic regurgitation. One patient underwent a repeat balloon dilation for recurrent aortic stenosis 3.5 years after her valvuloplasty. Freedom from reoperation (aortic valve replacement or re-repair) for late failure was 100%, while freedom from overall aortic valve reintervention was estimated to be 80% at three years (70% confidence interval = 68–92%). No variables including type of repair were found to be significantly associated with aortic valve reintervention in the Cox multivariate model. All patients were asymptomatic at last follow-up.

ECHOCARDIOGRAPHIC FOLLOW-UP

Intraoperative transesophageal echocardiography (TEE) postrepair revealed trace AR in 12 patients, mild AR in eight, and moderate AR in one. The median pull-back gradient, measured intraoperatively in eight patients, was 25 mmHg (range 10–45). All patients had echocardiographic assessment prior to discharge with no significant discrepancies with the intraoperative TEE findings.

At further follow-up, echocardiograms continued to reveal a significant reduction in AR grade (median AR grade = mild, $p < 0.001$). Mean left ventricular end diastolic diameter (LVEDD)–z scores were also significantly reduced (3.44 ± 1.97 (preoperative) versus 1.54 ± 2.27 (immediate follow-up), $p = 0.003$; 3.44 ± 1.97 (preoperative) versus 1.00 ± 1.73 (late follow-up), $p < 0.001$), as were proximal aortic regurgitation jet diameter to aortic annulus diameter ratios (0.53 ± 0.18 (preoperative) versus 0.17 ± 0.13 (immediate follow-up), $p < 0.001$; 0.53 ± 0.18 (preoperative) versus 0.28 ± 0.17 (late follow-up), $p < 0.001$). For both LVEDD–z scores and AR jet diameter to aortic annulus diameter ratios, immediate follow-up values were not significantly different from late follow-up values ($p = 0.84$ and $p = 0.09$, respectively). The freedom from increased AR was 100% at two years and 75% at three years. Preoperative Doppler maximal instantaneous gradient and at last follow-up did not change (43 ± 26 versus 43 ± 21 mmHg, $p = 0.95$). None of the variables listed above was significantly associated with increased AR in the Cox model ($p > 0.5$ for each).

Subsequent to the close of this series several of these patients have required reoperation most commonly because of progressive stenosis. At surgery the autologous pericardial patch was found to have calcified, particularly when relatively large patches were employed. Others have also reported satisfactory intermediate term results with aortic valve repair.[12–16] On the other hand, results of alternative procedures such as the Ross operation in this setting have been disappointing.[17]

MITRAL VALVE DISEASE

MITRAL VALVE STENOSIS

Isolated congenital mitral valve stenosis is a very rare entity. Most commonly mitral valve stenosis is associated with mitral valve hypoplasia and is part of Shone's syndrome, i.e. it is associated with left ventricular underdevelopment, left ventricular outflow tract obstruction, aortic valve stenosis as well as arch hypoplasia and coarctation.[18]

Anatomy

Structural problems of the mitral valve causing stenosis can occur at the level of the papillary muscles, at the level of the chords, as a result of leaflet abnormalities including commissural fusion or in the immediate supravalvar region. A parachute mitral valve is an entity in which there is usually a single papillary muscle into which all chords insert[19] (Figure 17.5). If the chords are thickened and fused as they often are in the setting of a single papillary muscle there will be obstruction to the entry of blood into the ventricle through the interchordal spaces. A supravalvar mitral web is a fibrous ring lying on the atrial surface of the mitral leaflets which usually restricts leaflet motion and may in itself be obstructive (Figure 17.6). Congenitally stenotic mitral valves usually display elements of obstruction at more than one level. The so-called 'mitral arcade' has fused commissures, thickened and immobile leaflets and shortened and thickened chords. The papillary muscles may give the appearance of inserting directly into the valve leaflets.[20] It is exceedingly rare that the patient with congenital mitral stenosis has relatively well developed commissures with fusion that can be easily broken down, either by a balloon or surgically, analogous to the situation with aortic or pulmonary valve stenosis. When this form of mitral stenosis is seen it is more likely to be rheumatic mitral stenosis.

The mitral valve can be structurally quite normal and yet functionally stenotic because of underdevelopment. In fact this is seen far more commonly than isolated structural mitral stenosis because this is usually the situation in hypoplastic left heart syndrome. If the z score of the mitral valve area is less than 2.5–3.0 it is highly unlikely that it will be a functionally useful valve even though it may be structurally perfect in every way other than its size.

Pathophysiology and clinical features

The pathophysiology of mitral stenosis is covered in detail in textbooks of acquired heart disease. One of the most notable findings in children is elevation of the pulmonary artery pressure and right ventricular pressure. This will be associated with failure to thrive. If the neonate has very severe stenosis it may not be possible for the left heart to support the systemic circulation alone and the child will be prostaglandin dependent. This is almost always in the setting of Shone's syndrome or hypoplastic left heart syndrome and is rarely seen with isolated structural mitral stenosis. The latter however will often become importantly symptomatic during the first year of life.

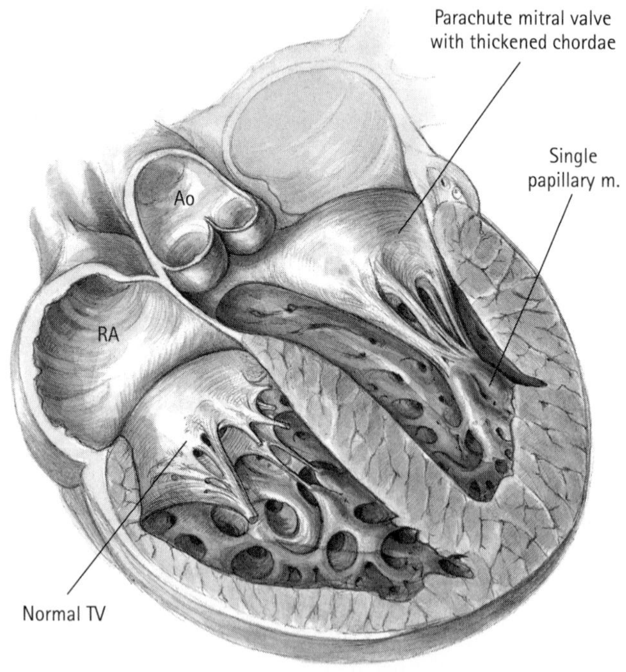

Figure 17.5 *The stenotic parachute mitral valve has thickened shortened chordae which insert into a single papillary muscle.*

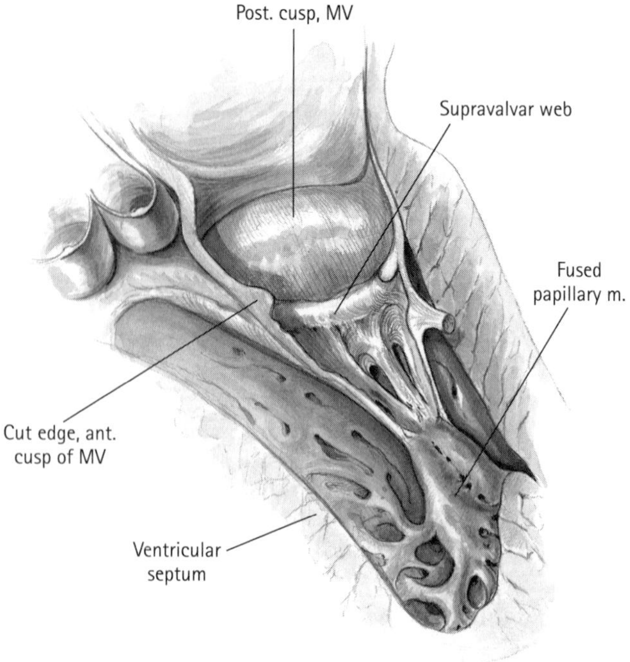

Figure 17.6 *A supravalvar mitral web is a fibrous ring lying on the atrial surface of the mitral leaflets, which usually restricts leaflet motion and may in itself be obstructive.*

The symptoms of mitral stenosis in the infant include all the usual features of congestive heart failure, particularly failure to thrive. Pulmonary congestion will mean that the child is prone to respiratory infections, such as RSV which have a real risk of being lethal. The child will be tachypneic and will feed poorly with sweating and irritability.

Diagnostic studies

The plain chest X-ray demonstrates pulmonary congestion and enlargement of the pulmonary arteries. The left ventricular size is not increased though the right ventricle may be prominent on the lateral film. The ECG demonstrates prominent right heart forces.

Echocardiography is diagnostic. The echo should define structural abnormalities at the valvar, subvalvar and supravalvar levels. Measurements of the diameter in two planes is important and calculation of the mitral valve area. These must be compared to normal dimensions for the child's size allowing calculation of z scores. A Doppler gradient should be estimated: a mean gradient of less than 4 or 5 mm can be considered to result from mild stenosis, 6–12 mm is likely to be moderate stenosis; whereas greater than 13 mm is severe. As with valve gradients in any situation however it is important to remember that the gradient is dependent on the flow through the valve which can be exaggerated by left to right flow through an associated VSD or reduced by left to right flow at atrial level.

A Doppler estimate of right ventricular pressure by interrogating any tricuspid regurgitant jet is helpful in confirming the degree of mitral stenosis. Severe stenosis is almost always associated with systemic pressure in the right heart. There will be corresponding right ventricular hypertrophy.

Cardiac catheterization is not particularly helpful in assessing mitral stenosis. Occasionally it is useful when echo is unable to obtain a reliable Doppler gradient or measurement of right sided pressure. Measurement of the pulmonary capillary wedge pressure to left ventricular end diastolic pressure gives a useful estimate of the degree of stenosis. However, ideally left atrial pressure should be measured directly.

Medical and interventional therapy

Mild and moderate mitral stenosis can be managed with the usual pharmacologic methods for treating congestive heart failure. However, if the child is not gaining weight and is suffering from frequent respiratory infections, consideration should be given to attempting balloon dilation of the valve.[21]

Before attempting dilation of the mitral valve a very careful assessment of the valve should be made jointly by the surgeon, interventional cardiologist and echocardiographer. The surgeon must be involved from the start because there is a much higher risk with this entity than with others that relatively urgent surgical intervention may be necessary if the dilation is unsuccessful. Over the longer term it is highly unlikely that surgery will be avoided if the child has come to the point of being considered for dilation.

Balloon dilation should not be attempted if the valve is parachute-like or if the valve leaflets are poorly defined with very thickened and shortened chords. Although the balloon may be able to reduce the degree of stenosis, almost certainly this will be at the price of important regurgitation. A controlled degree of regurgitation may be useful in encouraging growth of the hypoplastic annulus but our sense has been that this is much more difficult to achieve with the stenotic mitral valve in contrast to the stenotic aortic valve.

Indications for surgery

The most likely indication for surgery is the child who has been considered for balloon dilation but has been judged unsuitable because of anatomical considerations. The probability of achieving a successful surgical valvotomy is small and can be fairly accurately predicted by the structural appearance of the valve by echocardiography. However, if the valve appears suitable for surgical valvotomy it will also be suitable for balloon dilation which is our first preference.

Another likely indication for surgical management of the stenotic mitral valve is either a failed balloon dilation or balloon dilation complicated by the development of severe regurgitation.

Surgical management

TECHNICAL CONSIDERATIONS

Mitral valve repair

Resection of a supravalvar mitral ring or web is one of the most effective surgical interventions that can be performed for mitral stenosis. The web usually has the appearance and feel of being a secondary problem in much the same way that a subaortic membrane is usually not present at birth but develops secondary to other abnormalities of the outflow tract. Usually it is possible to peel the web away from the atrial surface of the mitral valve leaflets. This frees up the leaflets which are usually restricted in their motion by the web. In severe cases the web has a small central orifice which in itself is obstructive.

Commissurotomy is usually not possible other than over the most minimal distance of a millimeter or two. Great care must be taken to understand the chordal support anatomy so that a flail leaflet segment is not created.

Thickened and fused chords can be split apart and thinned by excision of interchordal fibrous tissue. When the papillary muscles insert directly into the leaflets it may be possible to increase the effective orifice area slightly by splitting the papillary muscles towards their base. Unfortunately the long-term results of splitting chords and papillary muscles have been disappointing so undue optimism should not

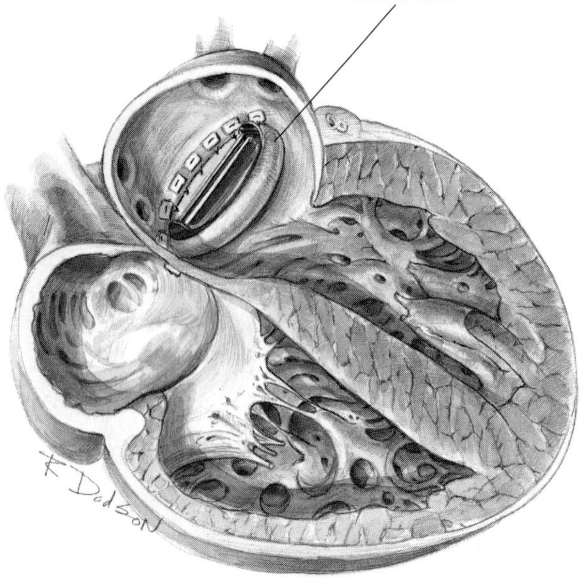

Figure 17.7 *Supra-annular mitral valve replacement is a useful technique in the child with a small mitral annulus which will not accommodate the smallest prosthesis. The valve is placed entirely within the left atrium between the inferior pulmonary veins and the true annulus.*

be felt and expressed to the family in spite of an encouraging intraoperative result as determined by TEE.[22]

Mitral valve replacement

Approach is by a median sternotomy. Continuous cardiopulmonary bypass is used with bicaval cannulation with right angle venous cannulas other than for neonates where circulatory arrest may be preferred. The mitral valve is exposed through a vertical incision in the atrial septum. In general, in small patients it is necessary to totally excise the entire mitral valve, including the subvalvar apparatus. It is important not to force too large a prosthesis into the true annulus, as this almost certainly contributes to a high incidence of complete heart block. If the annulus is smaller than the smallest prosthesis available, which is often the case in the infant with pure congenital mitral stenosis, the prosthesis should be inserted in a true supra-annular position.

Supra-annular mitral valve replacement

Standard everting, horizontal, pledgetted mattress sutures are used for supra-annular mitral valve placement (Figure 17.7). Posteriorly the sutures are placed as close as possible to the inferior right and left pulmonary veins, between the veins and the true annulus, without compromising these veins. Anteriorly sutures are passed through the atrial septum with the pledgets lying on the right atrial aspect of the septum. The valve lies above the level of the coronary sinus, which should decrease the risk of complete heart block.

The valve should be carefully checked for complete freedom of movement of the disk and if necessary (and if the valve design allows), the valve is rotated to a point where the greatest clearance from adjacent tissue is achieved. It is usually necessary to close the atrial septum with a patch of pericardium or polytetrafluoroethylene (PTFE). Before completion of the suture line on the atrial septal patch, the left heart is filled with saline, and air is vented through the cardioplegic infusion site in the ascending aorta.

Enlargement of the mitral annulus with preservation of the aortic valve

The mitral valve annulus can be enlarged by an incision through the left ventricular outflow tract in order to allow placement of a larger prosthesis at annular level. This is usually combined with enlargement of the aortic annulus with the same patch. However, on occasion we have performed a procedure where the aortic annulus is split between the right and noncoronary leaflets[23] (Figure 17.8a). A triangular patch is placed to enlarge the mitral annulus (Figure 17.8b). The aortic valve commissure is reconstructed at the apex of the patch usually with pericardial leaflet extension of the right and noncoronary leaflets to improve aortic valve competence.

Conduits from the left atrium to the left ventricle

One other option that has been reported for the difficult situation of congenital mitral stenosis in which hypoplasia of both the valve annulus and the left atrium does not permit an orthotopic valve replacement is the placement of a conduit from the left atrium to the left ventricle. In 1980 Laks and coworkers[24] described placement of a 12-mm porcine-valved Dacron conduit from the left atrium to the apex of the left ventricle in an eight week old male. Although the child was discharged from the hospital, he died eight months postoperatively. Corno and associates[25] described a similar operation in a three year old. We have successfully performed the same procedure in an 11 month old child with mitral stenosis and a hypoplastic left ventricle.[26] Interestingly, an allograft aortic conduit was used. Postoperatively the child remained ventilator dependent and, at catheterization, was found to have what was essentially a ventricular aneurysm because of systolic dilatation of the allograft. The child was returned to the operating room, where the allograft was wrapped with Dacron. The child subsequently did well. Nevertheless, in view of the well-recognized long-term problems with conduits, as well as the disadvantage of an apical left ventricular incision, this option should rarely, if ever, be used. Supra-annular valve replacement should be applicable in almost all cases in which this procedure might otherwise be contemplated.

Results of surgery

BALLOON ANGIOPLASTY OF CONGENITAL MITRAL STENOSIS

In 1990 Spevak et al[27] described the results of balloon angioplasty at Children's Hospital Boston in nine children with congenital mitral stenosis. In seven of the nine patients effective reduction in mitral gradient was achieved initially. Mean valve area increased from 1.1 to 1.8 cm/m^2. Poor gradient

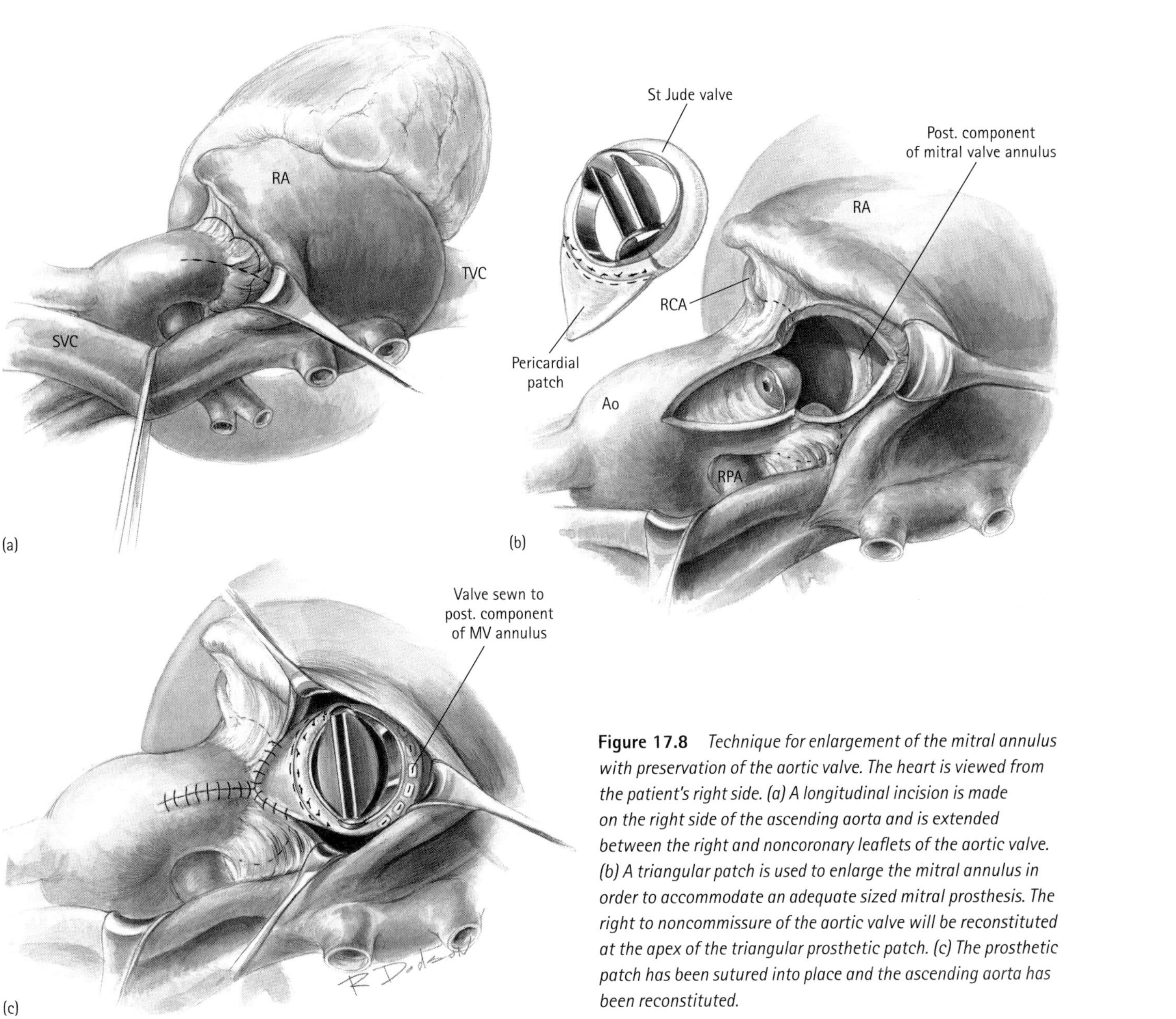

Figure 17.8 *Technique for enlargement of the mitral annulus with preservation of the aortic valve. The heart is viewed from the patient's right side. (a) A longitudinal incision is made on the right side of the ascending aorta and is extended between the right and noncoronary leaflets of the aortic valve. (b) A triangular patch is used to enlarge the mitral annulus in order to accommodate an adequate sized mitral prosthesis. The right to noncommissure of the aortic valve will be reconstituted at the apex of the triangular prosthetic patch. (c) The prosthetic patch has been sutured into place and the ascending aorta has been reconstituted.*

relief was seen in valves with unbalanced chordal attachments, with restriction to the valve apparatus as in mitral arcade and where the obstruction was not purely valvar as with the supravalvar mitral ring. No strokes, infection or deaths were caused by the procedure. The authors suggest balloon angioplasty should be considered for congenital mitral stenosis in younger patients and in patients in whom mitral valve replacement would be problematic.

SURGERY FOR CONGENITAL MITRAL STENOSIS

In 1987 Coles et al[28] from Toronto Canada described the surgical experience with 24 patients with predominant congenital mitral stenosis as well as 22 patients with congenital mitral incompetence other than complete AV canal. Most patients with mitral stenosis had abnormalities of all valve components. Virtual absence of chordal development was common. A supramitral ring with Shones complex was present in five patients, a parachute mitral valve in two, hypoplastic mitral annulus in three and rheumatic lesions in three. Overall the operative mortality was 19%. Actuarial freedom from death and reoperation was 44% at eight years.

In 1995 Uva et al[29] from Paris France described the results of surgery for 10 patients with congenital mitral stenosis and 10 with congenital regurgitation. Mean age at surgery was seven months. Four of the 10 patients with mitral stenosis had a parachute mitral valve, two had a hammock mitral valve and one had a supramitral ring. The operative mortality was zero. However, six early reoperations were required in five patients, five of whom required a mitral valve replacement. Actuarial freedom from reoperation was 58% at seven years.

In 1990 Kadoba et al[30] described the results of mitral valve replacement in the first year of life for 25 patients with either mitral stenosis or mitral regurgitation at Children's Hospital Boston. Five patients had congenital mitral stenosis, two had mitral arcade, two had supravalvar mitral stenosis and one had a parachute mitral valve. The actuarial survival at one year was 52% in this series that dated back to 1973. The report emphasizes the disadvantages of mitral valve replacement in the small infant. Supra-annular mitral valve replacement is often necessary in small babies who cannot avoid replacement. In this series four patients had the valve placed totally within the left atrium with no deaths. However, subsequent follow-up has suggested that the hemodynamic result with supra-annular mitral valve replacement is suboptimal.[31]

In 2000 Serraf et al[32] described the results of mitral valve surgery for 13 patients with isolated congenital mitral stenosis. Although there were no deaths in this group overall freedom from reoperation was 71% at 15 years and freedom from mitral valve replacement was 69%.

MITRAL VALVE REGURGITATION

Mitral valve regurgitation is very much more common than mitral valve stenosis. It is most commonly found in association with atrioventricular canal (septal) defects where it may be either a preoperative or postoperative problem.[30]

Anatomy

Mitral regurgitation associated with atrioventricular canal defects usually originates at one of two sites. The 'cleft' of the anterior leaflet is present naturally in the child with a partial atrioventricular canal while, in the child with a complete canal, a cleft is created as part of the repair. The cleft is the most common site for regurgitation.

Central regurgitation occurs when the valve annulus has dilated to the point where there is poor central apposition of the mural and anterior leaflets. Although the statement is often heard that a child has regurgitation because of 'inadequate leaflet tissue', we believe that a more common problem is that repair has been delayed too long allowing ventricular dilation secondary to the volume load of the left to right shunt. Once regurgitation of any cause is present it is likely to worsen over time because the regurgitation per se causes annular dilation resulting in worsening central regurgitation. Furthermore there are likely to be secondary changes in the valve leaflets such as thickening and rolling of the free edges which will also exacerbate regurgitation.

Mitral regurgitation can be a result of structural abnormalities of the valve that are similar to those causing mitral stenosis. Leaflets may be dysplastic and retracted, there may be thick and short chords and the papillary muscles may be abnormal. Other structural abnormalities include isolated cleft of the anterior leaflet, leaflet prolapse secondary to chordal elongation or rupture (usually in the setting of a connective tissue disorder such as Marfan's syndrome) or leaflet perforation or other injury by bacterial endocarditis.[33]

Pathophysiology and clinical features

Like mitral stenosis, mitral regurgitation increases left atrial pressure and therefore pulmonary artery pressure. However, mitral regurgitation imposes a volume load on the left ventricle in addition to imposing a pressure load on the right ventricle. The symptoms are the usual symptoms of congestive heart failure and are likely to be indistinguishable from the symptoms of mitral stenosis.

Diagnostic studies

The plain chest X-ray demonstrates the same features seen with mitral stenosis including an enlarged left atrium and prominence of the pulmonary vasculature. The distinguishing feature is that the left ventricle is also very enlarged. The ECG is likely to show increased left heart forces as well as the increased right heart forces resulting from pulmonary hypertension.

The echocardiogram is diagnostic. The degree of mitral regurgitation can be quantitated by assessment of the width of the jet at the level of the leaflets. It is important to do this in two planes as there may be a knife-thin jet coming through the cleft area. A central jet is more likely to be circular in shape.

As with mitral stenosis, the echocardiographer should analyse the mechanism of the regurgitation. Most commonly this will involve distinguishing regurgitation through the cleft versus central regurgitation.

Cardiac catheterization is not necessary or indeed useful in defining the degree or the mechanism of mitral regurgitation.

Medical and interventional therapy

Mitral regurgitation should be treated with the usual pharmacologic treatment for congestive heart failure. After-load reduction is particularly helpful in the setting of mitral regurgitation and should be maximized.

There are no interventional catheter methods that are useful in the management of mitral regurgitation.

Indications for surgery

The indications for mitral valve repair for mitral regurgitation should be quite a bit less stringent than those applied for mitral stenosis. This is because it is very likely that the valve can be significantly improved no matter what the cause of the regurgitation. On the other hand if surgery is delayed there will be secondary changes of the valve which will increase the difficulty of repair and reduce the probability that repair will be successful. It should be highly unlikely that valve replacement should be required at a first attempt to improve a regurgitant mitral valve surgically.

Surgical management

TECHNICAL CONSIDERATIONS

General setup

Mitral valve repair is most commonly performed in a reoperative setting beyond infancy and usually in a child who has previously undergone repair of complete AV canal. A TEE probe should be placed in all cases. Cardiopulmonary bypass is managed with bicaval cannulation, mild or moderate hypothermia and cardioplegia arrest. The valve is usually approached through the atrial septum.

Intraoperative valve assessment

The valve should be carefully studied by the surgeon and echocardiographer together before bypass using the TEE to confirm the preoperative assessment of the valve and to help plan the method of repair. Real-time three-dimensional echocardiography is a useful supplement to standard two-dimensional echocardiography.[10] When the valve has been exposed it should be tested by infusing cold cardioplegia into the left ventricle using a fine red rubber tube (the same as is used for tourniquets) attached to a 20 or 30 ml syringe. Care should be taken to avoid frothing as this can cause important left ventricular dysfunction postoperatively. Frothing will certainly occur if the cardioplegia is injected as a jet from a distance through the valve. This method should be avoided because the froth will enter the coronary arteries.

When the left ventricle has been distended with cardioplegia solution, the regurgitant jet should be carefully studied. Usually the predominant jet will be through the cleft though there may also be central regurgitation. The relative positions of the valve leaflets should be very carefully noted, particularly at the level of the cleft. The cleft must be very accurately approximated which can be achieved by very careful observation of how the subtle irregularities of the cleft margins fit together. Minor variations in the leaflet tissue can serve as landmarks to guide subsequent suturing of the cleft.

Cleft closure

In the reoperative setting the cleft margins are usually thickened and rolled and will hold sutures well. A continuous technique is probably the most secure method using running 6/0 or 5/0 Prolene. However, it can be more difficult to very accurately align the cleft margins as desired if a continuous suture is used. It may be preferable to use interrupted sutures which can be reinforced with fine pericardial pledgets if the valve leaflet tissue is fragile.

Annuloplasty for central regurgitation

If regurgitation through the center of the valve is noted after closure of the cleft it will be necessary to perform an annuloplasty. It is not appropriate to use annuloplasty rings in children because they will restrict growth potential. Therefore commissuroplasty sutures are placed at one or both commissures as originally described by Reed.[34] The lateral commissure is a safer location because it is further from the conduction bundle than the medial commissure. However, it is usually possible to determine that the central regurgitant jet is coming more towards one or other commissure and this should be the commissure preferred for the annuloplasty. Often commissuroplasty sutures will be required for both commissures. On occasion a third annuloplasty suture must be placed directly posteriorly to tighten the annulus further. It is important to remember that the circumflex coronary artery lies close to the annulus posteriorly and laterally.

Chordal shortening, chordal transfer

The various techniques popularized by Carpentier for rheumatic mitral valve disease and degenerative valve disease are rarely used for children with congenitally abnormal valves.

Repeat testing of the valve

Following each step of the repair it is a good idea to reassess the valve by repeat infusion of cardioplegia into the left ventricle. It should be possible to essentially eliminate any regurgitant jet with the low pressure testing that can be done in this way. The contraction of the annulus that occurs with ventricular systole should further tighten the valve and compensate for the higher pressure it will be exposed to when the heart is ejecting. The final test is the TEE assessment when the heart is ejecting off bypass. If there is a possibility that the valve can be significantly improved by further maneuvers such as an additional annuloplasty suture, then this is the best time to do it.

Mitral valve replacement for regurgitation

The technique for mitral valve replacement for regurgitation is the same as for stenosis. The important difference is that the annulus is very likely to be a generous size so that supra-annular positioning is unlikely to be necessary.

Results of surgery

In 1999 Yoshimura et al[35] described the results of surgery for 56 pediatric patients who underwent 36 mitral valve repairs and 30 mitral valve replacements. There were two hospital deaths and two late deaths in patients who underwent mitral valve repair. Reoperation was performed in four patients. Three of these four patients underwent mitral valve replacement because of residual mitral incompetence. There were no hospital deaths in the patients who underwent mitral valve replacement though there were two late deaths. Six patients had a total of 10 episodes of prosthetic valve thrombosis though in all cases thrombolytic therapy with urokinase was successful. The mean interval to re-replacement of the mitral valve was 78 months. Actuarial survival and freedom from cardiac events at 10 years after operation were 87% and 73% in children who underwent mitral valve repair and 90% and 67% for those who underwent replacement.

In 1999 Ohno et al[36] described the results of commissural plication annuloplasty in 49 patients managed at the Tokyo Women's Medical College. The cause of regurgitation was chordal anomalies in 69% of patients, annular dilation in 16% and leaflet anomalies in 14%. Of these patients, 88% had commissural plication annuloplasty, 11 had modified Devega procedures, five had cleft closure and three had plication of the anterior leaflet. Combined techniques were used in 19 of the 49 patients. There were no early or late deaths. The actuarial freedom from reoperation was 86% at 13 years. In 1988 Stellin et al[37] described the results of surgery for 30 patients with congenital mitral valve disease. Valve repair was possible in 87% of patients while the remainder required valve replacement. Three patients required late valve replacement but the remaining patients appear to have excellent mitral valve function on follow-up echocardiography. These authors like others emphasize the importance of attempting mitral valve repair whenever possible.

TRICUSPID VALVE DISEASE

TRICUSPID VALVE REGURGITATION

Ebstein's anomaly is by far the most important congenital cause of tricuspid valve regurgitation. Other causes are usually secondary to problems such as inaccurate placement of a VSD patch or pulmonary hypertension especially if accompanied by right ventricular volume overload and right ventricular dilation.

Ebstein's anomaly

Because Ebstein's anomaly is an exceedingly rare condition, few surgeons have the opportunity to deal with its complete anatomic spectrum. If a child with Ebstein's anomaly is seen by a cardiologist during the first year of life, he or she is usually seen within hours of birth and is both cyanotic and acidotic. On the other hand some individuals with Ebstein's anomaly do not present until adulthood with minor complaints of exercise intolerance.

Anatomy

Carpentier et al[38] described five anatomic characteristics that are relevant to the surgical management of this difficult condition (Figure 17.9).

- There is displacement of the septal and posterior leaflets of the tricuspid valve toward the apex of the right ventricle.
- Although the anterior leaflet is attached at the appropriate level of the tricuspid annulus, it is larger than normal and may have multiple chordal attachments to the ventricular wall.
- The segment of the right ventricle from the level of the true tricuspid annulus to the level of attachment of the septal and posterior leaflets is unusually thin and dysplastic and is described as 'atrialized.' The tricuspid annulus and the right atrium are extremely dilated.
- The cavity of the right ventricle beyond the atrialized portion is reduced in size, usually lacks an inlet chamber, and has a small trabecular component.
- The infundibulum is often obstructed by the redundant tissue of the anterior leaflet as well as by the chordal attachments of the anterior leaflet to the infundibulum.

Carpentier et al[38] described four grades of Ebstein's anomaly:

- type A: the volume of the true right ventricle is adequate
- type B: there is a large atrialized component of the right ventricle, but the anterior leaflet moves freely

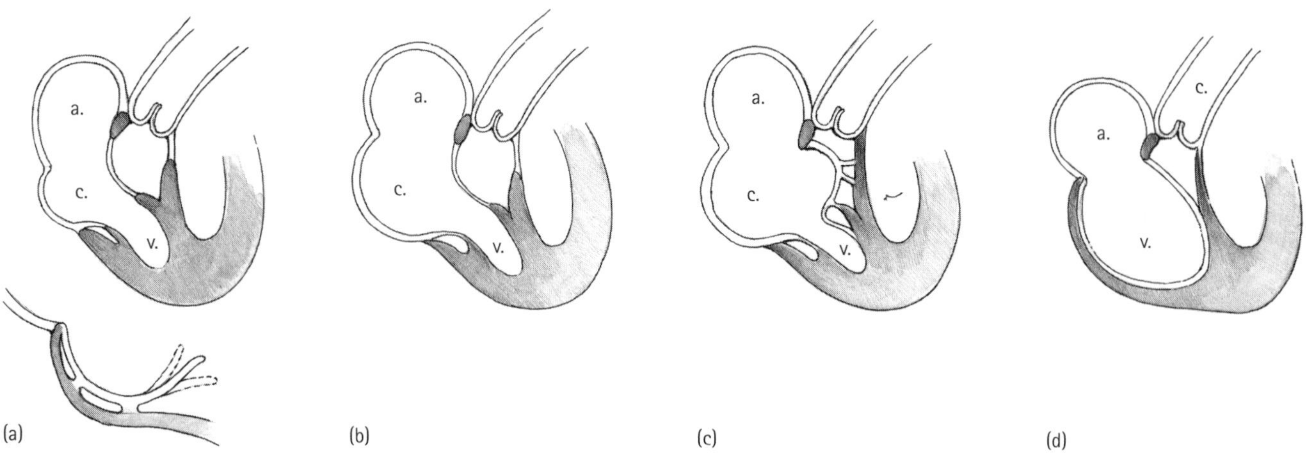

Figure 17.9 *Four anatomic types of Ebstein's anomaly. (a) Small, contractile atrialized chamber with mobile anterior leaflet, inset. (b) Large, noncontractile atrialized chamber with a mobile anterior leaflet. (c) Restricted motion of the anterior leaflet. (d) 'Tricuspid sac' leaflet tissue forms a continuous sac adherent to the dilated right ventricle.*

- type C: the anterior leaflet is severely restricted in its movement and may cause significant obstruction of the right ventricular outflow tract
- type D: there is almost complete atrialization of the ventricle with the exception of a small infundibular component. The only communication between the atrialized ventricle and the infundibulum is through the anteroseptal commissure of the tricuspid valve (Figure 17.10).

Associated anomalies

The most common associated anomaly is an atrial septal defect, which occurs in between 42% and 60% of cases.[39] In neonates at the severe end of the spectrum, survival is dependent on the presence of a patent ductus arteriosus. As already described, a variable degree of obstruction of the right ventricular outflow tract should be considered part of the basic anomaly. A Wolff-Parkinson-White type of accessory pathway, with associated pre-excitation, is present in approximately 10% of patients.[39] Other rare associations include ventricular septal defect, transposition of the great arteries, tetralogy of Fallot, and malformation of the mitral valve. An Ebstein-like malformation of the left sided tricuspid valve is commonly associated with (S, L, L) (corrected) transposition, ventricular septal defect and pulmonary stenosis, and is discussed in greater detail in Chapter 28.

Associated noncardiac anomalies include low-set ears, micrognathia, cleft lip and palate, absent left kidney, megacolon, undescended testes, and bilateral inguinal hernias.[40]

Pathophysiology

As might be anticipated from the wide spectrum of anatomic severity, there is a similar wide spectrum of pathophysiology. One fetal echocardiographic study revealed that this anomaly carries an extremely high rate of death in-utero.[41] Neonates who are symptomatic from the time of birth have massive cardiac enlargement with corresponding hypoplasia of both lungs. There is no forward flow from the ineffective right ventricle, so there is physiologic pulmonary atresia, and the child is dependent on ductal patency for survival. All systemic venous return must pass from right to left, across the atrial septum and through the foramen ovale. Because left ventricular output is also profoundly compromised in the sickest neonates, these children are both severely cyanosed and metabolically acidotic. It is speculated that the capacitance of the enormous right atrium and the 'to and fro' flow into the ineffective right ventricle prevent effective filling of the left ventricle. In addition the left ventricle is 'pancaked'

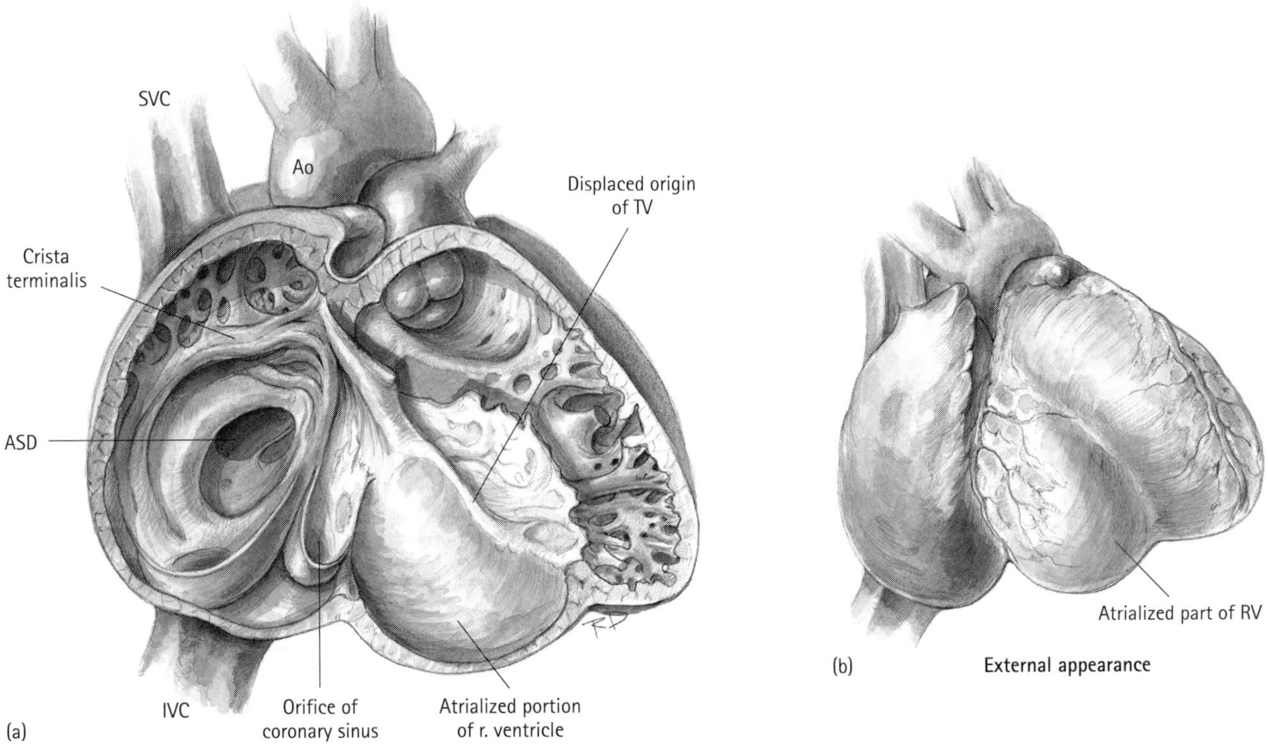

Figure 17.10 *Ebstein's anomaly, anatomic features. (a) Spiral displacement of particularly the septal as well as the posterior leaflet of the tricuspid valve into the right ventricle results in a large atrialized chamber and tricuspid valve regurgitation. (b) The atrialized component of the right ventricle can be visualized externally. Redrawn from Netter.*

flat by the enormous right ventricle. Considering this, it is hardly surprising that simple palliative procedures such as systemic to pulmonary artery shunts carry an unacceptable mortality. Neonates with less severe atrialization of the right ventricle and less pulmonary stenosis may have adequate pulmonary blood flow that will further improve as pulmonary resistance falls.[42] At the mildest end of the anatomic spectrum there may be only a very mild degree of cyanosis, which may not be noted until adult life and may result in few, if any, symptoms. In Watson's review of 505 cases only 35 children were seen in the first year of life.[39] Of these 35, more than half were neonates and were severely symptomatic.

Diagnostic studies

The plain chest X-ray of the neonate who is seen in extremis within hours of birth with cyanosis and acidosis is pathognomonic of Ebstein's anomaly. The cardiac silhouette almost completely fills the chest. Echocardiography should confirm the clinical diagnosis. Specific anatomic points of interest include the size of the right atrium and tricuspid annulus, the degree of atrialization of the right ventricle, the fixation of the anterior leaflet of the tricuspid valve, and the severity of pulmonary stenosis. Frequently, there is physiologic pulmonary atresia because of the inability of the right ventricle to generate sufficient pressure to open the pulmonary valve. The anatomy of the pulmonary artery should be examined, although it is unusual for there to be important distortion or hypoplasia of the central pulmonary arteries. It should not be necessary to undertake catheterization for anatomic definition of Ebstein's anomaly.

Hemodynamic assessment

Before the availability of echocardiography, many reports documented the hazards of cardiac catheterization for children with Ebstein's anomaly.[39,42] Supraventricular and ventricular arrhythmias were common and often fatal. In the presence of a patent ductus arteriosus, no useful information regarding the function of the right ventricle or the degree of pulmonary stenosis can be derived.

Medical and interventional therapy

The neonate who is in extremis within hours of birth requires extremely aggressive resuscitation if there is to be any chance of a successful surgical outcome. Pulmonary blood flow should be maintained by infusion of prostaglandin E1. The child should be anesthetized, intubated and paralysed. Pulmonary vascular resistance should be minimized by appropriate ventilation. Metabolic acidosis should be treated with bicarbonate infusion, and inotropic support should be given. The diagnosis of Ebstein's anomaly should be strongly suspected on the basis of the plain chest X-ray alone and then should be confirmed urgently by echocardiography. If it appears that the child is not responding to these supportive measures, it would seem reasonable to proceed immediately to the operating room, although because of the great rarity of this condition, there are no data to support such an approach.

Medical management of the older child or adult with a mild degree of cyanosis should be aimed at symptomatic relief only.

There are no useful interventional techniques in the management of critical Ebstein's anomaly in neonates. Balloon atrial septostomy serves to increase the right to left shunt, which would be inappropriate in a child who is excessively hypoxic.

The mechanism of right ventricular outflow tract obstruction suggests that balloon dilatation is unlikely to relieve this problem.

Indications for surgery

In older children and adults, surgery has been reserved traditionally for those with important symptomatic limitation (New York Heart Association class 3 or 4), progressive cyanosis, and/or arrhythmias. However, the introduction of intraoperative assessment by TEE means that it is likely that improved techniques with improved results are likely in the near future. Therefore it may be appropriate to loosen the indications. It is possible that as with other forms of valve repair, success is more likely with earlier surgery before secondary pathological changes including annular enlargement have progressed.

There are few useful reports to guide the decision regarding the need for and timing of surgery in the infant and neonate. As stated previously, the neonate who fails to respond to aggressive resuscitation with prostaglandin E1, intubation and ventilation, bicarbonate infusion, and inotropic support almost certainly will die without surgical intervention. However, the child who can be stabilized with this management has the possibility of improving over days and weeks as pulmonary resistance falls. Under such circumstances it might be reasonable to withdraw treatment with prostaglandin E1 on a trial basis and observe the effect of ductal closure, particularly if the child appears to have an anatomically milder form of the anomaly (Carpentier grade A or B).[42] In our limited experience with this condition, however, it is only the children with the anatomically unfavorable form who are seen in extremis during the neonatal period.

The gloomy natural history of Ebstein's anomaly during infancy was documented in the 1971 report from Children's Hospital Boston.[40] Among patients with isolated Ebstein's anomaly, there was a 70% rate of survival to two years and a 50% rate of survival to 13 years of age. When associated anomalies were present, only 15% of infants survived to two years of age. Nevertheless, in general, patients who survive beyond early childhood can expect relatively few limitations. In his review of 505 cases of Ebstein's anomaly, Watson[39] found that 73% of patients between 1 and 15 years of age had minimal disability, as did 69% of those between 16 and 25 years and 59% of those more than 25 years old. Thus, for this anomaly, early diagnosis alone should not be an automatic indication to proceed to surgery, as there is a reasonable probability that the asymptomatic patient will have relatively normal biventricular function for many years.

Surgical management

HISTORY

Ebstein's anomaly was first described by Wilhelm Ebstein in 1866.[43] The diagnosis was not made during life until 1949, by which time a total of only 26 cases had been described at autopsy.[44] In 1963 surgical management by tricuspid valve placement was first described by Barnard and Schrire.[45] In the following year Hardy and associates[46] reported successful tricuspid valve reconstruction using techniques previously described by Hunter and Lillehei.[47] The only large experience with the surgical management of Ebstein's anomaly has been described by Danielson and colleagues.[48] Carpentier et al[38] have contributed new insights into the management of this difficult anomaly.

TECHNICAL CONSIDERATIONS

Neonates

Severely symptomatic neonates present a serious challenge to the surgical team. Our experience has been that palliative procedures, such as closure of an atrial septal defect and Blalock shunt procedures, have been almost uniformly unsuccessful, particularly in the preprostaglandin era. In 1985, a 37-week-old fetus was delivered by cesarean section because of persistent fetal tachycardia following an in-utero echocardiographic diagnosis of severe Ebstein's anomaly. The child remained persistently acidotic after birth despite administration of prostaglandin E1, dopamine, and a bicarbonate infusion. The diagnosis of severe Ebstein's anomaly, including anatomic pulmonary atresia, was confirmed by two-dimensional echocardiography and was further verified by cardiac catheterization. It was concluded that the massive atrialization of the right ventricle was preventing effective flow into the left ventricle. Therefore, the child was taken urgently to the operating room, where the following procedure was performed.

The infant was placed on cardiopulmonary bypass using an ascending aortic cannula and a single venous cannula in the right atrium. The ductus was ligated immediately after beginning bypass. The child was cooled to a rectal temperature of less than 18°C, at which time the ascending aorta was cross clamped and crystalloid cardioplegic solution infused. Bypass was stopped and the venous cannula was removed. The right atrium was opened with an oblique incision, revealing the massively dilated tricuspid annulus. The foramen ovale was enlarged by excising the septum primum. A polytetrafluoroethylene (PTFE) baffle was sutured into the right atrium to direct blood from the superior vena cava, inferior vena cava, and coronary sinus exclusively to the left ventricle.

A 3-mm central shunt was constructed from the ascending aorta to the main pulmonary artery. Much of the redundant right atrial free wall was excised. Although the child initially did well after weaning from bypass, it became clear that the right ventricle was filling with blood, presumably from the Thebesian veins. This could be controlled by occasional aspiration of blood through an indwelling right ventricular catheter. However, over the first six hours in the intensive care unit, the child displayed worsening hemodynamic instability and eventually suffered a fatal cardiac arrest.

Postmortem examination confirmed that there was virtual valvar pulmonary atresia with only a pinhole opening in the valve. In retrospect it may have been sufficient to perform a limited pulmonary valvotomy to allow decompression of the right ventricle by enabling blood from the Thebesian veins to flow to the lungs. A similar concept has since been described and successfully executed by Pitlick and colleagues.[49] In 1988 and 1989, five neonates with a mean PO_2 of 30 mmHg and a pH of 7.20 ± 0.05 were all found to be prostaglandin E1 dependent. None of the neonates had *anatomic* pulmonary atresia, although all had *physiologic* pulmonary atresia. The mean age at the time of repair was five days. The procedure involved pericardial patch closure of the tricuspid valve, placing the coronary sinus on the ventricular side of the patch. The foramen ovale was enlarged, the right atrial free wall was plicated, and a 4-mm central shunt was placed between the ascending aorta and the main pulmonary artery. Interestingly, inotropic support with dopamine and epinephrine was required for right ventricular distention. Minimizing pulmonary vascular resistance with prostaglandin E1 and hyperventilation was also useful in decreasing the tendency for right ventricular distention. There were no perioperative or late deaths over a mean follow-up period of 14 months. All infants were asymptomatic at the time of follow-up, with growth at the 50th percentile for height and the 20th percentile for weight. Two children underwent successful Fontan procedures approximately two years after their initial palliative procedure, while one child had a Glenn shunt placed.

The dismal outlook for neonates who are seen in extremis soon after birth raises the issue of cardiac transplantation. However, we believe that few infants will be well served by this approach. For the neonate who cannot be stabilized by medical management, there is unlikely to be sufficient time in which to locate a suitable donor. Children who can be stabilized presumably have adequate left ventricular function. If, in addition, they have adequate right ventricular function, they are candidates for a biventricular repair. If the right ventricle does not function adequately, they require a Fontan operation.

Infants, children and adults

Many authors dealing with an elective population beyond early infancy have emphasized the importance of obliterating the paradoxic motion of the atrialized portion of the right ventricle in addition to correcting tricuspid valve regurgitation.[46–48] In 1958 Hunter and Lillehei[47] described the concept

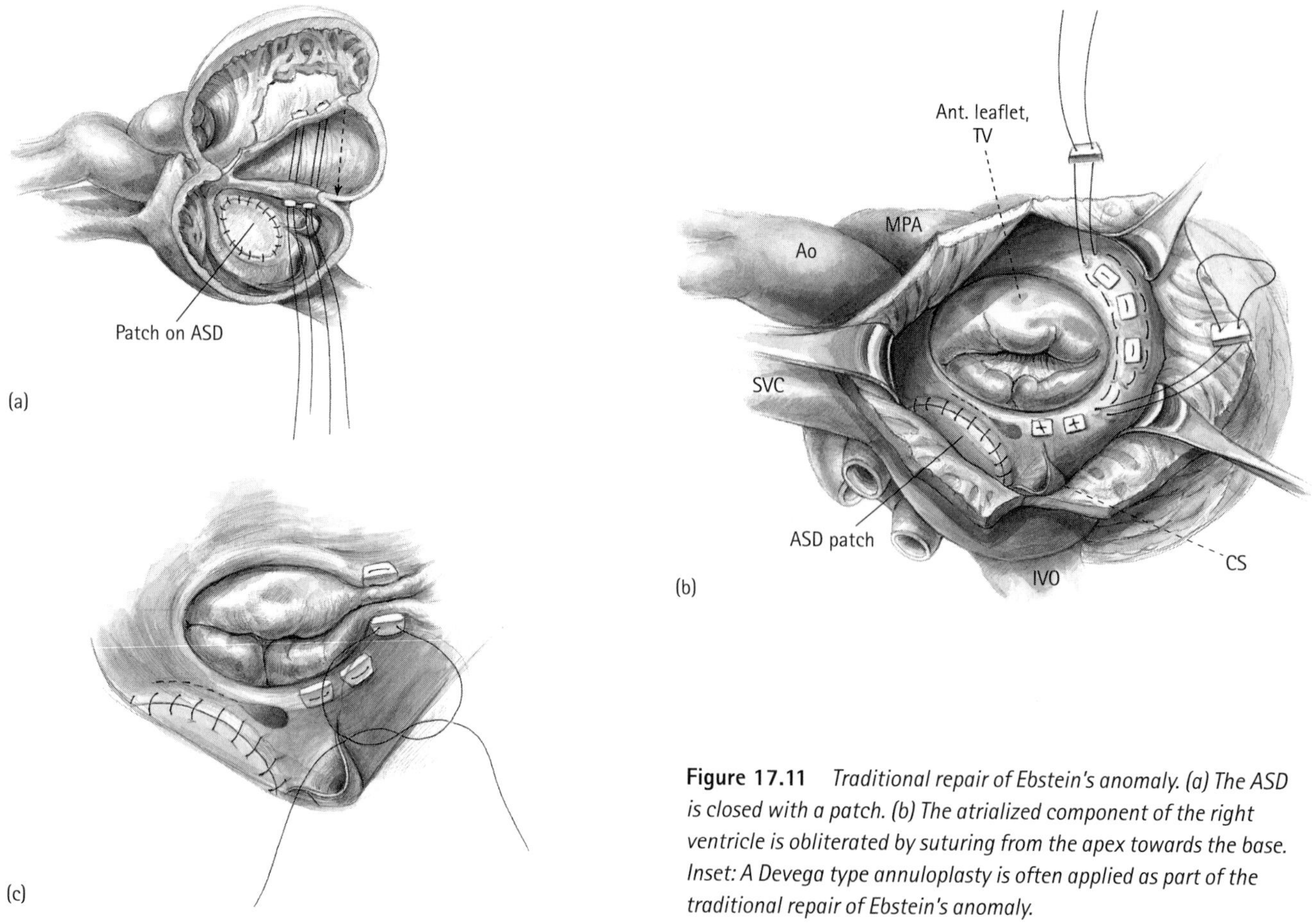

Figure 17.11 *Traditional repair of Ebstein's anomaly. (a) The ASD is closed with a patch. (b) The atrialized component of the right ventricle is obliterated by suturing from the apex towards the base. Inset: A Devega type annuloplasty is often applied as part of the traditional repair of Ebstein's anomaly.*

of tricuspid valve reconstruction for Ebstein's anomaly. This was further detailed by Hardy and colleagues,[46] who obliterated the atrialized portion of the right ventricle by transposing the displaced septal leaflet to the normal plane of the tricuspid valve and plicating the tricuspid annulus.

Danielson and colleagues have had considerable experience with a similar approach to tricuspid valve reconstruction.[48] By plicating the atrialized portion of the right ventricle from the apex toward the base (Figure 17.11), the displaced leaflets come to lie at a more appropriate level relative to the rest of the tricuspid annulus. The atrial septal defect is closed, and the redundant right atrial wall is plicated. In addition, accessory conduction pathways, causing ventricular pre-excitation, are mapped and divided.[50]

Valve replacement for Ebstein's anomaly carried a high risk of complete heart block in many early series.[51] In their classic paper, Barnard and Schrire[45] described placement of a prosthetic valve on the atrial side of the coronary sinus, leaving the coronary sinus to drain into the ventricle. This technique appears to minimize the risk of complete heart block. In a 1982 report, Westaby and associates described tricuspid valve replacement in 16 patients with Ebstein's anomaly.[52] Only two patients had plication of the atrialized ventricle. There was an early mortality rate of 25%. Complete heart block developed in one patient.

In 1988 McKay and colleagues[53] described successful replacement of the tricuspid valve with an unstented pulmonary homograft in a six month old child with Ebstein's anomaly. The technique was essentially the same as that described by Yacoub and Kittle in 1969 for replacement of the mitral valve.[54] The allograft pulmonary valve is mounted within a Dacron tube graft with a generous skirt of pericardium, creating a 'top hat' appearance. The coronary sinus is unroofed into the left atrium. The distal end of the homograft and the Dacron tube is anastomosed to the tricuspid annulus except in the region of the conduction bundle, where it is sutured directly to a remnant of septal leaflet tissue. The pericardial collar is sutured into the right atrium, creating a smooth pathway to the valve orifice.

Modifications of annuloplasty and plication procedures have been described by Carpentier et al[38] and Quaegebeur and coworkers.[55] These techniques are similar to the approach used for most patients at Children's Hospital Boston. Carpentier based his modifications on extensive anatomic studies of Ebstein's anomaly. The major difference relative to the more classic procedure is that plication is performed in a circumferential fashion (Figure 17.12), thereby preserving the apex-to-base dimension of the right ventricle. The circumferential plication sutures become progressively wider as they move from the apex of the wedge of atrialized ventricle towards the

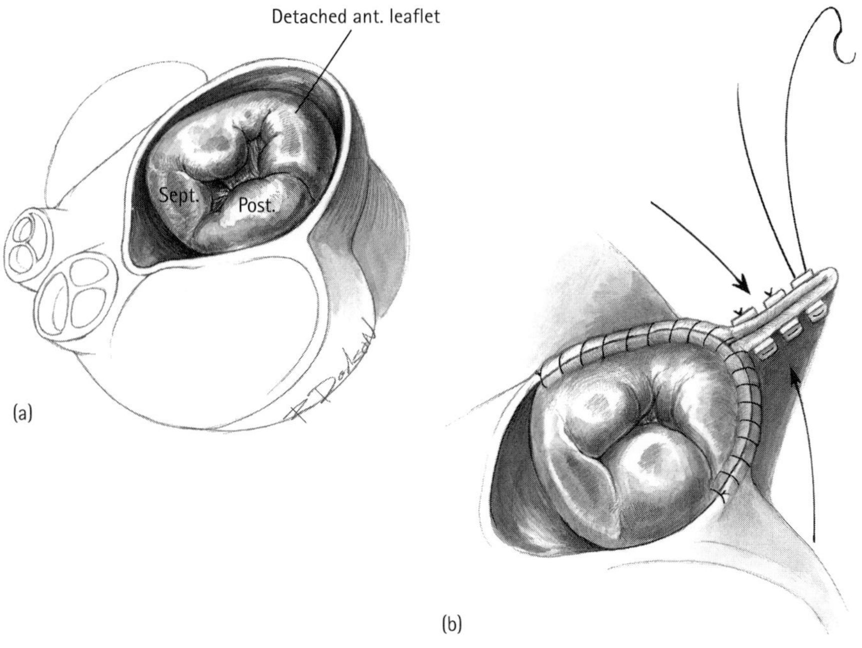

Figure 17.12 *Modifications of the traditional repair of Ebstein's anomaly described by Carpentier and Quaegebeur. (a) The anterior leaflet is detached from the tricuspid annulus. (b) An aggressive commisuroplasty is performed and the anterior leaflet is resuspended on the new tricuspid annulus.*

true annulus. The anterior and posterior leaflets may be detached and repositioned at the level of the tricuspid annulus. Finally, an annuloplasty ring is inserted in older patients to decrease the diameter of the dilated tricuspid annulus, thereby improving leaflet apposition and, therefore, competence of the valve.

Another manouevre that is important in some patients is to transfer the anterior papillary muscle towards the interventricular septum. Often the plication and annuloplasty procedures described result in improved apposition of the bellies of the leaflets but the free edges still fail to oppose. Either complete transfer of the papillary muscle or realignment of the chords by placement of appropriate PTFE sutures can help to improve free edge apposition.

POSTOPERATIVE MANAGEMENT

Points already emphasized that may be important in the management of the critically ill neonate include minimizing pulmonary vascular resistance with appropriate ventilation and sedation and support of the poorly functioning right ventricle with inotropic agents.

Results of surgery

In 1992 Danielson et al[48] from the Mayo Clinic described the results of 189 patients who underwent surgical repair of Ebstein's anomaly between 1972 and 1991. Tricuspid valve repair was possible in 58% of patients while in 36% of patients a prosthetic valve, usually a bioprosthesis, was inserted. In 5% of patients a modified Fontan procedure was performed. Overall hospital mortality was 6%. Twenty eight patients who had a Wolff Parkinson White type accessory conduction pathway underwent successful ablation. Ninety three percent of patients were in New York Heart Association class 1 or 2 at more than one year following surgery. There were 10 late deaths. Late postoperative exercise testing showed a significant improvement in performance. In 2003 Chavaud et al[56] from Carpentier's group in Paris, France, described the results of surgery for Ebstein's anomaly in 191 patients who underwent surgery between 1980 and 2002. A surgical repair was possible in 187 patients. In 60 patients an ancillary bidirectional cavopulmonary shunt was added. Only four patients had valve replacement. Hospital mortality was 9% secondary to right ventricular failure in 9 of the 18 patients who died. Actuarial survival was 82% at 20 years. Tricuspid valve insufficiency was 1 or 2+ in 80% of patients. Reoperation was necessary in 16 patients. In 10 of these a successful second repair was possible.

In 2002 Knott Craig et al[57] from Oklahoma described the results of surgery for eight severely symptomatic neonates with either Ebstein's anomaly or a closely related entity. Five patients had either anatomical or functional pulmonary atresia. Repair consisted of tricuspid valve repair, reduction atrioplasty, relief of right ventricular outflow tract obstruction, partial closure of atrial septal defect and correction of all associated cardiac defects. There was one hospital death. The authors suggest that a reparative approach is possible in the majority of severely symptomatic neonates and that the approach described by Pitlick from Starnes' group in which the right ventricle is excluded is rarely indicated.

TRICUSPID VALVE STENOSIS

Isolated congenital tricuspid valve stenosis is exceedingly rare. Tricuspid valve stenosis is almost always associated with hypoplasia of the valve annulus in association with underdevelopment of the right heart. This is usually in the setting of pulmonary atresia with intact ventricular septum (see Chapter 26: PA/IVS). Tricuspid stenosis is also occasionally seen in association with transposition of the great arteries usually with concomitant right ventricular outflow tract obstruction and arch hypoplasia.

PULMONARY VALVE DISEASE

PULMONARY VALVE STENOSIS

Isolated pulmonary valve stenosis is no longer an anomaly that is treated surgically. Balloon dilation at interventional catheterization is highly successful in managing the overwhelming majority of these children. Very occasionally there may be associated infundibular hypoplasia which will require management with an outflow patch. Pulmonary valve stenosis that is part of tetralogy of Fallot or is associated with a VSD is managed by surgical valvotomy as part of the corrective surgical procedure. It is important to remember that in the setting of a left to right shunt the gradient measured across the pulmonary valve is exaggerated. This is also often seen when an ASD is present. Although the valve is structurally normal and of adequate size for a normal cardiac output, it is not able to carry the increased pulmonary blood flow secondary to the left to right shunt without a gradient developing.

PULMONARY VALVE REGURGITATION

The most important anomaly that involves pulmonary valve regurgitation is the Absent Pulmonary Valve Syndrome. This is a variant of tetralogy of Fallot and is described in Chapter 16.

Pulmonary regurgitation secondary to placement of a transannular patch as part of tetralogy repair is a difficult entity both in terms of its assessment as well as decisions regarding management. The issue is also discussed in Chapter 16.

REFERENCES

1. Hoerstrup SP, Sodian R, Daebritz S et al. Functional living trileaflet heart valves grown in vitro. *Circulation* 2000; **102**(19 Suppl 3):III44–49.
2. Roberts WC, Morrow AG, McIntosh CL, Jones M, Epstein SE. Congenitally bicuspid aortic valve causing severe, pure aortic regurgitation without superimposed infective endocarditis. *Am J Cardiol* 1981; **47**:206–209.
3. Olson LJ, Subramanian R, Edwards WD. Surgical pathology of pure aortic insufficiency. A study of 225 cases. *Mayo Clin Proc* 1984; **59**:835–841.
4. Iglesias A, Oliver J, Munoz JE, Nunez L. Quadricuspid aortic valve associated with fibromuscular subaortic stenosis and aortic regurgitation treated by conservative surgery. *Chest* 1981; **80**:3.
5. Bacha EA, Satou GM, Moran AM et al. Valve-sparing operation for balloon-induced aortic regurgitation in congenital aortic stenosis. *J Thorac Cardiovasc Surg* 2001; **122**:162–168.
6. Tatsuno K, Konno S, Ando M, Sakakibara S. Pathogenetic mechanisms of prolapsing aortic valve and aortic regurgitation associated with VSD. *Circulation* 1973; **58**:1028–1037.
7. Van Praagh R, McNamara JJ. Anatomic types of ventricular septal defect with aortic insufficiency. *Am Heart J* 1968; **75**:604–619.
8. Newfeld EA, Muster AJ, Paul MH et al. Discrete subvalvular aortic stenosis in childhood. Study of 51 patients. *Am J Cardiol* 1976; **38**:53–61.
9. Grande-Allen KH, Cochran RP, Reinhall PG, Kunzelman KS. Mechanisms of aortic valve incompetence: Finite-element modeling of Marfan syndrome. *J Thorac Cardiovasc Surg* 2001; **122**:946-954.
10. Marx GR, Sherwood MC. Three-dimensional echocardiography in congenital heart disease: a continuum of unfulfilled promises? No. A presently clinically applicable technology with an important future? Yes. *Pediatr Cardiol* 2002; **23**:266–285.
11. Colan SD, Borow KM, Neumann A. Left ventricular end-systolic wall stress-velocity of fiber shortening relation: a load-independent index of myocardial contractility. *J Am Coll Cardiol* 1984; **4**:715–724.
12. Hawkins JA, Minich L, Shaddy RE et al. Aortic valve repair and replacement after balloon aortic valvuloplasty in children. *Ann Thorac Surg* 1996; **61**:1355–1358.
13. Caspi J, Ilbawi MN, Roberson DA, Piccione W, Monson DO, Wajafi H. Extended aortic valvuloplasty for recurrent valvular stenosis and regurgitation in children. *J Thorac Cardiovasc Surg* 1994; **107**:1114–1120.
14. Von Son JAM, Reddy VM, Black MD, Rajasinghe H, Haas GS, Hanley FL. Morphologic determinants favoring surgical aortic valvuloplasty versus pulmonary autograft aortic valve replacement in children. *J Thorac Cardiovasc Surg* 1996; **111**:1149–1157.
15. Smith PC, Barth MJ, Ilbawi MN. Pericardial leaflet extension for aortic valve repair: techniques and late results. *Semin Thorac Cardiovasc Surg Pediatr Card Surg Annu* 1999; **2**:83–93.
16. Frasier CD, Wang N, Mee RB et al. Repair of insufficient bicuspid aortic valves. *Ann Thorac Surg* 1994; **58**:386–390.
17. Laudito A, Brook MM, Suleman S et al. The Ross procedure in children and young adults: a word of caution. *J Thorac Cardiovasc Surg* 2001; **122**:147–153.
18. Shone RD, Sellers RD, Anderson RC, Adams PA, Lillehei CW, Edwards JE. The developmental complex of 'parachute mitral valve', supravalvular ring of left atrium, subaortic stenosis and coarctation of aorta. *Am J Cardiol* 1963; June: 714–725.
19. Oosthoek W, Wenink AC, Macedo AJ, Gittenberger-deGroot AC. The parachute-like asymmetric mitral valve and its two papillary muscles. *J Thorac Cardiovasc Surg* 1997; **114**:9–15.
20. Macartney FJ, Bain HH, Ionescu MI, Deverall PB, Scott O. Angiocardiographic/pathologic correlations in congenital mitral valve anomalies. *Eur J Cardiol* 1976; **4**:191–211.
21. Moore P, Adatia I, Spevak PJ et al. Severe congenital mitral stenosis in infants. *Circulation* 1994; **89**:2099–2106.
22. Barbero-Marcial M, Riso A, De Albuquerque AT, Atik E, Jatene A. Left ventricular apical approach for the surgical treatment of congenital mitral stenosis. *J Thorac Cardiovasc Surg* 1993; **106**:105–110.

23. Jonas RA, Keane JF, Lock JE. Aortic valve-preserving procedure for enlargement of the left ventricular outflow tract and mitral anulus. *J Thorac Cardiovasc Surg* 1998; **115**:1219–1222.
24. Laks H, Hellenbrand WE, Kleinman C, Talner NS. Left atrial-left ventricular conduit for relief of congenital mitral stenosis in infancy. *J Thorac Cardiovasc Surg* 1980; **70**:782–787.
25. Corno A, Giannico S, Leibovich S, Mazzera E, Marcelletti C. The hypoplastic mitral valve. *J Thorac Cardiovasc Surg* 1986; **91**:848–851.
26. Castaneda AR, Jonas RA, Mayer JE, Hanley FL. *Cardiac Surgery of the Neonate and Infant.* Philadelphia, WB Saunders, 1994, p 393.
27. Spevak PJ, Bass JL, Ben-Shachar G et al. Balloon angioplasty for congenital mitral stenosis. *Am J Cardiol* 1990; **66**:472–476.
28. Coles JG, Williams WG, Watanabe T et al. Surgical experience with reparative techniques in patients with congenital mitral valvular anomalies. *Circulation* 1987; **76**(3 Pt 2):III117–122.
29. Uva MS, Galletti L, Gayet FL et al. Surgery for congenital mitral valve disease in the first year of life. *J Thorac Cardiovasc Surg* 1995; **109**:164–174.
30. Kadoba K, Jonas RA, Mayer JE, Castaneda AR. Mitral valve replacement in the first year of life. *J Thorac Cardiovasc Surg* 1990; **10**:762–768.
31. Adatia I, Moore PM, Jonas RA, Colan SD, Lock JE, Keane JF. Clinical course and hemodynamic observations after supraannular mitral valve replacement in infants and children. *J Am Coll Cardiol* 1997; **29**:1089–1094.
32. Serraf A, Zoghbi J, Belli E et al. Congenital mitral stenosis with or without associated defects: An evolving surgical strategy. *Circulation* 2000; **102**(19 Suppl 3):III166–171.
33. Carpentier A, Branchini B, Cour JC et al. Congenital malformations of the mitral valve in children. Pathology and surgical treatment. *J Thorac Cardiovasc Surg* 1976; **72**:854–866.
34. Reed GE, Pooley RW, Moggio RA. Durability of measured mitral annuloplasty: seventeen-year study. *J Thorac Cardiovasc Surg* 1980; **79**:321–325.
35. Yoshimura N, Yamaguchi M, Oshima Y et al. Surgery for mitral valve disease in the pediatric age group. *J Thorac Cardiovasc Surg* 1999; **118**:99–106.
36. Ohno H, Imai Y, Terada M, Hiramatsu T. The long-term results of commissure plication annuloplasty for congenital mitral insufficiency. *Ann Thorac Surg* 1999; **68**:537–541.
37. Stellin G, Bortolotti U, Mazzucco A et al. Repair of congenitally malformed mitral valve in children. *J Thorac Cardiovasc Surg* 1988; **95**:480–485.
38. Carpentier A, Chauvaud S, Mace L et al. A new reconstructive operation for Ebstein's anomaly of the tricuspid valve. *J Thorac Cardiovasc Surg* 1988; **96**:92–101.
39. Watson H. Natural history of Ebstein's anomaly of tricuspid valve in childhood and adolescence. *Br Heart J* 1974; **36**:417–427.
40. Kumar AE, Fyler DC, Miettinen OS, Nadas AS. Ebstein's anomaly. *Am J Cardiol* 1971; **28**:84–95.
41. Hornberger LK, Sahn DJ, Kleinman CS, Copel JA, Reed KL. Tricuspid valve disease with significant tricuspid insufficiency in the fetus: Diagnosis and outcome. *J Am Coll Cardiol* 1991; **17**:167–173.
42. Radford DJ, Graff RF, Neilson GH. Diagnosis and natural history of Ebstein's anomaly. *Br Heart J* 1985; **54**:517–522.
43. Ebstein W. Uber einen sehr seltenen Fall von Insufficienz der Valvular tricuspidalis, bedingt durch eine angeborene hochgradige Missbildung deselben. *Arch Anat Physiol* 1866; **33**:238.
44. Tourniaire A, Deyrieux F, Tartulier M. Maladie d'Ebstein: Essai de diagnostic clinique. *Arch Mal Coeur* 1959; **42**:1211.
45. Barnard CN, Schrire V. Surgical correction of Ebstein's malformation with prosthetic tricuspid valve. *Surgery* 1963; **54**:302.
46. Hardy KL, May IA, Webster CA et al. Ebstein's anomaly: A functional concept and successful definitive repair. *J Thorac Cardiovasc Surg* 1964; **48**:927.
47. Hunter SW, Lillehei CW. Ebstein's malformation of the tricuspid valve with suggestions of a new form of surgical therapy. *Dis Chest* 1958; **33**:297.
48. Danielson GK, Driscoll DJ, Mair DD et al. Operative treatment of Ebstein's anomaly. *J Thorac Cardiovasc Surg* 1992; **104**:1195–1202.
49. Pitlick PT, Griffin ML, Bernstein D et al. Followup on a new surgical procedure for Ebstein's anomaly in the critically ill neonate. *Circulation* 1990; **83**:716.
50. Oh JK, Holmes DR, Hayes DL. Porter CB, Danielson GK. Cardiac arrhythmias in patients with surgical repair of Ebstein's anomaly. *J Am Coll Cardiol* 1985; **6**:1351–1357.
51. Lillehei CW, Kalke BR, Carlson RG. Evolution of corrective surgery for Ebstein's anomaly. *Circulation* 1967; **35**:111–118.
52. Westaby S, Karp RB, Kirklin JW, Waldo AL, Blackstone EH. Surgical treatment in Ebstein's malformation. *Ann Thorac Surg* 1982; **34**:388–395.
53. McKay R, Sono J, Arnold RM. Tricuspid valve replacement using an unstented pulmonary homograft. *Ann Thorac Surg* 1988; **46**:58–62.
54. Yacoub MH, Kittle CF. A new technique for replacement of the mitral valve by a semilunar valve homograft. *J Thorac Cardiovasc Surg* 1969; **58**:859–869.
55. Quaegebeur JM, Sreeram N, Fraser AG et al. Surgery for Ebstein's anomaly. The clinical and echocardiographic evaluation of a new technique. *J Am Coll Cardiol* 1991; **17**:722–728.
56. Chauvaud S, Berrebi A, d'Attellis N, Mousseaux E, Hernigou A, Carpentier A. Ebstein's anomaly: repair based on functional analysis. *Eur J Cardiothorac Surg* 2003; **23**:525–531.
57. Knott-Craig CJ, Overholt ED, Ward KE, Ringewald JM, Baker SS, Razook JD. Repair of Ebstein's anomaly in the symptomatic neonate: an evolution of technique with 7-year follow-up. *Ann Thorac Surg* 2002; **73**:1786–1792.

18

Left ventricular outflow tract obstruction: aortic valve stenosis, subaortic stenosis, supravalvar aortic stenosis

INTRODUCTION

The left ventricular outflow tract is a complex anatomic structure which includes subvalvular, valvular and supravalvular components. It lies centrally deep within the heart immediately adjacent to the two atrioventricular valves. Obstruction of the left ventricular outflow tract at one or more levels increases impedance to ejection from the left ventricle and promotes development of hypertrophy. In many instances obstruction occurs at multiple levels and although the degree of obstruction in any one area may not be severe, the combined effect of obstruction at multiple levels is clinically important.

Dealing with important obstruction in the left ventricular outflow tract is a significant challenge to the surgeon. Decision making as to the timing and extent of surgical intervention is complicated by the heterogenous makeup of patients with LV outflow obstruction. At one end of the spectrum are patients with isolated aortic valve stenosis, normal sized left heart structures and a normal aortic arch and isthmus. For these patients, relief of obstruction at the aortic valve level is all that is necessary to achieve a biventricular circulation. At the other end of the spectrum are patients with multiple sequential obstructive lesions that merge into the spectrum of hypoplastic left heart syndrome and severe Shone's anomaly. For these patients, a single ventricle approach commencing with a Norwood procedure may be the optimal approach.

AORTIC VALVE STENOSIS

INTRODUCTION

A bicuspid aortic valve is the most common of all the congenital cardiac anomalies occurring in 1–2% of the population, with an overwhelming majority of patients being male.[1]

Most patients do not have valvar stenosis in childhood and are asymptomatic. In later life as the valve leaflets become thickened and fibrotic aortic valve replacement may be indicated. At the other end of the spectrum there is such severe obstruction at valve level that the child is dependent on ductal patency for survival. This entity is termed 'critical neonatal aortic valve stenosis'. Overall congenital aortic valve stenosis represents about 3–5% of all patients with congenital heart disease.[2]

EMBRYOLOGY

Both semilunar valves appear as swellings of subendothelial tissue when septation of the bulbus cordis, the outflow tube from the embryonic heart, is completed by the spiral aortopulmonary septum. Three swellings guard the orifice both of the aorta and the pulmonary artery. These swellings consist of a covering of endothelium over loose connective tissue. They are soon excavated on the distal aspect to form the three cusps of the semilunar valve.[3]

Recent studies with zebrafish suggest that both the semilunar valves as well as the atrioventricular valves form as a result of invasion of the cardiac jelly or matrix by endocardial cells, hence the term endocardial cushion tissue.[4] In zebrafish mutants that specifically lack cardiac valves, the cardiac cushions fail to appear.[5] Studies are in progress to identify candidate genes responsible for this mutation. These studies will help to improve our understanding of cardiac valve embryogenesis.

ANATOMY

Critical neonatal aortic valve stenosis

Most patients who present with critical neonatal aortic valve stenosis have poorly defined leaflets that really cannot be classified as bicuspid or unicuspid.[6,7] The valve tissue is primitive, gelatinous or myxomatous in nature and appears immature and incompletely developed.[8] The orifice may be little more than a pinhole. The valve is almost always smaller than normal and may be severely hypoplastic. The ascending aorta is usually hypoplastic, often as small as 5–6 mm in diameter.

Associated anomalies

Critical neonatal aortic valve stenosis is almost always associated with some degree of underdevelopment of other left heart structures including the mitral valve, left ventricular cavity, left ventricular outflow tract, ascending aorta, arch, isthmus and periductal area.[9] There may also be important endocardial fibroelastosis which will have an important impact on left ventricular compliance.

Aortic valve stenosis and aortic valve hypoplasia are very commonly associated with a posterior malalignment VSD as is seen with interrupted aortic arch. Often the left ventricular outflow tract is also very small because of the posterior malalignment of the conal septum which projects towards the anterior leaflet of the mitral valve.

Aortic valve stenosis beyond the neonatal period

Patients who present beyond the neonatal period often have an adequate aortic annulus without associated cardiac anomalies. The valve is bicuspid in about 70% often with fusion at the intercoronary commissure.[10] There may be a fibrous raphe indicating the location of the vestigial commissure. There is a variable degree of commissural fusion at the anterior and/or posterior commissure. In about 30% of cases the valve is tricuspid with variable fusion at the commissures.

PATHOPHYSIOLOGY

Aortic valve stenosis increases impedance to LV ejection and produces a pressure gradient across the valve such that peak intraventricular pressure exceeds aortic systolic pressure. Under these circumstances LV wall stress (which equals $Pr/2h$, where P = peak intraventricular pressure, r = ventricular radius and h = LV wall thickness) is greatly elevated. This provides stimulus for LV concentric hypertrophy or wall thickening. The degree of thickening parallels the increase in ventricular pressure such that LV wall stress is normalized despite greatly elevated peak intraventricular pressure. This normalization of wall stress allows LV ejection fraction (EF) to be maintained despite increasing impedance to ejection. As aortic stenosis progresses eventually the valve orifice narrows to the point where stroke volume and EF can no longer be maintained. The development of LV concentric hypertrophy places the subendocardium at risk for hypoperfusion and the development of ischemia for a number of reasons:

- elevated LV end-diastolic pressure secondary to the diminished compliance which accompanies concentric hypertrophy
- an aortic diastolic blood pressure which is low relative to the elevated LV end-diastolic pressure
- compression of subendocardial vessels by the hypertrophied myocardium
- absence of any systolic coronary perfusion because the left ventricular systolic pressure greatly exceeds aortic systolic pressure.

Endocardial fibroelastosis may develop as a consequence of chronic in-utero subendocardial ischemia and infarction. The extent of fibrosis can be quite dramatic. A smooth, extremely thick layer can be seen to line the LV cavity and to encase the papillary muscles. As myocardium is lost and replaced by fibrous tissue systolic function will deteriorate. This process also severely impairs LV diastolic function and reduces compliance. When fibrosis is severe, left ventricular end diastolic pressure is likely to be markedly elevated even if complete relief of valvar stenosis is achieved. The severity of stenosis at the time of birth largely determines the subsequent pathophysiologic course. In neonates with mild stenosis there will be gradual development of hypertrophy over the course of years with essentially no fibrosis. In neonates with more severe stenosis there will have been development of in-utero hypertrophy and there may be some degree of fibrosis. Over the course of days to months it will become clear that hypertrophy has not progressed to the point of normalizing wall stress. This is a state of afterload mismatch, defined as the point where for a given level of contractility progressive increases in afterload result in progressive decreases in stroke volume. This point is reached when preload reserve is exhausted, when the sarcomeres are at their optimal length and there is no further preload recruitable stroke work. As a result LV end-diastolic pressure and left atrial pressure will be markedly elevated predisposing to pulmonary edema. In the neonate with critical aortic stenosis there will be severe afterload mismatch and very little antegrade ejection across the aortic valve. There will almost certainly be some degree of endocardial fibrosis. As a result the left ventricle will be more dilated than hypertrophied. The child will be dependent on right to left ductal blood flow to provide the majority of proximal and distal aortic blood flow. The brain and heart are thus dependent on retrograde aortic blood flow. If ductal closure occurs the child will sustain ischemic injury to the myocardium, brain, kidneys, and splanchnic bed. Unless prostaglandin E1 is rapidly instituted the child will not survive.

Beyond the neonatal period the pathophysiology of aortic valve stenosis primarily reflects the impact of left ventricular hypertrophy. There may be subendocardial ischemia during exercise causing angina. There also may be an ineffective increase in cardiac output with exercise leading to syncope.

CLINICAL FEATURES

Because there is often associated underdevelopment of left heart structures, critical neonatal aortic valve stenosis is frequently diagnosed prenatally by ultrasound. In this case prostaglandin can be begun immediately following birth. This will permit maintenance of systemic perfusion via the ductus during the first few days of life while pulmonary vascular resistance remains elevated. As pulmonary vascular resistance falls the tendency for $Q_p:Q_s$ to increase will jeopardize ductal dependent systemic perfusion. Neonates not diagnosed prenatally may present with signs of poor perfusion, cyanosis, and lethargy as the ductus begins to close. These children are often originally evaluated for sepsis. The presence of a murmur leads to an echocardiographic examination and the diagnosis. Occasionally a neonate will present with circulatory collapse following ductal closure. The extent of end organ damage will depend on the duration and severity of the systemic hypoperfusion as indicated by the degree of metabolic acidosis.

Neonates with severe, noncritical aortic stenosis in whom ductal blood flow is not essential for systemic perfusion are likely to present within weeks with respiratory distress secondary to pulmonary edema. Neonates with less severe aortic stenosis will be asymptomatic. Beyond infancy presentation may be similar to the adult with aortic valve stenosis including the classic symptoms of angina and syncope. A harsh systolic ejection murmur is noted on physical examination.

DIAGNOSTIC STUDIES

The echocardiogram is diagnostic. It is important however to understand that in the neonatal period when the ductus is patent, assessment of a gradient across the aortic valve either by catheter or Doppler-derived methods will underestimate the severity of the stenosis due to the low flow across the valve. Depressed contractility, high grade obstruction to transaortic flow, and ductal blood flow into the aorta all contribute to low flow across the aortic valve.

It is particularly important for the echocardiographer to measure all left heart structures in two planes. Cavity and valve dimensions should be measured and a z score for each calculated. Assessment of the mitral valve size and mobility is just as important as for the aortic valve. The long axis length of the left ventricle as a percentage of the total long axis length of the heart (atrioventricular valve annulus to apex) is also a valuable measurement. The decision whether to pursue a two ventricle or a one ventricle approach is largely guided by these calculations.[11,12] An assessment of the extent and severity of endocardial fibroelastosis should be made as well. In the older patient who is being followed for aortic valve stenosis serial echo studies should document the Doppler-derived valve gradient, left ventricular wall thickness and left ventricular volume. Calculations of left ventricular wall stress and other echocardiographic-derived methods for assessing left ventricular contractility allow informed decisions regarding the timing of intervention.[13,14]

MEDICAL AND INTERVENTIONAL THERAPY

Resuscitation of the child with critical neonatal aortic valve stenosis

The general principles of resuscitation are the same as those that apply to any child with obstruction to systemic outflow, such as hypoplastic left heart syndrome or interrupted aortic arch, and have been described in detail in Chapter 5.

Balloon dilation

Balloon dilation is the method of choice for management of critical neonatal aortic valve stenosis. The technique has been described in detail elsewhere.[15] The procedure should be undertaken by a highly skilled team with excellent imaging facilities. Surgical backup should be readily available throughout the procedure although in skilled hands complications such as acute severe aortic valve regurgitation or injury to the mitral valve are exceedingly rare. On occasion injury to a femoral or iliac vessel may necessitate reconstruction by the cardiovascular surgical team. In some instances this will necessitate Gortex tube graft replacement of the iliac artery from the aortic bifurcation to the femoral bifurcation. We generally use an extraperitoneal iliac fossa approach to undertake this procedure. Balloon dilation is also the preferred primary mode of therapy in the infant and child with aortic valve stenosis. Care must be taken to avoid oversizing the balloon which can lead to an unacceptable degree of valvar regurgitation.

INDICATIONS FOR AND TIMING OF INTERVENTION

These are unquestionably the most complicated issues in the management of the neonate, infant and child with aortic valve stenosis.

Neonatal aortic valve stenosis

A trial of discontinuation of prostaglandin can be undertaken if the left heart structures are well developed and the degree of aortic valve stenosis does not appear to be severe. Closure of the ductus must be documented by physical examination and echocardiography. No intervention is necessary if following ductal closure cardiac output is adequate, there is no respiratory distress, and the child can feed and grow.

PROSTAGLANDIN DEPENDENT CRITICAL NEONATAL AORTIC VALVE STENOSIS

If the child is prostaglandin dependent a decision must be made early in the neonatal period whether to proceed to a one ventricle (Norwood) or two ventricle pathway. At one end of the spectrum are infants who have an aortic root, left ventricle, and mitral valve of sufficient size such that they will clearly benefit from balloon valvotomy and can be expected to proceed to a two ventricle endpoint. At the other end of the spectrum are infants who have such severe hypoplasia of the aortic root, left ventricle and mitral valve that balloon valvotomy is unlikely to result in a viable two ventricle circulation. These patients will require a Norwood procedure within days. Those patients who do not clearly fall into either of these groups are the real management challenges. There are currently multivariable scoring systems (discussed below) to aid in this decision making process.

Unfortunately the option to try a two ventricle approach and to fall back to a single ventricle approach if necessary is not a good one and is not recommended. The usual scenario that results is that even though a satisfactory and successful balloon valvotomy procedure is performed with minimal residual gradient, the child remains ventilator dependent because of very high left atrial pressures. High left atrial pressure in this circumstance is usually the result of a combination of poor left ventricular compliance secondary to endocardial fibroelastosis and small left ventricular chamber size associated with a hypoplastic, stenotic mitral valve. When the child has been ventilator dependent for two or three weeks and the surgical and intensive care team realizes that a single ventricle approach will be necessary, by this time the pulmonary resistance is very high. This increases the risk of a Norwood procedure and may also eliminate the option of cardiac transplantation as well. Thus it is essential that the correct decision be made at the outset. Fortunately data analyses by several groups are now available to help guide this decision.

The Rhodes score

The scoring system published by Rhodes et al from Children's Hospital Boston[12] was developed using discriminate analysis to determine which of several echocardiographically measured left heart structures were independent predictors of survival after valvotomy for neonatal critical aortic stenosis. Clinical experience had suggested that a presumably adequate left ventricular size (end-diastolic volume) of more than 20 ml/m^2 did not correlate with survival following valvuloplasty. Using a scoring system based on mitral valve area (less than 4.75 cm^2/m^2), long axis dimension of the left ventricle relative to the long axis dimension of the heart (less than 0.8), diameter of the aortic root (less than 3.5 cm/m^2) and left ventricular mass (less than 35 g/m^2), it was possible to predict with 95% accuracy the likelihood of survival following a biventricular approach utilizing valvotomy. The presence of more than one of the 'Rhodes factors' noted above suggests a high probability of death if a two ventricle approach is pursued. While very useful in neonates with isolated aortic stenosis, the Rhodes score has proven to have lower accuracy in neonates with multiple left heart obstructive lesions. A more recent analysis included patients three months of age or less with two or more areas of left heart obstruction or hypoplasia. This analysis demonstrated the presence of a moderate/large VSD, unicommissural aortic valve, and hypoplastic mitral valve or left ventricle (z score less than -2.0) to be independent risk factors for failure of a biventricular repair.[16]

The CHSS calculator

The Congenital Heart Surgeon's Society has undertaken a multi-institutional study of 320 neonates with critical aortic stenosis.[11] These patients were enrolled at 24 institutions between 1994 and 2000. A total of 116 patients were directed towards a biventricular repair by having either a balloon valvotomy ($n = 83$) or surgery ($n = 33$) most commonly an open valvotomy. Survival was 82% at one month, 72% at one year and 70% at five years. Risk factors for death were a higher grade of endocardial fibroelastosis estimated by echocardiography, a lower z score of the aortic valve diameter at the level of the sinuses of Valsalva and younger age at entry. An initial Norwood procedure was performed in 179 patients with survival at five years of 60%. The risk factors for the Norwood approach are discussed in Chapter 19: Hypoplastic left heart syndrome. Because of the large number of patients in this study it was possible to use multiple logistical regression to develop a calculator which allows prediction for any individual patient as to whether a biventricular repair is more likely to result in survival than a Norwood procedure. The calculator can be accessed at the Congenital Heart Surgeons Society website (www.chssdc.org).

Intervention for aortic valve stenosis beyond the neonatal period

Balloon dilation of the aortic valve is a low risk procedure which serves both to reduce the transvalvular gradient and to promote growth of the aortic annulus. The latter is important as aortic stenosis in children is often associated with hypoplasia of the aortic valve. Balloon dilation of a stenotic valve early in life, particularly if it results in a mild degree of aortic regurgitation, provides an important stimulus for growth of the valve. If echocardiographic assessment indicates leaflet commissural fusion which is likely to be improved by balloon dilation, then intervention is indicated for a peak Doppler-derived gradient of more than 30–40 mmHg and a peak to peak catheter derived gradient of greater than 20–30 mmHg. These gradients are considerably lower than those previously used as the threshold for surgical intervention in children. Early aggressive intervention by balloon dilation allows the child to grow and exercise and promotes annular growth. At present there are essentially no indications for primary surgical intervention for a stenotic aortic valve with adequate annular dimensions.

SURGICAL MANAGEMENT

History

In 1910, Alexis Carrel performed experimental surgery using a conduit from the apex of the left ventricle to the aorta as a means of addressing left ventricular outflow obstruction.[17] In 1912, Tuffier approached the lesion directly, performing successful transaortic digital dilatation in a young man with aortic stenosis.[18] More than 40 years passed before any additional significant advance occurred. In 1953, Larzelere and Bailey performed a closed surgical commissurotomy.[19] In 1955, Marquis and Logan performed closed surgical dilatation of a stenotic aortic valve using antegrade introduction of dilators via an incision in the left ventricular apex.[20] Inflow occlusion with open valvotomy was reported in 1956 by both Lewis and Swan and their associates.[21,22] Also in 1956, Lillehei and colleagues performed an aortic valvotomy using cardiopulmonary bypass.[23] All of these milestones were achieved in patients well beyond infancy. In 1969, Coran and Bernhard, at Children's Hospital in Boston, reported surgical relief of critical aortic stenosis in neonates and infants, with cases dating back to 1960.[24]

Various surgical procedures have been described for enlargement of the hypoplastic aortic annulus. Posterior annular enlargement was the first of these techniques. It was reported by Nicks and colleagues from Sydney Australia in 1970.[25] A similar but more extensive technique was described in 1979 by Manougian, although there has been controversy regarding who should be credited with the original concept for the procedure.[26,27] Anterior enlargement of the hypoplastic annulus was described in 1975 by Konno from Tokyo, Japan.[28] Successful replacement of the aortic valve with a mechanical device was pioneered by Harken at the Brigham Hospital in Boston in 1960.[29] In 1962 Ross in London[30] and Barratt-Boyes in New Zealand[31] described successful implantation of an aortic allograft for replacement of the aortic valve. Ross later introduced the pulmonary autograft procedure[32] which has subsequently been combined with the Konno procedure for patients with annular hypoplasia and particularly those with associated tunnel subaortic stenosis.[33]

Percutaneous balloon aortic valvuloplasty in adults was described in 1984 by Lababidi and coworkers.[34] Use of this technique in infants was reported in 1985 by Rupprath and Neuhaus[35] and by Sanchez and associates.[36] Shortly thereafter use of the technique in neonates with critical aortic stenosis was described by Lababidi and Weinhaus.[37] At Children's Hospital Boston, percutaneous balloon valvuloplasty has been used in neonates and infants with critical aortic stenosis since 1985.[15] A comparison of surgical and percutaneous techniques reported from our institution in 1989 indicated comparable immediate and intermediate results.[38] At the present time, percutaneous balloon valvuloplasty is our procedure of choice.

Technical considerations

Percutaneous balloon dilation of the aortic valve is the procedure of choice for aortic valve stenosis. The outmoded technique of surgical valvotomy will not be described.

AORTIC VALVE REPLACEMENT WITH AORTIC ANNULAR ENLARGEMENT

Aortic valve replacement for pure aortic valve stenosis with a normal aortic annular diameter is almost never indicated in the pediatric age group. If an aggressive policy of balloon valve dilation is followed it will also be rare that the aortic valve needs replacement because of annular hypoplasia. When this situation does arise, however, a number of options are available.

Posterior enlargement of the aortic annulus: Manougian and Nicks procedures

These procedures are used when a modest degree of enlargement of the aortic annulus is required. They can be performed in conjunction with either mechanical aortic valve replacement or as part of an extended aortic root replacement using an aortic homograft. They are generally not performed in conjunction with the Ross procedure (see below).

Cardiopulmonary bypass setup: The Manougian and Nicks procedures are generally performed with ascending aortic cannulation, a single venous cannula in the right atrium and with a left ventricular vent inserted through the right superior pulmonary vein. Mild or moderate hypothermia is employed with standard cardioplegia arrest.

Nicks procedure

A standard reverse hockey stick incision is made extending the incision inferiorly towards the area between the left/non-commissure and the base of the noncoronary commissure. The membranous septum should be carefully visualized. It is usually below the more anterior half of the noncoronary sinus. The incision is not carried into the anterior leaflet of the mitral valve but is simply carried into the area of fibrous continuity between the aortic and mitral valves (see Figure 18.1). A collagen impregnated woven Dacron patch is used to supplement the annulus. The aortic valve leaflets are excised and horizontal mattress pledgetted sutures are placed except in the region of the patch where they are passed through the patch. Inverting sutures placed below the prosthesis allow a larger prosthesis to be placed relative to everting sutures placed above the prosthesis. Another option is to place all sutures from outside the aorta with care to avoid compromise of the coronaries.[39] The valve may be tilted slightly so that sutures are placed more distally on the Dacron patch than they are in the right and left coronary sinuses. We generally place a standard tilting disk (St Jude) valve with a standard sewing ring though the Regent rotatable model may be preferred. A number of alternative bileaflet carbon valves are available. The heart is de-aired in the usual fashion and when rewarming is completed discontinuation of bypass should be routine.

Manougian procedure

The incision is as for the Nicks procedure but is extended across the intervalvular fibrosa into the anterior leaflet of the mitral valve (see Figure 18.1). The roof of the left atrium is therefore entered. However, it can be easily picked up in the supplementing patch suture line and in fact serves a useful function in pledgetting the suture line. The Manougian procedure can be performed in conjunction with homograft replacement of the aortic root. In these circumstances the annulus is supplemented by the mitral valve component of the homograft. Great care should be taken in suturing the patient's mitral valve to the homograft mitral valve as breakdown in this area will result in mitral regurgitation. Consideration should be given to using Prolene sutures pledgetted with pericardium to buttress this suture line. If a prosthetic valve replacement is performed rather than a homograft root replacement it is probably best to use autologous pericardium treated with glutaraldehyde to close the defect in the mitral valve and to enlarge the aortic annulus and aortic root.

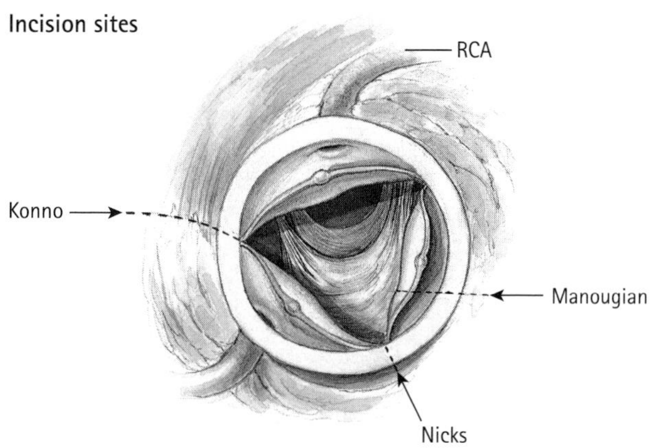

Figure 18.1 *The aortic annulus can be enlarged posteriorly by either a Nicks or Manougian incision. Anteriorly the annulus can be enlarged with a Konno incision which extends between the right and left coronary cusps of the aortic valve. If the subaortic area is to be enlarged the Konno incision is extended into the ventricular septum.*

Extended aortic root replacement with aortic homograft[40]

The cardiopulmonary bypass setup is as for the Nicks procedure. The aortic root and aortic valve leaflets are excised. The coronary arteries are mobilized on buttons of aortic wall. After extending the incision in the noncoronary sinus into the middle of the anterior leaflet of the mitral valve, the now enlarged aortic annulus is sized and an appropriate aortic homograft is selected. The mitral leaflet of the homograft is trimmed appropriately and is sutured into the patient's anterior leaflet of the mitral valve with fine Prolene sutures pledgetted with pericardium. The base of the homograft is now sutured to the supplemented aortic annulus using continuous 4/0 Prolene. A number of interrupted pledgetted horizontal mattress sutures are used as a second supporting row particularly across the muscular septal component of the homograft. Because the homograft is placed in the orthotopic position it is usually possible to excise the homograft left coronary artery origin and to reimplant the patient's left coronary button into this area using continuous 5/0 Prolene. Great care is taken to ensure that the suture line is meticulously constructed. Additional sutures should be placed as necessary as hemostasis in this area will be difficult when the procedure is completed. The distal ascending aortic anastomosis is fashioned after a marking suture has been placed externally to indicate the top of the anterior commissure of the homograft aortic valve. The root is distended with cardioplegia and the appropriate site for reimplantation of the right coronary artery is selected. Care is taken when excising this button to avoid injuring the homograft aortic valve, the location of which is indicated by the marking suture.

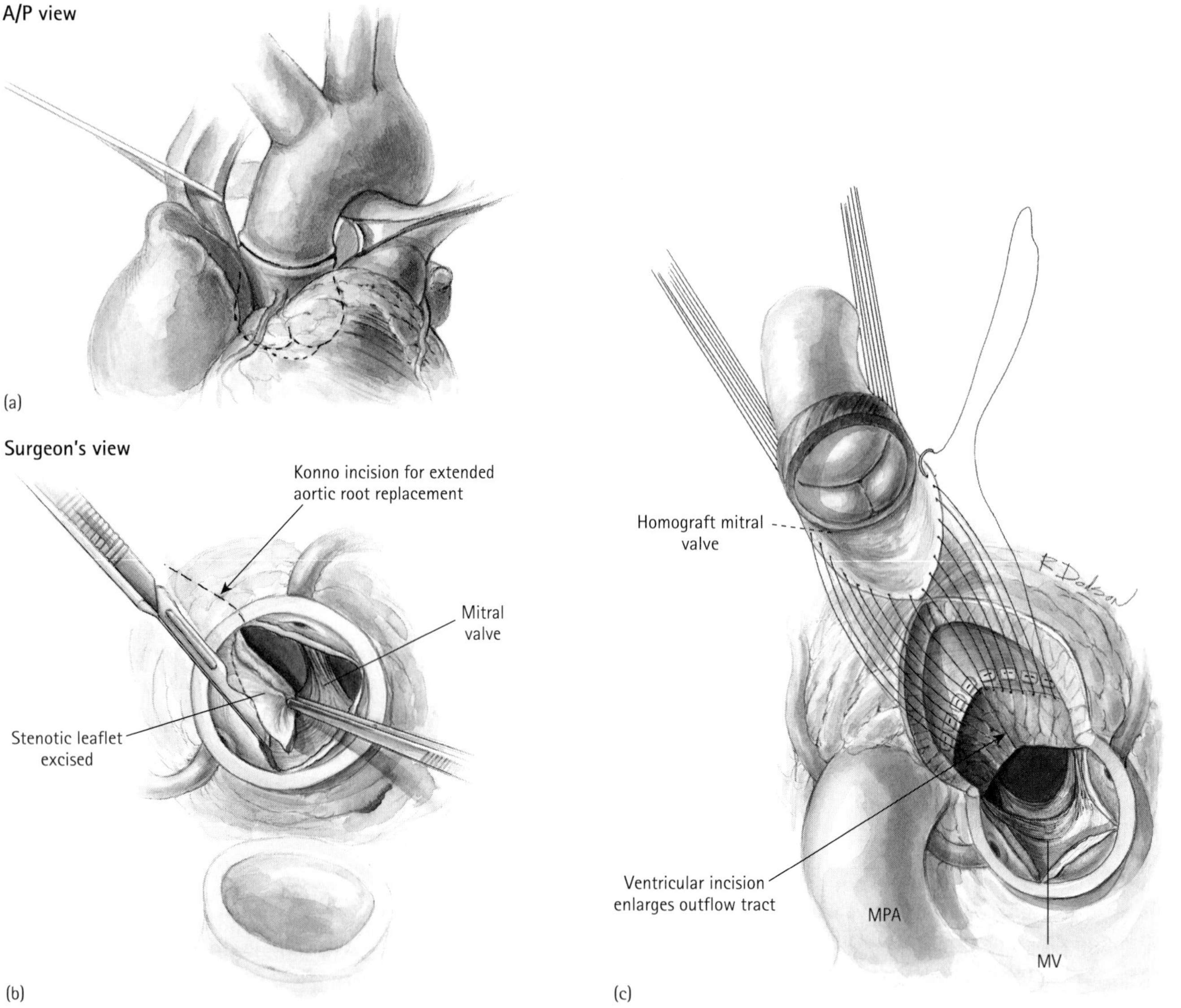

Figure 18.2 *Extended aortic root replacement with aortic homograft with Konno incision. (a) The ascending aorta is transected above the level of the sinotubular junction. (b) The stenotic aortic valve leaflets are excised. If the aortic annulus is to be enlarged a Konno type incision is made between the right and left coronary leaflets extending into the ventricular septum. (c) An aortic homograft is placed as a root replacement using the homograft mitral valve to supplement the annulus.*

ANTERIOR ENLARGEMENT OF THE AORTIC ANNULUS

When aortic annular hypoplasia is more severe the Konno procedure should be selected. The Konno procedure was originally described to allow insertion of an adequate size prosthetic aortic valve. The procedure carries significant disadvantages and risks in children including the need for permanent anticoagulation, a risk of paravalvar leak with associated hemolysis as well as a risk of projection of the rigid mechanical valve into the right ventricular outflow tract. For these reasons we avoided the classic Konno procedure for many years preferring a homograft root replacement with Konno (Figure 18.2) or the Ross/Konno procedure, i.e. replacement of the aortic valve with a pulmonary autograft in conjunction with anterior enlargement of the aortic annulus (see below). However, longer term follow-up of patients after homograft root replacement and after the Ross procedure when this is performed as a root replacement has caused us to reconsider use of the classic Konno procedure. Disadvantages of the Ross/Konno procedure include a need for lifelong homograft conduit changes in the right ventricular outflow tract, a risk of neoaortic root dilation with attendant neoaortic valve regurgitation as well as a risk of aneurysm formation of the subaortic patch. The principal disadvantages of aortic homograft root replacement are early calcification and valve failure.

Cardiopulmonary bypass setup: Two straight caval cannulas with caval tapes are employed with arterial cannulation of the ascending aorta. A left ventricular vent is inserted through the right superior pulmonary vein. Hypothermia down to at least 25°C is employed. Multiple infusions of cardioplegia are given throughout this relatively lengthy procedure.

Ross/Konno procedure

Excision of the aortic root: The aortic root and aortic valve are completely excised in the manner of an extended aortic root replacement. The coronary arteries are mobilized with generous buttons of aortic wall attached. The pulmonary autograft is harvested before the Konno septal incision is made (Figure 18.3a).

Harvesting the pulmonary autograft: It is important for the surgeon to understand that the incision used to harvest the autograft is different from the incision used to enlarge the left ventricular outflow tract. It is the support of the pulmonary valve by a ring of muscle, the subpulmonary conus, that makes the autograft procedure possible. The subpulmonary conus that is divided to harvest the autograft is subsequently used as the sewing ring to implant the pulmonary root (Figure 18.3b). The main pulmonary artery is divided just proximal to its bifurcation. The pulmonary valve is examined to be sure that it is suitable for the procedure. A right angle instrument is passed down through the valve and acts as a guide for the initial incision in the anterior wall of the infundibulum of the right ventricle. Failure to do this can result in placing the incision too close to the pulmonary valve. Consideration should be given to harvesting a little more infundibulum than for a standard Ross procedure if a Konno procedure is to be added as well. The autograft is now harvested with particular care being taken at the leftward extent of the incision which is always very close to the first septal perforator branch of the left anterior descending coronary artery. As a result, it is very common to expose the first septal perforator. We generally excise this portion of the autograft last after careful posterior mobilization with visualization of the left main coronary and its bifurcation. If the septal perforator is injured it is very important that it be repaired or at least oversewn. Failure to repair an injured perforator is likely to result in a steal of blood from the entire left coronary system. This has potential to cause considerably more ischemic injury than would be expected from injury to the perforator alone. The autograft is stored in a bowl which is clearly marked and separated from the pulmonary homograft which should be undergoing thawing and rinsing at this stage.

Konno incision: The aortic annulus is enlarged by incising the left ventricular outflow tract in a leftward direction rather than towards the apex. This will keep the incision well above the conduction area. The incision should not be extended too far into the anterior trabeculated ventricular septum as this will complicate closure of this end of the incision.

Insertion of pulmonary autograft: The pulmonary autograft is sutured into the aortic annulus and ventricular septal incision (Figure 18.3c). If necessary a triangular patch of Gortex can be used to close the Konno incision. In general, however, the pulmonary annulus is quite a bit larger than the aortic annulus and in conjunction with a small amount of supplementary infundibular muscle is adequate for closure of the entire outflow tract without a patch. It is important that the autograft be sutured to the Konno incision with interrupted pledgetted sutures with a second row of supporting sutures as needed to ensure that no VSD is created. The remainder of the procedure continues as for an extended aortic root replacement. The left coronary button is implanted. At this point an appropriate sized pulmonary homograft is anastomosed distally to the pulmonary bifurcation area. The ascending aortic anastomosis is performed subsequently (Figure 18.3d) followed by reimplantation of the right coronary artery. The pulmonary homograft is anastomosed proximally to the right ventricular outflow tract, usually with continuous 4/0 Prolene. Because this suture line passes very close to the left main coronary artery and the left anterior descending coronary artery most of this anastomosis should be performed with the aortic cross clamp still in place (Figure 18.3e). Towards the end of the suture line the left heart is allowed to fill with blood and air is vented through a site in the ascending aorta. The aortic cross clamp is released with the aortic vent site bleeding freely. During warming the usual monitoring lines are placed. It is a reasonable precaution to use TEE or to place a pulmonary artery monitoring line to check for any left to right shunt at the ventricular level. This will occur if there is breakdown of the suture line between the ventricular septum and the pulmonary autograft.

Classic Konno procedure

The classic Konno procedure contains many of the same elements as the Ross Konno procedure.[41] In the younger child a patch of glutaraldehyde treated autologous pericardium or in the older child Hemashield Dacron is used to enlarge the subaortic region and the aortic annulus as well as the aortic root. A second patch of pericardium is used to close the infundibular incision. The two junctions of points between the septal patch, the infundibular patch, the infundibular incision and the septal incision are two critical areas that must be carefully reinforced. Great care should be taken not to oversize the mechanical prosthesis. This can result in excessive projection into the right ventricular outflow tract necessitating a transannular patch. More importantly an oversized valve will cause distortion of the coronary arteries and may result in coronary ischemia.

COMBINED ANTERIOR AND POSTERIOR ANNULAR ENLARGEMENT WITH MECHANICAL VALVE REPLACEMENT

Enlargement of the aortic annulus both anteriorly and posteriorly allows for a more symmetrical enlargement and is less likely to cause coronary artery distortion or distortion of the right ventricular outflow tract. The procedure involves elements of both the Manougian and Konno procedures with patches placed anteriorly and posteriorly that are more modest in their width relative to what might otherwise be necessary.

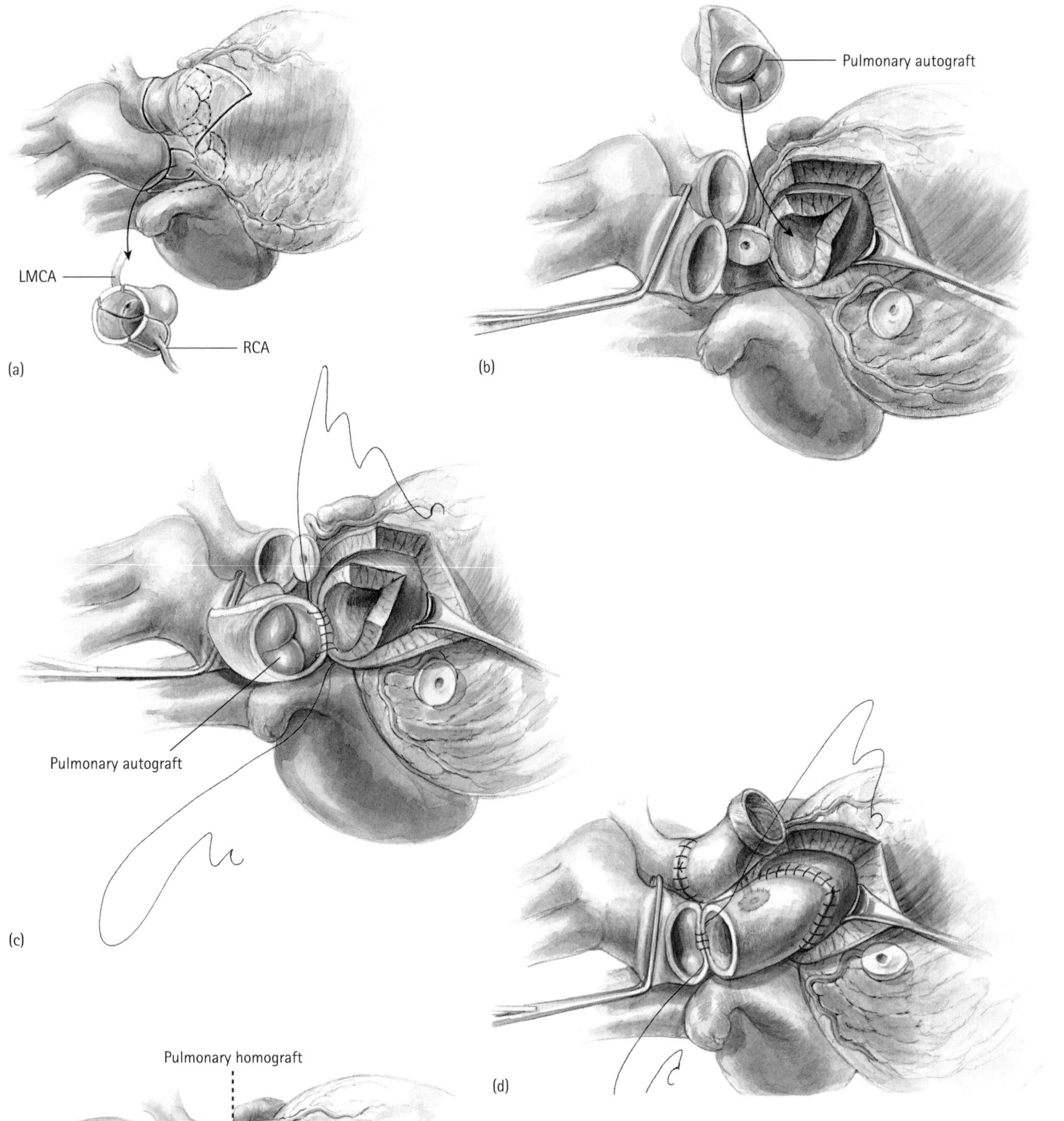

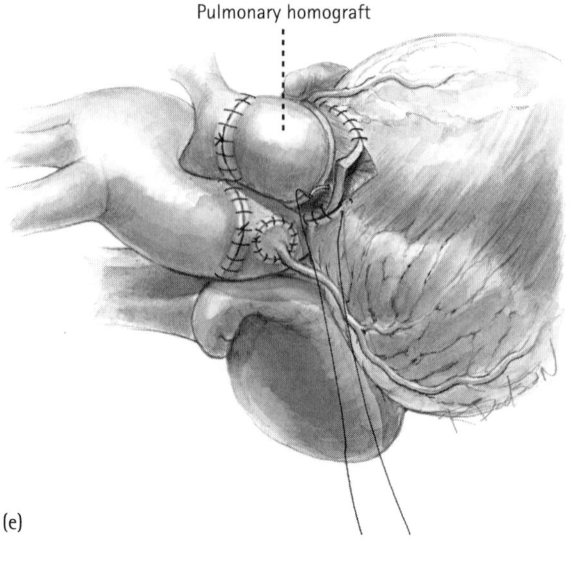

Figure 18.3 *Ross/Konno procedure. (a) The aortic root and aortic valve are completely excised. The coronary arteries are mobilized with generous buttons of aortic wall attached. The pulmonary autograft is harvested. (b) An incision has been made in the ventricular septum thereby opening the subaortic area and aortic annulus as described by Konno. (c) The pulmonary autograft is sutured to the base of the left ventricle using a continuous 4/0 Prolene suture reinforced externally with pledgetted interrupted sutures. (d) The left coronary artery has been implanted. The distal pulmonary homograft anastomosis has been fashioned to begin reconstruction of the right ventricular outflow tract. The distal aortic anastomosis is fashioned before reimplantation of the right coronary artery. (e) The right coronary artery has been implanted following distention of the aortic root with cardioplegia to obtain the site for reimplantation. The proximal anastomosis of the pulmonary homograft to the right ventricular infundibulum is undertaken.*

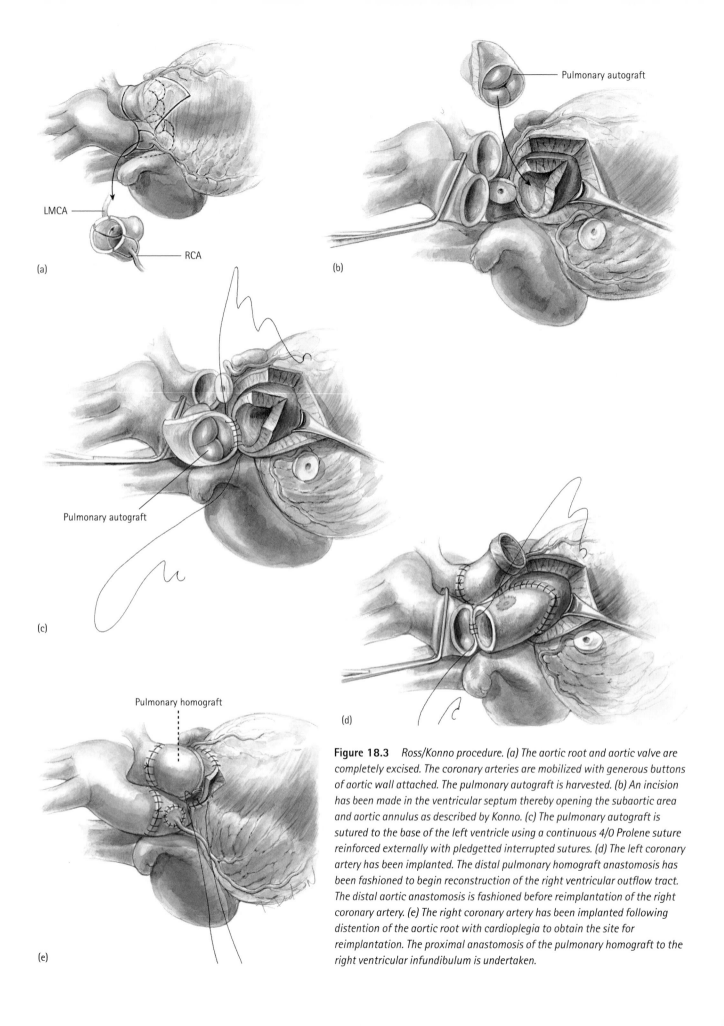

It is helpful to bring valve sutures from outside of the aortic wall so that pledgets lie externally. This allows for maximal use of the available internal circumference. The coronary arteries must be carefully assessed as to their height above the annulus. If the coronary ostia are placed relatively low great care must be taken in using supra-annular valve models such as the St Jude 'Hemodynamic Plus' or St Jude 'Regent' which project above the true annulus and can impinge upon the coronary ostia.

RESULTS OF SURGERY

Manougian procedure

A number of retrospective reviews have documented the effectiveness of the Manougian procedure in enlarging the aortic annulus.[42–44] The most common complication reported has been mitral regurgitation which ranged in frequency from 0% to 14%.

Classic Konno procedure

The largest series of classic Konno procedures has been reported from Tokyo Women's Medical College where the procedure originated.[41] Sixty patients have undergone a Konno procedure including mechanical valve replacement between 1984 and 2000. Mean age was 12 years. There were no hospital deaths and five late deaths. Freedom from reoperation for the mechanical valve was 80% at 10 years and 52% at 15 years.

Ross/Konno procedure

Katzuko and Spray have described the results of the Ross/Konno procedure at Children's Hospital of Philadelphia in 2002.[45] There was one death among 17 patients who underwent a Ross/Konno procedure between 1995 and 1998. Median age of patients was seven years. The most common morbidity was arrhythmia which occurred in 64% of the patients. However, none of the patients developed complete heart block. Other reports have described similar results.[46,47]

SUBAORTIC STENOSIS

INTRODUCTION

Subaortic stenosis can take a number of different forms. There may be a discrete thin subaortic membrane (Figure 18.4) or a long fibromuscular tunnel. There may be functional obstruction due to apposition of the anterior leaflet of the mitral valve against the hypertrophied ventricular septum as is found with the obstructive form of hypertrophic cardiomyopathy (HCM). This lesion is associated with varying degrees of systolic anterior motion of the mitral valve and mitral regurgitation. There may be organic structural subaortic stenosis due to projection of the conal septum into the outflow tract as seen with a posterior malalignment VSD or due to projection of accessory mitral valve tissue into the outflow tract. Decision-making regarding indications for and timing of surgery in these lesions is complicated. The technical aspects of their management also can be challenging.

EMBRYOLOGY AND ANATOMY

Subaortic stenosis may result from simple malseptation of the original common ventricle due to poor alignment of the conal septum with the muscular interventricular septum. If the

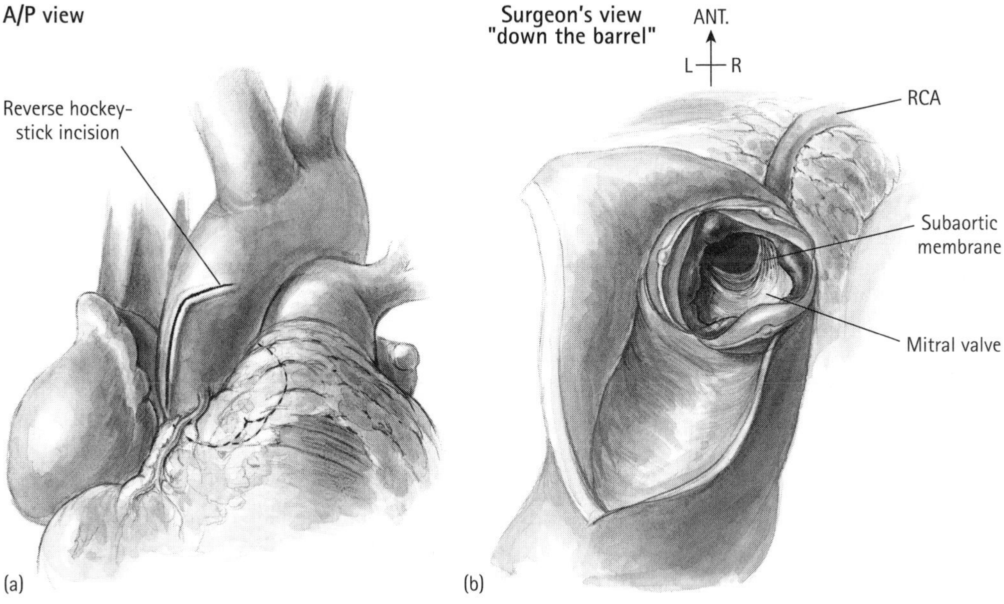

Figure 18.4 *Subaortic membrane. (a) A subaortic membrane is exposed through a reverse hockey stick incision extending into the middle of the noncoronary sinus. (b) A subaortic membrane is usually found a few millimeters below the aortic valve. It often extends onto the ventricular aspect of the anterior leaflet of the mitral valve.*

conal septum projects posteriorly into the left ventricular outflow tract this can result in a posterior malalignment conoventricular VSD. The conal septum itself causes obstruction to left ventricular outflow. Hypertrophic cardiomyopathy (HCM) is defined as left ventricular hypertrophy with a small left ventricular cavity which occurs in the absence of any increase in external load (afterload). Approximately 25% of patients with HCM exhibit left ventricular outflow tract obstruction. The genetic basis for HCM is now well established. It is a disease of sarcomeric proteins. More than 150 mutations in 10 genes each of which encodes a single sarcomeric contractile protein have been identified. Mutations in the genes encoding for three proteins (β-myosin heavy chain, myosin-binding protein C and troponin T) account for 70–80% of all cases of familial HCM. Familial HCM is inherited as an autosomal dominant disease with equal frequency in males and females.[48]

A discrete subaortic membrane is not a congenital lesion in the true sense of the term 'congenital'. It is thought to develop as the result of turbulence in an abnormally shaped left ventricular outflow tract. In these patients it has been demonstrated echocardiographically that the angle between the long axis of the left ventricle and the aorta is more acute than usual.[49] Turbulence in the left ventricular outflow tract causes endocardial injury and subsequent proliferation and fibrosis.[50,51] The membrane which results creates more turbulence and further perpetuates the process of injury and fibrosis. The turbulence can also cause injury to the aortic valve leaflets. The subsequent thickening and distortion can cause failure of leaflet coaption or frank prolapse resulting in aortic insufficiency.[52] In some instances the fibrous membrane may extend onto the undersurface of the aortic valve leaflets causing further distortion and worsening regurgitation. Tunnel-like subaortic stenosis is often a secondary lesion that is seen following earlier resection of a simple subaortic membrane. Scarring from the initial resection in conjunction with an abnormally shaped left ventricular outflow tract may result in progressive fibromuscular proliferation and the creation of a left ventricular outflow tract tunnel. The mitral valve also often contributes to the tunnel by being drawn anteriorly by contraction of fibrous bands which extend from the septum on to the ventricular surface of the anterior leaflet.

Rare causes of subaortic stenosis include septal chordal attachments of the mitral valve as well as accessory endocardial tissue which is attached to the ventricular surface of the anterior leaflet of the mitral valve and which billows into the outflow tract during systole. Both these forms of obstruction are more common in the setting of associated heart disease such as partial atrioventricular canal defect or l-loop (congenitally corrected) transposition.

PATHOPHYSIOLOGY

Subaortic stenosis results in a pressure load for the left ventricle which results in secondary ventricular concentric hypertrophy. In cases of severe concentric hypertrophy failure of coronary arterial bed neovascularization to keep pace with muscular hypertrophy will result in subendocardial ischemia and a predisposition to sudden death from ventricular fibrillation. In the obstructive form of HCM several factors combine to create a late peaking dynamic left outflow tract obstruction which results from contact of the anterior mitral valve leaflet with the ventricular septum. Patients with the obstructive form of HCM have an anatomic narrowing of the left ventricular outflow tract in the area between the ventricular septum and the anterior mitral valve leaflet. Anterior and central displacement of the papillary muscles, basal septal hypertrophy, and an elongated anterior mitral valve all contribute to narrowing of the left ventricular outflow tract (LVOT). In addition there is dynamic obstruction related to a variable degree of displacement of the anterior mitral valve leaflet into this narrowed area. This is known as systolic anterior motion of the mitral valve. The Venturi mechanism whereby accelerated flow over the anterior leaflet of the mitral valve lifts the anterior leaflet into the LVOT has been implicated in initiating the dynamic component of LVOT. However, the Venturi mechanism can not explain the systolic anterior motion occurring at the onset of systole when outflow velocities are low. It may however contribute to further motion in late systole. The anterior displacement of the papillary muscles produces chordal laxity in the anterior leaflet. This in combination with an abnormally long anterior leaflet is felt to be the initiating factor in systolic anterior motion and LVOT. The mitral insufficiency which accompanies obstructive HCM is the result of the coaptation point of the anterior and posterior leaflets moving from the tips to the body of the leaflets. The result is a posterior, laterally directed mitral regurgitation jet.

CLINICAL FEATURES

It is rare that subaortic stenosis is allowed to progress to the point where it becomes symptomatic. When it is very severe, obstruction can lead to exercise intolerance and angina. Syncope may also occur particularly in the setting of hypertrophic obstructive cardiomyopathy. Unfortunately sudden unheralded cardiac arrest resulting in death may be the first symptom that is encountered.

DIAGNOSTIC STUDIES

Unless obstruction is particularly severe the chest X-ray is not likely to demonstrate cardiomegaly. The ECG will show evidence of left ventricular hypertrophy when this is present. Echocardiography is usually diagnostic. It is particularly important to assess the competence of the aortic valve as new onset of aortic regurgitation is generally accepted as an indication for surgery. The Doppler-derived gradient across the outflow tract must also be assessed together with the degree of left ventricular hypertrophy. Cardiac catheterization is usually not helpful in the decision making regarding need for surgery.

MEDICAL AND INTERVENTIONAL THERAPY

It is unusual to allow subaortic obstruction to progress to the point where medical therapy for pulmonary congestion secondary to left atrial hypertension is necessary. Attempts to manage subaortic obstructive lesions with balloon dilation and/or stent placement have met with limited success. Short-term improvement may be possible but there is a risk of complete heart block and aortic valve damage.

INDICATIONS FOR AND TIMING OF SURGERY

Discrete subaortic membrane

Indications for removal of a thin discrete subaortic membrane remain unclear. Since this is usually a progressive lesion which may ultimately cause aortic regurgitation, some have argued that the mere presence of such a membrane is an indication for its removal.[53] Others require a relatively low pressure gradient such as 20 mmHg[54,55] while some argue for higher gradients such as 40–50 mmHg.[56] Most groups accept the fact that the onset of new aortic regurgitation is an important factor influencing the decision to proceed with surgery.

The risk of recurrence is not low and is higher in children under 10 years of age.[57] This has led some to recommend that where possible surgery should be deferred beyond 10 years of age. In general our own approach at present in a child less than 5–10 years of age with a thin discrete membrane and a peak Doppler gradient of less than 40–50 mmHg is to follow the membrane with regular (e.g. six month) echocardiographic evaluations. The onset of new aortic regurgitation, an increasing gradient across the outflow tract, or worsening left ventricular hypertrophy are generally accepted as indications to proceed with membrane removal.

Tunnel subaortic stenosis

Because this lesion must be dealt with by a more aggressive surgical procedure than simple removal of a subaortic membrane, we generally require a higher pressure gradient, moderate or severe left ventricular hypertrophy or the onset of new aortic regurgitation in order to recommend surgery. A peak Doppler gradient that is consistently greater than 50–60 mmHg is generally accepted as an indication to proceed with surgery.[58]

Obstructive hypertrophic cardiomyopathy

Many studies have demonstrated that a surgical myectomy procedure for the obstructive form of HCM is not associated with a reduced long-term mortality risk even with relief of an extremely high gradient.[59,60] In general therefore we reserve surgical intervention for children who have been symptomatic, usually with syncope, angina or exercise limitation.

Structural subaortic stenosis

Discrete projection of the conal septum into the left ventricular outflow tract can generally be dealt with quite successfully surgically. This is also true for projection of accessory mitral tissue causing a parachute-like effect on the ventricular aspect of the anterior leaflet of the mitral valve. As a result, there should be a low threshold for surgical intervention. A peak gradient of 30–40 mmHg, particularly if there has been progression in the severity of the gradient is sufficient indication for surgical intervention. Once again, the onset of new aortic regurgitation should be considered an absolute indication to proceed with surgery.

SURGICAL MANAGEMENT

Historical perspective

In 1956, Brock reported the surgical relief of subaortic membranous stenosis using closed transventricular dilatation.[61] This was followed by Spencer's report of surgical management using cardiopulmonary bypass in 1960.[62] Diffuse subaortic stenosis associated with aortic annular hypoplasia was addressed by Konno and coworkers in 1975.[28] Clarke and associates reported the use of aortic root replacement combined with ventricular septoplasty, using a valved aortic allograft with coronary transfer, for diffuse subaortic stenosis in infants.[63] Cooley introduced ventricular septoplasty with preservation of the native aortic valve in 1986.[64]

Technical considerations

DISCRETE SUBAORTIC MEMBRANE

Cardiopulmonary bypass method

We generally use a single venous cannula in the right atrium and arterial cannulation of the ascending aorta. The aorta is cross clamped and cardioplegia solution is infused into the aortic root in the routine fashion.

Exposure of membrane

A reverse hockey stick incision is carried into the noncoronary sinus of the aortic root (Figure 18.3a). A left ventricular vent may be inserted through the right superior pulmonary vein but usually this is not necessary. A nasal speculum is often useful to expose the subaortic region and also helps to protect the aortic valve leaflets. Alternatively an appropriate width malleable ribbon retractor is passed through the aortic valve. The membrane is carefully assessed, with particular attention to its relationship to the aortic valve leaflets. In more advanced cases fibrous tissue will extend onto the undersurface of one or more cusps of the aortic valve. The fibrous tissue may also extend onto the ventricular aspect of the anterior leaflet of the mitral valve. Very careful note is made of the relationship of the membrane to the membranous septum which is usually under the anterior half of the noncoronary cusp (Figure 18.3b). It is often useful to begin dissection of the membrane by making a radial incision into the membrane under the intercoronary commissure. At this point the membrane is furthest from the valve leaflet tissue and this area is safe with respect to injury to the mitral valve or the conduction system. Often it is useful to stabilize the membrane with a skin hook while the incision is being made. Using a Penfield dissector the membrane is now separated from the underlying endocardium by blunt dissection. It usually will shell out without too much difficulty. If the tissue extending onto the aortic valve begins to separate from the valve it is usually wise to complete the separation by sharp dissection. At all times great care must be taken in introducing instruments into the subaortic region such that no damage is done to the aortic valve leaflets. The membrane is separated from the ventricular surface of the anterior leaflet of the mitral valve. If there is fibrous tissue that is drawing the mitral valve anteriorly either at its lateral or medial edge it should be divided to release the mitral valve as has been emphasized by Yacoub.[65] It is important to look for evidence of a secondary membrane which may lie a few millimeters below the primary membrane.

Supplementary myectomy

Another unresolved issue in the management of simple subaortic membrane is the need for remodeling of the left ventricular outflow tract by a myectomy (often mislabeled myomectomy: this refers to resection of a myoma) procedure at the time of membrane removal. Some centers argue that myectomy reduces turbulence in the outflow tract by enlarging and reshaping the outflow tract.[66,67] These centers often recommend that a myectomy be undertaken in all patients who have developed a discrete membrane. On the other hand it can be argued that the resulting scarring can increase the risk of recurrent left ventricular outflow tract obstruction. In our practice we often excise a wedge of muscle under the intercoronary commissure with the excision extending under the left half of the right coronary cusp. Great care should be taken to avoid an excessively deep incision which can result in the creation of an iatrogenic VSD. Great care should also be taken to avoid resecting septal muscle under the right half of the right coronary leaflet and particularly under the anterior half of the noncoronary leaflet as this can result in complete heart block.

Discontinuation of bypass

Following routine closure of the aortotomy and exclusion of air, removal of the cross clamp and rewarming to normothermia the patient is separated from bypass. Intraoperative transesophageal echocardiography is useful in assessing the competence of the aortic valve as well as the adequacy of the resection. However, great care should be taken in interpreting any residual Doppler-derived gradient in the immediate post-bypass period. The gradient derived in a high output state secondary to early post-bypass hyperdynamic contraction and anemia will overestimate the severity of the residual obstruction and underestimate the area of the LVOT.

TUNNEL SUBAORTIC STENOSIS

Modified Konno procedure

Tunnel-like subaortic stenosis is best managed by the modified Konno procedure[58,65] (Figure 18.5). The alternative procedure of aggressive resection of subaortic fibrous tissue and muscle carries a considerable risk of complete heart block as well as creation of an iatrogenic VSD. In contrast, the modified Konno procedure has been demonstrated to carry a remarkably low risk of complete heart block.[68]

Cardiopulmonary bypass technique

Two straight caval cannulas with caval tapes are employed together with arterial cannulation of the ascending aorta. A left ventricular vent is inserted through the right superior pulmonary vein. Moderate hypothermia at 25–28°C is usually appropriate. After aortic cross clamping standard cardioplegic arrest is instituted.

Approach

The aorta is opened with a vertical incision which extends towards the intercoronary commissure of the aortic valve. An oblique incision is made in the infundibulum of the right ventricle with this incision also directed towards the intercoronary commissure (Figure 18.5a). The right ventricular aspect of the ventricular septum is exposed. A right angle instrument is passed through the aortic valve. The tip of the instrument is used as a guide for the transmural septal incision (Figure 18.5b). This incision can be challenging because of the extreme thickness of the ventricular septum in this condition. Once the incision has been carried through into the left ventricular outflow tract the right angle instrument is useful in separating the thickened septal edges. Working back and forth between the aortic incision and the septal incision, the septal incision is extended towards the intercoronary commissure of the aortic valve. Ideally the incision is carried superiorly into the intercoronary commissural triangle above the level of the bellies of the cusps of the right and left coronary leaflets. Great care is taken not to injure the valve leaflets. The incision is carried leftward as far as is necessary to get beyond the inferior end of the tunnel. It is important that the incision be carried more leftward than apically in order to avoid injury to the conduction bundle. It is also important that the right ventricular aspect of the incision not be carried into the trabeculated anterior muscular septum. Undermining the inferior edge places the conduction bundle at risk. The superior edge can be undermined by muscle excision. Accessory fibrous tissue is often present and can also be excised. This tissue may extend onto the anterior leaflet of the mitral valve.

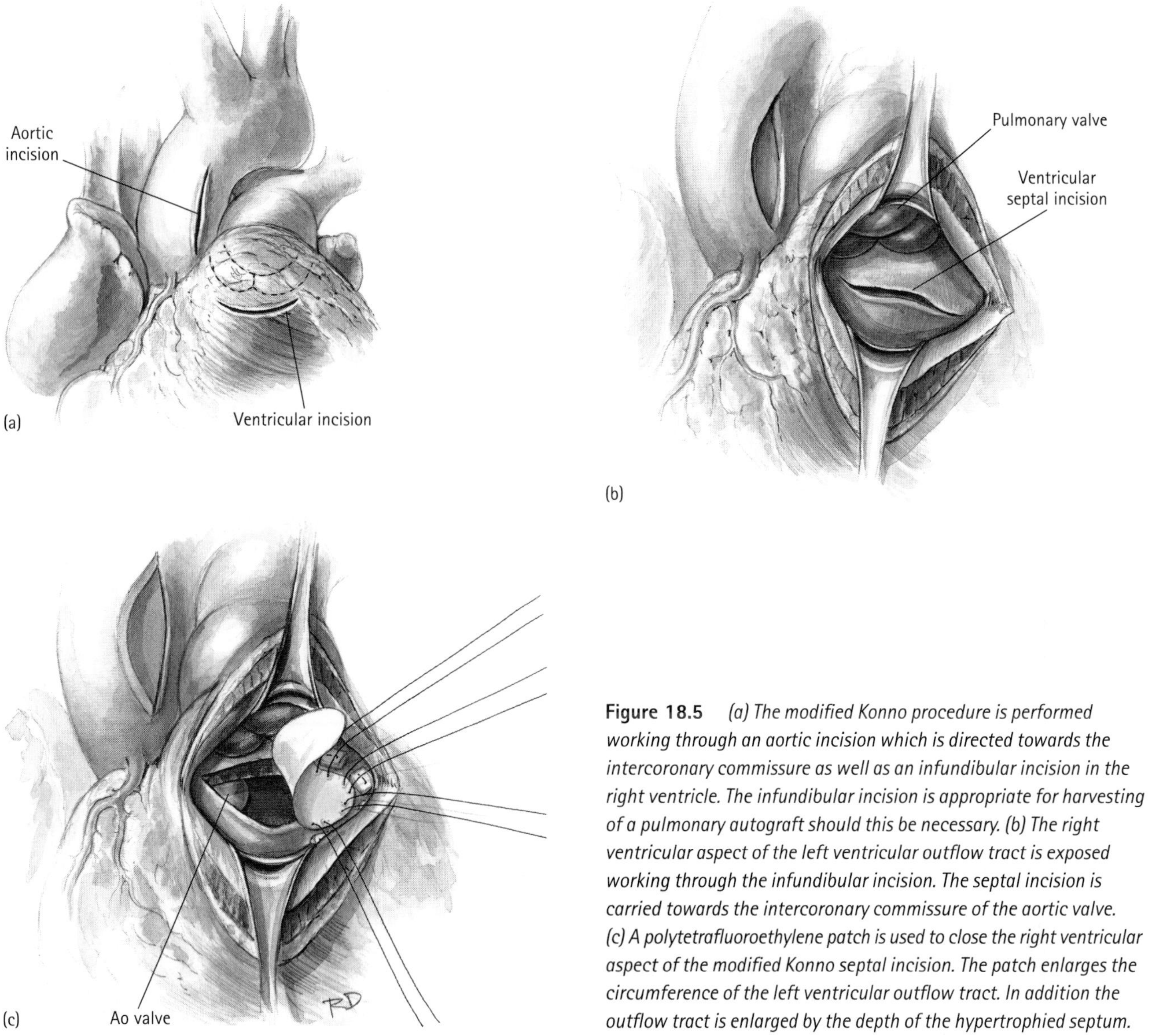

Figure 18.5 *(a) The modified Konno procedure is performed working through an aortic incision which is directed towards the intercoronary commissure as well as an infundibular incision in the right ventricle. The infundibular incision is appropriate for harvesting of a pulmonary autograft should this be necessary. (b) The right ventricular aspect of the left ventricular outflow tract is exposed working through the infundibular incision. The septal incision is carried towards the intercoronary commissure of the aortic valve. (c) A polytetrafluoroethylene patch is used to close the right ventricular aspect of the modified Konno septal incision. The patch enlarges the circumference of the left ventricular outflow tract. In addition the outflow tract is enlarged by the depth of the hypertrophied septum.*

Closure of the septal incision

A polytetrafluoroethylene (PTFE) patch which is square ended is used to close the right ventricular aspect of the septal incision (Figure 18.5c). This results in enlargement of the outflow tract by the thickness of the ventricular septum as well as adding to the circumference of the outflow tract by the width of the PTFE patch. The PTFE patch should be carefully anchored with interrupted pledgetted horizontal mattress sutures with particular care taken at the inferior end of the incision where it may be close to the trabeculated anterior muscular septum.

Closure of the aortic and infundibular incisions

The aortic incision is often supplemented with a patch of glutaraldehyde treated autologous pericardium which is sutured into position using continuous Prolene. The infundibular incision is also closed with autologous pericardium or possibly with a PTFE patch using PTFE suture.

Transaortic valve modification

The reason for using an incision which extends towards the intercoronary commissure is that on occasion it is useful to cut across the aortic annulus and separate the right and left leaflets of the aortic valve. However, this is only advisable when these leaflets are already somewhat thickened and suitable for subsequent supplementation with pericardial leaflet extenders following reconstitution of the annulus.

HYPERTROPHIC OBSTRUCTIVE CARDIOMYOPATHY

Hypertrophic obstructive cardiomyopathy can be managed in a similar fashion to tunnel subaortic stenosis using a modified

Konno approach. We have found that this is more effective than transaortic resection but it should be performed before the ventricular septum has become massively thickened (greater than 3 cm). If only a transaortic valve approach is used it is important that the channel that is cut into the left ventricular aspect of the bulging septum extend very deep beyond the tip of the anterior leaflet of the mitral valve.[69]

RESULTS OF SURGERY

Membranous subaortic stenosis

Lupinetti et al described the results of surgery for membranous subaortic stenosis at the University of Michigan in 1992.[54] Between 1978 and 1990 resection of membrane alone was performed in 16 patients and resection with myectomy was performed in 24 patients. Follow-up was approximately five years. There were no operative or late deaths. Recurrence occurred in 25% of the patients who had resection alone but only in 4% in patients who had an adjunctive myectomy.

In an earlier report from Children' Hospital Boston by Wright et al published in 1983,[57] 83 patients with subaortic stenosis were reviewed. Both this review as well as subsequent experience at Children's Hospital Boston suggest that the risk of recurrent subaortic stenosis is significantly greater in patients operated on before 10 years of age relative to those operated on after 10 years of age.

Tunnel subaortic stenosis

A review was undertaken of 46 patients who underwent surgery for complex and tunnel like subaortic stenosis at Children's Hospital Boston between January 1990 and November 1998.[68] Forty five of the 46 patients had tunnel like subaortic stenosis develop after repair of a primary congenital heart defect. Only one patient presented with de novo tunnel like subaortic stenosis. Fifteen of the 45 patients had previously undergone repair of double outlet right ventricle. The remaining 30 had undergone repair of a variety of defects. The median age at the time of surgery for subaortic stenosis was five years (range 3–10 years). The modified Konno procedure was performed in 15 patients, a classical Konno procedure with aortic valve replacement in three, Ross-Konno procedures in two, and transaortic valve resection in 12 patients. Five patients with double outlet right ventricle underwent replacement of the interventricular baffle and two patients underwent an aortic valve preserving procedure in conjunction with mitral valve replacement.

There were no hospital deaths. None of the patients had an exacerbation of aortic regurgitation and none developed complete heart block. The median follow-up was three years (range one month to 8.5 years). Two patients developed recurrent subaortic stenosis defined as a gradient of 40 mm or greater as diagnosed by transthoracic echocardiography. Freedom from recurrent subaortic stenosis at one, three and five years was 100%, 94% and 86%, respectively.

SUPRAVALVAR AORTIC STENOSIS

INTRODUCTION

Supravalvar aortic stenosis is a rare anomaly in which there is an exaggerated narrowing at the junction of the sinuses of Valsalva with the ascending aorta, i.e. at the sinotubular junction. This anomaly is often part of Williams syndrome[70] and may be associated with generalized hypoplasia of the ascending aorta and more distal arterial tree as well as with stenoses in the pulmonary artery tree. A recent analysis has demonstrated that even in children who have a relatively severe form of supravalvar aortic and pulmonic stenosis the long-term outlook can be quite satisfactory so long as an aggressive approach employing both surgical and interventional catheter procedures is undertaken.[71]

EMBRYOLOGY

Genetic aspects of Williams syndrome

A loss of function mutation of the elastin gene gives rise to this syndrome.[72] The great vessels, which normally have a large elastin content, are less elastic than usual. This exposes these vessels to considerably greater stresses than usual and contributes to progressive thickening and fibrosis of the medial smooth muscle and collagen layer. As the vessel narrows flow is accelerated resulting in increasing sheer stresses on the underlying endothelium. This in turn results in further thickening of the media, much as is seen with the development of pulmonary vascular disease.

ANATOMY

The principal feature of supravalvar aortic stenosis is severe thickening of the sinotubular ridge.[73] A longitudinal section of the ascending aorta extending into the sinuses of Valsalva demonstrates a wedge like projection at the junction of the sinuses of Valsalva with the ascending aorta. This corresponds with the tops of the commissures of the aortic valve. As a result the commissures are progressively drawn more closely together. There is also decreasing clearance between the free edges of the aortic valve leaflets and the sinotubular junction. On occasion the free edges of the aortic valve leaflets almost completely adhere to the sinotubular junction. Interestingly the aortic valve leaflets themselves are usually unaffected other than where they may have adhered to the sinotubular ridge. The coronary ostia may be narrow because of the thickening of the wall of the sinus of Valsalva.[74,75]

In more severe cases of Williams syndrome the entire ascending aorta is very thickened with a narrow lumen. The origins of the arch vessels may also have discrete stenoses. There may be supravalvar narrowing of the main pulmonary artery although this is much less common than aortic supravalvar stenosis. There may be narrowing of the main pulmonary artery extending into the mediastinal branch pulmonary arteries as well as peripheral pulmonary artery stenosis.[76]

PATHOPHYSIOLOGY

Supravalvar aortic stenosis results in left ventricular hypertension and secondary left ventricular hypertrophy. Coronary blood flow can be compromised by restriction of flow into the sinuses of Valsalva and coronary ostia as the result of limited clearance between the sinotubular junction and the right and left coronary cusps of the aortic valve. Further compromise may arise as the result of coronary ostial narrowing. The combination of increased myocardial substrate needs secondary to hypertrophy and restriction of coronary blood flow sets the stage for a high risk of sudden cardiac arrest secondary to ventricular fibrillation.[77] In this setting, cardiac catheterization is a high risk procedure, particularly if there are attempts at direct coronary angiography. In the case of pulmonary artery obstruction or supravalvar pulmonary stenosis there will be right ventricular hypertension and right ventricular hypertrophy. It is rare that this is isolated. Supravalvar pulmonary stenosis usually occurs in association with supravalvar aortic stenosis.

CLINICAL FEATURES

The association of supravalvar aortic stenosis with a distinctive elfin-like facies and mental retardation was first recognized by Dr Jim Lowe, Chief of Cardiology at Green Lane Hospital, Auckland, New Zealand. The syndrome was reported by Dr Lowe, with his colleague Williams as first author, so that the syndrome has come to be known as Williams syndrome.[70]

Only in the very late stages of Williams syndrome are cardiac symptoms likely to occur. As with other forms of severe left ventricular outflow tract obstruction, obstructive symptoms can include syncope, angina and an increased risk of cardiac arrest. Congestive heart failure with cardiomegaly is a late finding. A prominent systolic ejection murmur usually draws attention to the presence of the anomaly if the features of Williams syndrome are not present or have not been recognized.

DIAGNOSTIC STUDIES

The ECG will demonstrate evidence of left ventricular hypertrophy and if coronary flow is limited there may be signs of left ventricular strain. A chest X-ray is usually not helpful. Echocardiography is diagnostic although it may not be able to clarify the presence of more distal arch narrowing including stenoses at the origins of the arch vessels. Cardiac catheterization allows for accurate imaging of the arch vessels and more distal aorta. Great care should be taken in imaging the coronary arteries, particularly if there is a suggestion that coronary flow may be restricted because of adhesion of the valve leaflets to the sinotubular ridge. Magnetic resonance imaging is currently under investigation as a relatively new modality for assessing supravalvar aortic stenosis and may well prove to have all of the advantages of cardiac catheterization without the risk of ventricular fibrillation.

MEDICAL AND INTERVENTIONAL THERAPY

Supravalvar aortic stenosis is not amenable to medical or interventional catheter therapy. Because congestive heart failure is a very late finding, treatment for this entity should not be necessary. Agents to reduce afterload may decrease coronary perfusion and should be avoided. Balloon dilation is not effective therapy for supravalvar aortic or pulmonary stenosis. The only exception to this is peripheral pulmonary artery stenosis or perhaps mediastinal branch pulmonary artery stenosis, which can be treated successfully by balloon dilation with or without stenting.[78,79]

INDICATIONS FOR AND TIMING OF SURGERY

Supravalvar aortic stenosis is probably a progressive lesion in the majority of children and therefore should be treated before left ventricular hypertrophy has become severe. Early treatment will also decrease the risk of acute cardiac arrest and damage to the aortic valve. It may also decrease the probability of progressive coronary ostial stenosis. In general a Doppler-derived gradient of more than 40–50 mmHg in association with definite evidence by two-dimensional imaging of an important narrowing of the sinotubular junction should be an indication to proceed to surgery. If the gradient is less than 30–40 mmHg and there is no evidence of left ventricular hypertrophy it is reasonable to follow the child with regular, e.g. six monthly, echocardiographic evaluations.

If the child has evidence of Williams syndrome and the echocardiogram suggests that the lumen of the ascending aorta is small distally with stenoses extending into the arch vessels then magnetic resonance imaging or cardiac catheterization should be undertaken in order to determine the extent of reconstruction that will be required. Preoperative assessment should also carefully exclude the presence of associated supravalvar pulmonary stenosis or mediastinal branch or peripheral pulmonary artery stenoses.

SURGICAL MANAGEMENT

History

Both McGoon and Starr and their associates independently reported a series of patch enlargement for localized supravalvar aortic stenosis in 1961.[80,81] In 1976, Keane and coworkers reported a series of 18 patients who underwent operation at Children's Hospital Boston with the first procedure performed in 1956.[82] A major conceptual and therapeutic advance was made in 1976 when Doty and colleagues described the extended aortoplasty technique for this lesion.[83] Both Bernard and Colley and their collaborators each reported a technique for placing valved conduits from the left ventricle to the aorta for treatment of the diffuse form of this lesion in 1975.[84,85] Neither of these techniques is presently recommended. In 1993 Chard and colleagues[86] reported symmetric enlargement of all three aortic sinuses using autologous aortic tissue.

Technical considerations

SIMPLE REPAIR OF ISOLATED SUPRAVALVAR AORTIC STENOSIS OR EXTENDED REPAIR OF ASCENDING AORTA AND ARCH?

A careful assessment must be made preoperatively as to whether the repair should be limited to the area of the sinotubular junction or if a more extensive reconstruction of the ascending aorta and aortic arch is required. If there is obvious narrowing of the ascending aorta it is generally best to err on the side of extending a patch across the undersurface of the aortic arch. Failure to do this will transfer the supravalvar gradient to the distal ascending aorta. By extending a patch at least beyond the takeoff of the arch vessels the cardiac output can be decompressed into the arch vessels though there may still be some residual gradient at the toe of the patch.

COMBINED ASCENDING AND AORTIC ARCH PATCH PLASTY

This procedure should be performed at least in part under deep hypothermic circulatory arrest. The ascending aorta is cannulated on its rightward and superior aspect. A single venous cannula is placed in the right atrium and the patient is cooled to deep hypothermia. The aorta is cross clamped temporarily and cardioplegia solution is infused. With the patient in a slight Trendelenberg position bypass is discontinued. It is generally wise to remove the arterial cannula and the aortic cross clamp. A longitudinal incision is made on the anterior surface of the ascending aorta and is curved onto the lesser curve of the distal ascending aorta and then across the undersurface of the arch to a point just beyond the take off of the left subclavian artery. In smaller children it is appropriate to use a patch of glutaraldehyde treated autologous pericardium, whereas in larger children collagen impregnated woven Dacron is appropriate. The patch is sutured across the undersurface of the arch with a continuous Prolene technique. Once the patch has been placed below the level of aortic cannulation, a small amount of perfusate is run into the arch to allow for de-airing. The aortic cross clamp is applied and the remainder of the procedure is undertaken on continuous bypass. If necessary a left ventricular vent is inserted through the right superior pulmonary vein. Note that we generally avoid placement of tourniquets around the arch vessels because we believe that the risk of creating stenoses or exacerbating stenosis in the arch vessels exceeds the risk of air emboli being introduced during deep hypothermia. A similar practice is now employed in adults undergoing aortic arch reconstruction for atherosclerotic aneurysms under circulatory arrest.

MANAGEMENT OF DISCRETE SUPRAVALVAR AORTIC STENOSIS

A recent review of the experience at Children's Hospital by Stamm et al[71] has demonstrated that a single patch technique in the noncoronary sinus results in a significantly inferior outcome relative to a bifurcated patch or symmetric three patch technique. Therefore we limit use of a single patch extending into the noncoronary sinus to those instances where relief of mild to moderate supravalvar stenosis is being undertaken in conjunction with relief of left ventricular outflow tract obstruction at other levels.

Inverted bifurcated patch

This technique was originally described by Doty[83] and is appropriate for moderate or moderate to severe supravalvar aortic stenosis that does not involve important narrowing of the left coronary sinus of Valsalva (Figure 18.6). With ascending aortic cannulation and a single venous cannula in the right atrium and following the application of the aortic cross clamp and infusion of cardioplegia solution, a longitudinal incision is made on the anterior surface of the proximal ascending aorta. The incision is bifurcated into the middle of the noncoronary sinus as well as into the right coronary sinus to the left of the right coronary ostium and passes through the thickened sinotubular ridge (Figure 18.6a). It is important that the right coronary ostium be carefully visualized and that the incision has adequate clearance from the right coronary ostium to allow subsequent suturing. Following completion of the inverted bifurcated incision the right coronary ostium sits on a small triangle of tissue directly anteriorly. A generous pantaloon shaped patch is now sutured into the two sinuses of Valsalva (Figure 18.6b). It is important to understand that the goal is to create bulging sinuses of Valsalva similar to those seen normally so that the patch should appear quite a bit larger than one would initially anticipate. Interestingly in spite of placing very generous patches in the two anterior sinuses it is rare that sufficient distortion of the

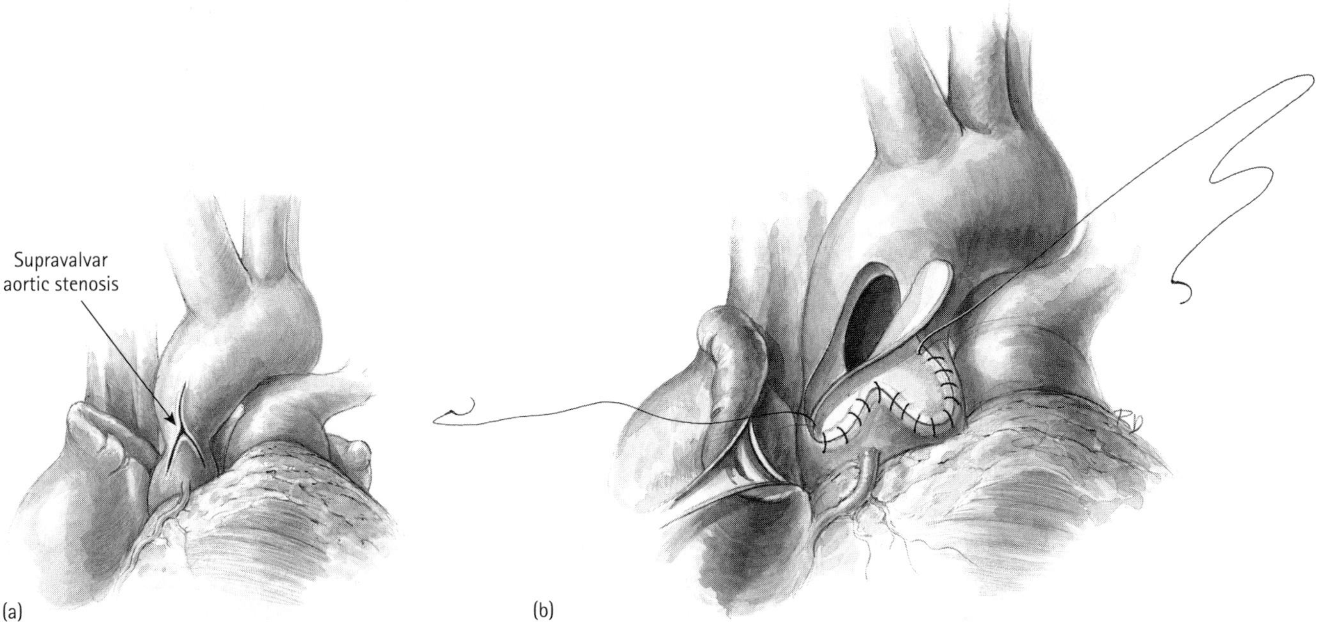

Figure 18.6 *Inverted bifurcated patch plasty repair of moderate supravalvar aortic stenosis. (a) The incision for this procedure begins as a longitudinal incision on the anterior surface of the mid-ascending aorta. The incision bifurcates above the sinotubular junction and extends into the right coronary sinus to the left of the right coronary ostium and into the noncoronary sinus to the right of the right coronary ostium. (b) A generous pantaloon-shaped patch of autologous pericardium is sutured into the two anterior sinuses of Valsalva.*

aortic valve is created that aortic regurgitation ensues. If this procedure is being undertaken in conjunction with patching of the ascending aorta and arch, one patch started in the arch and distal ascending aorta is used. The usual maneuvers are undertaken for de-airing the left heart including allowing an aortic vent site to bleed freely at the time of release of the aortic cross clamp.

Symmetric three patch approach

If there is important narrowing of the left coronary sinus as is often seen with severe forms of supravalvar stenosis, it is generally best to place three independent patches, one in each sinus of Valsalva.[83] Although this can be achieved by advancement of the ascending aorta as described by Chard et al[86] our preference is to use autologous pericardium. We believe that this provides improved compliance in the proximal aorta that can not be achieved with the use of ascending aortic tissue. Three independent teardrop shaped patches (Figure 18.7c) are sutured into three independent incisions that are extended into each of the sinuses of Valsalva following transection of the ascending aorta just distal to the sinotubular junction. Usually the distal ascending aorta is opened longitudinally on its anterior surface over at least half of its length. The anterior two patches are brought together superiorly and anteriorly to supplement this aortotomy.

Cardioplegic protection

It is important to remember that special attention should be focused on cardioplegia protection of the myocardium in view of the severe left ventricular hypertrophy that is often associated with supravalvar aortic stenosis. Regular direct administration of antegrade cardioplegia should be given into the coronary ostia every 20 minutes through the procedure. In general we use a systemic temperature of approximately 25°C for this procedure.

RESULTS OF SURGERY

A recent review described a 41 year experience with 75 patients undergoing operations to treat congenital supravalvar stenosis at Children's Hospital Boston up to 1998.[71] In 34 patients single patch enlargement of the noncoronary sinus was undertaken (almost all early in the series). Other procedures included an inverted bifurcated patch plasty in 35 patients and three sinus reconstruction of the aortic root in six patients. There were seven early deaths. Among early survivors 100% were alive at five years, 96% were alive at 10 years and 77% were alive at 20 years. Diffuse stenosis of the ascending aorta was a risk factor for both death and reoperation ($p < 0.01$ for each). Patients with multiple sinus reconstructions had a significantly lower probability of reoperation. Residual gradients were also lower after multiple sinus reconstruction of the aortic root as was the prevalence of moderate aortic regurgitation at follow-up. The authors concluded from this study that results of surgery for supravalvar aortic stenosis improved greatly after the introduction of more symmetric reconstruction of the aortic root. Multiple sinus reconstruction also resulted in superior hemodynamics and was associated with reductions in both mortality rate and the need for reparation. In 2001 Kang,

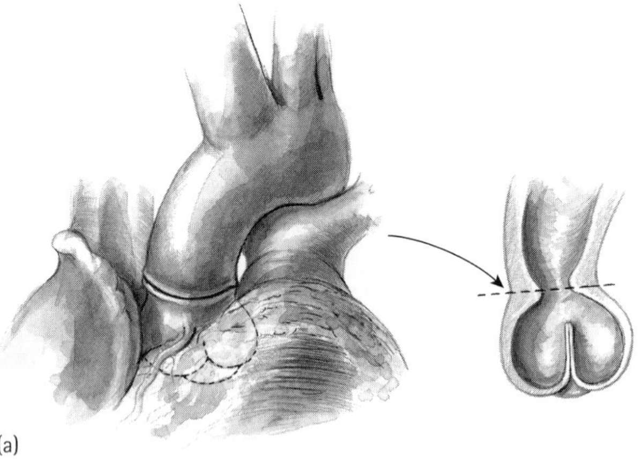
(a)

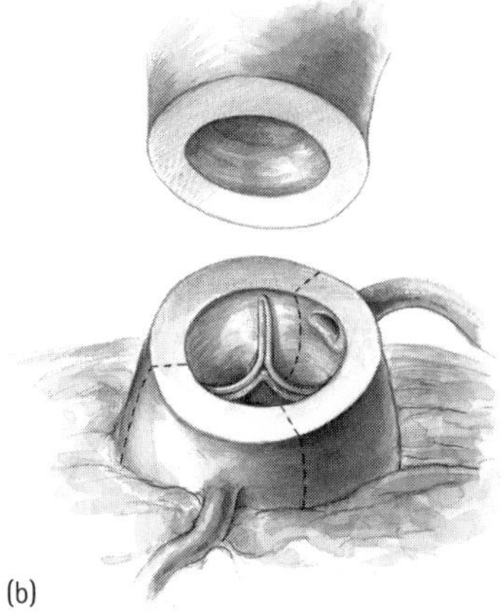
(b)

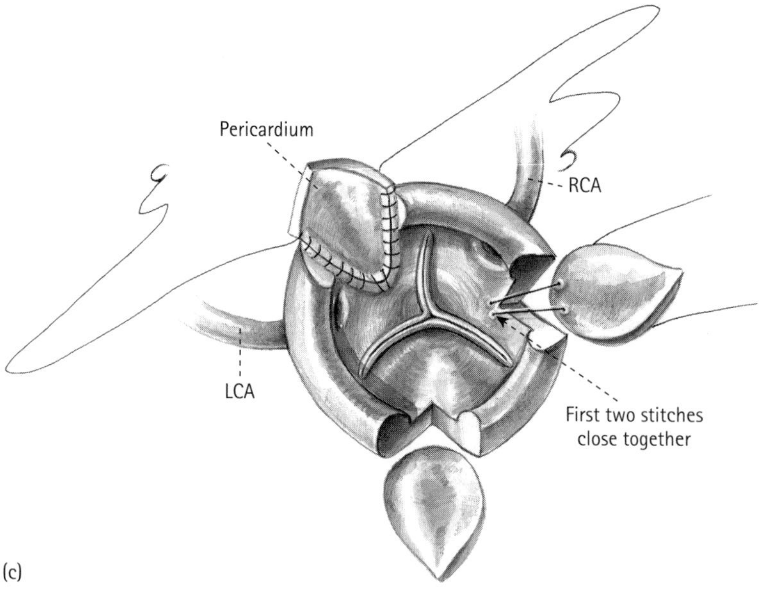

(c)

Figure 18.7 *Symmetric three patch repair of severe supravalvar aortic stenosis. (a) The ascending aorta is transected immediately above the sinotubular junction. (b) Three incisions are carried into each of the sinuses of Valsalva with great care to leave a sufficient margin clear of the coronary ostia. (c) Three independent teardrop-shaped patches of autologous pericardium are used to enlarge each of the sinuses of Valsalva and particularly the region of the sinotubular junction.*

Nunn, Andrews and Chard[87] updated the results of their experience with direct anastomosis repair of supravalvar aortic stenosis. One patient who had had a preoperative gradient of 120 mm and who underwent surgery at six months of age required subsequent surgery for subaortic stenosis. There was no residual gradient at the level of the supravalvar area. Another patient who underwent surgery at 2.5 years of age for a gradient of 100 mm had a residual gradient of 25 mm at age 7.5 years. The authors continue to believe that repair by direct end to end anastomosis is a useful technique in selected cases of discrete supravalvar aortic stenosis.

REFERENCES

1. Roberts WC. The congenitally bicuspid valve: A study of 58 autopsy cases. *Am J Cardiol* 1970; **26**:72–83.
2. Campbell M, Kauntze R. Congenital aortic valvular stenosis. *Br Heart J* 1953; **15**:179–190.
3. Hamilton WJ, Boyd JD, Mossman HW. *Human Embryology.* Cambridge, W Heffer & Sons, 1959, p 178.
4. Markwald R, Eisenberg C, Eisenberg L, Trusk T, Sugi Y. Epithelial-mesenchymal transformation in early avian heart development. *Acta Anat* 1996; **156**:173–186.
5. Stainier DYR, Fouquet B, Chen JN et al. Mutations affecting the formation and function of the cardiovascular system in the zebrafish embryo. *Development* 1996; **123**:285–293.
6. Dobell AR, Bloss RS, Gibbons JE, Collins GF. Congenital valvular aortic stenosis surgical management and long term results. *J Thorac Cardiovasc Surg* 1981; **81**:916–920.
7. Van Praagh R, Bano-Rodrigo A, Smolinsky A, Schuetz TJ, Fyler DC, Van Praagh S. Anatomic variations in congenital valvar, subvalvar and supravalvar aortic stenosis: A study of 64 postmortem cases. In Wells WJ, Lindesmith EE (eds). *Challenges in the Treatment of Congenital Cardiac Anomalies.* Mount Kisco, NY, Futura Publishing Company, 1986, pp 13–41.
8. Cheitlin MD, Fenoglio JJ, McAllister HA, Davia JE, DeCastro CM. Congenital aortic stenosis secondary to dysplasia of congenital bicuspid aortic valves without commissural fusion. *Am J Cardiol* 1978; **42**:102–107.
9. Hastreiter AR, Oshima M, Miller RA, Lev M, Paul MM. Congenital aortic stenosis syndrome in infancy. *Circulation* 1963; **28**:1084–1095.
10. Kirklin JW, Barratt-Boyes BG. *Cardiac Surgery,* 2nd edn. New York, Churchill Livingstone, 1993, p 1196.

11. Lofland GK, McCrindle BW, Williams WG et al. Critical aortic stenosis in the neonate: a multi-institutional study of management, outcomes, and risk factors. Congenital Heart Surgeons Society. *J Thorac Cardiovasc Surg* 2001; **121**:10–27.
12. Rhodes LA, Colan SD, Perry SB, Jonas RA, Sanders SP. Predictors of survival in neonates with critical aortic stenosis. *Circulation* 1991; **84**:2325–2335.
13. Borow KM, Colan SD, Neumann A. Altered left ventricular mechanics in patients with valvular aortic stenosis and coarctation of the aorta: effects on systolic performance and late outcome. *Circulation* 1985; **72**:515–522.
14. Colan SD, Borow KM, Neumann A. Left ventricular end-systolic wall stress-velocity of fiber shortening relation: a load-independent index of myocardial contractility. *J Am Coll Cardiol* 1984; **4**:715–724.
15. Lock JE, Keane JF, Perry SB. *Diagnostic and Interventional Catheterization in Congenital Heart Disease.* Boston, Kluwer Academic Publishers, 2000, p 151.
16. Schwartz ML, Gauvreau K, Geva T. Predictors of outcome of biventricular repair in infants with multiple left heart obstructive lesions *Circulation* 2001; **104**:682–687.
17. Carrel A. On the experimental surgery of the thoracic aorta and the heart. *Ann Surg* 1910; **52**:83.
18. Tuffier T. Etat actuel de la chirugie intrathoracique. *Transactions of the International Congress of Medicine.* London, 1913, section VII *Surgery*, pp 247–327.
19. Larzelere HB, Bailey CP. Aortic commissurotomy. *J Thorac Surg* 1952; **26**:31.
20. Marquis RM, Logan A. Congenital aortic stenosis and its surgical treatment. *Br Heart J* 1955; **17**:373.
21. Lewis FJ, Shumway NE, Niazi SA. Aortic valvulotomy under direct vision during hypothermia. *J Thorac Cardiovasc Surg* 1956; **32**:481.
22. Swan H, Kortz A. Direct vision trans-aortic approach to the aortic valve during hypothermia: Experimental observations and report of a successful clinical case. *Ann Surg* 1956; **144**:205.
23. Lillehei CW, Gott VL, Varco RL. Direct vision correction of calcific aortic stenosis by means of pump-oxygenator and retrograde coronary sinus perfusion. *Dis Chest* 1956; **30**:123.
24. Coran AG, Bernhard WF. The surgical management of valvular aortic stenosis during infancy. *J Thorac Cardiovasc Surg* 1969; **58**:401–408.
25. Nicks R, Cartmill T, Bernstein L. Hypoplasia of the aortic root (The problem of aortic valve replacement). *Thorax* 1970; **25**:339–346.
26. Rastan D. Aortic and aortic-mitral annular enlargement. *J Thorac Cardiovasc Surg* 1995; **109**:818–819.
27. Manouguian S, Kirchhoff PG. Aortic and aortic-mitral annular enlargement. *J Thorac Cardiovasc Surg* 1995; **112**:207.
28. Konno S, Imai Y, Iida Y, Nakajima M, Tatsuno K. A new method for prosthetic valve replacement in congenital aortic stenosis associated with hypoplasia of the aortic valve ring. *J Thorac Cardiovasc Surg* 1975; **70**:909–917.
29. Harken DC, Soroff HS, Taylor WJ, Lefemine AA, Gupta SK, Lunzer S. Partial and complete prostheses in aortic insufficiency. *J Thorac Cardiovasc Surg* 1960; **40**:744.
30. Ross DN. Homograft replacement of the aortic valve. *Lancet* 1962; **2**:487.
31. Barratt-Boyes BG. Homograft aortic valve replacement in aortic incompetence and stenosis. *Thorax* 1964; **19**:131.
32. Ross DN. Replacement of aortic and mitral valve with a pulmonary autograft. *Lancet* 1967; **2**:956.
33. Reddy VN, Rajasinghe HA, Teitel DF et al. Aortoventriculoplasty with the pulmonary autograft: The 'Ross Konno' procedure. *J Thorac Cardiovasc Surg* 1996; **111**:158–167.
34. Lababidi Z, Wu JR, Walls TJ. Percutaneous balloon aortic valvuloplasty: Results in 23 patients. *Am J Cardiol* 1984; **53**:194–197.
35. Rupprath G, Neuhaus KL. Percutaneous balloon valvuloplasty for aortic valve stenosis in infancy. *Am J Cardiol* 1985; **55**:1655–1666.
36. Sanchez GR, Metha AV, Ewing LL, Brickley SE, Anderson TM, Black IF. Successful percutaneous balloon valvuloplasty of the aortic valve in an infant. *Ped Cardiol* 1985; **6**:103–106.
37. Lababidi Z, Weinhaus L. Successful balloon valvuloplasty for neonatal critical aortic stenosis. *Am Heart J* 1986; **112**:913–916.
38. Zeevi B, Keane JF, Castaneda AR, Perry SB, Lock JE. Neonatal critical valvar aortic stenosis. A comparison of surgical and balloon dilation therapy. *Circulation* 1989; **80**:831–839.
39. Eghtesady P, Hanley F. Posterior aortic annular enlargement for mechanical aortic valve replacement. *Op Tech Thorac Cardiovasc Surg* 2002; **7**:181–187.
40. Hopkins RA. Left ventricular outflow tract reconstruction. In Hopkins RA (ed). *Cardiac Reconstructions with Allograft Valves.* New York, Springer-Verlag, 1989, p 131.
41. Kurosawa H. Konno procedure (anterior aortic annular enlargement) for mechanical aortic valve replacement. *Op Tech Thorac Cardiovasc Surg* 2002; **7**:181–187.
42. Kawachi Y, Tominaga R, Tokunaga K. Eleven year followup study of aortic or aortic-mitral annulus enlarging procedure by Manougian's technique. *J Thorac Cardiovasc Surg* 1992; **104**:1259–1263.
43. Sankar NM, Rajan S, Singh RKK, Cherian KM. Enlargement of small aortic annulus by modified Manougian's technique. *Asian Cardiovasc Thorac Ann* 1999; **7**:282–286.
44. Imanaka K, Takamoto S, Furuse A. Mitral regurgitation late after Manougian's annulus enlargement and aortic valve replacement. *J Thorac Cardiovasc Surg* 1998; **115**:727–729.
45. Pastuszko P, Spray TL. The Ross/Konno procedure. *Op Tech Thorac Cardiovasc Surg* 2002; **7**:195–206.
46. Kouchoukos NT, Davila-Roman BG, Spray TL, Murphy SF, Perrillo JB. Replacement of the aortic root with a pulmonary autograft in children and young adults with aortic valve disease. *N Eng J Med* 1994; **330**:1–6.
47. Erez E, Kanter KR, Tam VKH, Williams WH. Konno aortoventriculoplasty in children and adolescents: From prosthetic valves to the Ross operation. *Ann Thorac Surg* 2002; **74**:122–126.
48. Seidman JG, Seidman C. The genetic basis for cardiomyopathy: from mutation identification to mechanistic paradigms. *Cell* 2001; **104**:557–567.
49. Kleinert S, Geva T. Echocardiographic morphometry and geometry of the left ventricular outflow tract in fixed subaortic stenosis. *J Am Coll Cardiol* 1993; **22**:1501–1508.
50. Gewillig M, Daenen W, Dumoulin M, van der Hauwaert L. Rheologic genesis of discrete subvalvar aortic stenosis: A Doppler echocardiographic study. *J Am Coll Cardiol* 1992; **19**:818–824.
51. Cape EG, Vanauker MD, Sigfusson G, Tacy TA, del Nido PJ. Potential role of mechanical stress in the etiology of pediatric heart disease: Septal shear stress in subaortic stenosis. *J Am Coll Cardiol* 1997; **30**:247–254.
52. Newfeld EA, Muster AJ, Paul MH, Idriss RS, Riker WL. Discrete subvalvular aortic stenosis in childhood. Study of 51 patients. *Am J Cardiol* 1976; **38**:53–61.
53. Brauner R, Laks H, Drinkwater DC, Shvarts O, Eghbali K, Galindo A. Benefits of early repair of fixed subaortic stenosis. *J Am Coll Cardiol* 1997; **30**:1835–1842.
54. Lupinetti FM, Pridjian AK, Callow LB, Crowley DC, Beekman RH, Bove EL. Optimum treatment of discrete subaortic stenosis. *Ann Thorac Surg* 1992; **54**:467–471.

55. Coleman DM, Smallhorn JF, McCrindle BW, Williams WG, Freedom RM. Postoperative followup of fibromuscular subaortic stenosis. *J Am Coll Cardiol* 1994; **24**:1558–1564.
56. Rohlicek CV, del Pino SF, Hosking M, Miro J, Cote JM, Finley J. Natural history and surgical outcomes for isolated discrete subaortic stenosis in children. *Heart* 1999; **82**:708–713.
57. Wright GB, Keane JF, Nadas AS, Bernhard WF, Castaneda AR. Fixed subaortic stenosis in the young: Medical and surgical course in 83 patients. *Am J Cardiol* 1983; **52**:830–835.
58. Jonas RA. Modified Konno procedure for tunnel subaortic stenosis. *Op Tech Thorac Cardiovasc Surg* 2002; **7**:176–180.
59. Morrow AG, Koch JP, Maron BJ, Kent KM, Epstein SE. Left ventricular myotomy and myectomy in patients with obstructive hypertrophic cardiomyopathy and previous cardiac arrest. *Am J Cardiol* 1980; **46**:313–316.
60. Mohr R, Schaff HV, Danielson GK, Puga JR, Pluth JR, Tajik AJ. The outcome of surgical treatment of hypertrophic obstructive cardiomyopathy. *J Thorac Cardiovasc Surg* 1989; **97**:666–674.
61. Brock R. Aortic subvalvar stenosis. A report of 5 cases diagnosed during life. *Guys Hosp Rep* 1956; **105**:3491.
62. Spencer FC, Neill CA, Sank L et al. Anatomical variations in 46 patients with congenital aortic stenosis. *Am Surg* 1960; **26**:204.
63. Clarke DR. Extended aortic root replacement for treatment of left ventricular outflow tract obstruction. *J Card Surg* 1987; **2**:121–128.
64. Cooley DA, Garret JT. Septoplasty for left ventricular outflow obstruction without aortic valve replacement. A new technique. *Ann Thorac Surg* 1986; **42**:445–448.
65. Yacoub M, Onuzo O, Riedel B, Radley-Smith R. Mobilization of the left and right fibrous trigones for relief of severe left ventricular outflow obstruction. *J Thorac Cardiovasc Surg* 1999; **117**:126–132.
66. Ohye RG, Devaney EJ, Bove EL. Resection of discrete subaortic membranes. *Op Tech Thorac Cardiovasc Surg* 2002; **7**:172–175.
67. Rayburn ST, Netherland DE, Heath BJ. Discrete membranous subaortic stenosis: improved results after resection and myectomy. *Ann Thorac Surg* 1997; **64**:105–109.
68. Jahangiri M, Nicholson IA, del Nido PJ, Mayer JE, Jonas RA. Surgical management of complex and tunnel like subaortic stenosis. *Eur J Cardiothorac Surg* 2000; **17**:637–642.
69. Dearani JA, Minakata K, Nishimura RA. Extended septal myectomy for hypertrophic obstructive cardiomyopathy with anomalous mitral papillary muscles or chordae. Presented at the 83rd Annual Meeting of the American Association of Thoracic Surgery, Boston, May 7, 2003.
70. Williams JCP, Barratt-Boyes BG, Lowe JB. Supravalvar aortic stenosis. *Circulation* 1961; **24**:1311.
71. Stamm C, Kreutzer C, Zurakowski D et al. Forty-one years of surgical experience with congenital supravalvular aortic stenosis. *J Thorac Cardiovasc Surg* 1999; **118**:874–885.
72. Keating MT. Genetic approaches to cardiovascular disease: supravalvular aortic stenosis, Williams syndrome, and long-QT syndrome. *Circulation* 1995; **92**:142–147.
73. Stamm C, Li J, Ho SY, Redington AN, Anderson RH. The aortic root in supravalvular aortic stenosis: the potential surgical relevance of morphologic findings. *J Thorac Cardiovasc Surg* 1997; **114**:16–24.
74. van Son JA, Edwards WD, Danielson GK. Pathology of coronary arteries, myocardium, and great arteries in supravalvular aortic stenosis. *J Thorac Cardiovasc Surg* 1994; **108**:21–28.
75. Martin MM, Lemmer JH, Shaffer E, Dick M, Bove EL. Obstruction to left coronary artery blood flow secondary to obliteration of the coronary ostium in supravalvular aortic stenosis. *Ann Thorac Surg* 1988; **45**:16–20.
76. Perou ML. Congenital supravalvular aortic stenosis: morphological study with attempt at classification. *Arch Pathol Lab Med* 1961; **71**:453–466.
77. Doty DB, Eastham CL, Hiratzka LF, Wright CB, Marcus ML. Determination of coronary reserve in patients with supravalvular aortic stenosis. *Circulation* 1982; **66**(2 Pt 2):I186–192.
78. Lacro RV, Perry SB, Keane JF, Castaneda AR, Lock JE. Combined transcatheter and surgical therapy for severe bilateral outflow tract obstruction in Williams syndrome and familial supravalvar aortic stenosis. *Circulation* 1995; **92** (Suppl):I587.
79. Stamm C, Friehs I, Moran AM et al. Surgery for bilateral outflow tract obstruction in elastin arteriopathy. *J Thorac Cardiovasc Surg* 2000; **120**:755–763.
80. McGoon DC, Mankin HT, Vlad P et al. The surgical treatment of supravalvular aortic stenosis. *J Thorac Cardiovasc Surg* 1961; **41**:125.
81. Starr A, Dotter C, Griswold H. Supravalvular aortic stenosis: Diagnosis and treatment. *J Thorac Cardiovasc Surg* 1961; **41**:134.
82. Keane JF, Fellow KE, La Farge G, Nadas AS, Bernhard WF. The surgical management of discrete and diffuse supravalvar aortic stenosis. *Circulation* 1976; **54**:112–117.
83. Doty DB, Polansky DB, Jenson CB. Supravalvular aortic stenosis. Repair by extended aortoplasty. *J Thorac Cardiovasc Surg* 1977; **74**:362–371.
84. Bernhard WF, Poirier V, La Farge CG. Relief of congenital obstruction to left ventricular outflow with a ventricular-aortic prosthesis. *J Thorac Cardiovasc Surg* 1975; **69**:223–229.
85. Cooley DA, Norman JC, Mullins CE et al. Left ventricle to abdominal aorta conduit for relief of aortic stenosis. *Cardiovasc Dis* 1975; **2**:376.
86. Chard RB, Cartmill TB. Localized supravalvar aortic stenosis; A new technique for repair. *Ann Thorac Surg* 1993; **55**:782–784.
87. Kang N, Nunn GR, Andrews DR, Chard RB. Localized supravalvar aortic stenosis. A new technique for repair. *Ann Thorac Surg* 2001; **72**:661–662.

19

Hypoplastic left heart syndrome

INTRODUCTION

Hypoplastic left heart syndrome (HLHS) can be defined as an anomaly in which there is normal SDN segmental anatomy but the left heart structures are inadequately developed to support the systemic circulation. Because the right heart is usually normally developed it can be connected surgically to become the single functional systemic ventricle through application of the Norwood procedure.

Over the past two decades children with hypoplastic left heart syndrome have spurred advances in echocardiographic diagnosis, including in-utero diagnosis and intervention; they have presented the paradigm for early postnatal resuscitation of the acidotic neonate with a closing ductus; they have demonstrated that neonates can survive complex nonreparative surgical procedures; they have fundamentally changed the management of all children with a single ventricle pursuing the Fontan pathway through more widespread application of intermediate procedures such as the bidirectional cavopulmonary (Glenn) shunt and the development of the fenestrated Fontan procedure; and they have been the primary focus for the introduction of neonatal heart transplant programs. Finally they have been a stimulus for serious ethical and moral questioning regarding such issues as the use of anencephalic babies as heart donors and the concentration of expensive resources for the benefit of a relatively small number of babies at a time when the overall pool of resources for healthcare appears to be shrinking.

HLHS is not rare. The incidence among patients with congenital heart disease has been reported to be between 4 and 9%.[1–3] In the New England Regional Infant Cardiac Program (NERICP) report of 1980[1] the incidence of hypoplastic left heart syndrome was 7.5% among children with congenital heart disease. Before the advent of prostaglandin E1[4] and reconstructive surgery in the late 1970s, hypoplastic left heart syndrome was responsible for 25% of deaths from congenital heart disease in the first week of life.[5] In a report in 1990[6] the birth prevalence of hypoplastic left heart syndrome was 0.162 per 1000 live births, almost identical to the birth prevalence reported from the NERICP of 0.163 per 1000. Based on these estimates Morris et al[6] calculated that approximately 600 infants are born each year with hypoplastic left heart syndrome in the United States.

EMBRYOLOGY

Because the septum primum component of the atrial septum is often abnormally formed and tends to be leftward displaced in babies with HLHS, it has been speculated that this is the primary embryological defect that deflects the usual volume of blood away from the left heart and leads to its underdevelopment. There is no question that it is very rare to have underdevelopment of the mitral valve and normal development of the aortic valve (in the setting of an intact ventricular septum) which is consistent with the concept of flow driven development of downstream structures. If this is indeed the case there is hope that a fetal intervention that improves flow through the left heart might stimulate growth and avoid the development of HLHS.

ANATOMY

HLHS involves various degrees of underdevelopment of left heart structures. The mitral valve may be either stenotic or atretic, as may the aortic valve. Therefore, HLHS can be subcategorized into four anatomic subtypes based on the morphology of the left heart valves:

- aortic and mitral stenosis
- aortic and mitral atresia
- aortic atresia and mitral stenosis
- aortic stenosis and mitral atresia.

Among 78 consecutive patients with the HLHS who underwent surgery between 1983 and 1991 at Children's Hospital Boston, 35% had aortic atresia, mitral atresia and 20% had aortic stenosis, mitral stenosis. Aortic atresia tends to be associated with a more severe degree of hypoplasia of the ascending aorta than does aortic stenosis. Patients in the aortic stenosis subgroup of HLHS are part of a continuum with patients with critical neonatal aortic valve stenosis. Differentiating these two anomalies can be difficult and is discussed below.

Typically, the ascending aorta in a neonate with the aortic atresia form of HLHS is 2.5 mm in diameter, whereas in the neonate with aortic stenosis as part of the syndrome, the ascending aorta often is 4–5 mm in diameter. The ascending aorta is usually narrowest at its junction with the arch of the aorta and innominate artery, although it may be equally narrow at the sinotubular ridge, where it joins the small sinuses of Valsalva. The wall of the ascending aorta is usually thin and fragile.

The arch of the aorta is quite variable in length and is hypoplastic to various degrees. It may be interrupted. The diameter of the proximal arch is usually similar to that of the distal arch, usually between 3 and 5 mm. A coarctation shelf is present opposite the junction of the ductus with the proximal descending aorta in at least 80% of patients.[7,8] The ductus itself is large, often close to 10 mm in diameter. It is a direct extension of the main pulmonary artery, which is even larger (11–15 mm in diameter, and occasionally even larger). The right pulmonary artery arises very proximally from the main pulmonary artery, usually no more than 2–3 mm beyond the tops of the commissures of the pulmonary valve. It emerges from the posterior and rightward aspect of the main pulmonary artery. It is our impression that both pulmonary artery branches are often smaller in HLHS than in similar anomalies with a single ventricle and systemic outflow tract obstruction (e.g. tricuspid atresia with transposed great arteries and severe subaortic stenosis). The left pulmonary artery arises from the posterior and leftward aspect of the main pulmonary artery some distance from the takeoff of the right pulmonary artery. It runs parallel to the ductus and immediately adjacent to it for some distance. It often appears to be slightly smaller than the right pulmonary artery. The hypoplasia of the pulmonary artery branches may be a consequence of decreased in-utero pulmonary blood flow, which is itself a consequence of the left sided obstruction.

The left atrium is usually smaller than normal; this is exacerbated by the leftward displacement of the septum primum, which is often heavily muscularized. Occasionally the foramen ovale is severely restrictive. The left atrium may have a thickened and fibrotic endocardium analogous to that seen in endocardial fibroelastosis. Occasionally this process extends into the pulmonary veins, resulting in an obliterative, generalized stenosis of these veins. There is also generally increased muscularization of the walls of the pulmonary veins.

Associated cardiac anomalies

A number of associated cardiac anomalies are of surgical relevance. When a ventricular septal defect is present with aortic atresia as is the case in fewer than 5% of cases,[9] it is often associated with normal or near-normal size of the left ventricle, despite the presence of aortic atresia. This introduces the feasibility of biventricular repair in the neonate and perhaps therefore should exclude such variants from our definition of HLHS. Structural abnormalities of the tricuspid and pulmonary valves have been seen but appear to be rare. A bicuspid pulmonary valve was seen in 4% of 54 specimens reviewed by Hawkins and Doty.[10] Cleft tricuspid valve and tricuspid and pulmonary valve dysplasia were also seen in 4%. Other rare associated cardiac anomalies include total anomalous pulmonary venous connection, coronary sinus atresia, common pulmonary vein atresia, complete atrioventricular canal defect, quadricuspid pulmonary valve, double-orifice tricuspid valve, and interrupted aortic arch.[10] Sauer and coworkers[11] reported the presence of coronary artery stenoses in more than 50% of patients in the subgroup with aortic atresia and mitral stenosis, analogous to the situation with pulmonary atresia with intact ventricular septum. By contrast, coronary artery anomalies were rarely seen in patients with aortic atresia and mitral atresia.

Associated extracardiac anomalies, including chromosomal anomalies

In 1988, in a review of 83 autopsies of patients with HLHS at the Children's Hospital of Philadelphia, Natowicz et al[12] reported that nine had underlying chromosomal abnormalities, four had single gene defects and 10 had one or more major extracardiac anomalies without an identifiable chromosomal disorder. Overall, 28% had genetic disorders, major extracardiac anomalies, or both. Chromosomal abnormalities included Turner's syndrome and trisomies 18, 13 and 21. Anomalies not associated with chromosomal defects included diaphragmatic hernia, hypospadias and omphalocele. In a separate report from the same group in 1990,[13] congenital brain anomalies associated with HLHS were reviewed. The authors found that, overall, 29% of the 41 autopsies revealed either a major or minor central nervous system abnormality. Seventeen percent had specific recognizable patterns of malformations such as agenesis of the corpus callosum. Twenty-seven percent were found to have microcephaly, defined as brain weight at autopsy more than two standard deviations below the mean for age. The absence of dysmorphic physical features did not preclude overt or subtle central nervous system malformations.

PATHOPHYSIOLOGY

Before birth there is probably less pulmonary blood flow than is usual for the fetal circulation because of the obstruction to egress of blood from the left atrium. Right ventricular output is directed across the ductus, where it can pass antegrade down the descending aorta or retrograde around the aortic arch to the head vessels and the ascending aorta, which functions as a single coronary artery. After birth there is an immediate reduction in pulmonary vascular resistance, which reduces the proportion of right ventricular output passing to the systemic circulation. If the ductus remains patent, the child's continuing viability will be dependent on a reasonable balance between pulmonary and systemic vascular resistance and/or the capacity to produce an extremely high total cardiac output. Several pathologic studies have documented an increase in pulmonary arteriolar smooth muscle in neonates with HLHS.[14–16] This muscle is likely to be very sensitive to changes in the inspired oxygen concentration and the arteriolar pH. Thus, exposure of the neonate to supplemental oxygen or mechanical ventilation, thereby lowering the PCO_2, is likely to shift the balance of pulmonary and systemic flow adversely in favor of excessive pulmonary flow. This tendency to excessive pulmonary blood flow and inadequate systemic flow will be further exacerbated by even partial closure of the ductus. Complete closure of the ductus is incompatible with life.

CLINICAL FEATURES

Without intervention, HLHS is almost always fatal in the first weeks, if not the first days, of life, although there are occasional exceptions.[17] In 1992 we examined a nine year old child in China who had aortic atresia as part of HLHS and had remarkably few limitations. Generally, a child with this syndrome has a history of respiratory distress within the first 24–48 hours of life, usually while still in the newborn nursery. A mild degree of cyanosis may be noted. Prompt referral to a pediatric cardiologist should result in a rapid echocardiographic diagnosis of HLHS. The child can then be safely transported to a center specializing in neonatal and infant cardiac surgery while receiving a prostaglandin E1 infusion; supplemental oxygen should be avoided. Many transport teams prefer to electively intubate such children because of the risk of apnea induced by the prostaglandin. Facilities must be available to ventilate the child with room air when the child is intubated. Care should be taken to avoid hypocarbia.

Occasionally children are discharged from the nursery without any suspicion of congenital heart disease. This may be the result of insufficiently careful assessment of the child before discharge, but it may also be the result of continuing patency of the ductus and a spontaneously appropriate balance of pulmonary and systemic vascular resistance, resulting in a balance of pulmonary and systemic blood flow. Although when out of hospital the child is free of the risk of exposure to supplemental oxygen (which frequently results in deterioration while the child is in the hospital), there is a risk that the ductus will close precipitously or when the child is at a location geographically remote from medical attention. Under such circumstances the child is likely to develop serious metabolic acidosis and may be in a state of profound shock with cardiovascular collapse by the time the diagnosis is made and treatment with prostaglandin is begun. There may be multi-organ failure secondary to this acidotic insult, resulting in seizures, renal failure, hepatic failure, and depressed ventricular function.[18] The reversibility of these various organ deficits will depend on both the severity of the acidosis and its duration.

Very occasionally the foramen ovale is severely restrictive to left to right flow, thereby limiting pulmonary blood flow to the point where the child is profoundly cyanotic from the moment of birth. Under these circumstances the child will maintain adequate systemic blood flow initially, but metabolic acidosis will eventually develop secondary to the severe degree of hypoxia. This situation cannot be palliated medically but requires urgent intervention in the catheterization laboratory to open the atrial septum.

DIAGNOSTIC STUDIES

The diagnosis of HLHS is being made with increasing frequency by prenatal ultrasound. In many cases the diagnosis can be made confidently by 16–18 weeks of gestation. In a series of 6000 high-risk pregnancies reviewed by Allan and coworkers,[19] the diagnosis of HLHS was not missed once. Prenatal ultrasound is likely to provide fascinating new information regarding the normal development and natural history of the fetus with HLHS. In one case report, Maxwell, Allan, and Tynan[20] described identification of a dilated, poorly contractile left ventricle at 22 weeks of gestation. By 32 weeks the ventricle had not grown since the first study and had become hypoplastic and densely echogenic. Clearly the ability to diagnose this anomaly early in gestation invites prenatal intervention, either in the form of echocardiographically guided balloon dilatation of the aortic valve, as first reported by Maxwell and associates,[20,21] or by surgical means. However, it is important to remember that although prenatal echocardiography is quite sensitive for the diagnosis of HLHS it is not highly specific and can overdiagnose the problem. We have seen a number of cases where babies required only coarctation or aortic valve intervention and on occasion no intervention despite a prenatal diagnosis of HLHS.

Prenatal diagnosis allows time for counseling of the parents, hopefully by surgical as well as by cardiology personnel involved in the management of such children and familiar with the most current results; the fetal ultrasonography and obstetric team may not be in a position to answer more detailed inquiries posed by the parents. Prenatal diagnosis allows for expeditious transfer of the child to the tertiary care facility immediately after birth. Preferably the obstetric care should be undertaken in a facility immediately adjacent to the pediatric center.[22]

The diagnosis of HLHS after birth is made by echocardiography. The physical findings of a slightly cyanotic neonate in respiratory distress, with a variable degree of general circulatory collapse, are nonspecific. Likewise, the appearance on the chest X-ray of a slightly enlarged heart with congested lung fields does not help to distinguish this anomaly from many others. The electrocardiogram will show dominant right ventricular forces, as it does in any neonate. Echocardiography will generally provide excellent definition of the relevant features, including the annular diameters of the mitral and aortic valves, left ventricular volume, and any associated left sided anomalies. The investment of the aortic arch with the prominent thymus of the neonate usually guarantees excellent definition of this area, which may not be as clearly seen in an older infant or child. It is usually possible to define whether a shelf or coarctation is present opposite the insertion of the ductus; this is encountered in 80% of neonates with this anomaly. None of the morphologic features of HLHS is of particular importance to the surgeon in terms of planning the exact surgical strategy because the Norwood operation is a generic procedure that is not much influenced by individual anatomy.

The avoidance of cardiac catheterization when diagnosing the sick neonate with HLHS has been an important advance since the 1980s. Previously, to define the aortic arch it was necessary to pass a catheter either through or close to the ductus. This could result in injury to the ductus, with a subsequent need for emergency surgery if ductal patency was compromised. The osmotic load of angiographic dye was a further insult to the neonate, who may have already had compromised renal function. In addition, there were the general stresses inherent in any cardiac catheterization procedure (heat loss, blood loss and the catecholamine response to the stress of the procedure). Therefore, except in unusual circumstances, such as when intervention is required for a restrictive atrial septum, catheterization is avoided, and the diagnosis is based primarily on the echocardiogram.

Differentiation from critical aortic valve stenosis

The problem of distinguishing HLHS from critical stenosis of the neonatal aortic valve is the major diagnostic challenge with this spectrum of anomalies. The topic is covered in detail in Chapter 18. In summary the calculator developed by the Congenital Heart Surgeon's Society (available at www.chssdc.org)[23] is the most helpful tool for determining whether an individual child should be managed with a Norwood procedure or if the left heart structures are sufficiently well developed to attempt to achieve a biventricular circulation by performing an aortic valvotomy.

MEDICAL AND INTERVENTIONAL MANAGEMENT

The fundamental principle applied to the medical management of children with HLHS is that surgery should not be undertaken until the child is essentially normal with respect to all organ systems other than the cardiorespiratory system itself. Failure to achieve this goal will definitely jeopardize the outcome of surgery.

Transport to a tertiary center

The medical management by the referral obstetric hospital and the transport team is an essential key to the ultimate outcome for the child.[22] Early infusion of prostaglandin is currently practiced at most referral centers before definitive diagnosis is made, in the same way that antibiotics are begun before a diagnosis of sepsis is confirmed. Supplemental oxygen must be avoided. Medical management has been greatly simplified with the advent of reliable pulse oximeters. In fact, these instruments, which did not become widely available until approximately 1985, have improved the management of children with HLHS throughout all phases of their treatment. Metabolic acidosis must be aggressively treated. If the child continues to have poorly palpable pulses or if the blood pressure measured by an umbilical arterial line is low, a careful check should be made to ensure that the prostaglandin is being delivered into the bloodstream. Usually an umbilical venous line with excellent blood return is the safest venous access at this stage. If the team is sure that the prostaglandin is being delivered at an adequate dose (initially 0.1 μg/kg per minute), consideration should be given to supporting the child with a dopamine infusion, beginning at a dose of 5 μg/kg per minute up to 20 μg/kg per minute.

Children who have suffered a serious insult should be intubated before transport. This is often appropriate for any child receiving prostaglandin who may become apneic in the confined area of a transport vehicle, where intubation will be hazardous. Elective intubation before transport should be seriously considered for all patients. The general principles of neonatal resuscitation and transport, such as maintenance of adequate body temperature and blood glucose levels, should be carefully adhered to. Note, however, that a mild degree of hypothermia may be protective to the central nervous system exposed to an ischemic insult, and hyperthermia is deleterious under such circumstances; therefore, overly aggressive rewarming should be avoided. Likewise, there is evidence that hyperglycemia in mature animals exacerbates ischemic brain injury, although whether this applies in neonates is not clear. Nevertheless, it would seem wise to avoid very high levels of blood glucose.

Resuscitation in the cardiac intensive care unit

It is important that the child be managed preoperatively in an intensive care unit specializing in neonatal and infant cardiology and cardiac surgery. Cardiologists, cardiac surgeons and intensive care specialists should be aware of the child's arrival at the hospital so that they can collaborate in the child's resuscitation. Clear lines of communication are essential so that discussion can ensue regarding such issues as whether to pursue a univentricular or biventricular approach (balloon valvotomy in the catheterization laboratory), the timing of surgery, the need and timing of ancillary interventions (balloon dilatation of a restrictive atrial septal defect) and, perhaps, the decision to withhold medical or surgical therapy for the child who has been severely compromised or who has such serious associated anomalies that the consensus among all parties, including the child's parents, is that only general supportive measures should be given.

Counseling the child's parents

Prenatal diagnosis is an important benefit for many children with HLHS in that obstetric services can be provided close to a cardiac center, and the supportive measures previously outlined can be initiated expeditiously, including the immediate infusion of prostaglandin. In addition, there is an important psychological advantage for most prospective parents, who can prepare themselves logistically, intellectually, and emotionally for the hurdles that may lie ahead for them and that can be explained in detail several months before the delivery. On the other hand for some parents the worry induced by fetal diagnosis can be counterproductive and may even interfere with fetal growth and development. When the diagnosis is made after delivery, particularly if the child has been at home for some time and recognition of the child's deteriorating status may have been delayed, great care must be taken by the hospital team in carefully counseling the parents. For many families, parent support groups are of great help, particularly after the child has left the hospital and the parents are faced with the prospect of future hospital visits, cardiac catheterizations and surgery. Meeting children who are attending school and leading normal lives after completion of surgical treatment is a great emotional boost to parents who may be anticipating caring for a child who is chronically incapacitated.

Specific measures in the intensive care unit

Details are described in Chapter 5.

Catheter intervention

PRENATAL

Remarkable advances in obstetric ultrasound imaging and the development of interventional catheter hardware and techniques now allow balloon dilation of the stenotic aortic valve or restrictive atrial septum as early as 16–20 weeks' gestation. Anecdotal cases performed at Children's Hospital Boston in 2002 and 2003 suggest that early intervention may promote growth of left heart structures so as to allow a biventricular circulation when HLHS would otherwise have been present at birth.

POSTNATAL

If a child with HLHS presents at birth with severe hypoxia it is likely to be the result of restriction to left to right flow at the level of the atrial septum. This situation is best managed by urgent Brockenbrough puncture of the atrial septum in the catheterization laboratory with subsequent balloon dilation of the atrial septal puncture. The left atrium is usually too small and the atrial septum itself too heavily muscularized to allow a Rashkind type balloon septostomy.

In the child with a relatively well developed left heart but still inadequate to allow a biventricular circulation, the question may arise whether the left ventricle should be decompressed to reduce the risk of later malignant arrhythmias. It has not been our usual practice at Children's Hospital Boston to undertake dilation of the aortic valve under these circumstances because of concern that the valve might become regurgitant.

INDICATIONS FOR AND TIMING OF SURGERY

Because this anomaly is uniformly fatal without surgery, it is our practice to offer surgery to any child with HLHS who comes to Children's Hospital Boston, as long as the following contraindications do not apply. Prematurity (gestational age less than approximately 34 weeks) and low birth weight (<1500–1800 g) are generally, though not absolutely, considered to be contraindications to surgery because our experience suggests that the risks are very high in this setting. Likewise, serious chromosomal anomalies or serious extracardiac anomalies represent contraindications,[12] although in our experience, these have been exceedingly rare reasons for not undertaking surgery. Severe tricuspid or pulmonary regurgitation is an occasional contraindication to surgery, as is severe right ventricular dysfunction. Ventricular dysfunction is often present at the time of presentation, particularly if the child is still acidotic or is recovering from a recent acidotic insult. Ventricular function should be reassessed when the child has had a chance to be fully resuscitated, including a return to normal of all metabolic parameters, such as urea and creatinine levels and liver function test results. Occasionally a child does not recover from the initial insult and lapses into progressive renal or hepatic failure in spite of satisfactory cardiac output and appropriate distribution of blood flow between the pulmonary and systemic circulations. In our opinion, in the majority of cases, a failure to recover from the initial insult should also represent a contraindication to heart transplantation as well as to reconstruction. In contrast significant tricuspid or pulmonary regurgitation and isolated ventricular dysfunction represent contraindications only to reconstruction. Children with any of these problems should be fully assessed for possible heart transplantation after a complete discussion with the parents.

Although some centers may still consider no intervention appropriate for any child with HLHS including those at the mild end of the spectrum, we consider such an approach to be both ethically and logically inconsistent. There are many other congenital heart anomalies that today carry a prognosis that is just as bad if not worse; these include other forms of single ventricle with systemic outflow obstruction, single ventricle with heterotaxy, critical neonatal Ebstein's anomaly, and even severe forms of pulmonary atresia with intact ventricular septum. For some reason these anomalies are generally accepted as being part of a wide spectrum and treatment is almost never withheld for those at the more mild end of the spectrum. We maintain that a similar philosophy should hold for children with HLHS.

Timing of surgery

The average duration of resuscitation for neonates admitted with hypoplastic left heart syndrome at Children's Hospital Boston is two to three days. Occasionally there may be factors which result in a need for surgery sooner than this though more commonly there are likely to be factors which result in a greater delay of surgery. The child who presents at several days of age with signs of very high pulmonary blood flow despite a widely patent ductus, and who cannot be controlled by the measures to increase pulmonary vascular resistance described in Chapter 5, should undergo surgery within 12–24 hours of confirmation of the diagnosis by echocardiography. The child who is severely hypoxic because of a restrictive foramen ovale should undergo an urgent balloon procedure in the catheterization laboratory to open the atrial septum. Under these circumstances however there is concern that pulmonary vascular resistance will remain markedly elevated for at least several days resulting in the need for a large shunt at the time of surgery. Therefore it is advisable to wait for at least several days after the catheter procedure to allow pulmonary resistance to fall.

For the typical child who presents with mild elevation of serum creatinine and urea as well as liver function tests and in whom pulmonary blood flow can be controlled without great difficulty, the supportive measures outlined above should be continued until all indices of organ function have returned to normal. Although some centers have recommended routine balloon septostomy so that pulmonary vascular resistance will be as low as possible at the time of surgery, this has not been our practice. Not only does the catheter procedure itself carry significant risk, but in addition there is a chance that the child will develop grossly excessive pulmonary blood flow resulting in the need for relatively urgent surgery. Nevertheless there is certainly a gray area where pulmonary vascular resistance is importantly elevated preoperatively in part related to a restrictive foramen ovale which would be better dealt with preoperatively.

SURGICAL MANAGEMENT

History

There are a multitude of articles in the surgical literature describing various ingenious procedures that could enable survival of the neonate without a continuing requirement for prostaglandin. For example, in 1970 Cayler and colleagues[24] described anastomosis between the right pulmonary artery and ascending aorta with the placement of bilateral pulmonary artery bands. In a follow-up report,[25] this patient was said to be symptom free at three years of age. No report of a successful Fontan operation was published. Between 1977 and 1981, a number of authors, including Doty, Levitsky, Behrendt, Norwood, and their respective coworkers, described multiple modifications of possible surgical procedures.[26–29] While there were a few short-term survivors, there were no reports of a successful stage 1 procedure leading to a successful Fontan procedure until Norwood and coworkers' report in 1983.[30] Many of the alternative procedures to Norwood's first-stage operation suffer from inherent impediments to the successful development of a low-risk Fontan candidate. For example, banding of the main pulmonary artery distal to a conduit taken from the proximal main pulmonary artery fails to take into account the very short distance between the tops of the commissures of the pulmonary valve and the takeoff of the right pulmonary artery. Distortion of the right pulmonary artery takeoff will almost certainly ensue if the child survives the procedure. Many proposed procedures fail to take into account the restrictive nature of the aortic arch or the common occurrence of a coarctation. Procedures incorporating a permanent conduit fail to incorporate growth potential.

Technical considerations: stage 1 Norwood procedure

GENERAL AIMS

The goals of the first-stage reconstructive procedure for HLHS are identical to those of any palliative procedure that is preparatory to an ultimate Fontan operation. Ventricular function must be preserved by avoiding a pressure load (reconstructed aortic arch gradient) or excessive volume load (excessive pulmonary blood flow, e.g. a shunt that is too large), minimizing pulmonary vascular resistance (avoiding excessive pulmonary blood flow or pulmonary venous obstruction by a restrictive atrial septal defect), and maintaining optimal pulmonary artery growth (adequate size and freedom from distortion). In the absence of structural abnormalities of the tricuspid valve, this approach will also preserve tricuspid valve function by avoiding ventricular dilatation associated with excessive volume work by the ventricle.

CURRENT TECHNIQUE OF STAGE 1 PALLIATION

At present, the operative procedure in use at Children's Hospital Boston is based on the procedure described by Norwood et al in their 1983 report (Figure 19.1)[30] but now incorporates the modification described by Sano.[31] Attention to fine points of technique can mean the difference between a low-risk candidate for a Fontan operation and a nonsurvivor of the first stage. Meticulous coordination and communication between the anesthesia and surgical teams is an essential ingredient for the success of the procedure.[32] Inappropriate ventilatory, anesthetic, and inotropic manipulations substantially increase the risk of early mortality for this procedure though introduction of the Sano modification has unquestionably improved intraoperative and postoperative stability.

The child is transported to the operating room while receiving room air ventilation with a view to maintaining carbon dioxide levels close to normocarbia. Hyperventilation at this time is a common error and must be avoided. Monitoring of arterial pressure is continued using the umbilical arterial line and pulse oximetry is maintained. Central venous access is avoided at this time, as two atrial catheters will be placed by the surgical team during the procedure. Anesthesia is induced and maintained with a high-dose fentanyl technique. A urinary catheter is placed, and electrocardiographic monitoring is continued. The child is allowed to cool spontaneously somewhat during this phase related to the low ambient air temperature of the operating room.

Approach is through a median sternotomy. The thymus is partially excised to allow access to the aortic arch. It is not necessary to dissect the arch vessels at all. A 6/0 marking suture is placed on the right side of the tiny ascending aorta to help guide the aortotomy which will be made later. Following heparinization an 8 French Biomedicus arterial cannula is inserted in the mid-ductus and a 18 French venous cannula is placed in the right atrium through the atrial appendage (Figure 19.1a). Immediately after beginning bypass a 5/0 Prolene suture ligature is tied around the proximal ductus with care to avoid distortion of the takeoffs of the right and left pulmonary artery.

Although we previously controlled the branch pulmonary arteries with tourniquets during cooling, we found there were at least two important disadvantages with this approach. Firstly the tourniquets can cause intimal injury and subsequent stenosis in the branch pulmonary arteries. Secondly intermittent incompetence of the pulmonary valve as the heart is manipulated results in sudden and severe distention of the ventricle which is not well tolerated. The child is cooled over about 15–20 minutes to a rectal temperature of less than 18°C.

During cooling the proximal main pulmonary artery is divided 2–3 mm above the tops of the commissures of the pulmonary valve. Although in the past we used a patch to close the distal divided main pulmonary artery, today we usually close the artery by direct suture (Figure 19.1b). The closure is oblique in the sense that it is not in an anteroposterior plane or in a vertical plane. We believe that avoidance of a patch optimizes long-term growth of the central pulmonary arteries because the entire circumference has growth potential. It also avoids a central bulge of the pulmonary arteries which can result in torsion and kinking of the branch pulmonary artery origins.

The distal anastomosis of the Sano shunt should be constructed now (Figure 19.1b1). For the neonate between 2.0 and 3.5 kg a 5 mm stretch PTFE tube graft should be selected. The distal anastomosis can be incorporated in the oblique closure of the distal divided main pulmonary artery or can be made to a longitudinal arteriotomy between the left pulmonary artery takeoff and the main pulmonary artery closure. Continuous 6/0 Prolene is used.

By this time an appropriate homograft has been selected and thawed. It should be shaped appropriately for the arch reconstruction according to the length and diameter of the arch (Figure 19.1c). Bypass is now discontinued and cardioplegia is infused through a sidearm on the arterial cannula. During the infusion the head vessels and distal aorta are temporarily occluded with forceps. We no longer place tourniquets around the head vessels as we believe they can cause intimal injury and subsequent stenosis. There is also a risk that they will not be released at the appropriate time resulting in an unnecessary prolongation of circulatory arrest time. Furthermore it does not appear that air introduced into the carotid vessels presents a serious problem based on work in adults undergoing aortic arch reconstruction.

The arterial cannula is removed and the venous cannula is left open to drain. The ductus is divided at its junction with the descending aorta and redundant ductus tissue is excised. The resulting aortotomy is extended at least 5 mm distally (more if the isthmus and juxtaductal area are severely hypoplastic). Proximally, the arch and ascending aorta are filleted open to the level of the division of the main pulmonary artery. Because the arch vessels have not been dissected there is little risk that the arch incision will twist offline either anteriorly or posteriorly. The marking suture on the right side of the proximal ascending aorta ensures that the incision in the left side of the ascending aorta stays exactly on the left side and finishes at the correct level. An anastomosis is fashioned between the proximal portion of the divided main pulmonary artery and the filleted aorta with a supplementary cuff of homograft arterial wall (Figure 19.1d,e).[33] It is important that this neoaorta is not redundant and that it does not create a bowstring effect over the left pulmonary artery, which can be compressed between the neoaorta and the left main bronchus. These aims are best achieved by conceptualizing the more distal component of the homograft patch as a patch plasty for the distal part of the arch and proximal part of the descending aorta, while the more proximal component of the patch will create a tube that should be a little smaller in diameter than the original main pulmonary artery. Careful consideration must be given to the distensibility of the homograft

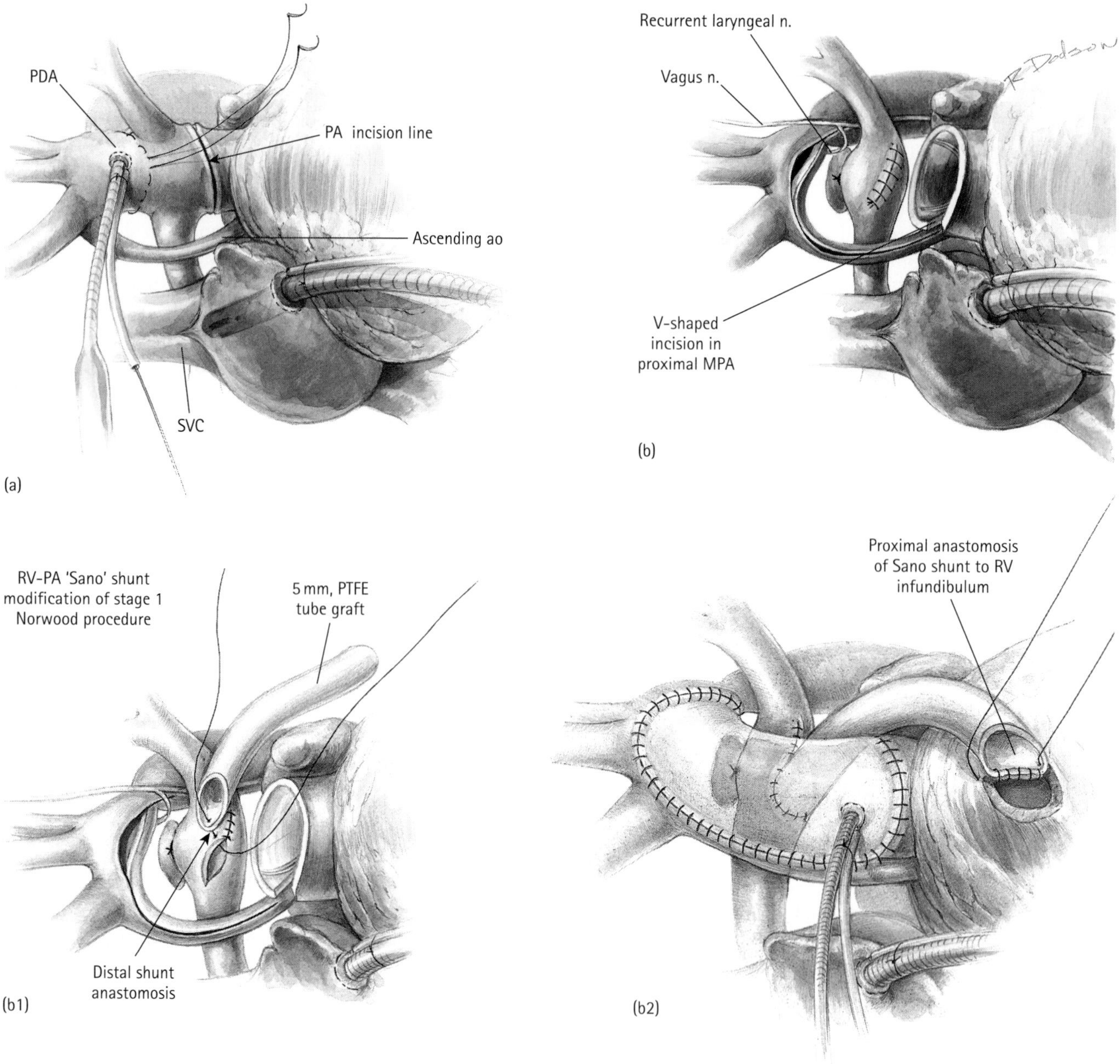

Figure 19.1a–b2 *Stage 1 Norwood procedure. (a) An 8 French arterial cannula is placed in the mid-ductus. A 5/0 Prolene suture ligature is tied around the proximal ductus immediately after commencing bypass. The main pulmonary artery is divided transversely a few millimeters distal to the pulmonary valve. (b) The distal divided main pulmonary artery is closed obliquely by direct suture. The ductus has been divided. The resulting aortotomy is extended distally as well as proximally across the undersurface of the arch and down the ascending aorta to the level of division of the main pulmonary artery. A V-shaped incision is made in the proximal divided main pulmonary artery. (b1) The distal anastomosis of the 5 mm Sano shunt is made to the distal divided main pulmonary artery. (b2) The proximal anastomosis of the Sano shunt is made to a short incision in the infundibulum of the right ventricle using 5/0 Gortex suture.*

tissue,[34] as well as to the contribution to the neoaorta by the original ascending aorta. An excessively large proximal neoaorta will compress the reconstructed pulmonary artery bifurcation, resulting in a central stenosis.

Avoiding coronary artery compromise

Great care must be taken to avoid obstructing flow to the coronary arteries when anastomosing the small ascending aorta to the proximal portion of the pulmonary artery. As noted above a marking suture placed on the ascending aorta while that vessel is distended is often useful to indicate placement of the anastomosis. After division of the main pulmonary artery a 2–3 mm V-shaped incision is made in the proximal pulmonary artery usually just anterior to the adjacent pulmonary valve commissure. At least three interrupted 7/0 sutures are placed at the apex of the ascending aortotomy

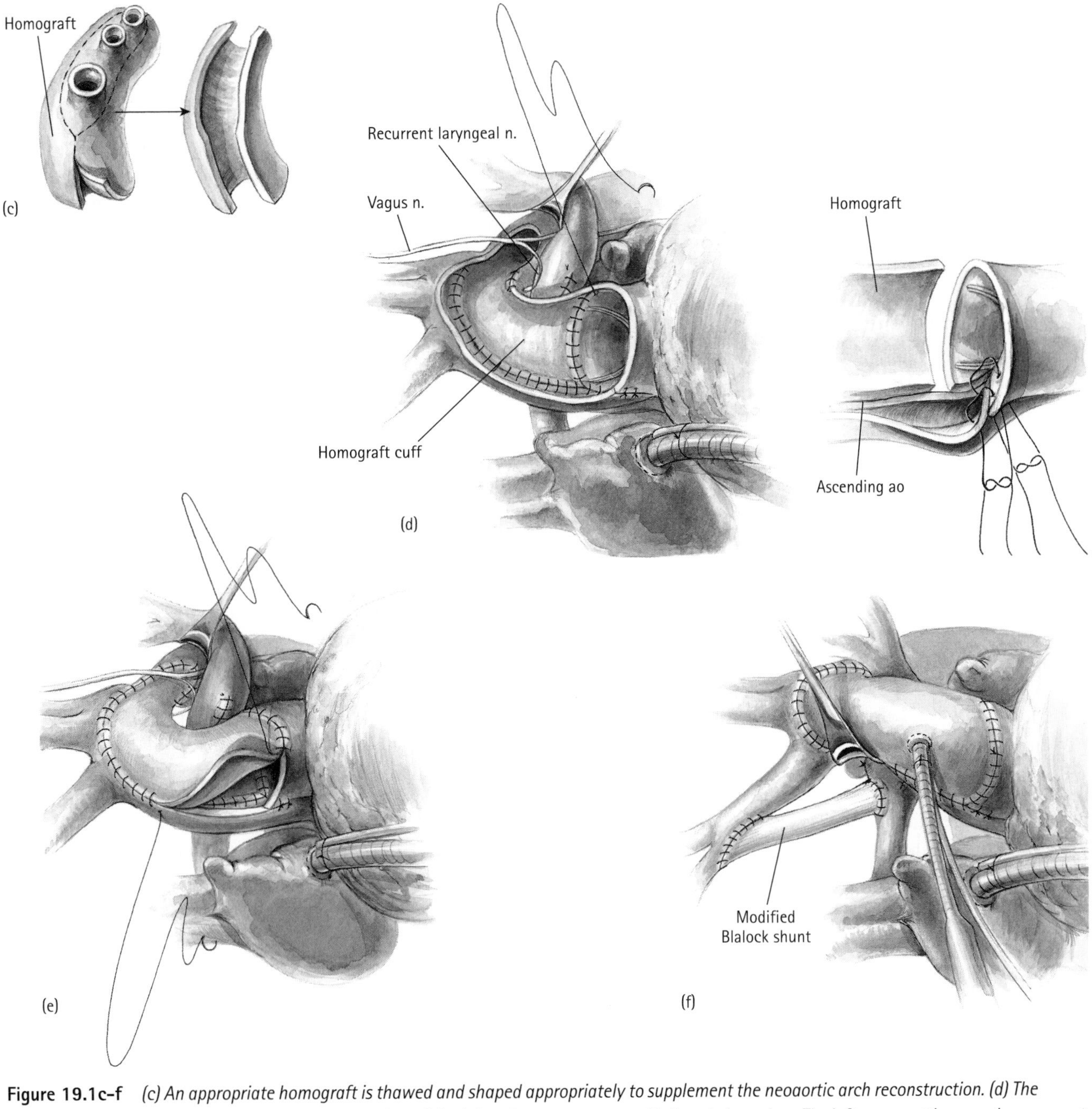

Figure 19.1c–f *(c) An appropriate homograft is thawed and shaped appropriately to supplement the neoaortic arch reconstruction. (d) The neoaortic arch is shaped so as to prevent compression of the left pulmonary artery and left main bronchus. The left recurrent laryngeal nerve must be carefully preserved. Inset: interrupted 7/0 prolene sutures are placed at the direct anastomosis of the proximal main pulmonary artery to the tiny ascending aorta in order to minimize the risk of coronary blood flow compromise. (e) Completion of the neoaortic arch reconstruction. (f) The neoaorta has been recannulated and de-aired. A modified Blalock shunt has been placed from the proximal right subclavian artery to the takeoff of the right pulmonary artery from the main pulmonary artery.*

(Figure 19.1d inset). In children in whom the ascending aorta is particularly small (less than 2 mm), we have, on occasion, divided the ascending aorta and implanted it end to side into a complete tube of homograft.

Atrial septectomy

The septum primum must be completely excised from the base of the foramen ovale down to the level of the inferior vena cava. Partial excision or simple incision, as practiced in the past, frequently led to later restriction at the atrial septal level. The septectomy can be performed through a very short incision low in the right atrial free wall or through the venous cannulation site in the right atrial appendage.

Shunts

We and others have used a number of different types of shunt over the 20 years that the Norwood procedure has been in use.[31,33,35] Our current preference is a Sano shunt from the right ventricle to the pulmonary bifurcation using stretch PTFE (Figure 19.1b2). The important advantage of the Sano shunt relative to the alternative Blalock shunt which we used for many years is that flow occurs only during systole (Figure 19.1f). There is no competition between pulmonary and coronary blood flow as is the case with the Blalock shunt. This is the most likely explanation for the very much improved stability of neonates with a Sano shunt relative to those with a Blalock shunt in the early postoperative period.

A 5 mm Sano shunt is used for neonates between 2.0 and 3.5 kg with either a 4 mm or 6 mm tube generally being used outside of this weight range. Many factors enter into the selection of appropriate shunt size in addition to the child's weight. For example, a judgment must be made as to the child's probable pulmonary vascular resistance, including consideration of the contribution of the atrial septum to total pulmonary resistance that will be eliminated by the septectomy. If the child is thought to have greater than average resistance it may be appropriate to use a 6 mm tube graft rather than the usual 5 mm. There does not appear to be any advantage in using a valved conduit because the branch pulmonary arteries have little capacitance and the pressure is usually not high so there is usually little pulmonary regurgitation.

Avoiding a homograft cuff

Norwood's original technique did not include use of a cuff to supplement the aortic to pulmonary anastomsosis.[30] This technique has been repopularized recently.[36] However, we continue to believe that it is important to avoid direct anastomosis of the proximal pulmonary artery to the arch in the majority of patients.[33] Direct anastomosis requires more distal division of the pulmonary artery. We prefer more proximal division of the pulmonary artery which allows direct closure of the distal pulmonary artery and therefore enhances growth potential of the critically important mid-pulmonary artery region. Another potential problem with direct anastomosis is a bowstring effect of the reconstructed aorta over the left main bronchus which can result in air-trapping in the left lung. Another objection that has been expressed to the use of a homograft cuff has been the risk of calcification of the homograft tissue. Interestingly it has been our observation that calcification is almost never a problem in the cuff of homograft tissue used for arch reconstruction in contrast to the heavy calcification that is frequently seen in homografts when they are used as a complete tube graft.

Minimizing or avoiding circulatory arrest

The technique described above usually allows the circulatory arrest time to be kept to less than 30–40 minutes. However, many ingenious technical variations have been described which permit the arrest time to be further reduced or even eliminated. As described in Chapter 9, our own studies of circulatory arrest have shown that it is not possible to detect any developmental advantage in avoiding less than 40–45 minutes of circulatory arrest.[37] Furthermore alternative techniques rely on novel and unproven perfusion methods such as retrograde perfusion through the Blalock shunt.[38] Studies of cerebral perfusion methods such as retrograde venous perfusion have demonstrated that perfusion is not homogeneous and in fact much of the flow does not go to the brain at all.[39] There is a real risk that the surgical team will have a false sense of safety and will extend the total repair time to a dangerous degree. There is also the problem that return of blood into the surgical field when novel perfusion methods are used increases the difficulty of the repair, particularly visualization of the distal arch reconstruction. Although clamps can be placed they can cause intimal injury with a risk of later stenosis. It will be important for the proponents of these intriguing new methods to demonstrate both with animal studies as well as with careful clinical neurodevelopmental outcome studies that their methods are as safe or safer as claimed than the technique of limited deep hypothermic circulatory arrest.

Proximal Sano shunt anastomosis

The proximal anastomosis of the Sano shunt may be constructed when bypass has been re-established (Figure 19.1b2). An oblique incision is made in the infundibulm of the right ventricle with care to avoid injury to coronary artery branches and the pulmonary valve. It is advisable to make the incision before the proximal neoaortic suture line is complete as this allows a right angle instrument to be passed into the ventricle through the neoaortic valve to guide the ventricular incision. The incision should point leftward and superiorly so as to direct the conduit into the left chest where it is less likely to be compressed by the sternum. It should be slightly longer than the diameter of the tube graft. The edges can be undermined a little if necessary. The anastomosis is performed with continuous 5/0 PTFE suture. It is helpful to suture most of the anastomosis from within to create an inverted suture line that is less problematic with needle hole bleeding than an everted suture line. Air is allowed to vent from the anastomosis before the suture is tied.

Weaning from bypass

Unlike the alternative Blalock shunt it is not necessary to control the Sano shunt during rewarming. A dopamine infusion is routinely employed at the time of discontinuation of bypass. This is administered via a catheter inserted through a purse-string suture into what is, at this point, a common atrium. The same catheter is used to monitor the filling pressure of the ventricle. Ventilation is begun and the filling pressure within the atrium is increased by the perfusionist so that the heart is ejecting relatively vigorously. Frequent arrhythmias at this stage, particularly when associated with discoloration of the ventricle may indicate coronary insufficiency. Reliable saturation sensing by a pulse oximeter must be established, once pulsatile flow is present, before the patient is weaned from bypass. Pulmonary vascular resistance is often elevated for the first 15–30 minutes after weaning from bypass, and thus it is often necessary to hyperventilate the child during this time. The arterial oxygen saturation may be as low as 50% to 60% during this period, but as long as adequate cardiac output appears to be maintained, these low saturations should be tolerated. If very low saturations persist or if ventricular function appears to be impaired, it may be necessary to revise the shunt. Of course, low arterial oxygen saturation may also represent inadequate cardiac output, in which case shunt revision would clearly be contraindicated. Only by careful observation of the chronologic sequence of the failure to wean from bypass can the primary cause of the low-output state be established. A sufficiently severe degree of hypoxia ultimately will always lead to myocardial failure, even when the myocardium itself, when well oxygenated, has excellent reserve.

The child who is weaned from bypass with a high oxygen saturation (>85–90%) may have excessive pulmonary blood flow, which may be associated with hypotension and the development of metabolic acidosis, particularly if a modified Blalock shunt has been used. However, it is important to consider that a high oxygen saturation may be the result of some forward flow through an open aortic valve in the patient with aortic stenosis and mitral stenosis. It may also be a reflection of excellent cardiac output with low oxygen extraction. Residual aortic arch obstruction will also be reflected in high oxygen saturation in a patient who has a Blalock shunt, as blood will be selectively directed into the shunt. If residual arch obstruction is suspected, it can be easily ruled out by measurement of the neoaortic root pressure relative to umbilical arterial pressure. Placement of both a pulse oximeter probe and a blood pressure cuff on a lower extremity is particularly important in the patient who does not have an umbilical arterial line. Detection of arterial pulsation by a pulse oximeter probe on the foot is often a useful indicator of at least adequate cardiac output.

Closure of the chest

If there is any doubt as to the child's stability, the sternum should not be approximated though this has been necessary only occasionally since we began using the Sano shunt in contrast to almost routinely leaving the chest open when we used the Blalock shunt. Chest tubes should be placed carefully where there is no possibility that they will impinge on the myocardium or the reconstructed vessels in the superior mediastinum. An elliptical Esmarch sheet should be sutured accurately to the skin edges and povidone-iodine ointment applied to the skin-Esmarch interface. An iodine impregnated adhesive plastic drape is applied to seal the closure.

Intensive care management after stage 1 reconstruction

The intensive care management of the child with a palliated 'in-parallel' circulation is described in Chapter 5.

Follow-up after stage 1 surgery

The principles of follow-up after stage 1 palliation for HLHS are identical to those applied to any child with single-ventricle physiology in whom a Fontan procedure is anticipated. Specifically, careful attention should be directed toward optimal pulmonary artery development, maintenance of ventricular function, and maintenance of low pulmonary vascular resistance, including absence of restriction at the level of the atrial septal defect. Because of the complexity of the neonatal surgery it is particularly important to have a high index of suspicion for the various problems which are not infrequently seen in patients after stage 1 surgery. It is also important to recognize that the infant is likely to outgrow a Sano shunt earlier than a Blalock because flow is limited to systole.

All patients should be catheterized by four to five months of age; this recommendation stands irrespective of clinical progress. A child may be feeding and growing well and yet have very severe stenosis in the area of the central pulmonary artery bifurcation. The lack of sensitivity of postoperative echocardiography to various problems observed in the first few months after stage 1 surgery is an additional reason catheterization should not be postponed beyond this age. Nevertheless, this is not to say that echocardiography should not be used as a screening tool early in the first few months of life. Clear demonstration of a problem developing in either the aortic arch or the pulmonary artery is an indication for earlier catheterization. Likewise obvious symptomatic indications for earlier investigation are the development of severe cyanosis or persistent signs of congestive heart failure, especially difficulty with feeding and failure to thrive.

If the 4–5-month catheterization demonstrates a problem, such as distortion of the central pulmonary artery area that is likely to compromise development of the left pulmonary artery, a bidirectional cavopulmonary shunt with an associated pulmonary arterioplasty should be undertaken. Other indications for early application of the cavopulmonary shunt have included the need for aortic arch reconstruction; the need for atrial septal defect enlargement; early outgrowth of the Sano shunt, resulting in unacceptably low oxygen saturation (<70–75%); and the development of tricuspid regurgitation or right ventricular dysfunction secondary to excessive volume load on the ventricle.

Attempts to perform a cavopulmonary shunt in the first weeks of life have been unsuccessful because of severe hypoxia, not because of excessively high superior vena caval pressures. However, cavopulmonary shunt procedures have been successfully performed in infants as young as 2.5–3 months of age, although there may be a higher incidence of pleural effusions, which are very rarely seen with this procedure in older infants and children. One other problem that is emerging as a possible long-term risk after the first-stage procedure is the development of regurgitation of the neoaortic valve (i.e. the original morphologic pulmonary valve). This finding, per se, is not a current indication to proceed to a bidirectional cavopulmonary shunt.

Two ventricle repair of aortic atresia with VSD

Aortic atresia with VSD is an anomaly that is closely related to hypoplastic left heart syndrome but does not strictly fall within the definition of hypoplastic left heart syndrome as applied at Children's Hospital Boston. The repair involves application of principles of both the Norwood procedure and the Rastelli procedure. The neoaorta is reconstructed utilizing a period of deep hypothermic circulatory arrest in exactly the same fashion as described above. However, the distal divided main pulmonary artery is not closed. Rather an appropriate sized homograft is anastomosed to the distal divided main pulmonary artery (Figure 19.2).

Bypass is recommenced when the neoaorta has been cannulated. Working through a vertical infundibular incision a baffle of autologous pericardium is placed so as to direct left ventricular blood through the VSD to the pulmonary valve and from there to the neoaorta. Interrupted pledgetted horizontal mattress 5/0 Tevdek sutures are used (Figure 19.2b).

The proximal anastomosis of the right ventricle to pulmonary artery homograft is fashioned to the infundibular incision supplemented with a hood of glutaraldehyde treated autologous pericardium (Figure 19.2c).

Bidirectional Glenn shunt, follow-up and fenestrated Fontan technique

These topics are covered in Chapter 20 because they are essentially generic for all patients traversing a single ventricle pathway including those with hypoplastic left heart syndrome.

RESULTS OF SURGERY

The largest and most comprehensive outcome analysis of patients undergoing a stage 1 Norwood procedure was reported by the Congenital Heart Surgeons Society in 2003.[40] Twenty nine institutional members of the Society enrolled 985 neonates between 1994 and 2000 who had either critical aortic stenosis or atresia. A total of 710 of the 985 patients underwent a stage 1 Norwood procedure. The survival was 76% at one month, 60% at one year and 54% at five years. Risk factors for death included patient specific variables such as lower birth weight, smaller ascending aorta and older age at the time of the Norwood procedure, institutional variables including institutions enrolling fewer than 10 neonates but also two institutions enrolling more than 40 neonates and procedural variables including shunt originating from the aorta, longer circulatory arrest time and the technique of management of the ascending aorta.

By 18 months from the time of the Norwood procedure 58% of patients had undergone a bidirectional Glenn shunt (Figure 19.3). Of patients who underwent a bidirectional Glenn shunt, 79% successfully achieved a third-stage Fontan circulation within six years of the bidirectional Glenn shunt. Mortality for the third stage was 9% and 3% of patients underwent cardiac transplantation. Risk factors for death after the bidirectional Glenn shunt included younger age at the time of the shunt and the need for right atrioventricular valve repair.

The Congenital Heart Surgeons Society study has documented that overall the outlook for babies with hypoplastic left heart syndrome has improved dramatically since the Norwood operation was initially introduced in 1983. Nevertheless as early as 1986[33] we described 25 neonates who had undergone various modifications of the first stage reconstructive procedure at Children's Hospital Boston between 1984 and 1995. There were six early deaths for an early mortality of 24%. Of those one was a preterm neonate weighing less than 2 kg and two were neonates who could not be adequately resuscitated with prostaglandin and who received cardiac massage immediately before surgery. Early deaths were related to excessive pulmonary blood in two patients and to a possible coronary embolus in one.

Seen in this light, therefore, the one month survival rate of the CHSS report of only 72% could be interpreted as a disappointing result. However, it is important to appreciate that the CHSS study includes a large number of institutions many of whom were quite early in their learning experience with the Norwood operation when the enrollment period opened in 1994.

Several reports suggest that the recent results for the Norwood procedure have improved markedly over the last five years. For example, Daebritz et al[41] reviewed 194 patients who underwent a stage 1 Norwood procedure between 1990 and 1998 at Children's Hospital Boston. A total of 131 patients had hypoplastic left heart syndrome while 63 patients had other forms of single ventricle with systemic outflow obstruction. The operative mortality decreased from 38.5% between 1990 and 1994 to 21.4% after 1994 ($p = 0.02$). Introduction of the Sano shunt at Children's Hospital Boston in 2002 has been associated with further reduction in stage 1 Norwood mortality which is now less than 10%.

The largest single institutional report has been by Mahle and colleagues from the Children's Hospital of Philadelphia.[42] A total of 840 babies underwent the Norwood procedure between 1984 and 1999. The hospital mortality between 1984 and 1988 was 44% while between 1995 and 1998 hospital mortality was 29%. Bove[43] described the outcomes for 253 patients who underwent the Norwood procedure at the University of Michigan between 1990 and 1997. Hospital mortality was 24%. Mortality was strongly influenced by the presence of associated noncardiac congenital conditions as well as severe preoperative obstruction to pulmonary venous return ($p = 0.03$). Survival following the second stage hemi-Fontan procedure or bidirectional Glenn was 97% and survival following the Fontan procedure was 88%. In 2002, Tweddell et al[44] described 115 patients who underwent the Norwood procedure in Milwaukee, Wisconsin between 1992 and 2001. Hospital mortality was 47% between 1992 and 1996 but between 1996 and 2001 hospital survival was 93%. The authors emphasize the value of continuous monitoring of systemic venous oxygen saturation as a factor which improves stage 1 Norwood survival. Improving results have also been reported by Azakie et al[45] from Toronto, Canada, as well as by Isihino et al[46] from Birmingham, UK.

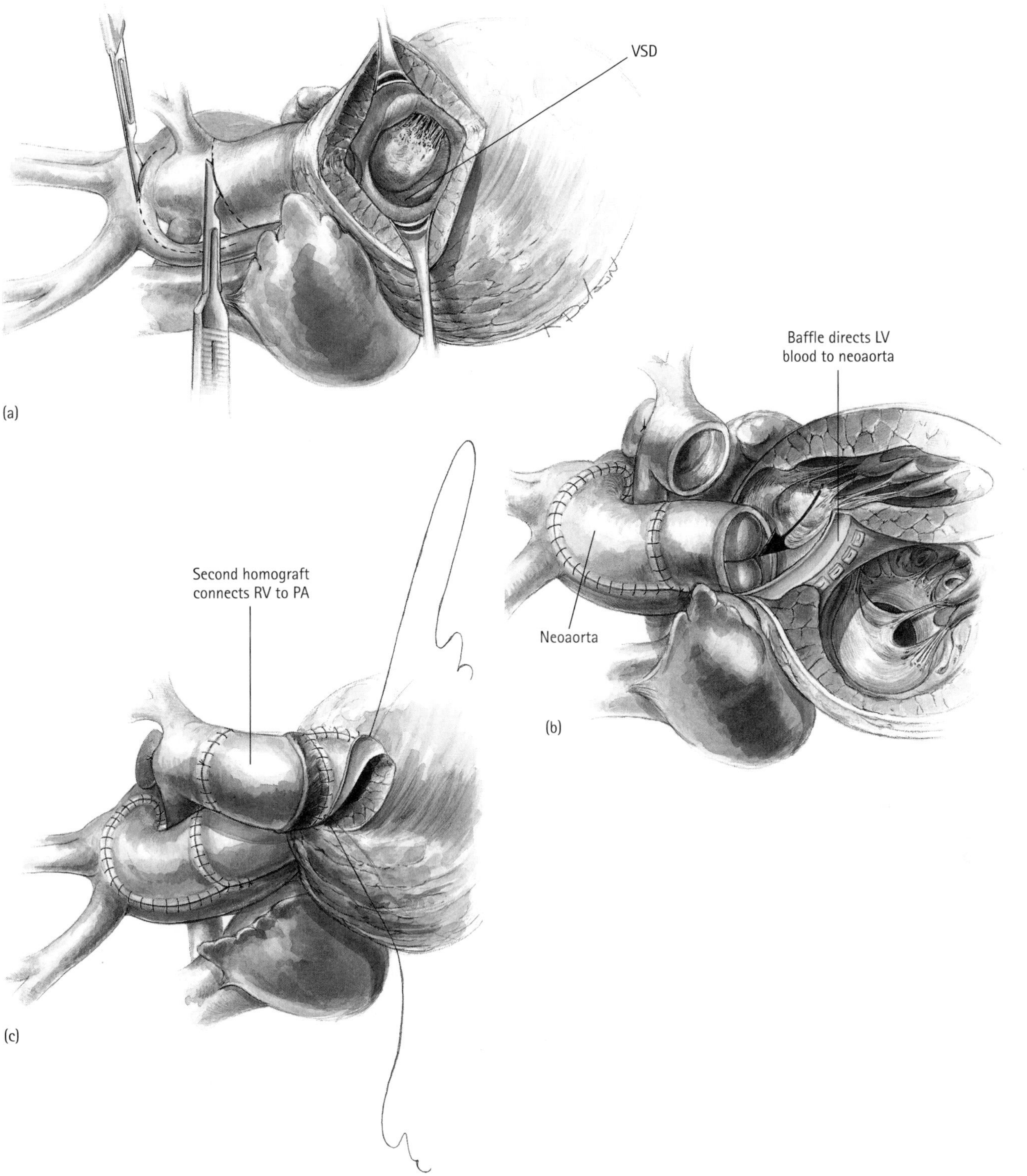

Figure 19.2 *Two-ventricle repair of aortic atresia with VSD. Aortic atresia with VSD is a rare anomaly that is related to hypoplastic left heart syndrome. The repair involves a combination of principles of the Norwood procedure and Rastelli procedure. (a) The infundibulum of the right ventricle is opened with a vertical incision to expose the VSD. The proximal main pulmonary artery is transected. The ductus will be ligated and divided and the proximal descending aorta, aortic arch and ascending aorta are opened as for the Norwood procedure. (b) A cutaway view illustrates the baffle which is placed within the right ventricle to direct left ventricular blood through the VSD into the pulmonary artery, i.e. neoaorta. (c) The neoaorta has been constructed as for a Norwood procedure. A homograft conduit is placed between the right ventricle and pulmonary artery bifurcation. The proximal anastomosis is supplemented with a hood of autologous pericardium.*

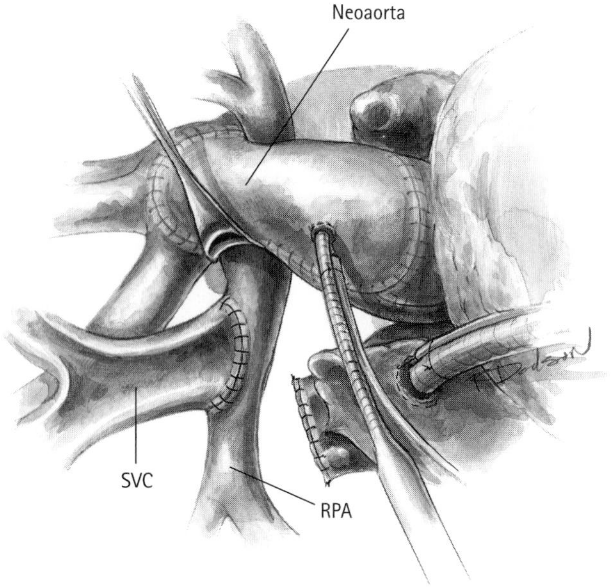

Figure 19.3 *The bidirectional Glenn shunt is the second stage of the reconstructive approach for hypoplastic left heart syndrome. The superior vena cava is divided and is anastomosed to the right pulmonary artery. The procedure is performed on cardiopulmonary bypass. Details are provided in Chapter 20.*

Outcome of Norwood procedure with Sano shunt

In 2003 Malec et al[47] from Krakow, Poland, described 68 children who underwent stage 1 Norwood procedures. The mortality for the 31 patients who had modified Blalock Taussig shunts was 35% while for patients who had the Sano shunt between the right ventricle and pulmonary arteries mortality was 5%. Sano et al and Norwood et al have also described improved results with the Sano modification relative to placement of a modified Blalock shunt.

Developmental outcome

Wernovsky et al[48] reviewed 133 patients who underwent developmental testing following the Fontan procedure at Children's Hospital Boston. The mean full scale IQ was 95.7 ± 17.4. The diagnosis of hypoplastic left heart syndrome as well as other complex anatomical forms of single ventricle were both associated with a worse outcome. The use of circulatory arrest was another factor associated with a lower IQ score. This study must be interpreted carefully with the understanding that many of these children underwent their stage 1 Norwood procedure during the 1980s when long periods of circulatory arrest were employed. Even more importantly the technique of circulatory arrest involved a very alkaline pH, severe hemodilution, rapid cooling and a relatively short period of cooling. Although it is possible that there is an inherent association between less good developmental outcome and hypoplastic left heart syndrome, a more likely explanation is that the technique of cerebral protection employed during the sequence of three reconstructive operations was suboptimal in the timeframe during which these patients were managed.

Goldberg et al[49] also studied the IQ of patients following a reconstructive approach to hypoplastic left heart syndrome at the University of Michigan. They found a mean full scale Wechsler score of 93.8 ± 7.3 which was significantly lower than patients with anomalies other than hypoplastic left heart syndrome who had undergone Fontan procedures who had a mean full scale IQ of 107.0 ± 7.0. The use of circulatory arrest and the occurrence of perioperative seizures were predictive of suboptimal neurodevelopmental outcome. Eke et al[50] reviewed the neurodevelopmental outcome in 38 patients who underwent cardiac transplantation mainly for hypoplastic left heart syndrome at Loma Linda California. The psychomotor development index of the Bayley scale was 91 and the mental developmental index was 88. Both of these scores should be greater than 100 in a normal population. Although the authors were not able to find a direct association between these suboptimal scores and technical aspects of the procedure it is important to recognize that the technique of hypothermic circulatory arrest involved an asanguineous prime resulting in a hematocrit of 5%. No surface precooling was used and the mean cooling time was 14 minutes. Mean duration of circulatory arrest was 56 minutes. Similar results following heart transplantation have been reported by Ilke et al[51] from Denver, Colorado. The median mental development index was 88 and the psychomotor development index was 86.5 among 26 children managed by heart transplantation for hypoplastic left heart syndrome.

REFERENCES

1. Fyler DC, Buckley LA, Hellenbrand WE et al. Report of the New England Regional Infant Cardiac Program. *Pediatrics* 1980; **65**:375–461.
2. Izukawa T, Mullholland C, Rowe RD et al. Structural heart disease in newborn, changing profile: comparison of 1975 with 1965. *Arch Dis Child* 1979; **54**:281–285.
3. Scott DJ, Rigby ML, Miller GAH, Shinebourne EA. The presentation of symptomatic heart disease in infancy based on 10 years experience (1973–1982): implications for the provision of service. *Br Heart J* 1984, **52**:248–257.
4. Freed MD, Heymann MA, Lewis AB et al. Prostaglandin E1 in infants with ductus arteriosus-dependent congenital heart disease. *Circulation* 1981; **64**:899–905.
5. Doty DB. Aortic atresia. *J Thorac Cardiovasc Surg* 1980; **79**:462–463.
6. Morris CD, Outcalt J, Menashe VD. Hypoplastic left heart syndrome: Natural history in a geographically defined population. *Pediatrics* 1990; **85**:977–983.
7. Elzenga NJ, Gittenberger-deGroot AC. Coarctation and related aortic arch anomalies in hypoplastic left heart syndrome. *Int J Cardiol* 1985; **8**:379–393.

8. von Rueden TJ, Knight L, Moller JH, Edwards JE. Coarctation of the aorta associated with aortic valvular atresia. *Circulation* 1975; **52**:951–954.
9. Roberts WC, Perry LW, Chandra RS, Myers GE, Shapiro SR, Scott LP. Aortic valve atresia. A new classification based on necropsy study of 73 cases. *Am J Cardiol* 1976; **37**:753–756.
10. Hawkins JA, Doty DB. Aortic atresia: Morphologic characteristics affecting survival and operative palliation. *J Thorac Cardiovasc Surg* 1984; **88**:620–626.
11. Sauer U, Gittenberger-de Groot AC, Geishauser M, Babic R, Buhlmeyer K. Coronary arteries in the hypoplastic left heart syndrome. *Circulation* 1989; **80**(suppl I): I168–176.
12. Natowicz M, Chatten J, Clancy R et al. Genetic disorders and major extracardiac anomalies with hypoplastic left heart syndrome. *Pediatrics* 1988; **82**:698–706.
13. Glauser TA, Rorke LB, Weinberg PM, Clancy RR. Congenital brain anomalies associated with the hypoplastic left heart syndrome. *Pediatrics* 1990; **85**:984–990.
14. Naeye RL. Perinatal vascular changes associated with underdevelopment of the left heart. *Chest* 1962; **41**:287–295.
15. Shone JD, Edwards JE. Mitral atresia associated with pulmonary venous anomalies. *Br Heart J* 1964; **26**:241–249.
16. Wagenvort CA, Edwards JE. The pulmonary arterial tree in aortic atresia with intact ventricular septum. *Lab Invest* 1961; **10**:924–933.
17. Ehrlich M, Bierman FZ, Ellis K, Gersony WM. Hypoplastic left heart syndrome: Report of a unique survivor. *J Am Coll Cardiol* 1986; **7**:361–365.
18. Glauser TA, Rorke LB, Weinberg PM, Clancy RR. Acquired neuropathologic lesions associated with the hypoplastic left heart syndrome. *Pediatrics* 1990; **85**:991–1000.
19. Allan LD, Sharland G, Tynan MJ. The natural history of hypoplastic left heart syndrome. *Int J Cardiol* 1989; **25**:341–343.
20. Maxwell D, Allan L, Tynan MJ. Balloon dilation of the aortic valve in the fetus: A report of two cases. *Br Heart J* 1991; **65**:256–258.
21. Yeager SB, Flanagan MF, Keane JF. Catheter intervention: Balloon valvotomy. In Lock JE, Keane JF, Perry SB (eds). *Diagnostic and Interventional Catheterization in Congenital Heart Disease*, Boston, Kluwer Academic Publishers, 2000, p 151.
22. Chang AC, Huhta JC, Yoon GY et al. Diagnosis, transport and outcome in fetuses with left ventricular outflow tract obstruction. *J Thorac Cardiovasc Surg* 1991; **102**:841–848.
23. Lofland GK, McCrindle BW, Williams WG et al. Critical aortic stenosis in the neonate: A multi-institutional study of management, outcomes, and risk factors. *J Thorac Cardiovasc Surg* 2001; **121**:10–27.
24. Cayler GG, Smeloff EA, Miller GE. Surgical palliation of hypoplastic left side of the heart. *N Engl J Med* 1970; **282**:780–783.
25. Cayler GG. Hypoplastic left heart syndrome. Letter. *Am J Cardiol* 1972; **30**:450.
26. Behrendt DM, Rocchini A. An operation for the hypoplastic left heart syndrome: Preliminary report. *Ann Thorac Surg* 1981; **32**:284–288.
27. Doty DB, Knott HW. Hypoplastic left heart syndrome. *J Thorac Cardiovasc Surg* 1977; **74**:624–630.
28. Levitsky S, van der Horst RL, Hastreiter AR, Eckner FA, Bennett EJ. Surgical palliation in aortic atresia. *J Thorac Cardiovasc Surg* 1980; **79**:456–461.
29. Norwood WI, Kirklin JK, Sanders SP. Hypoplastic left heart syndrome: Experience with palliative surgery. *Am J Cardiol* 1980; **45**:87–91.
30. Norwood WI, Lang P, Hansen DD. Physiologic repair of aortic-atresia-hypoplastic left heart syndrome. *N Engl J Med* 1983; **308**:23–26.
31. Sano S, Kawada M, Yoshida H et al. Norwood procedure to hypoplastic left heart syndrome. *Jpn J Thorac Cardiovasc Surg* 1998; **46**:1311–1316.
32. Hansen DD, Hickey PR. Anesthesia for hypoplastic left heart syndrome. Use of high dose fentanyl in 30 neonates. *Anesth Analg* 1986; **65**; 127–132.
33. Jonas RA, Lang P, Hansen D, Hickey P, Castaneda AR. First stage palliation of hypoplastic left heart syndrome: The importance of coarctation and shunt size. *J Thorac Cardiovasc Surg* 1986; **92**:6–13.
34. Kadoba K, Arminger LC, Sawatari K, Jonas RA. Mechanical durability of pulmonary allograft conduits at systemic pressure. *J Thorac Cardiovasc Surg* 1993; **105**:132–141.
35. Sade RM, Crawford FA, Fyfe DA. Symposium on hypoplastic left heart syndrome. *J Thorac Cardiovasc Surg* 1986; **91**:937–939.
36. Bu'Lock FA, Stumper O, Jagtap R et al. Surgery for infants with a hypoplastic systemic ventricle and severe outflow obstruction: early results with a modified Norwood procedure. *Br Heart J* 1995; **73**:456–461.
37. Bellinger DC, Wypij D, du Plessis AJ et al. Neurodevelopmental status at eight years in children with D-transposition of the great arteries: The Boston Circulatory Arrest Trial. *J Thorac Cardiovasc Surg* 2003; **126:**1385–1396.
38. Jonas RA. Deep hypothermic circulatory arrest: Current status and indications. *Sem Thorac Cardiovasc Surg Ped Card Surg Ann* 2002; **5**:76–88.
39. Duebener LF, Hagino I, Schmitt K et al. Direct visualization of minimal cerebral capillary flow during retrograde cerebral perfusion: An intravital fluorescence microscopy study in pigs. *Ann Thorac Surg* 2003; **75**:1288–1293.
40. Ashburn DA, McCrindle BW, Tchervenkov CI et al. Outcomes after the Norwood operation in neonates with critical aortic stenosis or aortic valve atresia. *J Thorac Cardiovasc Surg* 2003; **125**:1070–1082.
41. Daebritz SH, Nollert GD, Zurakowski D et al. Results of Norwood stage I operation: comparison of hypoplastic left heart syndrome with other malformations. *J Thorac Cardiovasc Surg* 2000; **119**:358–367.
42. Mahle WT, Spray TL, Wernovsky G, Gaynor JW, Clark BJ 3rd. Survival after reconstructive surgery for hypoplastic left heart syndrome: A 15-year experience from a single institution. *Circulation* 2000; **102**(19 Suppl 3):III136–141.
43. Bove EL. Current status of staged reconstruction for hypoplastic left heart syndrome. *Pediatr Cardiol* 1998; **19**:308–315.
44. Tweddell JS, Hoffman GM, Mussatto KA et al. Improved survival of patients undergoing palliation of hypoplastic left heart syndrome: lessons learned from 115 consecutive patients. *Circulation* 2002; **106**(12 Suppl 1):I82–89.
45. Azakie T, Merklinger SL, McCrindle BW et al. Evolving strategies and improving outcomes of the modified Norwood procedure: a 10-year single-institution experience. *Ann Thorac Surg* 2001; **72**:1349–1353.
46. Ishino K, Stumper O, De Giovanni JJ et al. The modified Norwood procedure for hypoplastic left heart syndrome: early to intermediate results of 120 patients with particular reference to aortic arch repair. *J Thorac Cardiovasc Surg* 1999; **117**:920–930.

47. Malec E, Januszewska K, Kolcz J, Mroczek T. Right ventricle-to-pulmonary artery shunt versus modified Blalock-Taussig shunt in the Norwood procedure for hypoplastic left heart syndrome – influence on early and late haemodynamic status. *Eur J Cardiothorac Surg* 2003; **23**:728–734.
48. Wernovsky G, Stiles KM, Gauvreau K et al. Cognitive development after the Fontan operation. *Circulation* 2000; **102**:883–889.
49. Goldberg CS, Schwartz EM, Brunberg JA et al. Neurodevelopmental outcome of patients after the Fontan operation: A comparison between children with hypoplastic left heart syndrome and other functional single ventricle lesions. *J Pediatr* 2000; **137**:646–652.
50. Eke CC, Gundry SR, Baum MF, Chinnock RE, Razzouk AJ, Bailey LL. Neurologic sequelae of deep hypothermic circulatory arrest in cardiac transplant infants. *Ann Thorac Surg* 1996; **61**:783–788.
51. Ikle L, Hale K, Fashaw L, Boucek M, Rosenberg AA. Developmental outcome of patients with hypoplastic left heart syndrome treated with heart transplantation. *J Pediatr* 2003; **142**:20–25.

20

Single ventricle

INTRODUCTION

The outlook for children with either one or two ventricles managed with a single ventricle pathway has improved dramatically over the past two decades. Today children who are managed carefully through infancy, so as to optimize their anatomy and physiology for a subsequent Fontan procedure, have a 90% probability of leading good quality lives with minimal if any restrictions. These children grow to become adults who continue to have a good quality of life including successful management of pregnancy. That is not to say that there are not ongoing challenges, which when overcome will allow even further improvement in the lives of patients managed with a single ventricle pathway. There are many unresolved controversies as described in this chapter that will require considerable effort, resources and multi-institutional collaboration and study if they are to be resolved.

EMBRYOLOGY

It is helpful to review the development of the ventricles in order to have an understanding of the embryological mechanisms resulting in a single functional ventricle.[1] Following looping of the primitive cardiac tube, septation of the primitive ventricle begins to separate the primordial left ventricle from the bulbus cordis. The bulboventricular foramen is the defect that remains, connecting the outflow chamber to the main ventricular cavity. As septation occurs the common AV canal is forming from endocardial cushion tissue. Many forms of single ventricle occur because there is poor alignment of the common AV valve with the ventricles. Another mechanism for development of a single functional ventricle is incomplete septation of the ventricular chambers.

ANATOMY

Classification of single ventricle using Van Praagh's segmental approach

The segmental approach developed by the Van Praaghs is a tremendously helpful shorthand method for classifying complex forms of cardiac anatomy such as occur in patients who have a single functional ventricle.[2] An important premise of the segmental approach is that almost all ventricles have a fundamental left ventricular or right ventricular morphology. For example the left ventricle has a smooth finely trabeculated endocardial surface with usually two papillary muscles on the free wall but not on the septum. In contrast the right ventricle is heavily trabeculated and there are multiple chordal attachments of the tricuspid valve to the right ventricular septal surface. The atrioventricular valve is an integral part of a ventricle so that the mitral valve is associated with the left ventricle while the tricuspid valve is associated with the right ventricle.

The segmental approach involves classification of each of the three main segments of the heart. The first of the three segments refers to the *situs* of the patient's heart. With normal *situs solitus* the inferior vena cava is right sided and enters a right sided right atrium. This will usually be associated with normal situs for the lungs so that there is a right sided branching pattern of the right main bronchus (early arising right upper lobe). There may or may not be situs solitus of the abdominal viscera, i.e. the liver being right sided and the stomach being left sided. If the situs is the opposite of usual it is described as *inversus*. Situs is therefore abbreviated as 'S' or 'I'.

The second of the two letters for the segmental classification refers to looping of the ventricles. Normally the primitive single ventricle loops to the right (dextro) so that the morphological left ventricle is left sided and the morphological right ventricle is right sided. If there is an l-loop (levo) the morphological right ventricle will be left sided and the morphological left ventricle will be right sided. Looping occurs independent of situs. The abbreviations *D* and *L* are used.

The final letter of the segmental approach refers to the location of the great vessels. If the aorta lies to the right of the pulmonary artery this is referred to as dextroposition of the aorta *D* while if the aorta is to the left of the pulmonary artery this is referred to as a levoposition of the aorta *L*.

A typical example of the segmental classification is the patient with transposition of the great arteries. If there is SDD transposition, the patient's right atrium is normally located on the right and is connected to a right sided right ventricle because of the d-loop. The aorta may be anterior and to the right of the pulmonary artery so that this patient will be classified as having SDD transposition of the great arteries. The physiology of this patient will be transposition type physiology since blue blood from the right atrium passes through the right ventricle to the aorta. On the other hand, a patient with SLL transposition has situs solitus of the atria. However, the right sided right atrium is connected to a right sided left ventricle while the left sided right ventricle connects to a left sided aorta. Even though this patient also has transposition of the great vessels, the physiology is normal, hence SLL transposition is also known as congenitally corrected transposition.

Single ventricle with obstruction to systemic outflow

Obstruction between a single functional ventricle and systemic outflow, i.e. the aorta, is one of the – if not *the* most – important factor in determining the long-term outlook for the patient with a single ventricle. Systemic outflow obstruction is almost certainly more important than the morphology of the single ventricle, e.g. whether the ventricle is morphologically a right or left ventricle. On the other hand so long as the presence of systemic outflow obstruction is identified early in infancy and so long as appropriate measures are taken in the early palliation of the child it is possible to minimize the impact of this otherwise very important risk factor.

Obstruction to systemic outflow is frequently associated with underdevelopment of the aortic arch and a coarctation of the aorta.[3,4] Even if obstruction does not appear to be present between a single functional ventricle and the ascending aorta at the time of neonatal presentation, the presence of a coarctation and/or hypoplastic aortic arch should almost always result in the patient being directed towards a management strategy that allows bypass of the potentially obstructed systemic outflow area, i.e. with the Damus-Kaye-Stansel or Norwood procedure.

The mechanism of obstruction to systemic outflow varies with different anomalies. The presence of transposition of the great arteries in association with tricuspid atresia for example means that the size of the VSD through which the single left ventricle communicates with the infundibular subaortic chamber is critically important. On the other hand in the setting of mitral atresia it is only when the great arteries are normally related that the size of the defects between a single right ventricle and hypoplastic left ventricular outflow chamber becomes the critical factor. Outflow tract obstruction can also occur when there is a subaortic conus as part of double outlet right ventricle or double inlet single ventricle. If the conus is long and if there is malalignment of the conal septum there may be functional obstruction between the single ventricle and the ascending aorta. Interestingly it is unusual that pure aortic valve stenosis results in obstruction between a single ventricle and ascending aorta.

Obstruction to pulmonary outflow

In general there is a reciprocal relationship between the pulmonary outflow and systemic outflow, i.e. when there is obstruction to systemic outflow, it is unusual that there is any obstruction to pulmonary outflow and vice versa. In fewer than 10% of patients with a single functional ventricle there is obstruction to both systemic and pulmonary outflow.[5]

As with obstruction to systemic outflow there are many anatomical variations that can result in obstruction to pulmonary outflow. There may be complete atresia of the main pulmonary artery and pulmonary valve. There may be muscular subpulmonary stenosis associated with valvar hypoplasia and pulmonary valve stenosis. Accessory atrioventricular valve tissue may crowd the subpulmonary area. Stenosis or atresia, particularly at the origin of the left or right pulmonary artery also complicates the management of the patient with single functional ventricle.

Major single ventricle anomalies

TRICUSPID ATRESIA AND STENOSIS INCLUDING PULMONARY ATRESIA WITH INTACT VENTRICULAR SEPTUM

SDN tricuspid atresia, i.e. tricuspid atresia with normally related great arteries, is generally considered to be the simplest form of single functional ventricle. This was the anomaly that was first successfully managed in the 1960s by Fontan using what has come to be called the Fontan procedure.[6] Fontan believed that there was an inherent advantage in having a normal left ventricle connected directly to the aorta though subsequent experience has not consistently identified an advantage for a single left ventricle versus a single right ventricle or common ventricle.[7]

The patient with tricuspid atresia has complete failure of development of the tricuspid valve. It may be replaced by muscular tissue, fibrofatty tissue or an atretic membrane.[8,9] There must be a patent foramen ovale to be consistent with life. Pulmonary blood flow is achieved by blood passing from the left ventricle through a VSD into an infundibular chamber that is connected to the main pulmonary artery. Alternatively there may be associated pulmonary atresia and under these circumstances the child is dependent on patency of the ductus or some other arterial level connection such as an aortopulmonary window for pulmonary blood flow.

When there is transposition of the great arteries associated with tricuspid atresia (i.e. SDD transposition of the great arteries with tricuspid atresia) the size of the defect becomes critically important as this will determine whether there is obstruction to systemic outflow. If there is a coarctation or hypoplasia of the aortic arch it is very likely that the size of the defect will be smaller than the size of the aortic annulus. Echocardiographic studies suggest that if the cross sectional area of the defect is less than $2\,cm^2/m^2$ then it is likely that the defect will become restrictive in the future, if it is not already restrictive.[10,11] If the tricuspid valve is patent but stenotic, i.e. there is tricuspid valve stenosis, an assessment must be made as to whether the valve is adequate to allow a two ventricle repair. Calculation of the z value for both the diameter as well as cross sectional area of the tricuspid valve is helpful. If the z value is smaller than -2 and particularly if smaller than -2.5 to -3 then almost certainly a single ventricle pathway should be pursued rather than a two ventricle repair. Some patients with pulmonary atresia and intact ventricular septum must ultimately be directed into a single ventricle pathway. Generally such patients will have a very small tricuspid valve in addition to having a small right ventricular cavity. These patients also frequently have coronary artery stenoses and may have dependence on the right ventricle for coronary perfusion of the left ventricle. These latter patients must pursue a single ventricle pathway even if it is suspected that the tricuspid valve may be of adequate size to allow a two ventricle repair. However, this is very rarely likely to be the case if the patient has right ventricular dependence of the coronary circulation.

DOUBLE INLET SINGLE VENTRICLE

As the name suggests the patient with double inlet single ventricle has two atrioventricular or inlet valves. The dominant ventricle is usually a morphological left ventricle[12] though there may be either a d-loop or l-loop. There may be stenosis usually with associated hypoplasia of one of the atrioventricular valves. There may be straddling of chords from either the tricuspid or the mitral valve to the contralateral ventricle. The following are some of the most common specific subtypes of double inlet single ventricle.

SLL double inlet single left ventricle

These patients have a dominant morphological left ventricle which is right sided. Both inlet valves enter the single left ventricle though the left sided tricuspid valve is likely to be at least in part associated with the left sided morphological right ventricular outflow chamber. There is frequently straddling of tricuspid chords into the single left ventricle.[13] The aorta is anterior and leftwards relative to the pulmonary artery and arises from the left sided right ventricular outflow chamber. The size of the bulboventricular foramen, i.e. the communication between the left ventricle and the outflow chamber is critically important. If this is smaller than the aortic annulus or smaller than $2\,cm/m^2$ then it should be anticipated that there either is or will be important obstruction to outflow between the single ventricle and the aorta.[10,11]

There may be subpulmonary and/or pulmonary valvar stenosis limiting pulmonary blood flow. This may in part be caused by AV valve tissue below the pulmonary valve.

SDD double inlet single left ventricle

These patients have normal d-looping so that the functional single ventricle is a left sided left ventricle. However, there is transposition of the great arteries so that the aorta arises from the right sided infundibular outflow chamber. Once again the size of the bulboventricular foramen is critically important. This is the most likely site of obstruction between the single ventricle and the ascending aorta. However, on occasion there may be obstruction within the infundibular chamber because of anterior malalignment of the conal septum.

SDN double inlet single ventricle (Holmes heart)

This variant of the double inlet single ventricle is less common than either the SLL or SDD variants but it happens to have an eponym.[14,15] Because the aorta connects normally to the single left ventricle it is less likely that there will be obstruction to systemic outflow than with the previously mentioned variant. This variant of double inlet single ventricle may be suitable for ventricular septation if there is some development of the ventricular septum and if the infundibular chamber and tricuspid valve are adequately developed. In fact it is reasonable to consider the Holmes heart as part of a spectrum which merges with the normal heart with very large ventricular septal defect.

SINGLE VENTRICLE WITH COMMON AV VALVE INCLUDING HETEROTAXY VARIANTS (ASPLENIA/POLYSPLENIA OR ATRIAL ISOMERISM)

There are a number of anatomical variants of single functional ventricle that have a common AV valve.

Unbalanced complete AV canal

If the common AV valve of a complete AV canal fails to align in a balanced fashion with the two ventricles there may be sufficient imbalance that the patient is best managed as though having a single ventricle. This is more likely to be the case if there is right ventricular dominance. Under these circumstances repair of the complete AV canal would result in an inadequate mitral valve and possibly inadequate left ventricle. Patients with right ventricular dominance may also have the potential for subaortic stenosis if the complete AV canal is repaired. These patients frequently have a coarctation and/or hypoplasia of the aortic arch. There must be extremely severe underdevelopment of the right ventricle and tricuspid component of the common AV valve before the left ventricular dominant complete AV canal requires management with a single ventricle pathway.

Heterotaxy[16]

There are a number of synonyms for heterotaxy including asplenia/polysplenia syndrome and atrial isomerism. The fundamental lesion in these patients is that there is poor differentiation into right and left side. This can result in bilateral right sidedness (asplenia syndrome) which may be associated with bilateral right lungs (i.e. an early rising upper lobe bronchus and three rather than two lobes bilaterally). In addition the atrial chambers may suggest bilateral right atria.[17] These patients are likely to have bilateral superior vena cavae and may have bilateral entrance of the hepatic veins into a common atrium. Because there is effective absence of the left atrium it is not uncommon to see anomalous pulmonary venous connection.[18] Patients with the polysplenia variant of heterotaxy tend to have bilateral left sidedness.[19] Not uncommonly there is interruption of the inferior vena cava with azygous extension of the IVC connecting either to a right sided or left sided superior vena cava. Patients with polysplenia also may have anomalous pulmonary venous connection although Van Praagh[20] has suggested that the connection to the atrium is normal and the appearance of abnormal pulmonary venous connection is due to malattachment of the atrial septum primum in an abnormally leftward position. In general in both polysplenia and asplenia there is minimal development of the atrial septum so that there is effectively a common atrium.

In both asplenia and polysplenia it is common to have subpulmonary or pulmonary valve stenosis. Pulmonary atresia is more common with asplenia and pulmonary stenosis is more common with polysplenia. Branch pulmonary artery anomalies are also not uncommon particularly when there is pulmonary atresia. The anatomy of the branch pulmonary arteries varies according to whether there is asplenia or polysplenia. Similar to the bronchial branching pattern when there is asplenia there tend to be bilateral right sided pulmonary arteries while with polysplenia there tend to be bilateral left sided pulmonary arteries.

Mitral atresia including hypoplastic left heart syndrome

Absence of the mitral valve as with marked absence of the tricuspid valve excludes the possibility of a biventricular repair. Mitral atresia or severe mitral stenosis is most commonly seen as part of hypoplastic left heart syndrome merging with Shone's syndrome. If there is associated atresia of the aortic valve and/or severe underdevelopment of the left ventricle then the decision to direct the patient to a single ventricle/Norwood pathway is an easy one. If the mitral valve is the only underdeveloped structure in the left heart an assessment must be made of the z scores for both the diameters and cross sectional area of the mitral valve. Generally a z score of smaller than -2 to -3 contraindicates a two ventricle repair.

In addition to its occurrence as part of hypoplastic left heart syndrome mitral atresia is not uncommonly associated with double outlet right ventricle.[21] Usually there is associated underdevelopment of the left ventricle. Even though the aorta arises directly from the functional single right ventricle in this anomaly, i.e. SDD double outlet right ventricle with mitral atresia, nevertheless this anomaly is not free of the risk of obstruction to systemic outflow. In general the aorta under these circumstances arises from a subaortic conus. This may be long and narrow and therefore cause significant obstruction to outflow into the systemic circulation.

PATHOPHYSIOLOGY AND CLINICAL FEATURES

Parallel versus in series circulation

In a normal biventricular circulation blood leaving the left ventricle has no choice other than to pass through the resistance bed of the systemic circulation. It then passes in series through the right ventricle and the resistance bed of the pulmonary circulation before returning to the left ventricle. This is an *in series* circulation. In contrast, the unoperated patient who has a single ventricle has parallel pulmonary and systemic circulations. Blood leaving the single ventricle has a choice of either passing to the pulmonary circulation or the systemic circulation. Therefore the relative resistances of the pulmonary and systemic vascular beds will determine the amount of flow which passes to each unless there is obstruction to pulmonary outflow or obstruction to systemic outflow. In the absence of either pulmonary or systemic outflow obstruction or pulmonary vascular disease there will be very much more pulmonary than systemic blood flow.

'Balanced' single ventricle

Occasionally an individual will have just the right amount of natural obstruction to pulmonary blood flow to achieve a reasonably equal distribution of blood to the lungs and to the systemic circulation. This will result in an arterial oxygen saturation of approximately 80% and is consistent with surprisingly good long-term survival with a satisfactory quality of life. The single ventricle under these circumstances is being asked to pump only double the normal cardiac output and generally this can be achieved for many years.

The single ventricle with obstruction to pulmonary outflow

Much more common than the long-term balanced single ventricle is the single ventricle with a progressive increase in obstruction to pulmonary outflow so that the patient becomes progressively more severely cyanosed. In time the patient will suffer the usual consequences of severe cyanosis including polycythemia, stroke, brain abscess, hemoptysis and ultimately death. At the other end of the spectrum the patient who has inadequate obstruction to pulmonary outflow will likely develop excessive pulmonary blood flow in the first weeks and months of life as pulmonary resistance falls and symptoms of congestive heart failure will develop. If the heart is able to cope with the massive volume load with which it is likely to be confronted there will subsequently be progressive development of pulmonary vascular disease. Although the patient's symptoms may abate for some time as pulmonary resistance itself comes to balance systemic resistance, with further progression of pulmonary vascular disease cyanosis worsens. The ultimate result is similar to the patient who has a severe fixed degree of obstruction to pulmonary outflow.

The single ventricle with obstruction to systemic outflow

As described in the anatomy section above there are many potential sites for obstruction to develop between the single functional ventricle and the ascending aorta. In most cases the obstruction is progressive in nature. If there is no obstruction to pulmonary outflow the consequence of increasing systemic outflow obstruction is increasing pulmonary blood flow. The single ventricle becomes progressively volume loaded and ultimately will fail unless pulmonary vascular disease intervenes. On the other hand if there is concomitant obstruction to pulmonary outflow, either natural or in the form of a surgically placed pulmonary artery band, the progressive obstruction to systemic outflow will result in an increasing pressure load for the single ventricle. The very serious consequence of a pressure load for the single ventricle is progressive ventricular hypertrophy with accompanying deterioration in compliance.

Clinical features of the patient with a single ventricle

The clinical presentation of the patient with a single ventricle is dependent on the balance of blood flow between the systemic and pulmonary circulation. For example the neonate who has a severe degree of fixed pulmonary outflow obstruction will present with profound cyanosis at the time of ductal closure. On the other hand the patient who has no obstruction to pulmonary outflow may initially appear to be free of symptoms but as pulmonary resistance falls in the first days and weeks of life there will be progressive onset of symptoms of congestive heart failure. Even though the patient has symptoms and signs of congestive heart failure, nevertheless mixing of pulmonary and systemic venous return usually at both atrial and ventricular level will mean that there is at least a modest degree of cyanosis. Auscultation of the chest will demonstrate the systolic murmur which results from either pulmonary or systemic outflow obstruction. If there is neither there may be little to be heard since it is unlikely that there will be a murmur generated within the single ventricle itself.

DIAGNOSTIC STUDIES

Assessment of pulmonary artery pressure and flow

The assessment of pulmonary blood flow with a consequent inference regarding pulmonary artery pressure is not difficult in the young infant. So long as there is no associated obstruction to systemic outflow the arterial oxygen saturation provides a helpful estimate of pulmonary blood flow. Generally an arterial oxygen saturation between 75% and 80% indicates that there is reasonable protection of the pulmonary vascular bed from excessive flow and pressure. This inference cannot be drawn in the older child who may initially have had excessive pulmonary blood flow and has now developed Eisenmenger's syndrome with a falling arterial oxygen saturation because of progressive pulmonary vascular disease. Nevertheless in the neonate and young infant there is generally no need to undertake cardiac catheterization for assessment of pulmonary blood flow and pressure.

The plain chest X-ray is a helpful adjunct to arterial oxygen saturation in the assessment of pulmonary blood flow. The patient with no obstruction to pulmonary outflow will have congested lung fields and an enlarged heart. Alternatively the child with a severe degree of obstruction to pulmonary outflow is likely to have oligemic lung fields and a relatively small heart size. One exception to these general guidelines to remember is that occasionally there can be streaming of blood flow within a single ventricle creating transposition type physiology, i.e. systemic venous return is preferentially directed through the single ventricle into the aorta while pulmonary venous return tends to be preferentially directed to the pulmonary circulation. However, this situation is highly unusual in the patient who has a true form of single ventricle.

The ECG is generally not helpful. Two-dimensional echocardiography with color Doppler mapping is usually diagnostic. It is important at the outset that the echocardiographer determine whether the ductus is patent. Patency of the ductus will complicate assessment of the degree of obstruction to pulmonary outflow. However, if the ductus is confirmed to be closed it is generally possible to make a reasonable assessment of pulmonary outflow obstruction by estimating the Doppler gradient between the single ventricle and the pulmonary arteries. Once again in the neonate and young infant however this information should be considered simply adjunctive to the systemic arterial oxygen saturation. It must be remembered the pulmonary vascular resistance is evolving, generally in a downward direction throughout the early weeks of life so there should not be undue concern if pulmonary artery pressure appears to be modestly elevated, e.g. at half systemic level in the young infant. This would clearly be of much greater concern in the older infant or young child.

The echocardiographer should determine the segmental classification of the patient's cardiac anatomy. The anatomy of the systemic veins and pulmonary veins must be carefully determined as this will have an important influence on the ultimate method of surgical reconstruction to be applied as well as having some influence on prognosis. In addition to assessing the degree of obstruction to pulmonary outflow the echocardiographer should determine the mechanism of obstruction as this may help to indicate whether obstruction is likely to be progressive. For example the patient who has a relatively small VSD in the setting of tricuspid atresia with normally related great arteries is likely to have progressive closure of the defect and therefore falling pulmonary blood flow and increasing cyanosis in the coming weeks.

Careful determination should be made as to whether the branch pulmonary arteries are in continuity and whether any origin stenoses are present. Fortunately it is uncommon for the patient with a single ventricle to have multiple peripheral pulmonary artery stenoses and even if these are present it is not important to define them at the time of the child's presentation in the neonatal period or early infancy.

Assessment of obstruction to systemic outflow

It is critically important that careful assessment be made at the time of presentation as to the presence or potential presence of obstruction to systemic outflow. A particularly helpful 'red flag' that obstruction may be present or is likely to develop is the presence of a juxtaductal coarctation of the aorta.[3,4] When the ductus is widely patent it is unlikely that there will be any gradient in the coarctation area. However, the presence of a prominent coarctation shelf should stimulate the echocardiographer to return for a repeat study within a day or two when the ductus has closed. In addition careful measurements must be taken of the proximal aortic arch, distal aortic arch and aortic isthmus and z values calculated. When the z value is smaller than -2 the arch segment should be considered hypoplastic and particularly careful study of the internal anatomy of the single ventricle must now be undertaken. As discussed in the anatomy section above, obstruction to systemic outflow can occur at a number of different levels. For example the patient with tricuspid atresia and transposition of the great arteries may have obstruction at the level of the VSD as well as obstruction within the infundibular outflow chamber. It is particularly important to remember that when the ductus is patent there will be no gradient across either of these areas even when relatively severe obstruction is present. The ductus allows equalization of pressure between the ascending and descending aorta so that the hypoplastic right ventricular outflow chamber contracts against the same pressure as the single left ventricle. The area should be reassessed when the ductus is closed. Even if the ductus is not closed or in the event that the ductus does not close a morphological assessment should be made of the size of the VSD. The defect is frequently not circular in shape and therefore must be assessed according to its area. Studies have suggested that a cross sectional area of less than $2\ cm^2/m^2$ is likely to be inadequate and either cause or lead to systemic outflow obstruction.[10,11]

MEDICAL AND INTERVENTIONAL THERAPY

Only a small percentage of patients with a single ventricle have a reasonable natural balance of pulmonary and systemic blood flow. Patients who have a severe degree of obstruction to pulmonary outflow are likely to suffer severe cyanosis when the ductus closes. These patients are ductally dependent and therefore require infusion of prostaglandin E1 until a systemic to pulmonary arterial shunt can be performed. Patients who have no obstruction to pulmonary outflow may have relatively few symptoms initially but gradually develop congestive heart failure as their pulmonary resistance falls. They will require treatment with the usual anti-congestive therapy and when their condition has been stabilized satisfactorily they should proceed to application of a pulmonary artery band assuming that there is no obstruction to systemic outflow.

There is usually no place for interventional catheter therapy for the patient presenting in the neonatal period or early infancy with a single ventricle. In rare circumstances where there is mitral atresia and an obstructive atrial septum it is important to open the atrial septum before surgery, not only to allow adequate pulmonary blood flow for reasonable oxygenation but also to lower the pulmonary resistance before surgery is undertaken. It is generally not advisable to consider balloon dilation of an obstructive pulmonary valve when there is a single ventricle with obstruction to pulmonary outflow. This might result in excessive pulmonary blood flow which can be just as problematic as inadequate pulmonary blood flow.

INDICATIONS FOR AND TIMING OF SURGERY

A basic premise of the management of single ventricle today is that the natural history of untreated single ventricle is so unlikely to be acceptable that the mere diagnosis of single ventricle alone is an indication to proceed along a pathway of surgical palliation. Although a small subset of patients with single ventricle physiology can have a balance of systemic and pulmonary blood flow over the long term, nevertheless there is an inherent volume loading (approximately twice normal) even in this type of mixed circulation which ultimately is likely to lead to premature ventricular failure. Furthermore there may be some increased risk of paradoxical embolus and sepsis when at least a part of the systemic venous return is allowed to bypass the lungs.

The optimal timing for the various steps that are presently applied for single ventricle palliation remains poorly defined. One thing that is clear is that particularly careful attention needs to be paid very early in infancy or ideally in the neonatal period to preventing excessive volume or pressure loading of the single ventricle. In addition great care must be taken to protect the pulmonary vascular bed as well as to prevent distortion of the central pulmonary arteries.

Following neonatal palliation most patients with single ventricle undergo a bidirectional Glenn shunt by six months of age. Although it is possible to defer the subsequent Fontan procedure for many years this is not always possible (see below). In general it is our preference at present to proceed to a fenestrated Fontan procedure within one to two years of a bidirectional Glenn shunt so long as the child is making satisfactory progress. It is critically important that the patient be monitored very closely during this time to ensure that the bidirectional Glenn circulation is functioning adequately and that the child is not developing an excessive degree of cyanosis.

SURGICAL MANAGEMENT

History of surgery

Laboratory studies were undertaken as early as the 1940s investigating potential means for surgically palliating patients with effectively only a single ventricle.[22–24] This was initially thought to be a potential problem in patients who might undergo repair of tetralogy of Fallot but whose right ventricle was thought to be inadequate to sustain the pulmonary circulation. Laboratory studies by William E Glenn at Yale led to the development of the classic Glenn shunt in 1958.[25] The classic Glenn shunt involves division of the right pulmonary artery with end to side anastomosis of the distal divided right pulmonary artery to the side of the superior vena cava. The atriocaval junction is subsequently ligated and the proximal divided right pulmonary artery is also oversewn. A variation of the classic Glenn shunt was the bidirectional Glenn shunt. In this operation the superior vena cava was divided. It was oversewn on its cardiac end. The cephalic end of the divided superior vena cava was anastomosed to the right pulmonary artery allowing flow to both the right and left lung. Many patients achieved surprisingly good palliation with both the classic Glenn shunt as well as the bidirectional Glenn shunt during the 1950s and 1960s. Glenn's early studies led him and others to the belief that it might be possible to completely bypass an inadequate right ventricle.[22–24]

During the 1960s homografts were introduced by Ross and Barratt-Boyes both as valves and as valved conduits (see Chapter 3). Fontan was the first to successfully clinically apply the principles established by William Glenn by combining a classic Glenn shunt with a homograft conduit to connect the right atrium to the left pulmonary artery.[6] Fontan believed the pulsatile assistance from the right atrium was important in achieving blood flow to the left lung. He therefore placed a homograft valve at the junction of the inferior vena cava and right atrium. In addition the ASD was closed. Fontan believed that the operation should be limited to patients who had tricuspid atresia. He and his cardiologist Choussat enumerated a list of 10 conditions which were felt to be important for patients undergoing the Fontan procedure.[26] Fontan published his work in 1970. Following description of the Ross procedure, i.e. use of the pulmonary valve as an autograft,[27] Kreutzer in Argentina[28] applied the concept of harvesting the pulmonary valve and in addition maintaining continuity with the main pulmonary artery and then connecting the pulmonary valve to the roof of the right atrium. This obviated the need for a nongrowing homograft conduit. In addition the posteriorly placed anastomosis was less prone to sternal compression. Kreutzer also found that it was not necessary to place a valve at the atriocaval junction.

The Fontan Kreutzer procedure was not widely applied during the 1970s. Many patients with tricuspid atresia had suffered the consequences of poor palliation, for example excessive pulmonary blood flow from a Waterston shunt with concomitant distortion of the pulmonary arteries. Patients who had excessive pulmonary blood flow were at risk of having developed pulmonary vascular disease. Gradually however various centers began to apply the Fontan procedure for more complex forms of single ventricle culminating in the successful publication by Norwood in 1983 of successful neonatal palliation of two children with hypoplastic left heart syndrome with a subsequent successful outcome following a Fontan procedure.[29]

The Fontan procedure for hypoplastic left heart syndrome not only demonstrated the feasibility of a successful outcome in the patient with a single right ventricle but in addition necessitated technical modifications of the Fontan procedure. No longer was it sufficient to close the atrial septum as had been the case for patients with tricuspid atresia. Patients with hypoplastic left heart syndrome required baffling of the pulmonary venous return to the tricuspid valve. This baffle proved to be particularly troublesome and was frequently a site of obstruction. A feedback loop was setup in which increasing right atrial pressure compressed the pulmonary venous baffle leading to even further elevation of right atrial pressure. This led Puga et al[30] and independently ourselves[31] to develop the concept of a lateral tunnel to direct inferior vena caval return to the pulmonary circulation for patients with left AV valve atresia or hypoplastic left heart syndrome. This concept appeared to be supported by the recently reported Kawashima procedure[32] in which it was found that a virtual Fontan type procedure could be achieved in patients with heterotaxy and interrupted IVC by direct connection of almost all of the systemic venous return to the pulmonary arteries without any atrial assistance. The lateral tunnel concept was most simply constructed in conjunction with a double cavopulmonary anastomosis. Interestingly, deLeval and colleagues[33] independently developed the concept of a lateral tunnel Fontan by studying the hydrodynamics of an atriopulmonary connection versus a lateral tunnel type connection. deLeval's studies suggested that the lateral tunnel had improved energy efficiency.

In the mid-1980s Hopkins[34] suggested that the bidirectional Glenn was a useful adjunct for palliating the patient with a single ventricle. Mazzera et al[35] and Lamberti et al[36] subsequently reported staging of patients with single ventricle using the bidirectional Glenn shunt as an intermediate step before proceeding to the completed Fontan procedure. In 1989 we reported the bidirectional Glenn as an interim step for patients with hypoplastic left heart syndrome.[37,38] Until this time the mortality for the Fontan procedure despite introduction of the lateral tunnel approach had been extremely high. Staging of the Fontan for patients with hypoplastic left heart syndrome was associated with a remarkable reduction in mortality.

In 1989 Bridges and Castaneda described the concept of baffle fenestration[39] which was an extension of the principle introduced by Laks et al.[40,41] This concept was analogous to the practice of leaving the patent foramen ovale open in patients following repair of tetralogy of Fallot as emphasized by Castaneda for many years.[42] By allowing a right to left shunt to maintain cardiac output after the Fontan procedure it was found that patients had a very much smoother and more rapid postoperative course. A relatively mild degree of cyanosis was well tolerated by these patients who had been chronically cyanosed preoperatively. On the other hand elevated right atrial pressure was poorly tolerated by young patients and frequently led to a syndrome of worsening fluid retention associated with deteriorating myocardial function.

In 1990 Marcelletti et al[43] introduced the concept of the extracardiac conduit allowing connection of the inferior vena cava to the pulmonary arteries. The possible advantage of this approach was to eliminate exposure of any atrial tissue to elevated pressure as well as minimizing suture lines within the right atrium. It was hoped that this would reduce the problem of late arrythmias which were being seen with increasing frequency in patients who had undergone the early atriopulmonary type of Fontan/Kreutzer procedure.

Goals of surgery

The ultimate goal of the sequence of surgical procedures that are undertaken for the patient with the single ventricle is to achieve optimal systemic oxygen delivery for as low a systemic venous pressure as possible. This goal is thought to be best achieved by optimizing compliance of the single ventricle as well as by minimizing the total resistance between the systemic veins and the ventricular chamber. Thus growth of the branch pulmonary arteries must be optimized and they must be kept free of distortion and scarring. Pulmonary vascular resistance must be minimized and the pulmonary venous pathway, which may include passage left to right across the atrial septum must also be free of obstruction. Ideally the procedures should minimize the probability of late tachyarrhythmias and late bradyarrythmias, should optimize late function of the AV valves and should incorporate growth potential.

OPTIMIZING VENTRICULAR COMPLIANCE

One of the most serious impediments to maintaining optimal compliance of the single ventricle is the development of ventricular hypertrophy.[44] This is most likely to be the result of a pressure load which is imposed by systemic outflow obstruction. Therefore the treatment strategy must not only carefully exclude the presence of outflow obstruction but also anticipate its potential development.

Ventricular compliance can also be impaired by a chronic excessive volume load. The premise that has evolved in managing patients with a single ventricle is that any volume loading of the ventricle should be minimized as early in life as possible in order to maintain long-term compliance. However, this premise has never been tested by clinical trials. It is interesting to conjecture whether a similar premise applies for patients with biventricular circulation. Surely regular exercise and frequent episodes of ventricular volume loading are considered an important component of a healthy lifestyle. Nevertheless there is no question that an excessive volume load, e.g. a $Q_p : Q_s$ of greater than 3 or 4 : 1 particularly in conjunction with a systemic pressure load as is the case for the single ventricle can in a relatively short time result in a dilated poorly contractile ventricle that has effectively gone over the top of the Starling curve.

OPTIMIZING TOTAL PULMONARY RESISTANCE

It is important to minimize exposure of the pulmonary arterioles to excessive pressure and flow as early in life as possible in order to minimize pulmonary arteriolar resistance. Growth of the pulmonary arteries must be optimized by eliminating central pulmonary artery stenoses and assuring that there is a balanced degree of blood flow passing to each lung. Surgical procedures on the pulmonary arteries should take place as centrally as possible to avoid injury to the hilar branches. Continuity of the central pulmonary arteries must be maintained and procedures such as the classic Glenn shunt should be avoided.

If there is anomalous pulmonary venous return with obstruction this must be repaired as early in life as possible. If there is restriction at the level of the atrial septum in the setting of obligatory left to right flow at the atrial septal level then the atrial septum must be surgically excised as early in life as possible. Balloon atrial septostomy is not adequate in this setting.[45]

Neonatal palliation

SURGERY FOR INADEQUATE PULMONARY BLOOD FLOW CAUSED BY PULMONARY OUTFLOW OBSTRUCTION

By far the commonest cause of inadequate pulmonary blood flow in the neonate or young infant with single ventricle physiology is obstruction to pulmonary outflow. If the ductus has closed and if the arterial oxygen saturation is consistently less than 75–80% then the neonate should undergo placement of a systemic to pulmonary arterial shunt.

Potential disadvantages of a systemic pulmonary arterial shunt

The most important risk of a systemic to pulmonary arterial shunt is that it will be excessively large and result in a degree of volume loading of the ventricle which subsequently impairs myocardial contractility. Therefore the shunt should be relatively small so as to achieve an arterial oxygen saturation of no more than 80–85% over a temporary period for the first several months of life during which time the child's pulmonary vascular resistance is undergoing its usual natural decline. Excessive shunt size can also result in an increase in pulmonary vascular resistance. A shunt can also result in scarring and distortion of the pulmonary arteries and if performed through a thoracotomy is likely to cause distortion of the lobar branches.[46]

Technique of placement of a systemic to pulmonary arterial shunt

It should rarely be necessary to employ cardiopulmonary bypass for shunt placement. If the child is duct-dependent, prostaglandin E1 should be continued and the distal anastomosis of the shunt should be placed on the branch pulmonary artery contralateral to the site of ductal insertion (Figure 20.1). If the child is moderately severely cyanosed, e.g. an arterial oxygen saturation of less than 70% and has presented beyond the neonatal period at a time when the ductus cannot be reopened, nevertheless it is usually possible to occlude a central branch pulmonary artery for shunt anastomosis with little change in arterial oxygen saturation. It is important that the approach is through a median sternotomy and not through the more traditional thoracotomy approach.[46] The most important advantage of the sternotomy approach for the patient with a single ventricle is that dissection of the pulmonary arteries occurs very centrally so that distortion of the lobar branches is highly unlikely to result from the surgery. The sternotomy approach has the cosmetic advantage of a single incision for all three stages of surgical palliation. There may be a lower risk of thoracotomy induced scoliosis. In our experience the incidence of Horner's syndrome is also decreased with the sternotomy approach.

It is important to avoid construction of a shunt which has growth potential such as the classic Blalock shunt, Waterston shunt or Potts shunt. All of these shunts can result in a progressive increase in pulmonary blood flow over time. They also have a higher risk of distortion of the pulmonary arteries relative to the modified Blalock shunt which uses a Gortex tube graft.

The shunt should be anastomosed to a central pulmonary artery where it is anticipated that the subsequent Fontan anastomosis will take place. Thus if there is a dominant right sided superior vena cava the Blalock shunt should be placed to the right pulmonary artery. In this way any distortion of the right pulmonary artery which results from the shunt can be incorporated later in the Fontan anastomosis. A left sided Blalock shunt performed through a thoracotomy is particularly problematic in that any distortion of the left pulmonary artery is quite distal and may be difficult to deal with surgically. Furthermore takedown of a left Blalock shunt increases the risk of a phrenic nerve injury relative to takedown of a right Blalock shunt.

The size of the Gortex tube graft selected as well as the site selected for the proximal anastomosis are critically important in avoiding excessive volume loading of the single ventricle. For the average sized neonate weighing between 3 and 4 kg, a 3.5 mm diameter shunt is generally appropriate. For smaller neonates it is appropriate that the proximal anastomosis be placed more distally, e.g. almost entirely on the right subclavian artery rather than on the innominate artery. This will also serve to lengthen the shunt which also helps to reduce the volume loading of the ventricle as originally suggested by

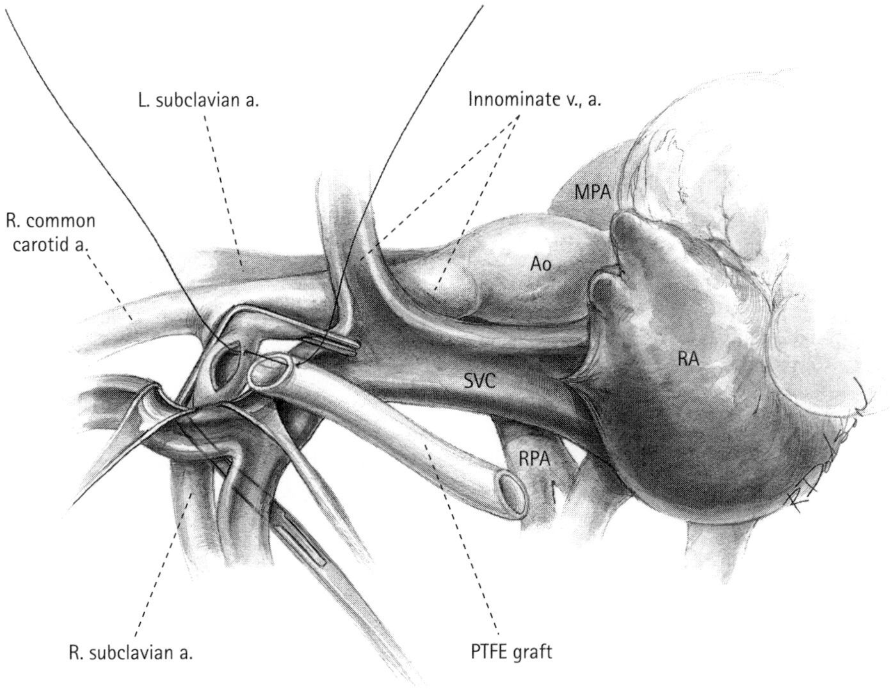

Figure 20.1 *A modified Blalock shunt is usually best placed on the same side as the dominant superior vena cava. Approach should be through a median sternotomy. The proximal anastomosis is placed to a longitudinal arteriotomy in the origin of the right subclavian artery which is controlled with a sidebiting clamp.*

de Leval when he introduced the modified Blalock shunt.[47] Neonates less than 3 kg in weight are often best served by a 3.0 mm shunt. On the other hand with larger neonates and young infants even up to 5 or 6 kg, a 3.5 mm shunt is often still appropriate. However, a child presenting at a weight of 5 or 6 kg is likely to be several months old. If there is a sufficient degree of cyanosis that a systemic to pulmonary arterial shunt has to be inserted then it is probable that the child has sufficiently low pulmonary resistance by that age, e.g. beyond two to three months that a more appropriate management strategy would be to proceed directly to a bidirectional Glenn shunt.

The child should be positioned supine with as much extension of the neck as can be tolerated. This is achieved by placing a relatively large roll behind the shoulders. This serves to draw the innominate and subclavian arteries out of the neck into the chest and improves exposure considerably. A standard median sternotomy incision is performed with the skin incision extending at least to the top of the sternal notch. The thymus is subtotally resected. Only small cervical remnants should be left. Even though it is possible to perform a shunt without opening the pericardium consideration should be given to the fact that the ventricle will need to dilate acutely to handle the additional volume load imposed by the shunt. If the pericardium is fully opened it is ideal to do this to the left or right side so that at a subsequent procedure a patch of anterior pericardium can be harvested if necessary.

The right pulmonary artery is dissected free between the superior vena cava and ascending aorta. The innominate artery and proximal right subclavian artery are dissected free being careful to avoid injury to the right recurrent laryngeal nerve which can be seen passing around the distal right subclavian artery. A sidebiting clamp is applied across the origin of the right subclavian artery and the distal innominate artery. A longitudinal arteriotomy is made either partially or completely on the right subclavian artery depending on the size of the child. An appropriate bevel is fashioned on the Gortex tube graft which has been selected. A direct anastomosis is fashioned. It is important to select as small a needle as possible, e.g. the BV1 needle supplied with Prolene in order to minimize needle hole bleeding. Prolene is considered preferable to Gortex suture because it distributes tension evenly between suture loops. Because it is not necessary to administer heparin during the clamping period as the child's vessels are not atherosclerotic, needle hole bleeding is not generally a problem. Following completion of the anastomosis the shunt is controlled with a bulldog clamp that is applied close to the anastomosis. The tube graft is cut to length. A sidebiting clamp is applied to the right pulmonary artery with appropriate rotation of the vessel so that an incision can be made on the superior surface. The anastomosis is fashioned once again with continuous Prolene. Upon release of the clamps there should be a decrease in diastolic pressure and an increase in arterial oxygen saturation.

The pericardium is loosely tacked together. A chest tube, usually 16 Fr, is placed carefully to avoid compression of the shunt anastomoses. The sternotomy incision is closed in the routine fashion.

Should the ductus be ligated? The question frequently arises in the duct dependent neonate whether the ductus should be ligated following opening of the shunt. Ligation of the duct avoids competitive flow and avoids the risk that there will be excessive pulmonary blood flow in the few hours before the duct closes spontaneously. There is also some risk that there will not be spontaneous closure of the ductus when prostaglandin is discontinued though this is rare. On the other hand if the shunt does subsequently thrombose there is a possibility of resuscitating the child through administration of prostaglandin. Although there is no clear answer to this conundrum it is our usual practice to ligate the ductus when it is clearly large or if there is an additional source of pulmonary blood flow, e.g. the child with forward pulmonary outflow through a stenotic pulmonary outflow, while in the setting of pulmonary atresia we generally do not ligate the ductus.

SURGERY FOR INADEQUATE PULMONARY BLOOD FLOW CAUSED BY OBSTRUCTED TOTAL ANOMALOUS PULMONARY VENOUS CONNECTION

Neonates with heterotaxy may present with a profound degree of cyanosis because of obstructed total anomalous pulmonary venous connection. If this is combined with obstruction to pulmonary outflow the degree of cyanosis will be further exacerbated by ductal closure. In our experience these children also tend to have branch pulmonary artery stenoses at the origin of either the right or left pulmonary artery or even discontinuity of the right and left pulmonary arteries. In order to optimize pulmonary artery development and to minimize pulmonary vascular resistance it is important that the total anomalous pulmonary connection be repaired shortly after presentation and that continuity be established between the branch pulmonary arteries. Pulmonary blood must be established with a systemic to pulmonary arterial shunt when there is associated obstruction to pulmonary outflow. The procedure for repair of total anomalous pulmonary venous connection is described in Chapter 22. Generally the repair, i.e. anastomosis of the pulmonary venous confluence to the posterior wall of the common atrium, will be performed under deep hypothermic circulatory arrest. During the rewarming period the systemic to pulmonary arterial shunt can be performed with the application of sidebiting clamps as described above.

SURGERY FOR INADEQUATE PULMONARY BLOOD FLOW CAUSED BY OBSTRUCTIVE ATRIAL SEPTUM

The patient who has mitral atresia has obligatory left to right flow at atrial septal level. If the ASD is not adequate in size there may be restriction to pulmonary blood flow because of pulmonary venous hypertension. It is unusual for this constellation to occur in the setting of obstruction to pulmonary outflow. In fact usually there is unrestrictive pulmonary blood flow and the child will require placement of a pulmonary artery band in addition to surgical atrial septectomy. It is particularly important to recognize that interventional catheter methods such as balloon atrial septostomy or balloon dilation of the atrial septum are at best temporizing that will decompress the left atrium for no more than few days to a few weeks. There is essentially always a recurrence of obstruction at atrial septal level unless a surgical septectomy is performed.[45]

Surgical atrial septectomy under normothermic caval inflow occlusion

Normothermic caval inflow occlusion is a technique that was used regularly at Children's Hospital Boston in the past for surgical valvotomy of the semilunar valves in the neonate presenting with critical semilunar valve stenosis.[48]

The procedure has become obsolete following the success of interventional catheter methods. However, the technique of inflow occlusion remains helpful for the patient who has a restrictive atrial septum and requires an atrial septectomy.[49] The advantage of avoiding cardiopulmonary bypass in this setting is in large part related to the impact of bypass on pulmonary resistance. Since a pulmonary artery band will generally be applied as part of this same surgical procedure the exacerbation of pulmonary hypertension that generally occurs with bypass can complicate accurate band placement. On the other hand it may be difficult to identify an anesthesiologist who feels comfortable with the technique and there is no question that the technique should be performed with an experienced anesthesiologist who is familiar with the technique. Therefore a brief period of cardiopulmonary bypass for performing the atrial septectomy is not an unreasonable alternative.

The patient is placed supine on the operating table. Following induction of general anesthesia, introduction of appropriate monitoring lines, prepping and draping a standard median sternotomy approach is employed. The thymus is subtotally resected. The pericardium is opened and supported with stay sutures. A small air vent controlled with a tourniquet (similar to a cardioplegia infusion site) is created at the highest point of the mid-ascending aorta. An appropriate sidebiting clamp (nested clamp is ideal) is placed obliquely on the right atrial free wall. An incision is made in the controlled segment of atrium. A suture line is begun at either end of the incision and will be used for supporting and closing the incision subsequent to the period of inflow occlusion. With careful communication with the anesthesia team vascular clamps are applied completely across the superior vena cava and inferior vena cava. The heart is allowed to empty for several beats, the vent site in the ascending aorta is opened to allow a small amount of bleeding and to vent any air that may be entrained and the nested clamp is released. Generally blood will be emerging vigorously from the restrictive atrial septum which allows immediate identification of the area to be excised. The septum primum is grasped with forceps and a generous wedge is excised. The two ends of the partial atrial suture line are lifted and the superior vena caval clamp is released. The atrium is allowed to fill with blood and the nested clamp is reapplied to control the atrial incision. The IVC clamp is released and the vent site in the ascending aorta is closed after a few beats when it is clear that there is no air in the heart. The atriotomy is closed with the sutures that were begun previously.

It is important that the anesthesia team hold ventilation during the period of inflow occlusion and that they be ready to give appropriate blood transfusion and bicarbonate at the end of the occlusion period. It is also important that the anesthesia team count out the time of occlusion which should be limited to less than two minutes. Generally no more than 60 seconds is required. However, unless the time has been called there is a tendency to rush and therefore to perform an inadequate or inaccurate septectomy. The child is allowed to stabilize for a few minutes before proceeding to application of the pulmonary artery band.

NEONATAL PALLIATION OF THE SINGLE VENTRICLE WITH EXCESSIVE PULMONARY BLOOD FLOW

The neonate or young infant with a single ventricle who has no obstruction to pulmonary outflow and no obstruction to pulmonary venous return either at the level of the veins themselves (obstructed total anomalous pulmonary venous connection) or at the level of the atrial septum will develop excessive pulmonary blood flow as pulmonary resistance falls in the first weeks of life. Excessive pulmonary blood flow is undesirable both from the perspective of minimizing pulmonary resistance as well as optimizing ventricular function. It is important to remember that a high oxygen saturation, e.g. greater than 85% or so, is quite undesirable for the child with a single ventricle since such a high level of arterial oxygen saturation can only be achieved by an extremely high pulmonary blood flow. It is important to eliminate the excessive volume loading of the single ventricle early in infancy as well as to reduce the pressure to which the pulmonary arterioles are exposed. These goals can be achieved by application of a pulmonary artery band.

Before proceeding with application of a pulmonary artery band it is particularly important to actively exclude the possibility of obstruction to systemic outflow from the single ventricle. If obstruction to systemic outflow is present or appears likely to occur in the near future (e.g. bulboventricular foramen area less than $2\,cm^2/m^2$)[10,11] then a band should not be applied but the patient should instead proceed to a Norwood or Damus-Kaye-Stansel procedure. In fact application of a pulmonary artery band where there is marginal systemic outflow obstruction is likely to precipitate obstruction. This occurs because of the immediate reduction in ventricular volume that occurs following application of the band because of the reduction in volume loading.[50]

Since the muscle mass of the ventricle cannot change instantaneously and the wall thickness must therefore necessarily be greater because of the smaller ventricular volume, this apparent 'hypertrophy' can narrow a marginally obstructed bulboventricular foramen. Over time the greater afterload presented by a combination of a pulmonary artery band and systemic outflow obstruction can result in a rapid progression in ventricular hypertrophy with a feedback loop in which increasing hypertrophy leads to increasing obstruction, increasing ventricular pressure and consequent increasing hypertrophy.[51]

Technique of pulmonary artery band insertion

A pulmonary artery band is best placed working through a median sternotomy (Figure 20.2). A band should almost never be placed working through a left thoracotomy in conjunction with repair of a coarctation for the patient with a single ventricle. The presence of a coarctation almost certainly indicates that systemic outflow obstruction is present or incipient and therefore a more appropriate procedure will be a Norwood type palliation.[3,4] There are also important advantages in placing a band through a median sternotomy. This approach allows the right side of the band to be tacked to the main pulmonary artery adventitia to prevent migration of the right side of the band which can cause stenosis at the origin of the right pulmonary artery. This is probably the most common complication of a pulmonary artery band that must be actively avoided by appropriate anchoring sutures. Use of the supine position and a median sternotomy allows both lungs to be fully inflated during the banding procedure so that a more accurate degree of band tightness can be achieved. In addition the same advantages that are present for placement of a shunt through a median sternotomy are relevant for the patient having a pulmonary artery band placed, i.e. the cosmetic advantage of a single incision as well as the reduced risk of scoliosis resulting from a neonatal thoracotomy. Following the induction of general anesthesia, introduction of monitoring lines, prepping and draping a standard median sternotomy incision is made. It is only necessary to open the superior third of the pericardium following subtotal resection of the thymus. It is important to exclude patency of the ductus before proceeding with banding. If the ductus is demonstrated to be patent it must be ligated. An extremely localized dissection is performed between the aorta and main pulmonary artery immediately proximal to the takeoff of the right pulmonary artery. Dacron impregnated silastic is an ideal material for banding. A narrow strip no more than 3 mm in width is cut to length. The band is initially passed around both great vessels through the transverse sinus. It is important not to attempt to pass a right angle instrument between the aorta and pulmonary artery from behind as this carries an important risk of injury to the right pulmonary artery. The right angle instrument should instead now be passed around the ascending aorta and the band is grasped at its rightward end. It is drawn between the aorta and pulmonary artery. This approach guarantees that the band will be placed proximal to the right pulmonary artery and minimizes the risk of injury to the right pulmonary artery.

The band is tightened so as to achieve approximately a 50% diameter reduction of the main pulmonary artery. Information regarding appropriate band tightness can be gained by monitoring distal pulmonary artery pressure though this can often be unhelpful because of various monitoring artifacts. Probably more useful is the judgment which incorporates assessment of the arterial oxygen saturation, change in systemic arterial pressure and absence of change of

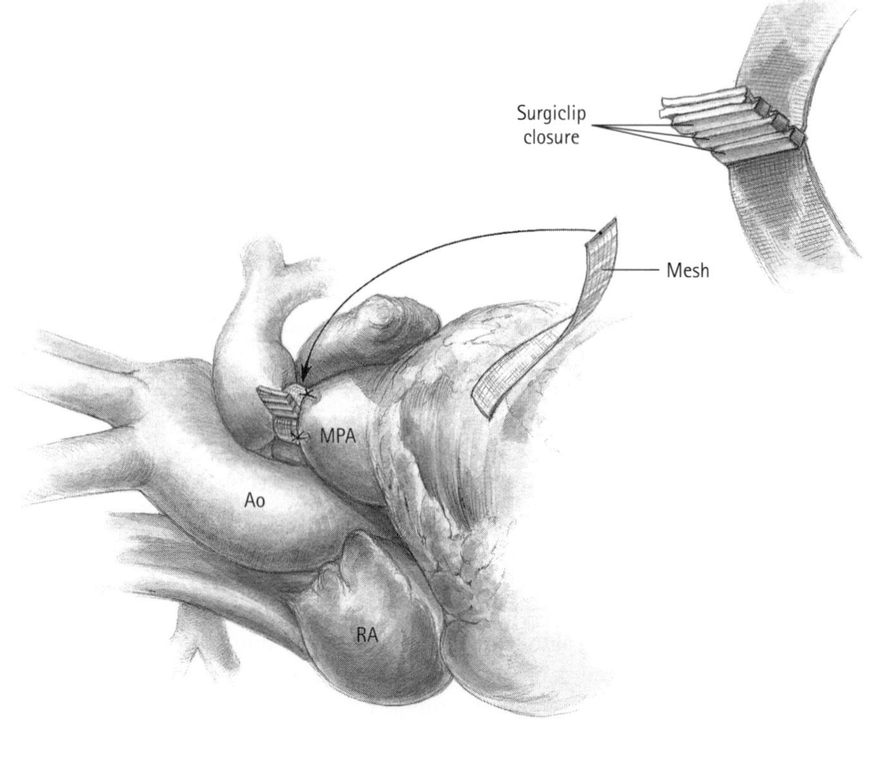

Figure 20.2 *Application of a pulmonary artery band. Approach is via a median sternotomy. The band tightness is adjusted by sequential placement of surgical clips. It is important that the band be anchored to the adventitia of the proximal pulmonary artery to prevent distal migration.*

heart rate. Important slowing of the heart rate, particularly when associated with a fall in arterial oxygen saturation to less than 70–75% almost certainly indicates excessive tightening of the band. In general appropriate tightening of the band will be accompanied by a 5–10 mm increase in systolic blood pressure (transiently) and a reduction in arterial oxygen saturation to between 80 and 85%. The surgeon must factor in an assessment of the patient's cardiac output which may be elevated under anesthesia because of an increased catecholamine level if the patient's level of anesthesia is relatively light. An increase in cardiac output will increase the arterial oxygen saturation. The effects of anesthesia in reducing pulmonary resistance, particularly if the inspired oxygen level is elevated and if the carbon dioxide level is low, may further increase the arterial oxygen saturation. There is no question that banding is an art form that requires considerable experience and judgment. There is no totally reliable scientific method including techniques that use pre-measurement of a band length.[52] The child's parents and the entire care team must work under the assumption that adjustment of the band may be necessary in the first few days following the procedure if it appears that the band is either excessively tight or loose.

The band is fixed at its selected diameter with three hemoclips. In fact the width of one hemoclip is an appropriate increment in band tightness and is a useful method for increasing band tightness, i.e. by placing an additional clip below the previous clip. It is also important to remember that the tacking sutures of 6/0 Prolene which must be placed both on the right side and left side of the main pulmonary artery to anchor the band and to prevent distal migration also have some impact in tightening the band and should be placed and tied before the final hemoclip is applied. The patient is observed for a period of 5–10 minutes to be sure that the hemodynamic situation is stable. The upper end of the pericardium is left open. A single chest tube is inserted extrapleurally from the right pleural cavity into the superior mediastinum. The sternotomy is closed in the usual fashion.

NEONATAL PALLIATION OF THE SINGLE VENTRICLE WITH SYSTEMIC OUTFLOW OBSTRUCTION

It is important that obstruction to systemic outflow between a single ventricle and the aorta is bypassed using the principle of the Norwood procedure or Damus-Kaye-Stansel procedure.[53] Both of these operations involve division of the main pulmonary artery and connection of the proximal main pulmonary artery to the aorta.

Damus-Kaye-Stansel procedure

The Damus-Kaye-Stansel procedure was described independently by Damus, Stansel and Kaye during the 1970s as an innovative method for managing transposition of the great arteries with intact ventricular septum[54–56] (Figure 20.3).

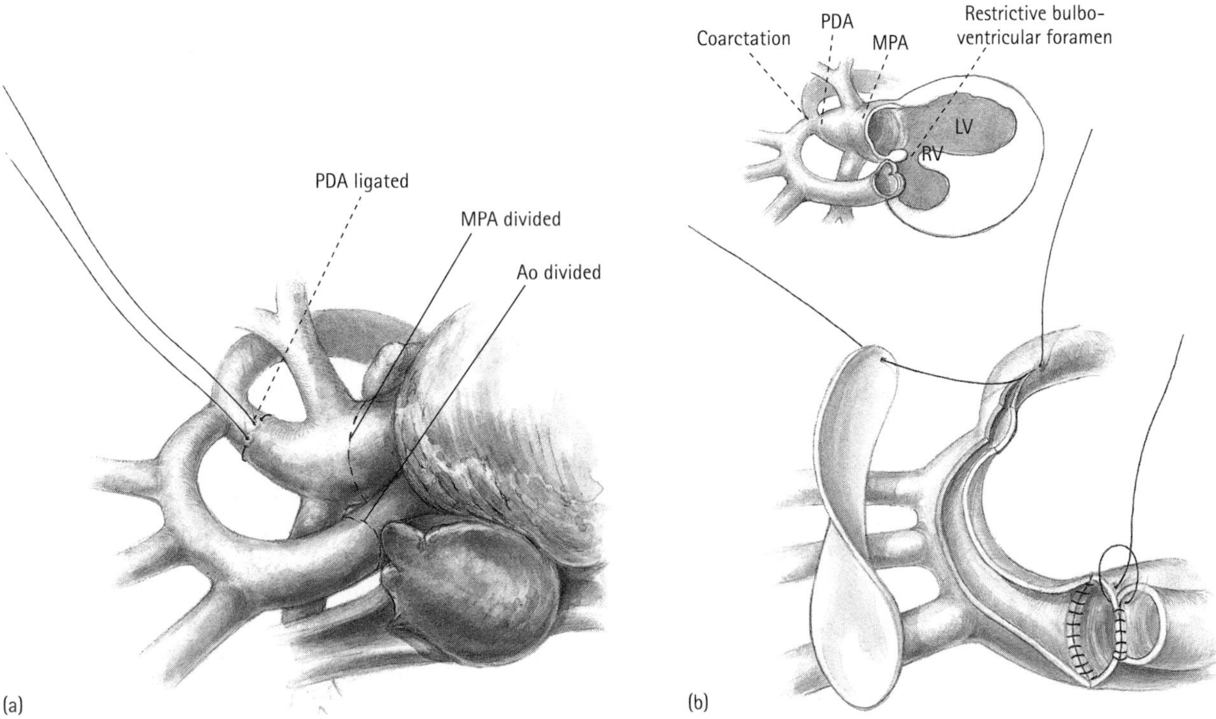

Figure 20.3 *The Damus-Kaye-Stansel procedure is a modification of the Norwood procedure that is used for patients with a single ventricle and systemic outflow tract obstruction. The patient illustrated has tricuspid atresia with transposed great arteries and a restrictive bulbo-ventricular foramen (inset). (a) The ductus will be ligated as indicated and the great vessels will be divided at the dashed lines. (b) The ascending aorta, arch and proximal descending aorta are enlarged with a patch of autologous pericardium or with homograft tissue. The proximal ascending aorta is anastomosed directly posteriorly to the proximal divided main pulmonary artery.*

There was some dispute regarding authorship priority so that all three names are now the eponymous descriptors of the technique though the acronym DKS is often applied. The procedure was described at a time when there was a naïve enthusiasm for congenital heart repairs incorporating conduits. In addition to placement of a conduit between the right ventricle and the pulmonary arteries the original DKS procedure involves division of the main pulmonary artery and connection to the ascending aorta so that the patient's left ventricle (connected to the pulmonary artery because of transposition) could eject into the systemic circulation. The DKS procedure as originally described was not applied for the patient with a single ventricle and also did not involve enlargement of the aortic arch. Today the procedure is most commonly used to describe a procedure in which systemic outflow obstruction within a single ventricle is bypassed by division of the main pulmonary artery and anastomosis of the proximal divided main pulmonary artery to the ascending aorta. It can be combined with a systemic to pulmonary artery (modified Blalock) shunt or single ventricle to pulmonary artery (Sano) shunt in the neonate or with a bidirectional Glenn shunt in the infant. It tends to be used for patients with single ventricle other than those with hypoplastic left heart syndrome. It also tends to be used when the aortic arch is adequately developed and does not require the extensive reconstruction that is implied by the Norwood procedure. Nevertheless the DKS procedure is conceptually the same as the Norwood procedure and since the aortic arch is frequently hypoplastic in the patient with a single ventricle and systemic outflow tract obstruction the procedures are not uncommonly essentially the same.

Norwood procedure

Like the DKS, the Norwood procedure uses the proximal divided main pulmonary artery as a means of bypassing obstruction between the patient's single functional ventricle and the systemic circulation. Of course in hypoplastic left heart syndrome that obstruction is total in that there is usually an intact ventricular septum and the patient's single functional right ventricle is connected only to the main pulmonary artery. Since there is almost always arch hypoplasia and a coarctation an essential part of the Norwood procedure involves reconstruction of the aortic arch and proximal descending aorta as well as connection of the main pulmonary artery to the neoaorta. Specific technical details of the Norwood procedure are described in Chapter 19.

Should the DKS/Norwood procedure be performed at the time of neonatal palliation?

There is ongoing controversy as to whether the child with potential or mild systemic outflow obstruction is better managed by a DKS/Norwood procedure in the neonatal period or alternatively if the DKS/Norwood should be deferred to the time of an early bidirectional Glenn shunt. Proponents of the latter approach point to the greater hemodynamic stability that is observed following the bidirectional Glenn shunt relative to neonatal palliation incorporating a systemic to pulmonary arterial shunt as had been the traditional source of pulmonary blood flow for a neonatal DKS or Norwood procedure.[57]

As the right ventricle to pulmonary artery 'Sano shunt' becomes more popular for the DKS and Norwood procedure it is apparent that hemodynamic instability is much less of a problem than with a standard systemic to pulmonary arterial shunt. Nevertheless delaying the DKS/Norwood procedure to the time of a bidirectional Glenn does allow avoidance of any incision in the ventricle.

The proponents of neonatal performance of the DKS/Norwood procedure point to the distortion of the pulmonary (neoaortic) valve that can be caused by a pulmonary artery band which must necessarily be placed in such patients in order to protect the pulmonary vascular bed and to prevent excessive volume loading of the single ventricle.[58] Application of a pulmonary artery band in the setting of mild systemic outflow obstruction is likely to increase the degree of obstruction for the reasons stated above. Because of the feedback loop that results with increasing hypertrophy causing increasing systemic outflow obstruction there may be a rapid progression of ventricular hypertrophy. There is a sense that the myocardium can be 'programmed for life' by exposure in the first months of life to high pressure and that ventricular compliance is not likely to be as low as will be achieved if the neonatal DKS/Norwood procedure is performed. Ideally a prospective trial, probably multi-institutional, will be performed in order to settle this controversy that has persisted for at least the past decade.

Results of neonatal palliation

SHUNTS

In 1995 Odim et al[46] described the results of surgery for 104 patients who had modified Blalock shunts placed at Children's Hospital Boston between 1988 and 1992. Fifty two of the shunts were constructed by the thoracotomy approach and 52 by the sternotomy approach. The overall hospital mortality was 8.7%. There was no difference in mortality whether the shunt was constructed through a thoracotomy or sternotomy. However, there was a significantly greater probability of shunt failure with the thoracotomy approach. It was the authors' opinion that the incidence of morbidity was also significantly less with the sternotomy approach relative to the thoracotomy approach. In 1997 Gladman et al[59] described the results of the modified Blalock Taussig shunt in 65 children with tetralogy managed at the Hospital for Sick Children in Toronto, Canada. Excluding noncardiac causes of death the overall survival was 90%. Patients who received shunts had significantly smaller distal right pulmonary arteries relative to a comparison group of patients with tetralogy who did not undergo shunt placement. Of patients who underwent palliation, 33% had angiographic evidence of pulmonary artery distortion. Shunt occlusion resulted in one death. This study highlights the disadvantages of shunt placement and contradicts the assertion by some that placement of a shunt facilitates pulmonary artery development and might even reduce the need for transannular patching.

BANDS

There are few large series in the modern era describing the results of pulmonary artery banding. In 1997 Pinho et al[60] described the results of pulmonary artery band placement in 135 consecutive patients managed in Capetown, South Africa over a 10 year period ending in 1992. Eighty nine of the patients had a VSD and 46 had more complex problems. The median age was three months and median weight was 3.5 kg. Mortality was 8.1% overall and in neonates was 22%. At follow-up the band was inadequate in 29% of patients, which was more probable if banding was necessary before three months of age. The mortality among the 60 patients who subsequently proceeded to definitive repair was 23% but if the band was inadequate at the time of repair, mortality was 44%. This report emphasizes that the general sense that placement of a palliative pulmonary artery band is a simple and therefore low risk procedure is incorrect. Both the mortality and morbidity of pulmonary artery banding is not insignificant.

In 1996, Jensen et al[61] described the results of banding in 26 patients managed at UCLA in California between 1984 and 1994. All patients had either a double inlet single ventricle or tricuspid atresia with transposed great arteries and were therefore at risk of developing subaortic stenosis. The band was placed at a mean age of two months. Nineteen patients subsequently underwent a Damus-Kaye-Stansel type procedure or VSD enlargement. The overall mortality was 19%. In spite of this high mortality, however, the authors believe that preliminary application of a pulmonary artery band is a reasonable approach for the patient with a single ventricle and potential subaortic stenosis. This position is also taken by the group from Southampton, UK. Weber et al in 1995[62] described the results of preliminary application of a pulmonary artery band in 18 infants with double inlet single left ventricle with transposition and aortic arch obstruction. Patients subsequently underwent a Damus-Kaye-Stansel type procedure at a later age. Overall mortality was 28%. Although these two groups have been encouraged by their results with early banding in the setting of a single ventricle with a potential for subaortic stenosis, the position at Children's Hospital Boston continues to be that the optimal management for these patients is an initial Damus-Kaye-Stansel or Norwood procedure which in the current era can be performed with a less than 20% mortality risk.

Dilatable pulmonary artery bands

There are a number of case reports and technical articles describing various ingenious methods for placing an adjustable pulmonary artery or a dilatable band. In one clinical series, Vince from Vancouver, Canada[63] described the results of banding in 11 patients who received dilatable bands and eight who received fixed bands. The authors found that the dilatable bands were easier to remove than the fixed bands but required greater surgical dexterity to place and adjust.

ATRIAL SEPTECTOMY

In 1985 we reported the use of normothermic caval inflow occlusion in 140 children managed at Children's Hospital Boston between 1972 and 1983.[49] Eleven of the patients had a surgical atrial septectomy. The mean age at the time of surgery was 11 months. Three patients had pulmonary artery bands placed at the same procedure and one had a Blalock shunt. There was one early death and no late deaths over a mean follow-up of 16 months. The importance of performing a surgical septecotomy rather than a balloon or blade septostomy in the setting of obligatory left to right flow in the patient with left AV valve atresia or stenosis was emphasized by Perry et al in a report from Children's Hospital Boston in 1986.[45] Results were unsatisfactory in five patients who underwent balloon septostomy and 12 who underwent blade septostomy with recurrence of a gradient across the atrial septum in the majority of patients. Even with surgical septectomy 78.5% were inadequate and 11% developed recurrent stenosis.

Management during the interval period between neonatal palliation and second stage palliation

The interval period between neonatal palliation of the child with a single ventricle and the second stage bidirectional Glenn shunt is a critically important period. There is an inherent instability of the parallel pulmonary and systemic circulations connected to a single ventricle. For example, any factor that increases pulmonary blood flow, e.g. exposure to a high inspired oxygen level or hyperventilation to a low carbon dioxide level will steal blood away from the systemic circulation and might result in a falling cardiac output with a fall in coronary perfusion pressure placing the child in a serious positive feedback loop. The early months of life are also a period where many factors that influence the balance of systemic and pulmonary blood flow are evolving. There is a progressive decrease in pulmonary vascular resistance with the normal transition from the fetal to mature circulation. There may be fibrosis and consequent constriction of a potential coarctation with a progressive increase in systemic afterload driving more blood flow into the pulmonary circulation. Obstruction to systemic outflow within the single ventricle may progress rapidly as may obstruction to pulmonary outflow. The child should be growing relatively rapidly during this period and may outgrow either the systemic to pulmonary artery shunt or pulmonary artery band in just three or four months leading to an excessive degree of cyanosis. For all these reasons the child needs to be monitored particularly closely during the interval period. If the child is becoming excessively cyanosed, e.g. resting arterial oxygen saturation of less than 75% then cardiac catheterization or a magnetic resonance imaging scan should be undertaken. If the child has signs of congestive heart failure and is growing poorly then evolving causes such as obstruction to systemic outflow or development of a coarctation should be sought. These issues, particularly the latter, can be difficult to define by echocardiography so that if there is any doubt cardiac catheterization should be undertaken. Cardiac catheterization also allows cineangiography to define the size and distribution of the pulmonary arteries as well as to define any central pulmonary artery stenoses. If the child has excessive pulmonary blood flow and if pulmonary artery pressure is elevated then a calculation of pulmonary resistance must be made. It may be necessary to consider tightening of a pulmonary artery band in order to prepare a child for a subsequent bidirectional Glenn shunt if the pulmonary resistance is markedly elevated, e.g. greater than five to six units. An MRI scan may be a reasonable alternative to catheterization if the child's situation is not particularly complex.

Stage 2 palliation: the bidirectional Glenn shunt or hemi-Fontan

Connection of the superior vena cava to the pulmonary arteries (bidirectional Glenn shunt, cavopulmonary shunt) eliminates the inherent inefficiency that is present with any type of circulation that is created by the neonatal palliative procedures described above (Figure 20.4). This inherent inefficiency cannot be avoided since the high neonatal resistance to pulmonary blood flow requires that a ventricle drive blood through the pulmonary circulation for the first months of life until the resistance has fallen sufficiently to allow venous pressure alone to be the driving force. Experience has suggested that beyond 2.5–3 months of age the pulmonary resistance is sufficiently low to allow progression to the second stage though the postoperative course tends to be smoother and more rapid if the second stage is deferred until four or five months rather than sooner.[64] There appears to be no advantage in further delaying the second stage beyond six months. Therefore in general cardiac catheterization should be scheduled by three to four months with a view to proceeding to surgery within a few weeks of catheterization.

SHOULD ALL PATIENTS UNDERGO A SECOND STAGE PROCEDURE?

Since the late 1980s when the bidirectional Glenn shunt was first introduced as an intermediate step between neonatal palliation and a completed Fontan procedure[38] it has progressively evolved to being considered essentially standard of care that all patients should undergo this second stage. Proponents of a mandatory three stage approach suggest that there is a disadvantage in an additional 6–12 months of volume loading for the single ventricle in waiting to 12–18 months which is generally considered the minimal age for a safe Fontan procedure. Furthermore in order for neonatal palliation to carry a child through until 12–18 months of age it is necessary to place a larger systemic pulmonary arterial shunt or a looser pulmonary artery band. Thus the pulmonary vasculature is exposed to greater blood flow and pressure during early infancy while the child is quite small and the ventricle is exposed to greater volume loading. Those who suggest selective avoidance of the second stage bidirectional Glenn shunt point to a higher mortality when one considers the additive mortality of two procedures (i.e. bidirectional Glenn second stage plus Fontan third stage) as well as the additional costs and impact on the quality of life for the child and family in undergoing two hospitalizations following neonatal palliation rather than one. As with many other controversies that are ongoing for patients with single ventricle physiology this one also will not be resolved until multi-institutional trials are organized.

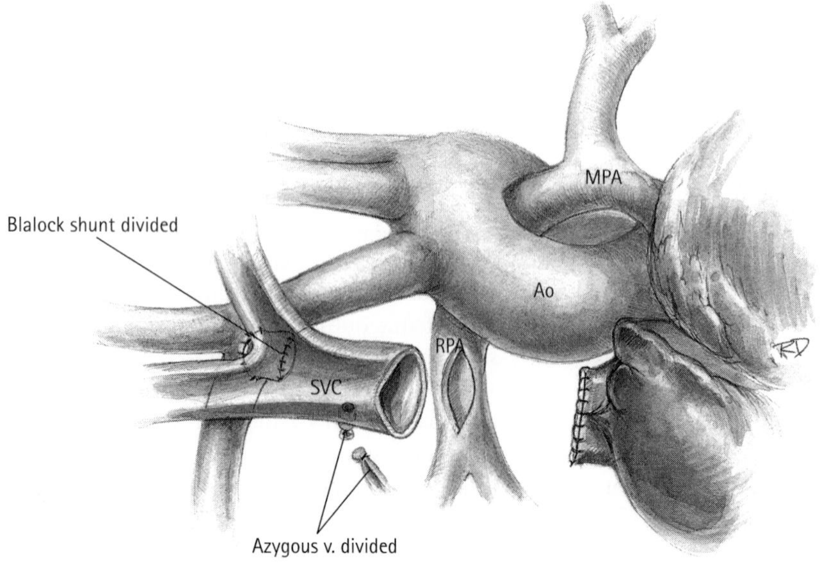

Figure 20.4 *When a right modified Blalock shunt has been placed for neonatal palliation it is taken down at the second stage. The bidirectional Glenn shunt (bidirectional cavopulmonary shunt) is constructed to the same distal anastomotic area as the Blalock shunt. In general it is preferable to disconnect the main pulmonary artery including excision of the pulmonary valve with oversewing of the main pulmonary artery proximally and distally (not shown).*

SURGICAL TECHNIQUE OF THE BIDIRECTIONAL GLENN SHUNT

The bidirectional Glenn shunt is performed through a standard median sternotomy approach using cardiopulmonary bypass.[65,66] This will usually be a reoperative sternotomy following previous neonatal palliation through a sternotomy approach (see Chapter 2 for details of the performance of a reoperative sternotomy). Purse-string sutures are placed in the ascending aorta, right atrium and left innominate vein. The purse-string suture in the left innominate vein should be a long narrow diamond which will minimize the risk of stenosing the vein when the purse-string is tied at the conclusion of the procedure. Following heparinization bypass is commenced with the arterial cannula in the ascending aorta and venous return via a right angle cannula in the left innominate vein and a straight cannula in the right atrium. If a systemic to pulmonary artery shunt is present it should be ligated immediately after commencing bypass. Dissection of a right sided modified Blalock shunt performed through a median sternotomy is simple and carries virtually no risk of injury to the right phrenic nerve. Dissection of a Sano shunt with subsequent excision and oversewing of the proximal and distal stumps can be performed at any convenient time during the procedure.

During cooling the dominant superior vena cava (a right sided SVC presumably, if a right sided modified Blalock shunt has been performed) is carefully dissected free, easing the right phrenic nerve away from the cava using scissors and blunt dissection rather than electrocautery. The azygous vein is doubly ligated and divided. The right pulmonary artery is dissected free between the aorta and superior vena cava. The heart continues to beat at a mild degree of hypothermia such as 30°C. A cross clamp is placed across the superior vena just inferior to the junction of the left and right innominate veins. A second vascular clamp is applied just above the atriocaval junction. The superior vena cava is divided just above the inferior clamp. The cardiac end of the divided SVC is oversewn with continuous 5/0 Prolene.

The distal anastomosis of the previous modified right Blalock shunt is taken down. The incision should be extended a few millimeters medially. It is generally not advisable to extend the arteriotomy laterally as this will bring the anastomosis too close to the upper lobe takeoff. Furthermore a more medial placement of the bidirectional Glenn shunt will help to achieve uniform distribution of flow to the right and left lung. An anastomosis is fashioned using continuous 6/0 absorbable Maxon suture. Maxon has the advantage that it does not slide as easily through tissue as Prolene and therefore is not likely to result in purse-stringing of the anastomosis. Furthermore the absorbable nature of Maxon guarantees optimal subsequent growth of the anastomosis.

Should all additional pulmonary blood be eliminated at the time of the bidirectional Glenn shunt?

Another ongoing controversy in the management of children with a single ventricle is the question as to whether all pulmonary blood flow other than the flow from the superior vena cava should be eliminated at the time of construction of the bidirectional Glenn shunt.[67,68] This is not as much of an issue for the child who has pulmonary atresia and the only source of pulmonary blood flow prior to the bidirectional Glenn shunt is a modified right Blalock shunt. Under these circumstances most surgeons prefer to take down the Blalock shunt and to use the distal anastomosis site of the Blalock shunt as the new distal anastomotic site for the bidirectional Glenn shunt. There are few reasons in support of placing a left sided modified Blalock shunt in the patient who has a right sided superior vena cava and the ability to leave supplementary pulmonary blood flow certainly should not be one of them. However, in the patient in whom a pulmonary artery band has been applied or who has a natural obstruction to pulmonary outflow, a reasonable argument can be made to allow continuing antegrade flow through the pulmonary outflow. The most important reason relates to subsequent development of pulmonary arteriovenous malformations following performance of a bidirectional Glenn shunt.[69] This phenomenon appears to be secondary to absence of hepatic venous blood passing through the pulmonary circulation. It is suspected that an angiogenic inhibitory factor is produced by the liver. When this factor is not seen by the lungs there is a tendency for new blood vessels to form, i.e. arteriovenous fistulas or arteriovenous malformations which bypass the gas exchanging units of the lungs. Leaving supplementary blood flow antegrade from the single ventricle allows hepatic venous blood to enter the lungs and probably reduces the likelihood of important pulmonary arteriovenous malformations forming.[70] Thus a longer period of palliation can be achieved with the bidirectional Glenn shunt than might otherwise be possible. In fact some proponents of this approach suggest that the bidirectional Glenn shunt with supplementary pulmonary blood flow can be considered the definitive palliation for the child with a single ventricle.

The principal argument against leaving supplementary pulmonary blood flow is that this additional blood flow is inherently inefficient in that some of the flow is recirculated pulmonary venous return which has no ability to pick up additional oxygen. Most importantly it is difficult to quantitate the amount of supplementary blood flow so that there is a risk of substantial over volume loading of the single ventricle. The amount of supplementary pulmonary blood flow will change over time as the child grows. For example a band will become progressively tighter, gradually reducing the amount of supplementary blood flow and likewise native obstruction to pulmonary outflow usually progresses over time. Another argument against leaving supplementary blood flow is that this will complicate the subsequent Fontan procedure. Although no formal randomized studies have been undertaken to investigate the question of supplementary pulmonary blood flow with the bidirectional Glenn shunt the one or two retrospective studies that have looked at this question suggest that there is a higher incidence of pleural effusions and probable longer hospitalization required if supplementary blood flow is left.[67]

The importance of excising or oversewing the native pulmonary valve

If a decision is made to eliminate all additional sources of pulmonary blood flow at the time of a bidirectional Glenn shunt it is particularly important that the proximal main pulmonary artery stump does not contain a pulmonary valve. For example, if a pulmonary artery band is taken down by simple ligation of the main pulmonary artery this will leave a proximal stump into which blood can flow through the pulmonary valve but cannot readily return into the ventricle. This pouch was found early in our experience to be an important source of thrombi which subsequently embolized into the systemic circulation and were a cause of strokes.[71] Furthermore simple ligation of the main pulmonary artery is frequently associated with recanalization and re-establishment of antegrade pulmonary blood flow. Therefore it is important that in addition to removing the pulmonary artery band the main pulmonary artery is divided. The distal divided main pulmonary artery is either closed by direct suture or if necessary with an autologous pericardial patch. The pulmonary valve leaflets are excised working through the proximal pulmonary stump. It is important to avoid allowing air to be entrained into the single ventricle if the aorta has not been cross clamped. If the heart is beating vigorously and the pulmonary annulus is large it may be wise to apply an aortic cross clamp. The proximal pulmonary stump is carefully oversewn. This area can be an important source of bleeding since the stump may be exposed to systemic ventricular pressure if there is no native obstruction to pulmonary outflow. Care should be taken in oversewing the proximal pulmonary stump to avoid incorporating the left main coronary artery which may be difficult to visualize because of adhesions secondary to the pulmonary artery band.

Pressure monitoring when weaning from bypass after the bidirectional Glenn shunt

An atrial monitoring catheter should be placed in the common atrium at a site separate from the venous cannula. When the patient has been almost fully rewarmed the right angle cannula in the left innominate vein is removed. By this time the heart should be ejecting and the patient should be ventilated. It is important to remember that venous return from the brain must now pass through the pulmonary vascular bed before returning to the heart. Therefore to leave the lungs in a collapsed state risks diverting blood away from the cerebral circulation particularly if the heart is not ejecting. A monitoring catheter is placed temporarily in the innominate vein cannulation site for measurement of SVC pressure. The patient is weaned from bypass usually with low dose inotropic support with dopamine. If the child has been well managed with appropriate neonatal palliation the common atrial pressure should be low at the time of weaning from bypass, e.g. no more than 5–6 mm and the innominate vein pressure, which should be equivalent to the superior vena caval pressure and pulmonary artery pressure, should generally be no more than 11 or 12 mm. Often the arterial oxygen saturation in the setting of anesthesia and a high inspired oxygen level will be greater than 90%. It is important to remember that cerebral vascular resistance has an inverse relationship to pulmonary vascular resistance with respect to carbon dioxide levels. Therefore it is likely to be counterproductive to hyperventilate the child since the alkalosis that ensues will reduce cerebral blood flow and therefore reduce pulmonary blood flow.[72]

THE HEMI-FONTAN PROCEDURE

The hemi-Fontan procedure is a modification of the bidirectional Glenn shunt that is used at a number of centers for second stage palliation of children with single ventricle physiology particularly those with hypoplastic left heart syndrome.[73] Proponents of this approach feel that it allows supplementation of the central pulmonary artery area so as to optimize flow to the left lung. This has been a particular concern in the past in patients with hypoplastic left heart syndrome where various technical issues can result in central pulmonary artery narrowing (see Chapter 19). The hemi-Fontan procedure also simplifies the subsequent Fontan procedure. In fact Norwood has recently demonstrated that the Fontan procedure can be completed after a hemi-Fontan in the catheterization laboratory by placement of a covered stent. The principal arguments against the hemi-Fontan procedure include the fact that it involves extensive surgery in the region of the sinus node and sinus node artery which might result in a higher incidence of late sinus node dysfunction. The procedure requires blood coming down the superior vena cava to take a 270° spiral turn in order to pass into the right pulmonary artery, rather than a simple 90° turn into the right lung as is the case with the bidirectional Glenn shunt. Opponents of the hemi-Fontan approach also suggest that if appropriate steps are taken at the time of a stage 1 Norwood procedure there should be a low incidence of central pulmonary artery stenosis. Finally the hemi-Fontan procedure through its name suggests that only 50% of the final palliation has been achieved that will ultimately be achieved by a Fontan procedure. In fact the name is misleading in that either the hemi-Fontan or the bidirectional Glenn shunt eliminates all recirculation of pulmonary venous blood. Following this second stage procedure the only blood flow passing into the pulmonary circulation is systemic venous blood (assuming that supplementary blood flow has been eliminated). Therefore the Fontan procedure does not improve the efficiency of the circulation by eliminating further volume loading though its does improve arterial oxygen saturation.

Surgical technique for the hemi-Fontan procedure

The hemi-Fontan procedure is not used at Children's Hospital Boston. In brief the technique involves construction of an atriopulmonary anastomosis posteriorly between an incision in the dome of the right atrium between the atrio-superior vena caval junction and the ascending aorta and a longitudinal incision on the inferior surface of the right pulmonary artery. A Gortex baffle or 'dam' as it has been labeled by Norwood who prefers this approach[74] is used to direct blood flow from the SVC atriocaval junction across the atriopulmonary anastomosis. The Gortex baffle extends into the left pulmonary artery behind the aorta thereby supplementing the central pulmonary artery area.

OTHER TECHNICAL VARIATIONS OF SECOND STAGE SINGLE VENTRICLE PALLIATION

A technical variation of the bidirectional Glenn shunt which has been incorrectly labeled by some as a hemi-Fontan procedure is to perform a double cavopulmonary anastomosis with internal patch closure of the cardiac anastomosis. The cephalic end of the divided SVC is anastomosed to the superior surface of the right pulmonary artery. The cardiac end of the divided SVC is anastomosed to the inferior surface of the right pulmonary artery. The internal orifice of the superior vena cava is closed with a Gortex patch. Proponents of this approach suggest that it simplifies the subsequent Fontan procedure in that the Gortex patch can be removed and a baffle constructed to direct blood from the inferior vena cava to the internal orifice of the superior vena cava.[75] Arguments against this approach include the fact that the Gortex baffle may leak resulting in early desaturation. The baffle may inhibit growth of the superior vena cava immediately superior to it. Furthermore even if growth is reasonable the segment of superior vena cava between the atrium and right pulmonary artery is not adequate in size to carry the total inferior vena caval return without obstruction. Finally removal of the Gortex patch results in a raw surface devoid of endocardium and may be a point of origin of thrombus formation.

Results of cavopulmonary shunt

In 1990 Bridges et al[38] described the results of bidirectional cavopulmonary anastomosis in 38 patients at Children's Hospital Boston who were considered to be at high risk for a Fontan procedure. Fontan risk factors included pulmonary artery distortion, pulmonary artery resistance greater than two units, atrioventricular valve regurgitation, systemic ventricular dysfunction, complex venous anatomy and subaortic obstruction. In spite of the high risks present in this group there were no deaths either early or late. Median arterial oxygen saturation increased from 79 to 84%. No patient had pleural effusions after seven days. These excellent results supported the concept of the bidirectional Glenn shunt as an intermediate step useful in staging patients between neonatal palliation and a subsequent Fontan procedure.

This report built on the work published by Hopkins et al[34] who described application of a bidirectional Glenn in 21 patients at Duke University. This was the first paper to suggest the concept of staging patients with single ventricle physiology with the bidirectional Glenn shunt before the Fontan procedure.

Another group which adopted the bidirectional Glenn shunt at an early stage was the group at Children's Hospital in San Diego. In 1999, Mainwaring, Lamberti et al[67] described the results of 149 patients who underwent a bidirectional Glenn between 1986 and 1998. Ninety three patients had elimination of all other sources of pulmonary blood flow while 56 patients had either a shunt or a patent right ventricular outflow tract to augment pulmonary blood flow. The operative mortality was 2.2% for those without accessory blood flow and 5.4% for those with additional blood flow. Actuarial analysis demonstrated a divergence of the Kaplan Maier survival curves in favor of the patients in whom there was no accessory blood flow ($p < 0.02$). The authors conclude that in general it is preferable to eliminate additional sources of pulmonary blood flow in patients undergoing placement of a bidirectional Glenn shunt.

Interval management between the second and third stages

The child's progress following second stage palliation is usually a remarkable contrast to progress following neonatal palliation. Generally growth is considerably more rapid once the inherent volume loading of the neonatal circulation has been eliminated. Initially the child's arterial oxygen saturation is likely to be quite satisfactory at approximately 85%. Interestingly in the first week or two following surgery systemic hypertension is very common and frequently requires treatment with an ACE inhibitor. The child is also likely to be quite irritable during this period but this usually settles. Presumably both the systemic hypertension and irritability are in some way centrally mediated by the abrupt increase in cerebral venous pressure that results from second stage palliation. Interestingly pleural effusions are remarkably rare even when central venous pressure in the superior vena cava is quite elevated. In the months following the second stage procedure the child is likely to show a gradual deterioration in arterial oxygen saturation. Children with heterotaxy who have undergone the *Kawashima procedure*, i.e. anastomosis of the superior vena cava which is receiving azygous return from an interrupted inferior vena cava[32] appear to have a particularly aggressive decline in arterial oxygen saturation.

There are three main factors that contribute to the deteriorating oxygen saturation. Growth of the child results in the head and upper half of the body contributing less to the total systemic venous return because of a change in the relative sizes of the head and body.[76] Secondly the differential venous pressure between the upper and lower body results in opening of venous collaterals which decompress the upper body and further reduce pulmonary blood flow. Finally, certain patients appear particularly prone to the development of pulmonary arteriovenous malformations which bypass the gas exchanging components of the lungs. As mentioned above this phenomenon may be related to absence of a hepatic inhibitory factor and has been cited as a reason to leave accessory pulmonary blood flow in addition to flow from a bidirectional Glenn shunt.[70]

Although it is possible to improve the child's oxygen saturation by interventional catheter techniques such as coil occlusion of venous collaterals it is generally preferable to proceed to a Fontan procedure in the child whose arterial oxygen saturation is consistently less than approximately 75%. It is important not to allow the child's oxygen saturation to deteriorate to very low levels such as less than 65–70% as this is likely to be due to profuse development of pulmonary arteriovenous malformations which will complicate the performance of the Fontan procedure. This is not to say that a diagnostic catheterization should not be undertaken in the child who has reached the point where cyanosis is indicating that it is time to proceed with the Fontan procedure. On occasion a simple explanation for the cyanosis will be found such as a previously unidentified left sided superior vena cava. Even a tiny left SVC can dilate dramatically and may decompress systemic venous return into the common atrium.[77] Coil occlusion of the left SVC is indicated both to increase arterial oxygen saturation before the Fontan procedure and also to reduce the need for dissection by the surgeon in the region of the left phrenic nerve. Occasionally systemic venous collateral vessels connect directly into the pulmonary venous system and must be coil occluded.

In the child who is making good progress following second stage palliation, cardiac catheterization is nevertheless indicated by 12 months from the time of the second stage. This allows assessment of issues such as growth and development of the pulmonary arteries, maintenance of excellent ventricular compliance and freedom from systemic outflow obstruction. Important hemodynamic measurements include the pulmonary artery pressure, pulmonary vascular resistance and ventricular end diastolic pressure. Ideally the pulmonary artery pressure should be less than 16–20 mm, pulmonary resistance should be less than four units and end diastolic pressure should be less than 12 mm. In the child who has been carefully managed from the neonatal period with appropriate neonatal palliation and a subsequent second stage procedure at approximately six months of age and who is making good progress with a satisfactory oxygen saturation at 18 months of age, it is highly improbable that any of these hemodynamic measurements is likely to contraindicate a Fontan procedure. In fact the observation that a child's arterial oxygen saturation is reasonable, e.g. greater than 75% when pulmonary blood flow is derived only from a bidirectional Glenn shunt is evidence in itself that a child will tolerate a Fontan procedure with no difficulty.

SHOULD DIFFUSE COLLATERALS BE COIL OCCLUDED AT THE TIME OF PRE-FONTAN CATHETERIZATION?

An ongoing controversy relates to the management of the diffuse systemic to pulmonary arterial collateral vessels which tend to form in patients subsequent to their bidirectional Glenn procedure. These so-called 'chest wall collaterals' are mainly derived from branches of the subclavian arteries, particularly the mammary arteries. Some centers believe that it is helpful to occlude both internal mammary arteries with coils to minimize volume loading following the Fontan procedure. Others have argued that since the child's arterial oxygen saturation is ultimately going to be close to normal following fenestration closure after the Fontan procedure, the stimulus for these chest wall collaterals to be maintained will be eliminated and therefore there is likely to be a natural regression. One report which has looked at this issue was unable to demonstrate that the course after a Fontan procedure was improved by preoperative coil embolization of chest wall collaterals.[78,79]

As with the many other controversies surrounding management of the patient with a single ventricle this question will be best answered by a multi-institutional trial.

Third stage palliation of single ventricle: the fenestrated Fontan

LATERAL TUNNEL INTRA-ATRIAL PTFE BAFFLE

The lateral tunnel Fontan procedure (also called total cavopulmonary connection) remains the procedure of first choice for the fenestrated Fontan procedure at Children's Hospital Boston (Figure 20.5). The technique has the important advantage of incorporating growth potential so that it can be applied in children who are 18 months to two years of age which is our usual age of election for performing this procedure. A decision as to whether a child is a suitable candidate to proceed to a Fontan procedure is no longer a difficult one. If the child is making reasonable progress with a bidirectional Glenn then almost certainly they will do well with a fenestrated Fontan procedure which is performed accurately. If an older child should present who has not undergone careful observation and palliation during infancy as described above and in whom there is doubt regarding the pulmonary resistance or ventricular function, e.g. pulmonary resistance is greater than four units or end disatolic pressure is greater than 12–14 mm, then an initial bidirectional Glenn should be performed. An initial bidirectional Glenn is also advisable in the older child who presents for the first time if ancillary procedures are required such as reconstruction of the pulmonary arteries.

Technical considerations for the lateral tunnel Fontan

The procedure is performed through the median sternotomy incision that was used for neonatal palliation and for the bidirectional Glenn shunt. The usual monitoring lines are placed with the patient in the supine position. Following skin preparation and draping a reoperative sternotomy is performed (see Chapter 2). It should be anticipated that dissection in the superior half of the mediastinum will be quite a bit more difficult than usual because of the increased venous pressure to which this tissue has been exposed. There may be a slightly edematous feel to the tissue and tissue planes are much less obvious than usual. The technique of cannulation for cardiopulmonary bypass is important. A right angle venous cannula should be placed in the left innominate vein (Figure 20.5a). The tip of the cannula should be small enough to allow flow to pass around the cannula so that the cannula drains both the right and left innominate vein. If a cannula is not placed at some point in the superior caval system there is a risk during the cooling phase of bypass that blood will preferentially flow to the lower half of the body which could result in cerebral ischemic injury. The blood returning from the brain must pass through the pulmonary vascular bed before reaching the common atrium.

One of the only cases of serious choreoathetosis that was seen at Children's Hospital Boston in the 1980s that was not a child with pulmonary atresia and multiple collateral vessels was a child with a bidirectional Glenn shunt in whom a single venous cannula was placed in the right atrium for cooling to deep hypothermia. Although the period of circulatory arrest was not prolonged the child clearly sustained an ischemic injury which in retrospect appeared to be related to imbalance of perfusion of the lower body versus the upper body.[80]

The inferior vena cava can be drained either with a flexible straight cannula or a right angle cannula. A straight cannula has the advantage that it can initially be placed so as to be draining the right atrium and is then advanced into the inferior vena cava after the aortic cross clamp has been applied. The IVC is encircled with a tourniquet. A very limited dissection is performed of the superior vena cava carefully teasing the phrenic nerve away from the cava with scissors and blunt dissection and minimizing use of electrocautery. Using a moderate degree of hypothermia, e.g. 28°C the ascending aorta is clamped and cardioplegia solution is infused into the root of the aorta. A second cross clamp is applied across the superior vena cava. The IVC cannula is advanced and the tourniquet is tightened. There is frequently considerable left heart return so that it is advisable at this point to insert a left atrial vent through the right pulmonary veins. The right atrial free wall is opened with vertical incision which superiorly is curved to the left of the SVC remnant which is indicated by the Prolene suture that was used to oversew the cava at the time of the bidirectional Glenn shunt. The incision should be limited at its superior extent to avoid injury to the sinus node artery (Figure 20.5a). A longitudinal incision is made on the inferior surface of the right pulmonary artery. The superior end of the atrial incision is anastomosed to the posterior edge of the pulmonary artery using continuous 5/0 Prolene (Figure 20.5b). A Gortex baffle is shaped appropriately. It is sutured into the right atrium so as to direct inferior vena caval blood to the atriopulmonary anastomosis (Figure 20.5c). The baffle roofs the atriopulmonary anastomosis. A 4 mm punch is used to create a fenestration at an appropriate site in the baffle that will be suitable for device closure at a later time (Figure 20.5d). The pulmonary venous atrium is reconstituted by suturing the anterior component of the original right atrial free wall obliquely over the anterior surface of the Gortex baffle (Figures 20.5e,f). The heart is de-aired in the usual fashion and the aortic cross clamp is released with the cardioplegia site bleeding freely as an air vent. During warming a monitoring catheter is placed in the original right atrial appendage to measure pulmonary venous atrial (left atrial) pressure. Two atrial and one ventricular pacing wire are placed. Towards the end of rewarming the right angle cannula is removed from the left innominate vein and is replaced with a monitoring catheter.

Weaning from bypass should be uncomplicated and is generally assisted with a low dose dopamine infusion. The monitoring catheter which had temporarily been placed in the left innominate vein cannulation site to assess SVC pressure is shifted to the IVC cannulation site. This enables an assessment of relative pressures in the SVC and IVC systems which should be identical. The arterial oxygen saturation can be quite variable in the early period after weaning from bypass. Saturation is influenced by many factors including the size of the child, the cardiac output and the pulmonary resistance. In the absence of profuse pulmonary arteriovenous malformations the oxygen saturation is generally in the region of 80–85%. Generally a fenestration will prevent a wide difference in pressure between the intra-baffle pressure which is usually no more than 12–14 mm and the left atrial pressure which is generally in the region of 6–8 mm.

COMPLICATIONS FOLLOWING THIRD STAGE PALLIATION

Fenestration thrombosis

Acute thrombosis of the fenestration may occur in the first hours following the Fontan procedure. This is usually signaled by a widening trans-pulmonary pressure gradient and an increase in the arterial oxygen saturation to greater than 95%. The risk of fenestration thrombosis may be increased by intraoperative use of aprotinin or antifibrinolytic agents or overly aggressive administration of coagulation factors including cryoprecipitate though it has not been possible to confirm this in a retrospective review.[81] It may be helpful to reduce the usual dose of protamine to half of the standard dose.

Although fenestration thrombosis is usually not associated with serious hemodynamic deterioration it is likely to be associated with a more prolonged postoperative course with a greater persistence of pleural effusion drainage. If a child has marginal hemodynamics then there may be acute hemodynamic deterioration. Therefore it is reasonable to assess fenestration patency by echocardiography. If thrombosis is confirmed the child is best taken to the catheterization laboratory where it is usually a simple matter to reopen the fenestration by passage of a small balloon catheter.[82] On occasion it is helpful to dilate the fenestration if it is inadequate in size. The fenestration can be dilated to the point where arterial oxygen saturation is as low as 75–80%.[83] This will generally be accompanied by an improved cardiac output.

Pleural effusions

It can be anticipated that most children will drain pleural effusions for at least three or four days following the Fontan procedure. Therefore chest tubes need to be placed in both

CPB setup for Fontan

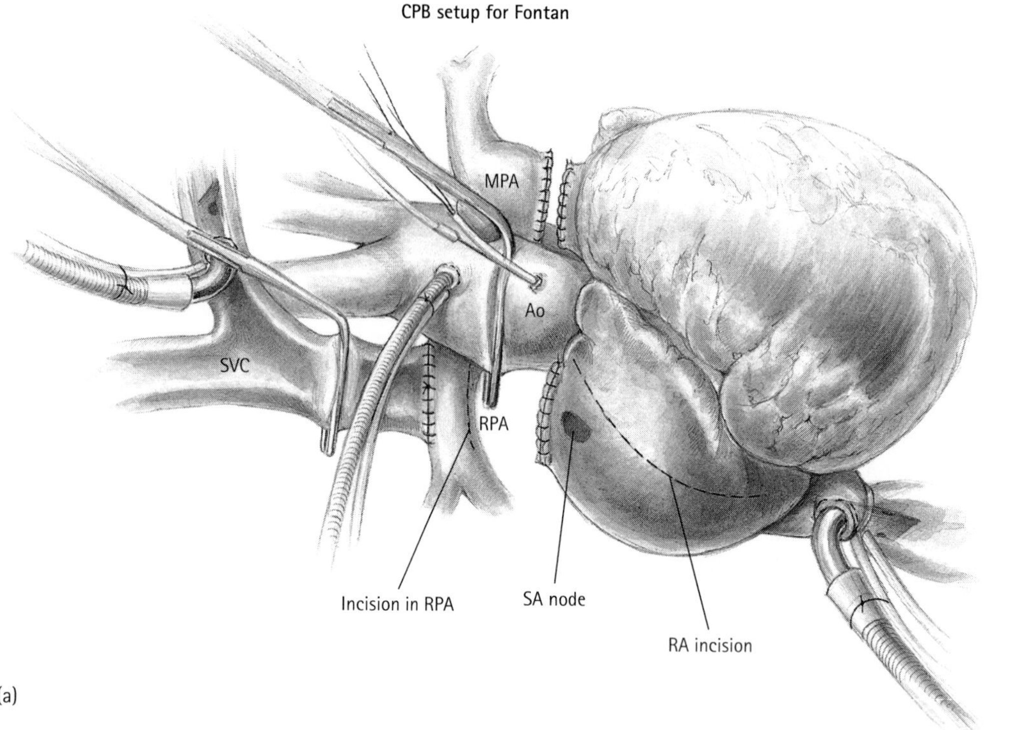

(a)

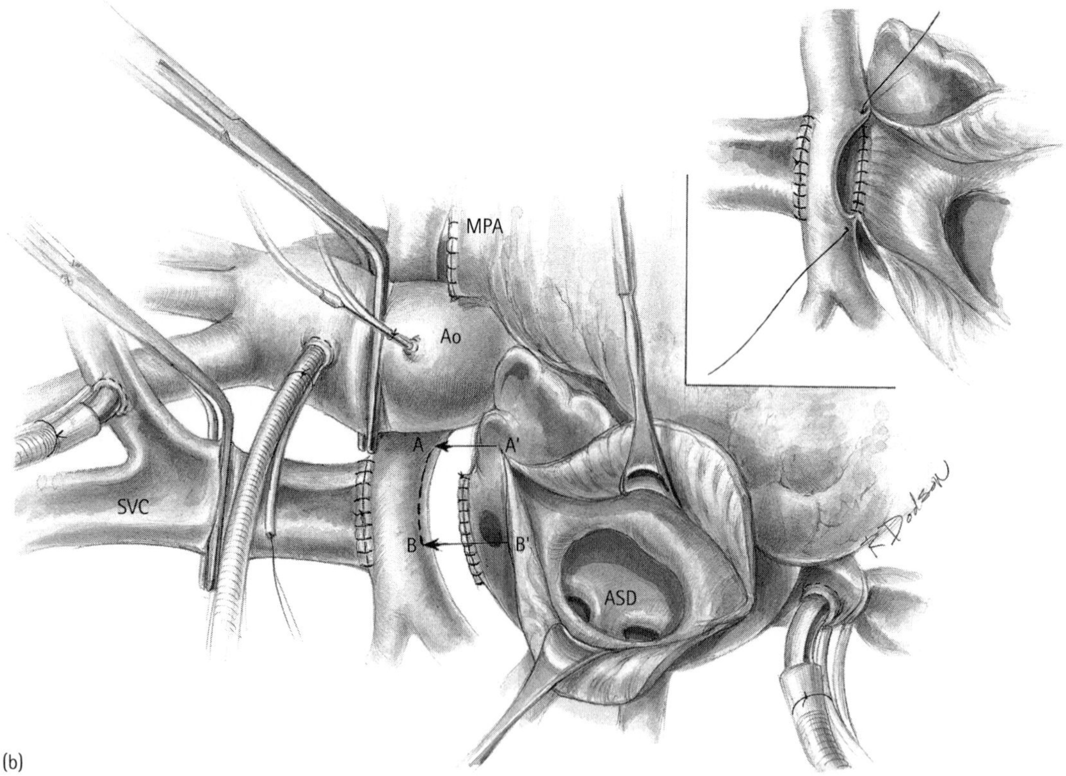

(b)

Figure 20.5a,b *Fenestrated Fontan procedure following previous bidirectional Glenn shunt. (a) Cardiopulmonary bypass setup includes a right angle cannula in the left innominate vein and either a straight or right angle cannula in the IVC. Previously the main pulmonary artery has been divided and oversewn at the time of the bidirectional Glenn shunt. Planned incisions on the undersurface of the right pulmonary artery and on the right atrial free wall are indicated. The atrial incision veers anterior to the sinus node. (b) The right atrium has been opened and direct anastomosis is fashioned posteriorly between the right atrium and right pulmonary artery.*

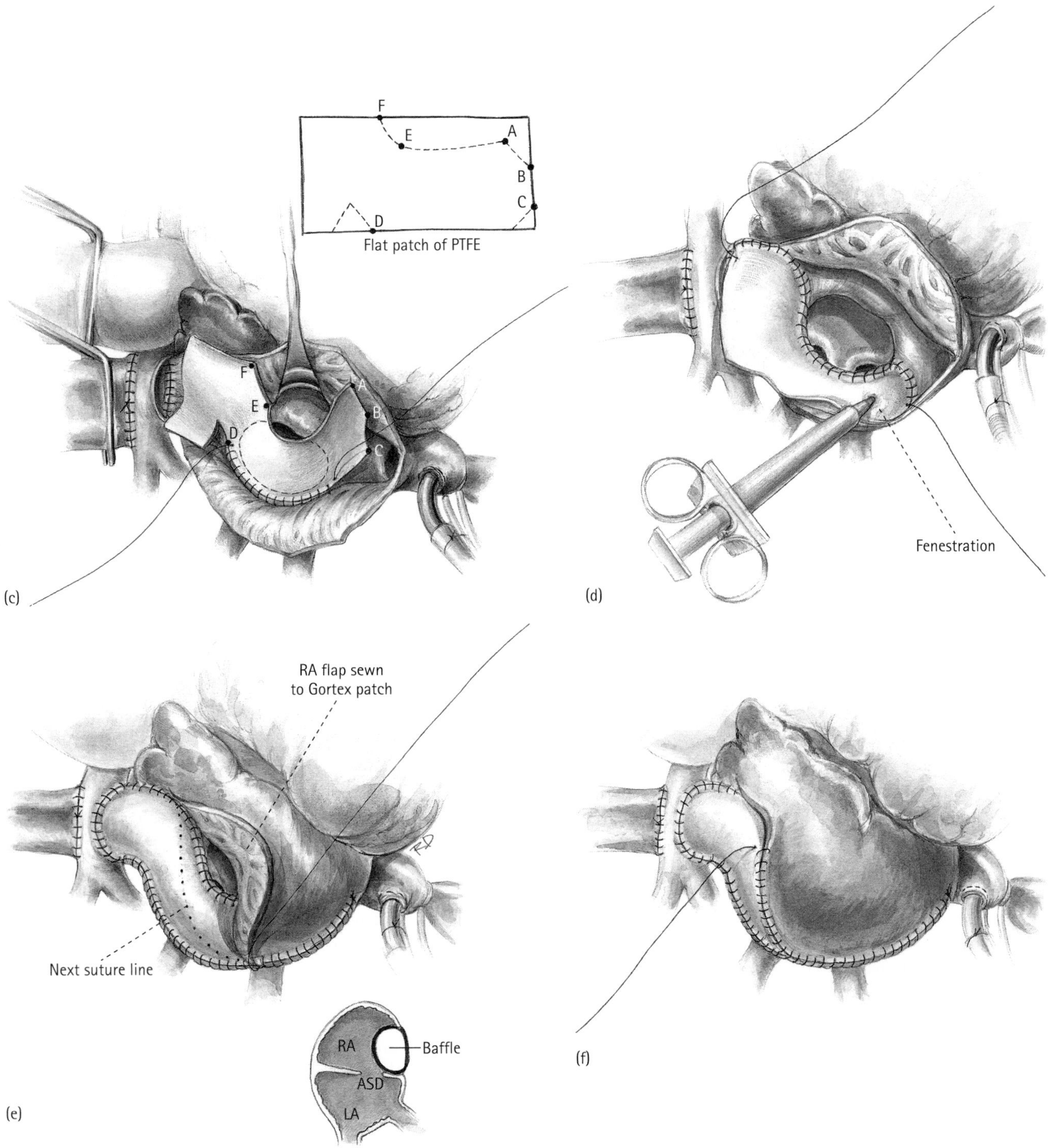

Figure 20.5c–f *(c) A PTFE baffle is sutured into the right atrium so as to direct IVC blood to the atriopulmonary anastomosis. The inset indicates the initial shape of the patch. (d) A 4 mm fenestration is punched in the baffle. (e) The pulmonary venous atrium is reconstituted by suturing the anterior component of the original right atrial free wall obliquely over the anterior surface of the baffle. (f) Completion of the pulmonary venous atrium. Inset indicates the lateral tunnel location of the baffle pathway.*

pleural cavities as well as in the mediastinum. It is unusual that pleural effusions drain for longer than one week so long as a child does not have important risk factors such as absence of one lung, important atrioventricular valve regurgitation that has not been repairable, elevated pulmonary resistance or compromised ventricular function. Although many interventions have been attempted in order to reduce the duration of persistent pleural effusions it is not considered that any of these is particularly helpful, including administration of a medium chain triglyceride, attempted pleurodesis through instillation of the usual agents or pleurectomy, ligation of the thoracic duct or administration of corticosteroids.

CLOSING THE FENESTRATION

Should the fenestration be closed? If so, when?

There is ongoing controversy as to whether the fenestration should be closed in the catheterization laboratory within a year or so of the Fontan procedure. This can be done very effectively with a small occluder device.[84] Current practice allows for temporary balloon occlusion of the fenestration with measurement of the change in cardiac output and increase in right atrial pressure. Generally a fall in cardiac output of up to 25% is tolerated. It must be remembered that this is the fall in cardiac output at rest. No assessment has been made of the impact of fenestration closure on cardiac output with exercise.

It is unclear what the natural history of fenestration closure is though clearly somewhere in the region of 20–30 or 40% of fenestrations will close spontaneously over the first year or two postoperatively. Although it has been argued that fenestration patency increases the risk of stroke from paradoxical embolus it can also be argued that the fall in cardiac output that accompanies fenestration closure also increases the risk of intra-atrial thrombosis. Exercise studies in the past have clearly demonstrated that patients who do not have a fenestration are unable to increase their cardiac output during exercise and in general simply increase their oxygen extraction so that venous oxygen saturation falls to very low levels.[85] It has been hypothesized that a fenestration may be helpful during exercise in that it will allow a substantial increase in cardiac output though this hypothesis has not been carefully tested. There is no question that these issues, which will clearly have a long-term impact on the quality of life of all patients undergoing the Fontan procedure, must be looked at in a systematic fashion.

THE FONTAN PROCEDURE INCORPORATING AN INTRA-ATRIAL CONDUIT

The child with heterotaxy is likely to have either complex systemic or pulmonary venous anatomy. For example the hepatic veins may enter the floor of the common atrium separate from the IVC. The pulmonary veins may enter the common atrium as a confluence relatively close to the entrance of one of the superior vena cavas. The surgeon must make a judgment as to whether it is possible to construct an intra-atrial baffle that will have a sufficient margin of clearance from appropriate structures particularly the pulmonary veins to allow undistorted growth. Often a preferable solution under these circumstances is to place an intra-atrial PTFE conduit which lies within the common atrium.[86] Depending on the specific anatomy the surgeon may choose to exit the conduit from the common atrium and to perform an anastomosis to an appropriate site on the pulmonary arteries separate from the atrium. This can be achieved simply by suturing the common atrium circumferentially around the conduit where it emerges. Fenestration of the intra-atrial component of the conduit is achieved quite simply.

THE EXTRACARDIAC CONDUIT MODIFICATION OF THE FONTAN PROCEDURE

It is interesting to note that Fontan's original technique involved placement of an extracardiac conduit (homograft) in order to connect the right atrium to the left pulmonary artery.[6] In an analysis performed by Dr John Kirklin from the University of Alabama and Professor Fontan it was found that use of a conduit as part of the Fontan procedure was a consistent risk factor.[87] However, the technique as originally described is quite a bit different from the current technique that has been popularized by Marcelletti and others.[43,88] The principal factor that stimulated the reintroduction of an extracardiac conduit for the Fontan procedure was the high incidence of late supraventricular arrythmias that was observed in patients who had undergone the original atriopulmonary type Fontan.[89] These patients tend to develop an extremely dilated and hypertrophied right atrium which not surprisingly is a source of arrythmias. Furthermore a laboratory study suggested that the suture line used for the lateral tunnel type Fontan resulted in a high risk of inducible supraventricular tachycardia in dogs.[90] Interestingly this has not proven to be the case with the lateral tunnel modification of the Fontan procedure used clinically. In fact the incidence of new late supraventricular arrhythmias in patients undergoing Fontan procedures over the last 10 years since the lateral tunnel Fontan was introduced has been remarkably low.[91] Nevertheless the extracardiac conduit has gained in popularity and is now a commonly used technique though it is rarely applied at Children's Hospital Boston.

The obvious disadvantage of an extracardiac conduit is that it does not incorporate growth potential. Even a gradient of 3 or 4 mm across a conduit will be important in the late development of complications following the Fontan procedure such as cirrhosis and protein losing enteropathy. Another important disadvantage of the extracardiac conduit is that it is difficult to place a fenestration. One technique which has been used is to punch a standard 4 mm fenestration and then to suture the atrial free wall several millimeters from the edge of the fenestration (Figure 20.6). However, this technique has been associated with a relatively high incidence of fenestration thrombosis. Other arguments in favor of the extracardiac conduit include the absence of prosthetic material within the atrium, particularly the pulmonary venous atrium, which might be a source of systemic emboli. It is also argued that the decreased suture load within the atria will minimize both brady- and tachyarrythmias. In fact in our experience the prosthetic material within the atrial chambers has been an exceedingly rare source of systemic emboli. Systemic emboli in the past have been traced to the pulmonary artery stump in the years before the pulmonary valve was excised. Systemic emboli also appear to be associated with a very low cardiac output state and with dilated atrial chambers. Furthermore humans are unable to extend an endothelial covering over a complete conduit beyond the first 5–10 mm. When an intra-atrial baffle is placed however there is almost no point that is more than 10 mm from

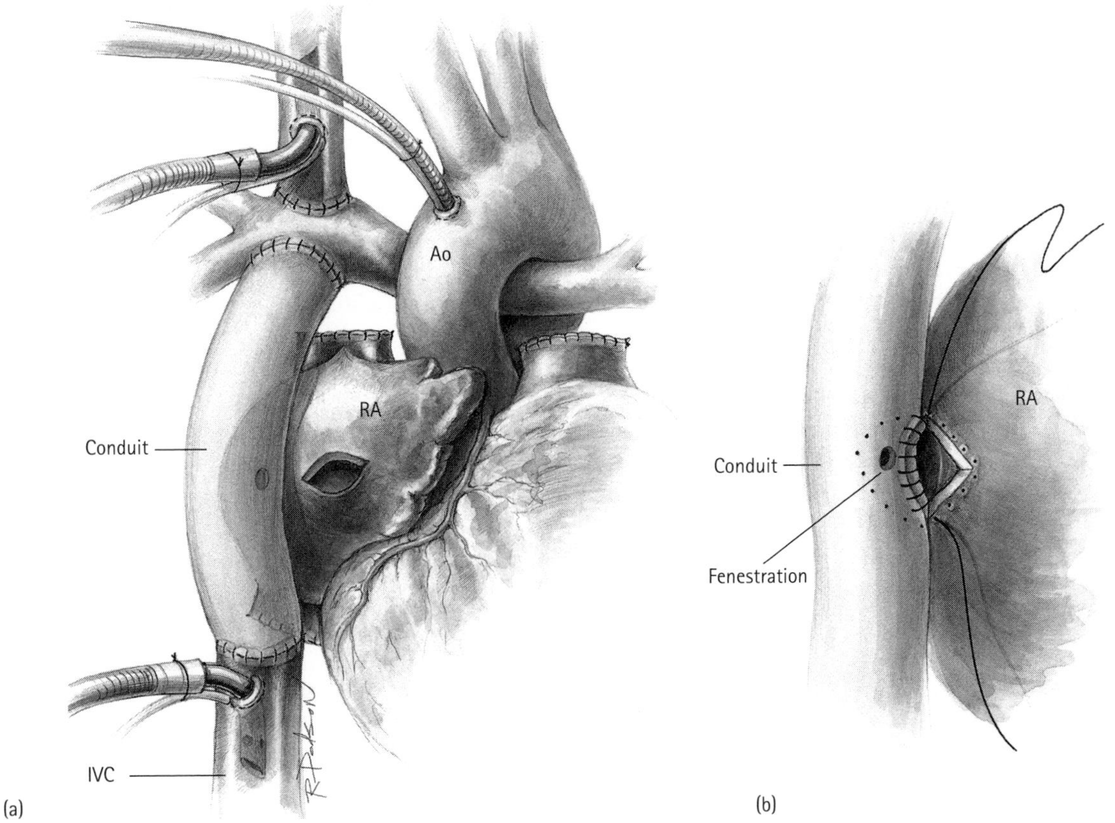

Figure 20.6 *Technique for fenestration creation with the extracardiac conduit modification of the Fontan procedure. (a) A 4 mm fenestration is punched in the midpoint of the PTFE extracardiac conduit. An adjacent incision is made in the right atrial (pulmonary venous atrial) wall. (b) The atrial tissue is sutured to the external wall of the PTFE baffle several millimeters from the fenestration itself. Suturing the atrial tissue directly to the fenestration narrows the fenestration and increases the probability of fenestration thrombosis.*

endocardium so that there is a reasonable probability that a baffle will become more completely endothelialized than a conduit. Thus it can be argued that the risk of baffle thrombosis is higher in an extracardiac conduit.

Avoidance of cardiopulmonary bypass in placing an extracardiac conduit

Some centers have adopted the practice of avoiding cardiopulmonary bypass when performing the extracardiac Fontan procedure.[88] Although this has been apparently associated with a lower incidence of pleural effusions (presumably related to avoidance of the inflammatory factors that are released by cardiopulmonary bypass) there must be concern that this technique will result in a less widely open anastomosis. Another serious concern with this technique is that application of sidebiting clamps in the region of a bidirectional Glenn anastomosis may complicate cerebral venous drainage and could result in brain injury. The technique therefore is not recommended.

Need for multi-institutional trial

As with so many other ongoing controversies in the management of patients with a single ventricle it will be necessary to perform a multi-institutional trial to settle the controversy as to whether there is a long-term advantage for any of the various techniques that are currently used to perform the Fontan procedure. Those trials must not only assess late survival and late quality of life but most importantly should include exercise studies with assessment of maximal oxygen consumption.

Results of the Fontan procedure

Numerous articles have been published describing the evolving results of the Fontan procedure at Children's Hospital Boston. The studies have been summarized by Mayer[92] in the *Pediatric Cardiac Surgery Annual* in 1998. In 2001, Stamm et al[91] reviewed the results of 220 patients who had at least 10 years of follow-up following a lateral tunnel type Fontan procedure at Children's Hospital Boston. Current follow-up information was available in 94% of patients so that the mean follow-up period was greater than 10 years. Despite the fact that these were the earliest lateral tunnel Fontan procedures performed between 1987 and 1991, early mortality was only 5%. Kaplan Meier survival was 93% at five years and 91% at 10 years. Freedom from new supraventricular tachyarrhythmia was 96% at five years and 91% at 10 years. Three patients had evidence of protein losing enteropathy. The most common problem was bradyarrhythmia with freedom from new bradyarrhythmias being 88% at five years and 79% at 10 years. Risk factors for development of supraventricular tachycardia included heterotaxy, atrioventricular valve abnormalities and preoperative bradycardia. Risk factors for bradycardia included systemic venous anomalies. The only risk factor for late failure was a previous coarctation repair.

The excellent late results of the lateral tunnel Fontan contrast sharply with the disappointing results of the older style Fontan procedures that allowed the right atrium to become massively distended. It will be particularly important in the future to distinguish clearly between reports which describe series of patients with the newer style lateral tunnel or total extracardiac conduit Fontan versus series that include the old style Fontan as was routinely performed before 1987.

In another report from Children's Hospital Boston Stamm et al[93] reviewed the results of the Fontan procedure for 135 patients with heterotaxy syndrome who underwent their Fontan procedure between 1981 and 2000. Ninety three patients had right isomerism and 42 had left isomerism. Many patients had anomalies of either systemic or pulmonary venous return. A total of 27% of patients had at least moderate AV valve regurgitation. Ten year survival was 70% for Fontan procedures before 1990 and 93% for Fontan procedures after 1990. At 10 years freedom from late bradyarrhythmia was 78% and from late tachyarrhythmia was 70%. The predictors of late arrhythmia were preoperative arrhythmias, older age at operation and anatomic features.

IS A FENESTRATION NECESSARY?

Although some groups continue to suggest that a fenestration is not helpful for the majority of patients undergoing a Fontan procedure such as the report by Thompson et al from San Francisco in 1999,[94] the majority of recent reports that have examined this issue suggest that a fenestration is helpful in reducing morbidity, particularly pleural effusions, shortening hospitalization and possibly reducing mortality.[95–97] For example Lemler et al performed a prospective randomized trial in which 25 patients were randomized to a fenestrated Fontan and 24 to a nonfenestrated Fontan procedure. The fenestrated and nonfenestrated groups were comparable with respect to age, body surface area, number of risk factors, bypass time, aortic cross clamping, preoperative oxygen saturation and dominant ventricular morphology. Patients in the fenestrated group had 55% less total chest tube drainage, 41% shorter total hospitalization and 67% fewer additional procedures in the postoperative period than those in the nonfenestrated group.

DEVELOPMENTAL OUTCOME

In 2000 Wernovsky et al[98] reviewed the developmental outcome in 133 patients following the Fontan procedure at Children's Hospital Boston. Mean full scale IQ was 95.7 ± 17.4 which was significantly below normal. After adjustment for socioeconomic status lower IQ was associated with the use of circulatory arrest before the Fontan procedure, the anatomic diagnosis of hypoplastic left heart syndrome and other complex anomalies as well as prior placement of a pulmonary artery band. The authors conclude that most individual patients palliated with the Fontan procedure in the 1970s and 1980s have cognitive outcome and academic function within the normal range but the performance of the cohort as a whole is lower than that of the general population. In a study of a more recent population, Forbess et al[99] reviewed the developmental outcome in 27 five year old children who had undergone the Fontan procedure at a mean age of two years four months during a more recent era than the cohort reviewed by Wernovksy et al. The more recent group of patients were not only younger at the time of their Fontan procedure but they were also more likely to have undergone the Norwood procedure, to have had a pre-Fontan bidirectional cavopulmonary anastomosis and to have undergone Fontan fenestration. The mean full scale IQ was 93 ± 16, mean verbal IQ was 95 ± 15 and mean performance (motor) IQ was 91 ± 17. There were no significant differences relative to the earlier cohort of patients. Once again the neurodevelopmental outcomes were in general within the normal range but overall somewhat lower than the general population. The addition of a fenestration and the performance of an additional staging procedure did not detrimentally affect developmental outcome.

Exercise testing after the Fontan procedure

One of the most comprehensive studies of exercise capacity after the Fontan procedure was reported by Gewillig et al in 1990.[86] There was a wide spectrum of exercise capacity. At the poor end of the spectrum the performance did not result from inadequate level of heart rate but from an inability to increase or maintain stroke volume. Multivariate analysis demonstrated that impairment of ventricular contractility had to be severe before it predicted limited performance. The authors were encouraged to note that of the 10 best performers compared with 10 age matched control subjects there were no differences found in cardiac index, stroke index, heart rate or blood pressure at any exercise level including maximal exercise.

REFERENCES

1. Van Praagh R. Embryology. In Fyler DC (ed). *Nadas' Pediatric Cardiology*, Philadelphia, Hanley & Belfus, 1992, pp 5–16.
2. Van Praagh R. Segmental approach to diagnosis. In Fyler DC (ed). *Nadas' Pediatric Cardiology*, Philadelphia, Hanley & Belfus, 1992, pp 27–35.
3. Freedom RM, Dische MR, Rowe RD. Pathologic anatomy of subaortic stenosis and atresia in the first year of life. *Am J Cardiol* 1977; **39**:1035–44.

4. Karl TR, Watterson KG, Sano S, Mee RB. Operations for subaortic stenosis in univentricular hearts. *Ann Thorac Surg* 1991; **52**:420–7.
5. Edwards JE. Congenital malformations of the heart and great vessels. C. Malformations of the valves. In Gould SE (ed). *Pathology of the Heart and Blood Vessels* 3rd edn, Springfield IL, Charles C Thomas, 1968, p 312.
6. Fontan F, Baudet E. Surgical repair of tricuspid atresia. *Thorax* 1971; **26**:240–8.
7. Mayer JE Jr, Bridges ND, Lock JE, Hanley FL, Jonas RA, Castaneda AR. Factors associated with marked reduction in mortality for Fontan operations in patients with single ventricle. *J Thorac Cardiovasc Surg* 1992; **103**:444–51.
8. Anderson RH, Wilkinson JL, Gerlis LM, Smith A, Becker AE. Atresia of the right atrioventricular orifice. *Br Heart J* 1977; **39**:414–28.
9. Scalia D, Russo P, Anderson RH et al. The surgical anatomy of hearts with no direct communication between the right atrium and the ventricular mass – so called tricuspid atresia. *J Thorac Cardiovasc Surg* 1984; **87**:743–55.
10. Matitiau A, Geva T, Parness IA, Spevak PJ, Sanders SP. Bulboventricular foramen size in single LV/tricuspid atresia: Relation to aortic outflow tract obstruction. *Circulation* 1990; **82**(Suppl):III353.
11. Matitiau A, Geva T, Colan SD et al. Bulboventricular foramen size in infants with double inlet left ventricle or tricuspid atresia with transposed great arteries. Influence on initial palliative operation and rate of growth. *J Am Coll Cardiol* 1992; **19**:142–8.
12. Van Praagh R, Plett JA, Van Praagh S. Single ventricle. *Herz* 1979; **4**:113–50.
13. Van Praagh R, Ongley PA, Swan HJC. Anatomic types of single or common ventricle in man. *Am J Cardiol* 1964; **13**:367.
14. Anderson RH, Lenox CC, Zuberbuhler JR, Ho SY, Smith A, Wilkinson JL. Double inlet left ventricle with rudimentary right ventricle and ventriculoarterial concordance. *Am J Cardiol* 1983; **52**:573–7.
15. Holmes AF. Case of malformation of the heart. *Trans Med Chir Soc Edin* 1824; **1**:252.
16. Van Praagh S, Santini F, Sanders SP. Cardiac malpositions with special emphasis on visceral heterotaxy (asplenia and polysplenia syndromes). In Fyler DC (ed). *Nadas' Pediatric Cardiology*, Philadelphia, Hanley & Belfus, 1992, pp 589–608.
17. Van Mierop LHS, Wiglesworth FW. Isomerism of the cardiac atresia in the asplenia syndrome. *Lab Invest* 1962; **11**:1303.
18. Van Praagh S, Kreutzer J, Alday L et al. Systemic and pulmonary venous connections in visceral heterotaxy with emphasis on the diagnosis of atrial situs. A study of 109 postmortem cases. In Clark E, Takao A (eds). *Developmental Cardiology: Morphogenesis and Function.* Mt Kisco, NY, Futura, 1990, pp 671–721.
19. Moller JH, Nakib A, Anderson RC, Edwards JE. Congenital cardiac disease associated with polysplenia: A developmental complex of bilateral 'left-sidedness'. *Circulation* 1967; **36**:789–99.
20. Van Praagh S, Kakou-Guikahue M, Kim HS et al. Atrial situs in patients with visceral heterotaxy and congenital heart disease: Conclusions based on findings in 104 postmortem cases. *Coeur* 1988; **19**:484–502.
21. Zamora R, Moller JH, Edwards JE. Double outlet right ventricle: Anatomic types and associated anomalies. *Chest* 1975; **68**:672.
22. Glenn WWL, Patino JF. Circulatory bypass of the right heart. I. Preliminary observations on the direct delivery of vena caval blood into the pulmonary arterial circulation. Azygous vein pulmonary artery shunt. *Yale J Biol Med* 1954; **27**:14.
23. Nuland SB, Glenn WWL, Guilfoil PH. Circulatory bypass of the right heart. III. Some observations on long-term survivors. *Surgery* 1958; **43**:184.
24. Patino JF, Glenn WWL, Guilfoil PH, Hume M, Fenn J. Circulatory bypass of the heart. II Further observations on vena caval pulmonary artery shunts. *Surg Forum* 1957; **6**:189.
25. Glenn WWL. Circulatory bypass of the right side of the heart. IV. Shunt between superior vena cava and distal right pulmonary artery – report of clinical application. *N Eng J Med* 1958; **259**:117.
26. Choussat A, Fontan I, Besse P, Vallot F, Chauve A, Bricand H. Selection criteria for Fontan's procedure. In RH Anderson, EA Shinebourne (eds). *Pediatric Cardiology 1977*, Edinburgh, Churchill Livingstone, 1978.
27. Ross DN. Replacement of aortic and mitral valve with a pulmonary autograft. *Lancet* 1967; **2**:956.
28. Kreutzer GO, Vargas FJ, Schlichter AJ et al. Atriopulmonary anastomosis. *J Thorac Cardiovasc Surg* 1982; **83**:427–6.
29. Norwood WI, Lang P, Hansen DD. Physiologic repair of aortic atresia-hypoplastic left heart syndrome. *N Engl J Med* 1983; **308**:23–6.
30. Puga FJ, Chiavarelli M, Hagler DJ. Modifications of the Fontan operation applicable to patients with left atrioventricular valve atresia or single atrioventricular valve. *Circulation* 1987; **76**(3 Pt 2):III53–60.
31. Jonas RA, Castaneda AR. Modified Fontan procedure: atrial baffle and systemic venous to pulmonary artery anastomotic techniques. *J Card Surg* 1988; **3**:91–6.
32. Kawashima Y, Kitamura S, Matsuda H, Shimazaki Y, Nakano S, Hirose H. Total cavopulmonary shunt operation in complex cardiac anomalies. *J Thorac Cardiovasc Surg* 1984; **87**:74–81.
33. de Leval MR, Kilner P, Gewillig M, Bull C. Total cavopulmonary connection: A logical alternative to atriopulmonary connection for complex Fontan operations. *J Thorac Cardiovasc Surg* 1988; **96**:682–95.
34. Hopkins RA, Armstrong BE, Serwer GA, Peterson RJ, Oldham HN. Physiological rationale for a bidirectional cavopulonary shunt. A versatile complement to the Fontan principle. *J Thorac Cardiovasc Surg* 1985; **90**:391–8.
35. Mazzera E, Corno A, Picardo S et al. Bidirectional cavopulmonary shunts: clinical applications as staged or definitive palliation. *Ann Thorac Surg* 1989; **47**:415–20.
36. Lamberti JJ, Spicer RL, Waldman JD et al. The bidirectional cavopulmonary shunt. *J Thorac Cardiovasc Surg* 1990; **100**:22–9.
37. Jonas RA. Intermediate procedures after first-stage Norwood operation facilitate subsequent repair. *Ann Thorac Surg* 1991; **52**:696–700.
38. Bridges ND, Jonas RA, Mayer JE, Flanagan MF, Keane JF, Castaneda AR. Bidirectional cavopulmonary anastomosis as interim palliation for high-risk Fontan candidates. Early results. *Circulation* 1990; **82**(5 Suppl):IV170–6.
39. Bridges ND, Lock JE, Castaneda AR. Baffle fenestration with subsequent transcatheter closure. Modification of the Fontan operation for patients at increased risk. *Circulation* 1990; **82**:1681–9.
40. Laks H, Pearl JM, Haas GS et al. Partial Fontan: Advantages of an adjustable interatrial communication. *Ann Thorac Surg* 1991; **52**:1084–94.
41. Laks H, Pearl J, Wu A, Haas G, George B. Experience with the Fontan procedure including use of an adjustable intra-atrial communication. In Crupi G, Parenzan L, Anderson RH (eds). *Perspectives in Pediatric Cardiac Surgery Pt 2.* Mt Kisco, NY, Futura Publishing Co, 1989, p 205.

42. Castaneda AR, Jonas RA, Mayer JE, Hanley FL. *Cardiac Surgery of the Neonate and Infant.* Philadelphia, WB Saunders, 1994, p 219.
43. Marcelletti C, Corno A, Giannico S, Marino B. Inferior vena cava-pulmonary artery extracardiac conduit. A new form of right heart bypass. *J Thorac Cardiovasc Surg* 1990; **100**:228–32.
44. Kirklin JK, Blackstone EH, Kirklin JW, Pacifico AD, Bargeron LM Jr. The Fontan operation. Ventricular hypertrophy, age, and date of operation as risk factors. *J Thorac Cardiovasc Surg* 1986; **92**:1049–64.
45. Perry SB, Lang P, Keane JF, Jonas RA, Sanders SP, Lock JE. Creation and maintenance of an adequate interatrial communication in left atrioventricular valve atresia or stenosis. *Am J Cardiol* 1986; **58**:622–6.
46. Odim J, Portzky M, Zurakowski D et al. Sternotomy approach for the modified Blalock-Taussig shunt. *Circulation* 1995; **92** (9 Suppl):II256–61.
47. de Leval MR, McKay R, Jones M, Stark J, Macartney FJ. Modified Blalock-Taussig shunt. Use of subclavian artery orifice as flow regulator in prosthetic systemic-pulmonary artery shunts. *J Thorac Cardiovasc Surg* 1981; **81**:112–9.
48. Jonas RA, Castaneda AR, Norwood WI, Freed MD. Pulmonary valvotomy under normothermic caval inflow occlusion. *Aust N Z J Surg* 1985; **55**:39–44.
49. Jonas RA, Castaneda AR, Freed MD. Normothermic caval inflow occlusion. Application to operations for congenital heart disease. *J Thorac Cardiovasc Surg* 1985; **89**:780–6.
50. Donofrio MT, Jacobs ML, Norwood WI, Rychik J. Early changes in ventricular septal defect size and ventricular geometry in the single left ventricle after volume-unloading surgery. *J Am Coll Cardiol* 1995; **26**:1008–15.
51. Freedom RM, Sondheimer H, Sische R, Rowe RD. Development of 'subaortic stenosis' after pulmonary arterial banding for common ventricle. *Am J Cardiol* 1977; **39**:78–83.
52. Albus RA, Trusler GA, Izukawa T, Williams WG. Pulmonary artery banding. *J Thorac Cardiovasc Surg* 1984; **88**(5 Pt 1):645–53.
53. Jonas RA, Castaneda AR, Lang P. Single ventricle (single- or double-inlet) complicated by subaortic stenosis: surgical options in infancy. *Ann Thorac Surg* 1985; **39**:361–6.
54. Damus PS. A proposed operation for transposition of the great vessels (correspondence). *Ann Thorac Surg* 1975; **20**:724.
55. Stansel HC Jr. A new operation for d-loop transposition of the great vessels. *Ann Thorac Surg* 1975; **19**:565–567.
56. Kaye MP. Anatomic correction of transposition of great arteries. *Mayo Clin Proc* 1975; **50**:638–40.
57. Odim JN, Laks H, Drinkwater DC Jr et al. Staged surgical approach to neonates with aortic obstruction and single-ventricle physiology. *Ann Thorac Surg* 1999; **68**:962–7.
58. Jenkins KJ, Hanley FL, Colan SD, Mayer JE Jr, Castaneda AR, Wernovsky G. Function of the anatomic pulmonary valve in the systemic circulation. *Circulation* 1991; **84**(5 Suppl):III173–9.
59. Gladman G, McCrindle BW, Williams WG, Freedom RM, Benson LN. The modified Blalock-Taussig shunt: clinical impact and morbidity in Fallot's tetralogy in the current era. *J Thorac Cardiovasc Surg* 1997; **114**:25–30.
60. Pinho P, Von Oppell UO, Brink J, Hewitson J. Pulmonary artery banding: adequacy and long-term outcome. *Eur J Cardiothorac Surg* 1997; **11**:105–11.
61. Jensen RA Jr, Williams RG, Laks H, Drinkwater D, Kaplan S. Usefulness of banding of the pulmonary trunk with single ventricle physiology at risk for subaortic obstruction. *Am J Cardiol* 1996; **77**:1089–93.
62. Webber SA, LeBlanc JG, Keeton BR et al. Pulmonary artery banding is not contraindicated in double inlet left ventricle with transposition and aortic arch obstruction. *Eur J Cardiothorac Surg* 1995; **9**:515–20.
63. Vince DJ, Culham JA, LeBlanc JG. Human clinical trials of the dilatable pulmonary artery banding prosthesis. *Can J Cardiol* 1991; **7**:339–42.
64. Chang AC, Hanley FL, Wernovsky G et al. Early bidirectional cavopulmonary shunt in young infants. Postoperative course and early results. *Circulation* 1993; **88**(5 Pt 2):II149–58.
65. Jahangiri M, Shinebourne EA, Keogh B, Lincoln C. Should the bidirectional glenn procedure be better performed through the support of cardiopulmonary bypass? *J Thorac Cardiovasc Surg* 2000; **119**:635.
66. Jahangiri M, Keogh B, Shinebourne EA, Lincoln C. Should the bidirectional Glenn procedure be performed through a thoracotomy without cardiopulmonary bypass? *J Thorac Cardiovasc Surg* 1999; **118**:367–8.
67. Mainwaring RD, Lamberti JJ, Uzark K, Spicker RL, Cocalis MW, Moore JW. Effect of accessory pulmonary blood flow on survival after the bidirectional Glenn procedure. *Circulation* 1999; **100** (19 Suppl):II151–6.
68. Mainwaring RD, Lamberti JJ, Uzark K, Spicer RL. Bidirectional Glenn. Is accessory pulmonary blood flow good or bad? *Circulation* 1995; **92**(9 Suppl):II294–7.
69. Duncan BW, Kneebone JM, Chi EY et al. A detailed histologic analysis of pulmonary arteriovenous malformations in children with cyanotic congenital heart disease. *J Thorac Cardiovasc Surg* 1999; **117**:931–8.
70. Marshall B, Duncan BW, Jonas RA. The role of angiogenesis in the development of pulmonary arteriovenous malformations in children after cavopulmonary anastomosis. *Cardiol Young* 1997; **7**:370–4.
71. du Plessis AJ, Chang AC, Wessel DL et al. Cerebrovascular accidents following the Fontan operation. *Pediatr Neurol* 1995; **12**:230–6.
72. Bradley SM, Simsic JM, Mulvihill DM. Hyperventilation impairs oxygenation after bidirectional superior cavopulmonary connection. *Circulation* 1998; **98**(19 Suppl):II372–6;
73. Douville EC, Sade RM, Fyfe DA. Hemi-Fontan operation in surgery for single ventricle: a preliminary report. *Ann Thorac Surg* 1991; **51**:893–9.
74. Jacobs ML, Norwood WI Jr. Fontan operation: influence of modifications on morbidity and mortality. *Ann Thorac Surg* 1994; **58**:945–51.
75. Castaneda AR, Jonas RA, Mayer JE, Hanley FL. *Cardiac Surgery of the Neonate and Infant*, Philadelphia, WB Saunders, 1994. p 263.
76. Gross GJ, Jonas RA, Castaneda AR, Hanley FL, Mayer JE Jr, Bridges ND. Maturational and hemodynamic factors predictive of increased cyanosis after bidirectional cavopulmonary anastomosis. *Am J Cardiol* 1994; **74**:705–9.
77. Rocchini A, Lock JE. Defect closure: Umbrella devices, In Lock JE, Keane JF, Perry SB (eds). *Diagnostic and Interventional Catheterization in Congenital Heart Disease.* Boston, Kluwer Academic Publishers, 2000, p 214.
78. Bradley SM. Management of aortopulmonary collateral arteries in Fontan patients: Routine occlusion is not warranted. *Semin Thorac Cardiovasc Surg Pediatr Card Surg Annu* 2002; **5**:55–67.
79. Bradley SM, McCall MM, Sistino JJ, Radtke WA. Aortopulmonary collateral flow in the Fontan patient: does it matter? *Ann Thorac Surg* 2001; **72**:408–15.
80. Wong PC, Barlow CF, Hickey PR et al. Factors associated with choreoathetosis after cardiopulmonary bypass in children with congenital heart disease. *Circulation* 1992; **86**(5 Suppl):II118–26.

81. Gruber EM, Shukla AC, Reid RW, Hickey PR, Hansen DD. Synthetic antifibrinolytics are not associated with an increased incidence of baffle fenestration closure after the modified Fontan procedure. *J Cardiothorac Vasc Anesth* 2000; **14**:257–9.
82. Kreutzer J, Lock JE, Jonas RA, Keane JF. Transcatheter fenestration dilation and/or creation in postoperative Fontan patients. *Am J Cardiol* 1997; **79**:228–32.
83. Nishimoto K, Keane JF, Jonas RA. Dilation of intra-atrial baffle fenestrations: results in vivo and in vitro. *Cathet Cardiovasc Diagn* 1994; **31**:73–8.
84. Goff DA, Blume ED, Gauvreau K, Mayer JE, Lock JE, Jenkins KJ. Clinical outcome of fenestrated Fontan patients after closure: the first 10 years. *Circulation* 2000; **102**:2094–9.
85. Gewillig MH, Lundstrom UR, Bull C, Wyse RK, Deanfield JE. Exercise responses in patients with congenital heart disease after Fontan repair: patterns and determinants of performance. *J Am Coll Cardiol* 1990; **15**:1424–32.
86. Vargas FJ, Mayer JE, Jonas RA, Castaneda AR. Anomalous systemic and pulmonary venous connections in conjunction with atriopulmonary anastomosis (Fontan-Kreutzer). Technical considerations. *J Thorac Cardiovasc Surg* 1987; **93**:523–32.
87. Fontan F, Kirklin JW, Fernandez G et al. Outcome after a 'perfect' Fontan operation. *Circulation* 1990; **81**:1520–36.
88. McElhinney DB, Petrossian E, Reddy VM, Hanley FL. Extracardiac conduit Fontan procedure without cardiopulmonary bypass. *Ann Thorac Surg* 1998; **66**:1826–8.
89. Ovroutski S, Dahnert I, Alexi-Meskishvili V, Nurnberg JH, Hetzer R, Lange PE. Preliminary analysis of arrhythmias after the Fontan operation with extracardiac conduit compared with intra-atrial lateral tunnel. *Thorac Cardiovasc Surg* 2001; **49**:334–7.
90. Gandhi SK, Bromberg BI, Rodefeld MD et al. Spontaneous atrial flutter in a chronic canine model of the modified Fontan operation. *J Am Coll Cardiol* 1997; **30**:1095–103.
91. Stamm C, Friehs I, Mayer JE Jr et al. Long-term results of the lateral tunnel Fontan operation. *J Thorac Cardiovasc Surg* 2001; **121**:28–41.
92. Mayer JE Jr. Late outcome after the Fontan procedure. *Semin Thorac Cardiovasc Surg Pediatr Card Surg Annu* 1998; **1**:5–8.
93. Stamm C, Friehs I, Duebener LF et al. Improving results of the modified Fontan operation in patients with heterotaxy syndrome. *Ann Thorac Surg* 2002; **74**:1967–77.
94. Thompson LD, Petrossian E, McElhinney DB et al. Is it necessary to routinely fenestrate an extracardiac fontan? *J Am Coll Cardiol* 1999; **34**:539–44.
95. Airan B, Sharma R, Choudhary SK et al. Univentricular repair: is routine fenestration justified? *Ann Thorac Surg* 2000; **69**:1900–6.
96. Lemler MS, Scott WA, Leonard SR, Stromberg D, Ramaciotti C. Fenestration improves clinical outcome of the fontan procedure: a prospective, randomized study. *Circulation* 2002; **105**:207–12.
97. Gaynor JW, Bridges ND, Cohen MI et al. Predictors of outcome after the Fontan operation: is hypoplastic left heart syndrome still a risk factor? *J Thorac Cardiovasc Surg* 2002; **123**:237–45.
98. Wernovsky G, Stiles KM, Gauvreau K et al. Cognitive development after the Fontan operation. *Circulation* 2000; **102**:883–9.
99. Forbess JM, Visconti KJ, Bellinger DC, Jonas RA. Neurodevelopmental outcomes in children after the fontan operation. *Circulation* 2001; **104**(12 Suppl 1):I127–32.

21

Complete atrioventricular canal

INTRODUCTION

Atrioventricular canal defect (also known as atrioventricular septal defect) includes a wide range of anomalies extending from simple ASD physiology to complex single ventricle physiology. This chapter will focus on AV canal defects that are suitable for a two ventricle repair, recognizing that there is a gray zone where it may be difficult to decide whether an anomaly should be more appropriately treated by a single ventricle approach.[1] Not only is there a wide spectrum under the rubric of AV canal defect but in addition there are important cardiac and noncardiac associated anomalies.

The most important associated cardiac anomaly is tetralogy of Fallot but left ventricular outflow tract obstruction may also be linked and unquestionably increases the risk of a less satisfactory long-term outcome. The most important noncardiac anomaly is Down's syndrome. Almost 50% of children with Down's syndrome have an AV canal defect, usually complete common AV canal.[2] Approximately 75% of patients with complete AV canal have Down's syndrome.[3] It is unusual for Down's patients with AV canal to have left ventricular outflow obstruction.[4]

As with other anomalies in which valve surgery is required AV canal defect has benefited tremendously from the development of improved echocardiographic techniques including transesophageal echocardiography and color Doppler mapping. The improved repair techniques that have resulted from the increased understanding of atrioventricular valve anatomy and physiology mean that the long-term outlook for the child with AV canal is now excellent.

EMBRYOLOGY

After the primitive cardiac tube has looped, usually in a dextro direction (d-loop), the next important step in intracardiac development is septation accompanied by the formation of two atrioventricular valves. These valves develop from endocardial cushion tissue which is primitive mesodermal tissue located at the crux of the heart.[5] Growth of the endocardial cushion tissue towards the posterior wall of the common atrial chamber results in creation of the atrial component of the atrioventricular septum. It is important to understand that this is not the septum primum which is the tissue that forms the base of the fossa ovalis. Absence of the septum primum therefore results in creation of a secundum ASD. It is absence of the atrioventricular component of the atrial septum that results in the formation of a primum ASD. A primum ASD is part of the spectrum of atrioventricular canal defect and can also be termed a partial AV canal defect.

Growth of the endocardial cushion tissue towards the apex of the heart results in formation of the ventricular component of the atrioventricular septum. It is the muscular tissue which lies immediately under the septal leaflet of the tricuspid valve. Failure of this component of the ventricular septum to form results in the creation of an inlet VSD. If it is also associated with a primum ASD and a single common AV valve rather than separate mitral and tricuspid valves then the defect is labeled complete common AV canal or complete atrioventricular septal defect (Figure 21.1). There may be a variable degree of underdevelopment of the inlet septum so that the VSD component of a complete AV canal anomaly

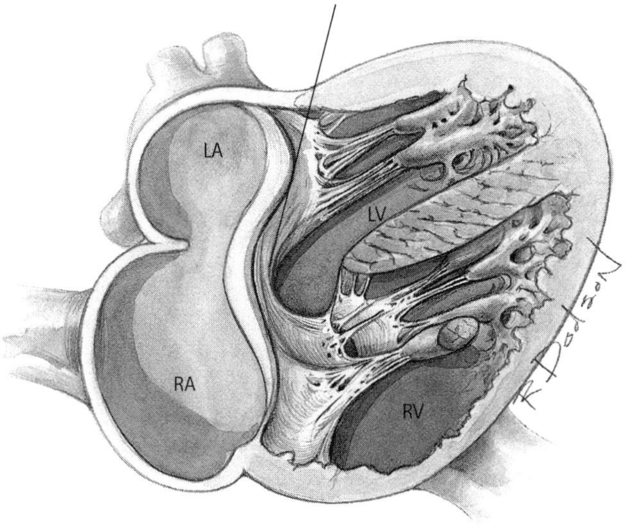

Figure 21.1 *Complete common atrioventricular canal (complete atrioventricular septal defect) consists of a primum ASD, an unrestrictive inlet VSD and a common AV valve in the place of separate mitral and tricuspid valves.*

can range from a pressure restrictive small VSD to a large unrestrictive VSD.

As the endocardial cushion tissue grows to the right and the left it results in formation of the septal leaflet of the tricuspid valve and the anterior leaflet of the mitral valve. Failure of the endocardial cushion tissue to contribute to normal valve development can result in a spectrum of abnormality ranging from a simple cleft of the anterior leaflet of the mitral valve to a common AV valve in which the septal components of the mitral and tricuspid valve fuse to form a superior common leaflet and an inferior common leaflet (termed by some the superior and inferior bridging leaflets).

ANATOMY OF ATRIOVENTRICULAR CANAL DEFECTS

Atrioventricular canal defects are classified as either partial, transitional or complete. The complete form of common AV canal is further subclassified into three anatomical subtypes as originally described by Rastelli.

Partial AV canal

A partial AV canal defect is synonymous with a primum ASD. It usually includes a complete cleft of the anterior leaflet of the mitral valve though the cleft may be partial or absent. A primum ASD is usually at least moderate in size and may be large though on occasion it can be quite small. Isolated cleft of the anterior leaflet of the mitral valve also occurs but generally would not be categorized as partial AV canal.

GOOSENECK DEFORMITY

Even though by definition there is no VSD component associated with partial AV canal there is usually an appearance suggestive of at least some deficiency of the ventricular component of the atrioventricular septum.[6] Thus the common hinge plane of the mitral and tricuspid valves is displaced in an apical direction. This serves to increase the length of the left ventricular outflow tract which results in a radiological appearance termed the 'gooseneck deformity'. Although elongation of the left ventricular outflow tract does not per se result in left ventricular outflow tract obstruction nevertheless if there are associated abnormalities such as multiple chordal attachments extending from the superior component of the cleft anterior leaflet of the mitral valve to the ventricular septum in the region of the left ventricular outflow then there is a significant risk that outflow tract obstruction will develop in time.[7,8] There is a tendency for accessory fibrous tissue to form on the ventricular surface of the superior component of the mitral valve which can become parachute like in nature and therefore rapidly result in an important left ventricular outflow tract gradient during systole. Septal chords also result in anterior movement of the anterior leaflet during systole and which results in accelerated flow and development of fibrosis and ultimate narrowing of the left ventricular outflow tract.[9] This problem is further exacerbated if there is overall underdevelopment of the left heart.

Transitional AV canal

The term transitional AV canal includes a partial AV canal defect and in addition there is a pressure restrictive VSD component. The VSD component may be limited to the point where the cleft of the septal leaflets of the mitral and tricuspid valve are in continuity. By color Doppler or angiography a small amount of blood can be seen to pass between the left ventricle and right ventricle at this point only. Further into the spectrum of severity there may be multiple dense chordal attachments from the crest of the ventricular septum to the undersurface of the superior and inferior common leaflets of the common AV valve. Because of the density and short length of the chordal attachments the VSD component is pressure restrictive. As with partial AV canal when there are multiple chordal attachments of the anterior leaflet of the mitral valve to the septum there is a risk that left ventricular outflow tract obstruction may develop.

Complete common AV canal

Complete common AV canal has been classified by Rastelli into three subtypes.[10]

RASTELLI TYPE A CAVC

This is the most common form of complete AV canal constituting approximately 75% of patients with the anomaly.

Classification as type A is determined by the anatomy of the superior common leaflet. In type A there is complete division of the superior common leaflet over the crest of the septum. By necessity therefore there are chordal attachments from the crest of the septum to the separate left and right septal components of the superior common leaflet. Division of the inferior common leaflet over the crest of the septum is almost never seen. However, the size of the VSD component can be quite variable under the inferior leaflet and is often quite small because of dense and short chordal attachments while the VSD component under the superior leaflet is often quite a bit larger because of longer and less dense chordal attachments.

RASTELLI TYPE B

This is a rare form of complete AV canal. It is almost never seen in the setting of balanced ventricles. Patients in this category have straddling chords which extend either from the tricuspid component into the left ventricle (usually seen when there is left ventricular dominance) or straddling of mitral chords into the right ventricle (usually when there is right ventricular dominance).

RASTELLI TYPE C

Approximately 25% of patients with complete common AV canal have the Rastelli type C form. These patients have a superior common leaflet which is undivided over the crest of the septum. There are usually no chords from the central part of the leaflet to the crest of the septum. The Rastelli type C form of complete AV canal is usually the form that is seen in association with tetralogy of Fallot.

Associated anomalies

TETRALOGY OF FALLOT

Complete AV canal is occasionally seen in association with tetralogy of Fallot. This is an unfortunate association, particularly when the degree of right ventricular outflow tract obstruction is severe and necessitates a transannular patch. The resultant obligatory pulmonary regurgitation is undesirable in the setting of a reconstructed tricuspid valve and can result in important right heart failure. As with all forms of tetralogy there is a wide spectrum ranging from a very mild degree of aortic override into the right ventricle (dextroposition) while at the severe end of the spectrum the anomaly merges into double right ventricle.

DOUBLE OUTLET RIGHT VENTRICLE AND TRANSPOSITION OF THE GREAT ARTERIES

When there is a sufficiently severe degree of aortic override such that the aorta is at least 50% over the right ventricle, the child should be considered to have complete AV canal with double outlet right ventricle rather than with tetralogy of Fallot. Reconstruction under these circumstances is quite a bit more difficult than for tetralogy with complete AV canal. If there is a sufficiently severe degree of aortic override of the right ventricle as well as posterior shift of the pulmonary valve so that it is predominantly over the left ventricle then transposition is present. Under these circumstances an arterial switch procedure will be required with a relatively standard AV canal repair. Thus the transposition end of the spectrum is less of a challenge than the middle of the spectrum where double outlet right ventricle is present.

LEFT VENTRICULAR OUTFLOW TRACT OBSTRUCTION

It is an interesting observation that left ventricular outflow tract obstruction is rarely seen in children with Down's syndrome.[4] In general left ventricular outflow tract obstruction is more common with partial AV canal than complete AV canal though when there is severe imbalance of the canal with right ventricular dominance, left ventricular outflow tract obstruction is common with either partial or complete AV canal. The presence of a coarctation with or without aortic arch hypoplasia is an indicator that left ventricular outflow tract obstruction is present or is incipient.

MULTIPLE VSDS

Additional VSDs can be seen anywhere in the muscular septum. When there is associated tetralogy of Fallot the usual inlet VSD of complete AV canal extends into the conoventricular area and is very large.

DOUBLE ORIFICE MITRAL VALVE

A secondary small completely formed orifice with its own chordal attachments is occasionally seen, usually in the inferior common leaflet. Usually this small secondary orifice is quite competent and does not interfere with the surgical repair.

SINGLE PAPILLARY MUSCLE

In the setting of underdevelopment of the left ventricle the usual two left ventricular papillary muscles tend to lie more closely together and on occasion may fuse to form a single papillary muscle. Concern has been expressed that when all chords attach into a single papillary muscle there might be a risk of creation of a parachute mitral valve if the cleft of the anterior leaflet is suture closed.[11] However, because the chords are usually thin and therefore the interchordal spaces are large this is not a situation that is truly analogous to parachute mitral valve. Nevertheless it is important to remember that a single papillary muscle is generally a marker of left ventricular hypoplasia.

PATHOPHYSIOLOGY

The presence of either partial, transitional or complete AV canal results in a left to right shunt and therefore increased pulmonary blood flow. When there is complete AV canal the VSD component is unrestrictive by definition and therefore pulmonary hypertension is present. With a transitional AV canal the VSD is restrictive and right ventricular pressure is therefore less than left ventricular pressure. With a partial AV canal the initial pathophysiology is similar to any ASD. As pulmonary resistance falls in the first weeks of life the left to right shunt increases and results in increasing dilation of the affected chambers. In the case of complete AV canal all four chambers of the heart are affected. As the heart dilates, the valve leaflets of the atrioventricular valves are likely to coapt less well and AV valve regurgitation will become apparent. This can lead to a positive feedback loop in which increasing ventricular dilation results in worsening AV valve regurgitation. AV valve regurgitation is often most prominent through the cleft of the anterior leaflet of the mitral valve though it can also be central through the tricuspid and mitral components of the common AV valve. Regurgitation through the cleft of the anterior leaflet of the mitral valve results in thickening and rolling of the cleft margins which is a further factor resulting in worsening AV valve regurgitation over time.

Pulmonary vascular disease

Children with Down's syndrome and complete AV canal appear to be at particular risk of accelerated pulmonary vascular disease.[12,13] Down's syndrome has been documented to be associated with reduced peripheral generations of bronchi and associated pulmonary vasculature. There is also increased formation of secretions and bronchiolar plugging. There is also a tendency to hypoventilation because of large airway obstruction in the pharynx. Chronic carbon dioxide retention, because of large airway obstruction and increased secretions, as well as variable lobar atelectasis, almost certainly explain in part the accelerated pulmonary vascular disease. However, if there is no pulmonary hypertension, either because the VSD component is small or there is no mitral regurgitation resulting in secondary pulmonary hypertension then the risk of accelerated pulmonary vascular disease is much less.

Impact of associated anomalies

LEFT VENTRICULAR OUTFLOW TRACT OBSTRUCTION AND COARCTATION

Left ventricular outflow tract obstruction and coarctation are often associated with some degree of underdevelopment of the left heart structures. The child is likely to have a greater left to right shunt and will present earlier in life with worse symptoms of congestive heart failure.

RIGHT VENTRICULAR OUTFLOW TRACT OBSTRUCTION, ASSOCIATED TETRALOGY OF FALLOT

The right ventricular outflow tract obstruction that occurs as part of tetralogy reduces the left to right shunt so that it is possible for the child to be in a relatively balanced state.

CLINICAL FEATURES

The clinical features of an AV canal defect depend on how much pulmonary blood flow is increased as well as the pulmonary artery pressure. Even if there is a large VSD component the child is likely to be relatively free of symptoms in the first weeks of life while pulmonary resistance remains relatively elevated. However, within four to six weeks the child is likely to develop the usual signs of pulmonary hypertension and a large left to right shunt with difficulty feeding, tachypnea, sweating and failure to thrive. Because of the high frequency of complete AV canal defect with Down's syndrome it is important that any child with Down's syndrome undergo careful cardiological assessment to exclude the presence of an AV canal defect. When mitral regurgitation is present, particularly when severe, the symptoms of cardiac failure are likely to be even more resistant to medical therapy than when symptoms are secondary to a left to right shunt alone. Symptoms are also more prominent and appear earlier in life when there is associated underdevelopment of the left heart or left ventricular outflow tract obstruction. As noted above, left ventricular outflow tract obstruction is much more likely if the child does not have Down's syndrome. If the child has a primum ASD and little or no mitral regurgitation the child may remain asymptomatic. If there is associated right ventricular outflow tract obstruction as part of tetralogy of Fallot with complete AV canal and if the degree of outflow tract obstruction is severe the child may present with cyanosis rather than failure.

DIAGNOSTIC STUDIES

Chest X-ray

The chest X-ray demonstrates evidence of increased pulmonary blood flow as well as dilation of the affected cardiac chambers. Particularly when mitral regurgitation is prominent the left atrium may be hugely distended and the left main bronchus is therefore elevated.

Electrocardiography

Because the bundle of His is displaced inferiorly due to absence of the inlet septum the electrical axis of the heart is usually shifted in a counterclockwise direction rather than the clockwise direction that is likely to be seen with a secundum ASD for example.[14] This may be helpful in differentiating a primum from a secundum ASD.[15] There will also be evidence of an increase in right heart forces secondary to the right ventricular hypertrophy which results from right ventricular hypertension when there is complete AV canal.

Echocardiography

Echocardiography is diagnostic. The echocardiographer should not only document the size of the ASD and VSD components as well as the degree of AV valve regurgitation but in addition should make a careful point to document the balance of the canal, i.e. the relative commitment of the common AV valve to the right ventricle and left ventricle. Other features to identify include the presence of one versus two papillary muscles, the presence of associated VSDs and the presence of double orifice mitral valve. If there is important AV valve regurgitation the location and mechanism should be carefully documented.

The presence of an important associated anomaly such as tetralogy of Fallot should also be documented.

MEDICAL AND INTERVENTIONAL THERAPY

The medical therapy for AV canal defect is the usual anticongestive measures. In addition an aggressive degree of afterload reduction is useful when AV valve regurgitation is prominent. There are no interventional catheter techniques that are useful for complete AV canal.

INDICATIONS FOR AND TIMING OF SURGERY

Complete AV canal

Because of the risk of accelerated pulmonary vascular disease it is important that surgery be undertaken at the latest by one year of age. However, a strong argument can be made for undertaking surgery early in infancy, i.e. in the first two to three months of life. If surgery is deferred beyond this time there is likely to be worse preoperative AV valve regurgitation secondary to chamber dilation and secondary pathological changes in the AV valve tissue including the cleft area. It is not uncommon to hear surgeons make the comment that there is 'inadequate AV valve tissue'. Another perspective on this observation, however, is that rather than there being inadequate valve tissue, the annulus has been allowed to dilate to the point where there is difficulty achieving good coaptation of the leaflet tissue. When there is an associated coarctation the child is likely to present with symptoms very early in infancy.[16] A careful assessment must be made of the left ventricular outflow tract and the size of the left ventricle. If the left heart appears to be inadequate to support the systemic circulation alone then consideration should be given to a single ventricle approach. If there is even a relatively minor degree of left ventricular outflow tract obstruction, very careful consideration should be given to undertaking a Norwood procedure rather than placing a pulmonary artery band. It is important to understand when assessing the left heart for adequacy that it is usual with complete AV canal for there to be greater dilation of the right ventricle than the left ventricle. Therefore structures should be referenced to normal values using *z* scores rather than simply relating the left heart structures to the relative size of the right heart structures. This assessment is further complicated by the fact that an extrapolation must be made as to where the ventricular septum will lie following repair[1] and a judgment must be made as to how the common AV valve will be divided into a left and right AV valve. Ventricular length should also be assessed. If the left ventricle fails to reach at least 80% of the total length of the heart it is quite likely that the left heart will be inadequate.

Partial and transitional AV canal

Because the pulmonary vasculature is protected in this setting there is less urgency about proceeding to repair. Nevertheless secondary pathological changes are likely to occur in the AV valve tissue and ventricular dilation may make reconstruction of the AV valves more difficult over time. On the other hand the margins of the cleft can be difficult to suture when the AV valve tissue is completely normal. The tissue is particularly thin and fragile and holds sutures poorly. Therefore it may be reasonable to observe the child during infancy and to operate towards the end of the first year of life when tissue integrity is somewhat greater. However, the older concept that surgery should be deferred until the child is large enough to accept a valve replacement should this be necessary is something of a self-fulfilling prophecy. If surgery is deferred for several years the heart may become so dilated from a combination of left to right shunt and AV valve regurgitation that the valve will not be reparable and indeed a mitral valve replacement will need to be undertaken.

TETRALOGY OF FALLOT WITH COMPLETE AV CANAL

If the child has balanced systemic and pulmonary blood flow it is probably reasonable to defer surgery until towards the end of the first year of life. This recommendation takes into consideration the fragility of the AV valve tissue in the young infant. On the other hand if the child is becoming symptomatic because of either excessive or inadequate right ventricular outflow tract obstruction our preference is perform a repair rather than a shunt. This applies because of all of the same considerations discussed in Chapter 16.

SURGICAL MANAGEMENT

History of surgery

The first repair of complete AV canal was performed by Lillehei and associates in 1954 using cross circulation.[17] The first report of successful repair of a partial AV canal appeared in 1955.[18,19] It is remarkable that successful surgical repair was possible for these lesions so early in the history of cardiac surgery because the complex anatomy of atrioventricular canal was very poorly understood at that time. Subsequent reports by Lev in 1958 describing the conduction system[14] as well as reports by Bharati[20,21] and Rastelli et al[10] contributed enormously to subsequent improvements in results for surgery. A number of different surgical techniques have been described for the management of atrioventricular canal and there is ongoing controversy regarding the optimal technique. Some authors prefer a single patch technique which has been the predominant technique applied at Children's Hospital Boston while others have emphasized the importance of two separate patches, one for the VSD closure and one for primum ASD closure.[22–24] The timing of surgery has progressively shifted to younger ages. Complete repair during infancy has been emphasized at Children's Hospital Boston since the 1970s.[25,26] In 1978, Carpentier suggested that the left AV valve in atrioventricular canal anomalies should be considered a 'trifoliate' valve and that the cleft should therefore not be closed.[27] This approach has not been followed at Children's Hospital Boston and the majority of subsequent reports as described later in this chapter emphasize the importance of cleft closure in avoiding late AV valve regurgitation.

In 1997, Wilcox et al described a technique in which the AV valve leaflets are brought down to the crest of the ventricular septum rather than placing a patch for VSD closure.[28] Wilcox used this technique selectively. In 1999, Nicholson and Nunn from Sydney, Australia, described application of a similar technique for routine repair of complete AV canal. We have termed this the 'Australian' technique.[29]

Partial AV canal

GENERAL SETUP INCLUDING TECHNIQUE OF CARDIOPULMONARY BYPASS

Approach is via a standard median sternotomy. The upper end of the skin incision can be quite low but in general we divide the entire sternum rather than using a mini-sternotomy approach. Arterial cannulation is standard ascending aortic cannulation while venous return is via two right angle caval cannulas inserted directly into the cavas. The patient is usually cooled to 25° or 28°C at which point the aortic cross clamp is applied and cardioplegia solution is infused. Caval tourniquets are tightened. It is generally not necessary to place a left atrial vent. It is important that the cannulas do not distort the AV valves.

CLEFT CLOSURE

The right atrium is opened with an oblique incision. After confirmation of the preoperative diagnosis the anatomy of the AV valve leaflets, particularly the mitral valve, is studied by floating the leaflets with injection of ice cold cardioplegia solution. It is important not to cause frothing by injection of a jet from a distance through the AV valve as the resultant fine froth can enter the coronary arteries and cause ventricular dysfunction. Instead, a small, red-rubber catheter is attached to a 30 ml syringe and is gently injected into the left ventricle. Careful note is taken of small variations in the leaflet tissue adjacent to the cleft. This provides information for subsequent accurate suturing of the cleft. The cleft should then be closed by direct suture. Although a continuous suture technique with 7/0 Prolene probably provides a more secure closure[30] it can be difficult to achieve accurate apposition using the landmarks previously observed. An alternative is to use very fine horizontal mattress 7/0 prolene sutures supported with small pericardial pledgets if the leaflet tissue is very delicate. If the leaflet tissue appears stronger simple 6/0 or 7/0 Prolene sutures can be employed (Figure 21.2b). The cleft is closed up to the free edge which is defined by the origin of chords. Repeat testing of the valve with injection of cardioplegia solution confirms there is now satisfactory competence of the valve.

COMMISUROPLASTY SUTURES

If the annulus is dilated there may be jet of central incompetence following cleft closure. The annulus can be decreased in size by placing commisuroplasty sutures at one or both commissures (Figure 21.2c). It is preferable to use the lateral commissure since this is further away from conduction tissue. However, there is a risk of injury to the circumflex coronary artery if deep bites are taken. A 5/0 Tevdek doubly pledgetted suture placed in the annulus as a horizontal mattress as indicated in the figure is generally effective (Figure 21.2c). If necessary an additional annuloplasty suture can be placed directly posteriorly midway between the two commissures. Once again, the valve is tested to confirm the efficacy of the commisuroplasty.

PRIMUM ASD CLOSURE

An autologous pericardial patch treated with 0.6% glutaraldehyde for 20 minutes is used for ASD closure. The patch is sutured directly to the region of continuity between the mitral and tricuspid valves using a simple continuous 6/0 or 5/0 prolene suture. Care is taken not to injure the underlying crest of the ventricular septum which could result in damage to the bundle of His. Inferiorly this suture line is brought inferior to the ostium of the coronary sinus so that postoperatively coronary sinus blood will drain to the left atrium (Figure 21.3b). The patch should be made somewhat redundant over the coronary sinus by gathering patch with the suture line in this area so that it is not tightly stretched over the ostium. It is probably not advisable to unroof the coronary sinus as it can be difficult to predict the location of the AV node. We no longer use the technique of suturing within the ostium of the coronary sinus which allows the coronary sinus to continue draining to the right atrium. This technique while generally effective in avoiding injury to the conduction system is not completely effective in this regard. If there is an associated secundum ASD or stretched patent foramen ovale it may be reasonable to bring the suture line around the secundum ASD so as to incorporate this under the same patch as is being used to close the primum ASD. Prior to completion of the suture line, which should occur at the highest point, the left heart is allowed to fill with blood or saline is injected into the left heart and air is vented through the cardioplegia site in the ascending aorta as well as through

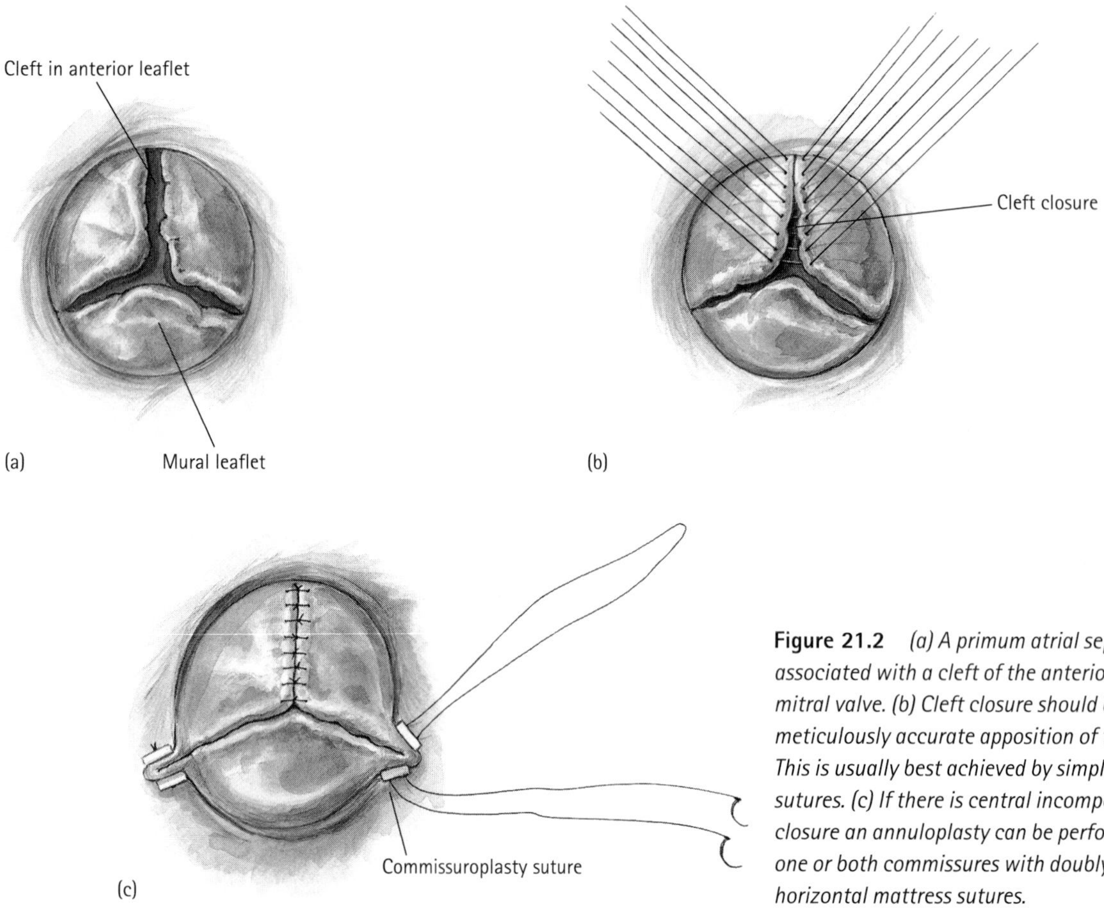

Figure 21.2 *(a) A primum atrial septal defect is usually associated with a cleft of the anterior leaflet of the mitral valve. (b) Cleft closure should be performed by meticulously accurate apposition of the cleft edges. This is usually best achieved by simple 6/0 or 7/0 Prolene sutures. (c) If there is central incompetence following cleft closure an annuloplasty can be performed by tightening one or both commissures with doubly pledgetted horizontal mattress sutures.*

the atrial septal suture line. When the suture has been tied the aortic cross clamp can be released with the cardioplegia site bleeding freely. During warming the right atriotomy is closed with continuous prolene. A left atrial monitoring line is inserted through the right superior pulmonary vein. Generally two atrial and one ventricular pacing wire are placed. With rewarming completed the child should wean from bypass with minimal inotropic support.

TRANSESOPHAGEAL ECHOCARDIOGRAPHY

Except in the very small infant it is advisable to undertake transesophageal echocardiography to confirm the adequacy of the valve repair. In small infants less than 3–4 kg in weight the presence of currently available probes in the esophagus can distort the left atrium and interfere with the reconstruction. The assessment of the valve is particularly affected by flexing of the probe which can project into the left atrium and distort the valve.

Transitional AV canal

VSD COMPONENT AT LEVEL OF CLEFT

The most common form of transitional AV canal occurs when there is an interventricular communication at the level of the cleft (Figure 21.3a). Generally a single pledgetted horizontal mattress suture can be placed at this level to both obliterate the VSD as well as to close the cleft over the crest of the septum (Figure 21.4b). This same suture can be used as a running suture to attach the pericardial patch to the atrial surface of the AV valve tissue as for partial AV canal repair. The remaining details of the closure are as for a partial AV canal as described above.

TRANSITIONAL AV CANAL WITH RESTRICTIVE VSD COMPONENT UNDER THE SUPERIOR AND INFERIOR COMMON LEAFLET

If the VSD component of a transitional AV canal extends under the superior common leaflet (Figure 21.4a) but is small because of multiple chords of short length the repair is best undertaken using the Australian technique as described below for complete AV canal.[29]

Complete AV canal

AUSTRALIAN TECHNIQUE

General setup and cardiopulmonary bypass

It is particularly important when performing complete AV canal repair that there be no distortion of the AV valve

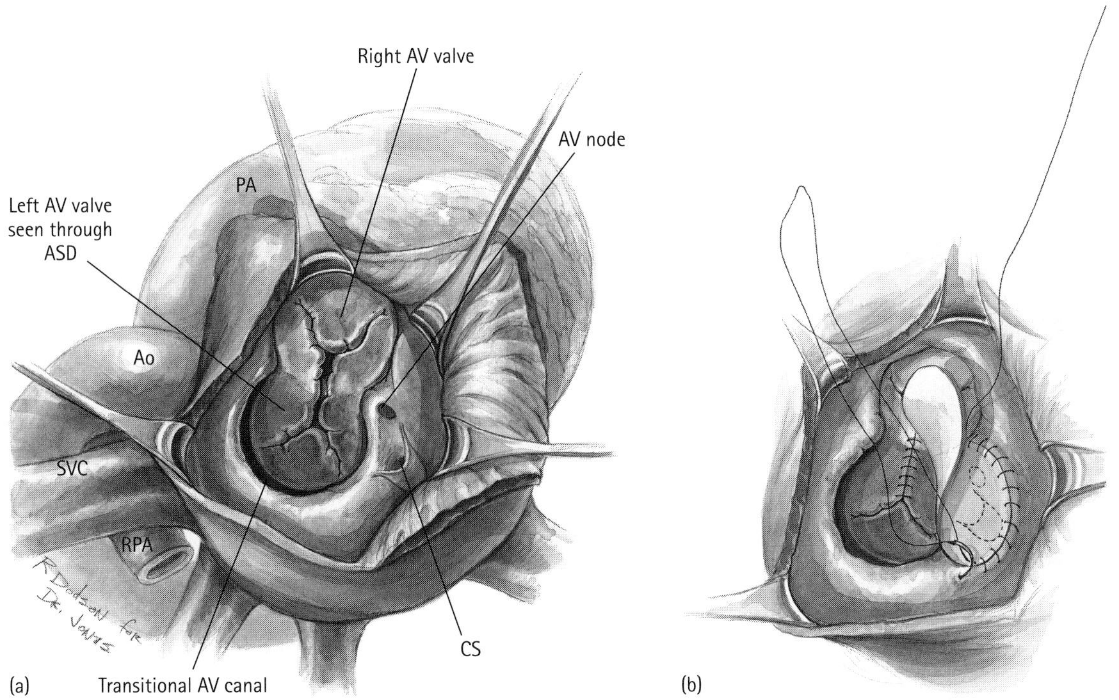

Figure 21.3 *(a) The transitional AV canal most commonly includes an interventricular communication at the level of the cleft. (b) Closure of the primum ASD component of all forms of AV canal should place the coronary sinus and AV node on the left atrial side of the autologous pericardial patch.*

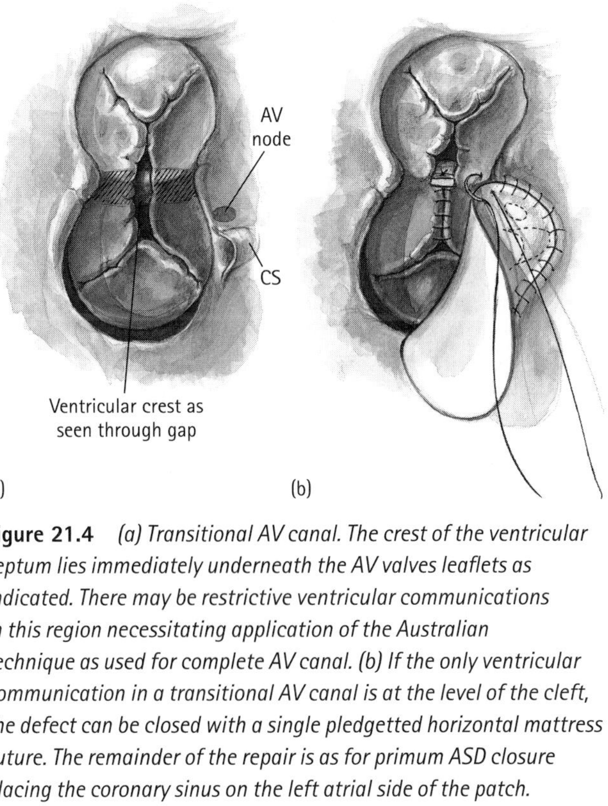

Figure 21.4 *(a) Transitional AV canal. The crest of the ventricular septum lies immediately underneath the AV valves leaflets as indicated. There may be restrictive ventricular communications in this region necessitating application of the Australian technique as used for complete AV canal. (b) If the only ventricular communication in a transitional AV canal is at the level of the cleft, the defect can be closed with a single pledgetted horizontal mattress suture. The remainder of the repair is as for primum ASD closure placing the coronary sinus on the left atrial side of the patch.*

annulus which can easily occur when multiple cannulas are present. For this reason we continue to use deep hypothermic circulatory arrest for infants who are less than 3–4 kg which is becoming our preferred age and size for repair (see Indications and timing). Thus a single venous cannula can be placed in the right atrial appendage and the child is cooled to deep hypothermia. At a rectal temperature of less than 18°C the ascending aorta is clamped and cardioplegia solution is infused into the root of the aorta. The venous cannula is removed. An oblique incision is made in the right atrium. The anatomy of the common AV valve is studied by floating the leaflets with ice cold cardioplegia solution injected gently through a small red rubber catheter attached to a 30 ml syringe. The superior and inferior common leaflet are very accurately approximated over the crest of the septum with a single 6/0 Prolene suture which is not tied. Multiple horizontal mattress 5/0 Tevdek sutures are passed through the crest of the septum and then through the superior and inferior common leaflet (Figure 21.5a). It is helpful to use a larger needle than is used for standard VSD closure. The sutures are subsequently passed through the edge of an autologous pericardial patch treated with 0.6% glutaraldehyde. When the sutures are tied the pericardial patch is brought down to the septum sandwiching the AV valve leaflet tissue between the patch and the crest of the septum (Figure 21.5b). It is useful as emphasized by Nicholson et al[29] to space the sutures across the crest of the septum in such a way that the patch acts as a partial annuloplasty at the level of the crest of the septum, i.e. the sutures are spaced closer on the pericardial patch than on the crest of the septum. We do not use a separate short strip of Dacron for this purpose as described by Nicholson et al. The pericardial patch is retracted anteriorly without tension to allow testing of the mitral valve. Careful note is made of minor features of the valve tissue adjacent to the cleft to allow

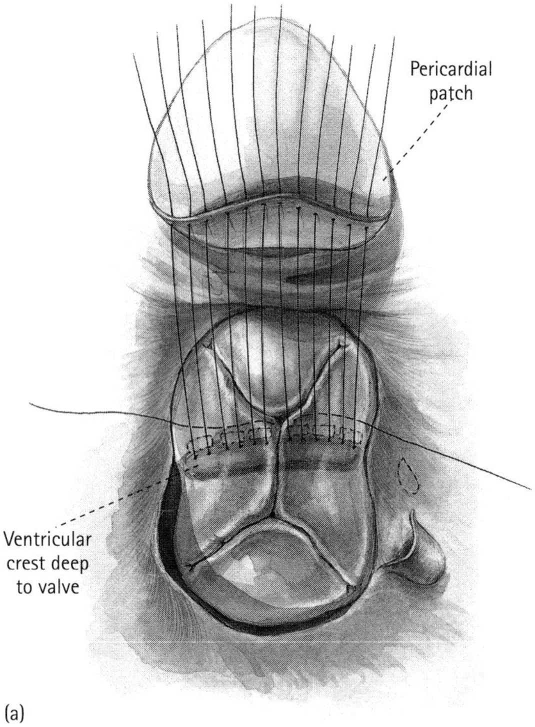

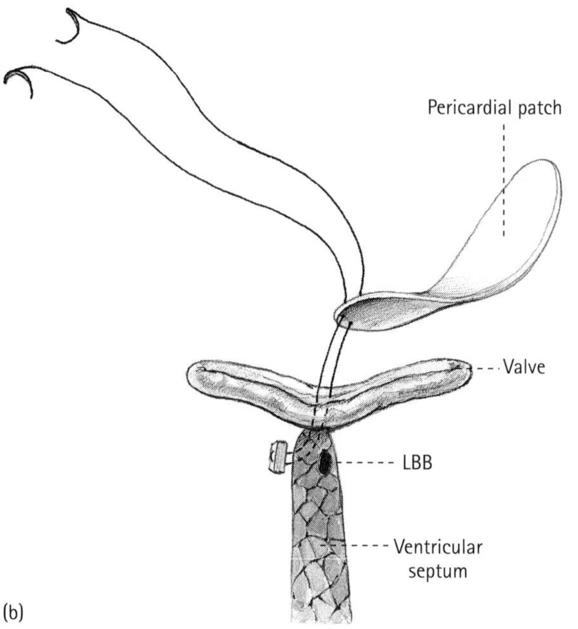

Figure 21.5 *(a) The Australian technique for repair of complete AV canal involves placement of multiple interrupted pledgetted sutures on the right side of the crest of the ventricular septum. These sutures are passed through the superior and inferior common leaflets and then through an autologous pericardial patch. (b) Tying the sutures placed in the ventricular crest as part of the Australian technique obliterates the VSD by bringing the common AV valve leaflets down to the crest of the septum.*

accurate approximation of the cleft with sutures as described for the cleft mitral valve associated with a primum ASD. If necessary additional commisuroplasty sutures are placed.

The primum ASD component of the complete AV canal is now repaired as for an isolated primum ASD. The coronary sinus ostium is placed on the left side of the patch. Prior to completion of this suture line it is possible to commence sucker bypass at a low flow rate of 10–20 ml/kg per minute. When the right atriotomy has been closed the venous cannula is reinserted and full bypass is recommenced. The aortic cross clamp is released after appropriate removal of air. The cardioplegia site is allowed to bleed freely. During warming a left atrial line is inserted through the right superior pulmonary vein. A pulmonary artery monitoring line is placed through the infundibulum of the right ventricle. Two atrial and one ventricular wire are placed. With rewarming completed it should be possible to wean from bypass with low dose dopamine support at 5 μg/kg minute.

Intraoperative assessment

In the small child who is less than 3–4 kg assessment by transesophageal echocardiography using current day probes can still cause hemodynamic compromise and is generally avoided. However, it should be anticipated that the left atrial pressure will be less than 10 mm without a prominent V wave. There should be excellent cardiac output though blood pressure will vary depending on the degree of vasodilation of the child. A pulmonary artery saturation and right atrial saturation can be drawn for assessment of residual left to right shunt. If there is any concern regarding possible presence of a residual shunt or poor valve function assessment can be undertaken by direct echocardiography using a hand-held transducer.

TRADITIONAL SINGLE PATCH TECHNIQUE

The general setup and technique of cardiopulmonary bypass is as for the Australian technique. After testing of the valve and placement of a single approximating suture over the crest of the septum between the superior and inferior leaflets (Figure 21.6a) both common leaflets are incised a little to the right of the middle of the crest of the septum (Figure 21.6b). The pericardial patch is sutured to the middle of the crest of the septum using continuous 5/0 Prolene (Figure 21.6c). It is important not to place the patch too far rightwards on the crest of the septum because this will tend to distract the left AV valve leaflets and prevent satisfactory central coaptation. Only at the inferior end of the ventricular septum should the suture line be brought a little more to the right side of the crest of the septum to avoid the bundle of His (Figure 21.6d). Continuous 5/0 Prolene is initially employed and is then reinforced with several interrupted pledgetted horizontal mattress 5/0 Tevdek sutures.

AV valve leaflet resuspension

The AV valve leaflets are resuspended on the pericardial patch using a continuous horizontal mattress 6/0 Prolene suture

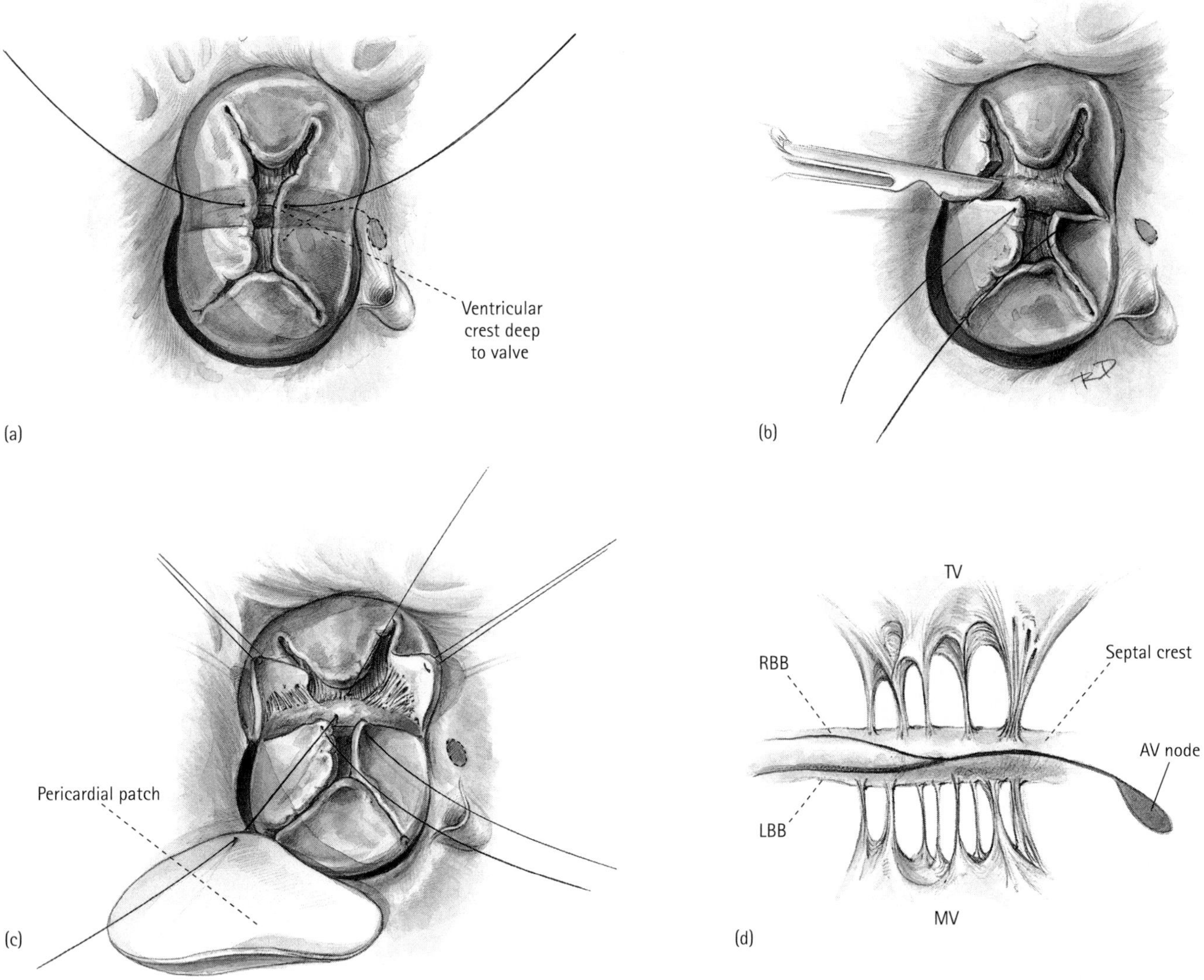

Figure 21.6a–d *Traditional single patch repair of complete AV canal. (a) The exact apposition of the superior and inferior common leaflets is determined by floating the leaflets with ice cold cardioplegia solution. A single 6/0 Prolene suture is placed through these leaflets over the crest of the ventricular septum to maintain accurate coaptation of the leaflets during incision of the superior and inferior common leaflets. (b) The superior and inferior common leaflets are incised a little to the right of the middle of the crest of the ventricular septum. (c) An autologous pericardial patch is sutured to the middle of the ventricular septum using continuous 5/0 Prolene reinforced with pledgetted sutures if necessary. (d) The bundle of His enters the ventricular septum close to the AV node and is vulnerable, particularly at the inferior end of the ventricular septal suture line. At this point the suture line should be kept to the right of midline.*

(Figure 21.6e,f). It is necessary to move the patch back and forward as the needle is passed successively through mitral valve tissue, pericardial patch, tricuspid valve tissue and then back in the reverse direction. It is important that the resuspension be reinforced with pledgetted horizontal mattress 5/0 Tevdek sutures with the pledgets lying on the mitral side of the suspension.[30] The pledgets should not consume an excessive amount of AV valve tissue which would reduce central coaptation.

Cleft closure

Following resuspension the competence of the mitral valve is tested with cardioplegia solution. The cleft is then closed as described for primum ASD (Figure 21.6g).

Primum ASD closure

The remainder of the repair is as for the Australian technique using the same pericardial patch as was used for VSD closure. The coronary sinus is routinely placed on the left atrial side of the patch (Figure 21.6h).

Tetralogy with complete AV canal

GENERAL SETUP AND BYPASS CONSIDERATIONS

Because the child undergoing repair of tetralogy of Fallot with complete AV canal is generally older and larger than the

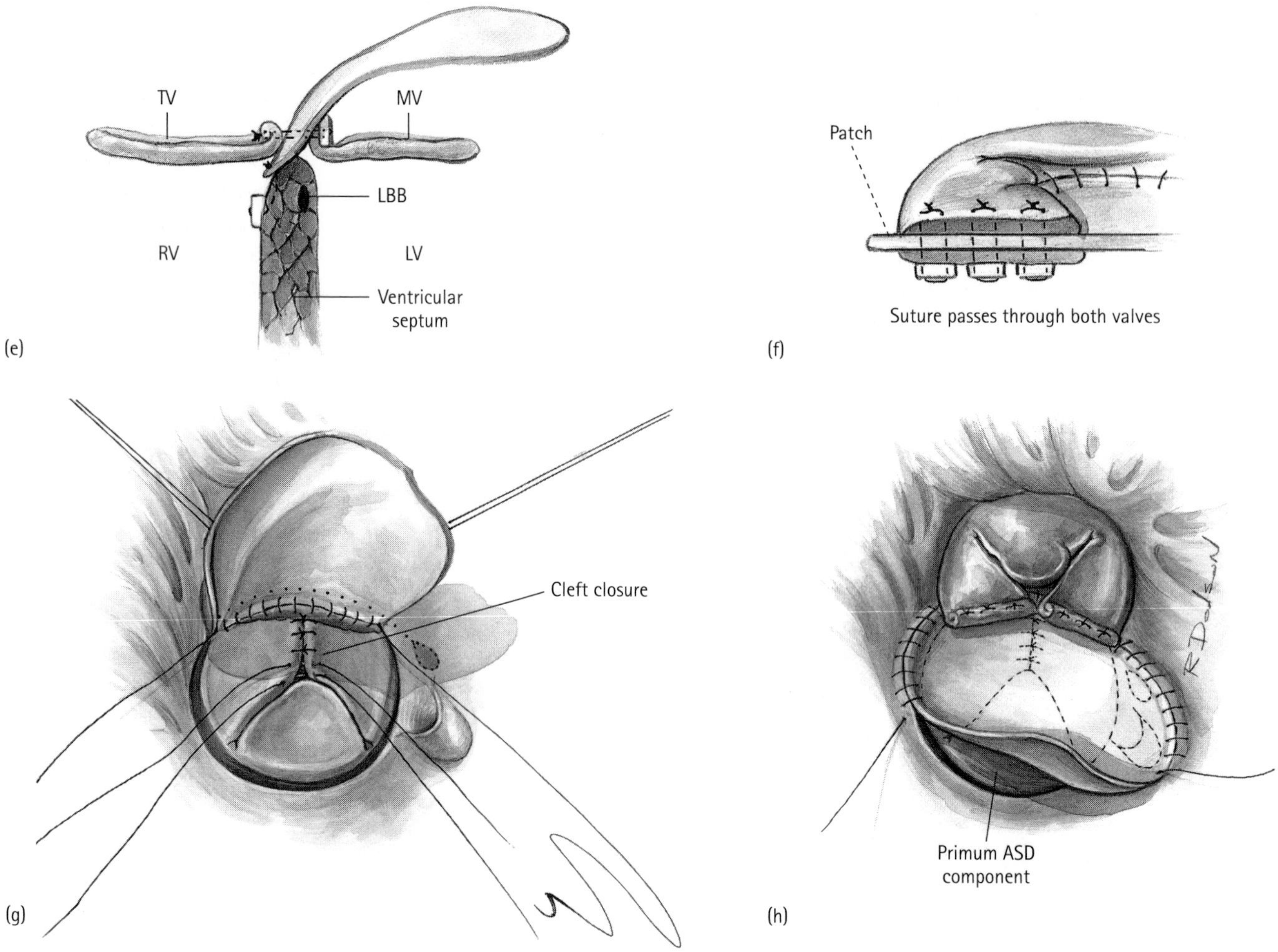

Figure 21.6e–h *(e,f) The superior and inferior common leaflets are resuspended on the pericardial patch using a continuous horizontal mattress 6/0 Prolene suture. In addition pledgetted sutures are placed with the pledgets lying on the mitral side. (g) Following resuspension of the superior and inferior common leaflets the cleft of the new mitral valve is closed as for the cleft associated with a primum ASD. (h) The primum ASD component of the complete AV canal is closed as for closure of an isolated primum ASD placing the coronary sinus on the left atrial side of the patch.*

child undergoing repair of regular complete AV canal the procedure is almost always performed using continuous cardiopulmonary bypass and moderate hypothermia. Right angle caval cannulas are employed together with cardioplegic arrest of the heart. Generally it is necessary to place a left atrial vent because collateral return is likely to be somewhat increased secondary to longstanding (months) cyanosis.

SINGLE PERICARDIAL PATCH REPAIR

Because the VSD component is very large with tetralogy of Fallot with complete AV canal it is usually necessary to employ the traditional single patch technique as described for standard complete AV canal. However, the patch should be cut to accommodate the extension into the anterior outlet septum. Depending on the degree of aortic override and the amount of extension of the VSD it may be necessary to perform part of the VSD closure working through an infundibular incision. The continuous 5/0 Prolene VSD suture which has been started working through the right atrium can be passed out through the infundibular incision and then suturing is continued working through the infundibular incision. When the suture line has been brought entirely around the aortic annulus the suture is once again passed back into the right atrium passing the suture through the superior common leaflet adjacent to the annulus. Once again, multiple interrupted pledgetted horizontal mattress 5/0 Tevdek sutures are important to reinforce this long VSD suture line. Resuspension of the AV valve leaflets is undertaken as for standard single patch complete AV canal repair. The primum ASD closure is also standard though it is particularly important to place a fenestration in the pericardial ASD patch in order to allow right to left decompression postoperatively as for regular tetralogy repair. In a child who is 5 or 6 kg in weight it is reasonable to place a 3 mm fenestration.

Transannular extension of the infundibular incision

Infundibular muscle bundles should be divided as for regular tetralogy with careful preservation of the moderator band. If the pulmonary annulus is smaller than two standard deviations below normal a transannular extension into the pulmonary artery should be made. A pericardial patch is sutured into the pulmonary arteriotomy and right ventriculotomy during rewarming and following clamp release. As with any tetralogy outflow patch it is important the patch not be excessively wide which would result in an excessive amount of pulmonary regurgitation. It is also important that conal coronary arteries are preserved whenever possible in making the right ventricular incision. The length of the incision should be just long enough to allow appropriate enlargement of the infundibulum. The incision should not extend into the body of the ventricle.

Tricuspid repair

Assessment should be made in any child undergoing repair of complete AV canal of the competence of the tricuspid valve. However, in the setting of tetralogy of Fallot with complete AV canal it is particularly important that meticulous attention be paid to reconstruction of the tricuspid valve. If there is important pulmonary regurgitation as well as tricuspid regurgitation postoperatively the child is likely to develop severe right heart failure postoperatively.

ANESTHETIC AND INTENSIVE CARE UNIT MANAGEMENT

The majority of patients undergoing two-ventricle repair of atrioventricular canal defects are medically managed as outpatients prior to surgery. These patients generally undergo outpatient preoperative evaluation and are admitted to the hospital the morning of surgery. Trisomy 21 is very common in this patient population and this syndrome presents some additional anesthetic challenges. Intravenous access tends to be poor and the peripheral arteries tend to be smaller than would be predicted by the child's age and weight. Intravenous and arterial access is further hindered by the increased quantity of subcutaneous fat present in these patients. The large tongue present in Trisomy 21 may predispose to airway obstruction; however, this is generally more of problem in older children than it is in infants. Similarly, difficulty with tracheal intubation is rarely an issue in infants but may be an issue in older children secondary to generalized obesity and the limits in neck extension dictated by the presence of atlanto-occipital insufficiency.

Induction of anesthesia should be directed toward avoiding the reductions in pulmonary vascular resistance (PVR) which will promote additional left to right physiologic shunting with subsequent systemic hypoperfusion. Mask induction of anesthesia with sevoflurane or halothane followed by placement of an intravenous catheter is feasible but only in patients where intravenous access can be expeditiously obtained. Given the limited cardiovascular reserve of these patients maintaining anesthesia with an inhalation agent for an extended period of time (more than 10 minutes) is likely to result in hypotension and systemic hypoperfusion. A more prudent approach may be an intramuscular induction or placement of an intravenous catheter using oral premedication and nitrous oxide.

In children with large atrial and ventricular level shunts without pulmonary hypertension hypercarbia to achieve a pH of 7.30–7.35 is utilized to increase PVR and reduce $Q_P:Q_S$. Reduced inspired oxygen concentrations can be utilized to increase PVR as well. However, in children with pulmonary V/Q mismatch this may result in a significant reduction in pulmonary venous and arterial saturation even in the absence of intracardiac right to left shunting. Hypotension prior to initiation of cardiopulmonary bypass is likely to be the result of excessive left to right shunting. If ventilatory manipulations to increase PVR fail to correct hypotension use of an inotropic agent should be considered. Volume infusion is unlikely to correct hypotension in this circumstance as preload reserve has likely already been exhausted.

Immediately prior to and following termination of cardiopulmonary bypass the extent, if any, of AV valve regurgitation should be assessed. Transesophageal echocardiography and observation of the right and left atrial pressure traces are invaluable in this regard. Because the atria of infants and young children with atrioventricular canal defects tend to be relatively small and noncompliant the height of the V wave correlates well with the severity of mitral and tricuspid regurgitation. It should be emphasized that the severity of mitral valve regurgitation is blood pressure dependent. High systemic afterload will increase the mitral regurgitant fraction by increasing the impedance to LV ejection. The extent of mitral regurgitation should be assessed at a time when blood pressure is in an age appropriate range. Functional impairment of AV valve leaflet apposition with concurrent regurgitation may result from annular dilation caused by ventricular dilation. Overzealous volume infusion or afterload mismatch (depressed ventricular systolic function for the degree of afterload) are the usual causes. In patients requiring both inotropic support and systemic vasodilation milrinone is a good choice.

RESULTS OF SURGERY

Australian technique

We adopted the Australian technique of single pericardial patch repair of complete AV canal in 1997. This technique was originally described by Wilcox and subsequently popularized by Nunn.[28,29] The AV valve leaflets are sutured directly to the crest of the ventricular septum thereby closing the VSD and obviating the need for leaflet division. Mora et al recently reviewed the 34 consecutive patients with complete AV canal who were repaired using this technique between December 1997 and October 2002 at Children's Hospital Boston.[31] Average age of the patients was 5.6 kg and median age was three years. A single papillary muscle was present in five patients. The canal was unbalanced and favored the left ventricle in three and right ventricle in six. Preoperatively the VSD was small in six, moderate in nine and large in 19. Three patients had had a pulmonary artery band placed elsewhere before reparative surgery. The mitral valve cleft was closed in 31 of the 34 patients. One patient had moderate intraoperative AV valve regurgitation requiring takedown and conversion to a classic single patch method. There were no perioperative deaths. No patient developed left ventricular outflow tract obstruction or required reoperation for AV valve regurgitation. Postoperative echocardiography both early and late demonstrated no patient with severe mitral regurgitation.

We concluded from this study that repair of complete AV canal using the modified single patch technique preserves AV valve leaflet integrity without reducing left ventricular outflow tract obstruction or compromising AV valve repair even in the presence of large VSDs or unbalanced complete AV canal with a single papillary muscle. One of the particular advantages of this technique is that it can be applied even in the neonatal period since there is no need to suture directly to leaflet tissue other than at the point of cleft closure. Cleft closure must be undertaken with great delicacy since the tissue in this area early in infancy can be particularly fragile. The results from Children's Hospital Boston using the Australian technique are similar to the results achieved by Nicholson, Nunn et al from Sydney, Australia, published in 1999.[29] The authors described 47 consecutive patients who underwent the Australian technique between 1995 and 1998. There were two deaths for a mortality of 4%. No patient developed heart block and there were no significant residual VSDs. Most importantly no patient developed left ventricular outflow tract obstruction either early or late. Mitral regurgitation was defined as absent in 28%, trivial in 40%, mild in 26% and moderate in 6%. The authors emphasize in their description of the technique the use of a Dacron strip to help to reduce annular size at the level of the ventricular septum. It will be important to review in longer term follow-up whether this results in any restriction to growth of the mitral annulus. The authors strongly endorse this technique and continue to use it as their primary method of repair of complete AV canal.

The report by Nicholson and Nunn built on the work of Wilcox et al who first described the technique of direct VSD closure in a report in 1997.[28] The authors used the technique in 12 of 21 patients who were undergoing repair of complete AV canal. The authors demonstrated that the Australian technique resulted in a significantly shorter bypass and cross clamp time. After a follow-up time of 34 months the results were equivalent to those of standard repair.

Standard repair of complete AV canal

One of the largest series ever reported describing results of the standard repair of complete AV canal was a report from Children's Hospital Boston by Hanley et al published in 1993.[32] The authors reviewed 301 patients with complete AV canal who underwent surgical repair between 1972 and 1992. Over this 20-year time period operative mortality decreased significantly from 25% before 1976 to 3% after 1987. The authors examined 46 patient related, morphologic, procedure related and postoperative variables for prediction of perioperative death and reoperation. The only risk factors for death identified by multivariate logistic regression analysis were earlier year of operation, the presence of double orifice left AV valve and postoperative residual regurgitation of the left AV valve. Reoperation for most residual lesions decreased over time and other than reoperation for left AV valve regurgitation were essentially eliminated in the years immediately prior to the study. However, reoperation for left AV valve regurgitation continued to be necessary in approximately 7% of patients even towards the end of the study period. However, in this series only 61% of patients had closure of the mitral cleft. The authors also were able to report in this series that earlier age at surgery was associated with a decreased incidence of postoperative pulmonary hypertension emphasizing the importance of earlier age at surgery, preferably in the first three months of life to minimize the risk of postoperative pulmonary hypertensive crises.

Cleft closure

In 2002, Boening et al[33] reviewed the results of surgical repair of complete AV canal in 121 consecutive patients undergoing surgery in Kiel, Germany, between 1975 and 1995. The mitral valve cleft was closed in 44% of patients. The early mortality was 15%. Actuarial survival at one year was 80%, at 10 years was 78% and at 20 years was 65%. The authors found that failure to close the mitral cleft was a predictor of both early and late deaths. They also found that pulmonary hypertension was a predictor of both early and late deaths and emphasized the importance of operating early in order to reduce the risk of mortality as well as postoperative pulmonary hypertension.

Another large series in which the importance of cleft closure is emphasized is the report by Crawford and Stroud from the Medical University of South Carolina published in 2001.[34] The authors described 172 patients who underwent repair of complete AV canal between 1981 and 2000. The mean age at surgery was 10.8 months. The mortality decreased from 16.4% in the first decade of the study to 3% in the second decade. Actuarial survival including operative deaths was 79% at 15 years. A total of 6.4% of operative survivors underwent reoperation for late mitral regurgitation. In nine patients mitral valve repair was possible and in one mitral valve replacement. Freedom from late reoperation for severe mitral regurgitation was 89.9% ± 3.1% over 15 years. Freedom from late reoperation from mitral regurgitation did not decrease in the second decade versus the first decade. The authors emphasize the importance of cleft closure.

Two patch technique

The results of the two patch technique which continues to be used by many centers are closely equivalent to the results of the single patch technique. For example, Bogers et al reported in 2000[35] the results of the two patch repair of complete AV canal in 97 patients undergoing repair of complete AV canal in Rotterdam, Netherlands, between 1986 and 1999. Of the 97 patients, 75 had Down's syndrome. The mean age at operation was 10.2 months. Early mortality was 4% with two late deaths. Survival at 10 years was 93%. The authors were unable to identify any predictors of mortality by multivariate analysis. Freedom from reoperation was 83% at 10 years. The need for preoperative diuretics and the presence of significant postoperative left AV valve regurgitation were the only predictors of need for late reoperation.

Mitral valve replacement or repair

In 2000, Moran et al[36] reviewed the results of 46 patients who underwent either mitral valve repair[37] or mitral valve replacement[9] at Children's Hospital Boston between 1988 and 1998 following previous surgery for either partial or complete AV canal. The median age at the time of the mitral valve operation was 2.8 years while the median age at the time of initial repair of AV canal was six years. The early mortality was 2.2% with survival at one year being 89.9% and at 10 years 86.6%. A high rate of complete heart block (37.5%) was noted within the mitral valve replacement group. Freedom from late mitral valve reoperation was similar for both groups. No significant morphological predictors necessitating mitral valve replacement were identified. Predictors of reoperation within the mitral valve repair group included the presence of moderate or worse mitral regurgitation in the early postoperative period. Following their mitral valve procedure patients demonstrated a decreased degree of mitral regurgitation as well as improved growth and decreased ventricular volume. The authors concluded mitral valve surgery following previous atrioventricular canal repair significantly improves clinical status with a sustained improvement in ventricular chamber size.

In a previous report from Children's Hospital Boston Kadoba et al[37] reviewed the results of mitral valve replacement in the first year of life. The majority of these patients had previously undergone repair of atrioventricular canal. Between 1973 and 1987, 25 infants underwent mitral valve replacement. Tissue valves performed particularly poorly in this situation in infancy. All six patients who had tissue valve replacement of the mitral valve died. Nine patients required a second mitral valve replacement for prosthetic stenosis 5–69 (mean 30) months after the original mitral valve replacement with one operative death. This report emphasizes the disadvantages of prosthetic mitral valve replacement in the infant in that there is inevitable outgrowth of the prosthesis and a lifelong need for anticoagulation. Meticulous attention to mitral valve construction at the initial repair of AV canal is essential since early function of the valve following repair predicts subsequent need for mitral valve intervention.

Other reports have described techniques and outcomes for mitral valve repair and replacement following AV canal surgery including the report by Ando and Fraser.[38] The authors describe a technique to enlarge the mitral annulus allowing a 17 mm prosthesis to be placed in an 11 mm annulus. An alternative technique for repair of the mitral valve following AV canal surgery was reported by Poirier et al from the Hospital for Sick Children in Toronto in 2000.[39] The authors estimated that 14% of patients require reoperation for mitral regurgitation within 10 years of initial repair. They describe a novel technique of leaflet augmentation using autologous pericardium to augment the bridging leaflets of the atrioventricular valve. This technique was applied in eight patients and was compared with 68 other patients who underwent either conventional repair[54] or valve replacement.[14] There were no early deaths or major complications following the patch repair technique. The authors believe that the results of the patch repair technique compare favorably with the 68 patients who underwent conventional surgery. An alternative method for dealing with severe and irreparable mitral valve regurgitation is to undertake supra-annular replacement of the mitral valve. The prosthesis is placed entirely within the left atrium. Although initial results with this technique were encouraging the late hemodynamic results have been less encouraging as documented in the paper by Adatia et al in 1997.[40]

Surgery for primum ASD

It is unwise to think of the primum ASD as being a simpler and more straightforward problem than a complete AV canal. Often these patients have complicating features that can result in a higher risk of late AV valve surgery or the development of left ventricular outflow tract obstruction. These features of partial AV canal are highlighted in a paper by Manning et al.[16] The authors reviewed 11 patients with primum ASD who presented with symptoms at Children's Hospital Boston between 1984 and 1992. This represented 10.5% of the 105 patients who underwent repair of primum ASD during this timeframe. The patients who presented with congestive heart failure in the first year of life had a high incidence of hypoplastic left sided cardiac structures including coarctation, abnormal mitral valve, left ventricular hypoplasia and subaortic stenosis. None of these patients had Down's syndrome versus an incidence of 19% in patients who did not present early. Elevated pulmonary artery pressure was common. There was a higher risk of need for reoperation. Mortality was high at 36%. The authors conclude that left sided obstructive lesions should be anticipated in children with primum ASD presenting in the first year of life and that the presence of these lesions alters prognosis and surgical management. In particular late appearance or progression of subaortic stenosis and deterioration of mitral valve function should be anticipated.

The largest review of surgery for primum ASD was reported by El Najdawi et al from the Mayo Clinic in 2000.[41] The authors studied 334 patients who underwent surgery up to 1995. The early mortality was 2%. Five year survival was 94% and 40-year survival was 76%. The authors emphasize the importance of closure of the cleft of the mitral valve. This was associated with improved survival. Surgery at age less than 20 years was also associated with improved survival. Reoperation was performed in 11% of patients, most commonly for mitral valve regurgitation. Left ventricular outflow tract obstruction occurred in 36 patients of whom seven required reoperation to relieve obstruction. Supraventricular arrhythmias were observed in 16% of patients after surgery and were more common with older age at the time of initial repair. Complete heart block occurred in 3% of patients.

Complete AV canal with tetralogy of Fallot

In 1986 Vargas et al[42] reviewed the results of 13 patients who underwent repair of complete AV canal with tetralogy of Fallot at Children's Hospital between 1975 and 1985. A transannular outflow patch was used in 10 of the 13 patients. There were no hospital deaths. However, three patients died late of either AV valve regurgitation, branch pulmonary artery stenosis or sepsis. Four patients required reoperation for mitral valve regurgitation. The authors also present in this paper the results of an autopsy study of 13 patients. They emphasize that in addition to infundibular stenosis other right sided obstructions are common.

In 1990 Ilbawi et al[43] reported the results of surgery for complete AV canal with tetralogy in Fallot in nine patients performed at Children's Memorial Hospital in Chicago. There was one early death for a hospital mortality of 11%. There was no late mortality and all patients were asymptomatic at follow-up. One patient required reoperation for relief of recurrent right ventricular outflow tract obstruction and one patient required reoperation for mitral valve regurgitation. The authors emphasize the importance of aggressive relief of right ventricular outflow tract obstruction with maintenance of pulmonary valve competence. They recommend use of two separate patches for closure of the septal defects.

REFERENCES

1. van Son JAM, Phoon CK, Silverman NH, Haas GS. Predicting feasibility of biventricular repair of right-dominant unbalanced atrioventricular canal. *Ann Thorac Surg* 1997; **63**:1657–1663.
2. Freeman SB, Taft LF, Dooley KJ et al. Population-based study of congenital heart defects in Down syndrome. *Am J Med Genet* 1998; **80**:213–217.
3. Wilson NJ, Gavalaki E, Newman CGH. Compete atrioventricular canal defect in presence of Down syndrome (letter to the editor). *Lancet* 1985; **1**:834.
4. Debiase L, Di Ciommo V, Ballerini L, Bevilacqua M, Marcelletti C, Marino B. Prevalence of left sided obstructive lesions in patients with atrioventricular canal without Down's syndrome. *J Thorac Cardiovasc Surg* 1986; **91**:467–472.
5. Van Mierop LHS, Alley RD, Kausel HW, Stranahan A. The anatomy and embryology of endocardial cushion defects. *J Thorac Cardiovasc Surg* 1962; **43**; 71–83.
6. Anderson RH, Neches WH, Zuberbuhler JR, Penkoske PA. Scooping of the left ventricular septum in atrioventricular septal defect. *J Thorac Cardiovasc Surg* 1988; **95**:146.
7. Ebels T, Meijboom EJ, Anderson RH et al. Anatomic and functional 'obstruction' of the outflow tract in atrioventricular septal defects with separate valve orifices ('ostium primum atrial septal defect'): An echocardiographic study. *Am J Cardiol* 1984; **54**:843.
8. Ebels T, Ho SY, Anderson RH, Meijboom EJ, Eijgelaar A. The surgical anatomy of the left ventricular outflow tract in atrioventricular septal defect. *Ann Thorac Surg* 1986; **41**:483–488.
9. Chang CI, Becker AE. Surgical anatomy of left ventricular outflow tract obstruction in complete atrioventricular septal defect. *J Thorac Cardiovasc Surg* 1987; **94**:897–903.
10. Rastellli GC, Kirklin JW, Titus JL. Anatomic observations on complete form of persistent common atrioventricular canal with special reference to atrioventricular valves. *Mayo Clin Proc* 1966; **41**:296–308.
11. David I, Castaneda AR, Van Praagh R. Potentially parachute mitral valve in common atrioventricular canal: Pathological anatomy and surgical importance. *J Thorac Cardiovasc Surg* 1982; **84**:178–186.
12. Haworth SG. Pulmonary vascular bed in children with complete atrioventricular septal defect: Relation between structural and hemodynamic abnormalities. *Am J Cardiol* 1986; **57**:833–839.
13. Clapp S, Perry BL, Farooki ZQ et al. Down's syndrome, complete atrioventricular canal, and pulmonary vascular obstructive disease. *J Thorac Cardiovasc Surg* 1990; **100**:115–121.
14. Lev M. The architecture of the conduction system in congenital heart disease. I. Common atrioventricular orifice. *AMA Arch Pathol* 1958; **65**:174.
15. Feldt RH, DuShane JW, Titus JL. The atrioventricular conduction system in persistent common atrioventricular canal defect. *Circulation* 1970; **42**:437–444.
16. Manning PB, Mayer JE Jr, Sanders SP et al. Unique features and prognosis of primum ASD presenting in the first year of life. *Circulation* 1994; **90**:II30–II35.
17. Lillehei CW, Cohen M, Warden HE. The direct vision intracardiac correction of congenital anomalies by controlled cross-circulation. Results in thirty-two patients with ventricular septal defects, tetralogy of Fallot and atrioventricularis communis defect. *Surgery* 1955; **38**:11–23.
18. Kirklin JW, Daugherty GW, Burchell HB et al. Repair of the partial form of persistent common atrioventricular canal: Ventricular communication. *Ann Surg* 1955; **142**:858.
19. Watkins E Jr, Gross RE. Experiences with surgical repair of atrial septal defects. *J Thorac Cardiovasc Surg* 1955; **30**:469.
20. Bharati S, Lev M. The spectrum of common atrioventricular orifice (canal). *Am Heart J* 1973; **86**:533–561.
21. Bharati S, Lev M, McAllister HA et al. Surgical anatomy of the atrioventricular valve in the intermediate type of common atrioventricular orifice. *J Thorac Cardiovasc Surg* 1980; **79**:884–889.
22. Maloney JV, Marable SA, Mulder DG. The surgical treatment of common atrioventricular canal. *J Thorac Cardiovasc Surg* 1962; **43**:84–91.
23. Rastelli GC, Ongley PA, Kirklin JW, McGoon DC. Surgical repair of complete form of persistent common atrioventricular canal. *J Thorac Cardiovasc Surg* 1968; **5**:299–308.
24. Rastelli GC, Weidman WH, Kirklin JW. Surgical repair of the partial form of persistent common atrioventricular canal, with special reference to the problem of mitral valve incompetence. *Circulation* 1965; **31**:I31.

25. Castaneda AR, Mayer JE, Jonas RA. Repair of complete atrioventricular canal in infancy. *World J Surg* 1985; **9**:590–597.
26. Chin AJ, Keane JF, Norwood WI, Castaneda AR. Repair of complete common atrioventricular canal in infancy. *J Thorac Cardiovasc Surg* 1982; **84**:437–445.
27. Carpentier A. Surgical anatomy and management of the mitral component of atrioventricular canal defects. In Anderson RH, Shinebourne EA (eds). *Pediatric Cardiology,* London, Churchill Livingstone, 1980, pp 477–490.
28. Wilcox BR, Jones DR, Frantz EG et al. Anatomically sound, simplified approach to repair of 'complete' atrioventricular septal defect. *Ann Thorac Surg* 1997; **64**:487–493.
29. Nicholson IA, Nunn GR, Sholler GF et al. Simplified single patch technique for the repair of atrioventricular septal defect. *J Thorac Cardiovasc Surg* 1999; **118**:642–646.
30. Katz NM, Blackstone EH, Kirklin JW, Bradley EL, Lemons JE. Suture techniques for atrioventricular valves: experimental study. *J Thorac Cardiovasc Surg* 1981; **81**:528–536.
31. Mora BN, Marx GR, Roth SJ, Lang P, Jonas RA. Modified single patch repair of complete atrioventricular canal defect. *J Thorac Cardiovasc Surg,* in press.
32. Hanley FL, Fenton KN, Jonas RA et al. Surgical repair of complete atrioventricular canal defects in infancy. Twenty-year trends. *J Thorac Cardiovasc Surg* 1993; **106**:387–394.
33. Boening A, Scheewe J, Heine K et al. Long-term results after surgical correction of atrioventricular septal defects. *Eur J Cardiothorac Surg* 2002; **22**:167–173.
34. Crawford FA Jr, Stroud MR. Surgical repair of complete atrioventricular septal defect. *Ann Thorac Surg* 2001; **72**:1621–1628.
35. Bogers AJ, Akkersdijk GP, de Jong PL et al. Results of primary two-patch repair of complete atrioventricular septal defect. *Eur J Cardiothorac Surg* 2000; **18**:473–479.
36. Moran AM, Daebritz S, Keane JF, Mayer JE. Surgical management of mitral regurgitation after repair of endocardial cushion defects: early and midterm results. *Circulation* 2000; **102**:III160–III165.
37. Kadoba K, Jonas RA, Mayer JE, Castaneda AR. Mitral valve replacement in the first year of life. *J Thorac Cardiovasc Surg* 1990; **100**:762–768.
38. Ando M, Fraser CD Jr. Prosthetic mitral valve replacement after atrioventricular septal defect repair: a technique for small children *Ann Thorac Surg* 2001; **72**:907–909.
39. Poirier NC, Williams WG, Van Arsdell GS et al. A novel repair for patients with atrioventricular septal defect requiring reoperation for left atrioventricular valve regurgitation. *Eur J Cardiothorac Surg* 2000; **18**:54–61.
40. Adatia I, Moore PM, Jonas RA, Colan SD, Lock JE, Keane JF. Clinical course and hemodynamic observations after supraannular mitral valve replacement in infants and children. *J Am Coll Cardiol* 1997; **29**:1089–1094.
41. El Najdawi E, Driscoll DJ, Puga FL et al. Operation for partial atrioventricular septal defect: A forty-year review. *J Thorac Cardiovasc Surg* 2000; **119**:880–889.
42. Vargas FJ, Coto EO, Mayer JE, Jonas RA, Castaneda AR. Complete atrioventricular canal and tetralogy of Fallot: surgical considerations. *Ann Thorac Surg* 1986; **42**:258–263.
43. Ilbawi M, Cua C, Deleon SY et al. Repair of complete atrioventricular septal defect with tetralogy of Fallot. *Ann Thorac Surg* 1990; **50**:407–412.

22

Anomalies of the pulmonary veins

TOTAL ANOMALOUS PULMONARY VENOUS CONNECTION

INTRODUCTION

Total anomalous pulmonary venous connection (TAPVC) is the most important anomaly of the pulmonary veins. When it is not an isolated anomaly in an otherwise normal biventricular heart, it is often an important component of heterotaxy syndrome where it is frequently found in conjunction with a single functional ventricle and anomalies of the systemic veins (see Chapter 20). In its most severe form total anomalous pulmonary venous connection is one of the only true surgical emergencies across the entire spectrum of congenital heart surgery. Unique to this anomaly is the absence of definitive means of medical palliation for the critically ill neonate. On the other hand, at the simple end of the spectrum, total anomalous pulmonary venous connection is a straightforward anomaly which can be managed with a low risk, relatively elective, technically simple procedure. The heterogeneous nature of total anomalous pulmonary venous connection can be explained by its embryologic origin.

EMBRYOLOGY

The lungs develop as an outpouching from the foregut. They carry with them a plexus of veins derived from the splanchnic (systemic) venous plexus, which drains to the heart through the cardinal and umbilicovitelline veins. TAPVC occurs when the pulmonary vein evagination or outpouching from the posterior surface of the left atrium fails to fuse with the pulmonary venous plexus surrounding the lung buds. In place of the usual connection to the left atrium, at least one connection of the pulmonary venous plexus to the splanchnic plexus persists. As a result the pulmonary veins drain anomalously to the heart through a systemic vein.[1]

ANATOMY

Persistent splanchnic venous connections can occur at almost any point in the central cardinal or umbilicovitelline venous systems. In the commonly used classification of Darling and coworkers,[2] TAPVC is described as *supracardiac* when the anomalous connection is to an 'ascending vertical vein', usually on the left and connected to the left innominate vein similar to a left sided superior vena cava; as *cardiac* when the pulmonary veins connect directly to the right atrium or to the coronary sinus; and as *infracardiac* when the connection is to intra-abdominal veins. In a large series of autopsies from Children's Hospital Boston, approximately 45% of the cases of TAPVC were supracardiac, 25% were cardiac, and 25% were infracardiac.[3] In 5% of the patients, pulmonary venous connection was *mixed*, with at least one of the main lobar pulmonary veins connecting to a different systemic vein relative to the remaining veins.

Pulmonary venous obstruction can occur at any point in the anomalous venous pathway, but is most commonly seen with an infracardiac connection, where it is almost always present to some degree. When pulmonary venous obstruction is present, there are usually morphologic changes in pulmonary arterioles with an increase in arterial muscularity and extension of muscle into smaller and more peripheral arteries. The pulmonary veins themselves are also likely to be thick walled with intimal fibrous hyperplasia when pulmonary venous obstruction has been present during in utero development. Small size of the pulmonary veins at the time of presentation is predictive of subsequent progressive obstruction of the pulmonary veins also through a process of intimal fibrous hyperplasia.[4]

Associated anomalies

Since all pulmonary venous return is to the right atrium, survival of the patient with total anomalous pulmonary venous connection is dependent on a right to left shunt, usually at atrial level through a stretched patent foramen ovale or an ASD. Although most patients with TAPVC other than those with heterotaxy have no associated major cardiac defects, many different associated anomalies have been reported, including tetralogy of Fallot, double-outlet right ventricle[5] as well as hypoplastic left heart syndrome. Associated anomalies, particularly a single functional ventricle, are much more likely to occur with heterotaxy syndrome (see Chapter 20).

In patients with TAPVC, the left atrial volume is small, and left ventricular volume is often at the lower limit of normal. This may be related to the leftward deviation of the ventricular septum that occurs secondary to right ventricular hypertension.[6–8] It may also be partially related to absence of pulmonary venous return directly to the left atrium during fetal development. Endocardial fibroelastosis of the left ventricle has also been reported.[9] The relative hypoplasia of the left ventricle is consistent with the low cardiac indices often seen in these patients postoperatively.[10]

PATHOPHYSIOLOGY

As noted above, because both pulmonary and systemic venous blood returns to the right atrium in all forms of TAPVC, survival of the child is dependent on the presence of a right to left intracardiac shunt. This almost always occurs through a patent foramen ovale that is rarely restrictive (i.e. there is no pressure gradient between the right and left atria).[11]

Mixing of systemic and pulmonary venous return results in at least some degree of cyanosis in all patients. The degree of cyanosis is determined by the amount of pulmonary blood flow relative to systemic blood flow, and this, in turn, is determined largely by the presence or absence of pulmonary venous obstruction. Pulmonary venous obstruction is almost always accompanied by pulmonary arterial and right ventricular hypertension. In fact, significant pulmonary venous obstruction is unlikely in the child with right ventricular pressure that is less than 85% of systemic pressure (Figure 22.1).[12]

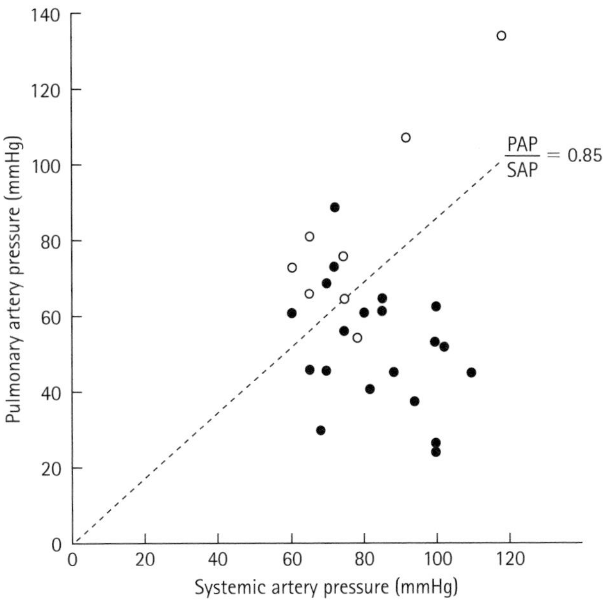

Figure 22.1 *Pulmonary venous obstruction (open circles), demonstrated either at surgical correction or at postmortem examination, is likely to be present in patients with TAPVC to the coronary sinus when right ventricular pressure is greater than 85% of systemic pressure at cardiac catheterization. (From Jonas RA et al. Obstructed pulmonary venous drainage with total anomalous pulmonary venous connection to the coronary sinus.* Am J Cardiol *1987;* ***59****:431–435, with permission.)*

When no pulmonary venous obstruction is present, pulmonary blood flow is often increased because pulmonary venous blood is returning to the compliant right heart analogous to the circulation with an ASD. The increase in pulmonary blood flow may result in pulmonary hypertension with pressure as high as systemic. However, suprasystemic right ventricular pressure is unlikely in the absence of pulmonary venous obstruction. The observed muscularity of pulmonary arterioles is reflected in a tendency for the patient to have labile pulmonary vascular resistance postoperatively, resulting in so-called 'pulmonary hypertensive crises'.

Both pulmonary venous obstruction and increased pulmonary blood flow are likely to cause an increase in extravascular lung water, which may be largely interstitial. At surgery very prominent lymphatic vessels can be seen on the surface of the lungs. In severe cases of pulmonary venous obstruction there may be frank pulmonary edema with fluid extravasation into the alveoli.

An interesting feedback loop can occur in some cases of supracardiac TAPVC. The anomalous vertical vein carrying the entire pulmonary venous return may pass between the left main bronchus and left pulmonary artery. Some degree of pulmonary venous obstruction will result in increased pressure within the left pulmonary artery, which further exacerbates the compression of venous return between the bronchus and the left pulmonary artery. Ultimately, a severe degree of obstruction may ensue from this so-called 'hemodynamic vise'.[13]

CLINICAL FEATURES AND DIAGNOSTIC STUDIES

The presenting features of the child with TAPVC are determined by the degree of pulmonary venous obstruction. If obstruction is severe, the child may be profoundly cyanosed and in respiratory distress within hours or even minutes of birth. Such a child will be tachycardic and hypotensive. In the absence of important pulmonary venous obstruction, clinical status is determined by the amount of pulmonary blood flow and the degree of pulmonary hypertension. The child with greatly increased pulmonary blood flow and pulmonary hypertension will fail to thrive and may have tachypnea and diaphoresis, particularly when feeding. The degree of cyanosis will be mild. If pulmonary artery pressure is only minimally elevated, the child may progress well for years with only a mild degree of cyanosis.

Obstructed neonatal TAPVC

In the child with serious obstruction, analysis of arterial blood gas reveals severe hypoxia (e.g. PO_2 less than 20 mmHg), often with associated metabolic acidosis. The chest X-ray shows a normal heart size with generalized pulmonary edema. The ECG demonstrates right ventricular hypertrophy, but this is to be expected in the neonate. Two-dimensional echocardiography is very reliable in establishing the diagnosis of TAPVC. Ventricular septal position and Doppler assessment of a tricuspid regurgitant jet if present will give a useful estimate of right ventricular pressure. Avoidance of cardiac catheterization in the desperately ill neonate with obstructed TAPVC has been an important advance in the preoperative management of this condition particularly because the osmotic load induced by angiography often exacerbated the degree of pulmonary edema.

Possibly obstructed TAPVC

In infants and children who present with less acute symptoms or possibly no symptoms, cardiac catheterization may occasionally be indicated in order to determine whether obstruction is present and to localize the level of obstruction. This may influence the technique of repair as for example with obstructed TAPVC to the coronary sinus. The important hemodynamic data to be collected include right ventricular and pulmonary artery pressures, as well as a measure of the degree of pulmonary venous obstruction as determined by the gradient between the pulmonary artery wedge pressure and right atrial pressure. Generally there is minimal or no gradient across the foramen ovale, and therefore, balloon or blade septostomy is not recommended. (Some centers do recommend balloon septostomy as a palliative procedure, although we prefer to proceed to early repair.) The point at which a step-up in oxygen saturation is observed within the systemic venous systems helps to localize the site of the pulmonary venous connection. Pulmonary arteriography demonstrates the anomalous pulmonary venous pathway during the levophase (which may be significantly delayed if obstruction is present). Cardiac magnetic resonance imaging is emerging as a helpful diagnostic modality particularly with atypical forms such as mixed total anomalous pulmonary venous connection.

MEDICAL AND INTERVENTIONAL MANAGEMENT

Obstructed TAPVC

Following the introduction of prostaglandin E1 obstructed TAPVC remained as perhaps the only true surgical emergency within the field of congenital heart disease. Other than intubation and positive-pressure ventilation with 100% oxygen, along with correction of metabolic acidosis, no medical measures have been demonstrated to palliate this problem adequately, although one report has suggested that maintenance of ductal patency with prostaglandin E1 may be useful.[14] Reopening the ductus with prostaglandin should provide some increase in cardiac output by allowing a right to left shunt through the ductus. However, in the child who is already profoundly hypoxic because of inadequate pulmonary blood flow, the increase in systemic cardiac output is achieved only at the expense of a further decrease in pulmonary blood flow. Nevertheless, if mixed venous saturation increases as the cardiac index increases, it is possible that there could be a net improvement in arterial saturation. However, it remains our preference to proceed with emergency surgery. This may necessitate direct transfer from the delivery room to the operating room where echocardiographic diagnosis can be confirmed on the operating table.

As noted above some groups frequently employ balloon atrial septostomy but this is very rarely done at Children's Hospital Boston. There are no other catheter interventions that are helpful for obstructed total anomalous pulmonary venous connection.

Nonobstructed TAPVC

As pulmonary vascular resistance decreases, there is a progressive increase in the volume load for the right heart. The child should be treated temporarily with standard decongestive measures. Optimally surgery should be undertaken early in infancy.

INDICATIONS FOR AND TIMING OF SURGERY

Because there is no possibility of spontaneous resolution of TAPVC, the diagnosis alone is an indication for surgery. The timing of surgery should be determined by the presence or absence of pulmonary venous obstruction.

OBSTRUCTED TAPVC

Because there is no effective means of medical palliation of obstructed TAPVC, the neonate with severe hypoxia and acidosis should be taken immediately to the operating room after echocardiographic diagnosis. Although extracorporeal membrane oxygenation has been described as a preoperative intervention[15,16] there is little advantage for most babies as standard cardiopulmonary bypass can be established just as quickly and allows immediate repair of the pulmonary venous obstruction. If necessary, extracorporeal membrane oxygenation can be applied postoperatively.[15,17]

NONOBSTRUCTED TAPVC

Surgical correction should be undertaken at a convenient time, early in infancy, before the deleterious pathologic changes in the heart and lungs and other organs secondary to cyanosis and a longstanding volume load have a chance to develop (see Chapter 1).

SURGICAL MANAGEMENT

History of surgery

TAPVC was first described by Wilson in 1798.[18] In 1951, Muller achieved surgical palliation by anastomosing the anomalous common pulmonary venous trunk to the left atrial appendage.[19] TAPVC was first corrected by Lewis et al in 1956, using hypothermia and inflow occlusion.[20] Correction using cardiopulmonary bypass was described in the same year by Burroughs and Kirklin.[21] The application of deep hypothermic circulatory arrest, as popularized by Barratt-Boyes and coworkers in the early 1970s[22] resulted in a marked improvement in surgical mortality among infants, including neonates in extremis because of obstructed TAPVC.

Technical considerations

ANESTHESIA FOR OBSTRUCTED TAPVC

The hypoxic, acidotic neonate with obstructed TAPVC requires meticulous anesthetic management. Pulmonary resistance should be minimized by hyperventilation with 100% oxygen. Anesthesia is induced with high dose fentanyl, which will decrease pulmonary vasoreactivity.[23] If an inotropic agent is required, isoproterenol may be helpful as long as the patient does not become unduly tachycardic. In view of the mildly hypoplastic nature of the left heart, however, a rapid heart rate of up to 200 beats per minute may, in fact, be necessary to maintain adequate cardiac output. Metabolic acidosis should be treated aggressively. There may be a large calcium requirement, and blood glucose may be labile. Occasionally, there is associated sepsis and renal failure. Digoxin is probably not useful, and it also lowers the threshold for ventricular fibrillation.

EMERGENCY SURGICAL MANAGEMENT OF OBSTRUCTED INFRACARDIAC TAPVC

Adequate venous access and a reliable arterial monitoring line, preferably in an umbilical artery, are essential. The pulse oximeter provides important information so that probes should be placed on several extremities to guarantee that oxygen saturation data will be available. It is best to avoid aggressive surface cooling, because these desperately ill children may fibrillate at a relatively high core temperature (greater than 30°C), particularly if large doses of digoxin have been given at the referral center. The chest is opened by a median sternotomy, and at least one lobe of the thymus, usually the left, is excised. A patch of anterior pericardium is harvested and treated with 0.6% glutaraldehyde for 20–30 minutes. It is essential that there be minimal disturbance of the myocardium after the pericardium is opened. Very slight retraction of the ventricular myocardium can result in ventricular fibrillation. After systemic heparinization, bypass is commenced with an arterial cannula in the ascending aorta and venous return via a single cannula inserted into the right atrial appendage. Immediately after bypass is begun, the ductus arteriosus is dissected free and ligated. This should be done in all cases in view of the presence of pulmonary hypertension which may have masked ductal patency on the preoperative echocardiogram. After 5 minutes or so of cooling so that myocardial temperature is less than 25°C, the aortic cross clamp is applied and cardioplegia is infused into the aortic root. With perfusion continuing the heart is gently retracted out of the chest to allow dissection of the anomalous descending vertical vein. It is preferable to cross clamp before lifting the heart because retraction often causes kinking of the coronary arteries and more importantly incompetence of the aortic valve. The myocardium must not be crushed by excessive retraction during this dissection. A suture ligature of 5/0 Prolene is tied around the vertical vein at the point where it pierces the diaphragm. The vertical vein is divided and filletted proximally to the level of the superior pulmonary veins (Figure 22.2a). The heart is then replaced in the pericardium. By the time the rectal temperature is less than 18°C, the esophageal temperature will be 13°C or 14°C, and tympanic temperature will be approximately 15°C. Bypass is discontinued and blood is drained from the child. The venous cannula is removed.

A transverse incision is made from the right atrial appendage and is carried posteriorly through the foramen ovale into the left atrium. Because the right pulmonary veins do not anchor the left atrium, excellent exposure of the previously dissected vertical vein is obtained. The incision in the posterior wall of the left atrium is carried inferiorly parallel to the vertical vein (Figure 22.2b). It may also be extended superiorly into the base of the left atrial appendage. Care should be taken to avoid incising too close to the mitral annulus which could result in injury to the circumflex coronary artery. The incision also should not be extended into the body of the left atrial appendage as this is usually very thin walled.

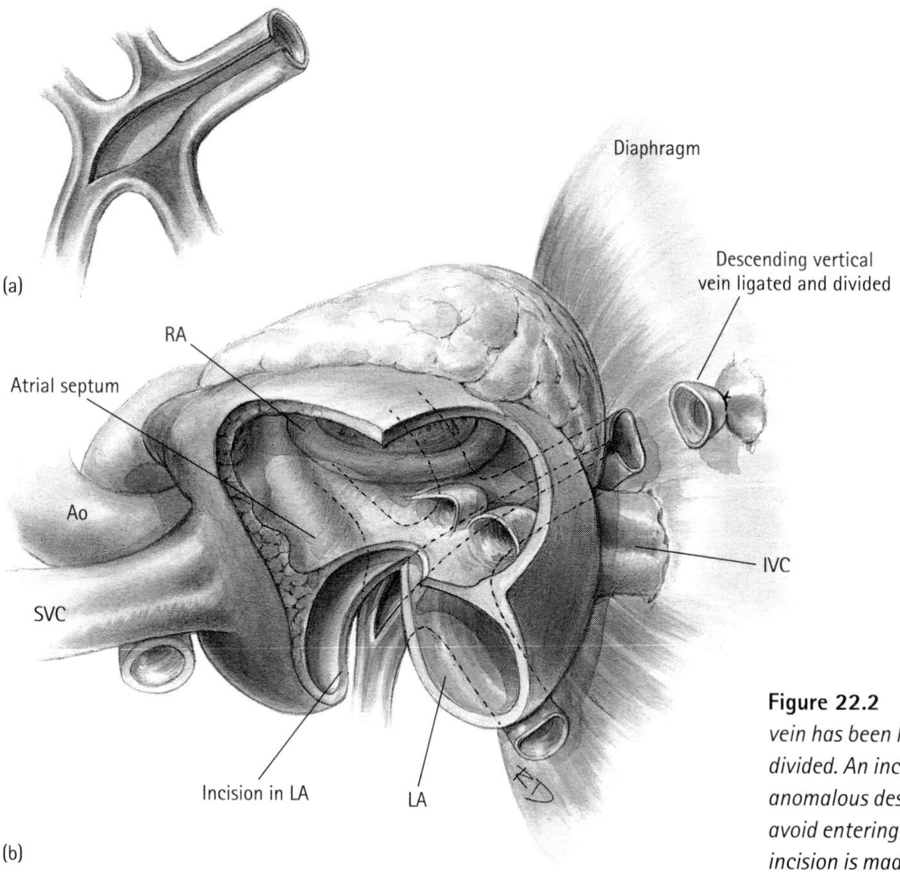

Figure 22.2 *(a) The anomalous descending vertical vein has been ligated at the level of the diaphragm and divided. An incision is made on the anterior surface of the anomalous descending vertical vein with care taken to avoid entering the individual pulmonary veins. (b) A parallel incision is made in the posterior surface of the left atrium.*

The vertical vein to left atrium anastomosis is performed using continuous 6–0 absorbable Maxon or polydioxanone suture. Excellent exposure is obtained by the approach described, and there is little possibility of kinking or malalignment, as may be the case with the alternative technique of performing the anastomosis with the heart everted from the chest. The foramen ovale and the more posterior part of the right atriotomy can be closed with a pericardial patch. Direct suture closure of the foramen ovale has a tendency to narrow the anastomosis and should be avoided. In addition the use of a patch to close the ASD allows the option of placing a graduated fenestration to allow right to left decompression in the early postoperative period. This is probably a wise maneuver if obstruction has been severe preoperatively and it is anticipated that the child will experience pulmonary hypertensive crises in the early postoperative period. In the average neonate a fenestration of approximately 3 mm is appropriate. Before the atrial septal defect is closed, the left heart should be filled with saline, and air is vented through the cardioplegia site in the ascending aorta. After closure of the right atriotomy, the left heart is filled with saline, the venous cannula is reinserted, and bypass is recommenced. The aortic cross clamp is released with the cardioplegia site bleeding freely. During rewarming a pulmonary artery monitoring line is inserted through a horizontal mattress suture in the infundibulum of the right ventricle and a right atrial monitoring line is inserted through a purse-string in the right atrial free wall. Insertion of a left atrial monitoring line through a pulmonary vein should be avoided because of the small size of the pulmonary veins. Although it is possible to insert a left atrial line through the left atrial appendage we do not recommend this. Apart from the increased risk of bleeding from this area it should be recognized that because of pulmonary hypertension and in spite of the slightly underdeveloped nature of the left heart, it is usually the right heart that is the limiting factor in determining cardiac output so that it is the right atrial pressure that should determine volume status both when weaning from bypass as well as in the ICU.

When the alternative approach of everting the apex of the heart from the chest is used, the pulmonary confluence to left atrial anastomosis is constructed by an external rather than an internal approach. Great care must be taken in retracting the heart with this technique. The heart is at risk of more rapid warming when removed from the pericardial well and there is also a risk of crush injury to the delicate neonatal myocardium if excessive retraction force is applied.

WEANING FROM CARDIOPULMONARY BYPASS

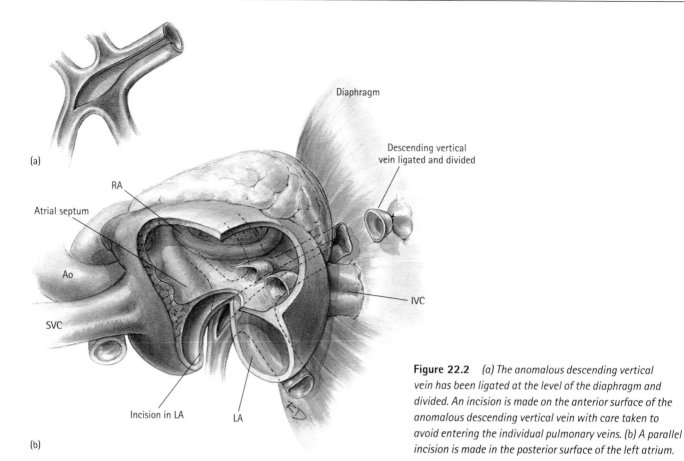

Once rewarming to a rectal temperature of at least 35°C is completed, the patient can be weaned from cardiopulmonary bypass. Although this should be uneventful in any patient after elective surgery, it can be a critical phase in the management of a patient who is acutely ill and has had severe obstruction preoperatively. Such patients tend to have markedly labile pulmonary vascular resistance. Their response to cardiopulmonary bypass is often a substantial, although brief, temporary increase in pulmonary resistance. Therefore, it is useful to monitor pulmonary artery pressure, in addition to aortic and right atrial pressure, at the time of weaning from bypass. It is not uncommon for pulmonary pressure to be close to systemic levels for the first 10–15 minutes after weaning from bypass. During this time, ventilatory management is critical. The patient should be maintained on 100% oxygen, nitric oxide and the PCO_2 should be lowered to at least 30 mmHg, though not lower than 25 mm which could impair cerebral perfusion. In the past isoproterenol was useful as an inotropic agent in further lowering pulmonary resistance but is rarely necessary today following the introduction of nitric oxide. In the presence of a widely open anastomosis, pulmonary pressure should fall to less than two thirds to one half systemic pressure within 15–30 minutes of weaning from bypass. If pulmonary artery pressure remains elevated, an obstructed anastomosis should be suspected. Intraoperative two-dimensional echocardiography with an epicardial transducer can give excellent visualization of this area. Transesophageal echocardiography in the small neonate carries a risk of compression of the anastomosis even when a very small transducer is employed. We generally avoid its use in this setting in babies of less than 3.5–4 kg.

ELECTIVE SURGICAL MANAGEMENT OF NONOBSTRUCTED SUPRACARDIAC TAPVC

The general operative approach to nonobstructed supracardiac TAPVC is similar to that for infracardiac TAPVC. Deep hypothermic circulatory arrest in the neonate and small infant provides optimal exposure and, therefore, the most consistently wide open anastomosis.

(In infants larger than 3–4 kg double venous cannulation is performed and the procedure is undertaken on continuous bypass with either moderate or deep hypothermia. It may be preferable to directly cannulate the left innominate vein with a right angle metal tipped cannula in order to optimize exposure of the area of anastomosis. Total cardiopulmonary bypass is achieved by tightening a tourniquet around the right angle cannula in the IVC and placing a clamp across the superior vena cava).

The horizontal pulmonary venous confluence is dissected free during the cooling period. Much of this dissection can be done from the right side working behind the left atrium without everting the heart out of the chest. The cross clamp is applied and cardioplegia is infused before retracting the heart out of the chest to complete dissection of the left end of the horizontal confluence. After cessation of cardiopulmonary bypass and removal of the venous cannula, the right atrial transverse incision is carried across the atrial septum at the level of the foramen ovale into the left atrium. It is then continued transversely, extending into the base of the left atrial appendage. A longitudinal incision is made in the horizontal pulmonary venous confluence parallel to the left atrial incision. A direct anastomosis is fashioned between the left atrium and the pulmonary venous confluence using continuous 6–0 Maxon suture (Figure 22.3). The anastomosis is begun at the most leftward point, using a continuous inverting suture technique and working toward the right within the anastomosis. Just as with obstructed infradiaphragmatic total anomalous pulmonary venous connection it is best to close the foramen ovale with a patch of autologous pericardium. This avoids any narrowing of the anastomosis and also helps to supplement the size of the small left atrium. It is unlikely that a fenestration will be useful for supracardiac TAPVC except in rare cases of important preoperative venous obstruction. The anomalous ascending vertical vein is always ligated but does not have to be divided. Pulmonary hypertension is rare after elective cases in which pulmonary artery pressure has usually been only mildly elevated before surgery.

ELECTIVE SURGICAL MANAGEMENT OF TAPVC TO THE CORONARY SINUS

It was previously thought that obstruction of TAPVC to the coronary sinus was extremely rare, but a review of TAPVC at Children's Hospital Boston revealed a surprisingly high incidence of 22% of such cases.[12] Therefore, two-dimensional echocardiography should carefully assess the point of junction between the pulmonary veins and the coronary sinus, which was the most common point of obstruction in this series. If there is any doubt about this area, a cardiac MRI scan, or occasionally cardiac catheterization should be performed. In the absence of obstruction, a simple unroofing procedure of the coronary sinus will suffice. The tissue between the foramen ovale and coronary sinus is incised (Figure 22.4a), and extended in the roof of the coronary sinus to the posterior wall of the heart. The resulting atrial septal defect is closed with an autologous pericardial patch (Figure 22.4b).

In an attempt to decrease the incidence of bradyarrythmias after this procedure, Van Praagh and colleagues suggested the 'fenestration' procedure, which includes unroofing of the coronary sinus toward the left atrium and separate closure of the coronary sinus ostium within the right atrium and foramen ovale. This technique allowed preservation of the tissue between the coronary sinus and the foramen ovale, where it was thought that important internodal conduction pathways may have existed. Experience with this operation at Children's Hospital Boston between 1972 and 1980 demonstrated that in the 10 patients in whom this procedure was used, there was no decrease in the incidence of bradyarrhythmias when compared with the more traditional procedure. Although no cases of restriction at the point of fenestration were observed at this hospital, there have been cases reported by others.[24]

If two-dimensional echocardiography reveals a potential site of obstruction at the junction of the coronary sinus with the horizontal confluence an operation similar to that described for supracardiac TAPVC should be performed. The horizontal confluence should be filletted and a parallel

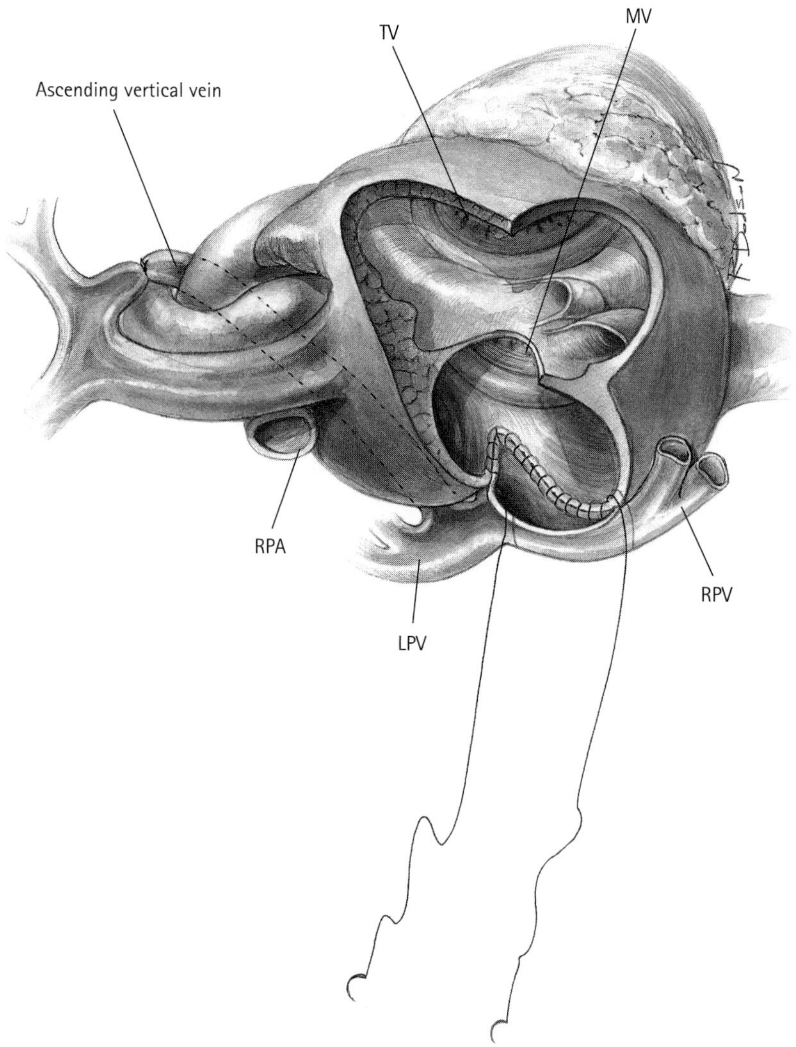

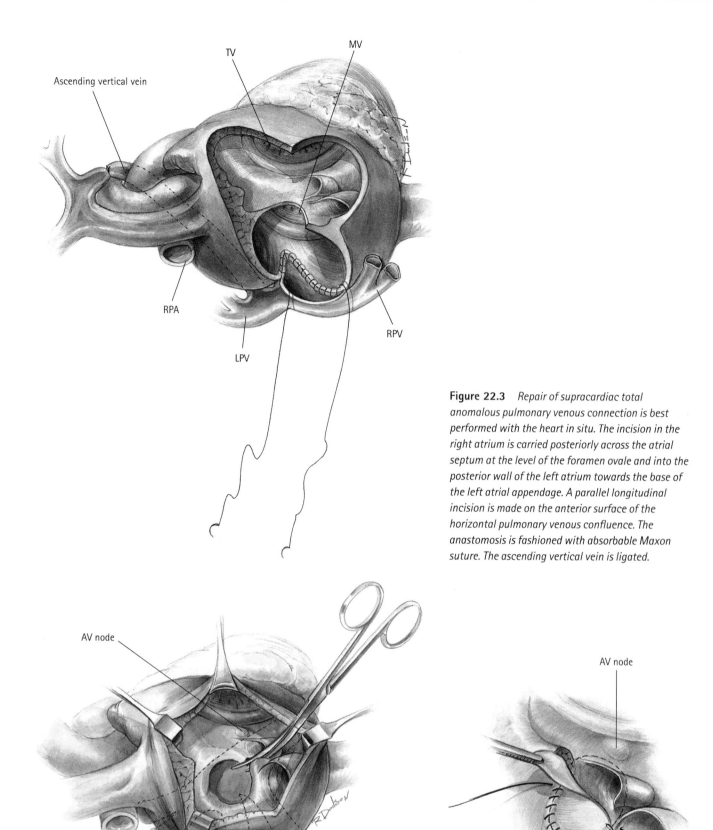

Figure 22.3 *Repair of supracardiac total anomalous pulmonary venous connection is best performed with the heart in situ. The incision in the right atrium is carried posteriorly across the atrial septum at the level of the foramen ovale and into the posterior wall of the left atrium towards the base of the left atrial appendage. A parallel longitudinal incision is made on the anterior surface of the horizontal pulmonary venous confluence. The anastomosis is fashioned with absorbable Maxon suture. The ascending vertical vein is ligated.*

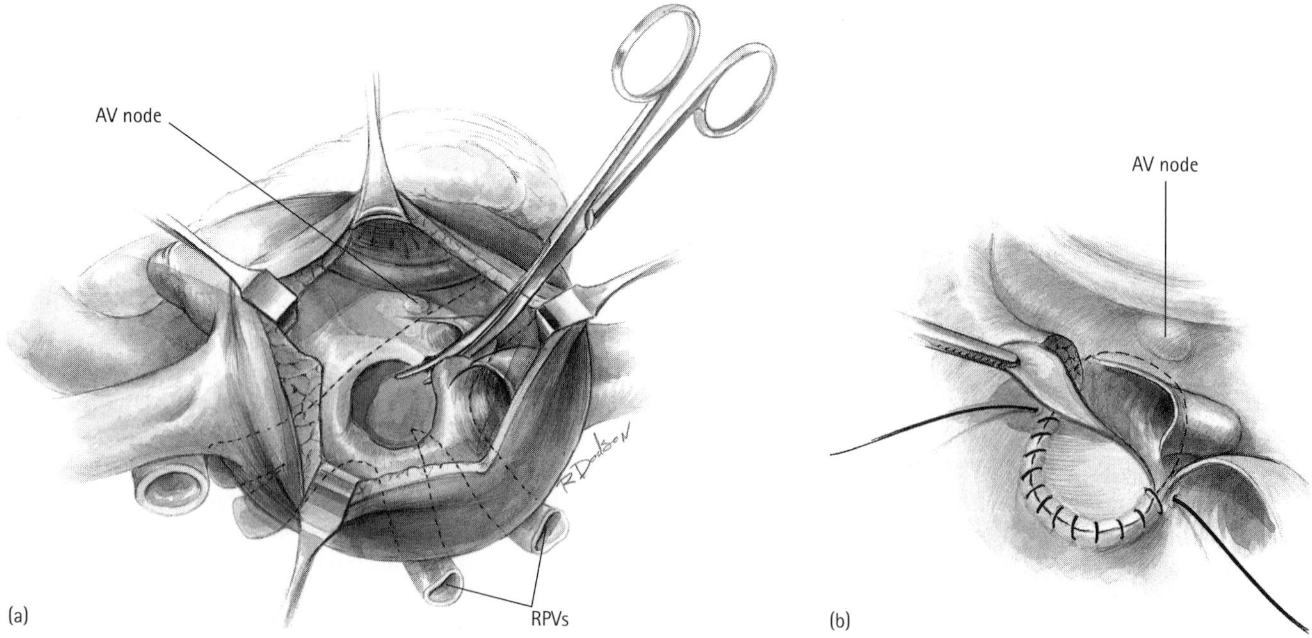

Figure 22.4 *Repair of TAPVC to the coronary sinus. (a) The tissue between the foramen ovale and coronary sinus is incised and extended in the roof of the coronary sinus to the posterior wall of the heart. It is important to note that obstruction between the confluence of pulmonary veins and coronary sinus must be excluded by appropriate preoperative studies. If obstruction is present an anastomosis between the horizontal confluence and left atrium is necessary. (b) The atrial septal defect resulting from unroofing of the coronary sinus is closed with an autologous pericardial patch.*

incision made in the posterior wall of the left atrium, extending into the left atrial appendage. A direct anastomosis can be fashioned using continuous absorbable Maxon suture.

ELECTIVE SURGICAL MANAGEMENT OF TAPVC TO THE RIGHT ATRIUM

Using deep hypothermic circulatory arrest for small neonates or double venous cannulation in larger infants, as described for the previous procedures, an autologous pericardial baffle can be used to direct the anomalous veins through the atrial septal defect, which may need to be surgically enlarged, into the left atrium.

FAILURE TO WEAN FROM CARDIOPULMONARY BYPASS

If the right ventricle appears to be incapable of generating the high pressures required in the early period after weaning from bypass, it may very occasionally be necessary to consider applying extracorporeal membrane oxygenation for a period of several days to allow a gradual decrease in pulmonary vascular resistance.[15,17] The same cannulas as used for the introperative procedure can be employed. The cannulas exit through the sternotomy incision which is not closed. An Esmarch patch is sutured to the skin edges and an iodine impregnated adhesive plastic drape is used to seal the closure.

INTENSIVE CARE MANAGEMENT

The heavily muscularized pulmonary arterioles of the child with obstructed TAPVC remain particularly labile for up to several days after corrective surgery. During this period, pulmonary resistance should be minimized by appropriate ventilatory management. The stress response of pulmonary vasoconstriction should be minimized by maintaining a constant state of anesthesia. Arterial PCO_2 should be maintained at approximately 30 mmHg, and the inspired oxygen and nitric oxide concentrations should be titrated so as to achieve a pulmonary pressure (as measured by the indwelling pulmonary artery line) that is less than two thirds of systemic pressure. A low-dose isoproterenol infusion of up to 0.1 μg/kg body weight per minute may also be continued for 24–48 hours for its pulmonary vasodilatory effects. After 24–48 hours of hemodynamic stability, the level of anesthesia may be lightened, with careful observation for pulmonary hypertensive crises. These are particularly likely to occur in response to the stress of endotracheal tube suctioning, which should be performed carefully after hyperventilation.

RESULTS OF SURGERY

Early results

Before 1970 repair of TAPVC in infancy generally carried a mortality rate greater than 50%.[25,26] Between 1970 and 1980 many centers reported mortality rates of between 10% and 20%. Between January 1, 1980 and June 31, 2000, 127 patients underwent repair of TAPVC at Children's Hospital Boston.[27] A total of 41 of these patients had a single functional ventricle while 86 had two ventricles. Overall 72 patients had some degree of obstructed pulmonary venous return and 55 underwent an emergency procedure. Among the 86 patients with two ventricles, pulmonary venous obstruction was present in 47 (55%).

Overall the early mortality was 17% (22 of 127), 34% for those with one ventricle and 9% for those with two ventricles. Supracardiac TAPVC made up 55% of the biventricular patients. The mortality for biventricular infracardiac TAPVC was 2/26 or 7.7%. Survival estimated by Kaplan Meier for the overall group was 74% at one year. Independent risk factors for early mortality were preoperative pulmonary venous obstruction ($p = 0.008$, hazard ratio 4.2) and single ventricle ($p < 0.001$, hazard ratio 4.1). Overall mortality was significantly associated with preoperative pulmonary venous obstruction ($p = 0.02$, hazard ratio 2.2), single ventricle anatomy ($p < 0.01$, hazard ratio 4.8) and intracardiac repair ($p = 0.009$, hazard ratio 2.8). Post-repair pulmonary vein stenosis occurred in 11 patients (8.7%). This was associated with the use of nonabsorbable suture ($p = 0.005$).

In a report from Children's Hospital of Philadelphia, Kirshbom et al[28] reviewed 100 patients who underwent repair of isolated TAPVC between 1983 and 2001. Overall hospital mortality was 14%, decreasing from 19% before 1995 to 5% after 1995. Multivariable logistic regression analysis demonstrated that associated chromosomal or noncardiac syndromes as well as pulmonary venous obstruction were significant predictors of overall health and school performance.

In a similar report from the Bambino Gesu Hospital in Rome Michielon et al[29] reviewed 89 patients who underwent surgery for nonheterotaxy TAPVC between 1983 and 2001. A total of 32% of patients underwent emergency surgery because of pulmonary venous obstruction. Overall early mortality was 8%. Kaplan Meier survival was 88% at 18 years with no difference according to anatomic subtype or surgical technique. Freedom from reintervention for pulmonary venous obstruction for operative survivors was 87% at 18 years. The presence of preoperative obstruction predicted a higher risk of reintervention for pulmonary vein stenosis ($p = 0.02$). The problem of pulmonary vein obstruction following repair of total anomalous pulmonary venous obstruction is the focus of a paper by Hyde et al from Birmingham, England.[30] The authors analysed 85 patients with nonheterotaxy TAPVC undergoing surgical correction between 1988 and 1997. Of 88 patients, 43 had supracardiac connection and 20 had infracardiac connection. Overall early mortality was 7%. The incidence of pulmonary vein stenosis requiring intervention postoperatively was 11% at a median follow-up of 64 months. A total of 56% of these patients survived. The authors also noted that patients who had recurrent obstruction because of endocardial sclerosis had a worse prognosis than patients who had an anatomical or extrinsic obstruction. Another large retrospective review by Bando et al from Riley Hospital Indianapolis[31] of 105 patients who underwent surgery between 1966 and 1995 also demonstrated that a small pulmonary confluence and diffuse pulmonary vein stenosis were both independent risk factors for early and late mortality as well as need for reoperation. This report published in 1996 confirmed a similar report by Jenkins et al published in 1993 describing the experience from Children's Hospital Boston.[4]

ARRHYTHMIAS AFTER REPAIR OF TAPVC

In a report from Dusseldorf, Germany, Korbmacher et al[32] described long-term follow-up of 52 patients operated on between 1968 and 1992. Early mortality was 35%. Mean follow-up was 10.7 years. All 24 long-term survivors underwent assessment of cardiac rhythm by 24-hour Holter monitoring. Significant arrhythmias were recorded in 11 of 24 cases including sinus node dysfunction in three patients. Multiform ventricular ectopic beats were noted in nine cases.

Important ventricular ectopy as well as supraventricular ectopy was noted in 25 patients from the All India Institute in Delhi who underwent Holter monitoring.[33] There was no correlation between the presence of arrhythmia and date of repair, anatomical subtype, operative approach or adequacy of repair. The authors conclude that long-term follow-up of rhythm after repair of TAPVC is important even in patients who are asymptomatic.

LIGATION OF THE ANOMALOUS VERTICAL VEIN

A number of reports have focused attention on the consequences of failure to ligate the vertical vein. For example, Shah et al[34] demonstrated the development of an important left to right shunt when the vertical vein was not ligated. Similarly, Kumar et al[35] found that the unligated vertical vein could be responsible for a left to right shunt. On the other hand Kron and Cope[36] support the original suggestion of Jegier et al[37] that it can be helpful to leave the vertical vein unligated to allow right to left decompression during the period of early hemodynamic instability.

REPAIR WITHOUT CARDIOPULMONARY BYPASS

Although there have been sporadic reports such as that by Ootaki et al[38] of the feasibility of repairing TAPVC without cardiopulmonary bypass, these have in general been isolated case reports. This technique is not recommended in the absence of long-term data from a reasonable number of patients.

IN-SITU PERICARDIAL REPAIR OF POSTOPERATIVE PULMONARY VEIN STENOSIS

Lacour-Gayet et al from Marie Lannelongue Hospital Paris[39] have popularized the concept of 'sutureless' repair of pulmonary vein stenosis, which occurs after repair of TAPVC. The authors describe 16 patients representing 9% of 178 patients who underwent correction of total anomalous pulmonary venous connection who experienced development of progressive pulmonary venous obstruction after a median interval of four months. In nearly half these patients the obstruction was bilateral. The obstruction was repaired by filleting open the obstructed pulmonary veins. The left atrium was disconnected from the pulmonary veins and was sutured to the pericardium in situ, avoiding direct suturing of the pulmonary veins. Early mortality was high at 27% with bilateral obstruction being the only risk factor for mortality. However, five of seven survivors had normal pulmonary artery pressure at a mean follow-up of 26 months. Nishi et al[40] from Osaka, Japan also described successful application of the in situ technique. On the other hand, van Son et al[41] from the Mayo Clinic described a satisfactory long-term result in six of eight patients with pulmonary vein stenosis managed with traditional plasty techniques. Five patients had developed this condition after repair of TAPVC. At follow-up extending to 16 years with a median follow-up of 6.5 years, six of seven surviving patients were in NYHA class 1. The problem of pulmonary venous obstruction after repair of TAPVC was described in a paper by Fujino et al from Tokyo Women's Medical College.[42] The authors analysed seven patients at a mean age of six years who had undergone surgical correction of TAPVC in early infancy. The authors found that infusion of isoproterenol resulted in a substantial increase in cardiac index without a change in pulmonary artery wedge pressure in all patients including one patient with mild pulmonary hypertension. They suggest that these results demonstrate that if no pulmonary venous obstruction is present within the first 12 months following correction then these patients do not have any hemodynamic impairment with infusion of isoproterenol.

PARTIAL ANOMALOUS PULMONARY VENOUS CONNECTION

The most common form of PAPVC is connection of one or several pulmonary veins from the right upper lobe to the superior vena cava in association with a sinus venosus ASD. This situation is often best dealt with by the Warden procedure, which is described in detail in Chapter 13.

CONGENITAL PULMONARY VEIN STENOSIS

This is an extremely rare anomaly that has a poor prognosis, either with or without surgical management. There is generally fibrous intimal hyperplasia, which most commonly affects the point of junction between the pulmonary veins and left atrium but as with post-repair obstruction in TAPVC often appears to be progressive in that with time the process extends upstream into the veins. The condition can progress to complete obliteration of the veins, which become fibrous cords.

Diagnosis is generally made in infancy when the child presents with respiratory distress and failure to thrive. Chest films reveal pulmonary venous hypertension, and right ventricular hypertrophy is seen on electrocardiogram because of pulmonary hypertension. Two-dimensional echocardiography can usually provide excellent visualization of the stenotic veins, making cardiac catheterization unnecessary. Cardiac magnetic resonance imaging may also be helpful.

Surgical management

Numerous surgical procedures have been attempted but success has been rare. Although early survival can be achieved with satisfactory decompression of the veins at the point of obstruction, there is usually an inexorable progression of the disease process. One procedure described by Pacifico involves the use of a vascularized flap of atrial septum, which is rotated into the orifices of the pulmonary veins. Lacour-Gayet[43] has described incision of the pulmonary veins, detachment of the left atrium and reanastomosis of the atrium to the pericardium. This procedure avoids direct suturing of the pulmonary veins but has generally only been successful when obstruction has been unilateral. The mechanism of pulmonary vein stenosis was analysed in a report by Sadr et al from Children's Hospital Boston.[44] The authors used microscopy, immunohistochemistry and cell culture to identify the mechanism of restenosis in four infants with isolated pulmonary vein stenosis. The authors found that recurrent obstruction was due to myofibroplastic proliferation. This finding no doubt explains the disappointing results obtained with placement of stents by interventional catheter methods. Stents covered with Gortex membrane have also been tried but success has usually been short lived because of recurrent stenosis at either end of the stent. Currently a trial of chemotherapy is under way with the hope that suppression of myofibroblast proliferation will reduce recurrent stenosis. However, preliminary results have been disappointing. Lung transplant remains the final option.

REFERENCES

1. Neill CA. Development of the pulmonary veins: With reference to the embryology of pulmonary venous return. *Pediatrics* 1956; **18**:880.
2. Darling RC, Rothney WB, Craig JM. Total pulmonary venous drainage into the right side of the heart. *Lab Invest* 1957; **6**:44.
3. Delisle G, Ando M, Calder AL et al. Total anomalous pulmonary venous connection: Report of 93 autopsied cases with emphasis on diagnostic and surgical considerations. *Am Heart J* 1976; **91**:99–122.
4. Jenkins KJ, Sanders SP, Orav J, Coleman EA, Mayer JE, Colan SD. Individual pulmonary vein size and survival in infants with totally anomalous pulmonary venous connection. *J Am Coll Cardiol* 1993; **22**:201–206.
5. DeLeon SY, Gidding SS, Ilbawi MN et al. Surgical management of infants with complex cardiac anomalies associated with reduced pulmonary blood flow and total anomalous pulmonary venous drainage. *Ann Thorac Surg* 1987; **43**:207–211.
6. Bove KE, Geiser EA, Meyer RA. The left ventricle in anomalous pulmonary venous return. Morphometric analysis of 36 fatal cases in infancy. *Arch Pathol* 1975; **99**:522–528.
7. Nakazawa M, Jarmakani JM,. Gyepes MT, Prochazka JV, Yabek SM, Marks RA. Pre and postoperative ventricular function in infants and children with right ventricular volume overload. *Circulation* 1977; **55**:479–484.
8. Hammon JW, Bender HW, Graham TP, Boucek RJ, Smith CW, Erath HG. Total anomalous pulmonary venous connection in infancy. Ten years' experience including studies of postoperative ventricular function. *J Thorac Cardiovasc Surg* 1980; **80**:544–551.
9. Leblanc JG, Patterson MW, Taylor GP, Ashmore PG. Total anomalous pulmonary venous return with left heart hypoplasia. *J Thorac Cardiovasc Surg* 1988; **95**:540–542.
10. Parr GV, Kirklin JW, Pacifico AD, Blackstone EH, Lauridsen P. Cardiac performance in infants after repair of total anomalous pulmonary venous connection. *Ann Thorac Surg* 1974; **17**:561–573.
11. Gathman GE, Nadas AS. Total anomalous pulmonary venous connection: Clinical and physiologic observations of 75 pediatric patients. *Circulation* 1970; **42**:143–154.
12. Jonas RA, Smolinsky A, Mayer JE, Castaneda AR. Obstructed pulmonary venous drainage with total anomalous pulmonary venous connection to the coronary sinus. *Am J Cardiol* 1987; **59**:431–435.
13. Burroughs JT, Edwards JE. Total anomalous pulmonary venous connection. *Am Heart* J 1960; **59**:913.
14. Yee ES, Turley K, Hsieh WR, Ebert PA. Infant total anomalous pulmonary venous connection: Factors influencing timing of presentation and operative outcome. *Circulation* 1987; **76**:III83–87.
15. Klein MD, Shaheen KW, Whittlesey GC, Pinsky WW, Arciniegas E. Extracorporeal membrane oxygenation for the circulatory support of children after repair of congenital heart disease. *J Thorac Cardiovasc Surg* 1990; **100**:498–505.
16. Ishino K, Alexi-Meskishvili V, Hetzer R. Preoperative extracorporeal membrane oxygenation in newborns with total anomalous pulmonary venous connection. *Cardiovasc Surg* 1999; **7**:473–475.
17. Weinhaus L, Canter C, Noetzel M, McAlister W, Spray TL. Extracorporeal membrane oxygenation for circulatory support after repair of congenital heart defects. *Ann Thorac Surg* 1989; **48**:206–212.
18. Wilson J. A description of a very unusual formation of the human heart. *Philos Trans R Soc Lond* 1798; **88**:346.
19. Muller WH. The surgical treatment of transposition of the pulmonary veins. *Ann Surg* 1951; **134**:683.
20. Lewis FJ, Varco RL, Taufic M et al. Direct vision repair of triatrial heart and total anomalous pulmonary venous drainge. *Surg Gynecol Obstet* 1956; **102**:713.
21. Burroughs JT, Kirklin JW. Complete surgical correction of total anomalous pulmonary venous connection. Report of three cases. *Proc Staff Meet Mayo Clin* 1956; **31**:182.
22. Barratt-Boyes BG, Simpson M, Neutze JM. Intracardiac surgery in neonates and infants using deep hypothermia with surface cooling and limited cardiopulmonary bypass. *Circulation* 1971; **43**:25–30.
23. Hickey PR, Hansen DD, Wessel DL, Lang P, Jonas RA, Elixson EM. Blunting of stress responses in the pulmonary circulation of infants by Fentanyl. *Anesth Analg* 1985; **64**:1137–1142.
24. Whight CM, Barratt-Boyes BG, Calder AL, Neutze JM, Brandt PW. Total anomalous pulmonary venous connection. Long term results following repair in infancy. *J Thorac Cardiovasc Surg* 1978; **75**:52–63.
25. Behrendt DM, Aberdeen E, Waterson DJ, Bonham-Carter RE. Total anomalous pulmonary venous drainage in infants. I. Clinical and

hemodynamic findings, methods and results of operation in 37 cases. *Circulation* 1972; **46**:347–356.

26. Mustard WT, Keon WJ, Trusler GA. Transposition of the lesser veins (total anomalous pulmonary venous drainage). *Prog Cardiovasc Dis* 1968; **11**:145.
27. Hancock-Friesen C, Zurakowski D, Jonas RA. Repair of total anomalous pulmonary venous connection. Presented at the Society of Thoracic Surgeons Meeting, San Antonio, Texas, Jan, 2004.
28. Kirshbom PM, Myung RJ, Gaynor JW et al. Preoperative pulmonary venous obstruction affects long-term outcome for survivors of total anomalous pulmonary venous connection repair. *Ann Thorac Surg* 2002; **74**:1616–1620.
29. Michielon G, Di Donato RM, Pasquini L et al. Total anomalous pulmonary venous connection: long-term appraisal with evolving technical solutions. *Eur J Cardiothorac Surg* 2002; **22**:184–191.
30. Hyde JA, Stumper O, Barth MJ et al. Total anomalous pulmonary venous connection: Outcome of surgical correction and management of recurrent venous obstruction. *Eur J Cardiothorac Surg* 1999; **15**:735–740.
31. Bando K, Turrentine MW, Ensing GJ et al. Surgical management of total anomalous pulmonary venous connection. Thirty-year trends. *Circulation* 1996; **94**:II12–16.
32. Korbmacher B, Buttgen S, Schulte HD et al. Long-term results after repair of total anomalous pulmonary venous connection. *Thorac Cardiovasc Surg* 2001; **49**:101–106.
33. Bhan A, Umre MA, Choudhary SK et al. Cardiac arrhythmias in surgically repaired total anomalous pulmonary venous connection: a follow-up study. *Indian Heart J* 2000; **52**:427–430.
34. Shah MJ, Shah S, Shankargowda S, Krishnan U, Cherian KM. L to R shunt: a serious consequence of TAPVC repair without ligation of vertical vein. *Ann Thorac Surg* 2000; **70**:971–973.
35. Kumar RNS, Dharmapuram AK, Rao IM et al. The fate of the unligated vertical vein after surgical correction of total anomalous pulmonary venous connection in early infancy. *J Thorac Cardiovasc Surg* **2001**:**122**:615–617.
36. Kron IL, Cope JT. Fate of the unligated vertical vein after surgical correction with total anomalous pulmonary venous connection in early infancy. *J Thorac Cardiovasc Sug* 2002; **123**:829.
37. Jegier W, Charrette E, Dobell ARC. Infradiaphragmatic anomalous pulmonary venous drainage. *Circulation* 1967; **35**:396–400.
38. Ootaki Y, Yamaguchi M, Oshima Y, Yoshimura N, Oka S. Repair of total anomalous pulmonary venous connection without cardiopulmonary bypass. *Ann Thorac Surg* 2001; **72**:249–251.
39. Lacour-Gayet F, Rey C, Planche C. Pulmonary vein stenosis. Description of a sutureless surgical procedure using the pericardium in situ. *Arch Mal Coeur Vaiss* 1996; **89**:633–636.
40. Nishi H, Nishigaki K, Kume Y, Miyamoto K. In situ pericardium repair of pulmonary venous obstruction after repair of total anomalous pulmonary venous connection. *Jpn J Thorac Cardiovasc Surg* 2002; **50**:338–340.
41. van Son JA, Danielson GK, Puga FJ, Edwards WD, Driscoll DJ. Repair of congenital and acquired pulmonary vein stenosis. *Ann Thorac Surg* 1995; **60**:144–150.
42. Fujino H, Nakazawa M, Momma K, Imai Y. Long-term results after surgical repair of total anomalous pulmonary venous connection – hemodynamic evaluation of pulmonary venous obstruction with isoproterenol infusion. *Jpn Circ J* 1995; **59**:198–204.
43. Lacour-Gayet F, Zoghbi J, Serraf AE et al. Surgical management of progressive pulmonary venous obstruction after repair of total anomalous pulmonary venous connection. *J Thorac Cardiovasc Surg* 1999; **117**:679–687.
44. Sadr IM, Tan PE, Kieran MW, Jenkins KJ. Mechanism of pulmonary vein stenosis in infants with normally connected veins. *Am J Cardiol* 2000; **86**:577–579.

23

Double outlet right ventricle

INTRODUCTION

Double outlet right ventricle encompasses a wide spectrum of pathophysiology from tetralogy of Fallot to transposition of the great arteries with quite different management at the two ends of the spectrum. Furthermore although DORV may be suitable for biventricular repair, many patients have a VSD which is remote from the aorta or pulmonary artery or they have severe underdevelopment of the left ventricle. In these circumstances a single ventricle/Fontan pathway should be pursued. DORV is a common cardiac anomaly in patients with heterotaxy and asplenia who have a common atrioventricular valve and transposed great arteries. DORV is also seen in conjunction with mitral atresia; in this setting the great vessels are usually normally related. Single ventricle forms of DORV are discussed in detail in Chapter 20.

EMBRYOLOGY

DORV, like tetralogy and transposition, is an anomaly of conotruncal development and in fact bridges the gap between tetralogy and transposition. There are two basic theories that attempt to explain the development of conotruncal anomalies.

Lev's theory of conotruncal malseptation

The conotruncus which will ultimately form the aorta and pulmonary artery forms as a single tube. A process of spiral septation divides the conotruncus into the two great vessels which should wrap around each other. If the septum does not 'spiral' in the usual fashion at all, the great vessels will be parallel to each other and there will be transposition of the great arteries. If the spiraling process is only slightly abnormal there will be dextroposition of the aorta relative to its usual location and tetralogy will result. DORV results when the spiraling anomaly is greater than the degree seen with tetralogy but less than the degree seen with transposition.[1,2]

Van Praagh's theory of conal underdevelopment

Usually the aortic, tricuspid and mitral valves are in fibrous continuity, united by the fibrous skeleton of the heart which also serves as an electrical insulator between the atria and the ventricles. Only the pulmonary valve is separate, being lifted superiorly from the other three valves by the subpulmonary conus (infundibulum) (Figure 23.1a). Van Praagh[3] has proposed the attractive hypothesis that tetralogy results when there is underdevelopment of the infundibulum. This results in a relative shift in the positions of the aortic and pulmonary valves such that the aortic valve is more anterior and rightward and more superior than its usual location relative to the pulmonary valve. The conal and ventricular septa no longer align and a conoventricular VSD results with anterior malalignment of the conal septum relative to the ventricular septum. This malalignment can cause obstruction to outflow from the right ventricle.

As an extension of Van Praagh's theory of tetralogy development it has been suggested that a greater degree of conal underdevelopment will result in the great arteries coming to lie in a side by side location, particularly if there is compensatory development of a subaortic conus. Now the aortic valve is lifted superiorly away from the atrioventricular valves and lies at the same height as the pulmonary valve and there are bilateral coni (Figure 23.1b).[4] Even further into

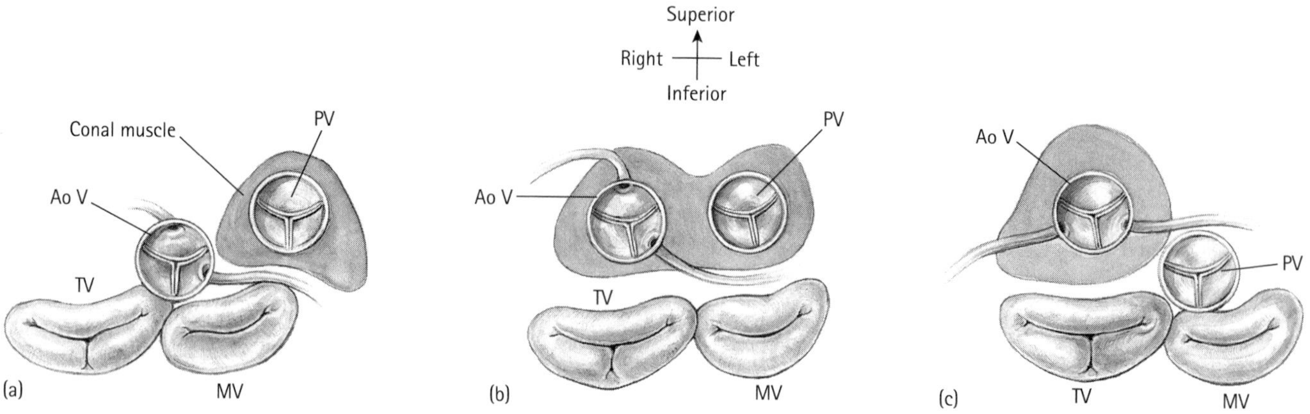

Figure 23.1 *(a) Usually the aortic (AoV), tricuspid (TV), and mitral (MV) valves are in fibrous continuity united by the fibrous skeleton of the heart. The pulmonary valve is separate, being lifted superiorly from the three other valves by the subpulmonary conus (infundibulum). (b) Double outlet right ventricle is characterized by bilateral coni. Both the aortic valve and pulmonary valve are lifted away from the atrioventricular valves by subvalvar coni. (c) When there is no subpulmonary conus the pulmonary valve is in fibrous continuity with the mitral and tricuspid valves. The aortic valve is lifted away from the other three valves by a subaortic conus. This is transposition of the great arteries.*

the spectrum there will be no subpulmonary conus and the aorta comes to lie anterior to the pulmonary artery. There is fibrous continuity between the pulmonary and mitral valves rather than the usual continuity between the aortic and mitral valves. Only the aortic valve is separate from the other three valves. This is transposition of the great arteries (Figure 23.1c).

ANATOMY

Defined simply, DORV is an anomaly in which both vessels arise from the right ventricle. However, to some extent this is also true of tetralogy of Fallot, as, by definition tetralogy includes override of at least some of the aorta over the right ventricle. How then can tetralogy of Fallot and DORV be differentiated? Once again, a simple definition would be that in DORV, at least 50% of the aortic annulus overlies the right ventricle, the so-called '50% rule'[5] For the surgeon this is probably as practically relevant as any definition, although in view of the curved nature of the ventricular septum and the presence of the subaortic ventricular septal defect that accompanies DORV at the tetralogy end of the spectrum, whether the aortic override is 40% or 60% may not be entirely clear. Pathologists have argued that the dividing line between tetralogy of Fallot and DORV can be defined by the presence of aortic to mitral fibrous continuity in tetralogy of Fallot,[4,6] and its absence in DORV. This is not something a surgeon can determine with the usual surgical exposure for DORV. Furthermore, in view of the variable length of the subaortic fibrosa, even in a normal heart, definition of fibrous continuity by two-dimensional echocardiography or angiography is only slightly more precise than assessment of the percentage of override by the surgeon. In any event, the definition is of little relevance to the surgical procedure, which is essentially the same for both tetralogy of Fallot and the tetralogy form of DORV, regardless of the terminology used. Nevertheless the definition is relevant when the results of surgery for DORV are analysed.

At the transposition end of the DORV spectrum, the aorta arises entirely from the right ventricle and the same problem regarding definition must be contemplated for the degree of override of the pulmonary artery over the left ventricle. If more than 50% of the pulmonary artery arises from the left ventricle, then by the 50% rule this is transposition and not DORV. Alternatively, fibrous continuity between the pulmonary valve and the mitral valve can also serve to distinguish transposition from DORV.

Classification of DORV by anatomy of the ventricular septal defect

DORV is virtually always associated with a ventricular septal defect. The classic pathologic classification of DORV centers on the location of the ventricular septal defect relative to the great vessels.[7] Although this is of some relevance to the surgeon, it does not focus on the critical anatomic features that determine the type of surgical procedure to select. Lev et al classified the ventricular septal defects associated with DORV as subaortic, subpulmonary, doubly committed, or noncommitted.[7] The anatomy and physiology of the DORV patient with a subaortic ventricular septal defect are likely to be similar to those of the patient with tetralogy of Fallot, who is also likely to have a subaortic ventricular septal defect (i.e. the ventricular septal defect is positioned immediately below the aortic valve). At the tetralogy end of the DORV spectrum, there is no subaortic conus, so the superior margin of the ventricular septal defect is the aortic annulus itself. Moving through the spectrum of DORV toward transposition there is progressive development of the subaortic conus so that the aortic valve moves cephalad, away from the ventricular septal defect, and the pulmonary valve becomes more intimately associated with the ventricular septal defect. Therefore, at the transposition end of the spectrum, the ventricular septal defect is

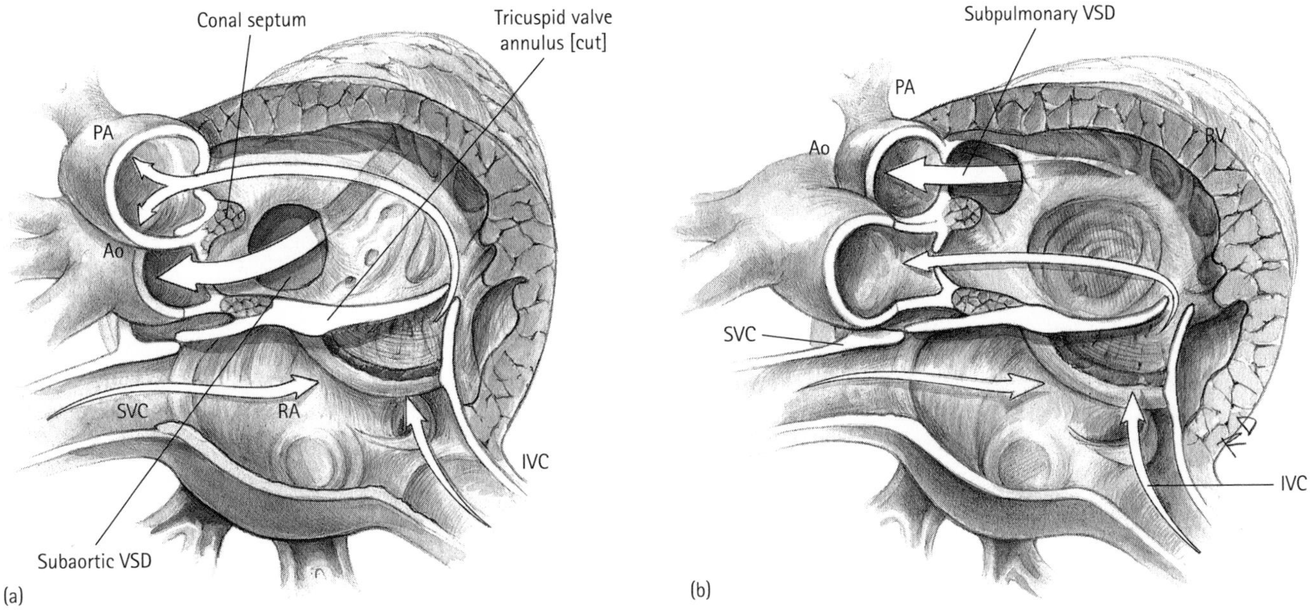

Figure 23.2 *(a) Double outlet right ventricle with subaortic VSD. Physiologically this anomaly is similar to tetralogy of Fallot. Left ventricular blood is predominantly directed to the aorta after passing through a subaortic VSD. (b) Double outlet right ventricle with subpulmonary VSD. Physiologically this anomaly is similar to transposition of the great arteries. Left ventricular blood passes through the subpulmonary VSD into the pulmonary arteries so that oxygen saturation is higher in the pulmonary artery than in the aorta.*

usually subpulmonary. Although this definition was originally designed as an anatomic definition, it probably more accurately serves as a physiologic definition (Figure 23.2) in that left ventricular blood is directed to the aorta after passing through a subaortic ventricular septal defect (Figure 23.2a) (i.e. pulmonary artery saturation will be lower than aortic saturation), while left ventricular blood is directed to the pulmonary artery by a subpulmonary ventricular septal defect (Figure 23.2b) (i.e. pulmonary artery saturation will be higher than aortic saturation, as in transposition).

At the midpoint of the DORV spectrum, a ventricular septal defect may appear to be equally committed to both the aorta and the pulmonary artery; this can be termed a doubly committed ventricular septal defect. As already stated, this does not help the surgeon determine the type of repair. Although this term implies that the surgeon might reasonably choose to use either a tetralogy or transposition type of repair, it is highly unlikely that the two forms of repair would be equally satisfactory.

Any ventricular septal defect that is not situated either within the conal septum (subpulmonary) or at the junction of the conal and muscular interventricular septa (conoventricular or subaortic) is likely to be so remote from the aorta that it will be difficult, if not impossible, to direct left ventricular blood to the aorta. Lev et al termed such ventricular septal defects noncommitted.[7] They frequently occur in the inlet septum (atrioventricular canal type); with an inlet VSD the surgeon must deal not only with the distance separating the aorta from the ventricular septal defect but also with the problem of negotiating a left ventricular baffle pathway around multiple tricuspid valve chordae. Midmuscular and apical muscular ventricular septal defects are also included in the category of noncommitted defects.

Anatomic determinants of method of repair

Despite the definitional problems encountered at both ends of the DORV spectrum, the transition from DORV to transposition, like the transition from tetralogy to DORV, does not interfere with the choice of surgical technique of repair. However, within the DORV spectrum there are points of transition in surgical technique. As stated previously, the type of ventricular septal defect does not help the surgeon select the optimal method of repair. The judgment as to which type of repair is best in a specific anatomic situation constitutes the fundamental complexity of the surgical management of DORV.

SEPARATION OF PULMONARY AND TRICUSPID VALVES

As one progresses from tetralogy into DORV, the repair is identical, whether 49% or 51% of the aorta overlies the right ventricle. The repair is intraventricular (i.e. entirely within the right ventricle); a baffle is constructed that creates a pathway from the left ventricle to the aorta, and the right ventricular outflow tract passes around the left ventricular baffle, but still within the right ventricle (Figure 23.3a). Further into the spectrum, the aorta lies even farther from the left ventricle as it moves cephalad, carried by the subaortic conus. This alone does not exclude an intraventricular repair although a longer tunnel baffle must be constructed. However, there is an associated anatomic shift that eventually precludes an

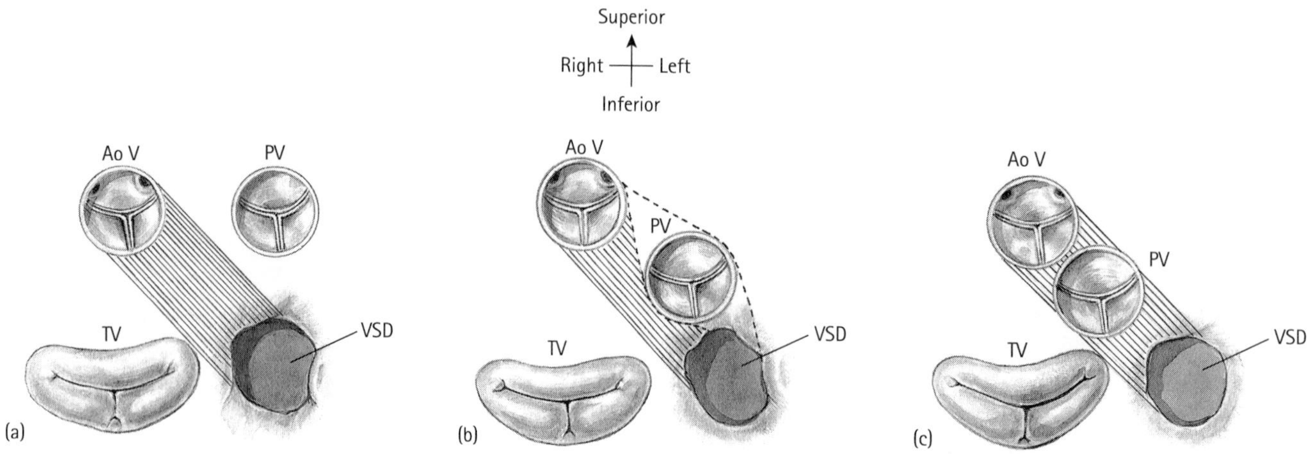

Figure 23.3 *Separation between the tricuspid and pulmonary valves is critical in determining anatomic suitability for an intraventricular baffle repair. (a) There is adequate separation between the pulmonary and tricuspid valves so that the pathway from the VSD to the aorta is unobstructed. (b) Separation of the tricuspid and pulmonary valve is less than the diameter of the aortic annulus. Intraventricular repair is highly likely to result in subaortic stenosis. (c) When the pulmonary valve is very close to the tricuspid valve a Rastelli procedure may be appropriate. The pulmonary valve lies within the baffle pathway necessitating division and oversewing of the main pulmonary artery.*

intraventricular repair. As the aortic valve moves superiorly away from the tricuspid valve, the pulmonary valve moves even closer to the tricuspid valve. Because both the tricuspid and pulmonary valves must, by definition, be within the right ventricle if there is to be an intraventricular repair, and because the baffle pathway from the left ventricle to the aorta must pass between the tricuspid and pulmonary valves, there is a point of transition where the tricuspid to pulmonary distance is significantly less than the diameter of the aortic annulus (Figure 23.3b). Beyond this point, more than 50% of the pathway from the left ventricle to the aorta is made up of the baffle, and although a satisfactory initial result can be achieved, there is a risk that the growth potential with such a repair will be insufficient. Late subaortic tunnel stenosis of the baffle is a difficult problem that should be strenuously avoided.

PROMINENCE OF THE CONAL SEPTUM

The length of the conal septum is largely determined by the degree of development of the subaortic conus, although it is also influenced by the development of the subpulmonary conus. If the ventricular septal defect is more leftward and anterior (i.e. more a subpulmonary than a subaortic ventricular septal defect), it will be necessary for the baffle pathway to follow a longer course around the inferior margin of the conal septum to reach the aortic annulus. A prominent conal septum, per se, does not exclude a tunnel repair, because it may be resected as long as there are not important chordal attachments of the mitral valve (tricuspid chordae may be detached and reattached) (Figure 23.4). However, a long conal septum may be associated with a shorter distance between the tricuspid and pulmonary valves and this may exclude intraventricular repair. A long conal septum – and therefore a long subaortic conus – may be associated with subaortic stenosis, which in turn is often associated with hypoplasia of the aortic arch and coarctation[8].

PRESENCE OF SUBPULMONARY STENOSIS

At the tetralogy end of the DORV spectrum, there is commonly some degree of subpulmonary stenosis. Intraventricular repair must include relief of this stenosis, usually by division of the hypertrophied septal and parietal ends of the conal septum as well as by placement of an infundibular outflow patch and, if necessary for pulmonary annular hypoplasia, a transannular patch. As one progresses toward the middle of the spectrum, there is less likely to be severe subpulmonary stenosis, although the left ventricular baffle pathway will protrude to some extent into the right ventricular outflow tract, necessitating at least an infundibular outflow patch in the right ventricle to prevent iatrogenic obstruction of the right ventricular outflow tract. At the transposition end of the DORV spectrum the left ventricular outflow tract may be stenotic for a number of reasons. There may be a bicuspid pulmonary valve, pulmonary valvar hypoplasia or subpulmonary stenosis. Subpulmonary stenosis can be secondary to posterior deviation of the conal septum or accessory fibrous tissue which may be intimately associated with the mitral valve.

When an intraventricular repair is no longer possible because of the proximity of the pulmonary valve to the tricuspid valve, and when there is important hypoplasia of the pulmonary annulus, a repair similar to the Rastelli repair for transposition must be undertaken (Figure 23.3c). The baffle pathway passes over the pulmonary annulus which is incorporated within the left ventricular pathway. The main pulmonary artery must be divided and is oversewn proximally and a conduit is placed from the right ventricle to the distal divided main pulmonary artery.

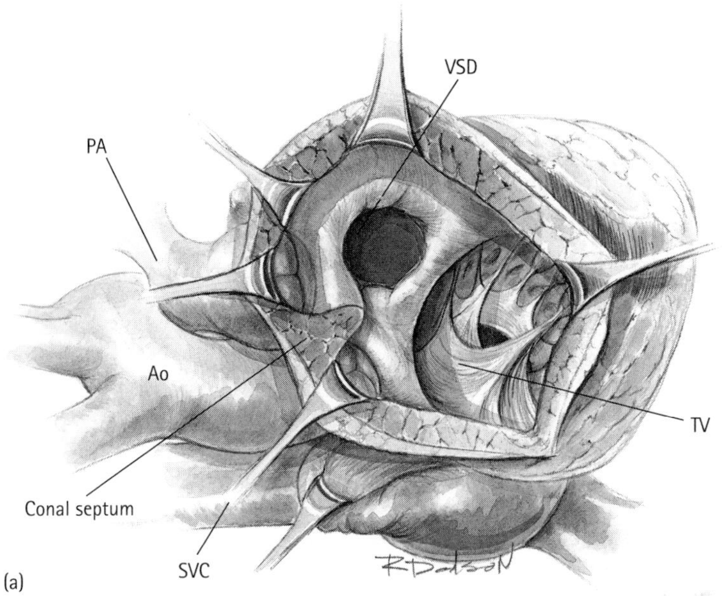

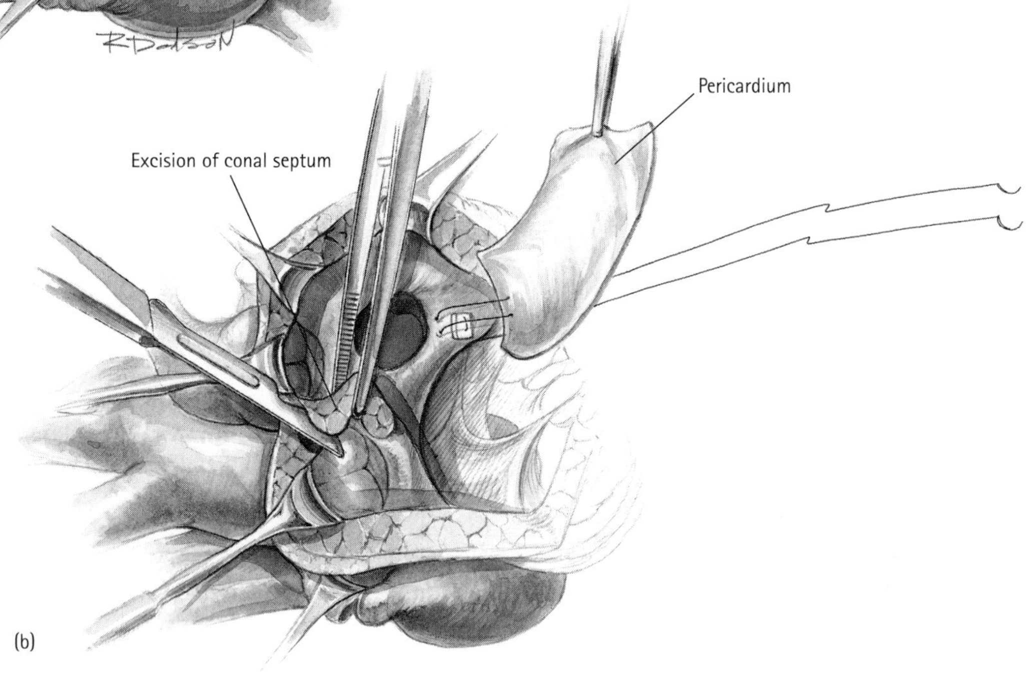

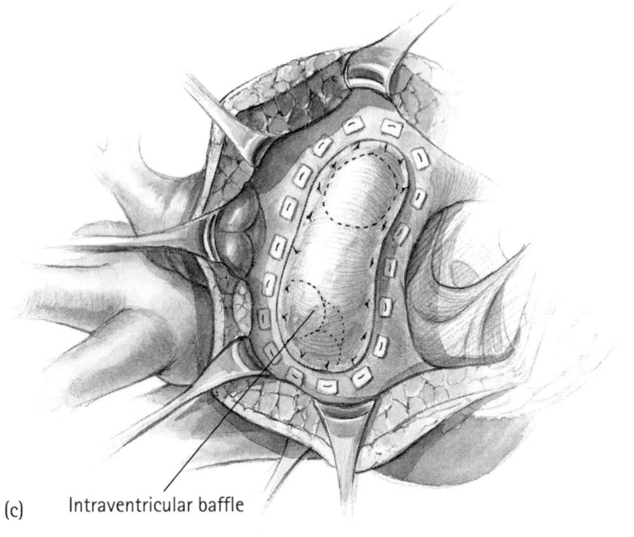

Figure 23.4 *(a) A prominent conal septum may project into the baffle pathway. (b) Resection of the conal septum may be necessary to prevent subaortic stenosis within the baffle pathway. (c) Completion of intraventricular repair with a baffle.*

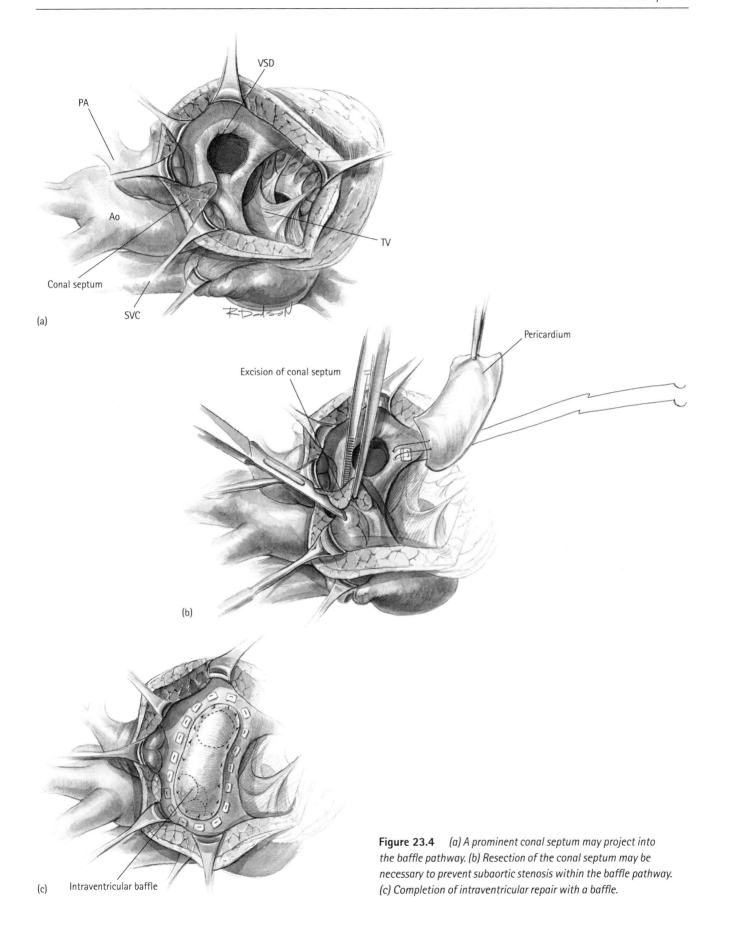

If there is no important subpulmonary or pulmonary annular hypoplasia and the distance between the pulmonary and tricuspid valves excludes an intraventricular repair, an arterial switch procedure should be performed, regardless of the relationship of the great vessels to one another (i.e. whether side by side or more anteroposterior) and regardless of coronary artery anatomy.

CORONARY ARTERY ANATOMY

There is an important difference between the coronary artery anatomy of tetralogy and that of transposition. In transposition, the left main coronary artery and the left anterior descending coronary artery usually pass anterior to the pulmonary root. Conversely, in tetralogy, the left anterior descending coronary usually passes posterior to the pulmonary artery. The presence of a left anterior descending coronary anterior to the pulmonary outflow will generally exclude an intraventricular repair without a conduit, and in any event, it is likely to signify that the defect is closer to the transposition end of the spectrum and that either an arterial switch (if there is no subpulmonary or pulmonary annular hypoplasia) or a Rastelli procedure should be selected.

The Taussig-Bing anomaly

The name 'Taussig-Bing' DORV is applied in at least two different ways and therefore may be confusing. When applied in a physiologic sense, it is a broad term that covers any form of DORV that is physiologically similar to transposition (i.e. the saturation is higher in the pulmonary artery than in the aorta because of a preferential flow pattern from the left ventricle to the pulmonary artery). If used in an anatomic sense, the name is restricted by most authors to a more limited entity that is similar to that originally described by Taussig and Bing in 1949.[9] Van Praagh summarized the anatomic definition in 1968.[4] Subaortic and subpulmonary coni separate both the aortic and the pulmonary valves from the atrioventricular valves. The semilunar valves lie side by side and are at the same height. There is a large subpulmonary ventricular septal defect above the septal band and the muscular ventricular septum. The ventricular septal defect, although subpulmonary, is not confluent with the pulmonary valve, the defect being somewhat separated from the valve by the subpulmonary conal free wall. There is a 'true' DORV, in that the aorta arises entirely above the right ventricle, while the pulmonary valve overrides the ventricular septum but does not override the left ventricular cavity.

ASSOCIATED ANOMALIES

At the transposition end of the DORV spectrum it is not uncommon to find associated coarctation, arch hypoplasia or interrupted aortic arch.[8]

Under these circumstances the ascending aorta is usually at least mildly hypoplastic as is the aortic annulus. The subaortic conus is usually also at least mildly hypoplastic and may be severely hypoplastic. At the tetralogy end of the DORV spectrum it is very unusual to find arch hypoplasia or coarctation.

PATHOPHYSIOLOGY

At the tetralogy end of the DORV spectrum, pathophysiology is similar to that in tetralogy. If there is only a mild degree of obstruction in the right ventricular outflow tract, there may be a left to right shunt, as in 'pink tetralogy.' If there is severe, fixed pulmonary stenosis, there will be a consistent right to left shunt, and the child may be severely cyanosed. Infundibular stenosis raises the possibility of intermittent, severe obstruction of the right ventricular outflow tract, causing spells similar to those seen with tetralogy.

At the transposition end of the DORV spectrum, pathophysiology resembles that in transposition (i.e. there are two parallel circulations, and the systemic saturation is determined by the degree of mixing between these circulations). Because there is almost always a nonrestrictive ventricular septal defect, the systemic arterial oxygen saturation is usually not a problem unless there is associated pulmonary stenosis. The presence of subaortic stenosis or coarctation will exacerbate the elevated pulmonary blood flow.

Just as for transposition with a nonrestrictive ventricular septal defect, there is a significant risk at the transposition end of the DORV spectrum of accelerated development of pulmonary vascular disease during the first year of life.[10] At the tetralogy end of the spectrum, the degree of subpulmonary stenosis will determine the risk of pulmonary vascular disease, which will clearly be low if the degree of obstruction is severe.

CLINICAL FEATURES AND DIAGNOSTIC STUDIES

The type of symptoms and the age at which they appear are largely determined by the degree of pulmonary stenosis. In most cases it will be evident that the child has a congenital heart anomaly during the neonatal period. Echocardiography can almost always provide adequate diagnostic information in the neonate and young infant. Only in the older infant or young child may catheterization be necessary to exclude the presence of pulmonary vascular disease although at the transposition end of the spectrum it is useful to undertake a balloon atrial septostomy preoperatively to improve mixing and, therefore, the oxygen saturation and stability of the child.

Preoperative studies should accurately determine the surgically relevant features that have already been described.

At the tetralogy end of the spectrum, the separation of the pulmonary valve from the tricuspid valve must be measured relative to the diameter of the aortic annulus. The location of the ventricular septal defect, including the degree of development of the conal septum, should be determined. Chordal attachments to the conal septum should be visualized, and the degree of subpulmonary and pulmonary stenosis should be assessed. A judgment should be made as to whether the subpulmonary stenosis might be dynamic rather than fixed. Coronary anatomy should be defined (by echocardiography), and the relative sizes of the great vessels and their relationship (whether side by side or anteroposterior) should be determined. The aortic arch should be inspected for the presence of hypoplasia or coarctation. Of course, preoperative studies should also exclude associated anomalies such as multiple ventricular septal defects and atrioventricular valve anomalies.

MEDICAL AND INTERVENTIONAL CATHETER MANAGEMENT

If pulmonary stenosis is minimal so that pulmonary blood flow is increased, it may be useful to begin giving the child decongestive medication and digoxin. However, there seems little point in aggressively pursuing medical therapy when surgical repair can be effectively undertaken early in infancy.

At the transposition end of the DORV spectrum balloon atrial septostomy is recommended. Not only does this improve mixing but in addition intraoperative management of the child is made easier if a preoperative balloon septostomy has been performed. The atrial septal defect allows decompression of the left side of the heart by placement of a single venous cannula in the right atrium; this provides a surgical field free from left heart return if the procedure is performed with continuous, low flow hypothermic bypass.

INDICATIONS FOR AND TIMING OF SURGERY

Because DORV does not resolve spontaneously, the diagnosis is sufficient indication for surgery. The usual arguments regarding the timing of surgery can be applied and have been described in detail in Chapter 1. Currently we prefer to undertake repair during the neonatal period, regardless of the specific form of DORV. This also applies in situations where a conduit will be necessary, for example, when there is pulmonary annular hypoplasia and an intraventricular repair is not feasible. Although a systemic-to-pulmonary shunt is a reasonable alternative in this setting, it does not reduce the total number of operations that will be necessary, and it does impose a period of abnormal physiology that has been demonstrated, in some circumstances, to prejudice the quality of the final outcome.

SURGICAL MANAGEMENT

History

Repair of a DORV with a subaortic ventricular septal defect (tetralogy type) was first performed by Kirklin and associates in 1957[11] and shortly thereafter in 1958 by Barratt-Boyes and coworkers.[12] For some time the transposition end of the DORV spectrum was confused with transposition; therefore, it is difficult to determine when the first repairs of this anomaly were undertaken. Early reports include those by Kirklin, Kawashima, and Patrick and their associates.[11,13,14] Other important contributors to the understanding of the surgical management of DORV were Pacifico and Lecompte.[15,16]

Technical considerations

INTRAVENTRICULAR REPAIR FOR TETRALOGY TO MID-SPECTRUM DORV

The general setup and approach to this form of DORV are the same as those used for tetralogy of Fallot. After a median sternotomy, a generous patch of anterior pericardium is harvested and treated with 0.6% glutaraldehyde solution for 20–30 minutes. Either circulatory arrest or continuous bypass may be selected, although for more complex intraventricular baffles, it is generally wise to use continuous bypass to avoid an excessively long period of circulatory arrest. After application of the aortic cross clamp and administration of cardioplegic solution, an infundibular incision is made (Figure 23.5a; note that the figures exaggerate the length of the ventriculotomy to allow visualization of intracardiac structures). As in tetralogy, great care is taken to preserve as many coronary arteries as possible. Often, there is a long conal coronary artery that may reach well toward the apex of the heart. It is important that the infundibular incision is carefully planned to preserve this artery.

The relationship of the aortic annulus to the ventricular septal defect is carefully defined, and the length of the conal septum is assessed with respect to both the aortic and pulmonary valves. The presence of tricuspid chordal attachments to the conal septum is noted. The anatomy of the subpulmonary stenosis is also defined. Usually, excision of the conal septum helps to relieve the subpulmonary stenosis to some degree (Figure 23.4b). If there are chordal attachments, these may be reattached to the patch on the ventricular septal defect at a later time. Close to the tetralogy end of the spectrum, simple division of the septal and parietal extensions of the conal septum will relieve subpulmonary stenosis when performed with subsequent placement of an infundibular outflow patch. Until reaching the mid-point of the DORV spectrum, there should be a sufficient distance separating the pulmonary and tricuspid valves to allow a tunnel repair to be constructed.

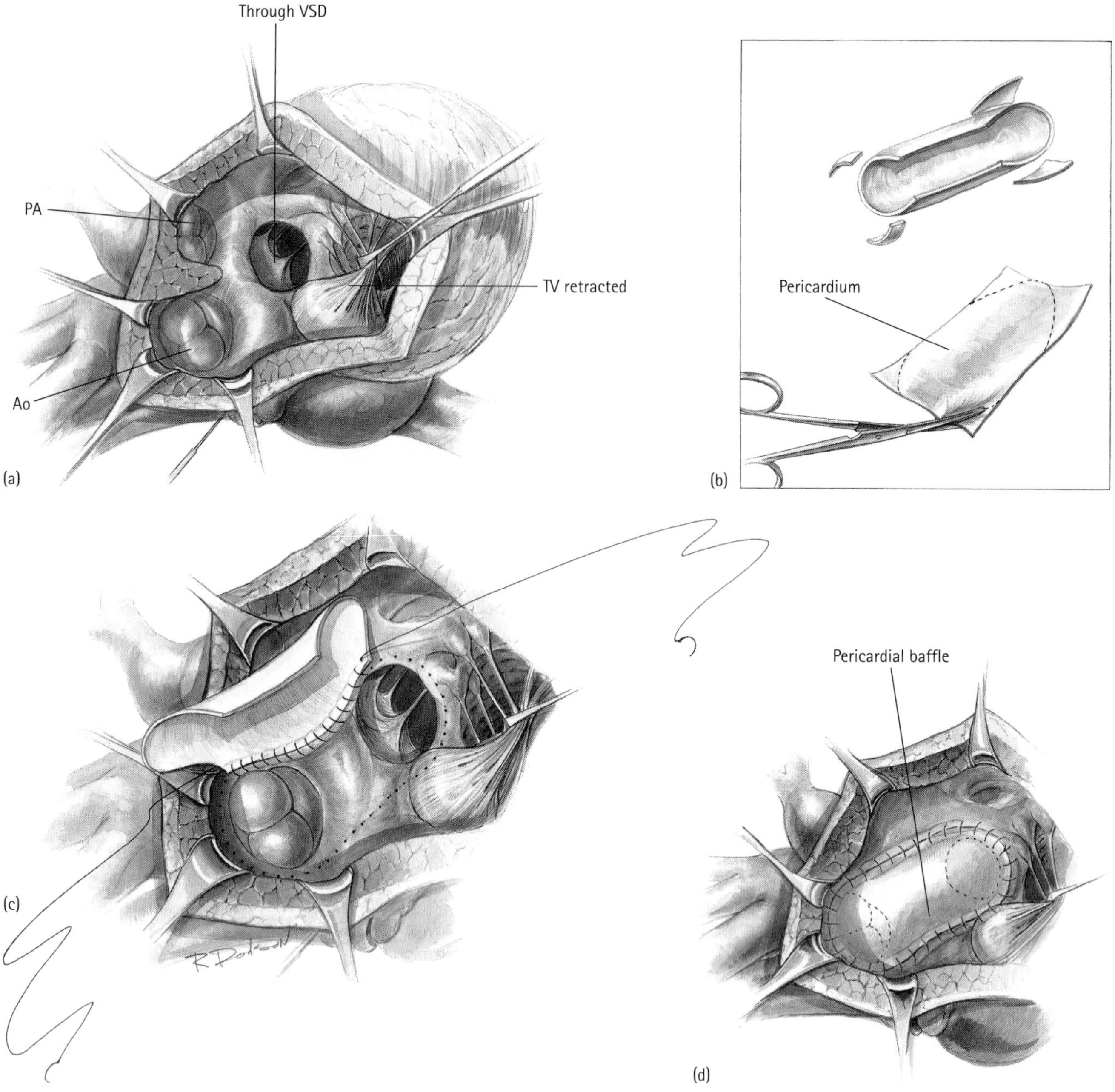

Figure 23.5 *(a) Intraventricular repair of double outlet right ventricle with a subaortic VSD that is moderately distant from the aortic annulus. (b) Autologous pericardium is preferred for baffle construction (or 'stretch' PTFE). Both these materials are less likely to acquire a thick fibrous pseudointima than Dacron. There is also greater pliability of the baffle so that a kink is less likely to project into the central point of the pathway. (c) Beyond infancy the baffle pathway may be so long that it is impractical to use interrupted pledgetted sutures. A running technique is a reasonable alternative. (d) The completed left ventricle to aorta baffle pathway as part of an intraventricular repair of DORV.*

Sutures are placed around the circumference of the baffle pathway using the standard pledgetted, horizontal mattress technique that we generally prefer in neonates and infants. In older children the circumference of the baffle is so great that it is generally impractical to use all interrupted sutures, and a continuous suture technique is necessary (Figure 23.5c). In infants the friability of the muscle may result in an unacceptable incidence of residual ventricular septal defect if a continuous suture technique is used, and in any event, the circumference is very much shorter than in the older child.

Although a flat patch of knitted Dacron velour is used when the ventricular septal defect is closely related to the aortic annulus, i.e. close to the tetralogy end of the spectrum, consideration should be given to the use of autologous pericardium when the patch becomes a baffle creating a tunnel rather than a simple flat patch (Figure 23.5b). PTFE is also a better option than Dacron for a long baffle.

Particular care must be taken at the mid-point of the baffle tunnel to ensure that a 'waist' is not created where the pulmonary valve begins to approach the tricuspid valve. Care must also be taken at the site of excision of the conal septum, where lack of the endocardium may increase the risk that sutures will tear out of the raw muscle surface. As is the case with closure of the anterior malalignment ventricular septal defect of tetralogy, great care should be taken with the placement of sutures as one passes around the aortic annulus. Muscle trabeculations often extend up to the annulus, creating 'ridges and valleys.' Failure to place sutures virtually in the annulus (taking great care not to injure the leaflets) may result in a residual ventricular septal defect through the 'valleys.'

Relief of subpulmonary stenosis is largely achieved by division of the septal and parietal extensions of the conal septum with or without excision of the conal septum itself. The ventricular incision should virtually never be closed by direct suture, as such closure will necessarily consume some of the circumference of the right ventricular outflow tract. A patch of autologous pericardium is used to close the incision, employing a continuous Prolene suture. If the pulmonary annulus is too small, it may be necessary to place a transannular patch. The decision process used for DORV is the same as that used for tetralogy (see Chapter 16).

THE RASTELLI AND REV REPAIRS FOR MID-SPECTRUM TO TRANSPOSITION-LIKE DORV WITH SUBPULMONARY STENOSIS AND/OR INADEQUATE PULMONARY TO TRICUSPID VALVE SEPARATION

When the pulmonary valve is so close to the tricuspid valve that there is a significant risk that either early or late subaortic stenosis may be created within a tunnel repair (Figure 23.3b), it is necessary to place the baffle over both the pulmonary and aortic valves, as described by Rastelli[17] for transposition with a ventricular septal defect and pulmonary stenosis (Figure 23.6b). The main pulmonary artery should be divided (not ligated) and may be connected distally to the right ventricle using either a pulmonary or aortic allograft conduit (Rastelli repair) (Figure 23.6c). The pulmonary valve should be excised and the proximal divided main pulmonary artery oversewn.

An alternative to the use of an allograft or synthetic conduit for the Rastelli type of repair is wide mobilization of the pulmonary arteries, as for the arterial switch repair, followed by direct suture of the main pulmonary artery to the right ventriculotomy (Figure 23.7c). This technique was first described by Lecompte and the group from Hopital Laennec, Paris,[18] and has been termed *reparation a l'etage ventriculaire* (REV). Anteriorly the repair is completed by placement of a generous patch of pericardium (Figure 23.7d). To achieve the so-called 'Lecompte maneuver' as part of the REV repair, it is necessary to divide the ascending aorta (Figure 23.7a). The aorta is reconstituted by direct anastomosis with continuous polydioxanone sutures. When the great arteries are related directly anterior a nd posterior, it is useful to bring both pulmonary artery branches anterior to the aorta, using the Lecompte maneuver (Figure 23.7b).[19] If this is not done, either the right or the left pulmonary artery must traverse an excessively long course around the aorta, depending on whether the main pulmonary artery is brought around the left side or the right side of the aorta once the aorta has been moved posteriorly. The advantage of the Lecompte maneuver – less distance that the pulmonary artery branch must reach – is considerable for anteroposterior great arteries, being at least $\pi/2 \times$ aortic diameter.

When the great vessels take up a more side by side relationship (as one moves from the transposition end of the DORV spectrum toward the tetralogy end), the advantage of the Lecompte maneuver decreases, but it is probably still useful until the aorta lies in a plane posterior to the main pulmonary artery. It is not possible to establish a rule as to when to apply the Lecompte maneuver, because not only are the pulmonary arteries being translocated in an anteroposterior direction, but there is also translocation in a superoinferior plane onto the anterior right ventricular free wall. The amount of superoinferior movement necessary will be determined by the development of the right ventricular infundibulum, as well as the distribution of the coronary arteries, which will determine the location of the right ventriculotomy. In addition, careful consideration must be given to the relationship of the anterior coronary artery (usually the right coronary artery as it arises from the aorta) to the main pulmonary artery. Because the pulmonary artery will be under some degree of tension, it must not lie directly on the coronary artery, as this may cause unacceptable compression. In a report of 40 cases of REV by Vouhe et al,[20] the mortality rate was 12.5%, highlighting the additional risks that may be inherent in this procedure.

CORONARY ARTERY ANTERIOR TO THE INFUNDIBULUM

If the anterior descending coronary artery passes across the infundibulum at its narrowest point, this may present a contraindication to the standard intraventricular repair of DORV without a conduit. The right ventricular incision must be placed lower in the right ventricular free wall. Continuity between the right ventricle and the pulmonary arteries is generally established by the placement of a conduit – usually an aortic allograft, as a pulmonary allograft is unlikely to be sufficiently long. The REV procedure usually is not feasible in this setting because of the long distance separating the ventriculotomy from the pulmonary arteries. In addition, the severe tension that would result from the distance required for translocation might cause serious compression of the anteriorly placed coronary.

AORTIC TRANSLOCATION (NIKAIDOH PROCEDURE)

An alternative procedure for DORV or transposition with pulmonary stenosis, including pulmonary annular hypoplasia, is aortic translocation with reconstruction of the right ventricular outflow tract.[21] The aortic root, including the aortic valve, is excised from the right ventricular outflow tract in a manner analogous to that applied for the Ross pulmonary autograft operation. In addition, it is usually necessary to

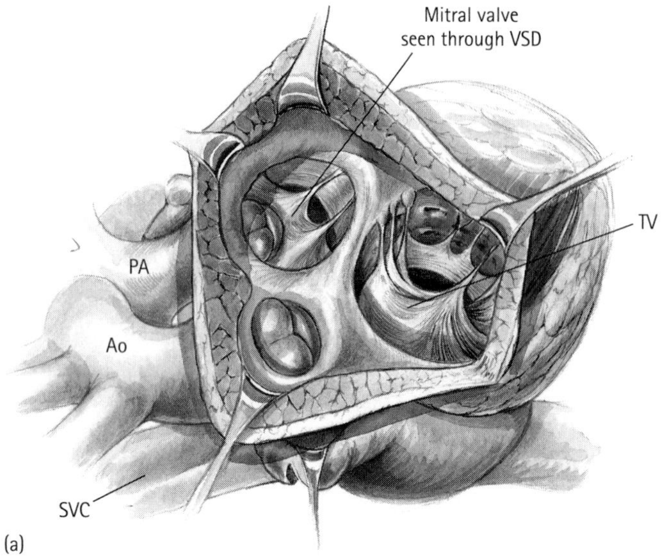

(a)

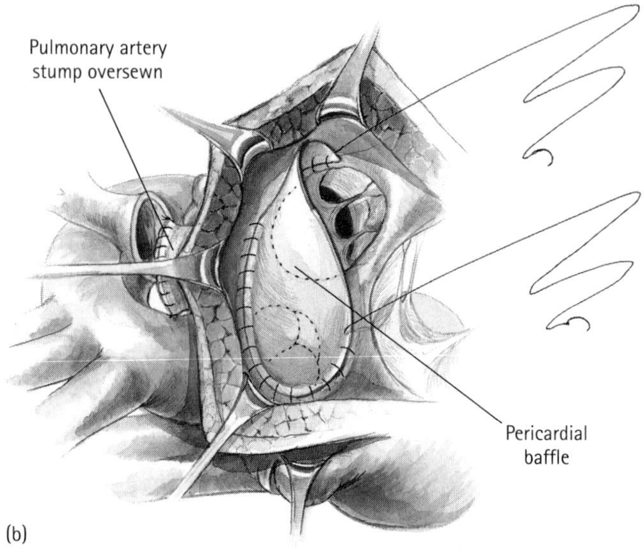

(b)

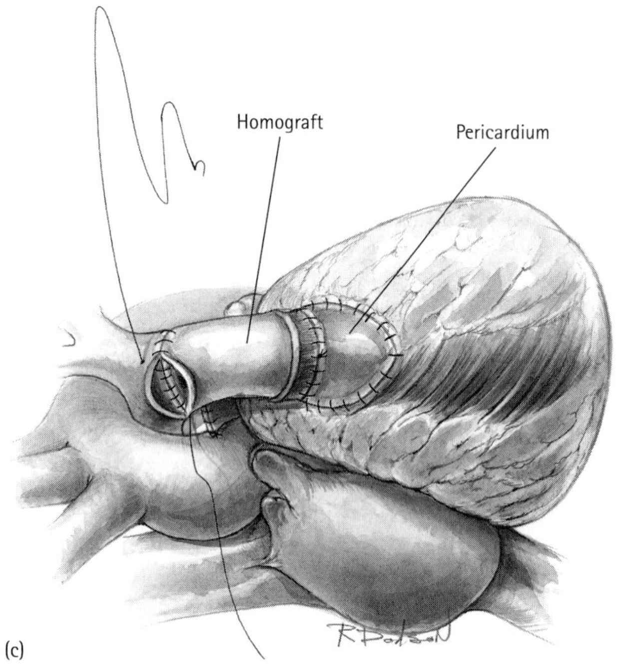

(c)

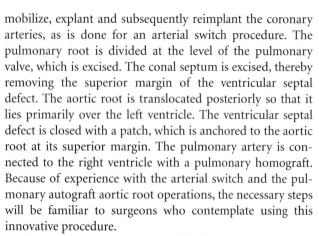

Figure 23.6 *Rastelli repair for DORV. (a) This patient is close to the transposition end of the DORV spectrum so that the pulmonary valve is almost in fibrous continuity with the mitral valve. (b) The main pulmonary artery has been divided, the pulmonary valve has been excised and the stump of the proximal main pulmonary artery has been oversewn. A pericardial or stretch PTFE baffle is being sutured into place to direct left ventricular blood through the VSD to the aorta. The former pulmonary outflow is incorporated under the baffle. (c) The Rastelli repair is completed by placing a homograft conduit between the right ventricle and distal divided main pulmonary artery.*

mobilize, explant and subsequently reimplant the coronary arteries, as is done for an arterial switch procedure. The pulmonary root is divided at the level of the pulmonary valve, which is excised. The conal septum is excised, thereby removing the superior margin of the ventricular septal defect. The aortic root is translocated posteriorly so that it lies primarily over the left ventricle. The ventricular septal defect is closed with a patch, which is anchored to the aortic root at its superior margin. The pulmonary artery is connected to the right ventricle with a pulmonary homograft. Because of experience with the arterial switch and the pulmonary autograft aortic root operations, the necessary steps will be familiar to surgeons who contemplate using this innovative procedure.

The principal advantage of the Nikaidoh procedure is that the homograft is placed more posteriorly than is the case for the Rastelli procedure and is therefore less prone to sternal compression. However, there is some risk of late deterioration of aortic valve function and coronary artery patency.

ARTERIAL SWITCH PROCEDURE

In view of the consistent association of DORV with a ventricular septal defect, as well as the known poor results of atrial inversion procedures such as the Senning and Mustard operations when combined with ventricular septal defect closure (see Chapter 15), it is highly unlikely that circumstances could arise in which an atrial inversion procedure would be indicated for the management of DORV at the transposition end of the DORV spectrum. In contrast to the poor results achieved with atrial inversion procedures, excellent results have been achieved with the arterial switch procedure for DORV, although many institutions experienced a learning curve in translating this procedure to the specific anatomic requirements of DORV.

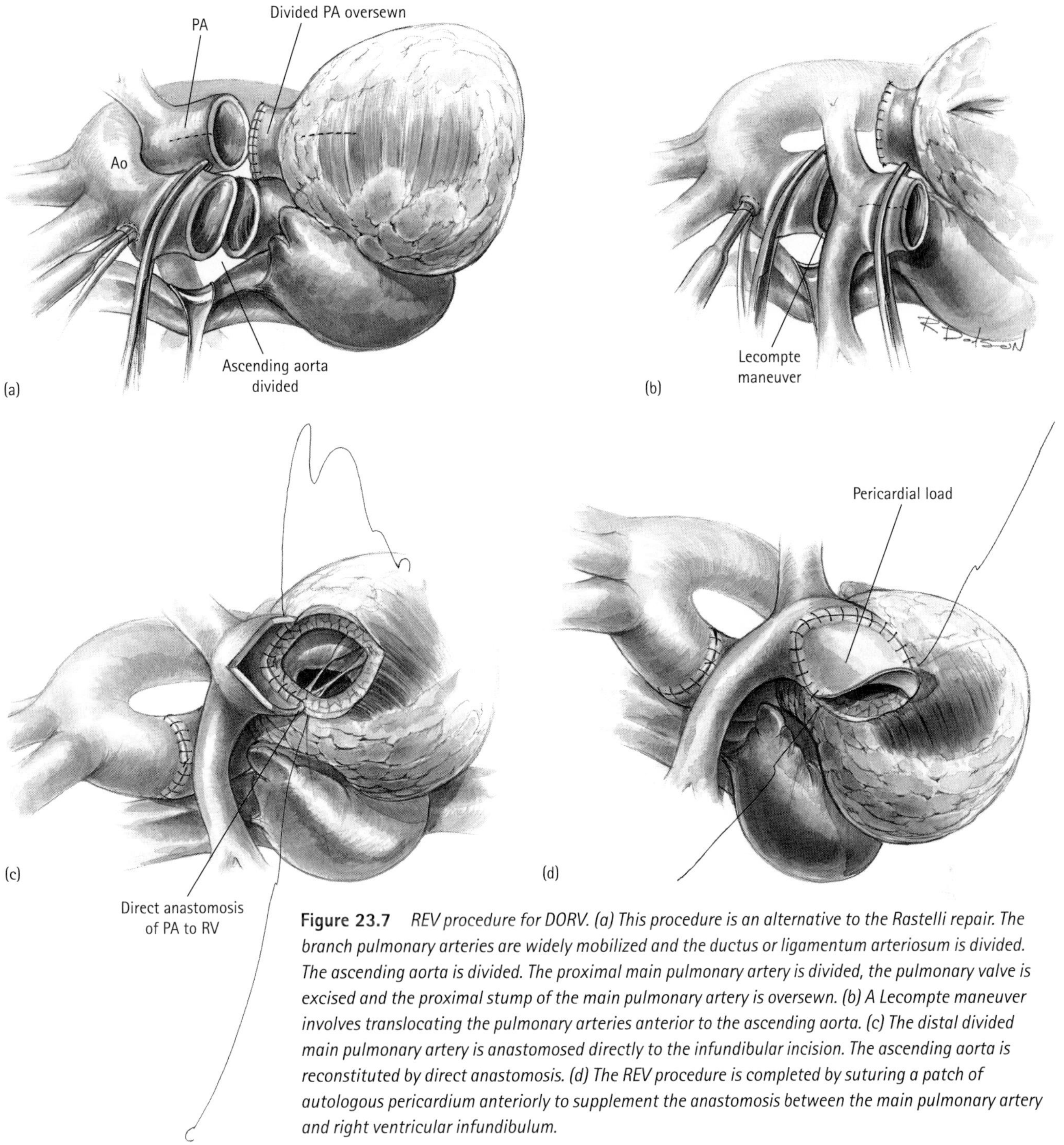

Figure 23.7 *REV procedure for DORV. (a) This procedure is an alternative to the Rastelli repair. The branch pulmonary arteries are widely mobilized and the ductus or ligamentum arteriosum is divided. The ascending aorta is divided. The proximal main pulmonary artery is divided, the pulmonary valve is excised and the proximal stump of the main pulmonary artery is oversewn. (b) A Lecompte maneuver involves translocating the pulmonary arteries anterior to the ascending aorta. (c) The distal divided main pulmonary artery is anastomosed directly to the infundibular incision. The ascending aorta is reconstituted by direct anastomosis. (d) The REV procedure is completed by suturing a patch of autologous pericardium anteriorly to supplement the anastomosis between the main pulmonary artery and right ventricular infundibulum.*

An arterial switch procedure is indicated at the transposition end of the DORV spectrum when there is little or no pulmonary or subpulmonary stenosis. It may be possible to resect muscular or fibrous tissue including accessory mitral valve tissue from the subpulmonary region as long as there are no important chordal attachments of the mitral valve to the narrow area, thereby allowing an arterial switch even when moderate subpulmonary stenosis is present. Similarly, a bicuspid pulmonary valve should not be considered an absolute contraindication to an arterial switch, particularly if the alternative procedures carry significant short-term or long-term risks, such as a high early and late mortality risk for an atrial inversion procedure or the lesser quality of life dictated by the use of a conduit.

The general principles of the arterial switch operation for DORV are identical to those employed in the operation for transposition. The procedure is generally performed using low flow hypothermic bypass though the intracardiac steps (i.e. closure of the atrial and ventricular septal defects) may on occasion be performed during a period of circulatory arrest, which can be kept to less than 30–40 minutes.

Division of the great arteries is followed by inspection of the pulmonary valve and left ventricular outflow tract to ensure that there is no important outflow tract obstruction

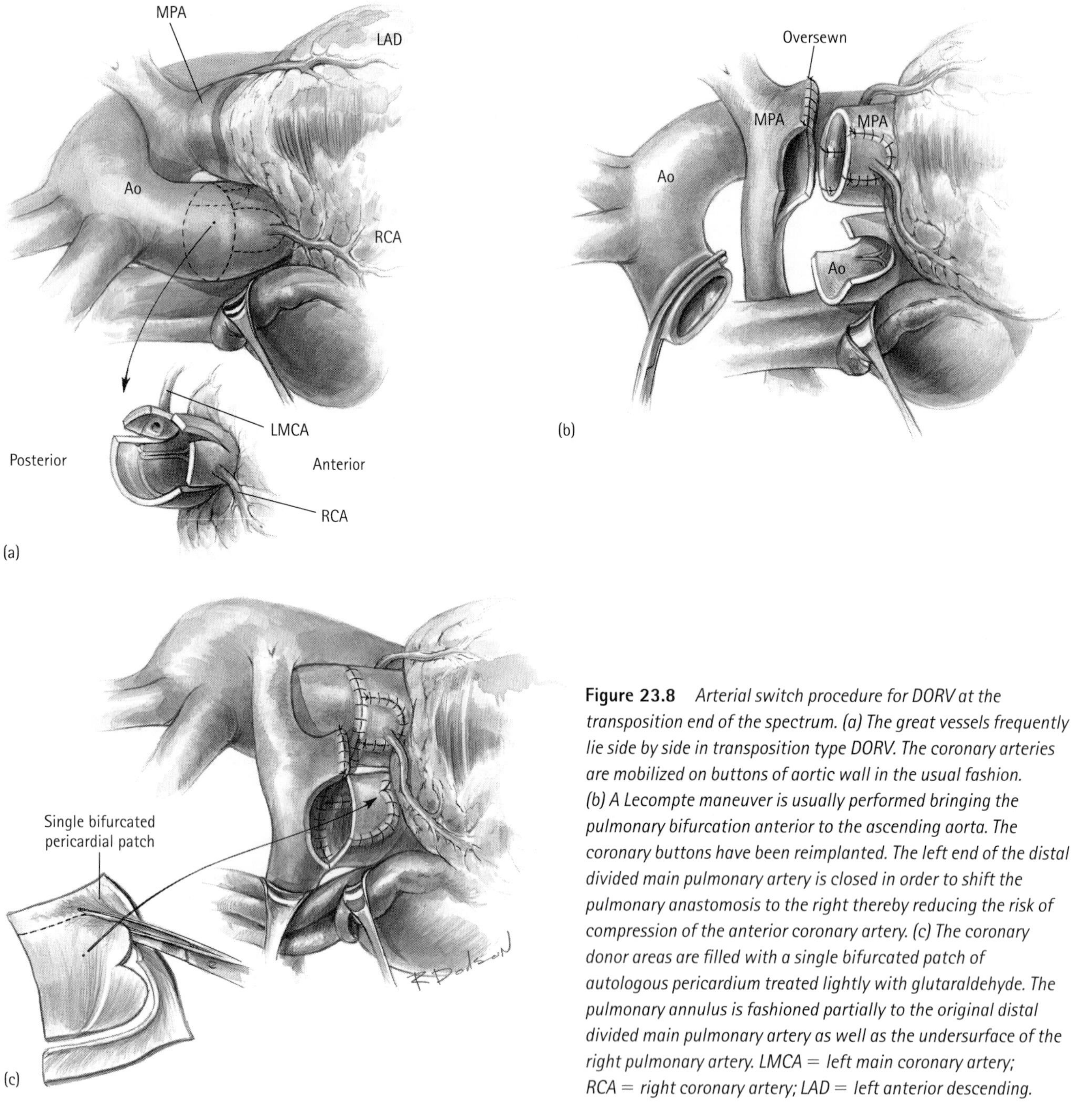

Figure 23.8 *Arterial switch procedure for DORV at the transposition end of the spectrum. (a) The great vessels frequently lie side by side in transposition type DORV. The coronary arteries are mobilized on buttons of aortic wall in the usual fashion. (b) A Lecompte maneuver is usually performed bringing the pulmonary bifurcation anterior to the ascending aorta. The coronary buttons have been reimplanted. The left end of the distal divided main pulmonary artery is closed in order to shift the pulmonary anastomosis to the right thereby reducing the risk of compression of the anterior coronary artery. (c) The coronary donor areas are filled with a single bifurcated patch of autologous pericardium treated lightly with glutaraldehyde. The pulmonary annulus is fashioned partially to the original distal divided main pulmonary artery as well as the undersurface of the right pulmonary artery. LMCA = left main coronary artery; RCA = right coronary artery; LAD = left anterior descending.*

that might increase the risks of an arterial switch. Coronary mobilization and transfer are performed, followed by the aortic anastomosis (Figure 23.8b). It is preferable not to undertake closure of the intracardiac communications before these steps are taken, as the ASD and VSD will allow venting of left heart return to the single right atrial cannula. A single venous cannula is thus preferred to two caval cannulas.

The ventricular septal defect may be approached through the anterior semilunar valve, through the right atrium, or occasionally through a right ventriculotomy, as determined by the specific anatomic situation. Often there is some element of subaortic narrowing, so a right ventricular infundibular incision serves a dual purpose: access for closure of the ventricular septal defect as well as for placement of an infundibular outflow patch to relieve outflow tract obstruction. Approach through the semilunar valve or ventriculotomy usually allows continuation of bypass throughout closure of the ventricular septal defect. The atrial septal defect is closed through a short, low, right atriotomy. The left heart is filled with saline to exclude air before tying the suture.

With bypass re-established, the aortic cross clamp is released. Perfusion of all areas of the myocardium is checked. A single large pericardial patch is used to reconstruct the coronary donor areas, although to obtain optimal exposure, this step may be performed before the intracardiac steps (Figure 23.8c). It is important that the pericardial patch actually supplement the neopulmonary artery (i.e. the patch needs to be quite a bit larger than the excised coronary buttons, because the aorta is frequently somewhat smaller than the pulmonary artery, particularly if there is a long and somewhat narrow subaortic conus). The pulmonary anastomosis is fashioned, and the patient is weaned from bypass.

VARIATIONS OF THE ARTERIAL SWITCH OPERATION FOR DORV

Coronary patterns

Unusual coronary patterns are much more common with side by side great arteries than in standard transposition with anteroposterior great arteries.[22] A common pattern is an anterior origin of the right main coronary and left anterior descending coronary arteries from a single ostium, with the circumflex originating from a posterior facing sinus. Extensive mobilization of the right coronary is necessary to prevent tethering of the anterior coronary, which must be transferred directly away from the line of the right coronary. Conal and right ventricular free wall branches of the right and anterior descending coronaries should be extensively mobilized from their epicardial beds to prevent tension on the arteries and on the anastomosis. On occasion, we have used an autologous pericardial tube extension of the coronary artery to avoid excessive tension (see Chapter 15). Excessive tension will be manifested by persistent bleeding from the coronary anastomosis and early or late coronary insufficiency. Another common coronary pattern with side by side great arteries is origin of the right and circumflex coronaries from the posterior sinus, with the left anterior descending artery originating from the anterior-facing sinus. As will be discussed below (see 'Pulmonary artery anastomosis'), it is important to guard against compression of the anteriorly transferred coronary by the posterior wall of the main pulmonary artery.

Closure of the ventricular septal defect

Exposure of the ventricular septal defect associated with DORV may present special difficulties. The defect may be quite leftward and anterior in what almost appears, from the surgeon's perspective, to be a separate, leftward, blind-ending infundibular recess. Exposure through the anterior semilunar valve and right atrium is particularly difficult, and even through a right ventriculotomy may not be easy. Although exposure may be achieved of the left ventricular aspect of the VSD through the original pulmonary valve (neoaortic), this is usually not recommended because of the risk of damage to the conduction system and the neoaortic valve. An additional complication to ventricular septal defect closure in this setting is the tendency for the very leftward ventricular septal defect to extend into the anterior trabeculated septum, i.e. there appears to be no clear leftward anterior margin to the defect. However, by taking large bites with pledgetted sutures, the size of any residual ventricular septal defect can be minimized. Catheter-delivered devices have been useful for ultimate closure of residual ventricular septal defects in this area.[23,24]

Multiple ventricular septal defects

Surgical closure of multiple muscular ventricular septal defects as well as of the large subpulmonary ventricular septal defect may be difficult and may consume an excessive amount of circulatory arrest time. One approach to this problem is intraoperative delivery of a double-clamshell device[25].

After division of the two great vessels, an excellent view is obtained of both sides of the ventricular septum. The sheath loaded with the device is introduced through the right atrium and tricuspid valve into the right ventricle. A right-angled instrument is passed through the original pulmonary valve into the left ventricle, through the ventricular septal defect, and into the right ventricle, where it grasps the delivery pod. The pod is drawn into the left ventricle, and the left ventricular arms are released under direct vision.

The pod is then carefully pulled back into the right ventricle, and, viewing through the original aortic valve into the right ventricle, the right ventricular arms are released. If necessary, multiple devices may be placed. Although this system has worked well for children weighing more than 4–5 kg, the delivery pod requires further modification for neonates and infants weighing less than 4 kg.

Pulmonary artery anastomosis

Although the Lecompte maneuver is uniformly useful for patients with standard transposition in which the great arteries are positioned anteroposteriorly (or relatively close to this), for side by side great arteries judgment is required in deciding whether translocation of the right pulmonary artery anterior to the aorta will be useful in decreasing tension on the right pulmonary artery. In general, if the aorta is the slightest bit anterior to the pulmonary artery, a Lecompte maneuver should be performed. Another consideration in this decision, other than just the tension on the right pulmonary artery, is the relationship of the transferred coronary arteries to the pulmonary artery. Care must be taken to ensure that there is no compression of the coronary arteries.

A useful maneuver to minimize the risk of coronary compression, as well as to decrease the tension on the pulmonary artery anastomosis, is to shift the anastomosis somewhat from the original distal divided main pulmonary artery into the right pulmonary artery. The leftward end of the main pulmonary artery is closed (usually by direct suture, although the pericardial patch used to fill the coronary donor areas may be extended here), and the orifice is extended into the right pulmonary artery (Figure 23.8b,c). In other respects the anastomosis is performed in the usual fashion. This maneuver has the effect of shifting the main pulmonary artery rightward so that it will not lie anterior to the aorta, where it would likely cause compression of the anteriorly transferred coronary artery.

Repair with noncommitted ventricular septal defect

The most common form of noncommitted ventricular septal defect is the atrioventricular canal type, which extends under the septal leaflet of the tricuspid valve. Some authors[26,27] have suggested that when this defect occurs with pulmonary stenosis (which precludes an arterial switch), the procedure of choice is patch closure of the ventricular septal defect with creation of a generous anterior and superior extension. The ventricular septal defect extension is then baffled to the aorta as for the standard intraventricular repair described previously. In view of the known tendency for surgically created ventricular septal defects to close spontaneously, as well as the inherent risk of creating subaortic stenosis with the tunnel repair, we have generally avoided this approach. If the child's hemodynamics are ideal for a Fontan procedure as they usually are because of the presence of natural pulmonary stenosis, we often choose that approach rather than an atrial-level repair or other complex bi-ventricular repairs employing a conduit.

Repair of associated subaortic stenosis and arch anomalies

The long subaortic conus associated with DORV toward the transposition end of the spectrum may cause some degree of subaortic stenosis pre-repair. Not surprisingly, aortic arch hypoplasia and coarctation often accompany such subaortic stenosis. There is likely to be considerable disparity between the diameters of the great vessels. The coronary transfer should be undertaken in the usual fashion, using low flow bypass. The circulation is then arrested, and the aortic cross clamp is removed. An incision is made along the lesser curve of the ascending aorta and arch, extending across the coarctation. (We no longer place tourniquets around the arch vessels but place the patient in a mild Trendelenberg position to avoid cerebral air.) A long patch of pericardium is sutured into this aortotomy, which serves to minimize the disparity between the proximal neoaorta and the distal ascending aorta. The aortic cross clamp is reapplied, and bypass may be recommenced. The remainder of the procedure is undertaken as described previously. We do not favor coarctation repair with pulmonary artery banding as a preliminary palliative procedure.

RESULTS OF SURGERY

In 2001 Takeuchi et al[28] reported the results of a seven-year experience at Children's Hospital between 1992 and 1999 of patients with double outlet right ventricle and subpulmonary VSD. Twelve of the 32 patients were considered unsuitable for an arterial switch procedure and underwent a bidirectional Glenn procedure followed by a modified Fontan. There were no deaths in the single ventricle group. Four patients in the arterial switch group died early. Two of them had a single coronary artery, one had a straddling mitral valve and one had a hypoplastic aortic arch and one had multiple VSDs. Actuarial survival for the entire group at five years was 87%. The authors concluded that although the arterial switch procedure is the operation of first choice for patients with DORV and a subpulmonary VSD, nevertheless there are a number of important anatomical risk factors which should be taken into account in choosing between the arterial switch and a single ventricle pathway. The results of the single ventricle pathway for these patients who have two well developed ventricles is excellent.

In 1994 Aoki et al[29] reviewed the 10 year experience between 1981 and 1991 at Children's Hospital Boston with biventricular repair of double outlet right ventricle. A total of 73 patients underwent surgery during this timeframe. The authors classified patients using the Lev method of ventricular septal defect location. Figure 23.9 illustrates the types of VSD and their frequency as well as associated anomalies. Normal coronary anatomy was found in the majority of patients with subaortic and doubly committed VSDs. Patients with subpulmonary and noncommitted VSDs had a wide variety of coronary anatomy. Patients with subpulmonary and noncommitted VSDs also had a higher prevalence of aortic arch obstruction. A tricuspid to pulmonary annulus distance equal to or greater than the diameter of the aortic annulus was a useful predictor of the possibility of achieving a conventional intraventricular tunnel type repair. A tricuspid to pulmonary annular distance sufficient for intraventricular tunnel repair was most likely in patients with a rightward and posterior or rightward side by side aorta. Five different types of biventricular repair were undertaken during the 10 year study period: intraventricular tunnel type repair, arterial switch with VSD to pulmonary artery baffle, Rastelli type extracardiac conduit repair, Damus-Kaye-Stansel repair and atrial inversion with VSD to pulmonary artery baffle. Overall actuarial survival was 81% at eight years. Risk factors for early mortality were the presence of multiple VSDs and patient weight lower than median. Reoperation was less likely in patients who had a subaortic VSD. On the other hand patients with a noncommitted VSD were at a significantly higher risk for reoperation during the study period.

The difficult problem of double outlet right ventricle with noncommitted VSD was reviewed in a paper by Lacour-Gayet in 2002.[27] Although the VSD was described as noncommitted the specific anatomical location of the VSDs was described as perimembranous with inlet or trabecular extensions. Some might argue with this definition and would limit noncommitted VSD to apply to an inlet type VSD under the septal leaflet of the tricuspid valve or a mid-muscular or apical muscular VSD. Using the definition applied by the authors they found that they were able to baffle the VSD to the pulmonary artery and perform an arterial switch procedure in all 10 patients. There was one early death and at follow-up no patient had a subaortic gradient of greater than 15 mm.

In 2001 Brown et al[30] reviewed a 20-year experience with surgery for double outlet right ventricle at Indiana University. The 120 patients were divided into three groups: 47 noncomplex patients with a subaortic VSD, 39 with a subpulmonary VSD and 38 with complex anomalies including straddling AV valves, noncommitted VSD or hypoplastic ventricle. A total of 53 of the patients had an intraventricular repair, 20 had a Rastelli type repair, 16 had an arterial switch with baffling of the left ventricle to the neoaorta and 33 patients entered a single ventricle pathway. There were six early

Subaortic VSD

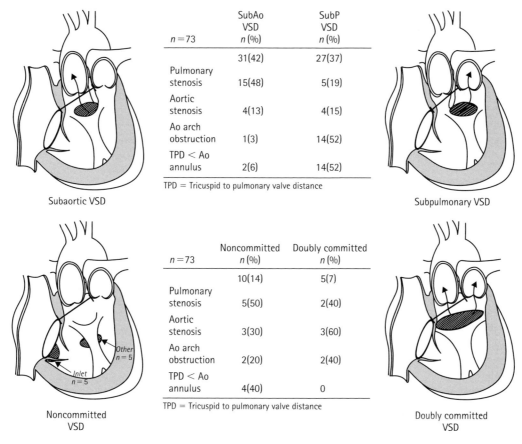

n = 73	SubAo VSD n (%)	SubP VSD n (%)
	31(42)	27(37)
Pulmonary stenosis	15(48)	5(19)
Aortic stenosis	4(13)	4(15)
Ao arch obstruction	1(3)	14(52)
TPD < Ao annulus	2(6)	14(52)

TPD = Tricuspid to pulmonary valve distance

Subpulmonary VSD

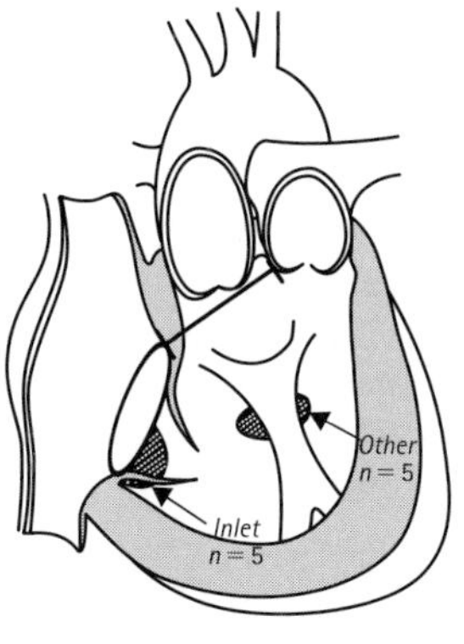

Noncommitted VSD

n = 73	Noncommitted n (%)	Doubly committed n (%)
	10(14)	5(7)
Pulmonary stenosis	5(50)	2(40)
Aortic stenosis	3(30)	3(60)
Ao arch obstruction	2(20)	2(40)
TPD < Ao annulus	4(40)	0

TPD = Tricuspid to pulmonary valve distance

Doubly committed VSD

Figure 23.9 *Important anatomic features of VSD groups in a review of 73 patients who underwent biventricular repair of DORV between 1981 and 1991 at Children's Hospital Boston. (From Aoki* et al. *Results of biventricular repair for double outlet right ventricle.* J Thorac Cardiovasc Surg, *1994;* ***107****:340, with permission from Elsevier.)*

deaths (4.8%). Fifteen year survival was 95.8% for patients with a subaortic VSD, 89.7% for patients with a subpulmonary VSD and 89.5% for patients with complex anomalies. Risk factors for mortality included location of the largest VSD, the presence of multiple VSDs, the presence of ventricular outflow obstruction or hypoplasia and the presence of a previous palliative procedure as well as the specific definitive procedure. Eleven percent of patients required reoperation. The authors emphasize the importance of careful selection of the individual patient for an optimal surgical approach. Masuda et al[31] described the results of the arterial switch procedure for double outlet right ventricle with subpulmonary VSD in 27 patients who underwent surgery at Kyushu University, Japan, between 1986 and 1997. There was one operative death (3.7%). Actuarial survival was 83 ± 8% at nine years. However, the operation free rate was only 46 ± 20% at nine years.

In 1997, Kleinert et al[32] reviewed the results of surgery for double outlet right ventricle of 193 patients who were managed at Royal Children's Hospital in Melbourne, Australia between 1978 and 1993. The patients were divided into two groups: a noncomplex group of 117 patients and a complex group of 76 patients with features such as multiple VSDs, straddling AV valve and ventricular hypoplasia. Of the 193 patients, 148 had a biventricular repair. Early mortality in the complex group was 22% versus 3.6% for the noncomplex patients. Risk factors for mortality were multiple VSDs, operation before 1985 and aortic arch obstruction. Overall 10-year survival probability was 81% though probability of survival free from reoperation was only 65% at 10 years.

The results of surgery for double outlet right ventricle reported over the past 10 years illustrate the tremendous improvement in outlook that has occurred for these children over the past two to three decades. Probably one of the most important steps forward was the introduction of the arterial switch procedure in the mid-1980s. This is documented by Musumeci et al from the Brompton Hospital, London in their 1988 report.[33] In their review of 120 consecutive patients undergoing surgical management of double outlet right ventricle between 1973 and 1986 the introduction of the arterial switch procedure was the event with the greatest effect on hospital mortality in patients with a subpulmonary VSD. The poor outlook for patients with double outlet right ventricle before the mid-1980s is well documented in the landmark paper by Kirklin et al from 1986.[34] In their review of 127 patients undergoing repair of double outlet right ventricle between 1967 and 1984 at the University of Alabama the overall actuarial survival rate at 12 years was only 38%. The 10-year survival rate for patients with double outlet right ventricle and a noncommitted VSD was only 22%. Unlike other anomalies where the introduction of prostaglandin E1 was exceedingly important in improving outcome after the late 1970s, double outlet right ventricle is generally not a ductus dependent lesion. The dramatic improvement that has occurred in surgical outcomes can be attributed to many other factors including an improved understanding and diagnosis of the complex anatomy of double outlet right ventricle, improved bypass techniques and improved surgery.

REFERENCES

1. Lev, M. The conotruncus. I. Its normal inversion and conus absorption. *Circulation* 1972; **46**:634–636.
2. Pexieder T. Conotruncus and its septation at the advent of the molecular biology era. In Clark EB, Markwald RR, Takao A (eds). *Developmental Mechanisms of Heart Disease*. Armonk, NY, Futura Publishing Company, 1995, pp 227–248.
3. Van Praagh R, Van Praagh S, Nebesar RA, Muster AJ, Sinha AJ, Paul MH. Tetralogy of fallot: underdevelopment of the pulmonary infundibulum and its sequelae. *Am J Cardiol* 1970; **26**:25–33.
4. Van Praagh R. What is Taussig-Bing malformation? *Circulation* 1968; **38**:445–449.
5. Walters HL 3rd, Mavroudis C, Tchervenkov CI, Jacobs JP, Lacour-Gayet F, Jacobs ML. Congenital Heart Surgery Nomenclature and Database Project: double outlet right ventricle. *Ann Thorac Surg* 2000; **69**:S249–263.
6. Howell CE, Ho SY, Anderson RH, Elliott MJ. Variations within the fibrous skeleton and ventricular outflow tracts in tetralogy of Fallot. *Ann Thorac Surg* 1990; **50**:450–457.
7. Lev M, Bharati S, Meng CC, Liberthson RR, Paul MH, Idriss, F. A concept of double-outlet right ventricle. *J Thorac Cardiovasc Surg* 1972; **64**:271–281.
8. Sondheimer HM, Freedom RM, Olley PM. Double outlet right ventricle: clinical spectrum and prognosis. *Am J Cardiol* 1977; **39**:709–714.
9. Taussig HB, Bing RJ. Complete transposition of the aorta and a levoposition of the pulmonary artery. Clinical, physiological and pathological findings. *Am Heart J* 1949; **37**:551–559.
10. Stewart RW, Kirklin JW, Pacifico AD, Blackstone EH, Bargeron LM Jr. Repair of double outlet right ventricle: An analysis of 62 cases. *J Thorac Cardiovasc Surg* 1979; **78:**502–514.
11. Kirklin JW, Harp RA, McGoon DC. Surgical treatment of origin of both vessels from right ventricle, including cases of pulmonary stenosis. *J Thorac Cardiovasc Surg* 1964; **48**:1026–1036.
12. Barratt-Boyes BG, Lowe JB, Watt WJ, Cole DS, Williams JCP. Initial experience with extracorporeal circulation in intracardiac surgery. *Br Med J* 1960; **2**:1826–1835.
13. Kawashima Y, Fujita T, Miyamoto T, Manabe H. Intraventricular rerouting of blood for the correction of Taussig-Bing malformation. *J Thorac Cardiovasc Surg* 1971; **62**:825–829.
14. Patrick DL, McGoon DC. Operation for double outlet right ventricle with transposition of the great arteries. *J Cardiovasc Surg* 1968; **9**:537–542.
15. Pacifico AD, Kirklin JK, Colvin EV, Bargeron LM Jr. Intraventricular tunnel repair for Taussig-Bing heart and related cardiac anomalies. *Circulation* 1986; **74**:153–160.
16. Sakata R, Lecompte Y, Batisse A, Borromee L, Durandy Y. Anatomic repair of anomalies of ventriculoarterial connection associated with ventricular septal defect. I. Criteria of surgical decision. *J Thorac Cardiovasc Surg* 1988; **95**:90–95.
17. Rastelli GC. A new approach to "anatomic" repair of transposition of the great arteries. *Mayo Clin Proc* 1969; **44**:1–12.
18. Borromee L, Lecompte Y, Batisse A et al. Anatomic repair of anomalies of ventriculoarterial connection associated with ventricular septal defect. *J Thorac Cardiovasc Surg* 1988; **95**:96–102.
19. Lecompte Y, Neveux JY, Leca F, Zannini L, Tu TV, Duboys Y, Jarreau MM. Reconstruction of the pulmonary outflow tract without prosthetic conduit. *J Thorac Cardiovasc Surg* 1982; **84**:727–733.
20. Vouhe P, Tamisier D, Leca F, Ouaknine R, Vernant F, Neveux JY. Transposition of the great arteries, ventricular septal defect, and pulmonary outflow obstruction. *J Thorac Cardiovasc Surg* 1992; **103**:428–436.
21. Nikaidoh H. Aortic translocation and biventricular outflow tract reconstruction. *J Thorac Cardiovasc Surg* 1984; **88**:365–372.
22. Uemura H, Yagihara T, Kawashima Y et al. Coronary arterial anatomy in double-outlet right ventricle with subpulmonary VSD. *Ann Thorac Surg* 1995; **59**:591–597.
23. Lock JE, Block PC, McKay RG, Baim DS, Keane JF. Transcatheter closure of ventricular septal defects. *Circulation* 1988; **78**:361–368.
24. Perry SB, van der Velde ME, Bridges ND, Keane JF, Lock JE. Transcatheter closure of atrial and ventricular septal defects. *Herz* 1993; **18**:135–142.
25. Fishberger SB, Bridges ND, Keane JF, Hanley FL, Jonas RA, Mayer JE, Castaneda AR, Lock JE. Intraoperative device closure of ventricular septal defects. *Circulation* 1993; **88**:II205–II209.
26. Barbero-Marcial M, Tanamati C, Atik E, Ebaid M. Intraventricular repair of double-outlet right ventricle with noncommitted ventricular septal defect: advantages of multiple patches. *J Thorac Cardiovasc Surg* 1999; **118**:1056–1067.
27. Lacour-Gayet F, Haun C, Ntalakoura K et al. Biventricular repair of double outlet right ventricle with non-committed ventricular septal defect (VSD) by VSD rerouting to the pulmonary artery and arterial switch. *Eur J Cardiothorac Surg* 2002; **21**:1042–1048.
28. Takeuchi K, McGowan FX Jr, Moran AM et al. Surgical outcome of double-outlet right ventricle with subpulmonary VSD. *Ann Thorac Surg* 2001; **71**:49–52.
29. Aoki M, Forbess JM, Jonas RA, Mayer JE, Castaneda AR. Results of biventricular repair for double outlet right ventricle. *J Thorac Cardiovasc Surg* 1994; **107**:338–350.
30. Brown JW, Ruzmetov M, Okada Y, Viyaj P, Turrentine MW. Surgical results in patients with double outlet right ventricle: a 20-year experience. *Ann Thorac Surg* 2001; **72**:1630–1635.
31. Masuda M, Kado H, Shiokawa Y et al. Clinical results of arterial switch operation for double-outlet right ventricle with subpulmonary VSD. *Eur J Cardiothorac Surg* 1999; **15:**283–288.
32. Kleinert S, Sano T, Weintraub RG, Mee RB, Karl TR, Wilkinson JL. Anatomic features and surgical strategies in double-outlet right ventricle. *Circulation* 1997; **96**:1233–1239.
33. Musumeci F, Shumway S, Lincoln C, Anderson RH. Surgical treatment for double-outlet right ventricle at the Brompton Hospital, 1973 to 1986. *J Thorac Cardiovasc Surg* 1988; **96**:278–287.
34. Kirklin JW, Pacifico AD, Blackstone EH, Kirklin JK, Bargeron LM Jr. Current risks and protocols for operations for double-outlet right ventricle. Derivation from an 18 year experience. *J Thorac Cardiovasc Surg* 1986; **92**:913–930.

24

Truncus arteriosus

INTRODUCTION

Truncus arteriosus, like tetralogy and transposition, is an anomaly of the conotruncus. There is a single semilunar 'truncal' valve which has the appearance of being a fused aortic and pulmonary valve often with more than three leaflets. There is almost always a large subarterial VSD directly below the truncal valve. The pulmonary arteries arise directly from the truncus so that they are exposed not only to systemic ejection from both ventricles but also to the diastolic pressure within the systemic arterial bed. Associated interruption of the aortic arch is not rare. In spite of the serious challenges presented by the child with truncus arteriosus, this is an anomaly which today can be managed with an exceedingly low risk of early and late mortality.

EMBRYOLOGY

Truncus arteriosus results from malseptation of the conotruncus.[1] Unlike transposition where the fundamental problem is failure of the septation process to spiral in the usual fashion, truncus arteriosus results from complete failure of septation. An interesting observation is that the ductus arteriosus is rarely present when the aortic arch is intact.

Truncus blends into the spectrum of aortopulmonary window. An extremely large aortopulmonary window results in there being only a tiny conotruncal septum separating the aortic and pulmonary valves. When the septum is completely absent and the aortic and pulmonary valves fuse there is a single semilunar (truncal) valve and the pulmonary arteries arise from the truncus. Further details of the embryology of truncus have been described elegantly by the Van Praaghs.[2]

ANATOMY

Pulmonary arteries

Collett and Edwards have classified truncus arteriosus according to the origin of the pulmonary arteries from the truncus.[3] In type 1 truncus there is a discrete main pulmonary artery segment which arises from the left side of the truncus and then bifurcates into a right and left pulmonary artery. In type 2 truncus the right and left pulmonary artery arise as separate orifices from the leftward and posterior aspect of the truncus. In type 3 truncus the right and left pulmonary artery arise from the opposite sides of the truncus. It has been our observation that the most common form of truncus lies somewhere between types 1 and 2 and is colloquially labeled 'type one and a half'. Generally the branch pulmonary arteries are well developed without central or peripheral stenoses.

Truncal valve

The truncal valve has a variable number of leaflets and variable morphology. There may be as few as two or as many as six leaflets though it is very rare to find more than four well-formed leaflets.[2] Often one or two leaflets are poorly formed with inadequate commissural support which can result in important regurgitation.[4] The poorly formed leaflets tend to be somewhat myxomatous and thickened and can hold sutures even in the neonatal period unlike normal semilunar valve tissue. It is rare for a truncal valve to be structurally stenotic.

Ventricular septal defect

The VSD in truncus arteriosus can be described as 'subarterial'. It lies immediately under the truncus and is usually separated from the tricuspid valve by the posterior limb of the septal band so that the risk of complete heart block at the time of surgical closure is small.[5] On occasion the truncal valve appears to lie predominantly over the right ventricle and the VSD can appear small so that there is a chance of restriction to left ventricular outflow at VSD level following repair.

Coronary arteries

Although the distal branching of the coronary arteries is usually normal it is not uncommon for one or both ostia to be abnormally positioned.[6,7] The left ostium for example may be extremely close to the takeoff of the right or more commonly the left pulmonary artery.[2,4] As with tetralogy there may be an anomalous anterior descending coronary artery which arises from the right coronary artery and passes across the infundibulum of the right ventricle.

ASSOCIATED ANOMALIES

A right aortic arch is present in approximately 25% of patients and an aberrant subclavian artery is seen in 5–10%.[8] As noted above under embryology, a ductus is rarely present if the aortic arch is intact. However, in 10–15% of patients the aorta is interrupted, either between the left carotid and left subclavian or beyond the left subclavian[9,10] and the descending aorta gives the appearance of being a direct continuation of the main pulmonary artery. The observation has been made by us and others (BG Barratt-Boyes, personal communication) that the ductus under these circumstances rarely closes and rarely requires a prostaglandin infusion to maintain patency.

PATHOPHYSIOLOGY

So long as pulmonary resistance remains at the high levels of the neonate the child with truncus arteriosus will have relatively balanced pulmonary and systemic circulations and may be free of symptoms. However, as pulmonary resistance falls in the first days and weeks of life there will be an increasing amount of pulmonary blood flow and the child is likely to develop signs of congestive heart failure. Heart failure can be quite pronounced in the child with truncus because pulmonary blood flow occurs not only during systole but also during diastole. There is often retrograde flow in the abdominal aorta during diastole stealing blood flow from the hepatic, renal and mesenteric circulation.

Retrograde flow is further exacerbated by the presence of truncal valve regurgitation. Generally a gradient across the truncal valve is a reflection of massively increased total flow across the valve secondary to both high pulmonary blood flow in combination with the systemic blood flow passing across the valve as well as the regurgitant fraction passing across the valve. After repair including repair of the regurgitant valve the gradient is usually eliminated.

Both right ventricular and left ventricular blood are ejected through the truncal valve resulting in at least a mild degree of cyanosis. The degree of cyanosis is influenced by the total pulmonary blood flow which as mentioned above is usually increased. Thus truncus is like transposition in that it is a cyanotic anomaly but pulmonary blood flow is increased. However, the degree of cyanosis in truncus is usually much less severe than with transposition. The massively increased pulmonary blood flow and exposure of the pulmonary arteries to both systolic and diastolic systemic arterial pressure results in accelerated development of pulmonary vascular disease. Thus if the child is able to survive the congestive heart failure which can be severe by one or two months of age, there is an important risk of irreversible pulmonary vascular disease as early as six months of age.[11]

DIAGNOSTIC STUDIES

Generally a murmur is detected shortly after birth. A chest X-ray will demonstrate evidence of increased pulmonary blood flow though arterial blood gases reveal at least mild cyanosis. Echocardiography is diagnostic. A careful assessment should be made of the aortic arch as well as the truncal valve. Cardiac catheterization is rarely if ever indicated in the neonatal period. If a child presents beyond two or three months of age, cardiac catheterization may be necessary to assess pulmonary resistance.

MEDICAL MANAGEMENT

Truncus arteriosus is not a prostaglandin dependent anomaly. Even when interrupted aortic arch is present it is rare for the ductus to close acutely so that it is rare for the neonate to present in shock or acidotic. Generally symptoms and signs of congestive heart failure appear gradually over the first weeks of life as pulmonary resistance falls. It is only in the rare circumstance that a child has been allowed to lapse into a severe degree of failure that aggressive medical stabilization will be required before surgery. In general, however, no attempt should be made to manage truncus medically for any extended period of time but only in the immediate preoperative period perhaps for a day or two to optimize the child's status before surgery. This should hold true even when the child is born prematurely.[12]

In the past deferral of surgery with aggressive medical management led to a high risk of problems with pulmonary hypertension including pulmonary hypertensive crises in the early postoperative period.[13]

INDICATIONS FOR AND TIMING OF SURGERY

The diagnosis of truncus arteriosus is an indication in itself for surgical treatment. Ideally diagnosis should be made within hours of birth if it has not been made prenatally. The child should be stabilized in the intensive care unit for 24–48 hours during which time diagnostic studies can be carefully analysed. Ideally surgery should be undertaken within the first week of life. If diagnosis is delayed the child should undergo a brief period of medical stabilization usually for no longer than two or three days and then surgery should be undertaken.

SURGICAL MANAGEMENT

History

Truncus arteriosus was managed in the 1950s and early 1960s by pulmonary artery banding.[14,15] The first documented repair of truncus arteriosus was performed in 1962, as reported by Behrendt and colleagues in 1974.[16] This involved a valveless conduit from the right ventricle to the pulmonary artery and closure of the ventricular septal defect. In 1967 McGoon first used a valved allograft conduit to repair truncus arteriosus, basing the operation on the experimental work of Rastelli.[17] In the 1960s and 1970s results of repair in infancy were poor, with the mortality rate being well over 50%. During this time valved allografts fell out of favor, a development that increased the technical risks of the repair, especially in small infants. However, results of repair in older infants, who were managed medically for the first six months of life before referral for surgical correction, were equally poor because of the morbidity secondary to pulmonary vascular disease. In 1984 Ebert and associates described a series of 100 infants repaired mainly before the age of six months with a remarkably low mortality rate for the time of only 11%, emphasizing that repair early in infancy was critical in avoiding the development of pulmonary vascular obstructive disease.[18]

In the 1980s a number of groups including our own recommended elective neonatal repair with encouraging results.[13,19] The availability of cryopreserved valved allografts in the US in the mid-1980s including very small sizes such as 7 and 8 mm allowed primary repair even in the youngest and smallest infants.

Technical considerations

ANESTHESIA

Pre-cardiopulmonary bypass

Routine anesthesia and monitoring procedures are described in detail in Chapter 4, while anesthetic considerations specific to patients with truncus arteriosus will be addressed here. Maintaining a balanced circulation in these patients in the pre-bypass period is a real challenge. Diastolic runoff from the aorta into the pulmonary arteries reduces aortic diastolic blood pressure and coronary perfusion pressure. Truncal valve regurgitation will exacerbate this reduction. Ventricular end-diastolic and subendocardial pressure will be elevated secondary to ventricular volume overload. Subendocardial perfusion is thus compromised and as a result these patients are prone to myocardial ischemia and ventricular fibrillation.

The association of this lesion with DiGeorge syndrome presents additional management issues. Specifically, patients with this syndrome are at risk for hypocalcemia and immune deficiencies. This requires that blood products be irradiated and that additional vigilance be directed toward maintenance of serum calcium levels particularly when citrated blood products are given. The majority of patients (90%) with DiGeorge syndrome have a microdeletion of chromosome 22q11 or CATCH 22 syndrome.[20,21] This is the same chromosomal region involved in velo-cardio-facial or Shprintzen syndrome. As a result some patients with DiGeorge syndrome will present with a characteristic facies consisting of a cleft palate, a long narrow face with maxillary excess and a retruded mandible/chin deficiency. Obviously, careful airway evaluation is necessary.

Induction and maintenance

Some infants will be transported to the operating room from the ICU having undergone preoperative intubation and stabilization. These infants will be ventilated with an FiO_2 of 17–21% and will have a $PaCO_2$ of 45–50 mmHg with an arterial pH of 7.25–7.35. Transport to the operating room should be with an FiO_2 of 21% and appropriate hypoventilation. Anesthesia can be maintained with fentanyl and a nondepolarizing muscle relaxant. Pancuronium should be used with caution if the heart rate is elevated (>160–170 bpm) and the diastolic blood pressure is low (<25 mmHg) as a further increase in heart rate will almost certainly compromise diastolic coronary perfusion. Vecuronium or cis-atracurium will be a better choice.

The induction of the nonintubated infant must be managed carefully. Intravenous induction is preferred. Induction can then be carried out with a synthetic opioid such as fentanyl or sufentanyl in combination with pancuronium. The dose of fentanyl is titrated to effect but is generally in the range of 10–25 μg/kg. Alternatively ketamine, etomidate, or a combination of etomidate and an opioid could be used. Pancuronium is given in a dose of 0.1–0.2 mg/kg. Prior to intubation during mask ventilation 100% oxygen should be administered. Once intubation of the trachea has been confirmed the infant should be ventilated with an FiO_2 of 21% to maintain an SaO_2 of 75–80%. There will be a tendency to induce hypocarbia due to the increased efficacy of ventilation and the reduction in metabolic rate/CO_2 production which accompanies anesthesia/paralysis. Minute ventilation should be adjusted to maintain $PaCO_2$ of 45–50 mmHg with an arterial pH of 7.25–7.35.

As the infant cools prior to bypass, minute ventilation will have to be adjusted to match decreased metabolic rate and CO_2 production. Minute ventilation is reduced by decreasing respiratory rate and maintaining tidal volume. This preserves functional residual capacity and prevents atelectesis. It is not unusual to have a tidal volumes of 12–15 ml/kg, I : E ratio of 1 : 2.5–1 : 3, and a respiratory rate of 4–5 per minute just prior to bypass.

Myocardial ischemia

Detection of myocardial ischemia is best accomplished with simultaneous display of ECG leads II and V5. Factors which predispose to ischemia should be anticipated and treated early. Elevated HR (>160) combined with decreasing diastolic blood pressure particularly when diastolic blood pressure is less than 20–25 mmHg is likely to result in myocardial ischemia and ST segment changes. Ventilation should be altered to assure that the circulation is balanced and that pulmonary overperfusion is not the cause. An adequate depth of anesthesia will help prevent increases in heart rate. The hematocrit should be maintained >35%. This is best accomplished by avoiding unnecessary fluid administration.

Volume infusion to increase diastolic blood pressure and reduce heart rate is rarely effective unless substantial volume has been lost from the surgical field. These patients have ventricular volume overload and exhausted preload reserve (no preload recruitable stroke work). Volume infusion is unlikely to increase diastolic blood pressure and will certainly further elevate ventricular end-diastolic pressure, further compromising subendocardial perfusion. Dopamine 3–5 μg/kg per minute is a better strategy to elevate blood pressure and reduce ventricular dimensions. Heart rate can be expected to remain constant or fall.

If surgical exposure permits the RPA can be looped with a vessel loop and occluded. This drastically reduces runoff into the pulmonary bed, elevates systolic and diastolic blood pressure and generally reduces ventricular dimensions. Adjustments in minute ventilation are usually not necessary despite the fact that the right lung is ventilated but not perfused (dead space ventilation). End tidal carbon dioxide ($ETCO_2$) will fall markedly and will not be an accurate reflection of $PaCO_2$. As a result adjustments in minute ventilation cannot be made on the basis of $ETCO_2$. FiO_2 may have to be increased slightly (FiO_2 30–50%) to maintain an SaO_2 of 75–80%.

Post-cardiopulmonary bypass

CPB can usually be terminated with dopamine at 3–5 μg/kg minute and a left atrial pressure of 5–10 mmHg. Residual truncal regurgitation should not compromise separation from bypass unless the regurgitation is severe.

Elevated pulmonary vascular resistance with subsequent impairment of RV ejection (afterload mismatch) can be a problem particularly in patients who are repaired beyond the neonatal period. Ventilatory maneuvers to normalize or reduce PVR should be undertaken. Ventilation should be with an FiO_2 of 100% with a PCO_2 in the range of 30–35 mmHg with a pH of 7.50–7.60. A deep level of anesthesia should be maintained as well. Low levels of PEEP can improve pulmonary gas exchange without elevating mean airway pressure to any significant degree.

As with tetralogy of Fallot repair right to left shunting should be expected at the level of the patent foramen ovale (see Chapter 16). Transient RV systolic and diastolic dysfunction following ventriculotomy and conduit placement will elevate right atrial pressure above left. The presence of pulmonary hypertension will exacerbate this elevation. Right to left shunting across this communication will provide an important contribution to systemic cardiac output (at the expense of SaO_2) in the presence of RV dysfunction and elevated pulmonary artery pressures. The SaO_2 will be determined by the relative volumes and saturations of systemic and pulmonary venous blood that mix in the left atrium. As such it is important that pulmonary venous saturation be optimized with appropriate ventilation and that systemic venous saturation be optimized by maintaining high systemic oxygen delivery in conjunction with a low oxygen consumption. High systemic delivery is achieved by maintaining high alveolar PO_2 (100% O_2), hematocrit (35–40%), and cardiac output. Cardiac output is optimized by maintaining stroke volume and heart rate. Output will be compromised if heart rate is low (<140 bpm) given the reduced compliance of the RV. Increased heart rates will also minimize the hemodynamic consequences of truncal valve regurgitation. In general dopamine will augment stroke volume and heart rate but atrial pacing may on occasion be necessary. Low oxygen consumption is best achieved by maintaining a deep level of anesthesia and avoiding hyperthermia (>37°C). If these objectives are achieved an SaO_2 >85–90% is possible even with substantial shunting at the atrial level.

TECHNIQUE OF CARDIOPULMONARY BYPASS

Although many groups choose to use bicaval cannulation and continuous cardiopulmonary bypass at moderate hypothermia it is our preference to use a single right atrial venous cannula and deep hypothermia. Deep hypothermia in the neonate provides excellent myocardial protection and allows for single dose cardioplegia infusion. Multi-dose cardioplegia requires direct coronary ostial perfusion and is cumbersome. Some reports have suggested that multidose cardioplegia causes important myocardial edema in the neonate and therefore should be avoided.[22]

A single right atrial cannula optimizes access to the superior mediastinum and most importantly ensures that there is no possibility of SVC obstruction and therefore differential perfusion away from the brain.

Control of pulmonary arteries

Because the pulmonary arteries arise directly from the truncus it is necessary to snare both pulmonary arteries coincident with beginning cardiopulmonary bypass. Failure to snare the pulmonary arteries would result in runoff through the lungs back to the left heart resulting in inadequate systemic perfusion as well as the potential for left heart distention and pulmonary injury. It is often helpful to tighten one of the tourniquets during preliminary dissection as this will increase diastolic perfusion and improve myocardial perfusion before beginning bypass.

Management of truncal valve regurgitation

If the truncal valve is severely regurgitant it is important to cross clamp the aorta shortly after commencing cardiopulmonary bypass to avoid left heart distention as myocardial action weakens with cooling. Truncal valve regurgitation should not be managed by placement of a left ventricular vent as this will simply steal from systemic perfusion. Also reliable function of a left ventricular vent is difficult in a small neonate. It may be possible to manage the first half of the cardioplegia infusion directly into the truncal root with massage of the left ventricle. The remainder of the infusion can then be undertaken directly into the coronary ostia.

SURGICAL APPROACH

The surgical approach is through a standard median sternotomy. A patch of anterior pericardium is harvested and treated with 0.6% glutaraldehyde for at least 20 minutes. Careful note is made of the size of the thymus which may be hypoplastic if there is associated Digeorge syndrome. The thymus is subtotally resected. The arterial cannula is placed distally in the ascending aorta following heparinization. A single venous cannula is introduced through the right atrial appendage. Immediately after commencing bypass tourniquets which had previously been placed around the right and left pulmonary artery are tightened. Usually there is no ductus present but if one is present it is doubly suture ligated and divided at the onset of bypass.

The child is cooled to a rectal temperature of less than 18°C using the pH stat strategy and a flow rate of 150 ml/kg per minute for the average size neonate. Hematocrit is maintained above 30%. During cooling the branch pulmonary arteries are thoroughly mobilized. After at least 5–10 minutes of cooling the ascending aorta is clamped distally and cardioplegia solution is infused into the truncal root. If there is truncal regurgitation the left ventricle is gently massaged to avoid distention.

Excision of pulmonary arteries

In the past we preferred to excise the pulmonary arteries from the left side of the truncus leaving the right side intact. More recently our approach has been one of transection of the truncus at the level of the pulmonary arteries in all cases (Figure 24.1a). This has at least three important advantages. Firstly the distal ascending aorta is usually very much smaller than the truncal root. If the proximal truncus is tailored down uniformly to the size of the distal ascending aorta this is useful in limiting the diameter of the sinotubular junction and probably aids in maintaining truncal valve competence. Secondly and more importantly, if the pulmonary arteries are excised from the left side of the truncus and this area is closed either directly or with a patch it can result in distortion of the left coronary ostium causing coronary ischemia. Finally, direct anastomosis of the proximal truncus to the distal ascending aorta results in a more symmetrical reconstruction (Figure 24.1e). Direct closure or patch closure results in a bulge which projects into the path of the right ventricle to pulmonary artery homograft conduit.

Ventricular septal defect closure

A vertical incision is made in the infundibulum of the right ventricle (Figure 24.1b). Great care is taken to preserve as many conal coronary arteries as possible. The incision should be sufficiently far from the left anterior descending to be sure that there will be no compromise of the vessel due to close suturing when the homograft is placed. The incision should be approximately the same length as the diameter of the homograft so that in general for a neonate it should be no more than 10 mm in length. By this time the child's rectal temperature should be less than 18°C and low flow can be begun at a rate of 50 ml/kg per minute. Usually the single venous cannula in the right atrium provides excellent exposure within the right ventricle because competence of the tricuspid valve prevents air entrainment. The VSD can be well visualized and is closed with interrupted pledgetted horizontal mattress 5/0 Tevdek sutures (Figure 24.1c). Because the posterior limb of the septal band separates the VSD from the tricuspid valve and conduction bundle, sutures can be placed across the posterior and inferior aspect of the VSD without difficulty and with minimal risk to the bundle of His. A knitted velour Dacron patch is threaded over these sutures and is tied into place.

Distal homograft anastomosis

By this time an appropriate sized homograft should have been selected and thawed. For the average neonate the internal diameter of the homograft is generally in the region of 9–11 mm. The homograft is cut to length and the distal anastomosis is fashioned using continuous 6/0 Prolene. Exposure of this anastomosis is facilitated by the fact that the truncus has not yet been reconstituted (Figure 24.1d).

Ascending aortic anastomosis

The proximal truncus is anastomosed to the distal ascending aorta using continuous 6/0 Prolene (Figure 24.1e). Because of the disparity in size, it is necessary to aggressively tailor down the proximal truncus by taking wide bites on the truncus with close bites on the ascending aorta. If the disparity is greater than 2:1 which is not uncommon, it is preferable to take a tuck on the rightward and posterior aspect in what would usually be the noncoronary sinus. It is important both in forming this dog-ear as well as in running the suture across the posterior wall to avoid any tension or distortion of

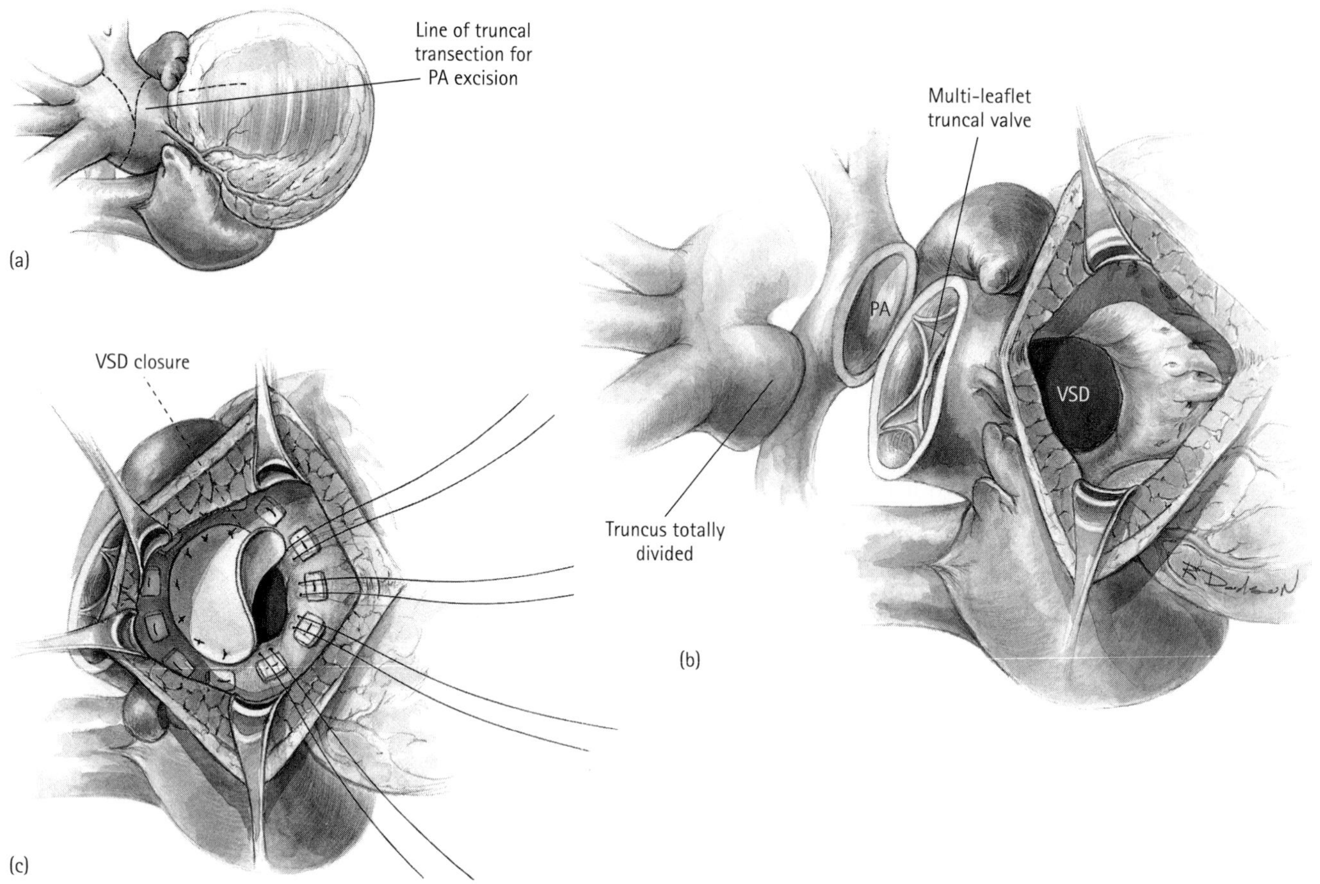

Figure 24.1a–c *(a) The pulmonary arteries are best excised from the truncus by complete division of the truncus at the level of the pulmonary arteries as indicated. (b) VSD closure is performed through a right ventriculotomy. The length of the ventriculotomy is exaggerated in this figure to allow visualization of intracardiac structures. The top end of the incision should be several millimeters from the truncal valve and right coronary artery. As many conal coronary arteries as possible should be preserved. (c) The subarterial VSD is closed with a knitted velour Dacron patch using interrupted pledgetted horizontal mattress 5/0 polyester sutures. Because the posterior limb of the septal band separates the VSD from the conduction bundle sutures can be placed safely across the posterior and inferior aspect of the VSD.*

the left coronary ostium which should be carefully visualized. Prior to tying the suture anteriorly the left heart should be allowed to fill with blood and air should be vented through the suture line. Any remaining air is then vented through the original cardioplegia site.

PROXIMAL HOMOGRAFT ANASTOMOSIS

The homograft is anastomosed to the infundibular incision using continuous 6/0 or 5/0 Prolene (Figure 24.1e,f). The homograft is sutured directly to the superior half of the ventriculotomy. The autologous pericardium which was harvested initially is used to roof the proximal anastomosis. Towards the inferior end of the ventriculotomy there should be considerable gathering of the pericardium by taking very wide bites of the pericardium and very close bites on the myocardium so that the hood adopts a curved shape with depth to it rather than lying taut and flat. Before completion of this suture line the left heart is once again de-aired and the aortic cross clamp is released with gentle compression of the right coronary artery to minimize air passing into the right coronary system. Rewarming is begun and flow is gradually increased. The open proximal homograft anastomosis allows venting of blood from the right heart before cardiac action is regained. It is also possible to pass a sucker through the homograft valve to vent the left heart if there is evidence of left heart distention. Distention of the homograft is a useful indicator of left heart distention.

MONITORING LINES

During rewarming a left atrial line is inserted through the right superior pulmonary vein in the routine way. Two atrial and one ventricular pacing wire are placed. A pulmonary artery line is inserted through the infundibulum of the right ventricle.

WEANING FROM BYPASS

When the rectal temperature has reached 35°C the child is weaned from bypass. Generally no more than 5 μg/kg per minute of dopamine support should be necessary. Following removal of the cannulas, protamine is given. Hemostasis is assisted with thrombin soaked gelfoam. A right atrial line is inserted through the right atrial appendage. Chest tubes are placed and the chest is closed in the routine fashion.

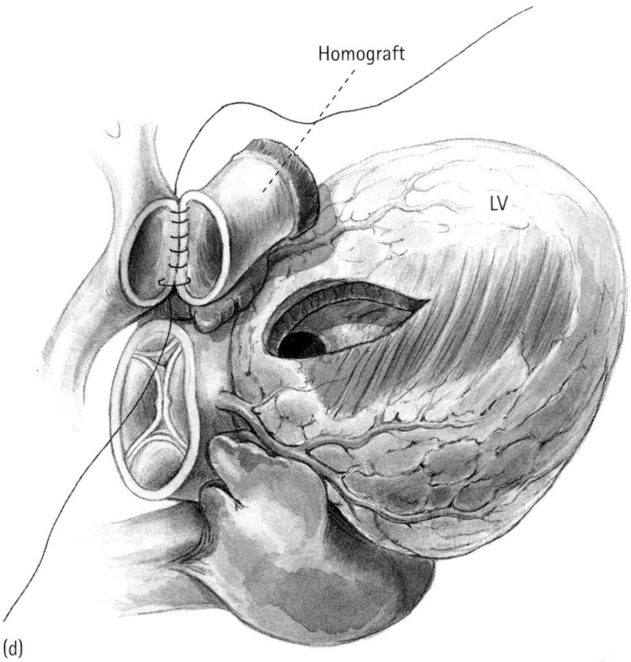

(d)

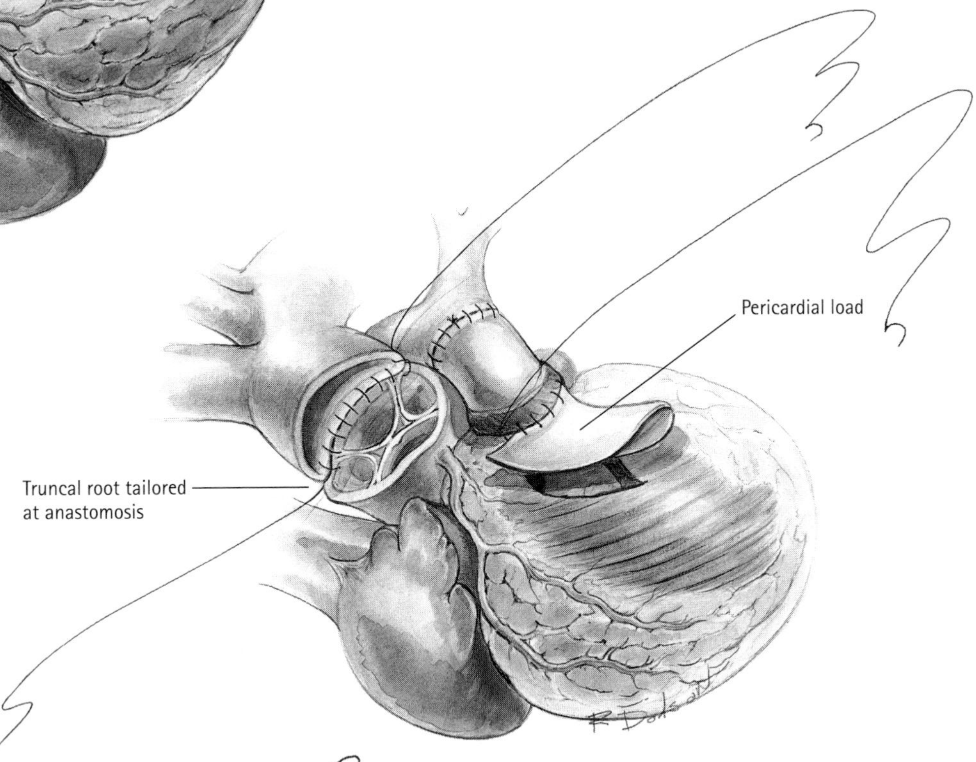

(e)

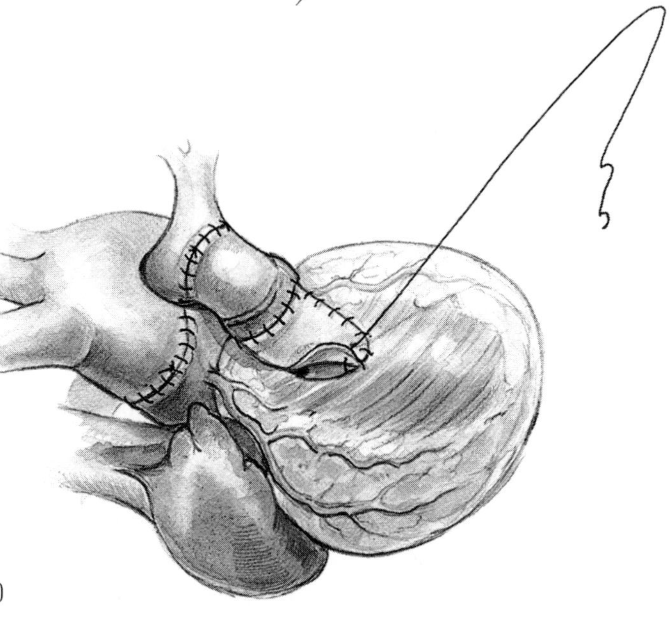

(f)

Figure 24.1d–f *(d) The distal anastomosis of a homograft to the pulmonary bifurcation is performed before the ascending aorta is reconstituted. (e) The proximal truncus is anastomosed to the distal ascending aorta using a running suture technique. There is usually considerable disparity in size between the ascending aorta and original truncus necessitating aggressive tailoring of the anastomosis to match the two vessels. (f) The proximal anastomosis of the homograft to the right ventricle is supplemented with a hood of autologous pericardium lightly tanned with glutaraldehyde.*

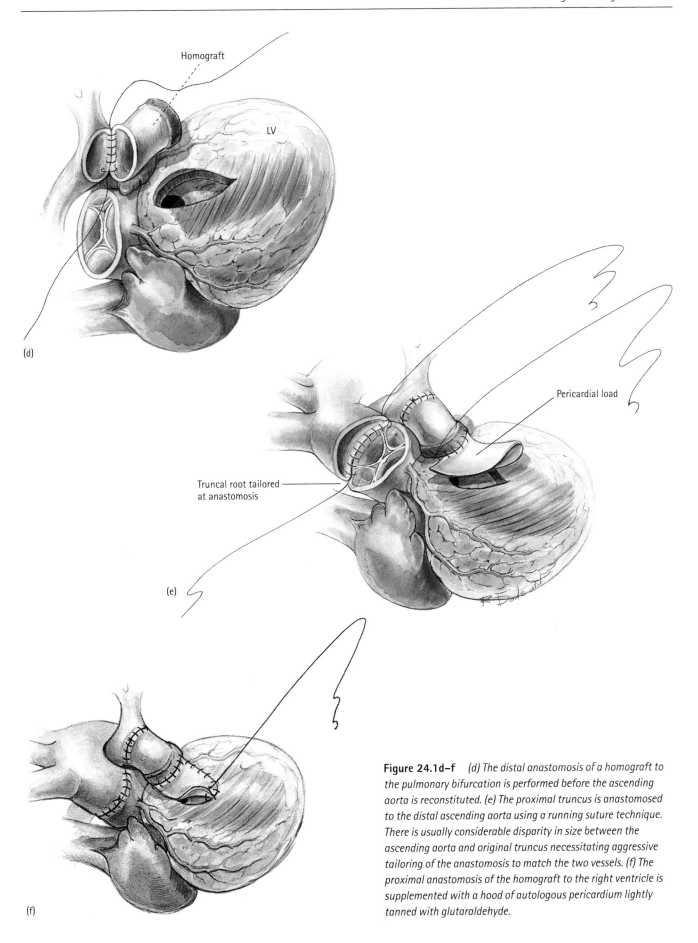

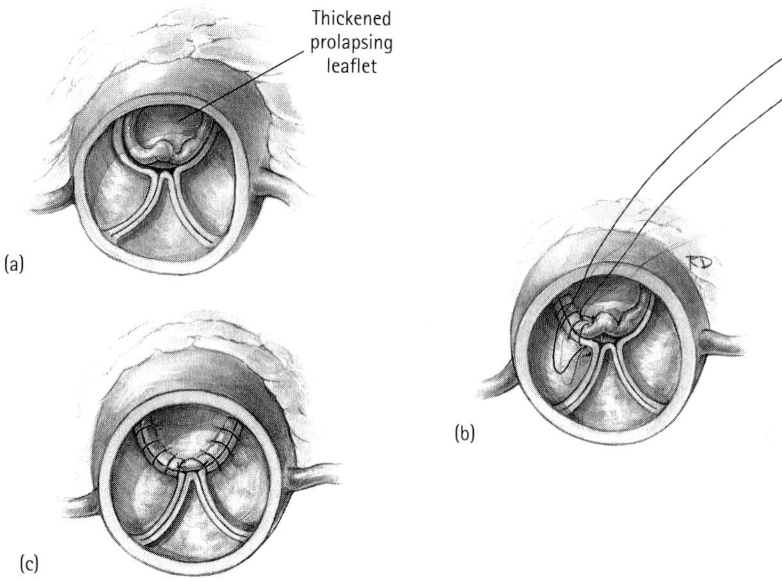

Figure 24.2 *(a) The regurgitant truncal valve often has a vestigial leaflet which prolapses. (b) A prolapsing vestigial leaflet can be supported by closure of one commissure. (c) When there is severe prolapse of a vestigial leaflet, two commissures can be closed to provide support for the prolapsing leaflet. The valve is effectively converted to a bicuspid valve.*

MANAGEMENT OF THE REGURGITANT TRUNCAL VALVE

The regurgitant truncal valve is almost always amenable to various repair techniques. Replacement should rarely if ever be necessary in the neonatal period. One of the most useful techniques is to support a prolapsing leaflet by suturing it to adjacent leaflets (Figure 24.2a, b, c). This is generally facilitated by the fact that the prolapsing leaflet is thickened and the adjacent leaflet edges are also relatively thickened and hold sutures surprisingly well for a neonatal valve. Regurgitation is often exacerbated by splaying of the tops of the commissures secondary to dilation of the sinotubular junction. This can be improved by wedge excisions taken into the sinuses of Valsalva. It is even possible to completely excise leaflets including the adjacent sinus of Valsalva with reconstitution of the annulus and truncal root by direct anastomosis.[23]

As with any valve reconstruction intraoperative TEE is invaluable in understanding the mechanism of regurgitation pre-repair as well as analysing the effectiveness of repair.

MANAGEMENT OF ASSOCIATED INTERRUPTED AORTIC ARCH

Repair of an associated interruption of the aortic arch should be undertaken with an initial brief period of hypothermic circulatory arrest. As described for the standard repair of truncus the child is cooled with a single arterial cannula in the distal ascending aorta. The pulmonary arteries are occluded with tourniquets. Flow to the descending aorta passes from the truncus through the ductus arteriosus into the descending aorta. When the rectal temperature is less than 18°C, the ascending aorta is clamped and cardioplegia solution is infused into the truncal root while the ductus is controlled with forceps. With the flow rate reduced to 50 ml/kg per minute or less the pulmonary arteries are excised from the truncus and the descending aorta is excised from the pulmonary arteries (Figure 24.3a). It is usually very difficult to distinguish ductal tissue but if this is apparent it should be excised. Circulatory arrest is now begun.

The proximal divided ductus and ascending aorta are oversewn (Figure 24.3b). Although it is tempting to anastomose the descending aorta to the site of excision of the pulmonary arteries, particularly if this has been done without transecting the truncus, this is not generally advisable. The arch anastomosis will be too proximal on the truncus and will interfere with the course of the homograft conduit. Instead, a longitudinal anastomosis should be made on the ascending aorta immediately proximal to the takeoff of the head vessels and perhaps extending a little on to the left common carotid artery if this is a type B interruption (Figure 24.3c). The descending aorta can be controlled with a C-clamp in order to reduce tension on the anastomosis as this is fashioned. The aortic cross clamp should be removed in order to improve exposure for the anastomosis. Tourniquets are no longer used on the head vessels as is the practice for adult arch surgery. The anastomosis is fashioned with continuous 6/0 Prolene. Upon completion of the anastomosis air is displaced by running the arterial cannula at an extremely low flow rate and then the aortic cross clamp is reapplied. The remainder of the procedure can be undertaken as for a standard repair.

RESULTS OF SURGERY

In 2000, Jahangiri et al reported the results of 50 patients who had undergone surgical repair of truncus arteriosus at Children's Hospital Boston between 1992 and 1998.[10] The median age at surgery was two weeks. Nine of the patients had associated interrupted arch. Of the 14 patients in whom truncal valve regurgitation was diagnosed preoperatively, five had mild regurgitation, five had moderate regurgitation and

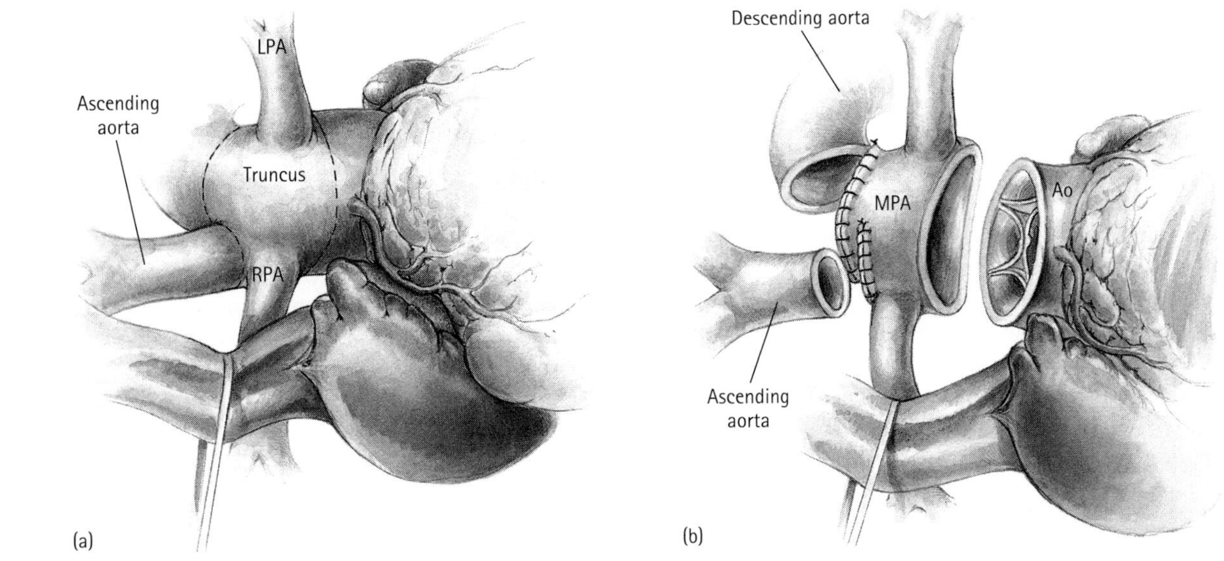

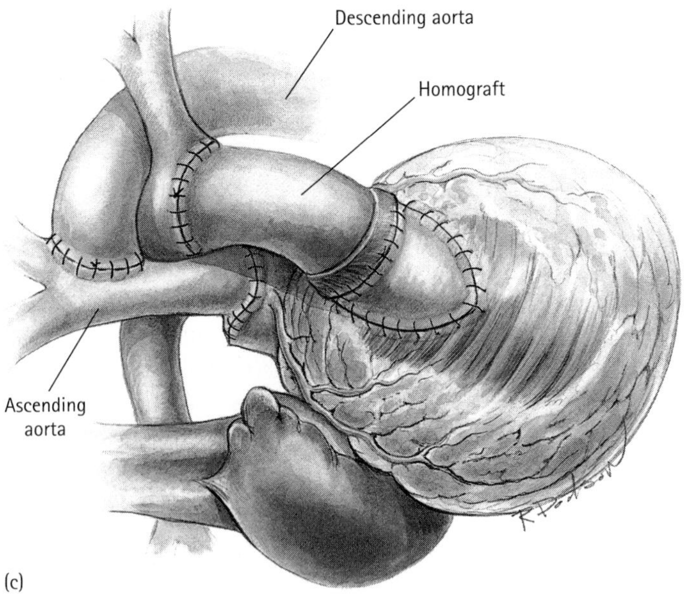

Figure 24.3 *(a) Truncus arteriosus with interrupted aortic arch. The pulmonary arteries are excised from the truncus by transection as indicated. In addition the ductus is divided a few millimeters distal to the left pulmonary artery. The ascending aorta is divided at its takeoff from the truncus. (b) The proximal divided ductus and ascending aorta are oversewn. (c) The proximal descending aorta is anastomosed to the left side of the ascending aorta distally extending on to the origin of the left common carotid artery. Because of the marked disparity between the proximal truncus and the distal ascending aorta it is necessary to reduce the size of the proximal truncus by taking a tuck on the rightward and posterior aspect of the truncal root thereby creating a dog-ear. The ascending aorta is sutured to the left side of the truncal root which improves the lie of the homograft conduit.*

four had severe regurgitation. Five patients underwent truncal valve repair and one underwent homograft replacement of the truncal valve with coronary reimplantation. The actuarial survival overall was 96% at 30 days, 1 and 3 years. There were no deaths in patients with associated interrupted aortic arch. The two deaths in the series occurred in patients with truncal valve regurgitation, neither of whom underwent repair. Postoperative transthoracic echocardiography in patients who underwent valve repair showed minimal residual valvar regurgitation. None of the patients required reoperation because of truncal valve problems or aortic arch stenosis at a median follow-up of 23 months though conduit replacement was necessary in 17 patients after a mean duration of two years. Freedom from reoperation for those who had an aortic homograft was four years and for those who had a pulmonary homograft was three years. We concluded from this series that despite the magnitude of the operation excellent results can be achieved in complex forms of truncus arteriosus and that in the current era interrupted arch is no longer a risk factor for repair of truncus. Aggressive application of truncal valvuloplasty methods has neutralized the traditional risk factor of truncal valve regurgitation.

Jahangiri's report was a follow-up on a previous report from Children's Hospital Boston by Hanley et al published in 1993.[13] The previous report reviewed results of surgery for 63 patients with truncus arteriosus who underwent repair between 1986 and 1991. During this timeframe management evolved from elective repair at three months to elective primary repair in the early neonatal period. In this earlier timeframe truncal valve regurgitation, interrupted aortic arch, coronary artery anomalies and age at repair greater than 100 days were risk factors for perioperative death. Pulmonary hypertensive episodes were fewer and duration of ventilator dependence as well as absolute pulmonary artery pressure were significantly less in patients undergoing correction before 30 days of age.

Other centers have confirmed the effectiveness of aggressive truncal valve repair. In 2001 Mavroudis and Backer[23] described the results of surgery for eight patients who underwent intervention for severe truncal valve insufficiency between 1995 and 2000. In addition to valve suture technique the authors employed leaflet excision and annular remodeling. Among the three patients who had valve suture techniques only there was one death with two patients requiring acute valve replacement. However, the patients who had more aggressive techniques were doing well at follow-up.

A number of other authors have described various techniques and results of surgery for truncal valve repair.[24–27] In 2001 Thompson et al[28] described the results of surgery for 65 patients less than one month of age who underwent primary repair of truncus arteriosus at UCSF between 1992 and 1999. A total of 23% of patients had moderate or severe truncal valve regurgitation and 12% had interrupted aortic arch. Early mortality was 5%. During a median follow-up of 32 months there were two deaths resulting in a Kaplan Meier estimate of survival at one year of 92%. The only factors significantly associated with poorer survival over time were operative weight of 2.5 kg or less ($p = 0.01$) and truncal valve replacement ($p = 0.009$). Actuarial freedom from conduit replacement among early survivors was 57% at three years.

A number of authors have focused attention on the relatively disappointing durability of homografts used for the conduit aspect of the repair of truncus arteriosus. Perron et al reviewed the results of valved homograft repair in neonates and young infants in 84 patients undergoing surgical repair with a homograft conduit at Children's Hospital Boston between 1990 and 1995.[29] Although the early mortality was satisfactory at 4.7% for anomalies which did not include interrupted aortic arch or absent pulmonary valve syndrome the durability of homografts was disappointing. A total of 47% of the patients underwent conduit replacement after a mean follow-up of 34 months. The median time to reoperation was 3.1 years. Univariate analysis revealed that patients with a homograft with an internal diameter of 8 mm or less were most likely to suffer early graft failure and reoperation. Survival was unaffected. Simple cases had improved long-term survival relative to complex cases. Age, weight, pathology, type of homograft (aortic versus pulmonary), length of homograft and source of the homograft from different tissue banks did not influence early graft failure. At least one recent report has suggested that failure of homografts in infants is not simply related to somatic outgrowth.[30] The authors reviewed imaging studies of 40 patients who had undergone homograft conduit replacement between 1996 and 2000. They found that 53% of patients had shrinkage of the homograft relative to the original size. This is most commonly observed at the annular area. The authors have speculated that this may be related to immune mechanisms.

A number of authors have described the use of conduits other than homografts for repair of truncus. For example Schlicter et al[31] described the use of fresh autologous pericardial valve conduits in 82 patients. Freedom from reintervention at 5 and 10 years was 92% and 76% and was 100% at 10 years in conduits larger than 16 mm at the time of implantation.

Danton et al[32] reviewed 61 infants who underwent repair of truncus arteriosus in Birmingham, England between 1988 and 2000. A total of 23 of these patients had direct anastomosis of the pulmonary arteries to the right ventricle augmented anteriorly with a monocusp in 15 patients or a simple pericardial patch in eight. The remaining 38 patients had either a homograft conduit (28 patients) or a xenograft containing conduit (10 patients). The authors reported that patients who had direct anastomosis had an 89 ± 10% freedom from reintervention for the right ventricular outflow tract at 10 years versus 56 ± 10% for patients who had a conduit ($p = 0.023$). They found that the use of a xenograft conduit was an independent risk factor for reintervention ($p < 0.001$). In spite of these results some centers have recently begun to recommend the use of xenograft conduits as an alternative to homografts. For example Chard et al[33] reported use of the Medtronic freestyle xenograft conduit as an alternative to a homograft conduit and suggested that short-term results were satisfactory. Aupecle[34] described use of a composite stented porcine valved conduit constructed from bovine pericardium in 55 patients between 1996 and 2000. Twenty of the patients had truncus arteriosus. Actuarial freedom from conduit dilation or reoperation was 94% at one year and 54% at four years. Other conduits that have been suggested for repair of truncus arteriosus include the bovine jugular vein conduit ('Contegra')[35] as well as a Gortex conduit containing a stented bovine pericardial valve.[36]

A number of centers are presently extending the durability of right ventricle to pulmonary artery conduits by stent implantation. For example Powell et al[37] described 44 patients who underwent implantation of 48 stents in obstructed RV to PA conduits at Children's Hospital Boston. The authors found that actuarial freedom from reoperation was 65% at 30 months after the procedure. The authors concluded that stent implantation results in significant immediate hemodynamic and angiographic improvement and in a subgroup of patients prolongs conduit lifespan by several years. Nevertheless the role of stent implantation in heavily calcified homograft conduits needs to be further defined.

REFERENCES

1. Pexieder T. The conotruncus and its septation at the advent of the molecular biology era. In Clark EB, Markwald RR, Takao A (eds). *Developmental Mechanisms of Heart Disease*. Armonk NY, Futura Publishing Co, 1995, pp 227–248.
2. Van Praagh R, Van Praagh S. The anatomy of common aortico-pulmonary trunk (truncus arteriosus communis) and its embryonic implications. A study of 57 necropsy cases. *Am J Cardiol* 1965; **16**:406–425.

3. Collett RW, Edwards JE. Persistent truncus arteriosus: A classification according to anatomic types. *Surg Clin North Am* 1949; **29**:1245–1257.
4. Suzuki A, Ho SY, Anderson RH, Deanfield JE. Coronary arterial and sinusal anatomy in hearts with a common arterial trunk. *Ann Thorac Surg* 1989; **48**:792–797.
5. Bharati S, McAllister HA, Rosenquist GC, Miller RA, Tatooles CJ, Lev M. The surgical anatomy of truncus arteriosus communis. *J Thorac Cardiovasc Surg* 1974; **67**:501–510.
6. Lenox CC, Debich DE, Zubebuhler JR. The role of coronary artery abnormalities in the prognosis of truncus arteriosus. *J Thorac Cardiovasc Surg* 1992; **104**:1728–1742.
7. delaCruz MV, Cayre R, Angelini P, Noriega-Ramos N, Sadowinski S. Coronary arteries in truncus arteriosus. *Am J Cardiol* 1990; **66**:1482–1486.
8. Calder L, Van Praagh R, Van Praagh S et al. Truncus arteriosus communis. Clinical angiographic and pathologic findings in 100 patients. *Am Heart J* 1976; **92**:23–38.
9. Sano S, Brawn WJ, Mee RB. Repair of truncus arteriosus and interrupted aortic arch. *J Cardiac Surg* 1990; **5**:157–162.
10. Jahangiri M, Zurakowski D, Mayer JE, del Nido PJ, Jonas RA. Repair of the truncal valve and associated interrupted arch in neonates with truncus arteriosus. *J Thorac Cardiovasc Surg* 2000; **119**:508–514.
11. Marcelletti C, McGoon DC, Mair DD. The natural history of truncus arteriosus. *Circulation* 1976; **54**:108–111.
12. Reddy VM, McElhinney DB, Sagrado T, Parry AJ, Teitel DF, Hanley FL. Results of 102 cases of complete repair of congenital heart defects in patients weighing 700 to 2500 g. *J Thorac Cardiovasc Surg* 1999; **117**:324–331.
13. Hanley FL, Heinemann MK, Jonas RA et al. Repair of truncus arteriosus in the neonate. *J Thorac Cardiovasc Surg* 1993; **105**:1047–1056.
14. Armer RM, DeOliveira PF, Lurie PR. True truncus arteriosus. Review of 17 cases and report of surgery in 7 patients. *Circulation* 1961; **24**:878–890.
15. Smith GW, Thompson WM, Damman JF et al. Use of pulmonary artery banding procedure in treating type II truncus arteriosus. *Circulation* 1964; **29**(Suppl 1):108.
16. Behrendt DM, Kirsh MM, Stern A, Sigmann J, Perry B, Sloan H. The surgical therapy for pulmonary artery-right ventricular discontinuity. *Ann Thorac Surg* 1974; **18**:122–137.
17. McGoon DC, Rastelli GC, Ongley PA. An operation for the correction of truncus arteriosus. *JAMA* 1968; **205**:69–73.
18. Ebert PA, Turley K, Stanger P, Hoffman JI, Heymann MA, Rudolph AM. Surgical treatment of truncus arteriosus in the first six months of life. *Ann Surg* 1984; **200**:451–456.
19. Bove EL, Beekman RH, Snider AR et al. Repair of truncus arteriosus in the neonate and young infant. *Ann Thorac Surg* 1989; **47**:499–505.
20. Momma K, Ando M, Matsuoka R. Truncus arteriosus communis associated with chromosome 22q11 deletion. *J Am Coll Cardiol* 1997; **30**:1067–1071.
21. Goldmuntz E, Clark BJ, Mitchell LE et al. Frequency of 22q11 deletions in patients with conotruncal defects. *J Am Coll Cardiol* 1998; **32**:492–498.
22. Jonas RA. Myocardial protection for neonates and infants. *Thorac Cardiovasc Surg* 1998; **46**(Suppl 2):288–291.
23. Mavroudis C, Backer CL. Surgical management of severe truncal insufficiency: experience with truncal valve remodeling techniques. *Ann Thorac Surg* 2001; **72**:396–400.
24. Elami A, Laks H, Pearl JM. Truncal valve repair: initial experience with infants and children. *Ann Thorac Surg* 1994; **57**:397–401.
25. McElhinney DB, Reddy VM, Rajasinghe HA, Mora BN, Silverman NH, Hanley FL. Trends in the management of truncal valve insufficiency. *Ann Thorac Surg* 1998; **65**:517–524.
26. Black MD, Adatia I, Freedom RM. Truncal valve repair: initial experience in neonates. *Ann Thorac Surg* 1998; **65**:1737–1740.
27. Imamura M, Drummond-Webb JJ, Sarris GE, Mee RB. Improving early and intermediate results of truncus arteriosus repair: A new technique of truncal valve repair. *Ann Thorac Surg* 1999; **67**:1142–1146.
28. Thompson LD, McElhinney DB, Reddy VM, Petrossian E, Silverman NH, Hanley FL. Neonatal repair of truncus arteriosus: continuing improvement in outcomes. *Ann Thorac Surg* 2001; **72**:391–395.
29. Perron J, Moran AM, Gauvreau K, del Nido PJ, Mayer JE, Jonas RA. Valved homograft conduit repair of the right heart in early infancy. *Ann Thorac Surg* 1999; **68**:542–548.
30. Wells WJ, Arroyo H, Bremner RM, Wood J, Starnes VA. Homograft conduit failure in infants is not due to somatic outgrowth. *J Thorac Cardiovasc Surg* 2002; **124**:88–96.
31. Schlichter AJ, Kreutzer C, Mayorquim RC et al. Five to fifteen year follow-up of fresh autologous pericardial valved conduits. *J Thorac Cardiovasc Surg* 2000; **119**:869–879.
32. Danton MH, Barron DJ, Stumper O et al. Repair of truncus arteriosus: a considered approach to right ventricular outflow tract reconstruction. *Eur J Cardiothorac Surg* 2001; **20**:95–103.
33. Chard RB, Kang N, Andrews DR, Nunn GR. Use of the Medtronic Freestyle valve as a right ventricular to pulmonary artery conduit. *Ann Thorac Surg* 2001; **71**:S361–364.
34. Aupecle B, Serraf A, Belli E et al. Intermediate follow-up of a composite stentless porcine valved conduit of bovine pericardium in the pulmonary circulation. *Ann Thorac Surg* 2002; **74**:127–132.
35. Brown JW, Ruzmetov M, Okada Y, Vijay P, Turrentine MV. Truncus arteriosus repair: outcomes, risk factors, reoperation and management. *Eur J Cardiothorac Surg* 2001; **20**:221–227.
36. Allen BS, El-Zein C, Cunco B, Cava JP, Barth MJ, Ilbawi MN. Pericardial tissue valves and gore-tex conduits as an alternative for right ventricular outflow tract replacement in children. *Ann Thorac Surg* 2002; **74**:771–777.
37. Powell AJ, Lock JE, Keane JF, Perry SB. Prolongation of RV-PA conduit life span by percutaneous stent implantation. Intermediate-term results. *Circulation* 1995; **92**:3282–3288.

25

Tetralogy of Fallot with pulmonary atresia

INTRODUCTION

Patients with tetralogy of Fallot with pulmonary atresia may fall anywhere within an extremely wide spectrum of severity ranging from simple valvar atresia to complete absence of the true pulmonary arteries. In the past this anomaly was thought of as being part of a spectrum with tetralogy with pulmonary stenosis and would have been described in the same chapter. Although there is no question that the two entities share a common embryological background and are part of a spectrum anatomically, nevertheless the management of these patients and the results of management are so different that tetralogy with pulmonary atresia will be considered here as a separate chapter. Many centers prefer the terminology 'pulmonary atresia with VSD' to recognize the differences between the two anomalies. There is probably no entity which better illustrates the collaborative role that can be played by the interventional cardiologist and the congenital cardiac surgeon than tetralogy with pulmonary atresia. The child at the severe end of the spectrum with hypoplastic true pulmonary arteries and multiple aortopulmonary collaterals requires a carefully coordinated team approach in order to achieve optimal outcome. Even with optimal management these children require so many interventions that there is a significant impact on their quality of life. Indeed many would consider that the quality of life for children at the severe end of the spectrum including ultimate exercise capacity may be more limited than for children with hypoplastic left heart syndrome and heterotaxy. Certainly the total financial cost of treatment of these children is at the very far end of the entire spectrum of congenital heart disease.

EMBRYOLOGY

The basic embryology for the development of tetralogy of Fallot has been described in Chapter 16.[1] During normal development there is fusion of the right and left sixth dorsal aortic arch with the plexus of systemic arteries carried by the lung buds from the primitive foregut. If there is failure of this normal process of fusion pulmonary atresia results and there is a persistence of connections from the aorta. These abnormal vessels are termed 'aortopulmonary collaterals' (also referred to as 'bronchial collaterals' or 'major aortopulmonary collateral arteries' or 'MAPCAs'). There is variable development of the true pulmonary arteries, presumably depending on the point in gestation at which connection of the lumen of the true pulmonary arteries with the right ventricle is completely lost.

ANATOMY

Intracardiac anatomy

The intracardiac anatomy of tetralogy of Fallot with pulmonary atresia is very similar to that of tetralogy with pulmonary stenosis.[2] There is an anterior malalignment VSD which is essentially identical to the VSD seen in tetralogy with pulmonary stenosis. There is usually some development of the right ventricular infundibulum although it ends blindly. The lumen of the infundibulum may be very small and difficult to locate.

True pulmonary arteries

There is great variability in the anatomy of the true pulmonary arteries until one gets to the severe end of the spectrum where there is surprising uniformity. In this instance the right and left pulmonary arteries are usually 1.5–2 mm in diameter and are frequently in continuity, although they may be discontinuous. They are usually also in continuity with a vestigial main pulmonary artery that is also approximately 2 mm in diameter and usually extends to the atretic infundibulum (Figure 25.1).

At the most mild end of the spectrum of tetralogy of Fallot with pulmonary atresia the branch pulmonary arteries are normally developed and are supplied by a normally positioned ductus arteriosus. The main pulmonary artery may also be relatively well developed and extend to the atretic infundibulum. At the mildest end of the spectrum there is even development of the pulmonary valve so that the patient may be considered to have 'valvar' pulmonary atresia. Moving further across the spectrum there may be a segment of discontinuity between the infundibulum and the main pulmonary artery. Even further across the spectrum there is complete absence of development of the main pulmonary artery so that the right and left pulmonary arteries connect to each other as a continuous tube-like structure.

At any point in the spectrum of pulmonary artery development these anomalies may be further complicated by discontinuity of the right and left pulmonary arteries.

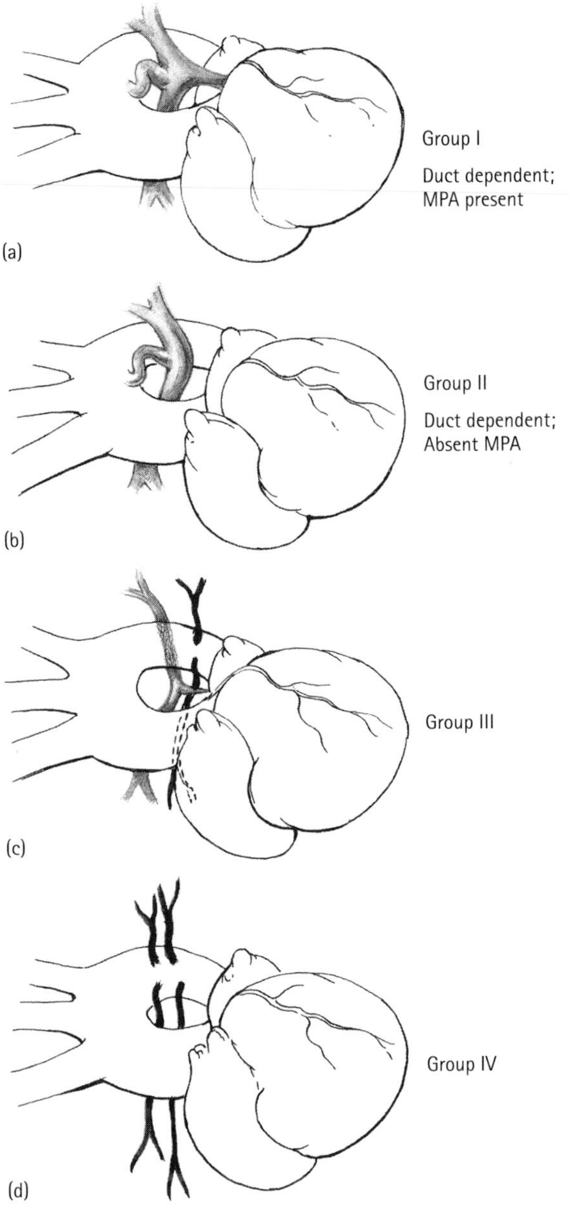

Figure 25.1 *Tetralogy of Fallot with pulmonary atresia exists in a wide spectrum of severity according to the development of the true pulmonary arteries and the presence of aortopulmonary collateral vessels. In group 1 there is simple valvar or infundibular atresia. In group 2 there is absence of the main pulmonary artery though the branch pulmonary arteries are in continuity and the pulmonary artery circulation is duct dependent. In group 3 the true pulmonary arteries are severely hypoplastic and multiple aortopulmonary collaterals are present. In group 4 the true pulmonary arteries are absent and the entire blood supply is from aortopulmonary collateral vessels.*

Aortopulmonary connections: ductus arteriosus and aortopulmonary collaterals

At the mild end of the spectrum of tetralogy of Fallot with pulmonary atresia pulmonary blood flow is usually supplied by a patent ductus arteriosus which connects in the usual location at the distal end of the main pulmonary artery adjacent to the takeoff of the left pulmonary artery. Occasionally there are bilateral ducti with the right sided ductus usually arising from the innominate or right subclavian artery. There may or may not be discontinuity between the right and left pulmonary arteries.[3]

Aortopulmonary collateral vessels most commonly arise from the proximal descending aorta at approximately the level of the tracheal carina, i.e. T4, similar to the level of origin of bronchial arteries (hence the term 'bronchial collaterals').[4] It is unusual for them to arise more than one or two vertebral spaces above or below this level. On the other hand there is a considerable variability as to the level in the lungs where the aortopulmonary collaterals connect into the pulmonary circulation (Figure 25.2). In fact in many cases there may be no connection to the true pulmonary circulation. Under these circumstances collaterals may form a 'duplicate supply' if the relevant bronchopulmonary segments are also supplied by a branch of the true pulmonary artery. Collateral vessels may connect fairly proximally into a macroscopic lobar pulmonary artery. They may connect more distally at arteriolar level or alternatively there may be a diffuse connection which is almost at capillary level. In addition to discrete collateral vessels there may also be diffuse distal small vessel connections to the lungs from the systemic circulation most commonly from the chest wall particularly if there are adhesions from previous surgery.

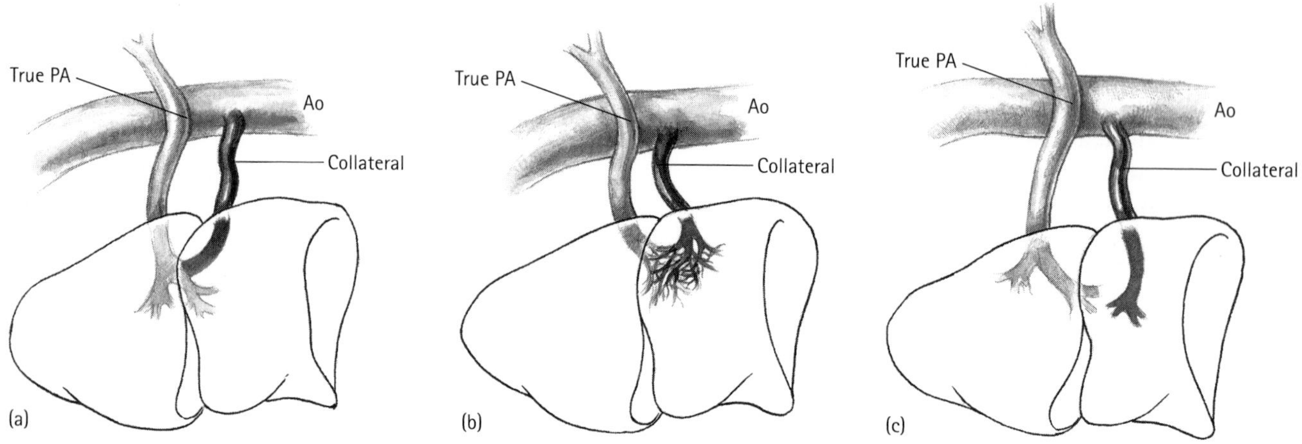

Figure 25.2 *Aortopulmonary collateral vessels may connect to the true pulmonary arteries at one of several levels. (a) Connection of an aortopulmonary collateral to a lobar branch pulmonary artery. (b) Very peripheral connection of a collateral to the true pulmonary circulation. (c) There is no connection between the aortopulmonary collateral and true pulmonary circulation.*

Multiple stenoses of true pulmonary arteries and aortopulmonary collaterals

Aortopulmonary collaterals have the characteristics of muscular arteries until they penetrate the lung parenchyma where they assume characteristics that are more similar to pulmonary arteries (Figure 25.3). The segments that are muscular are particularly prone to the development of severe stenoses which are often progressive. On the other hand if there are no proximal stenoses and the distal vascular bed supplied directly from the aorta is exposed to aortic pressure then there is likely to be rapid development of pulmonary vascular obstructive disease in the distribution of the collateral vessels.

Like collateral vessels the true pulmonary arteries in tetralogy of Fallot with pulmonary atresia are particularly likely to develop multiple peripheral stenoses. These stenoses are frequently but not always adjacent to points of bifurcation such as the takeoff of the right upper lobe.

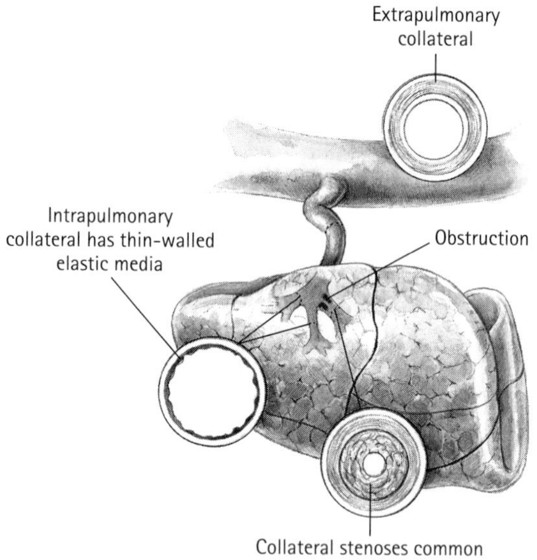

Figure 25.3 *Aortopulmonary collaterals have the characteristics of muscular arteries until they penetrate the lung parenchyma where they assume characteristics that are more similar to pulmonary arteries. The segments of collaterals that are muscular are particularly prone to the development of severe stenoses which are often progressive.*

Associated anomalies

The same cardiac anomalies that may be associated with tetralogy of Fallot with pulmonary stenosis including coronary anomalies and multiple VSDs may also be associated with pulmonary atresia. It is important to appreciate that *pulmonary atresia*, i.e. failure of connection between a ventricle and the true pulmonary arteries occurs as a component of many anomalies including double outlet right ventricle and many forms of single ventricle but these anomalies are considered to be distinct and separate entities from tetralogy with pulmonary atresia even though there may be a common embryological origin.

EXTRACARDIAC ANOMALIES

A cluster of congenital anomalies which may include tetralogy of Fallot with pulmonary atresia (or pulmonary stenosis) is the VACTERL association. In addition to vertebral and anal anomalies these babies most importantly have a tracheoesophageal fistula associated with esophageal atresia. The combination of a severe airway problem (tracheoesophageal fistula) with the complex cardiac and pulmonary vascular anomalies is a serious complicating factor in the management of these patients.[5]

PATHOPHYSIOLOGY AND CLINICAL FEATURES

It is an unfortunate paradox that babies at the most severe end of the spectrum of tetralogy of Fallot with pulmonary atresia are often remarkably free of symptoms and signs of heart disease. On the other hand, at the mild end of the spectrum where there is simple valvar atresia babies are duct dependent and will present with a profound degree of cyanosis shortly after birth when the ductus closes.

Duct dependent tetralogy of Fallot with pulmonary atresia

Because there is an unrestrictive VSD the pressure in the right ventricle is the same as the pressure in the left ventricle. So long as ductal patency is maintained by infusion of prostaglandin E1 there is usually an appropriate amount of pulmonary blood flow so that the child's oxygen saturation can be maintained reasonably stable in the range of 80–90%. It is unusual under these circumstances for the child to have an excessive amount of pulmonary blood flow resulting in the development of congestive heart failure. Occasionally the ductus does not close early in life and the child may remain relatively free of symptoms and perhaps even undiagnosed for several years.

Hypoplastic true pulmonary arteries and multiple aortopulmonary collateral vessels

These children are not duct dependent and therefore may not present with obvious signs and symptoms at birth. If there are few stenoses in the aortopulmonary collateral vessels there may be a progressive increase in pulmonary blood flow in the early weeks and months of life resulting in congestive heart failure but only a mild degree of cyanosis. In time, however, there is likely to be development of pulmonary vascular disease in lung segments that are supplied by collaterals without proximal stenoses. There is also likely to be progression of stenoses within the collateral vessels themselves. Either way there is likely to be a gradual deterioration in oxygen saturation over the coming months and years. Nevertheless many individuals with tetralogy of Fallot with pulmonary atresia with multiple aortopulmonary collateral vessels achieve a remarkably balanced circulation such that they can function free of symptoms for many years.

Cyanotic spells with pulmonary atresia?

Rather surprisingly it is not unheard of for patients with tetralogy of Fallot with pulmonary atresia to suffer from cyanotic spells. Although spells in tetralogy with pulmonary stenosis are attributed to spasm in the infundibulum of the right ventricle thereby increasing the dynamic component of right ventricular outflow tract obstruction, nevertheless the fact that patients with pulmonary atresia also may have spells illustrates that there is an alternative important mechanism causing spells. All blood leaves the heart through the aorta and has a choice or either perfusing systemic vessels or pulmonary vessels. Thus a balance must be maintained between systemic and pulmonary vascular resistance. Any situation that results in a decrease in systemic resistance will result in a fall in pulmonary blood flow which will become evident as cyanosis.

Late consequences of tetralogy with pulmonary atresia

If children have not succumbed because of ductal closure in the neonatal period or congestive heart failure because of excessive blood flow through large collaterals they may live with a reasonably well balanced circulation to their teenage years or twenties. At this stage it is common for progressive chronic cyanosis to result in the usual long-term consequences resulting from polycythemia including cerebral thrombosis and cerebral abscess. Clubbing of the extremities and nose may be prominent.

DIAGNOSTIC STUDIES

Pulse oximetry

Pulse oximetry is helpful in determining the balance of pulmonary and systemic blood flow. The child who has an excessive degree of collateral formation and who is at risk of developing congestive heart failure will usually have a resting oxygen saturation by pulse oximetry of greater than 85–90%. If there is inadequate pulmonary blood flow because of ductal closure, progression of collateral stenoses, progression of true pulmonary artery stenoses or development of pulmonary vascular disease then the pulse oximeter will demonstrate a falling oxygen saturation of less than 75–80%.

Chest X-ray and electrocardiography

If there is excessive pulmonary blood flow the lung fields will appear congested and plethoric. The heart size is likely to be large as congestive heart failure develops. If pulmonary blood flow is inadequate the lung fields will appear dark and oligemic. The heart size may be normal or smaller than normal.

Because some lung segments may be supplied with excessive blood flow while others may have inadequate blood flow there may be regional differences in lung perfusion apparent on the chest X-ray. Overall, however, the child's oxygen saturation can still achieve a reasonable balance at 75–85%.

The ECG, as with tetralogy of Fallot with pulmonary stenosis, is normal at birth but in time will demonstrate an abnormal degree of right ventricular hypertrophy secondary to the systemic pressure in the right ventricle which results from the unrestrictive anterior malalignment VSD.

Two-dimensional echocardiography

In contrast to the situation with tetralogy of Fallot with pulmonary stenosis, it is generally unwise to rely on echocardiography alone for definition of the anatomical features of the child with tetralogy of Fallot with pulmonary atresia. Perhaps at the mildest end of the spectrum, i.e. the neonate with duct dependent valvar or short segment pulmonary atresia in whom the branch pulmonary arteries can be seen to be of good size and in continuity it may be reasonable to rely on echocardiography alone. However, even in this situation it is important that the descending aorta be carefully interrogated for aortopulmonary collaterals.[6] Echocardiography is a reasonably sensitive method for detecting aortopulmonary collateral vessels but is not helpful in defining the specific anatomy of such collaterals or for defining peripheral pulmonary artery stenoses which are so commonly seen with tetralogy of Fallot with pulmonary atresia. In spite of these limitations in defining collaterals and peripheral pulmonary artery anatomy nevertheless echocardiography is helpful in defining intracardiac anatomy particularly the presence of multiple VSDs.[7] Echocardiography can also alert the management team to the presence of unusual coronary anatomy or the presence of a secundum ASD rather than a patent foramen ovale.

Cardiac catheterization

At the initial cardiac catheterization an attempt should be made to define the anatomy of all aortopulmonary collateral vessels. It may be difficult to define the anatomy of the true pulmonary arteries unless they are duct dependent and in continuity or if there is a proximal connection between a collateral vessel and the true pulmonary arteries. However, frequently it is necessary to use retrograde venous wedge angiography and even this may afford only a glimpse of the tiny true central pulmonary arteries. The angiographer will need to look carefully in either a lateral or left anterior oblique view for the characteristic 'seagull' appearance of the true pulmonary arteries. The right and left pulmonary artery represent the wings of the seagull while the body and head of the seagull are represented by the tiny main pulmonary artery. With each cardiac contraction the main pulmonary artery will bob inferiorly and the wings will appear to flap. The angiographer should be looking for a vessel that is no more than 1–2 mm in diameter which is frequently similar to the diameter of the catheter. At the initial catheterization it is generally not necessary to define features of intracardiac anatomy unless there has been a question on the initial echocardiogram of multiple VSDs or other rare associated anomalies.

SUBSEQUENT DIAGNOSTIC CATHETERIZATIONS

After continuity has been achieved between the right ventricle and true pulmonary arteries (see 'Surgical management' below) it is possible to advance a catheter from the right ventricle into the true pulmonary arteries. It is now essential to define the blood supply of each of the 20 bronchopulmonary segments of the lungs, i.e. whether a segment is supplied by a branch of the true pulmonary arteries, by a collateral vessel, or whether there is duplicate supply. In addition an attempt should be made to define the level at which the true pulmonary arteries communicate with collateral vessels if indeed there is communication. Finally it is important for the surgeon in particular to understand the relationship of the collateral vessels to other mediastinal structures, especially the trachea and esophagus. Some collateral vessels pass posterior to the esophagus, some pass between the trachea and esophagus and some pass anterior to the trachea and bronchi. It is even possible for a single collateral to bifurcate into two branches, one of which passes between the trachea and esophagus and the other behind the esophagus or in front of the trachea. This must be carefully studied on the lateral or anterior oblique views since a review of the AP projection alone may mislead the surgeon into believing that a simple unifocalization procedure can be achieved.

HEMODYNAMIC DATA

In addition to the important anatomical information derived from cineangiography, cardiac catheterization also allows the determination of important hemodynamic information. An assessment should be made regarding distal pressure within collateral vessels. If the distal pressure is importantly elevated, for example greater than a mean pressure of 20–25 mm, it is likely that pulmonary vascular disease either has already developed or will develop within the lung segments supplied. Cardiac catheterization is also helpful in determining when VSD closure is appropriate. When a left to right shunt is present following dilation of peripheral pulmonary artery stenoses and appropriate unifocalization procedures then it can be assumed by definition that the pulmonary artery tree is able to carry at least one cardiac output. Therefore closure of the VSD should not result in greater than systemic pressure within the right ventricle. In fact the pressure within the right ventricle is an important endpoint in assessing the success of the overall management strategy for an individual with tetralogy of Fallot with pulmonary atresia. Ideally right ventricular pressure should eventually be less than 50% of systemic pressure or at least less than 75% of systemic pressure. Unfortunately this goal can be very difficult to achieve.

Magnetic resonance imaging

MRI is emerging as a particularly helpful diagnostic tool for the patient with complex tetralogy of Fallot with pulmonary atresia. It can be extremely difficult using angiography alone to understand the inter-relationship of collateral vessels and true pulmonary arteries. The ability to perform three-dimensional reconstruction using MRI is particularly helpful in understanding complex collateral and pulmonary artery anatomy and aids in the planning of unifocalization procedures.[8]

MEDICAL AND INTERVENTIONAL THERAPY

The management of complex tetralogy of Fallot with pulmonary atresia, i.e. the child with hypoplastic true pulmonary arteries and multiple aortopulmonary collateral vessels, is the paradigm for close collaborative management between the interventional cardiologist and the congenital cardiac surgeon. The child must also be very carefully managed with appropriate medical therapy while in the ICU as well as on an outpatient basis.

Prostaglandin E1

Babies who are ductally dependent will require infusion of prostaglandin E1 to maintain ductal patency until pulmonary blood flow can be achieved through an appropriate intervention.

Beta-blockers, vasoconstrictors

Although cyanotic spells can be seen occasionally in the child with tetralogy of Fallot with pulmonary atresia their mechanism is at least in part different from patients with tetralogy of Fallot with pulmonary stenosis. Long-term prophylactic therapy with a beta-blocker is definitely not indicated. Occasionally severe cyanosis can be managed temporarily in the ICU setting with a vasoconstrictor such as phenylephrine. As noted for tetralogy of Fallot with pulmonary stenosis it is important to avoid vasoconstricting the child immediately before cardiopulmonary bypass.

Anticongestive therapy

The child who has excessive pulmonary blood flow and who therefore develops congestive heart failure will need to be managed with digoxin and diuretics. These children are at risk of developing pulmonary vascular disease.

Interventional catheterization procedures

Skilful interventional catheterization procedures are an essential component of the overall management of the child with pulmonary atresia.[9] Delicate steel or titanium coils with protruding tufts of thrombogenic Dacron fabric are used to occlude collateral vessels that provide duplicate blood supply to bronchopulmonary segments. Balloon dilation catheters are used to dilate the multiple peripheral stenoses that are frequently present in the true pulmonary arteries. Balloon dilation is also necessary for the stenoses that occur in collateral vessels including anastomotic stenoses after unifocalization has been performed surgically. Because the stenoses that occur in tetralogy of Fallot with pulmonary atresia are frequently difficult to dilate because of the thick walled and fibrous nature of these stenoses it is not uncommon for techniques such as cutting balloons and stent placement to be required. The sequencing of these various interventions will be discussed under 'Surgical management' below.

CATHETER PERFORATION OF VALVAR ATRESIA

Unlike neonates with pulmonary atresia and intact ventricular septum who often have a well developed annulus and main pulmonary artery, the neonate with valvar atresia in the setting of tetralogy of Fallot with pulmonary atresia (i.e. with a nonrestrictive anterior malalignment VSD rather than an intact ventricular septum) rarely has a normal sized pulmonary annulus and main pulmonary artery. Thus it is unusual that such babies will be suitable for catheter perforation of the atretic valve. Furthermore, as discussed under interventional therapy for tetralogy of Fallot with pulmonary stenosis (Chapter 16), there is a risk that successful opening of the right ventricular outflow tract will result in an unrestricted left to right shunt which may precipitate serious congestive heart failure. Since surgical management of the VSD is required even if there is successful dilation of the outflow tract, it is probably best to avoid interventional catheterization under these circumstances and to proceed directly to surgical management.[10]

INDICATIONS FOR AND TIMING OF SURGERY

The indications and timing of surgery at the simple end of the spectrum of tetralogy of Fallot with pulmonary atresia are simple. Since the neonate is ductally dependent it is essential that a surgical procedure be undertaken in the newborn period. On the other hand the child who has hypoplastic true pulmonary arteries and whose blood supply is derived from multiple aortopulmonary collateral vessels will remain relatively free of symptoms so long as there is a balanced degree of pulmonary blood flow. If there is excessive pulmonary blood flow the child will develop congestive heart failure. Under these circumstances it is important to proceed to catheterization and coil occlusion of duplicate collateral vessels. However, even if the child is free of symptoms it is important to establish a connection between the right ventricle and true pulmonary arteries as early in life as possible. Work by Rabinovitch and others[11–13] has demonstrated that children with pulmonary atresia have fewer generations of both the bronchoalveolar tree as well as the pulmonary vascular tree. Presumably earlier establishment of normal antegrade pulmonary blood flow is associated with more normal development of alveolar number as well as a more normal total cross sectional area of pulmonary capillaries. Experience has also demonstrated that there is remarkable potential for tiny central pulmonary arteries to enlarge very rapidly during the first year of life.[14]

On the other hand failure to establish antegrade pulmonary blood flow results in arrested development of the central pulmonary arteries which continue to remain at 1.5–2 mm in diameter even in the older child or adult. If antegrade blood flow is not established until later childhood there is clearly much less potential for rapid development of the true pulmonary arteries.

An ethical dilemma: the teenager and young adult with balanced circulation

A number of individuals with tetralogy of Fallot with pulmonary atresia will survive into their teenage years and even young adulthood with remarkable balance of pulmonary and systemic blood flow.[15] This results from development of proximal collateral stenoses as well as the development of vascular disease in a limited number of bronchopulmonary segments. These individuals can function with a surprising degree of normality and on occasion may not even be diagnosed until their teenage years or young adulthood. Because almost by definition there must be many bronchopulmonary segments with vascular disease or supply from collaterals with relatively severe proximal stenoses, it can be particularly challenging in such individuals to achieve a corrected circulation. Furthermore multiple interventions will be necessary. Since it seems very likely that the potential for development of a normal capillary cross sectional area and normal alveolar development is unlikely by this age many have questioned the advisability of proceeding with any interventions. It will be important in the future to analyse carefully the results of multiple catheter and surgical interventions in patients who present with a well balanced circulation in their teenage years or young adulthood and compare these to the natural history of the disease. On the other hand it is important not to confuse these individuals with the neonate, infant or young child less than 5–10 years of age who retains the potential for development of the pulmonary vascular tree and bronchoalveolar tree and in whom the multiple catheter and surgical interventions can achieve extremely good results.

SURGICAL MANAGEMENT

History of surgery

Tetralogy of Fallot with pulmonary atresia is the prime example of an anomaly which must be managed by interposition of a conduit between the right ventricle and pulmonary arteries. The history of development of conduits including their application for tetralogy with pulmonary atresia has been covered in Chapter 3. All of the various systemic to pulmonary artery shunts have been applied for tetralogy of Fallot with pulmonary atresia. The history of development of systemic to pulmonary artery shunts has been covered in Chapter 16.

Technical considerations

DECISION MAKING REGARDING ALTERNATIVE STRATEGIES FOR MANAGEMENT

Shunt or no shunt

The advantages of early primary repair have been described in detail in Chapters 1 and 16. Even when the branch pulmonary arteries are relatively well developed dissection in the region of the pulmonary arteries as well as suturing for a distal shunt anastomosis will interfere with the normal compliant nature of the branch pulmonary arteries. Furthermore in the setting of tetralogy of Fallot with pulmonary atresia the branch pulmonary arteries may be quite hypoplastic. It will be particularly difficult under these circumstances to maintain shunt patency because of poor runoff through the shunt. In addition there is a high risk of creating an important branch pulmonary artery stenosis.

One stage or multi-stage management

There is considerable confusion regarding the circumstances under which it is appropriate to proceed to one stage repair of tetralogy of Fallot with pulmonary atresia. An important principle to bear in mind is that if the true pulmonary arteries are providing most or all of the pulmonary blood flow and if the child's oxygen saturation is at least 75–80% then it is highly probable that the pulmonary artery tree will be able to carry a full cardiac output with acceptable subsystemic right ventricular pressure. It is not necessary under these circumstances to assess the anatomical size of the branch pulmonary arteries using indices such as the Nakata or McGoon indices.[16,17] In fact such indices can be quite misleading since the branch pulmonary arteries may be exposed to a low perfusion pressure preoperatively at the time of their assessment. Thus the child who presents with ductally dependent pulmonary arteries in continuity who has an arterial oxygen saturation of 85% with the duct maintained open with prostaglandin E1 can definitely proceed to one stage repair as *long as there are no other important sources of pulmonary blood flow*. If additional sources of pulmonary blood flow are identified, i.e. important aortopulmonary collateral vessels, the child should undergo cardiac catheterization. If the aortopulmonary collateral vessels are demonstrated to be duplicate then they should be test occluded to assess the impact on oxygen saturation. If the oxygen saturation remains adequate, i.e. greater than 70–75% then the duplicate collateral vessels should be coil occluded. Since the child is now being maintained alive only by the true pulmonary artery tree a reasonable inference can be made that repair can be undertaken. In fact repair will be undertaken more safely following elimination of collaterals which would otherwise have stolen important flow from the cardiopulmonary bypass perfusion.

If the true pulmonary arteries are very hypoplastic, i.e. usually 1.5–2 mm in diameter, then there will definitely be multiple other sources of pulmonary blood flow derived from aortopulmonary collateral vessels. Although it is theoretically possible to proceed to a one stage unifocalization procedure including closure of the VSD,[18] a preferable approach is to undertake an initial palliative procedure which will promote development of the true pulmonary arteries. This will allow for safer subsequent unifocalization procedures which are less likely to distort or even occlude the true pulmonary arteries. An initial palliative procedure connecting the right ventricle to the hypoplastic true pulmonary arteries also allows for a subsequent diagnostic catheterization procedure to define more accurately the distribution of the true pulmonary arteries. A more informed decision can be made regarding duplicate supply or lack of supply to all bronchopulmonary segments.[14]

ONE STAGE REPAIR

One stage repair of tetralogy of Fallot with pulmonary atresia is usually performed in the neonate with duct dependent pulmonary circulation. Many of the same principles apply as are used for repair of tetralogy of Fallot with pulmonary stenosis. For example, in neonates less than 3.5–4 kg in weight a single venous cannula in the right atrium is employed. With appropriate cannula placement tricuspid valve competence will prevent air being entrained into the cannula. The child should be cooled to deep hypothermia so that a brief period of circulatory arrest can be employed for placement of VSD sutures in the region of the tricuspid valve. In neonates weighing less than 2–2.5 kg hypothermic circulatory arrest is often employed for most of the VSD closure.

Management of the patent ductus arteriosus

Following full heparinization, placement of the arterial cannula in the ascending aorta and a single venous cannula in the right atrium bypass is commenced. Immediately after commencing bypass it is important to ligate the ductus arteriosus. Failure to ligate the ductus will result in a steal of blood from the systemic circulation into the pulmonary circulation. Not only will this result in hypoperfusion of the body but in addition it will cause serious left heart distention. The duct can be ligated with a simple 2/0 Ethibond ligature or alternatively with a 5/0 Prolene suture ligature. Care should be taken to avoid overtightening the ligature as the ductal tissue is quite friable and can be easily cut through.

Preparation of the pulmonary arteries for anastomosis

During the cooling phase of bypass to deep hypothermia the right and left pulmonary arteries should be dissected free together with the main pulmonary artery if this is present. The vestigial main pulmonary artery should be divided proximal to its bifurcation. The resulting arteriotomy is extended over an appropriate length into the right and left pulmonary artery (more on the left than the right) so as to achieve an arteriotomy that will be similar in diameter to the homograft conduit that has been selected.

Length and location of the ventriculotomy

Unlike tetralogy of Fallot with pulmonary stenosis there is no possibility of avoiding an incision in the infundibulum of the right ventricle. The infundibular incision will form the proximal anastomosis of the conduit from the right ventricle to the pulmonary arteries. It is also the most convenient access for VSD closure. The ventriculotomy incision is made after the aortic cross clamp has been applied and cardioplegia has been infused. The length of the ventriculotomy should be no more than 1 or 2 mm greater than the internal diameter of the conduit. It should be located in the infundibulum of the right ventricle with adequate clearance on the left from the left anterior descending coronary artery, superiorly from the left main coronary artery and on the right from the conal branch of the right coronary artery. Great care must be taken during VSD closure to avoid excessive retraction resulting in lengthening of the ventriculotomy by muscle tearing that can leave inadequate clearance from any of these coronary arteries.

Other technical considerations

A number of other relevant technical considerations are essentially identical to those applied for repair of tetralogy of Fallot with pulmonary stenosis (see Chapter 16). For example, care should be taken to avoid excessive division of infundibular muscle bundles. In fact it is rarely necessary to divide any accessory muscle bundles in the setting of tetralogy of Fallot with pulmonary atresia. The moderator band should be carefully preserved. The technique of VSD closure is the same as the technique described for tetralogy of Fallot with pulmonary stenosis. Also it is important to leave the foramen ovale patent so that it will be able to allow right to left decompression in the early postoperative period.

Conduit selection

Until recently the only conduit suitable for neonatal repair of tetralogy of Fallot with pulmonary atresia has been either an aortic or pulmonary homograft. Even the smallest porcine valve containing Dacron conduits (12 mm) are too large and rigid for neonatal repair. With such conduits there is a risk of left main coronary artery compression. The rigid Dacron does not suture well to the delicate pulmonary arteries of the neonate. Finally, rapid calcification of the porcine valve and rapid accumulation of pseudointima within the low porosity Dacron conduit results in early failure of such conduits. There is presently no long term clinical information regarding the performance of bovine jugular vein conduits for this application.[19] Xenograft conduits even when treated with an anticalcification process have not performed well.[20]

Both aortic and pulmonary homografts can be applied for neonatal repair of tetralogy of Fallot with pulmonary atresia. There is no convincing evidence that pulmonary homografts perform better than aortic homografts in this setting perhaps because even aortic homografts at this size are quite thin walled and less prone to the heavy calcification that is seen in larger aortic homografts.[21] Nevertheless with either an aortic or pulmonary homograft there may be accelerated stenosis with failure in as short a time as 12 months perhaps caused by immune factors.[22] On the other hand many homografts inserted in the neonatal period or early infancy can last many years, on occasion as long as 12–14 years. The size of homograft that is selected for neonatal application will depend on a number of factors including most importantly homograft availability. For an average sized neonate of 3.5 kg a homograft with an internal diameter of 9–10 mm is generally appropriate.[23] It is rarely appropriate to select more than an 11–13 mm diameter homograft as there is likely to be inadequate retrosternal space and there will be important compression of the homograft. On the other hand a small homograft of 7–9 mm can produce a very satisfactory short term hemodynamic result, presumably because the length of the ventriculotomy is limited.

Technique of homograft conduit insertion

The distal homograft anastomosis to the branch pulmonary arteries is performed following VSD closure. It is generally preferable to leave the aortic cross clamp in place during this part of the procedure. The patient should be maintained at deep hypothermia with either low flow perfusion or a continuation of deep hypothermic circulatory arrest if there is excessive blood return from the pulmonary arteries. The homograft which by this time has been thawed and rinsed and carefully inspected must be cut to length. An excessively long homograft can kink causing right ventricular outflow tract obstruction. Because the branch pulmonary arteries have been well mobilized they are able to accommodate a homograft that has been cut slightly short: therefore it is generally best to err on the side of cutting the homograft slightly too short rather than too long. A simple end to side anastomosis is fashioned using continuous 6/0 Prolene. Usually it is preferable to use a smaller needle such as the BVI needle because of the delicacy of the pulmonary artery tissue. The proximal anastomosis of the homograft to the right ventricle should always be supplemented with a hood (see Chapter 2). Generally it is preferable to use autologous pericardium. However, initially direct anastomosis is fashioned posteriorly between both sides of the cephalad one third of the ventriculotomy and the posterior circumference of the homograft. If the homograft is aortic it should be rotated so that the homograft mitral valve lies posteriorly. It is a mistake to place the muscle shelf resulting from the homograft ventricular septum in the posterior location. This will result in a ridge which can accelerate stenosis of the homograft. The posterior direct anastomosis of the homograft to the right ventriculotomy is generally performed with continuous 5/0 Prolene using a larger needle such as the RB2.

The hood of autologous pericardium which roofs the proximal anastomosis must be created with depth using a careful gathering technique as described in Chapter 2 under 'Creating patches with depth'.

It is generally preferable to leave the aortic cross clamp in place throughout most of the performance of the proximal anastomosis. This suture line is generally within 2–3 mm of coronary arteries which must not be encircled by sutures. Because the distances to be sutured are quite short it should be possible to maintain the total cross clamp time at well under one hour and circulatory arrest time at less than 30–40 minutes. However, the aortic cross clamp should be released before the hood suture line is completed. This allows the right heart to decompress through the suture line before cardiac action is fully regained. Furthermore a sucker can be passed across the homograft valve to decompress the left heart if necessary. It is not uncommon to see some increase in left heart return in these patients even if macroscopic collateral vessels have not been identified. At all times great care must be taken to anticipate increased left heart return and to avoid left heart distention with its consequent injury to both the left ventricle and the lungs.

Other technical aspects of the repair of tetralogy of Fallot with pulmonary atresia are very similar to those for tetralogy of Fallot with pulmonary stenosis. For example weaning from bypass should be uncomplicated. If there is a problem right ventricular outflow tract obstruction, residual VSD or coronary obstruction or compression should be sought.

MULTISTAGE REPAIR OF COMPLEX TETRALOGY OF FALLOT WITH PULMONARY ATRESIA WITH HYPOPLASTIC PAs AND MAPCAs

Stage 1 surgery: establishing continuity between right ventricle and hypoplastic pulmonary arteries

When it has been determined that one stage complete repair will not be possible because of the hypoplastic nature of the true pulmonary arteries an initial palliative procedure must be performed to connect the right ventricle to the branch pulmonary arteries. Although it is theoretically to perform this procedure without cardiopulmonary bypass it has become apparent that the proximal anastomosis of the homograft to right ventricle is best achieved using a brief period of CPB. Because the branch pulmonary arteries are generally no more than 1.5–2 mm in diameter a relatively small homograft conduit, either aortic or pulmonary, should be selected. Generally an internal diameter of 6–8 mm is appropriate. Approach is via a median sternotomy. The thymus is subtotally resected. A patch of anterior pericardium is harvested and treated with 0.6% glutaraldehyde for 20–30 minutes. The branch pulmonary arteries and vestigial main pulmonary artery are dissected free using great care since these vessels are very small and quite fragile (Figure 25.4a). Generally no ductus is present. A single C-clamp is applied to control both the right and left pulmonary arteries. The main pulmonary artery is transected quite proximally. The presence of pulmonary atresia is confirmed because no forward flow emerges from the right ventricle. The tiny main pulmonary artery is filleted open bilaterally (Figure 25.4a inset). It is very important not to extend this incision into the bifurcation itself and certainly not into either right or left pulmonary artery. The small homograft having previously been thawed and rinsed is cut to length with appropriate beveling of the distal end. A direct anastomosis is fashioned to the arteriotomy and the vestigial main pulmonary artery using continuous 6/0 or 7/0 Prolene (Figure 25.4b).

Creation of the proximal homograft anastomosis maintaining a beating heart on warm CPB: Prior to making the ventriculotomy the posterior third of the proximal circumference of the homograft is anastomosed to the infundibulum of the right ventricle using continuous 5/0 or 6/0 Prolene (Figure 25.4c). A careful note must be taken as to where the suture lies deep to the surface of the infundibulum. A generous patch of autologous pericardium which will form the hood of the anastomosis is sutured to the homograft itself and partially to the infundibulum of the right ventricle parallel to the

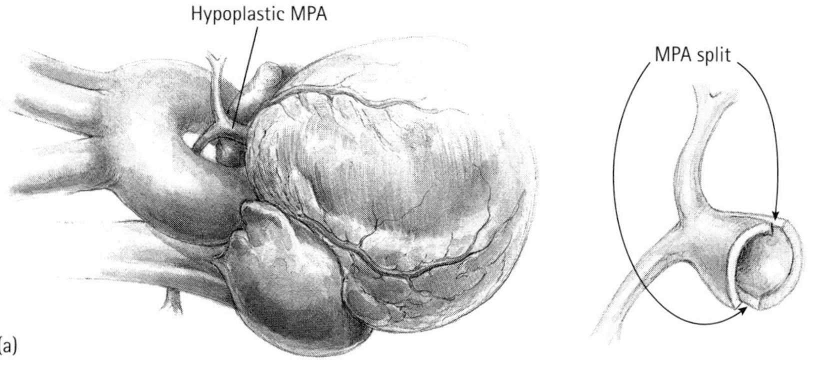

(a)

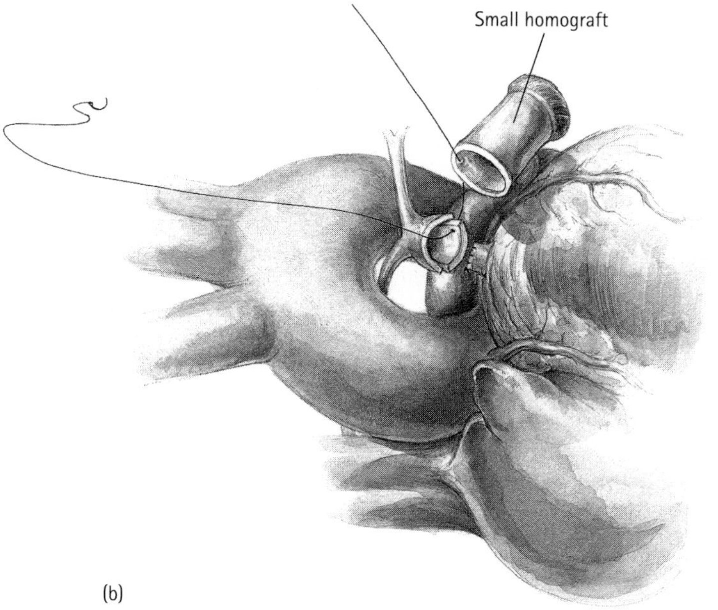

(b)

Figure 25.4a,b *Stage 1 surgery for tetralogy of Fallot with pulmonary atresia with hypoplastic central pulmonary arteries and multiple aortopulmonary collaterals. (a) The vestigial main pulmonary artery and tiny branch pulmonary arteries are carefully dissected free. Inset: the tiny main pulmonary artery is split bilaterally following proximal division. (b) A very small pulmonary homograft, e.g. 6–8 mm, is thawed and cut to length. The distal anastomosis is fashioned to the vestigial main pulmonary artery.*

anticipated ventriculotomy. By this point the patient has been fully heparinized and cannulas are inserted. Bypass is commenced. It is important that the prime of the bypass circuit be at normothermia and that the calcium concentration has been normalized. In this way the heart should be beating normally within one to two minutes of commencing bypass. An air vent is created in the proximal ascending aorta similar to a cardioplegia infusion site. This small needle hole is allowed to bleed in order to vent any air that may be entrained during the performance of the ventriculotomy and completion of the hood suture line. With the aortic vent bleeding appropriately a longitudinal incision is made inferior to the homograft to right ventricle suture line (Figure 25.4d). Because the heart is continuing to beat through this period blood will be ejected through the ventriculotomy though this can be controlled by careful communication between the surgeon and perfusionist regarding the flow rate and amount of venous drainage. In a matter of a minute or two the remainder of the pericardial hood suture line can be completed around the ventriculotomy (Figure 25.4e). As the final sutures are tightened it is important to avoid air being entrained into the ventricle as this will be ejected either into the pulmonary or systemic circulation.

Weaning from bypass should be uncomplicated because the homograft should make little difference to the patient's hemodynamics. The true pulmonary arteries are so hypoplastic in this setting that they initially carry very little pulmonary blood flow. There is little likelihood of excessive pulmonary perfusion and consequent inadequate systemic perfusion in spite of the fact that multiple aortopulmonary collateral vessels are present. Furthermore there has been no myocardial ischemia as no aortic cross clamp is applied. In fact application of an aortic cross clamp would create the need to insert a left heart vent which would steal from the systemic circulation because of the presence of multiple collateral vessels. By maintaining the heart beating throughout the procedure the blood returning to the heart from collaterals is ejected back into the systemic circulation.

Stage 2 management of complex TOF/PA: interventional catheterization

The timing of the first catheterization following connection of the right ventricle to the hypoplastic pulmonary arteries will be determined to some extent by the evolution of the child's arterial oxygen saturation. Ideally at least three to six weeks should be allowed to pass to allow for adequate healing

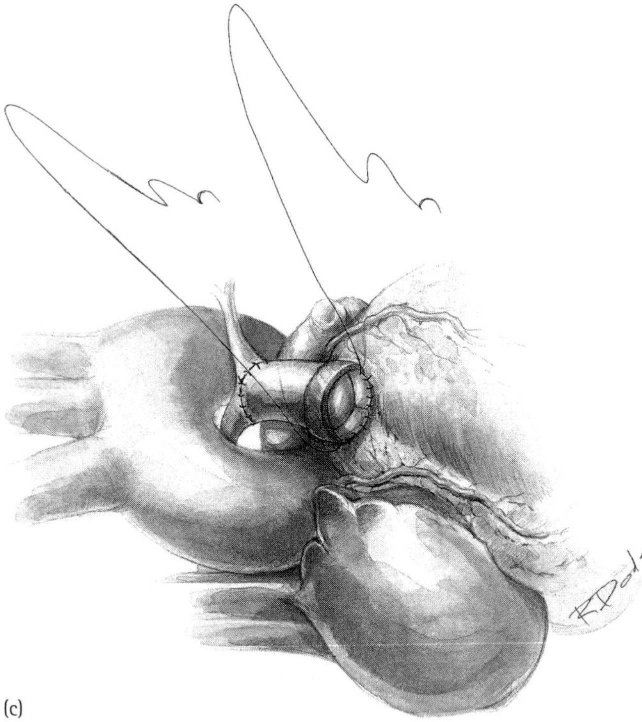

(c)

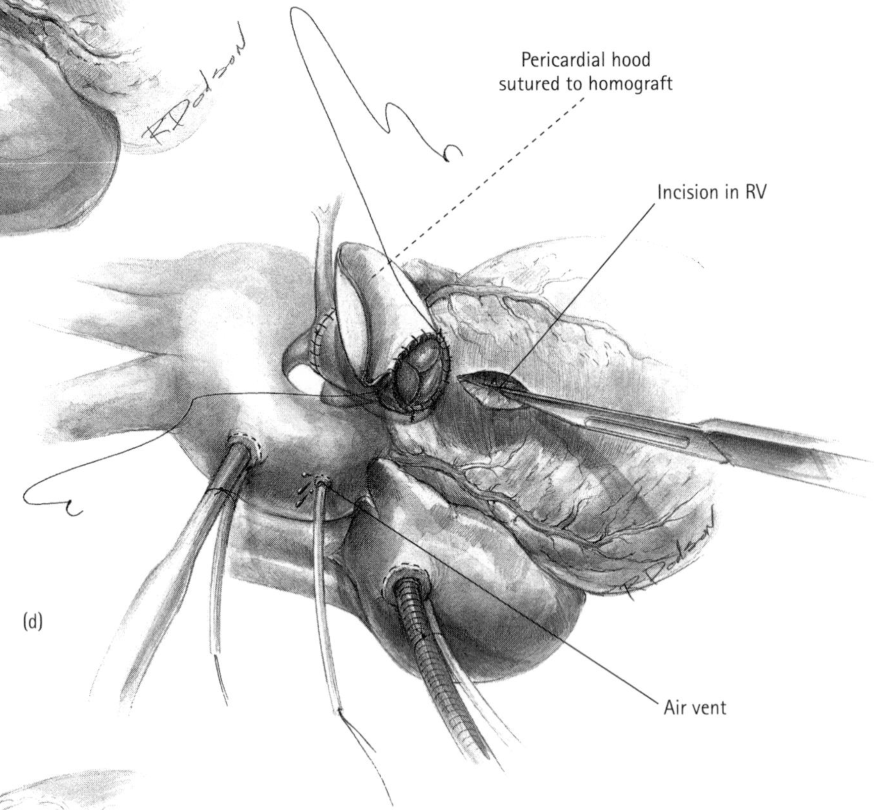

(d)

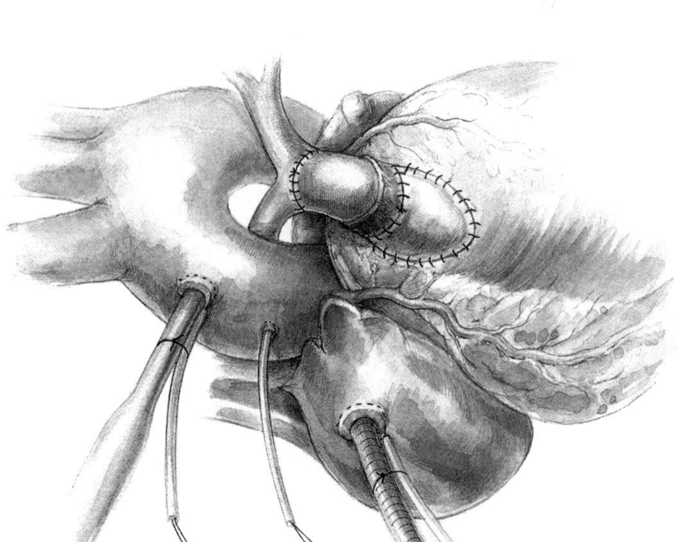

(e)

Figure 25.4c–e *(c) Part of the posterior circumference of the proximal homograft is sutured to the infundibulum of the right ventricle before the infundibular incision is made. (d) Warm normocalcemic bypass is established and an air vent is created in the proximal ascending aorta. A longitudinal incision is made in the infundibulum below the homograft after a pericardial hood has been partially sutured to the homograft and right ventricle. The pericardial hood supplementing the proximal homograft anastomosis has been completed and the patient is weaned from bypass.*

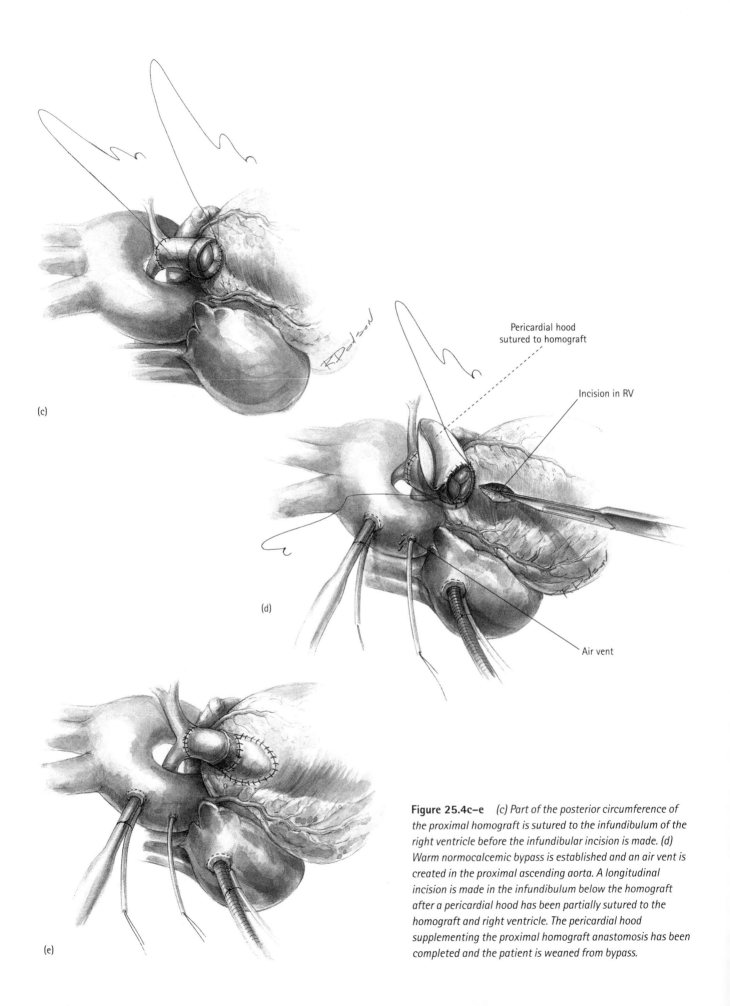

of all anastomoses before balloon dilation is attempted. In general the catheterization procedure will be undertaken three to six months following homograft conduit insertion. Hopefully by this time there will have been an increase in arterial oxygen saturation perhaps from a level such as 80% preoperatively to 90% at three to six months postoperatively. This increase in arterial oxygen saturation suggests satisfactory growth of the true pulmonary arteries that are now able to carry an increasing amount of pulmonary blood flow. It will also allow a satisfactory safety margin that will permit coil occlusion of aortopulmonary collateral vessels.

Definition of true pulmonary artery distribution: The most important diagnostic information that should be obtained at this catheterization is the segmental distribution of the true pulmonary arteries. In general it will not have been possible to determine this at the preoperative catheterization when visualization of the true pulmonary arteries was only possible indirectly (by retrograde venous wedge angiography). When the information regarding distribution of the true pulmonary arteries is collated with previous information regarding collateral distribution a decision can be made whether certain bronchopulmonary segments are receiving duplicate supply from both a true pulmonary artery segmental branch as well as aortopulmonary collaterals. Any duplicate aortopulmonary collateral vessels are then temporarily occluded by balloon occlusion. The fall in arterial oxygen saturation that results is observed. So long as a reasonable oxygen saturation of greater than 75% or so is maintained it is reasonable to proceed to permanent coil occlusion of these duplicate aortopulmonary collaterals. In addition to occluding duplicate collaterals the first postoperative catheterization allows for planning regarding unifocalization of nonduplicate collaterals. Usually this will apply to at least two or three collaterals but there may be as many as five or six which need to be unifocalized. Balloon dilation procedures are usually undertaken at this catheterization both within the true pulmonary arteries as well as within collateral vessels.

Unifocalization of collateral vessels to the true pulmonary arteries

The term 'unifocalization' is employed to describe a surgical procedure in which aortopulmonary collateral vessels are divided from their aortic origin and are anastomosed to the true pulmonary arteries. Although the traditional approach has been through a thoracotomy more recently most groups have favored a central approach working through a median sternotomy.[18,24]

Unifocalization via median sternotomy: Hanley has popularized the central approach to aortopulmonary collaterals working through a median sternotomy. Because the majority of large aortopulmonary collateral vessels arise in the subcarinal region they can be approached through the posterior wall of the transverse sinus. It is essential that the surgeon has a clear understanding of the origin and distribution of the multiple collateral vessels before embarking on the procedure. MRI is very helpful in this regard. The ascending aorta is retracted leftward and using electrocautery the posterior wall of the transverse sinus is opened. There are multiple subcarinal lymph nodes in this area which must be carefully excised. The esophagus and vagus nerves must be carefully preserved. The descending aorta is generally identified without difficulty and then careful identification of the collateral anatomy must be undertaken (Figure 25.5a). When collateral vessels run directly from the aorta into the lung substance they can

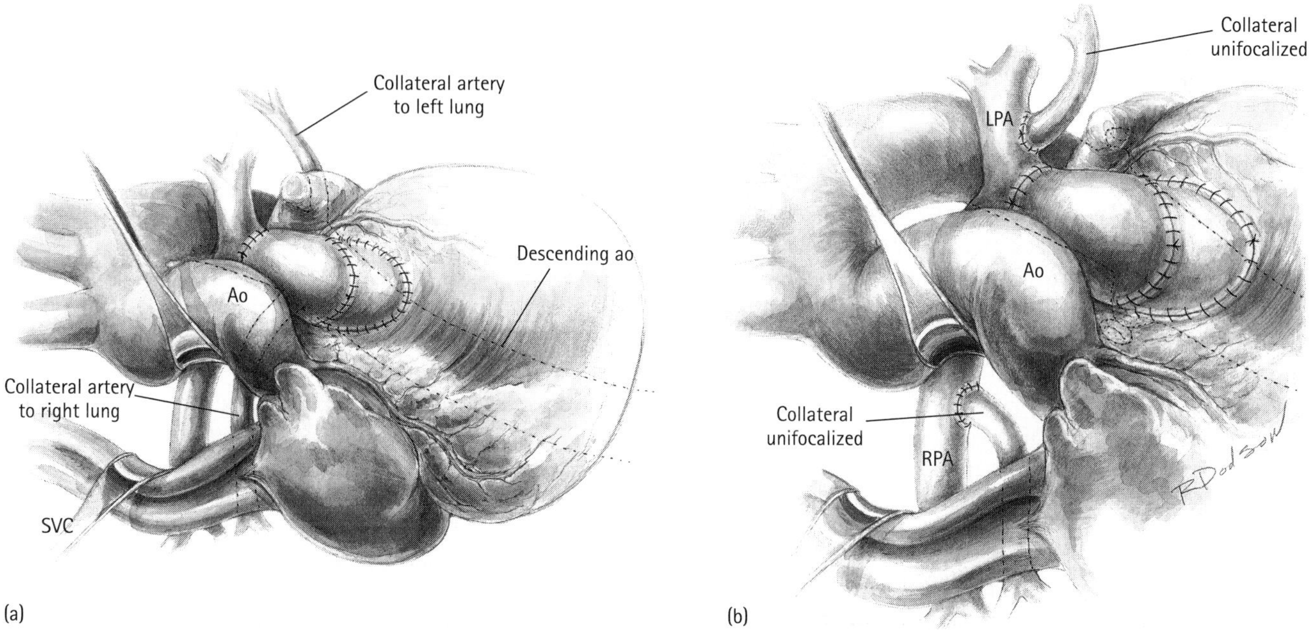

Figure 25.5 *Unifocalization of collateral vessels to true pulmonary arteries via median sternotomy. (a) A collateral artery to the right lung is identified posterior to the transverse sinus with retraction of the ascending aorta leftwards. (b) One collateral vessel has been unifocalized to the true right pulmonary artery and a second collateral vessel has been unifocalized to the left pulmonary artery.*

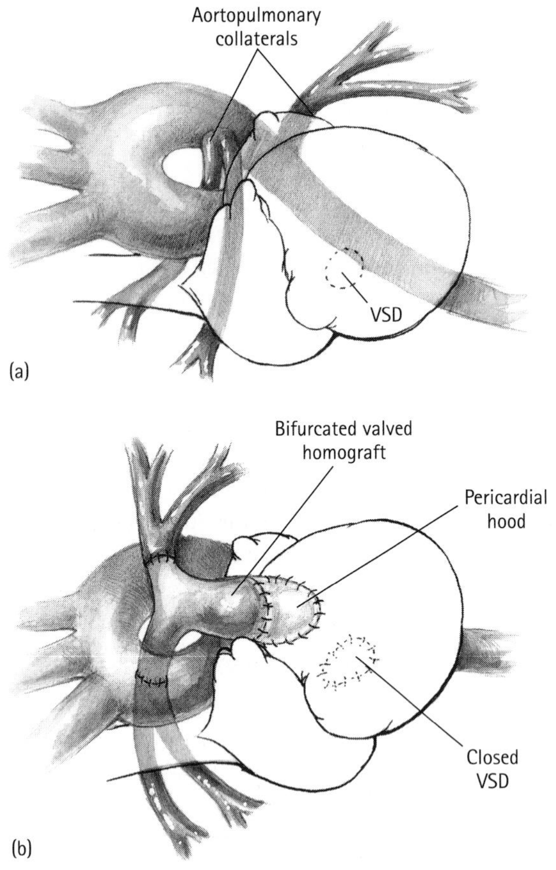

Figure 25.6 *One stage unifocalization may be appropriate if the true pulmonary arteries are completely absent though this is exceedingly rare. (a) Patient has absent true pulmonary arteries and pulmonary blood flow is derived from two very large aortopulmonary collateral vessels. (b) One stage unifocalization with end to end anstomoses between the collaterals and homograft branch pulmonary arteries. VSD closure is possible so long as distal pulmonary resistance is not severely elevated.*

be easily unifocalized directly to the true pulmonary arteries by end to side anastomosis or to the homograft conduit also by end to side anastomosis (Figure 25.5b). However, if the collaterals bifurcate and pass in different directions around mediastinal structures such as the esophagus then unifocalization is more difficult. Occasionally a decision will have to be made to divide a bifurcating collateral and to perform two separate anastomoses though the collateral branches are likely to be very small.

If the true pulmonary arteries are absent a one stage unifocalization procedure may be appropriate including end to end anastomoses to the homograft branch pulmonary arteries (Figure 25.6). It may be possible to proceed to VSD closure at the same operation if adequate unifocalization is possible and the peripheral resistance is sufficiently low.

VSD closure at the first unifocalization procedure? It is rarely possible to proceed to either partial or complete VSD closure at the time of the initial unifocalization procedure.[25] Generally even at this time the true pulmonary arteries are still quite small, e.g. 4–5 mm in diameter, so that even with satisfactory anastomosis of all collateral vessels there is still inadequate pulmonary arterial cross sectional area to allow VSD closure. However, if the VSD is not closed and there is difficulty weaning from cardiopulmonary bypass consideration should be given to the possibility that there is an excessive left to right shunt at VSD level. This should be apparent because the child will be fully saturated.

Unifocalization by thoracotomy: A number of authors have popularized the thoracotomy approach for unifocalization of multiple aortopulmonary collateral vessels including Puga from the Mayo Clinic[26] and Imai from Tokyo Women's Medical College.[27] Although Puga's earlier approach was to place small caliber Gortex grafts to facilitate unifocalization more recently he has recommended direct anastomosis whenever possible.[28] Imai has popularized the concept of anastomosing multiple collateral vessels working through a thoracotomy to a blind ending tube constructed from pericardium which acts like a manifold. Initially he recommended equine pericardium but more recently has used autologous pericardium because of problems with calcification of equine pericardium.[29] The mediastinal end of the pericardial 'roll' is tacked to the mediastinum where it will be retrieved at a subsequent sternotomy procedure and anastomosed to a right ventricle to pulmonary artery conduit. In the meantime the blood supply to the pericardial roll with its attached collaterals is derived from a modified Blalock type shunt using a Gortex tube graft taken from the right or left subclavian artery. In addition to describing the pericardial roll concept, Imai has emphasized the advantage of intra-pulmonary unifocalization whenever possible. Because the extrapulmonary collateral vessels are muscular arteries that are very susceptible to stenosis it is preferable to unifocalize more distally where the vessels are thin walled and more similar to true pulmonary arteries. By dissecting into the lobar fissures Imai believes it is generally possible to identify points where the collateral vessels are close to the true pulmonary arteries and can be anastomosed by side to side anastomosis. However, it is important to understand that this concept is more applicable to the older child and is very difficult to apply in the neonate or infant in the first year or two of life.

Post unifocalization catheterization

Following the unifocalization procedure a follow-up catheterization should be performed within three to six months to determine the success of the procedure. Once again, the child's oxygen saturation is helpful in determining the timing of the catheterization. If the oxygen saturation steadily increases over the three to six months following surgery this may be a sign that satisfactory growth is occurring of both the true pulmonary arteries as well as the unifocalized collaterals. Even without any change in arterial oxygen saturation, however, it is advisable to undertake catheterization within three to six months. Almost certainly there will be multiple peripheral stenoses in both the true pulmonary arteries as well as the unifocalized collaterals that will require balloon dilation with or without stenting. This may include anastomotic stenoses. There is also a significant risk that unifocalized vessels will be demonstrated to have become occluded. These vessels often have quite a tortuous course through the mediastinum, they have an abnormal wall structure and the anastomosis may have been undertaken under tension.

Assessment of need for further unifocalization procedures: The post-unifocalization catheterization may demonstrate that not all collateral vessels have been unifocalized. If the remaining vessels arising from the aorta supply an important number of bronchopulmonary segments another surgical unifocalization procedure may be advisable. Perhaps these may be vessels that could not be reached through a median sternotomy approach and will require a thoraocotomy approach.

Assessment of timing of VSD closure: VSD closure is indicated when a net left to right shunt can be documented by oxygen saturation data, i.e. there is a step up between SVC saturation and pulmonary artery saturation. Usually this will mean that at least 10–12 bronchopulmonary segments are now supplied by the true pulmonary arteries. Often, however, the situation is complicated by the fact that the child is now a year or 18 months beyond the initial surgical procedure at which a small right ventricle to pulmonary artery homograft was placed. There may now be a moderate degree of stenosis across the conduit, e.g. a gradient of 30–50 mm. If there is equal systemic and pulmonary blood flow under this circumstance then it can be anticipated that following conduit change there will be a net left to right shunt. Perhaps there may also be one final aortopulmonary collateral vessel that can be unifocalized at the time of conduit change. With the expectation that this will further increase any left to right shunt it may be reasonable to proceed to VSD closure.

VSD closure with or without fenestration

If the sequence of procedures described above has been begun in the neonatal period or early infancy the child will generally be in the range of one to three years of age by the time VSD closure is undertaken. The previous median sternotomy is reopened. The child is cannulated with the arterial cannula in the ascending aorta and venous return via two straight caval cannulas inserted through the right atrium. By this time essentially all collateral vessels have been unifocalized so there should not be a problem with excessive left heart return. Generally the procedure is undertaken at a temperature of 25–28°C with aortic cross clamping and cardioplegia infusion. If the homograft conduit is to be replaced as is likely to be necessary it is removed following application of the aortic cross clamp. Working through the proximal homograft conduit anastomosis the VSD is closed in the usual fashion using a knitted velour Dacron patch and interrupted pledgetted horizontal mattress sutures. If there is serious concern that in spite of changing the homograft the pulmonary vasculature is only just adequate to accept a full cardiac output then a fenestration can be placed in the VSD patch at this time. More commonly, however, the VSD is totally closed and the homograft is replaced with a new larger homograft. The patient is de-aired, the aortic cross clamp is released and the patient is rewarmed to normothermia. After weaning from bypass right ventricular pressure is carefully measured and compared with central aortic pressure (not radial arterial pressure). If right ventricular pressure is more than 10–20% greater than systemic pressure then the patient should be returned onto cardiopulmonary bypass. The patient is cooled to 32°C, the aortic cross clamp is reapplied and once again cardioplegia solution is infused. The proximal homograft anastomosis is partially taken down by releasing part of the pericardial hood. Using a skin hook the central part of the VSD patch is tented up and a 3–4 mm fenestration is cut in the central part of the patch. It is important to place the fenestration away from the aortic valve so there will be no risk of aortic valve damage when the fenestration is later closed with a catheter delivered device. However, the fenestration also must be well clear of tricuspid chordal apparatus. Thus a central fenestration is usually appropriate. Once again the heart is de-aired, the aortic cross clamp is released and the patient is separated from bypass after rewarming to normothermia.

Catheterization subsequent to VSD closure: device closure of fenestration

It is likely that further rehabilitation procedures for the pulmonary arteries will be helpful even following VSD closure. The goal should be to reduce right ventricular pressure to less than half systemic if possible. Multiple ballooning and stenting procedures are often necessary. Eventually, however, it is hoped that a net left to right shunt will be detectable across the fenestrated VSD patch. At this time an appropriate catheter delivered device can be used to close the fenestration.

RESULTS OF SURGERY

An assessment of the results of management of tetralogy of Fallot with pulmonary atresia is a particularly difficult undertaking. Not only is there is an extremely wide spectrum of severity but in addition many different approaches have been applied by different groups. The aggressiveness of interventional catheter techniques used in conjunction with surgery is another important variable.

Multi-stage repair including unifocalization

The largest report of traditional multi-stage treatment of tetralogy of Fallot with pulmonary atresia was published in 2002 by Cho et al from the Mayo Clinic.[28] A total of 495 patients had surgery for tetralogy with pulmonary atresia between 1977 and 1999. A total of 160 patients failed to achieve complete repair including VSD closure. Of these, 28% had preliminary surgical stages such as unifocalization or right ventricular outflow tract reconstruction and 21% had all surgical stages but were rejected for complete repair. Early mortality was 16% and late mortality was 23%. The presence of major aortopulmonary collateral vessels was a risk factor for late mortality.

Complete repair was achieved in 335 patients. In 30% this was done in a single stage while 69% had staged reconstruction. A total of 6.6% of patients required reopening of their ventricular septal defect because of right ventricular hypertension. Early mortality was 4.5%. Risk factors for mortality were a peak right ventricular to left ventricular pressure ratio of greater than 0.7 and a need for reopening of the VSD. Late mortality was 16% over a mean follow-up of 11 years. Risk factors for late mortality included male gender, nonconfluent central pulmonary arteries, reopening of the VSD and post-repair conduit change. Twenty-year survival was 75% and freedom from reoperation at 20 years was 29%.

In 1989, Sawatari, Imai et al[27] from Tokyo Women's Medical College described in detail their technique of unifocalization of multiple aortopulmonary collateral vessels with an equine pericardial tube initially connected to a modified Blalock shunt. The authors described 34 patients with a mean age of seven years who underwent first stage unifocalization with a mortality of 6%. Second stage repair carried a mortality of 12%. In 2001 Metras et al[30] from Marseille, France, described a multi-stage approach to tetralogy with pulmonary atresia in patients with extremely hypoplastic pulmonary arteries and major collaterals. There were 10 such patients among 63 with pulmonary atresia and VSD. Complete correction was achieved in seven patients after multiple stages including an initial connection between the true pulmonary arteries and right ventricle, subsequent interventional catheterizations including pulmonary artery dilation and stent placement as well as coil occlusion of collaterals and then subsequent VSD closure. There was one early death and one late death. The right ventricular to left ventricular pressure ratio at follow-up of 83 months was 0.6.

In 1995, Hadjo et al[31] from Bordeaux, France, described 52 patients who underwent staged surgical management of tetralogy of Fallot with pulmonary atresia. In 50% of these patients the pulmonary arteries were confluent and were supplied by a ductus arteriosus. The remaining 26 patients were either partially or completely dependent on systemic collateral vessels. In this latter group severe arborization defects with fewer than 10 pulmonary vascular segments connected to the true pulmonary arteries were present in eight patients. Corrective surgery was possible in 23 of 26 patients with confluent duct dependent pulmonary arteries but only in 9 of the 26 patients who were collateral dependent. Overall there was one early death and two late deaths. Also in 1995, Dinarevic et al[32] from the Brompton Hospital in London described 54 patients who were managed between 1972 and 1992. A total of 56% of the patients had duct dependent confluent pulmonary arteries, 31% were entirely dependent on collaterals and 15% were predominantly dependent on collaterals. In patients with confluent duct dependent pulmonary arteries corrective surgery was performed in 27% of patients. Only 17% of patients with collateral dependent pulmonary circulation achieved complete repair. In the first decade of the study mortality was 42% while in the second decade, i.e. between 1983 and 1993 mortality was 26%. Results from this early era were sufficiently disappointing that not surprisingly some authors, e.g. Bull, Somerville et al suggested that the natural history of this condition is as good or better than surgery. For example, in 1996 Bull, Somerville et al[15] reviewed 218 patients with tetralogy with pulmonary atresia. The authors concluded from their review that they could not be sure that the multiple operations and interventions that have been recommended for this complex anomaly have a positive impact on the outlook for most patients.

Catheter rehabilitation of the pulmonary artery tree

In 1993, Rome et al[14] from Children's Hospital Boston described the experience with 91 patients with tetralogy with pulmonary atresia managed between 1978 and 1988. A total of 48 of the patients had diminutive pulmonary arteries with a Nakata index between 38 and 104 mm^2/m^2. Of nine patients managed conservatively with no intervention before five years of age, four died and only one had a satisfactory hemodynamic result after repair. Of 10 patients who had shunts, three died and three had satisfactory repairs. Of 20 patients managed with an initial connection between the right ventricle and pulmonary arteries, subsequent balloon dilation of pulmonary artery stenoses and embolization of collaterals and subsequent VSD closure, 10 of 20 had complete repairs though seven died after various stages. The authors concluded that a combined catheter and surgery approach begun at an early age is ideal for this most challenging patient subgroup with diminutive pulmonary arteries and multiple collaterals.

One stage repair

In 2000, Reddy et al from San Francisco[33] updated their experience with one stage repair of tetralogy of Fallot with pulmonary atresia. The authors described 85 patients managed after 1992 who had pulmonary atresia with multiple collaterals. Of these, 56 patients underwent complete one stage unifocalization and intracardiac repair. A total of 23 patients underwent unifocalization in a single stage with the VSD left open and six underwent staged unifocalization. There were nine early deaths and seven late deaths with actuarial survival at three years being 80%. Despite their early enthusiasm for one stage repair of tetralogy with pulmonary atresia, in a more recent publication from San Francisco Rodefeld et al[34] suggest that a certain subgroup of patients should undergo an initial creation of aortopulmonary window. The authors described 18 patients with centrally confluent true pulmonary arteries which were 1–2.5 mm in diameter with a well developed peripheral arborization pattern. Most of these patients were markedly cyanotic and had aortopulmonary collaterals which communicated with the true pulmonary arterial system. There were no early deaths and the two late deaths were unrelated to the procedure. Fifteen of the 17 patients who had follow-up angiography demonstrated good growth of the true pulmonary arteries. These patients subsequently proceeded along a similar protocol as described earlier in this chapter. Nevertheless others, e.g. Lofland[35] as well as Tchervenkov et al[24] have recommended one stage repair. As Reddy et al have now acknowledged this approach fails to capitalize on the developmental potential of the tiny central pulmonary arteries, particularly when these have satisfactory arborization.

Neonatal repair

Two reports from Children's Hospital Boston, one from Pigula et al[36] and one from an earlier era from DiDonato[37] described the experience with neonatal repair of tetralogy of Fallot with pulmonary atresia. In Pigula's report from 1999 early mortality was 3% among 99 patients who underwent repair of tetralogy either with pulmonary stenosis or pulmonary atresia in the first 90 days of life. A total of 59 of the 99 patients were prostaglandin dependent. These patients did not include the subgroup with diminutive central pulmonary arteries and dependence on multiple aortopulmonary collateral vessels. The results from Pigula's series represent a substantial improvement over the early report by DiDonato. DiDonato's report from 1991 of neonatal repair of tetralogy of Fallot with and without pulmonary atresia extended back to a time period before the introduction of prostaglandin. Between 1973 and 1988, 27 neonates with either symptomatic tetralogy of Fallot with pulmonary stenosis or with pulmonary atresia underwent repair. There were five hospital deaths, three of which were considered due to avoidable technical problems. Actuarial survival at five years was 74%. The contrasting outcomes from the Pigula and DiDonato reports emphasize the tremendous advances that have occurred in neonatal surgery in the past 10–15 years.

REFERENCES

1. Barratt-Boyes BG, Neutze JM. Primary repair of tetralogy of Fallot in infancy using profound hypothermia with circulatory arrest and limited cardiopulmonary bypass. A comparison with conventional two-stage management. *Ann Surg* 1973; **178**:406–411.
2. Anderson RH, Devine WA, del Nido P. The surgical anatomy of tetralogy of Fallot with pulmonary atresia rather than pulmonary stenosis. *J Cardiac Surg* 1991; **6**:41–58.
3. Formigari R, Vairo U, de Zorzi A, Santoro G, Marino B. Prevalence of bilateral patent ductus arteriosus in patients with pulmonic valve atresia and asplenia syndrome. *Am J Cardiol* 1992; **70**:1219–1220.
4. Shimazaki Y, Maehara T, Blackstone EH, Kirklin JW, Bargeron LM. The structure of the pulmonary circulation in tetralogy of Fallot with pulmonary atresia. *J Thorac Cardiovasc Surg* 1988; **95**:1048–1058.
5. Iuchtman M, Brereton R, Spitz L, Kiely EM, Drake D. Morbidity and mortality in 46 patients with the VACTERL association. *Isr J Med Sci* 1992; **28**:281–284.
6. Mackie AS, Gauvreau K, Perry SB, del Nido PJ, Geva T. Echocardiography predictors of aortopulmonary collaterals in infants with tetralogy of Fallot and pulmonary atresia. *J Am Coll Cardiol* 2003; **41**:852–857.
7. Spevak PJ, Mandell VS, Colan SD et al. Reliability of Doppler color flow mapping in the identification and localization of multiple ventricular septal defects. *Echocardiography* 1993; **10**:573–581.
8. Geva T, Greil GF, Marshall AC, Landzberg M, Powell AJ. Gadolinium-enhanced three-dimensional magnetic resonance angiography of pulmonary blood supply in patients with complex pulmonary stenosis or atresia: comparison with x-ray angiography. *Circulation* 2002; **106**:473–478.
9. Lock JE, Keane JF, Perry SB. *Diagnostic and Interventional Catheterization in Congenital Heart Disease*. Boston, Kluwer Academic Publishers, 2000, pp 230–232.
10. Hausdorf G, Schulze-Neick I, Lange PE. Radiofrequency-assisted 'reconstruction' of the right ventricular outflow tract in muscular pulmonary atresia with ventricular septal defect. *Br Heart J* 1993; **69**:343–346.
11. Rabinovitch M, Herrera-deLeon V, Castaneda AR, Reid LM. Growth and develoment of the pulmonary vascular bed in patients with tetralogy of Fallot with or without pulmonary atresia. *Circulation* 1981; **64**:1231–1249.
12. Reid LM. Lung growth in health and disease. *Br J Dis Chest* 1984; **78**:113–134.
13. Haworth SG. Pulmonary vascular development. In Long WA (ed). *Fetal and Neonatal Cardiology*. Philadelphia, WB Saunders, 1990, pp 51–63.
14. Rome JJ, Mayer JE, Castaneda AR, Lock JE. Tetralogy of Fallot with pulmonary atresia. Rehabilitation of diminutive pulmonary arteries. *Circulation* 1993; **88**:1691–1698.
15. Bull K, Somerville J, Ty E, Spiegelhalter D. Presentation and attrition in complex pulmonary atresia. *J Am Coll Cardiol* 1995; **25**:491–499.
16. Piehler JM, Danielson GK, McGoon DC, Wallace RB, Fulton RE, Mair DD. Management of pulmonary atresia with ventricular septal defect and hypoplastic pulmonary arteries by right ventricular outflow construction. *J Thorac Cardiovasc Surg* 1980; **80**:552–567.
17. Nakata S, Imai Y, Takanashi Y et al. A new method for the quantitative standardization of cross-sectional areas of the pulmonary arteries in congenital heart diseases with decreased pulmonary blood flow. *J Thorac Cardiovasc Surg* 1984; **88**:610–619.
18. Reddy VM, Liddicoat JR, Hanley FL. Midline one-stage complete unifocalization and repair of pulmonary atresia with ventricular septal defect and major aortopulmonary collaterals. *J Thorac Cardiovasc Surg* 1995; **109**:832–844.
19. Scavo VA Jr, Turrentine MW, Aufiero TX, Sharp TG, Brown JW. Valved bovine jugular venous conduits for right ventricular to pulmonary artery reconstruction. *ASAIO J* 1999; **45**:482–487.
20. Pearl JM, Cooper DS, Bove KE, Manning PB. Early failure of the Shelhigh pulmonary valve conduit in infants. *Ann Thorac Surg* 2002; **74**:542–548.
21. Stark J, Bull C, Stajevic M, Jothi M, Elliott M, de Leval M. Fate of subpulmonary homograft conduits: determinants of late homograft failure. *J Thorac Cardiovasc Surg* 1998; **115**:506–514.
22. Wells WJ, Arroyo H Jr, Bremner RM, Wood J, Starnes VA. Homograft conduit failure in infants is not due to somatic outgrowth. *J Thorac Cardiovasc Surg* 2002; **124**:88–96.
23. Perron J, Moran AM, Gauvreau K, del Nido PJ, Mayer JE Jr, Jonas RA. Valved homograft conduit repair of the right heart in early infancy. *Ann Thorac Surg* 1999; **68**:542–548.
24. Tchervenkov CI, Salasidis G, Cecere R et al. One-stage midline unifocalization and complete repair in infancy versus multiple-stage unifocalization followed by repair for complex heart disease with

major aortopulmonary collaterals. *J Thorac Cardiovasc Surg* 1997; **114**:727–735.
25. Reddy VM, Petrossian E, McElhinney DB, Moore P, Teitel DF, Hanley FL. One-stage complete unifocalization in infants: when should the ventricular septal defect be closed? *J Thorac Cardiovasc Surg* 1997; **113**:858–866.
26. Puga FJ. Unifocalization for pulmonary atresia with ventricular septal defect. *Ann Thorac Surg* 1991; **51**:8–9.
27. Sawatari K, Imai Y, Kurosawa H, Isomatsu Y, Momma K. Staged operation for pulmonary atresia and ventricular septal defect with major aortopulmonary collateral arteries. New technique for complete unifocalization. *J Thorac Cardiovasc Surg* 1989; **98**:738–750.
28. Cho JM, Puga FJ, Danielson GK et al. Early and long-term results of the surgical treatment of tetralogy of Fallot with pulmonary atresia, with or without major aortopulmonary collateral arteries. *J Thorac Cardiovasc Surg* 2002; **124**:70–81.
29. Toyoda Y, Yamaguchi M, Ohashi H et al. Unifocalization and systemic-to-pulmonary shunt using internal mammary artery for tetralogy of Fallot and pulmonary atresia with diminutive pulmonary artery and arborization anomaly. *J Cardiovasc Surg* 1997; **38**:527–529.
30. Metras D, Chetaille P, Kreitmann B, Fraisse A, Ghez O, Riberi A. Pulmonary atresia with ventricular septal defect, extremely hypoplastic pulmonary arteries, major aorto-pulmonary collaterals. *Eur J Cardiothorac Surg* 2001; **20**:590–596.
31. Hadjo A, Jimenez M, Baudet E et al. Review of the long-term course of 52 patients with pulmonary atresia and ventricular septal defect. Anatomical and surgical considerations. *Eur Heart J* 1995; **16**:1668–1674.
32. Dinarevic S, Redington A, Rigby M, Shinebourne EA. Outcome of pulmonary atresia and ventricular septal defect during infancy. *Pediatr Cardiol* 1995; **16**:276–282.
33. Reddy VM, McElhinney DB, Amin Z et al. Early and intermediate outcomes after repair of pulmonary atresia with ventricular septal defect and major aortopulmonary collateral arteries: experience with 85 patients. *Circulation* 2000; **101**:1826–1832.
34. Rodefeld MD, Reddy VM, Thompson LD et al. Surgical creation of aortopulmonary window in selected patients with pulmonary atresia with poorly developed aortopulmonary collaterals and hypoplastic pulmonary arteries. *J Thorac Cardiovasc Surg* 2002; **123**:1147–1154.
35. Lofland GK. The management of pulmonary atresia, ventricular septal defect, and multiple aorta pulmonary collateral arteries by definitive single stage repair in early infancy. *Eur J Cardiothorac Surg* 2000; **18**:480–486.
36. Pigula FA, Khalil PN, Mayer JE, del Nido PJ, Jonas RA. Repair of tetralogy of Fallot in neonates and young infants. *Circulation* 1999; **100**:II157–161.
37. DiDonato RM, Jonas RA, Lang P, Rome JJ, Mayer JE Jr, Castaneda AR. Neonatal repair of tetralogy of Fallot with and without pulmonary atresia. *J Thorac Cardiovasc Surg* 1991; **101**:126–137.

26

Pulmonary atresia with intact ventricular septum

INTRODUCTION

As recently as the mid-1980s pulmonary atresia with intact ventricular septum had a surprisingly high early mortality in the neonatal period. By this time the Fontan procedure could be performed for patients with tricuspid atresia with quite a low early mortality. Even the Norwood procedure at an early stage in its development carried only a 30–40% mortality in some series.[1] So it was difficult to understand why a condition that appeared to be morphologically related to tricuspid atresia should carry such a high risk. What many centers did not appreciate at the time had already been emphasized by Freedom and others.[2,3] Pulmonary atresia and intact ventricular septum is frequently accompanied by important anomalies of the coronary arteries – including, most importantly – proximal coronary artery stenoses and coronary artery fistulas with distal supply of the coronary arteries from the right ventricle. Under these circumstances any attempt to decompress the right ventricle will result in massive infarction of the left ventricle leading to the patient's death.[4] Now that coronary angiography has become a routine part of the diagnostic workup of patients with pulmonary atresia and intact ventricular septum the mortality is much less than 15–20 years ago. That is not to say, however, that the management of this condition has become simple. Because there is a wide spectrum of right ventricular size and morphological development, a relatively complex algorithm for management options must be followed in order to optimize outcome for the individual patient.

EMBRYOLOGY

The specific embryological mechanisms that result in failure of the pulmonary valve leaflets to separate during development remain unknown. Presumably the fact that blood flow through the tricuspid valve and right ventricle is markedly reduced is the cause of the tricuspid valve hypoplasia and right ventricular hypoplasia that almost always accompanies the pulmonary valvar atresia to some degree.[5]

It seems likely that the coronary artery anomalies that are seen with pulmonary atresia with intact ventricular septum result from the fact that much of the normal coronary venous drainage of the right ventricle is via Thebesian veins directly into the right ventricle itself rather than to the coronary sinus. Because pressure in the right ventricle is markedly elevated since there is inflow but no outflow to the ventricle, the only potential egress for blood is through the Thebesian veins retrograde into the coronary arterial circulation. Enlarged Thebesian veins which do not obviously communicate with the coronary arterial circulation are termed coronary *sinusoids*. When gross communications can be seen with the coronary arterial circulation these connections are termed coronary *fistulas*. It remains unclear why coronary fistulas are frequently associated with coronary arterial stenoses though some have speculated that the jets of retrograde blood passing into the coronary arteries result in turbulence with consequent endothelial injury and subsequent stenosis formation.[4]

ANATOMY

The sine qua non of pulmonary atresia intact ventricular septum is atresia of the pulmonary valve. Usually the main pulmonary artery is normally developed or mildly hypoplastic. The sinuses of Valsalva of the pulmonary valve are often normally formed. However, the three valve cusps are fused along their usual lines of separation (Figure 26.1).[6] The cusps are often quite thickened and sometimes cartilaginous in

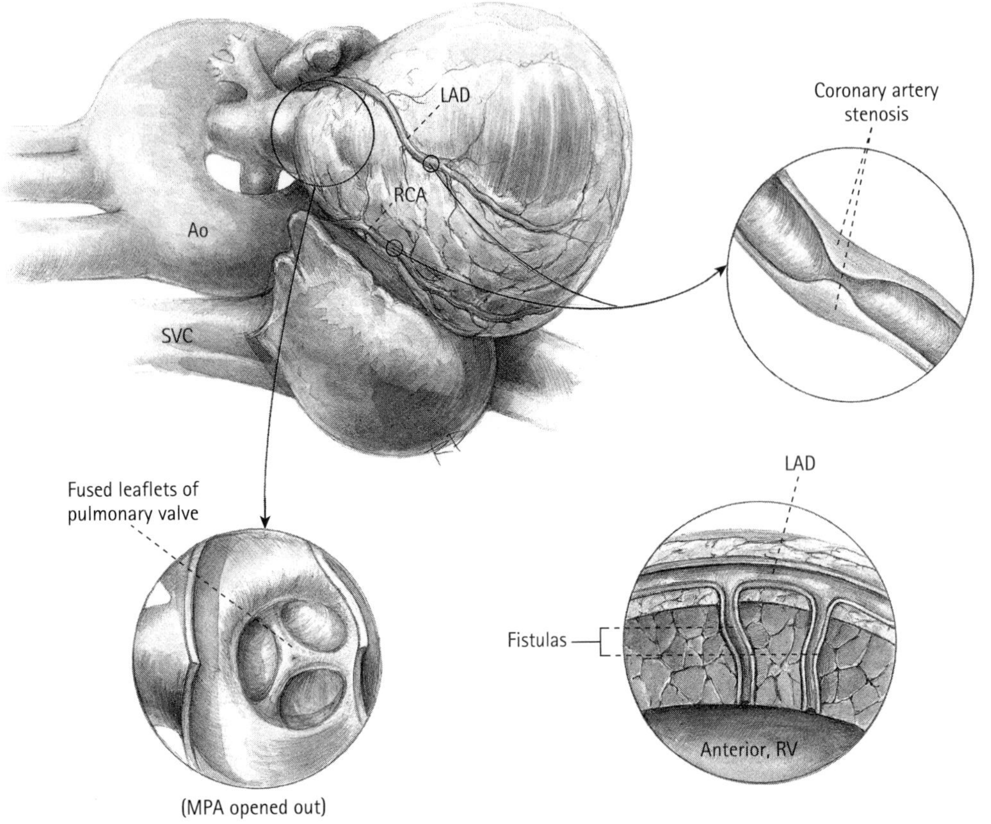

Figure 26.1 *(Inset, bottom left) Obstruction to outflow from the right ventricle in pulmonary atresia with intact ventricular septum is usually a cartilaginous-like valve with fusion along the usual lines of leaflet separation. (Inset, top right) Coronary artery stenoses are frequently present when fistulous communications exist between coronary arteries and the right ventricular chamber. (Inset, bottom right) Fistulous communication between the right ventricular chamber and the left anterior descending coronary artery.*

nature.[7] It is important to distinguish patients in whom there is some patency of the pulmonary valve as the decompression which this affords is important in preventing the development of coronary artery anomalies. Furthermore the development of the tricuspid valve as well as the size of the right ventricle are more likely to be close to normal.

Tricuspid valve

The tricuspid valve is usually morphologically normal with normal leaflet consistency as well as normal chordal and papillary muscle development. However, the valve is almost always hypoplastic to some degree. In situations where the tricuspid valve is larger than normal it is usually Ebstein-like in nature and the anomaly should more properly be classified under Ebstein's anomaly with associated pulmonary atresia.

Morphology of the right ventricle

It is useful to classify the morphology of the right ventricle into three components, namely the inflow, the trabeculated apical component and the infundibular outflow component as originally described by Bull et al.[8] With a mild to moderate degree of hypoplasia the apical trabeculated component of the right ventricle is most likely to be poorly developed or even absent. With a more severe degree of hypoplasia the infundibulum may also be absent. Occasionally the right ventricle may be miniscule, usually in association with a miniscule tricuspid valve.

Associated anomalies

As stated above it is usual for the main pulmonary artery to be normally developed. The branch pulmonary arteries also are almost always in continuity and normally developed. It is extremely rare to see peripheral pulmonary artery stenoses.[9] There is usually a large patent ductus arteriosus. It is extremely uncommon for important aortopulmonary collateral vessels to be present.

Approximately 10% of patients have either major stenoses or atresia of one or more of the major coronary arteries (Figure 26.1).[7] The coronary vascular bed distal to such stenoses usually receives its blood supply from fistulous communications with the right ventricle (Figure 26.1). Calder and Sage[10] found that such fistulas were present in more than 60% of autopsy cases. Satou et al[11] found that an echocardiographically derived tricuspid valve z score of less than −2.5 is a helpful predictor of coronary fistulas and right ventricle dependent coronary circulation. Either a stretched patent foramen ovale or secundum ASD is almost always present.

As mentioned above there may be an Ebstein-like malformation of the tricuspid valve but this anomaly should be classified under Ebstein's anomaly, rather than as pulmonary atresia with intact ventricular septum.[12] Occasionally the right ventricular wall may be very thin as for Uhl's anomaly, usually in the setting of Ebstein's anomaly of the tricuspid valve.[13]

PATHOPHYSIOLOGY

Because there is complete occlusion at the level of the pulmonary valve and aortopulmonary collateral vessels are rarely if ever present, pulmonary blood flow is entirely dependent on patency of the ductus arteriosus. Furthermore, there is an obligatory right to left shunt at atrial septal level so that systemic venous return can pass to the normally developed left ventricle after mixing with pulmonary venous return.

The pressure in the right ventricle is usually at least systemic and is often markedly suprasystemic, often as high as two to three times systemic pressure. When there are important proximal coronary artery stenoses and large coronary fistulas from the body of the right ventricle to the distal coronary arteries, the myocardium which is perfused by the distal coronary arteries is dependent on a continuing high pressure in the right ventricle for perfusion. When there are no proximal coronary artery stenoses but large fistulas present there is a potential for a steal from the coronary arteries into the right ventricle. However, presumably because of lack of egress from the right ventricle as well as the small size of the right ventricle it is our impression that a coronary steal through fistulas to the right ventricle is not an important mechanism of coronary ischemia. This appears to be true even when the right ventricle has been decompressed.

Right ventricular compliance

Because of the severe degree of right ventricular hypertension the right ventricle is usually markedly hypertrophied. Perhaps because of the abnormal coronary artery supply it is also common for the right ventricle to be quite fibrotic. This is very apparent to the surgeon when an incision is made into the right ventricular infundibulum. Interestingly the right ventricle does not usually develop the thick porcelain-like endocardial fibroelastosis that is seen in the left ventricle with severe obstruction to left ventricular outflow. Nevertheless the combination of ventricular hypertrophy and intramyocardial fibrosis results in a poorly compliant right ventricle.

CLINICAL FEATURES AND DIAGNOSTIC STUDIES

The neonate who presents with cyanosis because of a closing ductus will have minimal murmur. The chest X-ray demonstrates poorly perfused lung fields with a relatively normal cardiac silhouette. The ECG shows underdeveloped right heart forces.

The two-dimensional echocardiogram is diagnostic. However, it may be difficult for the echocardiographer when ductal patency has been re-established by prostaglandin infusion to distinguish a very severe degree of pulmonary stenosis from pulmonary atresia with intact ventricular septum. If the right ventricle does not generate any more than systemic pressure, the retrograde flow through a widely patent ductus will minimize or even eliminate forward flow even through the patent pulmonary valve.

The echocardiographer should carefully measure the dimensions of the tricuspid valve in two planes. The dimensions of the main pulmonary artery and pulmonary annulus should also be measured. A careful assessment should be made of the morphology of the right ventricle including the degree of development of the inflow, the apical trabeculated component and the outflow. It is particularly important from the surgeon's perspective to confirm that the infundibulum extends to the valve plate and that the main pulmonary artery also extends to the valve plate so that a transannular patch will allow decompression of the right ventricle.

It is exceedingly rare that the ASD is limiting so that it is not necessary to focus undue attention on the Doppler gradient across the atrial septum.[14] Likewise, it is highly improbable that there are either mediastinal branch pulmonary artery stenoses or peripheral pulmonary artery stenoses.

Coronary artery fistulas are usually easily demonstrated by color Doppler flow mapping and confirm the need for coronary angiography which should be undertaken in almost all patients with pulmonary atresia and intact ventricular septum. It will only be in the rare patient with almost normal development of the tricuspid valve and a tripartite well developed right ventricle without evidence of coronary fistulas that coronary angiography can be avoided.

Coronary angiography

Coronary angiography should be undertaken in order to define the presence of proximal coronary artery stenoses as well as the amount of left ventricular and septal myocardium supplied by the right ventricle.[4] Although it is not possible to be completely sure that the left ventricle is totally dependent on the right ventricle, a useful rule of thumb is to determine how many of the three main coronary arteries (right coronary, left anterior descending, circumflex coronary) are supplied predominantly from the right ventricle. If two of the three main coronary arteries are right ventricular dependent we consider right ventricular decompression to be contraindicated.[15]

MEDICAL AND INTERVENTIONAL THERAPY

Neonates with pulmonary atresia and intact ventricular septum are by definition prostaglandin dependent at birth.

However, it is extremely rare that the atrial septum is sufficiently restrictive that balloon atrial septostomy is indicated. In fact it can be argued that it is useful to maintain a gradient of up to 6–7 mm across the atrial septum in order to encourage flow into the right ventricle and therefore to optimize right ventricular and tricuspid valve growth either with or without decompression of the right ventricle. Although this has been the philosophy at Children's Hospital Boston for many years, the practice at some other centers has been different in that at these centers the majority of patient with pulmonary atresia and intact ventricular septum undergo a balloon atrial septostomy.[16]

Over recent years there has been increasing enthusiasm amongst cardiologists for catheter perforation of the pulmonary valve with subsequent balloon dilation with or without stent placement.[17] It remains unclear whether this approach provides adequate long-term decompression of the right ventricle and optimizes right ventricular growth in the critical early months of life when the myocardium still has the potential for hyperplasia. Fifteen to twenty years ago the surgical approach for this condition was pulmonary valvotomy or valvectomy. These procedures were almost always followed by recurrent right ventricular outflow tract obstruction within two to three months necessitating repeat surgical intervention. Because we believe that the first months of life are the most important for optimizing tricuspid valve and right ventricular growth, we believe that as complete decompression of the right ventricle as can be achieved should be done as early in life as possible. Thus we continue to believe that a surgically placed transannular patch extending well down into the body of the right ventricle is the most appropriate operation in patients in whom right ventricular decompression is indicated (see below).

INDICATIONS FOR SURGERY

Since by definition all neonates with pulmonary atresia with intact ventricular septum are prostaglandin and ductal dependent, either a surgical shunt or right ventricular decompression or most commonly both will be required. It is unusual that a patient will have an adequate tricuspid valve and an adequately compliant right ventricle in order to allow balloon valvotomy of the pulmonary valve alone to adequately decompress the right ventricle and provide sufficient pulmonary blood flow. It is important to remember when reviewing reports that take a different position on this issue, however, that in some patients it can be difficult to distinguish pulmonary valvar stenosis with a tiny orifice versus true pulmonary atresia.

The majority of patients will benefit from a shunt and right ventricular outflow tract patch in the neonatal period. The complex decision tree as to which procedure to undertake both in the neonatal period as well as subsequently is outlined in the surgical techniques section below.

SURGICAL MANAGEMENT

History

The first description of pulmonary atresia with intact septum was probably by the great anatomist John Hunter in 1783 as described by Peacock in 1839 who added seven patients of his own.[18] In 1955 Greenwold at the Mayo Clinic described the wide spectrum of severity of this condition and suggested that a pulmonary valvotomy would be adequate only at the most mild end of the spectrum with a well-developed right ventricle.[19] In 1961 Davignon et al, also at the Mayo Clinic, suggested that if the right ventricle was underdeveloped a systemic to pulmonary shunt should be added to the valvotomy.[20] Successful application of these principles was subsequently reported in 1962 from the University of Minnesota.[21] In 1971 Bowman et al from Columbia University, New York described combination of a shunt with a right ventricular outflow patch for pulmonary atresia with intact septum.[12]

Technical considerations

TWO VENTRICLE REPAIR

Right ventricular decompression procedure only

Fewer than 10% of patients with pulmonary atresia with intact ventricular septum have at birth a sufficiently well developed tricuspid valve (morphologically normal, z score greater than -2 to -3) as well as a tripartite well-developed right ventricle, such that a right ventricular decompression procedure only is adequate. Many of these patients merge into the spectrum of critical pulmonary valve stenosis and have miniscule patency of the pulmonary valve. Under these circumstances it may be possible to decompress the right ventricle adequately with a balloon dilation procedure.

Right ventricular decompression procedure plus shunt

Different reports suggest that between 30% and 60% of patients will have sufficient potential for development of the tricuspid valve and right ventricle that they will ultimately be able to maintain a two ventricle circulation with no shunts either at atrial septal or arterial level.[22,23] However, right ventricular compliance in the neonatal period is often so poor that the right ventricle is unable to maintain adequate pulmonary blood flow in the first weeks and months of life. Although one approach is to wait expectantly while right ventricular compliance improves following a decompression procedure, this often entails subjecting the child to a severe degree of cyanosis ($PO_2 < 30$–35 mm) for many weeks or months. Thus our preference has evolved to take a more aggressive approach in the placement of a shunt as an adjunct to the right ventricular decompression in the neonatal period (Figure 26.2). If the child's right ventricular compliance improves rapidly and the child begins to develop congestive heart failure, it is possible to close the shunt in the catheterization laboratory with coils. It may be possible to close the foramen ovale with a device at the same catheterization though the foramen is often large with elastic margins that may not be suitable for device closure.

Technique of modified right Blalock-Taussig shunt, right ventricular outflow patch and ductus ligation

The approach is through a median sternotomy. The thymus is subtotally resected. A patch of anterior pericardium is harvested and treated with 0.6% glutaraldehyde for 20–30 minutes. The shunt is constructed first. The innominate artery and origin of the right subclavian artery are dissected free with careful preservation of the right recurrent laryngeal nerve which passes around the more distal subclavian artery. The right pulmonary artery is dissected free between the aorta and superior vena cava. A bed for the shunt is created behind the left innominate vein resecting one or two of the mediastinal paratracheal lymph nodes above the right pulmonary artery if necessary. The shunt is constructed with a longitudinal arteriotomy at the origin of the right subclavian artery for the proximal anastomosis and on the superior surface of the proximal right pulmonary artery for the distal anastomosis. The proximal anastomosis should not be placed on the proximal innominate artery as this will almost certainly result in excessive pulmonary blood flow. The vessels are controlled with a side-biting clamp during the performance of each anastomosis and the shunt is controlled with a bulldog clamp after construction of the proximal anastomosis while the distal anastomosis is being constructed. Continuous 6/0 Prolene suture is generally used. Heparin is not usually given at this stage so that bleeding through the suture holes in the Goretex soon stops.

It is advisable to ligate the patent ductus arteriosus in most patients undergoing combined placement of a Blalock shunt and right ventricular outflow tract patch for pulmonary atresia with intact ventricular septum. Although it is generally our policy to leave the ductus patent when placing a Blalock shunt (for example, for patients with single ventricle and pulmonary atresia) because this allows restarting of prostaglandin if there should be thrombosis of the shunt in the early postoperative period, nevertheless in the setting of pulmonary atresia with intact ventricular septum it appears that the ductus is often quite large. The combination of three sources of pulmonary blood flow, i.e. a Blalock shunt, patent ductus arteriosus and forward pulmonary blood flow from the outflow patch not infrequently results in excessive pulmonary blood flow and inadequate systemic perfusion leading to cardiac arrest. For this reason the ductus is routinely ligated in this particular setting.

The ductus is dissected free following careful identification of the left pulmonary artery. It may be ligated with a 5/0 Prolene suture ligature with care not to place the suture too proximally on the ductus such that it might cause stenosis of the origin of the right or left pulmonary arteries. Following ligation of the ductus arteriosus preparations are made for cardiopulmonary bypass.

Placement of transannular right ventricular outflow tract patch on cardiopulmonary bypass

Usually the aorta and right atrium are normally developed so that cannulation can be safely carried out with a 10 French Bard arterial cannula in the ascending aorta and an 18 or 20 French Bard venous cannula inserted through the right atrial appendage. Systemic heparin is not given until shortly prior to cannulation and following opening of the shunt and closure of the ductus. This allows a few minutes for the needle holes in the Gortex tube graft to stop bleeding. Immediately after commencing bypass the shunt is controlled with a bulldog clamp. A mild degree of hypothermia is usually chosen, e.g. 34–35°C but the ionized calcium level is not normalized so that the heart will not beat aggressively during the procedure.

A longitudinal incision is made in the main pulmonary artery and is carried inferiorly to the level of the valve plate. The incision is then carried through the valve plate which leads to the infundibular chamber. Because the infundibulum may be very hypertrophied it is important to progress from above downwards with the incision as described rather than attempting to locate the infundibular cavity with an initial incision in the infundibulum itself. The infundibular muscle usually is quite fibrotic. The incision is carried well down into the body of the right ventricle. This incision is usually quite a bit longer than would be used for standard repair of tetralogy of Fallot for example (Figure 26.2a). It may be useful to divide some of the muscle bundles within the right ventricle with excision of dense trabeculations from the apical region in order to encourage right ventricular growth. However, it is important that septal chords supporting the tricuspid valve are not divided. An autologous pericardial patch is sutured into the pulmonary arteriotomy and right ventriculotomy (Figure 26.2b).

Completion of the two ventricular repair

The growth and development of the right ventricle and tricuspid valve should be carefully followed over the first 6 to 12 to 18 months of life. If the tricuspid valve is within a normal size range (z score > -2) and the child's arterial oxygen saturation is remaining stable or perhaps is even increasing in spite of body growth then these are indications that the child may be able to move to an in-series two ventricle circulation. Cardiac catheterization should be undertaken. Temporary balloon occlusion of the shunt as well as of the ASD allows confirmation that the right ventricle is now adequate. It is hoped that it is possible to coil occlude the shunt and to close the ASD with a device. If the ASD is too large to allow device closure the child will need to undergo surgical closure of the ASD. The shunt can be ligated and divided at the same time.

If cardiac catheterization does not confirm that the right ventricle is adequate then a decision must be made as to whether to persist in the hope of ultimately establishing a two ventricle repair or whether to move to a one and a half ventricle repair as described below. This decision will be influenced by factors such as the rate of growth of the tricuspid valve and right ventricle as well as the degree of severity

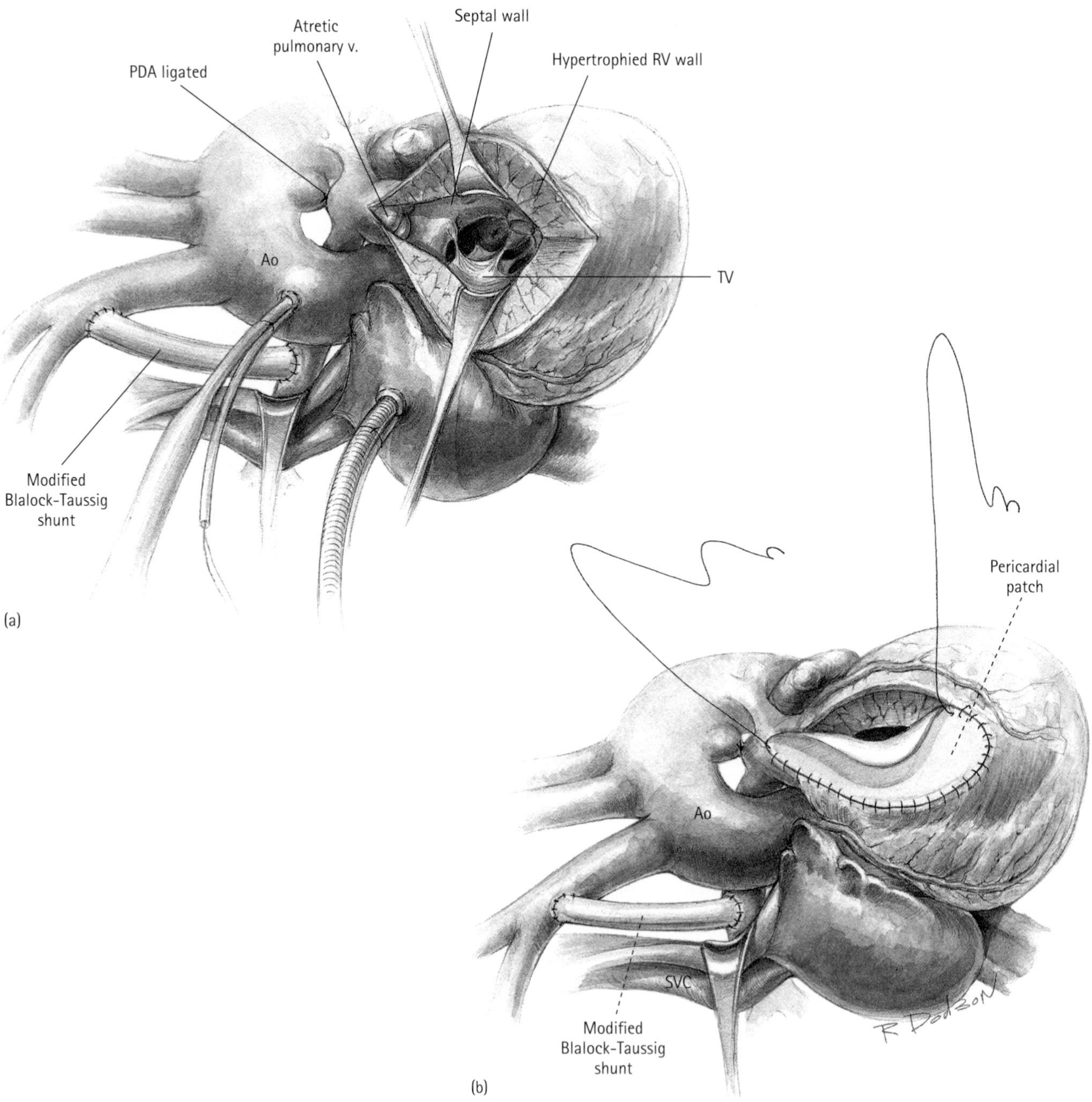

Figure 26.2 *(a) The majority of neonates with pulmonary atresia and intact ventricular septum are managed by placement of a modified right Blalock-Taussig shunt, ligation of the patent ductus arteriosus and placement of a transannular patch to open the atretic right ventricular outflow tract. The incision should be carried further into the body of the right ventricle than the standard incision for repair of tetralogy of Fallot. (b) An autologous pericardial patch is sutured into the pulmonary arteriotomy and right ventriculotomy. Not only does the patch allow decompression of the right ventricle but in addition the pulmonary regurgitation which results probably improves right ventricular compliance and accelerates growth of the right ventricle.*

of failure with balloon occlusion of the shunt and ASD. For example, if right atrial pressure increases to 25–30 mm and cardiac output falls dramatically upon successful occlusion of the shunt and the ASD and if there is no recurrent right ventricular outflow tract obstruction that could be more effectively relieved, then it would seem prudent to move at this point to a one and a half ventricle repair approach.

ONE AND A HALF VENTRICLE REPAIR

The one and a half ventricle repair is a useful intermediate state between a completed two ventricle repair and the Fontan procedure (Figure 26.3). Not only does it allow the right ventricle to contribute some degree of pulsatile flow to the pulmonary circulation, it also has the added advantage of

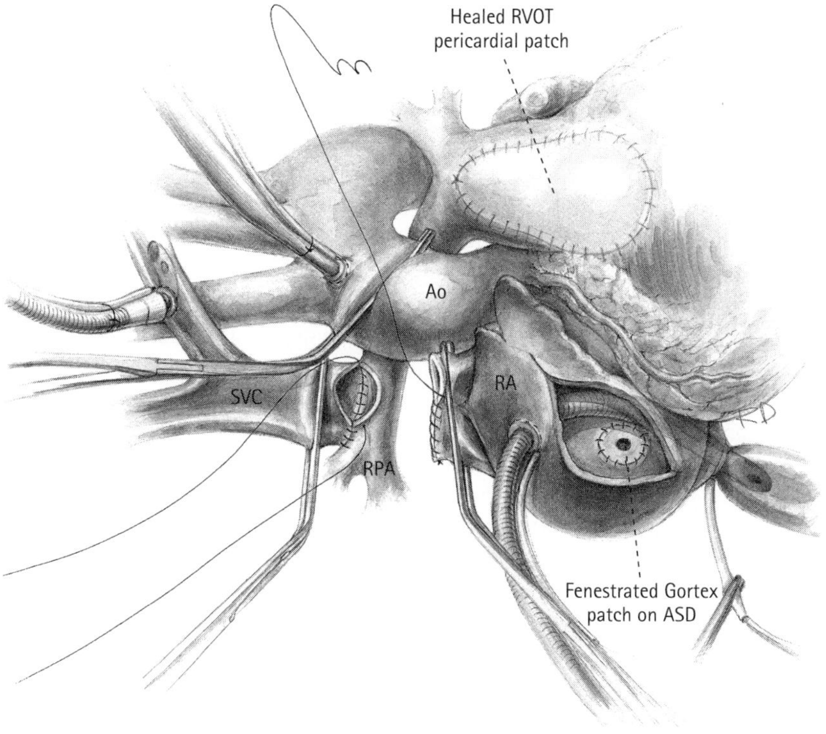

Figure 26.3 *The one and a half ventricle repair is performed on cardiopulmonary bypass with a right angle cannula in the left innominate vein and a straight cannula in the inferior vena cava. A bidirectional Glenn shunt is constructed with the distal anastomosis placed at the same site as the previous Blalock shunt anastomosis. The cardiac end of the divided superior vena cava is oversewn. If the right ventricle appears to be sufficiently well developed and is close to allowing a two ventricle repair then the atrial septal defect can be closed with a fenestrated Gortex patch.*

allowing complete decompression of the right ventricle. Furthermore it also allows for the continuing possibility of right ventricular and tricuspid valve growth.

The one and a half ventricle repair is generally undertaken between 6 and 18 months of age. The usual indication is that a child has failed the test of right ventricular adequacy at cardiac catheterization including temporary occlusion of the Blalock shunt and ASD. Although the right ventricle is not capable of pumping the entire cardiac output to the pulmonary circulation it may nevertheless be quite capable of managing the venous return from the inferior vena cava. After the procedure the superior vena caval flow will bypass the right ventricle and right atrium by being connected directly to the pulmonary arteries. This is accomplished by constructing a bidirectional Glenn shunt.

Although some have suggested that it is on occasion possible to place a bidirectional Glenn shunt without the use of cardiopulmonary bypass[24] we believe that there are significant risks to the brain in taking this approach. Following heparinization the arterial cannula is placed in the ascending aorta and venous return is accomplished with a small right angle cannula in the left innominate vein and a straight cannula in the right atrium. Cardiopulmonary bypass is maintained at a temperature of 34–35°C with the heart beating throughout the procedure. Immediately after commencing bypass the right Blalock shunt is ligated. The distal shunt anastomosis is taken down and the resulting right pulmonary arteriotomy is extended a few millimeters in either direction with great care not to compromise the origin of the right upper lobe pulmonary artery. The superior vena cava is divided between clamps at the level of the right pulmonary artery. The cardiac end of the divided SVC is oversewn with continuous 5/0 Prolene. The azygous vein is doubly ligated and divided. An end to side anastomosis is fashioned between the cephalic end of the divided SVC and the right pulmonary artery using continuous absorbable 6/0 Maxon suture. The use of Maxon suture is preferred in this setting not only because it allows for growth but more importantly because it prevents purse-stringing of the anastomosis as can happen when Prolene is employed.

While rewarming to a rectal temperature of 35°C the venous cannula in the left innominate vein is replaced with a monitoring catheter. The heart is allowed to eject and ventilation is begun to optimize venous return through the lungs to the remaining venous cannula. A second monitoring catheter is placed in the right atrium. The child is weaned from bypass in the routine fashion. After establishing satisfactory hemodynamics the monitoring catheter is moved from the innominate vein to the right atrial appendage.

In children in whom it appears that the right ventricle is very close to allowing a two ventricle repair but nevertheless catheterization has demonstrated that it is inadequate despite perhaps a year or two of potential growth, it is possible to close the ASD partially to encourage ongoing growth of the right ventricle (Figure 26.3). However, this does require cross clamping of the aorta, infusion of cardioplegia solution and snaring of the inferior vena caval cannula. A Gortex patch is sutured into the secundum ASD. It is perforated with a fenestration, generally 4 mm in diameter. During weaning from bypass careful note is made of the right atrial pressure as well as the superior vena caval pressure. It is probably unwise to accept a right atrial pressure of greater than 17–20 mm. This will place the child at risk of developing ascites, hepatomegaly and of having poor renal function. If these problems should appear postoperatively consideration can be given to balloon dilation of the fenestration in order to lower right atrial pressure.[25]

Whether a fenestrated ASD patch has been placed or the foramen ovale has been left open, the child can be serially assessed in the coming years for complete atrial septal closure thereby creating a completed one and a half ventricle repair. In the case of the fenestrated ASD patch, closure with a device almost always will be technically possible assuming that temporary balloon occlusion has indicated satisfactory hemodynamics. This hemodynamic assessment will primarily involve measurement of right atrial pressure and cardiac output as the arterial saturation is likely to be reasonably well maintained by flow through the bidirectional Glenn shunt. However, an increase in right atrial pressure to greater than 17–20 mm and a fall in cardiac index to less than 2–2.5 l/min/m^2 should suggest that the atrial septum should be left open.

ONE AND A QUARTER VENTRICLE REPAIR

The one and a quarter ventricle repair is an option for patients whose right ventricle and tricuspid valve are large enough to raise concern that performance of a standard lateral tunnel Fontan procedure will leave the right ventricle at high pressure and a potential source of malignant arrhythmias. On the other hand the one and a quarter ventricle repair does have the disadvantages of the old style modified Fontan procedure in which the right atrium can become excessively dilated.

The one and a quarter ventricle repair may be undertaken at the time of construction of a bidirectional Glenn shunt when it is concluded fairly early in the child's management, i.e. at the 6–18 month catheterization, that even a one and a half ventricle repair will not be possible because of inadequate development of the tricuspid valve and right ventricle. Alternatively the procedure may be chosen when a child has failed to progress from the initial stage of a one and a half ventricle repair, i.e. with the ASD widely open, and despite up to several years of further observation it is clear that ASD closure will not be possible. In either situation cannulation is undertaken for cardiopulmonary bypass with a right angle cannula in the left innominate vein and a second cannula placed initially in the right atrium and subsequently advanced into the IVC and snared. Following cross clamping of the aorta and infusion of cardioplegia solution the right atrium is opened with an oblique incision. A Gortex patch fenestrated with a 4 mm fenestration is used to close the ASD partially if this has not been done previously at the time of the bidirectional Glenn shunt (Figure 26.4). In addition an atriopulmonary connection is fashioned between the roof of the right

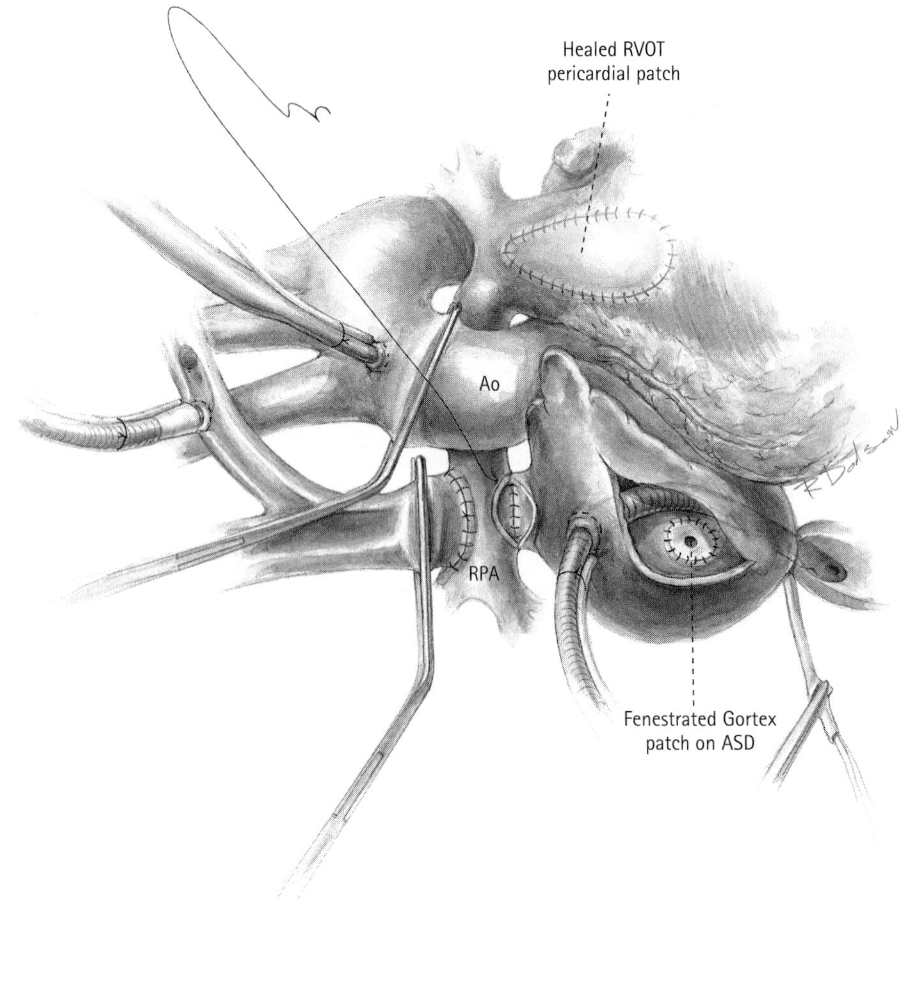

Figure 26.4 *A one and a quarter ventricle repair is an option for patients whose right ventricle and tricuspid valve are sufficiently large to require ongoing decompression into the pulmonary arteries. An atriopulmonary anastomosis is fashioned and a fenestrated Gortex patch is used to close the atrial septal defect. This approach should not be used if the right atrial pressure is likely to be importantly elevated because it will result in an excessively large right atrial chamber. Concern that this approach might result in a circular shunt from right ventricle to right pulmonary artery to right atrium and back to right ventricle appears to be unfounded.*

atrium and the undersurface of the right pulmonary artery opposite the bidirectional Glenn shunt anastomosis.

After a year or two of observation the child should undergo cardiac catheterization including temporary balloon occlusion of the fenestration. Using the same criteria proposed for the one and a half ventricle repair a decision is made regarding suitability of the fenestration for device closure. Thus the child has a circulation that is close to a completed Fontan circulation with blood from the inferior vena cava and from the superior vena cava being able to pass directly into the pulmonary circulation. However, there is the continuing option for blood from either cava to pass to the tricuspid valve and to be ejected into the main pulmonary artery. Although some have expressed concern that this modification might allow for a circular shunt with the blood that is ejected into the right pulmonary artery passing back into the right atrium through the atriopulmonary anastomosis and then once again into the right ventricle and pulmonary artery, we have not observed this complication.[26] Once again it is important to emphasize that this modification should only be used in the setting of a very small right ventricle which is not likely to contribute much forward flow to the pulmonary circulation. On the other hand if pulmonary resistance is elevated or the pulmonary arteries are not well developed or if left ventricular compliance is not excellent, serious consideration should be given to performing a standard lateral tunnel Fontan procedure because exposure of the entire right atrium to high pressure as is the case with the one and a quarter ventricle repair, may lead to an increased risk of late complications such as supraventricular arrhythmias, thrombus formation and right pulmonary vein obstruction.

SINGLE VENTRICLE APPROACH

There are several indications for adopting a single ventricle approach in the neonatal period. The most important of these is the identification by coronary angiography that the neonate has a right ventricular dependent coronary circulation. Under these circumstances decompression of the right ventricle will cause massive infarction of the left ventricle and is likely to be fatal. Other indications for adopting a single ventricle approach from the neonatal period are extremely small size of the tricuspid valve, e.g. a tricuspid valve z score of less than -4 to -5 as well as absence of the infundibular component of the right ventricle. This is usually accompanied by absence of development of the trabeculated apical component of the right ventricle.

When it is apparent that a single ventricle approach must be employed the child should undergo placement of a modified right Blalock shunt. We prefer to place the shunt through a median sternotomy approach as described in Chapter 20. Unlike the situation described above where the shunt will provide additional blood flow in conjunction with forward flow through the open right ventricular outflow tract this is not the case in the single ventricle setting. Therefore we do not ligate the patent ductus arteriosus under these circumstances unless the ductus is clearly very large. Generally a 3.5 mm right Blalock shunt is selected for neonates ranging in weight from 2.5 to 4 kg.

Because the neonatal Blalock shunt is the only source of pulmonary blood flow when a single ventricle approach is being pursued it is likely that the child will outgrow the shunt by approximately six months of age. At about this time cardiac catheterization should be undertaken in order to demonstrate pulmonary arterial anatomy and to confirm satisfactory hemodynamics. The technique of the bidirectional Glenn shunt is identical to that described under the one and a half ventricle repair though no consideration is given to partial closure of the ASD.

The technique of the modified fenestrated Fontan procedure is the standard technique used for any child with a single ventricle. In addition to constructing an atriopulmonary anastomosis as well as placing a lateral tunnel of Gortex with a 4 mm fenestration it is probably also useful to excise the remnants of the atrial septum. This will ensure that oxygenated pulmonary venous blood will pass into the pulmonary venous component of the original right atrium and from there can pass into the tricuspid valve and right ventricle to perfuse the myocardium in the setting of right ventricular dependent coronary circulation.

RESULTS OF SURGERY

Improving outlook

In 2000 Jahangiri et al[27] described the outcomes for 47 patients with pulmonary atresia and intact ventricular septum who underwent surgery at Children's Hospital Boston between 1991 and 1998. There was one early death among the 31 patients who did not have a right ventricular dependent coronary circulation. Ten of these patients achieved a two ventricle repair, six a one and a half ventricle repair and eight had a Fontan procedure. Sixteen (34%) of the patients were identified as having a right ventricular dependent coronary circulation. The tricuspid valve z score for these patients was -3.0 ± 0.66 versus -2 ± 0.95 for those who did not have right ventricular dependent circulation. All patients with a right ventricular dependent coronary circulation had a systemic to pulmonary artery shunt with one death. At the close of the series, 14 of the 16 patients had undergone a bidirectional Glenn shunt at a median of nine months after their first operation and nine had progressed to a Fontan procedure with no deaths. We concluded from this analysis that the outcome for patients with pulmonary atresia with intact ventricular septum had improved dramatically subsequent to careful identification of right ventricular dependent coronary circulation and appropriate stratification according to this finding.

RIGHT VENTRICULAR DEPENDENT CORONARY CIRCULATION

In 1992 Giglia et al[28] described the evolution in understanding of the importance of right ventricular dependent coronary circulation at Children's Hospital Boston. Of 82 patients who presented between 1979 and 1990, 32% were found to have right ventricular to coronary artery fistulas. Of the 23 patients with adequate preoperative coronary angiograms, 16 had undergone right ventricular decompression in the neonatal period. All 7 of the 16 who had fistulas but not coronary artery stenosis survived right ventricular decompression. Four of six patients who had stenosis of a single coronary artery survived, while the three patients with stenosis of two main coronary arteries all died shortly after right ventricular decompression because of acute left ventricular dysfunction.

The authors concluded that the potential for steal from a coronary artery into the decompressed right ventricle through a fistula should not be a contraindication to decompression. Fistulas associated with stenosis of a single coronary artery also do not preclude decompression but the presence of stenosis in two coronary arteries should be considered to be a contraindication to right ventricular decompression. In 1993 Gentles et al[15] reviewed the effect of less extensive coronary anomalies than had been described in the previous report by Giglia at Children's Hospital Boston. The authors reviewed 24 patients with pulmonary atresia and intact ventricular septum, 12 of whom had fistulas with no more than one coronary artery stenosis. They found that regional left ventricular dysfunction was rare on echocardiography in patients without coronary artery abnormalities. In patients with no more than one coronary artery stenosis, regional left ventricular dysfunction was common before and increased after right ventricular decompression but severe global left ventricular dysfunction was unusual.

A further report of the experience at Children's Hospital Boston with right ventricular dependent coronary circulation was published by Powell et al in 2000.[29] Twelve patients with right ventricular dependent coronary circulation who underwent staged surgery directed towards a Fontan procedure had an 83% five-year actuarial survival. Both deaths in the study appeared to be related to coronary ischemia and occurred in the first four months of life. This study confirmed our clinical impression that long-term patient survival and quality of life can be surprisingly good despite severe coronary abnormalities including virtual complete dependence on myocardial perfusion by the right ventricle through fistulas.

Other surgical reports

The most extensive recent analysis of the results of surgery for pulmonary atresia with intact ventricular septum has been undertaken by the Congenital Heart Surgeons Society.[22] This retrospective review analysed 408 neonates who were managed by 33 institutions between 1987 and 1997. Like the Boston report by Jahangiri[27] this study documents the considerable improvement in outlook that has occurred over the timeframe of the study. Although survival overall was 60% at five years and 58% at 15 years it appears probable that in the current era 85% of neonates are likely to reach a definitive endpoint such as biventricular circulation, one and a half ventricle repair or Fontan procedure. In this review 33% of patients achieved a two ventricle repair, 20% a Fontan procedure, 5% a one and a half ventricle repair, 2% heart transplant, 38% death before a definitive endpoint and 2% were alive without having achieved a definitive endpoint.

Patient related factors that determined whether patients were directed to a single ventricle, one and a half ventricle or two ventricle endpoint included adequacy of right sided heart structures, coronary artery abnormalities, low birth weight and tricuspid valve regurgitation. Institutional factors also contributed importantly to outcome with two institutions being predictive of a two ventricle repair, one institution predictive of a Fontan endpoint and six institutions predictive of death before definitive repair. The two institutions which were predictive of both a two ventricle and a Fontan repair achieved a higher risk adjusted prevalence of definitive endpoint and a lower prevalence of pre-repair mortality. Institutions which attempted to achieve a two ventricle endpoint for a greater proportion of patients paid the price of a higher mortality and the converse was also true.

The report from the Congenital Heart Surgeons Society[22] built on a previous analysis of 171 neonates who were enrolled by the CHSS between 1987 and 1991.[30] In that study coronary artery fistulas were present in 45% of patients with severe right ventricular dependency in 9%. The z value of the tricuspid valve diameter was negatively correlated with the presence of both fistulas and right ventricular dependency. Survival was 81% at one month and 64% at four years in this early phase of the study. Multivariate analysis showed that small diameter of the tricuspid valve, severe right ventricular coronary dependency, birth weight and the date and type of initial procedure were risk factors for death.

In 1994 Bull et al from Great Ormond Street Hospital in London[31] described the outcome for 135 patients with pulmonary atresia and intact ventricular septum. The total mortality for patients who underwent an initial closed valvotomy was 50% with only 22% of patients being alive and suitable for a biventricular repair at five years. Only half of decompressed ventricles achieved growth of the tricuspid valve disproportionate to somatic growth as a result of the neonatal procedure. This report by Bull et al built on a previous report from the same group which emphasized right ventricular morphology as a determinant of outcome rather than coronary anatomy.[8,32]

Pawade et al[23] from Royal Children's Hospital Melbourne, Australia like Bull have emphasized the importance of infundibular development as a predictor of outcome. Forty eight neonates were managed between 1980 and 1992. In 31 neonates with a well-formed infundibulum the initial palliation was a pulmonary valvotomy without bypass and a PTFE shunt from the left subclavian artery to the main pulmonary artery. There was one death after this initial palliation in this subgroup. If necessary the right ventricular cavity was later enlarged by excision of hypertrophic muscle within the trabecular and infundibular portions before attempting biventricular repair. The actuarial probability of achieving a biventricular repair at 40 months was 60%. There was one late death among 13 patients who underwent a biventricular repair. Seventeen patients without a well formed infundibulum were directed to a single ventricle pathway. These patients had an initial modified Blalock shunt only. There were four early deaths in this subgroup. Actuarial survival in this subgroup was 77% at nine years while for patients entering a biventricular pathway survival was greater than 90%.

In 1998, Rychik et al[33] from Children's Hospital of Philadelphia described the outcome for 67 patients managed between 1981 and 1998. Right ventricular dependency of the coronary circulation was noted in eight patients (12%). Severity of coronary abnormality did not influence survival. One third of patients achieved a biventricular repair. These patients had a mean z score of the tricuspid valve of -0.5 versus a mean tricuspid valve z score of -3.0 for patients who either underwent a single ventricle strategy or heart transplantation.

In 1992, Laks et al[34] described the use of an adjustable ASD device to achieve partial biventricular repair for patients with pulmonary atresia and intact ventricular septum. Of 39 patients managed between 1982 and 1991, 19 underwent biventricular repair. In 12 of these patients an adjustable ASD device was used. The authors emphasize the utility of this device which allows a controlled right to left shunt at atrial level thereby reducing the risk of low cardiac output and severe venous hypertension following partial biventricular repair. It was the introduction of this concept by Laks et al that subsequently led to the development of the fenestrated baffle for patients undergoing a Fontan procedure for various forms of single ventricle.

In 1997 Mair et al[35] from the Mayo Clinic described the outcome of 40 patients who had a nonfenestrated Fontan procedure for pulmonary atresia with intact ventricular septum. Forty patients underwent surgery between 1979 and 1995 with three early deaths and three late deaths. Of the 34 survivors, 33 were in NYHA class 1 or 2 and all but three were either fulltime students or working fulltime. More than half of the patients were not receiving any cardiovascular medication. This study adds further weight to the contention that, despite a hypertensive right ventricle and coronary fistulas and stenoses, patients can achieve a satisfactory long-term outcome with a single ventricle approach.

Fetal diagnosis and interventions

In 2002 Tulzer et al[36] described the outcome of two fetuses who had undergone in-utero dilation of the pulmonary valve at 28 and 30 weeks' gestation. A balloon catheter was introduced through a needle inserted through the mother's abdominal wall, uterus, the child's chest wall and right ventricle. Both babies had evidence of improved circulation following the procedure though both required a repeat valvuloplasty following birth. Ultimately both children achieved a biventricular circulation. In 1998, Daubeney et al[37] reviewed the impact of fetal echocardiography on the incidence of pulmonary atresia with intact ventricular septum at birth as well as impact on postnatal outcome in the UK and Eire. There were 183 live births with this anomaly between 1991 and 1995 for an incidence of 4.5 per 100 000 live births. Eighty six fetal diagnoses were made at a mean of 22 weeks which led to 53 terminations of pregnancy, four intrauterine deaths and 29 live births. The incidence at birth would have been 5.6 per 100 000 births in the absence of fetal diagnosis. The probability of survival at one year of age was 65% and was the same for live born infants whether or not a fetal diagnosis had been made.

One and a half ventricle repair

In 1999 Kreutzer et al[38] from Buenos Aires, Argentina, described 30 patients who underwent a one and a half ventricle repair between 1986 and 1996. The most common diagnosis was pulmonary atresia with intact ventricular septum which comprised 15 patients. Overall there were two early deaths and one late death. Mean oxygen saturation was 94%, which was unchanged at one year of follow-up. Mean early postoperative SVC pressure was 14 and mean right atrial pressure was 10. The authors conclude that the one and a half ventricle repair is a valid alternative for management of right ventricular hypoplasia or dysfunction with favorable early and intermediate follow-up. Stellin et al[39] have also described encouraging intermediate follow-up on a smaller group of eight patients who underwent a one and a half ventricle repair in Padova, Italy, between 1994 and 2001.

In 1994 Gentles et al[26] described surgical options other than a one and a half ventricle repair which fall between a biventricular repair and a Fontan procedure. Eight patients underwent such procedures at Children's Hospital Boston between 1988 and 1993. There were no deaths either early or late with a median follow-up of 24 months. At postoperative catheterization right atrial mean pressure ranged from 7 to 13 mm and mixed venous saturation from 62% to 70%. The authors concluded that these procedures allow right atrial decompression as well as incorporation of a small right ventricle into the pulmonary circulation with excellent results.

Interventional catheter perforation of the pulmonary valve

A complete description of interventional catheter results for the management of pulmonary atresia with intact ventricular septum is beyond the scope of this book. However, in the recent report by Agnoletti et al from Paris[40] 39 newborns with a favorable anatomical subtype underwent attempted perforation of the pulmonary valve. Perforation was successful in 33 of the 39 patients. Among these 17 subsequently required neonatal surgery, 13 did not require any surgery and three had elective surgery after the first month of life. There were two procedure related deaths, seven non fatal procedural complications and four postsurgical deaths. At a median follow-up of 5.5 years freedom from surgery was 35%. Although conceding that the technique is 'burdened by non-negligible mortality and morbidity', the authors believe that it is effective in selected patients with a normal sized right ventricle.

In 2000 Alwi et al[41] published a report of 33 patients who underwent either percutaneous radiofrequency valvotomy and balloon dilation or surgical valvotomy with concomitant Blalock shunt based on right ventricular morphology. Among the 19 patients who underwent interventional catheter procedures there was one early death and two late deaths. Of the remaining 16 survivors, 12 achieved a biventricular circulation but only seven required no further intervention. In the surgical group of 14 patients there were three early deaths with one late death at four months. All survivors required a second right ventricular decompression after which two patients died.

Although the authors believe that this experience supports the safety of the interventional catheter procedure it must be remembered that this was a selected series where patients with more favorable anatomy underwent the catheter procedure. One of the earliest groups to endorse the use of catheter management of pulmonary atresia with intact ventricular septum described a follow-up of their results in 1998. Ovaert et al[42] from Guys Hospital, London, UK described 12 neonates and infants who underwent either laser or radiofrequency assisted balloon valvotomy after 1990. The atretic pulmonary valve was successfully perforated and dilated in nine of 12 patients. However, five of these nine patients required additional catheter or surgical procedures to augment pulmonary blood flow. Of the six long-term survivors, five have a two ventricle circulation.

REFERENCES

1. Jonas RA, Lang P, Hansen D, Hickey P, Castaneda AR. First stage palliation of hypoplastic left heart syndrome. The importance of coarctation and shunt size. *J Thorac Cardiovasc Surg* 1986; **92**:6–13.
2. Freedom RM, Harrington DP. Contributions of intramyocardial sinusoids in pulmonary atresia and intact ventricular septum to a right sided circular shunt. *Br Heart J* 1974; **36**:1061–1065.
3. Essed CE, Klein HW, Kredict P. Coronary and endocardial fibroelastosis of the ventricles in the hypoplastic left and right heart syndromes. *Virchows Arch* 1975; **368**:87.
4. Gittenberger-De Groot AC, Sauer U, Bindl L, Babic R, Essed CE, Buhlmeyer K. Competition of coronary arteries and ventriculo-coronary arterial communications in pulmonary atresia with intact ventricular septum. *Int J Cardiol* 1988; **18**:243–258.
5. Kutsche LM, Van Mierop LHS. Pulmonary atresia with and without ventricular septal defect: a different etiology and pathogenesis for the atresia in the two types? *Am J Cardiol* 1983; **51**:932–935.
6. Zuberbuhler JR, Anderson RH. Morphological variations in pulmonary atresia with intact ventricular septum. *Br Heart J* 1979; **41**:281–288.
7. Van Praagh R, Ando M, Van Praagh S, Senno A, Hougen TJ, Novack G, Hastreiter AR. Pulmonary atresia: Anatomic considerations. In Kidd BSL, Rowe RD (eds). *The Child with Congenital Heart Disease After Surgery.* Mt Kisco, NY, Futura Publishing Co., 1976, p 103.
8. Bull C, deLeval MR, Mercanti C, Macartney FJ, Anderson RH. Pulmonary atresia and intact ventricular septum. A revised classification. *Circulation* 1982; **66**:266–272.
9. Elliott LP, Adams P, Edwards JE. Pulmonary atresia with intact ventricular septum. *Br Heart J* 1963; **25**:489.
10. Calder AL, Co EE, Sage MD. Coronary arterial abnormalities in pulmonary atresia with intact ventricular septum. *Am J Cardiol* 1987; **59**:436–442.
11. Satou GM, Perry SB, Gauvreau K, Geva T. Echocardiographic predictors of coronary artery pathology in pulmonary atresia with intact ventricular septum. *Am J Cardiol* 2000; **85**:1319–1324.
12. Bowman FO, Malm JR, Hayes CJ, Gersony WM, Ellis K. Pulmonary atresia with intact ventricular septum. *J Thorac Cardiovasc Surg* 1971; **61**:85–95.
13. Cote M, Davignon A, Fouron JC. Congenital hypoplasia of right ventricular myocardium (Uhl's anomaly) associated with pulmonary atresia in a newborn. *Am J Cardiol* 1973; **31**:658–661.
14. Edwards JE, Carey LS, Neufeld HN, Lester RG. Pulmonary atresia with intact ventricular septum. In *Congenital Heart Disease.* Philadelphia, WB Saunders, 1965, p 576.
15. Gentles TL, Colan SD, Giglia TM, Mandell VS, Mayer JE, Sanders SP. Right ventricular decompression and left ventricular function in pulmonary atresia with intact ventricular septum. *Circulation* 1993; **88**:183–188.
16. Freedom R (ed). *Pulmonary Atresia with Intact Ventricular Septum.* Mt Kisco, NY, Futura Publishing Co., 1989.
17. Parsons JM, Reese MR, Gibbs JL. Percutaneous laser valvotomy with balloon dilatation of the pulmonary valve as primary treatment for pulmonary atresia. *Br Heart J* 1991; **66**:36–38.
18. Peacock TB. Malformation of the heart: Atresia of the orifice of the pulmonary artery. *Trans Pathol Soc Lond* 1869; **20**:61.
19. Greenwold WE. *A Clinico-Pathologic Study of Congenital Tricuspid Atresia and of Pulmonary Stenosis or Pulmonary Atresia with Intact Ventricular Septum.* Thesis, University of Minnesota, November 1955.
20. Davignon AL, Greenwold WE, DuShane JW, Edwards JE. Congenital pulmonary atresia with intact ventricular septum. Clinicopathologic correlation of two anatomic types. *Am Heart J* 1961; **62**:591.
21. Benton JW, Elliott LP, Adams P, Anderson RC, Hong CY, Lester RG. Pulmonary atresia and stenosis with intact ventricular septum. *Am J Dis Child* 1962; **104**:83.
22. Ashburn DA, Blackstone EH, Wells WJ et al. Determinants of mortality and type of repair in neonates with pulmonary atresia and intact ventricular septum. *J Thorac Cardiovasc Surg*, in press.
23. Pawade A, Capuani A, Penny DJ, Karl TR, Mee RB. Pulmonary atresia with intact ventricular septum: surgical management based on right ventricular infundibulum. *J Card Surg* 1993; **8**:371–383.
24. Jahangiri M, Keogh B, Shinebourne EA, Lincoln C. Should the bidirectional Glenn procedure be performed through a thoracotomy without cardiopulmonary bypass? *J Thorac Cardiovasc Surg* 1999; **118**:367–368.
25. Nishimoto K, Keane JF, Jonas RA. Dilation of intra-atrial baffle fenestrations: results in vivo and in vitro. *Cathet Cardiovasc Diagn* 1994; **31**:73–78.

26. Gentles TL, Keane JF, Jonas RA, Marx GE, Mayer JE. Surgical alternatives to the Fontan procedure incorporating a hypoplastic right ventricle. *Circulation* 1994; **90**(Suppl II): 1–6.
27. Jahangiri M, Zurakowski D, Bichell D, Mayer JE, del Nido PJ, Jonas RA. Improved results with selective management in pulmonary atresia with intact ventricular septum. *J Thorac Cardiovasc Surg* 1999; **118**:1046–1055.
28. Giglia TM, Mandell VS, Connor AR, Mayer JE, Lock JE. Diagnosis and management of right ventricle-dependent coronary circulation in pulmonary atresia with intact ventricular septum. *Circulation* 1992; **86**:1516–1528.
29. Powell AJ, Mayer JE, Jahangiri M et al. Improved results with selective management in pulmonary atresia with intact ventricular septum. *J Thorac Cardiovasc Surg* 1999; **118**:1046–1055.
30. Hanley FL, Sade RM, Blackstone EH, Kirklin JW, Freedom RM, Nanda NC. Outcomes in neonatal pulmonary atresia with intact ventricular septum. A multiinstitutional study. *J Thorac Cardiovasc Surg* 1993; **105**:406–423.
31. Bull C, Kostelka M, Sorensen K, de Leval M. Outcome measures for the neonatal management of pulmonary atresia with intact ventricular septum. *J Thorac Cardiovasc Surg* 1994; **107**:359–366.
32. de Leval M, Bull C, Stark J, Anderson RH, Taylor JF, Macartney FJ. Pulmonary atresia and intact ventricular septum: surgical management based on a revised classification. *Circulation* 1982; **66**:272–280.
33. Rychik J, Levy H, Gaynor JW, DeCampli WM, Spray TL. Outcome after operations for pulmonary atresia with intact ventricular septum. *J Thorac Cardiovasc Surg* 1998; **116**:924–931.
34. Laks H, Pearl JM, Drinkwater DC et al. Partial biventricular repair of pulmonary atresia with intact ventricular septum. Use of an adjustable atrial septal defect. *Circulation* 1992; **86**(Suppl 5): II159–166.
35. Mair DD, Julsrud PR, Puga FJ, Danielson GK. The Fontan procedure for pulmonary atresia with intact ventricular septum: operative and late results. *J Am Coll Cardiol* 1997; **29**:1359–1364.
36. Tulzer G, Arzt W, Franklin RC, Loughna PV, Mair R, Gardiner HM. Fetal pulmonary valvuloplasty for critical pulmonary stenosis or atresia with intact septum. *Lancet* 2002; **360**:1567–1568.
37. Daubeney PE, Sharland GK, Cook AC, Keeton BR, Anderson RH, Webber SA. Pulmonary atresia with intact ventricular septum: impact of fetal echocardiography on incidence at birth and postnatal outcome. UK and Eire Collaborative Study of Pulmonary Atresia with Intact Ventricular Septum. *Circulation* 1998; **98**:562–566.
38. Kreutzer C, Mayorquim RC, Kreutzer GO et al. Experience with one and a half ventricle repair. *J Thorac Cardiovasc Surg* 1999; **117**:662–668.
39. Stellin G, Vida VL, Milanesi O et al. Surgical treatment of complex cardiac anomalies: the one and one half ventricle repair. *Eur J Cardiothorac Surg* 2002; **22**:1043–1049.
40. Agnoletti G, Piechaud JF, Bonhoeffer P et al. Perforation of the atretic pulmonary valve. Long-term follow-up. *J Am Coll Cardiol* 2003; **41**:1399–1403.
41. Alwi M, Geetha K, Bilkis AA et al. Pulmonary atresia with intact ventricular septum percutaneous radiofrequency-assisted valvotomy and balloon dilation versus surgical valvotomy and Blalock Taussig shunt. *J Am Coll Cardiol* 2000; **35**:468–476.
42. Ovaert C, Qureshi SA, Rosenthal E, Baker EJ, Tynan M. Growth of the right ventricle after successful transcatheter pulmonary valvotomy in neonates and infants with pulmonary atresia and intact ventricular septum. *J Thorac Cardiovasc Surg* 1998; **115**:1055–1062.

27

Interrupted aortic arch

INTRODUCTION

Interrupted aortic arch (IAA) is a complete interruption of the aorta that, unlike coarctation, most commonly occurs between the left common carotid and left subclavian arteries. It is frequently associated with small left heart structures, especially the left ventricular outflow tract which leads to a high incidence of need for reoperation after successful repair in the neonatal period. Although the mortality for this anomaly was very high in the early years of cardiac surgery, the introduction of prostaglandin E1 resulted in a dramatic improvement in the outlook for these children. However, a common association with microdeletion of chromosome 22 does mean that many of these children subsequently demonstrate features of DiGeorge syndrome including developmental delay.

EMBRYOLOGY

The development of the aortic arch is a fascinating example of the way in which the developing fetus assembles modules that had a useful purpose in our phylogenetic past (see also Chapter 29). Modules which have become redundant are then eliminated by the process of apoptosis leaving only those components that are useful to the present day individual. Thus early in fetal development there are six aortic arches forming the six 'branchial' arches as used by gill breathing organisms (branchial = gill). These six arches connect with the right and left dorsal aortas distally (descending aorta) and with the conotruncus (ascending aorta) proximally. The first to third arches regress to become minor facial and skull vessels. The proximal aortic arch is derived from the aortic sac from the conotruncus, the distal arch from the fourth embryonic arch (usually the left giving a left aortic arch as the usual) and the isthmus is derived from the junction of the sixth embryonic arch (ductus) with the left dorsal aorta and the fourth embryonic arch.[1] Not surprisingly this complex composite of segments introduces a risk of developmental anomalies in the form of interruptions or stenoses at the various junction points.

ANATOMY

The arch of the aorta is described as having a proximal component, the proximal aortic arch, which extends from the takeoff of the innominate artery to the left common carotid artery. The distal component, the distal aortic arch, extends from the left common carotid to the takeoff of the left subclavian artery. The segment of aorta which connects the distal aortic arch to the juxtaductal region of the descending aorta is termed the 'isthmus'.

A useful classification of interrupted aortic arch was introduced by Celoria and Patton in 1959 (Figure 27.1).[2] Type A interruption occurs at the level of the isthmus. Not uncommonly it is seen in a milder form in which a short fibrous chord connects across the interruption even though there is no luminal continuity. This has been termed aortic arch 'atresia' and generally represents less of a surgical challenge than a long segment discontinuity. Type B interruption occurs between the left common carotid artery and the left subclavian artery. It is the most common type seen. In a review of the experience at Children's Hospital Boston between 1974 and 1987 by Sell et al[3] 69% of the 71 patients had type B interruption. In a more recent multi-institutional study by the Congenital Heart Surgeon's

Society,[4] 79% of 183 neonates with interrupted aortic arch and associated VSD had type B interruption. Type B interruption is often associated with an aberrant origin of the right subclavian artery from the descending aorta. This is important because in this subtype more flow must pass through the ductus arteriosus during fetal development and less flow through the left ventricular outflow tract and ascending aorta than with the standard type B interruption, i.e. with normal origin of the right subclavian from the innominate artery. Thus it is not surprising to find that the risk of subaortic stenosis is increased when the right subclavian artery arises aberrantly.

Type C interruption occurs between the innominate artery takeoff and left common carotid. It is extremely rare having been described in less than 4% of most large clinical and pathological series. There were no cases among the entire series of 250 patients with interrupted aortic arch reviewed by the CHSS.[4]

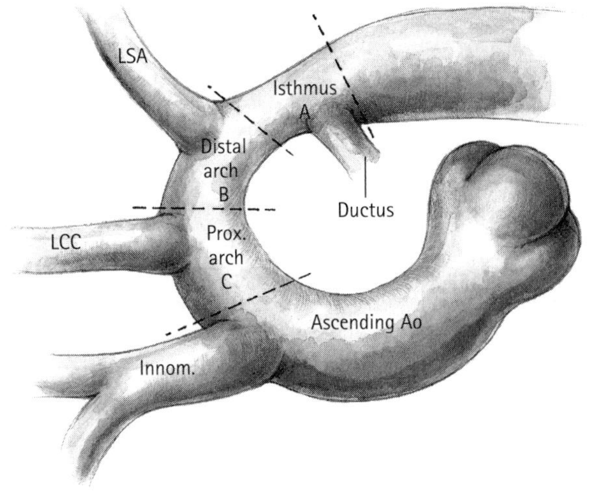

Figure 27.1 *Interrupted aortic arch has been classified by Celoria and Patton[2] as type A: interruption at the isthmus between the left subclavian artery and ductus; type B: interruption of the distal aortic arch between the left common carotid and left subclavian arteries; and type C: interruption of the proximal aortic arch between the innominate artery and left common carotid artery.*

ASSOCIATED ANOMALIES

Isolated interrupted aortic arch is exceedingly rare. Apart from patent ductus arteriosus, a single VSD is the most common associated anomaly. In the CHSS study, 73% of 250 patients had an isolated VSD as the only associated anomaly.[4] There is frequently posterior malalignment of the conal septum relative to the ventricular septum which contributes to left ventricular outflow tract obstruction[5,6] (Figure 27.2a). Other anatomic features that may contribute to left ventricular outflow tract obstruction include the aortic annulus itself which is usually at least moderately hypoplastic. The aortic valve is

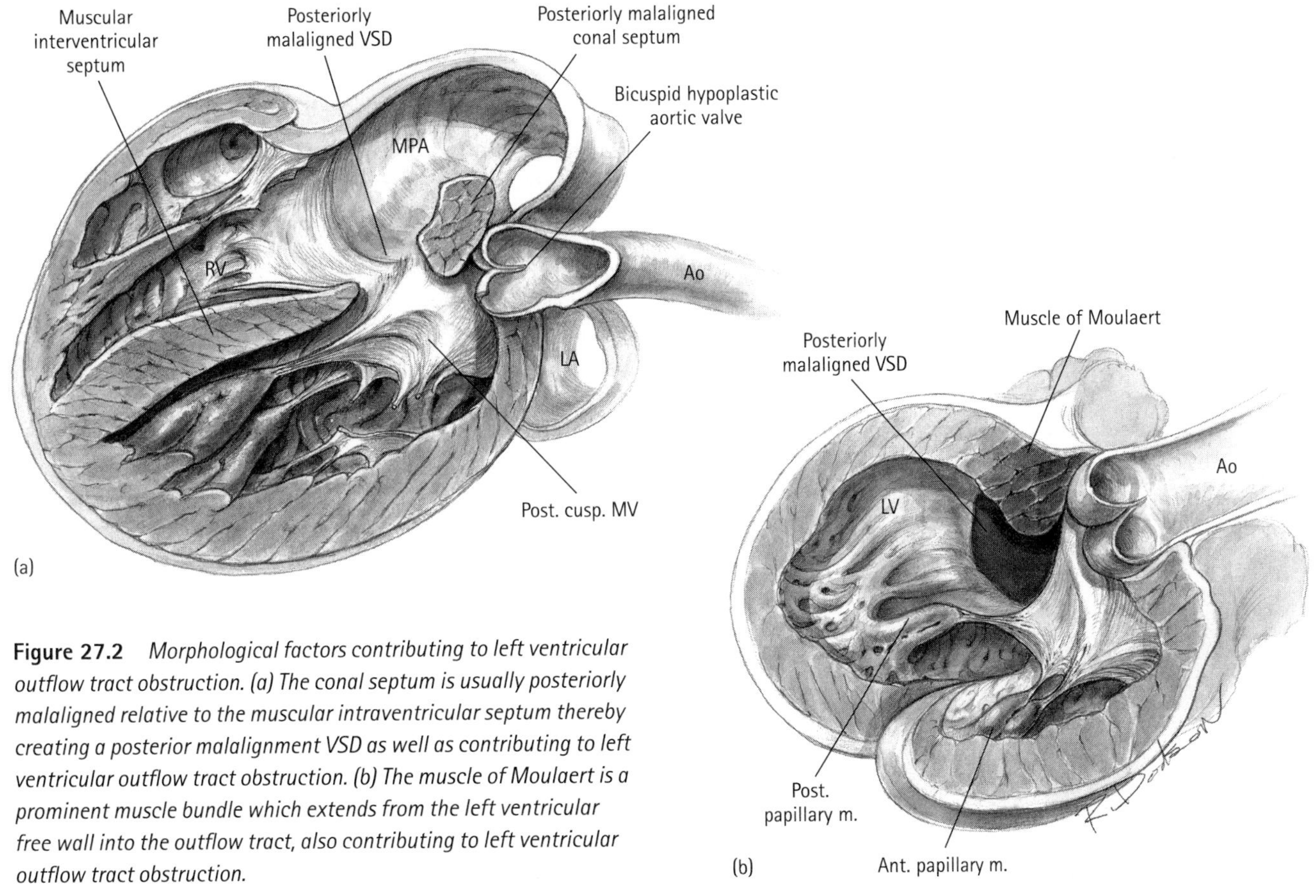

Figure 27.2 *Morphological factors contributing to left ventricular outflow tract obstruction. (a) The conal septum is usually posteriorly malaligned relative to the muscular intraventricular septum thereby creating a posterior malalignment VSD as well as contributing to left ventricular outflow tract obstruction. (b) The muscle of Moulaert is a prominent muscle bundle which extends from the left ventricular free wall into the outflow tract, also contributing to left ventricular outflow tract obstruction.*

frequently bicuspid and there may be commissural fusion.[7,8] Opposite the septum there may be a prominent muscle bundle on the left ventricular free wall which projects into the outflow tract, the so-called 'muscle of Moulaert'[9] (Figure 27.2b). A fibrous subaortic membrane is almost never seen in the neonate with interrupted aortic arch but not uncommonly develops within a year or two of repair.[10] An atrial septal defect is frequently seen in conjunction with interrupted aortic arch. This is usually in the form of a stretched patent foramen ovale but can be quite large and therefore hemodynamically important. Perhaps this results from the left to right shunt which results during in-utero development because of the left sided obstruction due to the interruption itself as well as associated left ventricular outflow tract obstruction.

Other anomalies seen in association with interrupted aortic arch are listed in Table 27.1.[2] It can be seen that various forms of single ventricle are seen in 11% of patients with IAA and truncus arteriosus in 10%.

PATHOPHYSIOLOGY

Interruption of the aortic arch of any type has no important impact on the fetal circulation. This is not surprising in light of the fact that less than 10% of the fetal cardiac output is usually distributed through the isthmus.[11] Following birth the lower body continues to be adequately perfused so long as the ductus remains patent and pulmonary resistance remains high. Ductal closure in the first day or two of life is a common reason for presentation because it leads to a profound degree of ischemia of the lower body and in the case of the common type B interruption, the left subclavian artery territory also becomes ischemic.

CLINICAL FEATURES

Prenatal diagnosis by ultrasound is becoming increasingly common. Prostaglandin E1 is started immediately after birth and an acidotic insult is avoided. For the patient who is not diagnosed prenatally with the most common form of IAA, that is with an associated patent ductus arteriosus and conoventricular VSD, there may be little suspicion of serious heart disease during the early neonatal period until ductal closure begins. If that should occur abruptly or is not recognized rapidly, the child will soon become profoundly acidotic and anuric as perfusion of the lower body becomes entirely dependent on collateral communications between the two separate aortic systems. The distribution of palpable pulses will depend on the anatomical subtype. For example with the common type B interrupted aortic arch, the right arm pulse will remain palpable when the left arm pulse and femoral pulses become impalpable secondary to ductal closure. Ischemic injury to the liver will be reflected in a marked elevation of hepatic enzymes (transaminases, lactate dehydrogenase) and ischemic injury to the gut may be followed by evidence of necrotizing enterocolitis such as bloody stools. Renal injury can be quantitated to some extent by the elevation observed in serum creatine. A very severe degree of systemic acidosis (prolonged pH less than 7.0) will result ultimately in injury to all tissues of the body including the brain and the heart itself. The child may have seizures and become flaccid and poorly responsive. Myocardial injury will be manifest as a low cardiac output state despite correction of acidosis. Since pulmonary blood flow is preserved during ductal closure it is rare to see evidence of pulmonary insufficiency so that the child is not likely to become cyanotic.

Occasionally the ductus will not close during the neonatal period and diagnosis may be delayed for several weeks. As pulmonary resistance falls there will be an increasing left to right shunt and the child will present with evidence of congestive heart failure including failure to thrive.

DIAGNOSTIC STUDIES

Anatomy

Accurate anatomical diagnosis can be made using echocardiography alone. This is an important advantage for the

Table 27.1 *Anomalies seen in association with interrupted aortic arch*

		Type of IAA *n* (%)		
Associated cardiac anomalies	*n*	**Type A**	**Type B**	**Type C**
VSD (isolated)	44	7 (35)	35 (71)	2 (100)
'Single ventricle'	8	5 (25)	3 (6)	NA
Truncus arteriosus	7	2 (10)	5 (10)	NA
DORV	5	2 (10)	3 (6)	NA
TGA + VSD	2	2 (10)	NA	NA
Complete AV canal	2	1 (5)	1 (2)	NA
DOLV	1	NA	1 (2)	NA
Isolated v. inversion + VSD	1	1 (5)	NA	NA
None (PDA present)	1	NA	1 (2)	NA
Total	71	20 (100)	49 (100)	2 (100)

neonate who presents in extremis and in whom invasive cardiac catheterization would be a serious additional insult. In addition to localizing the site of the interruption, the echocardiographer should provide the following information: the length of the discontinuity should be measured: the narrowest dimension of the left ventricular outflow tract (generally secondary to posterior displacement of the conal septum and therefore best assessed in the parasternal long-axis view): the diameter of the aortic annulus and the diameter of the ascending aorta should also be measured. It is unusual for segments of the arch which are present to be so hypoplastic that they cause hemodynamic compromise. The features of associated anomalies must be carefully defined. For example, the location of an associated VSD should be defined in relation to its margins. The conal septum is often severely hypoplastic rendering approach to the superior margin of the defect through the tricuspid valve particularly difficult. Additional VSDs are very rare. The presence or absence of the thymus can usually be ascertained by echocardiography. An absent thymus has important implications because of its association with microdeletion of chromosome 22 and DiGeorge syndrome.

The role of magnetic resonance angiography is yet to be defined though presently it would appear to have little advantage in the unrepaired neonate over echocardiography.

Hemodynamic assessment

Because diagnosis will generally be made after ductal patency has been re-established using prostaglandin E1, pressure data will be of little use in formulating a plan for surgical management. The question which most commonly arises is the adequacy of the left ventricular outflow tract. Attempts to quantitate the degree of obstruction by measuring a pressure gradient are hampered by lack of information regarding the amount of flow passing through this area. The VSD will usually be nonrestrictive. There is no evidence that multiple VSDs are more accurately identified by angiography than color flow Doppler echocardiography.[12]

MEDICAL AND INTERVENTIONAL MANAGEMENT

The introduction of prostaglandin E1 in 1976 revolutionized the management of IAA. Before this time, which also predated the introduction of two-dimensional echocardiography, it was necessary to manage acidotic neonates symptomatically as they underwent emergency cardiac catheterization and were then rushed from the catheterization laboratory to the operating room. Not surprisingly few survived this sequence.

Prostaglandin E1 must be infused through a secure intravenous line. If ductal patency does not become apparent in any neonate less than one week of age within one hour, it should be assumed until proven otherwise that there is a technical problem with delivery of the medication into the central bloodstream. Establishing ductal patency represents just the first step in medically resuscitating the neonate with IAA. Because the lower half of the body is dependent on perfusion through the ductus and because blood in the ductus also has the choice of passing into the pulmonary circulation, it is important that pulmonary resistance be maximized. This can be achieved by avoiding a high level of inspired oxygen (usually room air is appropriate) as well as avoiding respiratory alkalosis caused by hyperventilation. In fact, control of ventilation is best achieved by anesthetizing and intubating the neonate and inducing paralysis. A peak inspiratory pressure and ventilatory rate should be selected which will achieve a PCO_2 level of 40–50 mm. Metabolic acidosis should be aggressively treated with boluses of sodium bicarbonate though care must be taken to avoid producing an overall alkalotic pH. Because myocardial function is likely to be depressed at the time of presentation and it may be necessary for the heart to handle a moderate volume load (dependent on the success with which pulmonary resistance is maximized), an inotropic agent such as dopamine is usually employed. Dopamine has the added advantage of maximizing renal perfusion in this setting of an ischemic renal insult. It is not uncommon to persist with medical resuscitation in the manner described for two to three days before surgery is undertaken. It should be very unusual that a child is taken to the operating room with any abnormalities of acid/base, renal or hepatic indices.[3]

There are no catheter interventions that are helpful in the unrepaired neonate. Balloon angioplasty is often very helpful for postoperative anastomotic stenosis of the aortic arch repair site.

INDICATIONS FOR AND TIMING OF SURGERY

The presence of IAA is incompatible with life unless ductal patency is maintained (i.e. it is a duct dependent anomaly), so that the diagnosis alone is the indication for surgery. Surgery should be undertaken when metabolic resuscitation is complete using the techniques described previously.

SURGICAL MANAGEMENT

History of surgery

IAA was first described by Steidele in 1778.[13] Celoria and Patton reported their anatomical classification as noted above in 1959.[2] Successful surgical repair was first described by Samson et al in 1955[14] in a patient with short segment type A IAA. A direct anastomosis was possible. However, the associated VSDs were not closed at the time of the arch repair. One stage repair was first accomplished by Barratt-Boyes.[15] In the procedure he described, arch continuity was established using a synthetic conduit. One stage repair incorporating direct arch anastomosis was first described by Trusler in 1975.[16] Interrupted aortic arch carried an extremely high mortality risk until the introduction of prostaglandin E1 by Neutze, Starling and Elliott in 1976.[17] Over the next 5–10 years it became apparent that careful resuscitation of the neonate, often over a time span of days before proceeding to surgery was associated with a dramatic improvement in surgical outcome.

Technical considerations

The ideal method of surgical management has become less controversial over the last decade. There is now widespread agreement that primary one stage repair in the neonatal period is optimal management though minor controversy persists regarding some of the details. Palliative options were commonly used in the past but are used infrequently today as more units have become familiar with corrective neonatal surgery. Noncorrective procedures used in the past include application of a pulmonary artery band during the neonatal period with closure of the associated VSD at some time beyond infancy and usually before five years of age. Rather than a corrective direct anastomosis, arch continuity was achieved previously by insertion of a synthetic conduit.[18] Both these palliative options are generally undertaken working through a left thoracotomy though some surgeons prefer to use a combined thoracotomy and sternotomy approach for placement of an ascending to descending aortic conduit. Our current preference is to undertake one stage repair during the neonatal period including a direct aortic arch anastomosis.[4]

During transport to the operating room and while preparing and positioning the child, it is important to continue applying the management principles which have been employed during the resuscitation of the child over the previous few days in the intensive care unit. In particular a high level of inspired oxygen and hyperventilation must be avoided. In addition to the usual monitoring equipment, careful consideration must be given to monitoring of arterial pressure. It is preferable to be able to measure blood pressure both above and below the forthcoming arch anastomosis. Often this is achieved by placement of a right radial arterial line in addition to an umbilical arterial line. Not only does this allow one to assess immediately any pressure gradient across the anastomosis, but in addition the adequacy of perfusion of the separate upper and lower body circulation can be assessed during the cooling phase on cardiopulmonary bypass.

Approach is via a median sternotomy alone. If a thymus is present it is subtotally excised. Pericardium is not usually harvested. Accurate arterial cannulation is an essential key to the success of the procedure. Although a single arterial cannula will usually ultimately achieve complete cooling, we currently believe that cannulation of both the ascending aorta and pulmonary artery optimize tissue perfusion, particularly of the brain and heart in the critical early phase of cooling when all organs are still warm. Generally an 8 French thin walled wire-wrapped (e.g. Biomedicus) arterial cannula is used for the ascending aorta. As indicated by Figure 27.3a, this cannula should be inserted on the right lateral aspect of the ascending aorta exactly opposite the anticipated location of the arch anastomosis. The tip of the cannula should not extend more than 1.5–2 mm into the lumen of the ascending aorta. This will decrease the chance that either retrograde flow to the coronary arteries or antegrade flow to the brain will be compromised. The second arterial cannula is connected to the arterial tubing by a Y connector and is inserted in the anterior surface of the main pulmonary artery (Figure 27.3a). Because of the larger size of the main pulmonary artery relative to the ascending aorta (often 10–12 mm versus 5–6 mm), a larger cannula, e.g. 10Fr Bard arterial cannula can be employed. Immediately after beginning bypass it is necessary to tighten tourniquets around the right and left pulmonary arteries so that flow from the cannula in the pulmonary artery will be directed through the ductus arteriosus to the descending aorta (prostaglandin E1 infusion must be continued during the cooling phase of cardiopulmonary bypass). Alternatively the ductus is cannulated distally and is ligated proximally immediately after commencing bypass. Venous cannulation is routine with a single straight cannula in the right atrium.

ARCH ANASTOMOSIS

During cooling the ascending aorta and its branches are thoroughly mobilized. The ductus and descending aorta are also mobilized to minimize tension on the arch anastomosis. If an aberrant right subclavian artery is present it should be ligated and divided at its origin from the descending aorta also to reduce tension on the arch anastomsois. It is also often useful to divide the left subclavian artery in a type B interruption to further minimize anastomotic tension as well as simplifying the anastomosis, thereby decreasing the risk of bleeding and stenosis.

When both rectal and tympanic temperatures are less than 18°C, bypass is discontinued. Tourniquets may be tightened around the right and left common carotid arteries though this is not essential so long as care is taken in de-airing the aorta before perfusion is recommenced. The pulmonary artery tourniquets are removed. Cardioplegia is infused through a sidearm on the ascending arterial connector. Both arterial cannulas are then removed together with the venous cannula.

The ductus is ligated and divided at its junction with the descending aorta. Any residual ductal tissue is excised from the descending aorta (Figure 27.3b). A C-clamp is applied across the descending aorta and helps to draw the descending aorta to the level of the anastomosis which can be performed with the opposing tissues under no tension. The anastomosis should be sited on the ascending aorta where it is most mobile where tension will be minimized. Although many surgeons believe that this requires siting the anastomosis partially on the left common carotid artery, we generally prefer to site the anastomosis completely on the ascending aorta. The distal limit of the ascending aortotomy is usually close to the bifurcation of

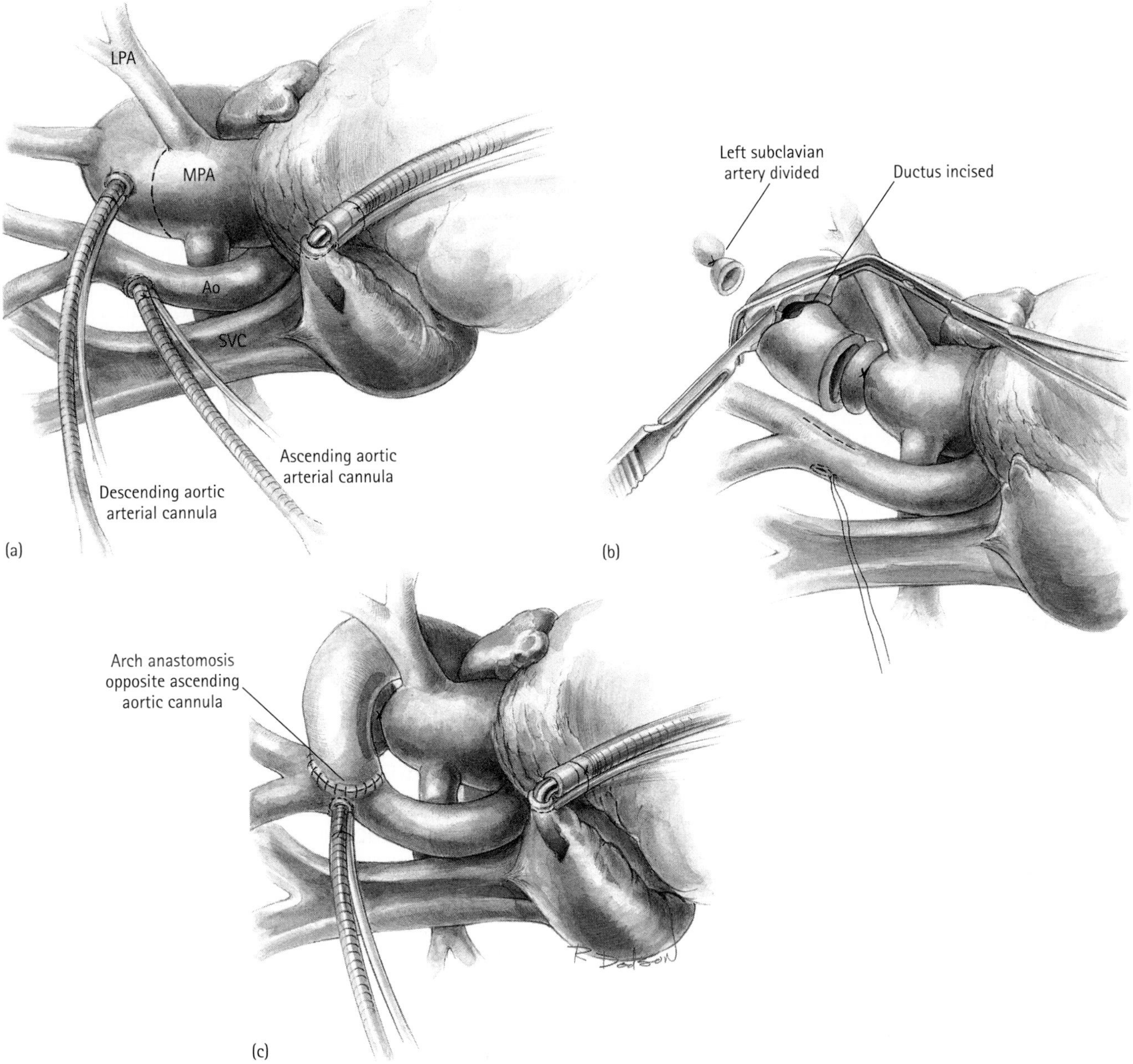

Figure 27.3 *(a) Arterial cannulation is a critically important component of the repair of interrupted aortic arch in the neonate. For type B interruption two arterial cannulas are employed connected by a Y. Generally an 8 French thin walled cannula is inserted in the small ascending aorta. The cannula should be positioned on the right side of the ascending aorta opposite the intended site of aortic anastomosis. A single venous cannula is placed in the right atrium. Either the branch pulmonary arteries are controlled with separate tourniquets or alternatively the second arterial cannula can be placed in the ductus and a ligature tightened around the proximal ductus immediately after commencing bypass. (b) After the onset of hypothermic circulatory arrest both arterial cannulas are removed. The ductus is ligated proximally. Ductal tissue is excised up to the level of the descending aorta opposite the left subclavian artery. It may be helpful to divide the left subclavian artery to reduce tension on the arch anastomosis. The intended site of the anastomosis on the ascending aorta is indicated. A cross clamp is helpful in minimizing tension on the anastomosis as it is performed. (c) The ascending aortic cannula has been reinserted after carefully de-airing the aorta and arch vessels. A period of cold reperfusion of five minutes may be employed if a second period of hypothermic circulatory arrest is necessary for transatrial approach to the VSD. However, commonly the VSD is approached through the main pulmonary artery.*

the aorta into the innominate and left common carotid arteries. The anastomosis should be exactly opposite the ascending aortic cannulation site. Continuous absorbable polydioxanone or Maxon 6–0 suture may be used though there is no evidence that use of this suture results in a lower incidence of anastomotic stenosis. Many surgeons continue to prefer polypropylene suture. Its lesser tissue drag distributes tension more evenly through the suture line which appears to enhance hemostasis relative to the absorbable sutures. We have not generally supplemented the anastomosis and/or the ascending aorta with a patch of pericardium or arterial allograft tissue though this is practiced by some. Data from the CHSS study supports this practice when left ventricular outflow tract obstruction is present.[4]

RECANNULATION AND COLD REPERFUSION

The aorta is carefully filled with saline through the ascending aortic cannulation site in order to displace air from the ascending aorta, arch, head vessels and descending aorta. One arterial cannula (the 8Fr thin walled cannula) is carefully reinserted (in the ascending aorta only). A cross clamp is applied proximal to the cannula, the venous cannula is reinserted and bypass is recommenced. A period of cold reperfusion is maintained for a minimum of five minutes at a flow rate of 100 ml/kg per minute before reducing flow to 50 ml/kg per minute for the VSD closure if this is to be done through the pulmonary artery. If the approach is to be through the right atrium, a second period of circulatory arrest is begun.

VENTRICULAR SEPTAL DEFECT CLOSURE

The approach to the VSD will depend on the preoperative echocardiographic assessment which must be carefully viewed by the surgeon preoperatively. Frequently there will be marked hypoplasia of the conal septum. In such cases the optimal approach for VSD closure is via a transverse incision in the proximal main pulmonary artery immediately distal to the pulmonary valve (Figure 27.4). It is usually possible to continue low flow hypothermic bypass throughout VSD closure even when using a single venous cannula in the right atrium. The VSD is closed in the routine fashion for a subpulmonary VSD.[19] At the superior margin sutures are passed through the pulmonary annulus with the pledgets lying above the pulmonary valve leaflets. Although this has the potential to distort the pulmonary valve thereby excluding its use for a Ross procedure, there is at least one report of a successful Ross procedure after transpulmonary approach to the VSD.[20] Consideration should be given to using autologous pericardium rather than Dacron in order to minimize fibrotic distortion of the pulmonary valve.

ATRIAL SEPTAL DEFECT CLOSURE

A decision should be made preoperatively regarding the need to close an atrial septal defect which will be present in most patients. Because of the poor left sided compliance which is often present with interrupted aortic arch with VSD, even a small atrial septal defect can result in a large left to right shunt postoperatively. The ASD can usually be closed by direct suture working through a short low right atriotomy during a brief period of hypothermic circulatory arrest.

REWARMING AND SEPARATING FROM BYPASS

After VSD and ASD closure rewarming is begun. The left heart is de-aired in the usual fashion and the aortic cross clamp is released. Routine monitoring lines, i.e. a left atrial, pulmonary artery and right atrial line are placed during rewarming. Separating from bypass and early postoperative management should be uncomplicated since a biventricular repair has been achieved. If problems are encountered a residual VSD or anastomotic stenosis must be excluded. It is unusual for left ventricular outflow tract obstruction to result in hemodynamic compromise early after surgery.

INTERRUPTED AORTIC ARCH WITH VSD AND LEFT VENTRICULAR OUTFLOW TRACT OBSTRUCTION

Very occasionally left ventricular outflow tract obstruction in the neonatal period may be sufficiently severe to justify a radical alternative primary procedure described by Yasui et al.[21]

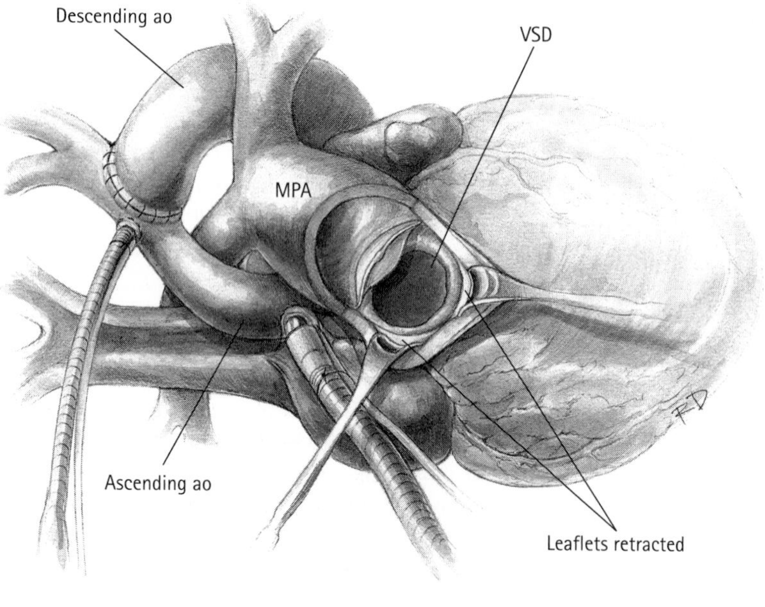

Figure 27.4 *Because there is frequently severe hypoplasia of the conal septum the best approach for VSD closure for interrupted aortic arch is often through a transverse incision in the main pulmonary artery. This can usually be performed with hypothermic bypass continuing. An aortic cross clamp is usually applied to the ascending aorta during this period (not shown).*

Although others have felt it necessary to employ such a procedure relatively frequently, we did not do so even once in 71 patients with IAA between 1974 and 1987 although several patients had a narrowest dimension of the left ventricular outflow tract of only 3.5–4 mm.[3] However, we have subsequently seen a very occasional neonate with a subaortic diameter of only 1 or 2 mm and under these circumstances agree that this area must be bypassed. The principle employed is analogous to the Damus-Kaye-Stansel procedure described for transposition (Figure 27.5). Left ventricular output is directed through the VSD to the proximal divided main pulmonary artery by a baffle patch constructed of autologous pericardium. The main pulmonary artery is divided proximal to its bifurcation. The proximal divided main pulmonary artery is anastomosed to the side of the ascending aorta. A tube graft bridges the arch interruption itself if direct anastomosis is not possible.[21] A conduit, preferably an aortic or pulmonary homograft is placed between the right ventricle and the distal divided main pulmonary artery. Another variation on this theme is to supply pulmonary blood flow with a shunt following the pulmonary to aortic anastomosis and arch repair. This is essentially a Norwood procedure with the addition of arch repair.[22] However, since two ventricles are present we do not recommend this palliative procedure though satisfactory results have been reported with this approach from centers very familiar with the Norwood procedure.[22]

INTERRUPTED ARCH WITH OTHER ANOMALIES

The general principle should be applied that if two ventricles are present a biventricular repair incorporating growth potential should be undertaken during the neonatal period. For example, the child with transposition of the great arteries, VSD and interrupted arch should undergo an arterial switch procedure with VSD closure and direct arch anastomosis. Although this complex procedure requires a long cross-clamp time, it is generally well tolerated so long as an accurate repair is achieved.[23] Transfer of the aorta posteriorly as part of the arterial switch in fact helps to reduce tension on the arch anastomosis. Various technical modifications have been proposed.[24] Similarly with truncus arteriosus and interrupted arch, the large size of the truncus decreases the difficulty with which aortic cannulation is achieved relative to the child with simple interrupted arch where the ascending aorta is often very hypoplastic. An analysis published in 2000 of the results of surgery at Children's Hospital Boston between 1992 and 1998 revealed that interrupted aortic arch is no longer a risk factor for early death after repair of truncus with interrupted aortic arch.[25]

Management of the child with a single functional ventricle and interrupted arch remains a significant challenge, presenting many of the same problems experienced with management of hypoplastic left heart syndrome. There is almost always important obstruction present within the single ventricle,

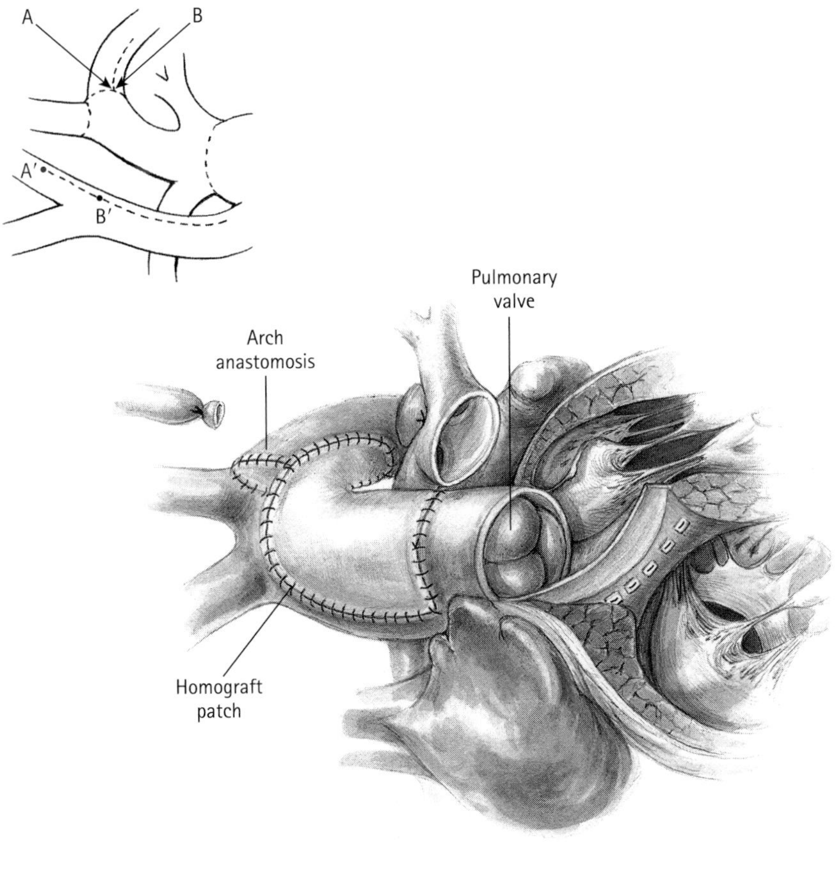

Figure 27.5 *When the subaortic diameter is exceedingly small, e.g. 1–2 mm, a radical alternative primary procedure described by Yasui et al[21] can be performed. Left ventricular output is directed through the VSD to the proximal divided main pulmonary artery by a baffle patch constructed of autologous pericardium. Point A is sutured to point A′, point B to B′. The proximal divided main pulmonary artery is anastomosed to the side of the ascending aorta as well as to the proximal divided descending aorta supplemented with a homograft patch. A homograft conduit is placed between the right ventricle and the distal divided main pulmonary artery to complete the repair.*

often in the form of an obstructive bulboventricular foramen. This must either be bypassed using a pulmonary to aortic anastomosis (Damus-Stansel-Kaye, Norwood) or must be relieved by resection of the bulboventricular foramen. Residual arch obstruction is very poorly tolerated with either a shunt dependent circulation (following a pulmonary-aortic anastomosis) or with a pulmonary artery band if bulboventricular foramen enlargement is undertaken. Such obstruction will result in excessive pulmonary blood flow unless the band itself is very tight. This creates a highly labile situation. Application of the Sano modification of the Norwood procedure, i.e. a ventricle to pulmonary artery shunt may be just as helpful in improving stability in this setting as it is for hypoplastic left heart syndrome.

Postoperative management of interrupted aortic arch

Following biventricular repair of simple interrupted aortic arch with VSD, postoperative management should be routine. Failure to progress appropriately, e.g. minimal inotropic requirement within 24–48 hours and satisfactory progress towards extubation within two to three days (depending largely on preoperative status) should stimulate an aggressive search for residual hemodynamic lesions. A residual VSD should be excluded by oxygen saturation data collected from the pulmonary artery line on the first postoperative morning. An anastomotic gradient should have been excluded both intraoperatively and in the early postoperative period by appropriate blood pressure determination. Echocardiography including intraoperative transesophageal echocardiography and if there is any doubt, cardiac catheterization, can exclude important left ventricular outflow tract obstruction. A left to right shunt at atrial level should also be excluded. If an important residual hemodynamic lesion is identified, the child should be expeditiously returned to the operating room for correction of the problem.

RESULTS OF SURGERY

Advantages of one stage primary repair, direct anastomosis

There was a dramatic improvement in both early and late results of surgery for interrupted aortic arch with VSD at Children's Hospital Boston between 1974 and 1987.[3] The risk of death within two weeks of surgery in 1974 was greater than 50% while by 1987 the risk was less than 10%. There were many changes in the management of neonates during this timeframe which may have contributed to this improvement. The importance of complete preoperative resuscitation, for example, is illustrated by Figure 27.6. This effect is apparent for children with complex associated anomalies such as single ventricle and truncus arteriosus as well as for patients with VSD as the only associated anomaly. Our analysis in 1988 did not conclusively demonstrate that one stage repair during the neonatal period or that direct arch anastomosis rather than placement of a conduit contributed to the reduction in mortality. This was also the case in the analysis by the CHSS.[4] Nevertheless our current results as well as recent reports from other large neonatal centers[26–31] have encouraged us to continue an approach of one stage direct anastomotic repair because of the multiple psychosocial, economic and logistical advantages relative to a staged procedure employing a tube graft.

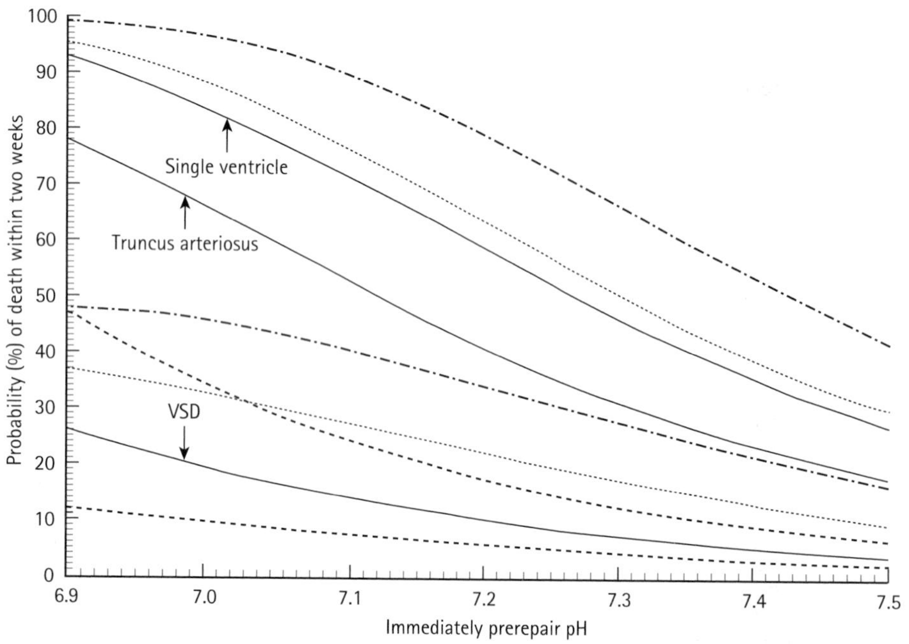

Figure 27.6 *Probability of death within two weeks of surgery for patients with a single ventricle, truncus arteriosus and VSD in association with interrupted aortic arch relative to the arterial pH sampled immediately before surgery at Children's Hospital Boston from 1974 to 1987. The important influence of complete preoperative resuscitation is demonstrated: 70% confidence intervals are shown. (From Sell et al. The results of a surgical program for interrupted aortic arch.* J Thorac Cardiovasc Surg *1988; **96**:871, with permission from Elsevier.)

Complications

EARLY

Potential technical complications have been enumerated above under postoperative management. In addition bleeding can be troublesome. Bleeding is more likely if the arch anastomosis is performed under excessive tension which will result if there is inadequate mobilization of the ascending and descending aorta. Extreme friability of tissue also contributes to the risk of bleeding. Friability can result from severe preoperative acidosis but is also apparent if ductal tissue is incorporated in the anastomosis. Including ductal tissue presumably also increases the risk of late anastomotic stenosis. As with all neonatal surgery, hemostasis must be accelerated by appropriate use of blood replacement with truly fresh blood representing the optimal choice. In the absence of fresh blood, judicious but nevertheless aggressive transfusion of concentrated factors including cryoprecipitate as well as platelet concentrates is indicated. The selection of a perfusion hematocrit of at least 30% is also an important factor in achieving rapid hemostasis. Crystalloid hemodilution to 20% is likely to result in inadequate levels of fibrinogen and other coagulation factors. Both conventional and modified ultrafiltration have a role to play in maintaining an ideal hematocrit. Aprotinin is very effective in improving hemostasis in the neonate after interrupted arch repair. Even if it has not been infused prebypass and during the bypass period it appears still to be effective when begun postoperatively. The use of deep hypothermic circulatory arrest is not a contraindication to the use of aprotinin; in fact in a study undertaken in piglets at Children's Hospital Boston animals treated with aprotinin had an improved recovery after circulatory arrest as determined by magnetic resonance spectroscopy.[32]

Both the left recurrent laryngeal and phrenic nerves are at risk during repair of IAA. Phrenic nerve injury in our experience was particularly common following placement of an ascending to descending aortic conduit despite meticulous care of the nerve itself. We have speculated that direct compression of the nerve by the synthetic material may have been the cause of this problem. Phrenic nerve palsy has been rare following direct arch anastomosis.

LATE

Pressure gradient across arch

Ultimately all patients who have a tube graft inserted during the neonatal period will develop obstruction (defined as a pressure gradient greater than 30 mm) across the graft secondary to somatic growth alone. In addition synthetic grafts have a variable rate of accumulation of a pseudointima which may accelerate the rate of obstruction. The actuarial freedom from tube graft obstruction in our early experience was 55% by five years. In contrast patients who had a direct arch anastomosis were more likely to have obstruction with only 40% having less than a 30 mm gradient within 18 months of surgery.[3] However, balloon dilation can successfully relieve such gradients in the majority of children who have had a direct arch anastomosis[33] while conduit replacement is inevitable for those with conduits. In the experience analysed by the Congenital Heart Surgeons Society the freedom from reintervention for arch obstruction was approximately 86% at three years for patients who had undergone a direct anastomosis, with a trend to a higher rate of reintervention for those patients who had undergone some other form of arch reconstruction including placement of a tube graft ($p = 0.15$).[4] It is likely that the lower rate of reintervention in the more recent timeframe reflects increasing familiarity with wide mobilization of the ascending aorta, arch vessels and the descending aorta.

Left ventricular outflow tract obstruction

Left ventricular outflow tract obstruction is one of the most important late problems after repair of interrupted aortic arch. Salem et al found that the diameter of the aortic valve was the most sensitive predictor of subsequent outflow tract obstruction. All patients with an aortic annulus less than 4.5 mm developed late left ventricular outflow obstruction.[34] In contrast Apfel et al found that the indexed cross sectional area of the subaortic area was the most useful predictor of subsequent obstruction[35].

The large CHSS experience suggested that performance of conal septal resection or performance of a pulmonary to aortic (DKS) anastomosis during the neonatal period carried a greater risk of early death than simple repair.[4] This was true by multivariate analysis of either the entire group or by analysis of just the subgroup with important left heart hypoplasia in addition to interrupted aortic arch. It is important to remember, however, that this report describes a multi-institutional experience in which there was a very wide range of patient volume and outcomes. Reports by Jacobs[36] and Bove[37] suggest that the Norwood procedure or conal septal resection can be performed with an acceptable mortality but probably should not be attempted at centers unfamiliar with these approaches. Another approach described by Luciani et al[38] involves anchoring VSD sutures on the left side of the conal septum hopefully resulting in a rightward and anterior shift of the posteriorly displaced septum when the left ventricle is pressurized. There is no evidence, however, that this approach has any advantage from this perspective than the usual placement of sutures on the right side of the conal septum.

Although left ventricular outflow tract is rarely sufficiently severe to justify an alteration in surgical strategy during the neonatal reparative procedure, it is by contrast not uncommon for surgical intervention to be required for left ventricular outflow tract obstruction late postoperatively.[10] Among 33 patients reviewed by Sell et al[3] who underwent repair of a conoventricular VSD as the only associated anomaly with IAA, only 58% were free of evident left ventricular outflow tract obstruction (defined as a gradient of greater than 40 mm) by three years postoperatively. In the CHSS report 77% were free from reintervention at three years (Figure 27.7).

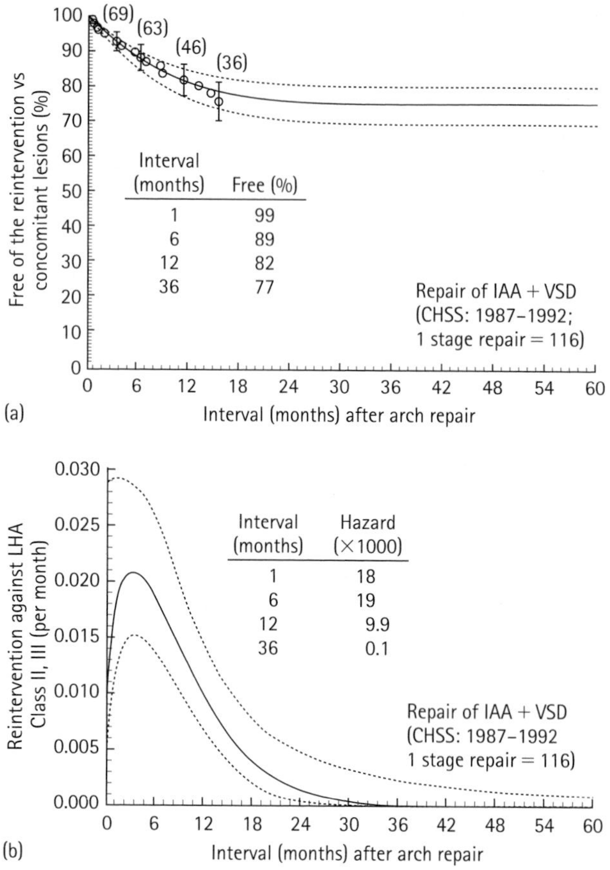

Figure 27.7 *(a) Time related percent freedom from reintervention for one or more levels of obstruction in the left ventricular outflow tract following primary one stage repair of interrupted aortic arch with VSD. (b) Hazard function for the first reintervention against left ventricular outflow tract obstruction following an initial primary one stage repair of interrupted aortic arch with VSD. (From Jonas et al. Outcomes in patients with interrupted aortic arch and ventricular septal defect.* J Thorac Cardiovasc Surg, *1994; 107:1106, with permission from Elsevier.)*

Since the morphology of left ventricular outflow tract obstruction with IAA is variable, surgical management beyond the neonatal period will vary according to the specific circumstances. In some cases it is possible to resect the posteriorly deviated conal septum working through the aortic valve. An aortic valvotomy may also be required if there is valvar stenosis. If there is tunnel subaortic stenosis we perform a modified Konno procedure, i.e. ventricular septoplasty.[39] Working through a right ventricular infundibular incision, an incision is made in the ventricular septum into the left ventricular outflow tract. The incision is carried up to the aortic valve. A patch is placed on the right ventricular aspect of the surgically created VSD. If there is also aortic annular hypoplasia as well as tunnel subaortic stenosis and if the pulmonary valve is undistorted by the previous VSD closure, we may perform a Ross/Konno procedure, i.e. placement of a pulmonary autograft in the aortic position with an anterior incision into the ventricular septum[40] (see also Chapter 18). Often it is necessary to perform the classic Konno procedure incorporating replacement of the aortic valve with a mechanical prosthesis.[41] Today there is no place for use of a left ventricular apical to descending aortic conduit although this procedure was popular in the past for complex left ventricular outflow obstruction.

DiGeorge syndrome

Absence or severe hypoplasia of the thymus was commonly seen in the Boston series with IAA but was limited to patients with type B interruption.[3] Comprehensive testing of lymphocyte function was undertaken in only a small number of patients so that no concrete inferences can be drawn regarding the incidence of the complete syndrome. Although a large calcium requirement is often seen during the early postoperative period, it is rarely necessary for children to leave hospital receiving oral calcium supplements (fortunately since these are often poorly tolerated). Occasionally vitamin D supplements are useful to maintain serum calcium levels during the first few postoperative weeks. We are not aware that serious problems with immune function have been encountered among long-term survivors of IAA surgery though it must be recognized that there were very few survivors before the early 1980s. The association of interrupted aortic arch with microdeletion of chromosome 22 has been confirmed by FISH testing. There are important implications for the developmental potential with respect to both cognitive and motor abilities of these children.[42]

Left bronchial obstruction

The left main bronchus usually passes under the arch of the aorta. If a direct anastomosis is performed without adequate mobilization, a bow string effect over the left main bronchus may result. This will cause air trapping in the left lung with hyperexpansion seen on plain chest X-ray. The diagnosis can be confirmed by bronchoscopy together with CT scan or MRI. Surgical management may entail placement of an ascending to descending aortic conduit following division of the arch though occasionally an aortopexy procedure with retrosternal suspension will suffice. With adequate initial mobilization of the ascending and descending aorta, however, this should rarely be necessary.

CONCLUSIONS

Prostaglandin E1 has revolutionized the management of IAA. Complete resuscitation should proceed over several days if necessary before surgery is undertaken. One stage primary neonatal repair with direct arch anastomosis and VSD closure is the preferred surgical approach. Although this procedure is physiologically corrective it should not be viewed as fully corrective because of the high incidence of important late left ventricular outflow tract obstruction. This may respond to a simple surgical reintervention such as subaortic resection but in some cases an extensive procedure to enlarge the left ventricular outflow tract will be necessary. However, procedures directed against subaortic stenosis should rarely be employed as part of the initial surgical management during the neonatal period.

REFERENCES

1. Van Mierop LHS. Diseases – congenital anomalies. In Netter FH (ed). *The CIBA Collection of Medical Illustrations.* Vol 5, New York, Ciba Pharmaceutical, 1969, pp 160–163.
2. Celoria GC, Patton RB. Congenital absence of the aortic arch. *Am Heart J* 1959; **48**:407.
3. Sell JE, Jonas RA, Mayer JE, Blackstone EH, Kirklin JW, Castaneda AR. The results of a surgical program for interrupted aortic arch. *J Thorac Cardiovasc Surg* 1988; **96**:864–877.
4. Jonas RA, Quaegebeur JM, Kirklin JW, Blackstone EH, Daicoff G. Outcomes in patients with interrupted aortic arch and ventricular septal defect. *J Thorac Cardiovasc Surg* 1994; **107**:1099–1109.
5. Freedom RM, Bain HH, Esplugas E, Dische R, Rowe RD. Ventricular septal defect in interruption of aortic arch. *Am J Cardiol* 1977; **39**:572–582.
6. Ho SY, Wilcox BR, Anderson RH, Lincoln JC. Interrupted aortic arch – Anatomical features of surgical significance. *Thorac Cardiovasc Surg* 1983; **31**:199–205.
7. Immagoulou A, Anderson RC, Moller JH. Interruption of the aortic arch. *Circulation* 1962; **26**:39.
8. Van Praagh R, Bernhard WF, Rosenthal A, Parisi LF, Fyler DC. Interrupted aortic arch: Surgical treatment. *Am J Cardiol* 1971; **27**:200–211.
9. Moulaert AJ, Oppenheimer-Dekker AO. Anterolateral muscle bundles of the left ventricle, bulboventricular flange, and subaortic stenosis. *Am J Cardiol* 1976; **37**:78–81.
10. Jonas RA, Sell JE, Van Praagh R et al. Left ventricular outflow obstruction associated with interrupted aortic arch and ventricular septal defect. In Crupi G, Parenzan L, Anderson RH (eds). *Perspectives in Pediatric Cardiology.* New York, Futura, 1989, pp 61–65.
11. Rudolph AM. The changes in the circulation after birth. Their importance in congenital heart disease. *Circulation* 1970; **41**:343–359.
12. Spevak PJ, Mandell VS, Colan SD et al. Reliability of Doppler color flow mapping in the identification and localization of multiple ventricular septal defects. *Echocardiography* 1993; **10**:573–581.
13. Steidele RJ. *Samml Chir u Med Beob*, Vienna 1778; **2**:114.
14. Merrill DL, Webster CA, Samson PC. Congenital absence of the aortic isthmus. *J Thorac Surg* 1957; **33**:311–320.
15. Barratt-Boyes BG, Nicholls TT, Brandt PW, Neutze JM. Aortic arch interruption associated with patent ductus arteriosus, ventricular septal defect, and total anomalous pulmonary venous connection. *J Thorac Cardiovasc Surg* 1972; **63**:367–373.
16. Trusler GA, Izukawa T. Interrupted aortic arch and ventricular septal defect. Direct repair through a median sternotomy incision in a 13-day-old infant. *J Thorac Cardiovasc Surg* 1975; **69**:126–131.
17. Elliott RB, Starling MB, Neutze JM. Medical manipulation of the ductus arteriosus. *Lancet* 1975; **1**:140–142.
18. Mainwaring RD, Lamberti JJ. Mid- to long-term results of the two-stage approach for type B interrupted aortic arch and ventricular septal defect. *Ann Thorac Surg* 1997; **64**:1782–1785.
19. Castaneda AR, Jonas RA, Mayer JE, Hanley FL. *Cardiac Surgery of the Neonate and Infant*, Philadelphia, WB Saunders, 1994, p 194.
20. Luciani GB, Starnes VA. Pulmonary autograft after repair of interrupted aortic arch, ventricular septal defect and subaortic stenosis. *J Thorac Cardiovasc Surg* 1998; **115**:266–267.
21. Yasui H, Kado H, Nakano E et al. Primary repair of interrupted aortic arch with severe aortic stenosis in neonates. *J Thorac Cardiovasc Surg* 1987; **93**:539–545.
22. Ilbawi MN, Idriss FS, Deleon SY, Muster AJ, Benson DW, Paul MH. Surgical management of patients with interrupted aortic arch and severe subaortic stenosis. *Ann Thorac Surg* 1988; **45**:174–180.
23. Wernovsky G, Mayer JE, Jonas RA et al. Factors influencing early and late outcome of the arterial switch operation for transposition of the great arteries. *J Thorac Cardiovasc Surg* 1995; **109**:289–302.
24. Liddicoat JR, Reddy VM, Hanley FL. New approach to great-vessel reconstruction in transposition complexes with interrupted aortic arch. *Ann Thorac Surg* 1994; **58**:1146–1150.
25. Jahangiri M, Zurakowski D, del Nido PJ, Mayer JE, Jonas RA. Repair of the truncal valve and associated interrupted aortic arch in neonates with truncus arteriosus. *J Thorac Cardiovasc Surg* 2000; **119**:508–514.
26. Fulton JO, Mas C, Brizard CPR, Cochrane AD, Karl TR. Does left ventricular outflow tract obstruction influence outcome of interrupted aortic arch repair. *Ann Thorac Surg* 1999; **67**:177–181.
27. Serraf A, Lacour-Gayet F, Robotin M et al. Repair of interrupted aortic arch: A ten year experience. *J Thorac Cardiovasc Surg* 1996; **112**:1150–1160.
28. Schreiber C, Eicken A, Vogt M et al. Repair of interrupted aortic arch: results after more than 20 years. *Ann Thorac Surg* 2000; **70**:1896–1899.
29. Tlaskal T, Hucin B, Hruda J et al. Results of primary and two-stage repair of interrupted aortic arch. *Eur J Cardiothorac Surg* 1998; **14**:235–242.
30. Hirooka K, Fraser CD Jr. One-stage neonatal repair of complex aortic arch obstruction or interruption. Recent experience at Texas Children's Hospital. *Tex Heart Inst J* 1997; **24**:317–321.
31. Sandhu SK, Beekman RH, Mosca RS, Bove EL. Single-stage repair of aortic arch obstruction and associated intracardiac defects in the neonate. *Am J Cardiol* 1995; **75**:370–373.
32. Aoki M, Jonas RA, Nomura F et al. Effects of aprotinin on acute recovery of cerebral metabolism in piglets after hypothermic circulatory arrest. *Ann Thorac Surg* 1994; **58**:146–153.
33. Sato S, Akiba T, Nakasato M, Suzuki H, Sato T. Percutaneous balloon aortoplasty for restenosis after extended aortic arch anastomosis for type B interrupted aortic arch. *Pediatr Cardiol* 1996; **17**:275–277.
34. Salem MM, Starnes VA, Wells WJ et al. Predictors of left ventricular outflow obstruction following single-stage repair of interrupted aortic arch and ventricular septal defect. *Am J Cardiol* 2000; **86**:1044–1047.
35. Apfel HD, Levenbraun J, Quaegebeur JM, Allan LD. Usefulness of preoperative echocardiography in predicting left ventricular outflow obstruction after primary repair of interrupted aortic arch with ventricular septal defect. *Am J Cardiol* 1998; **82**:470–473.
36. Jacobs ML, Chin AJ, Rychik J, Steven SM, Nicolson SC, Norwood WI. Interrupted aortic arch. Impact of subaortic stenosis on management and outcome. *Circulation* 1995; **92**(Suppl II): II128–131.

37. Bove EL, Minich LA, Pridijan AK et al. The management of severe subaortic stenosis, ventricular septal defect, and aortic arch obstruction in the neonate. *J Thorac Cardiovasc Surg* 1993; **105**:289–296.
38. Luciani GB, Ackerman RJ, Chang AC, Wells WJ, Starnes VA. One-stage repair of interrupted aortic arch, ventricular septal defect and subaortic obstruction in the neonate: A novel approach. *J Thorac Cardiovasc Surg* 1996; **111**:348–355.
39. Jahangiri M, Nicholson IA, del Nido PJ, Mayer JE, Jonas RA. Surgical management of complex and tunnel-like subaortic stenosis. *Eur J Cardiothorac Surg* 2000; **17**:637–642.
40. Starnes VA, Luciani GB, Wells WJ, Allen RB, Lewis AB. Aortic root replacement with the pulmonary autograft in children with complex left heart obstruction. *Ann Thorac Surg* 1996; **62**:442–448.
41. Konno S, Imai Y, Lida Y et al. A new method for prosthetic valve replacement in congenital aortic stenosis associated with hypoplasia of the aortic valve ring. *J Thorac Cardiovasc Surg* 1975; **70**:909.
42. Rauch A, Hofbeck M, Leipold G et al. Incidence and significance of 22q11.2 hemizygosity in patients with interrupted aortic arch. *Am J Med Genet* 1998; **78**:322–331.

28

Congenitally corrected transposition of the great arteries

INTRODUCTION

Congenitally corrected transposition of the great arteries is very much rarer than dextro (d-) transposition representing only 0.7% of all congenital anomalies.[1] It is unique in that the circulation is physiologically normal with no shunts, no pressure load and no cyanosis. Early in life, in the absence of associated anomalies, there are usually no symptoms. However, the right ventricle and tricuspid valve must function at systemic pressure and ultimately can fail. Frequently, however, associated anomalies are present including abnormalities of atrioventricular conduction, pulmonary valvar and subvalvar stenosis, a large conoventricular or inlet VSD and often an Ebstein-like malformation of the tricuspid valve. Dextrocardia is also present in approximately 25%. Corrected transposition is a common form of single ventricle in which the left sided right ventricle is hypoplastic and often little more than an infundibular outflow chamber. This form of corrected transposition is discussed in Chapter 20. The past decade has seen important changes which are discussed below in the surgical strategy for management of biventricular congenitally corrected transposition.

EMBRYOLOGY

During normal cardiac development the primitive cardiac tube loops to the right such that the morphological left ventricle comes to lie leftward and posterior while the morphological right ventricle is rightward and anterior. If the cardiac tube loops to the left rather than to the right (i.e. l-loop rather than d-loop) the ventricles will be laterally inverted, i.e. they will be mirror-images of normal ventricles and their location also is inverted relative to the usual. If there is also malseptation of the conotruncus, the aorta will arise from the morphological right ventricle and the pulmonary artery from the left ventricle. Assuming there is situs solitus (i.e. normal position of the atria), systemic venous blood will flow through the right atrium into the mitral valve (atrioventricular discordance) and is pumped by the morphological left ventricle to the lungs. Pulmonary venous blood returns to the left atrium and passes through the tricuspid valve to the (systemic) right ventricle to be pumped to the body.

ANATOMY OF CORRECTED TRANSPOSITION

There are two forms of corrected transposition, S,L,L and I,D,D depending on whether situs is normal (solitus, S) or inverted (inversus, I). The solitus form is much more common than the inversus form.[2] The ventricles carry their usual inlet valve to their inverted location as well as their usual coronary artery distribution.[3] The ventricles should be described according to their underlying morphology rather than their location though it is helpful to confirm that this convention is being followed by specifying 'morphological right or left ventricle' or if necessary 'right or left sided ventricle'. It is important to understand that these ventricles are indeed mirror images of the usual in the same way that the left hand is a mirror image of the right hand. In fact the Van Praagh's have developed a useful method using the hands to help distinguish an l-loop heart from a d-loop heart which is particularly helpful in hearts with complex anatomy and positioning.

Associated anomalies

VENTRICULAR SEPTAL DEFECT

Approximately 80% of hearts with corrected transposition have an associated VSD.[4] It is usually not a perimembranous defect but rather a large, nonrestrictive conoventricular defect. There may be some malalignment of the conal septum towards the right sided left ventricle which may contribute to subpulmonary stenosis.[5] Not uncommonly the VSD extends somewhat under the septal leaflet into the inlet septum. There may be associated multiple muscular VSDs though these are rare.

LEFT VENTRICULAR OUTFLOW OBSTRUCTION (PULMONARY AND SUBPULMONARY STENOSIS)

Hemodynamically important obstruction to pulmonary blood flow is present in at least 25% of patients with corrected transposition[6] and perhaps as many as 40%.[7] It occurs both as an isolated associated anomaly as well as in association with a VSD. The mechanism of obstruction is often multifactorial including pulmonary valvar stenosis (bicuspid pulmonary valve), pulmonary annular hypoplasia and subpulmonary stenosis. The mechanism of the subpulmonary stenosis itself also can be multi-factorial including accessory atrioventricular valve tissue (usually mitral though occasionally tricuspid prolapsing through the VSD), membranous subpulmonary stenosis and tunnel subpulmonary stenosis due to a long subpulmonary conus with malalignment of the conal septum.[8–10]

EBSTEIN-LIKE LEFT ATRIOVENTRICULAR VALVE

The tricuspid valve becomes incompetent over time in up to 30% of patients with corrected transposition. While the valve is often described as being Ebstein-like, it is rare to see a severe degree of spiral displacement of the septal leaflet, enlargement of the anterior leaflet or atrialization of the right ventricle as is seen with true Ebstein's anomaly.[11]

CONDUCTION SYSTEM

Since the right atrium must connect with the left ventricle when there is situs solitus and an l-loop (i.e. atrioventricular discordance), it is not surprising that the conduction system is abnormal. Pioneering work in this area was undertaken by Anderson and colleagues.[12,13] In (S,L,L) corrected transposition (C-TGA), the functional atrioventricular node arises anteriorly and superiorly and is usually lodged between the annulus of the mitral valve and the superior and anterior aspect of the limbus of the fossa ovalis. This functional AV node is therefore superior to the usual location of the AV node which may be present as an accessory node. After penetrating the fibrous trigone that is present at the point of mitral to pulmonary fibrous continuity, the elongated, nonbranching portion of the atrioventricular bundle traverses the anterior wall of the morphologic left ventricular outflow tract just over the pulmonary valve annulus and remaining on the left ventricular aspect of the septum (Figure 28.1a). It then continues subendocardially to descend still within the left side of the ventricular septum, where it trifurcates into the left anterior, left posterior, and right bundle branches. When there is a conoventricular ventricular septal defect, the proximal conduction system is in close proximity to its anterosuperior and anteroinferior borders, unlike the usual relationship in (S,D,S) hearts, in which the proximal conduction system travels along the posteroinferior margin of the septal defect. Often there is a posterior atrioventricular node in its usual position within the triangle of Koch, but it is usually disconnected from the remainder of the conduction tissue. In contrast when there is situs inversus, i.e. (I,D,D) C-TGA hearts, the atrioventricular bundle arises from the posterior atrioventricular node to follow a conventional path along the posteroinferior margin of the ventricular septal defect if one is present.[14–16]

The conduction system in C-TGA is more tenuous than that of normal hearts. Fibrosis of the junction between the atrioventricular node and the atrioventricular bundle has been seen in older patients with spontaneously occurring complete heart block in patients with this anomaly[13] and there may be congenital absence of connection between the AV node and bundle of His.[17]

PATHOPHYSIOLOGY AND CLINICAL FEATURES

As the name 'corrected transposition' implies, the physiology of SLL transposition is normal. In the absence of associated anomalies there are no abnormal shunts, no pressure load and no cyanosis. Therefore there is no murmur, no symptoms of congestive heart failure and no cyanosis is detectable and the condition is likely to be undetected for decades. Several reports have suggested that only 1–2% of patients have absolutely no associated anomalies.[4,6,18] It still remains unclear what percentage of these patients will become symptomatic in later life and if so when. Although some patients do present in middle age with failure of the systemic right ventricle, there are many case reports where SLL transposition has been found as an incidental finding following death in the seventh, eighth or ninth decade.[19]

The most common symptom in the patient with corrected transposition is cyanosis because of associated LV outflow obstruction and VSD. It is probable that LV outflow obstruction progresses over time because most neonates and young infants do not have sufficiently severe cyanosis to mandate surgery in the first year of life. Interestingly it is also unusual for the patient with an isolated VSD as the only associated anomaly to present with uncontrollable heart failure in the first year of life despite the usual unrestrictive nature of the VSD. It may be that there is sufficient mild functional subpulmonary stenosis secondary to ventricular septal shift so that pulmonary blood flow and pressure are not sufficiently increased to cause symptoms.

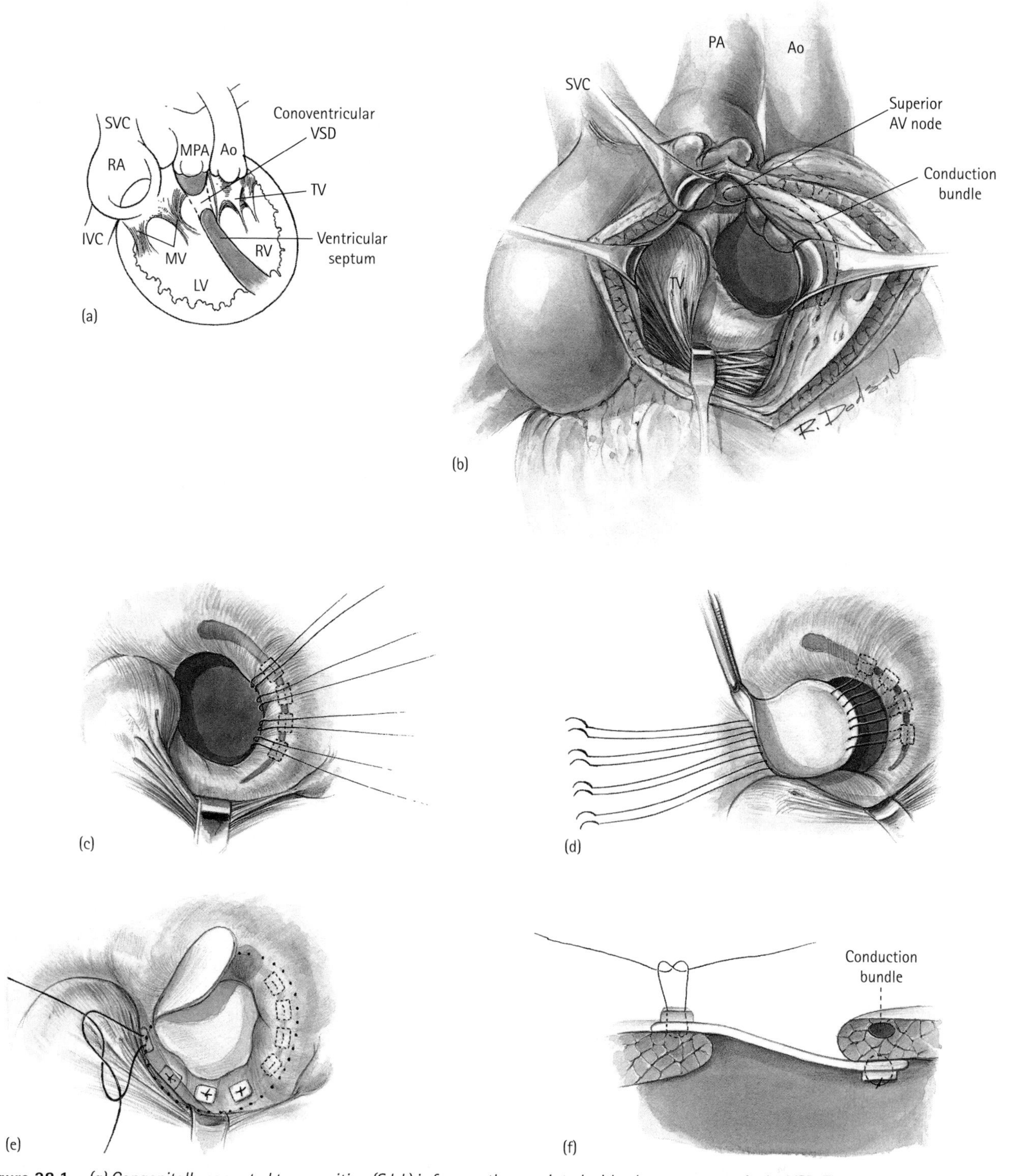

Figure 28.1 *(a) Congenitally corrected transposition (S,L,L) is frequently associated with a large conoventricular VSD. The aorta arises anteriorly and to the left of the main pulmonary artery from the morphological right ventricle while the pulmonary artery arises from the right sided morphological left ventricle. (b) Exposure of the conoventricular VSD through an incision in the morphological left ventricle as depicted here should rarely if ever be employed. The aortic valve can be seen through the large conoventricular VSD. The mitral valve in the morphological left ventricle is seen. The conduction bundle arises from an AV node which lies more superiorly than the usual location of the AV node. The conduction bundle runs on the right side of the ventricular septum, i.e. on the morphological left ventricular side. (c) The traditional surgical management of the VSD in corrected transposition involves placement of sutures on the morphological right ventricular aspect of the septum to reduce the risk of injury to the bundle of His. (d) The pledgetted VSD sutures are passed through the VSD patch. (e) One of the serious disadvantages of traditional management of corrected transposition was that sutures lie close to the left sided tricuspid valve unless they are transitioned to the right side of the septum. (f) The VSD patch lies partially on the morphological right ventricular aspect of the septum and partially on the left ventricular aspect.*

DIAGNOSTIC STUDIES

The diagnosis of corrected transposition is not uncommonly first suspected on the basis of an abnormal chest X-ray. Dextrocardia is present in 25%[20] and mesocardia is also common. Even if there is levocardia the leftward and anterior location of the aorta creates an abnormal cardiac silhouette. A chest X-ray may also demonstrate evidence of reduced or increased pulmonary blood flow according to the presence of associated anomalies.

The definitive diagnosis of corrected transposition is made by two-dimensional echocardiography. Careful assessment must be made of the size and location of the VSD, the severity and nature of any left ventricular outflow tract obstruction and the morphology and function of the left sided tricuspid valve. Right ventricular function should also be assessed. Real-time 3D-echocardiography is emerging as a useful modality in planning biventricular repair of corrected transposition. It is particularly helpful in assessing complex left ventricular outflow tract obstruction as well as the feasibility of baffling difficult VSDs (e.g. with inlet extension) to the aorta as part of a Senning/Rastelli repair. Cardiac magnetic resonance imaging is also useful in assessing these issues but has the disadvantage that general anesthesia is required.

Cardiac catheterization is usually not indicated except in the older child in whom there is concern that pulmonary vascular disease may be present.

MEDICAL AND INTERVENTIONAL THERAPY

Standard decongestive therapy with digoxin and diuretics is used for heart failure in the setting of a VSD with minimal LV outflow obstruction. It might be possible to delay surgery in the child with excessive cyanosis by balloon dilation or stenting of the outflow tract but in general we prefer to proceed with surgical repair.

INDICATIONS FOR AND TIMING OF SURGERY

The patient with symptoms

Surgery is indicated for the child who has an unacceptable degree of cyanosis or whose congestive heart failure cannot be controlled with medical therapy. If a child is suitable for a true double switch procedure, i.e. atrial plus arterial switch, there is little point in deferring surgery beyond early infancy. However, if there is LV outflow obstruction and a conduit will be necessary as part of an atrial switch plus Rastelli procedure, it is not unreasonable to defer surgery until the child is older and larger, though care must be taken that the child is not developing pulmonary vascular disease because of excessive pulmonary flow and pressure. If the VSD is unrestrictive it is probably advisable to perform surgery by 12 months of age and earlier than this if symptoms are not easily controlled with medical therapy.

In some children it is unclear if a two ventricle repair will be possible for one of several reasons. The VSD may be an inlet VSD associated with LV outflow obstruction. It may not be possible to baffle the LV to the aorta as part of an atrial switch/Rastelli. Under these circumstances it is wise to perform a modified Blalock shunt on the side of the dominant SVC. The presence of dextrocardia may also complicate an atrial switch/Rastelli because of difficulty placing a homograft conduit in a location where it will not be compressed by the sternum. This is also influenced by the exact anatomy of the coronary arteries on the surface of the right ventricle which will influence the location of the ventriculotomy. Once again a shunt is a reasonable option that does not exclude the possibility of a two ventricle repair at a later time.

The asymptomatic patient

It will be several decades before there is adequate information regarding the indications for surgery in the child who is found to have corrected transposition but who has no associated anomalies and therefore no symptoms. The probability of the right ventricle failing at systemic pressure in early middle age remains to be determined. Also the long-term results of the double switch and switch-Rastelli must be carefully analysed. At present, however, it would seem reasonable to proceed in the asymptomatic patient who has documented evidence of deteriorating right ventricular function with RV dilation and especially if there is associated tricuspid regurgitation or at least morphological abnormalities of the tricuspid valve.

SURGICAL MANAGEMENT

History of surgery

Von Rokitansky first described corrected transposition in 1875.[21] After Monckeberg's description in 1913[22] of the anteriorly positioned atrioventricular node, the next most surgically relevant report on C-TGA came in 1957 when Anderson and colleagues described the clinical, radiologic, electrocardiographic, and cardiac catheterization features of this syndrome and reviewed their surgical experience with 10 patients with C-TGA.[23] They suggested, among other things, closure of the ventricular septal defect through the right atrium and mitral valve. De Leval et al added the important technical innovation of suturing on the morphological right ventricular side of the septum in order to reduce the risk of damaging the conduction tissue during closure of the ventricular septal defect.[24] Although isolated reports of the differences in the conduction system in patients with (SLL) C-TGA had been published before, much is owed to Lev et al[25] and Anderson[13] and their colleagues, who substantiated and carefully documented the position of the anteriorly located atrioventricular node and the anterosuperior trajectory of the conduction bundle. Later, Dick and associates, through intraoperative mapping, further outlined the anatomy of the conduction system in cases of (IDD) C-TGA.[14]

In 1990 Ilbawi and associates described a conceptually new approach to the management of corrected transposition.[26] This was driven by the disappointing results of the traditional management, i.e. VSD closure and if necessary placement of a conduit from the left ventricle to the pulmonary arteries[27] (see also 'Results of surgery' below). Furthermore by this time it had become clear that the arterial switch could be performed at low risk as could the Senning or Mustard procedure and Rastelli procedure. Ilbawi suggested that these procedures be combined thereby both anatomically and physiologically correcting the anomaly.

Technical considerations

TRADITIONAL SURGICAL MANAGEMENT

The traditional surgical approach to corrected transposition should rarely if ever be used today. Although methods have been developed which can reduce the probability of complete heart block they suffer from the fundamental limitation that a VSD patch must be placed close to the systemic (tricuspid) atrioventricular valve. Furthermore, the systemic morphological right ventricle must assume a spherical shape on cross section which results in the chordal attachments of the tricuspid valve to the ventricular septum tending to interfere with tricuspid competence. The combination of distortion by the VSD patch and septal chord traction is likely to result in early systemic atrioventricular valve regurgitation with subsequent right ventricle dilation and failure. This problem is further exacerbated if complete heart block occurs either spontaneously or following surgery. The child is likely then to require frequent reoperations for pacemaker revision, tricuspid valve replacement and conduit replacement if there is important subpulmonary stenosis. Ultimately this leads to need for heart transplantation. Nevertheless these procedures will be described for completeness sake.

Simple VSD closure

It is critically important to understand that the main conduction bundle lies on the morphological left ventricular aspect of the ventricular septum (Figure 28.1b). An approach described by de Leval et al[24] involves a right atriotomy and exposure of the VSD through the right sided mitral valve. The VSD sutures are carefully placed on the morphological right ventricular aspect of the VSD margins (Figure 28.1c–f). As one passes clockwise around the circumference of the VSD and approaches the posterior and inferior corner there may be tricuspid valve tissue immediately adjacent to the VSD margin. Although in theory one should be able to at this point begin to place sutures on the morphological left ventricular aspect of the septum in our experience this resulted in a high probability of complete heart block. It is equally undesirable to place sutures within the tricuspid valve tissue itself because of the potential for distortion of the tricuspid valve by fibrosis in this area (Figure 28.1e). A preferable approach to the right atrial approach is the transaortic approach to VSD closure. Using continuous cardiopulmonary bypass with bicaval cannulation, cross clamping and cardioplegic arrest the large ascending aorta is opened with a transverse incision a few millimeters distal to the aortic valve. Working through the aortic valve, sutures are conveniently placed on the morphological right ventricular aspect of the ventricular septal defect margin. This approach allows much more accurate placement of sutures since the appropriate side of the septum is viewed directly. In our experience the incidence of complete heart block was reduced with this approach relative to a trans-mitral valve approach. On the other hand there is a risk of distortion of the aortic valve which can lead to later aortic regurgitation. It is important to avoid a morphological right ventricular incision. A morphological left ventricular incision does not provide any advantage over a trans-right atrial/trans-mitral valve approach.

VSD closure, LV to PA conduit

When there is important morphological left ventricular outflow tract obstruction it is necessary to place a conduit from the left ventricle to the pulmonary arteries because of the presence of the right sided coronary artery in the right sided atrioventricular groove which contraindicates placement of a transannular patch. It remains unclear what degree of obstruction necessitates conduit placement since it can be argued that the left ventricle is designed to function at systemic pressure. Certainly a higher level of pulmonary ventricular hypertension can be tolerated in this setting than for a normal right ventricle. Using continuous cardiopulmonary bypass, bicaval cannulation, aortic cross clamping and cardioplegic arrest an incision is made in the anterior surface of the morphological left ventricle towards the atrioventricular groove. Although it is possible to close the VSD working through the left ventriculotomy it was our preference in the past when we used this strategy to close the defect transaortically as described above. An appropriate sized cryopreserved homograft is thawed and cut to length. The distal anastomosis is fashioned to the pulmonary bifurcation area leaving the main pulmonary artery intact. Thus, the left ventricle will have a double outlet, i.e. through the native left ventricular outflow tract as well as through the homograft conduit. The proximal homograft is sutured to the left ventriculotomy supplemented with a hood of glutaraldehyde treated autologous pericardium or PTFE. Prior to completion of this suture line the systemic ventricle is allowed to fill with blood and air is vented through the cardioplegia site. The aortic cross clamp is released with the cardioplegia site bleeding freely. During rewarming the usual monitoring lines are placed, i.e. a left atrial line through the right superior pulmonary vein as well as a pulmonary artery line inserted through a stab in the left ventricle into the homograft conduit.

Pacing wires

It is advisable to place a permanent ventricular pacing wire at the time of surgery even if the patient is in sinus rhythm after removing the aortic cross clamp. It is also important to place two temporary atrial and two temporary ventricular pacing wires in the routine fashion.

DOUBLE SWITCH PROCEDURE

This is the procedure of choice for the child who has only functional left ventricular outflow tract obstruction or a mild degree of fixed left ventricular outflow tract obstruction or no left ventricular outflow tract obstruction. It is important to be sure that the left ventricle has been exposed to a sufficiently high pressure that it will be able to take over acutely at systemic pressure. Generally this will be the case if a VSD is present since the VSD is almost always unrestrictive. However, if left ventricular pressure has been less than approximately two thirds right ventricular pressure a preliminary banding procedure is necessary to prepare the left ventricle as described in the section regarding 'rapid two stage arterial switch' for d-transposition of the great arteries (see Chapter 15). The double switch procedure is a technically demanding procedure that requires a long cross-clamp time that in many surgeons hands will approach 2.5 hours. Thus very careful attention to myocardial protection is necessary. Cardioplegia should be reinfused every 20–30 minutes. It is probably advisable to use deep hypothermia since periods of circulatory arrest may be necessary. Deep hypothermia will also help to supplement the myocardial protection afforded by cardioplegia.

Cannulation

A metal tip right angle venous cannula is placed in the left innominate vein or high in the superior vena cava. A second right angle venous cannula is placed as low in the inferior vena cava as possible. The ascending aorta is cannulated as far distally as possible. A vent is inserted through the right atrial appendage. Frequently a stretched foramen ovale or secundum ASD will be present so that the right atrial vent will allow drainage of the left heart. If necessary the tip of the vent can be directed through the mitral valve to drain both ventricles.

Senning procedure

An incision is made in the right atrial free wall as shown in Figure 28.2a. The right atrial tissue posterior to this incision will become the anterior wall of the systemic venous baffle. The atrial septum when present is developed as a flap by incising the three sides other than the right side where the septum meets the right atrial free wall (Figure 28.2b). A vertical incision is made in the left atrium immediately posterior to the right side of the atrial septum and just anterior to the right pulmonary veins (Figure 28.2a).

The posterior wall of the systemic venous baffle is now fashioned using either the atrial septum alone, the atrial septum supplemented with a small patch of pericardium or with pericardium alone (Figure 28.2d). The suture line is begun anterior to the left sided pulmonary veins and posterior to the left atrial appendage. As the suture line passes posterior to the SVC and IVC orifices great care should be taken to avoid purse-stringing the caval orifices. The anterior wall of the systemic venous baffle is now completed by suturing the appropriate segment of right atrial free wall to the edge of the excised atrial septum between the mitral and tricuspid valves (Figure 28.2f). If there is dextrocardia which is often associated with small size of the right atrium it may be necessary to supplement the anterior as well as the posterior wall of the systemic venous baffle with a patch of autologous pericardium. However, it is important that the systemic baffle not be too large. Ideally it should have a waist centrally so that pulmonary venous return from the left pulmonary veins will be able to pass around the baffle to the tricuspid valve. The pulmonary venous atrium is completed by suturing the anterior component of the original right atrial free wall either directly to the pulmonary veins or more commonly to a pericardial flap (Figure 28.2g, h) or to the pericardium in situ.[28] It is necessary that the pericardial reflection around the inferior vena cava be intact if the pericardium in situ technique is used. The pericardium in situ technique for completing the pulmonary venous atrium is similar to the technique described by Lacour Gayet and others for dealing with pulmonary vein stenosis.[29,30]

It is particularly important as the suture line is brought across the superior vena cava that the suture line is kept superior to the area of the sinus node and the sinus node artery. In addition, great care should be taken to avoid purse-stringing the superior vena cava by taking wider bites on the atrial free wall than on the SVC (see Chapter 2).

Arterial switch procedure and VSD closure

The left atrial vent should be left in the original right atrial appendage and continues to drain left heart return through the remainder of the procedure. The coronary sinus now drains to the pulmonary venous atrium so that the vent will also remove cardioplegia effluent during the remainder of the procedure. The ascending aorta is divided at its midpoint opposite the pulmonary bifurcation as for a standard arterial switch procedure. The coronary buttons are developed in the usual fashion (Figure 28.3a). When the coronary buttons have been excised the aortic root can be splayed open to allow access for VSD closure. The VSD should be closed working through the left sided semilunar valve (neopulmonary valve) with care taken to keep the sutures on the morphological right ventricular aspect of the septum as described above. However, because the tricuspid valve will function at pulmonary pressure there need be no concern if it is necessary to place sutures within tricuspid tissue to anchor the patch in the posterior and inferior corner of the VSD. Although the conduction bundle is described as running anteriorly and superiorly our experience suggests that great care should be taken to avoid placing sutures in the

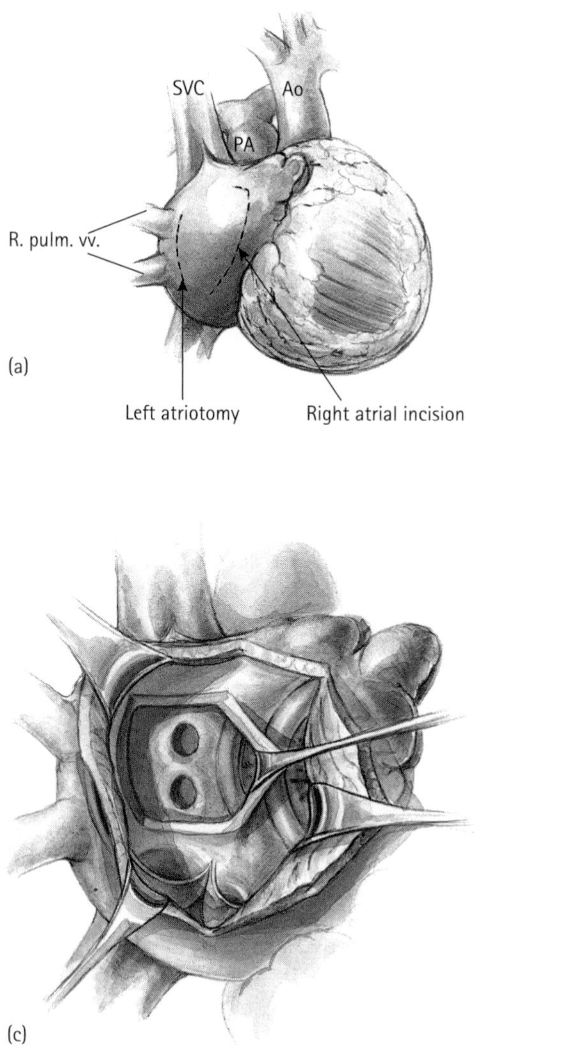

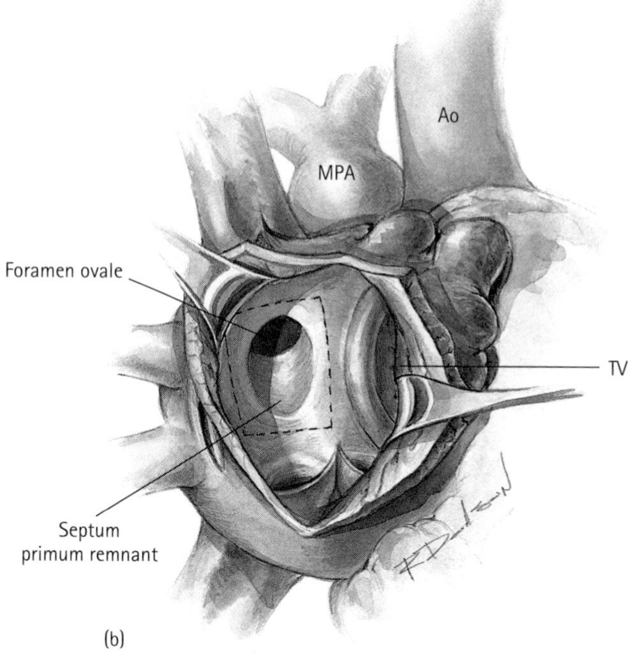

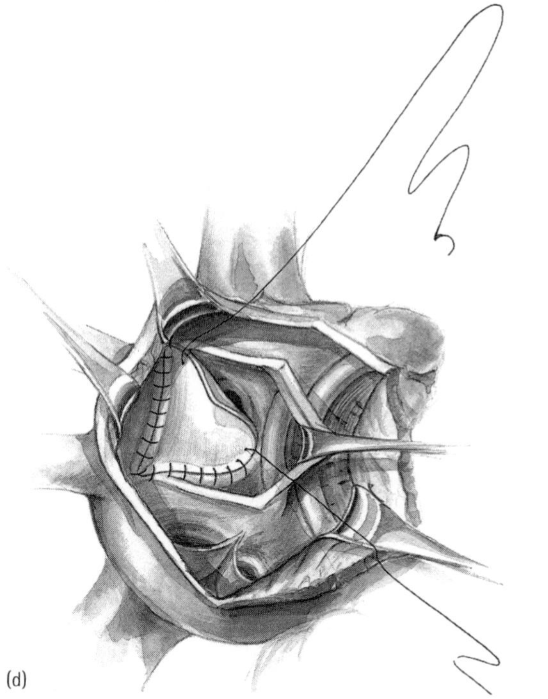

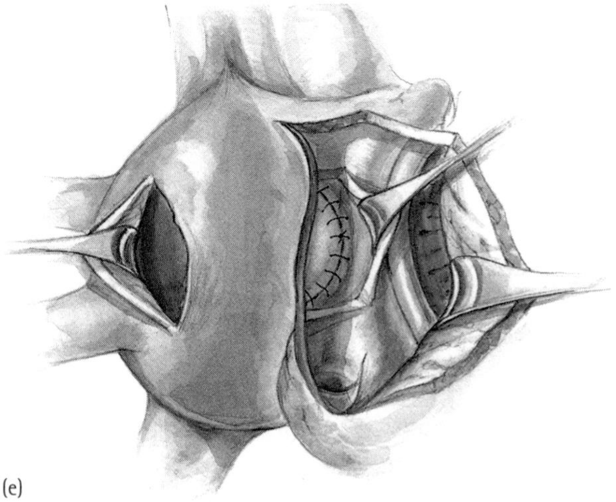

Figure 28.2a–e *Senning procedure as a component of the double switch for congenitally corrected transposition. (a) Incisions in the right atrium and left atrium. (b) The atrial septum when not well developed is totally excised. Alternatively it may be developed as a flap by incising the three sides other than the right side where the septum meets the right atrial free wall. (c) The atrial septum has been totally excised. (d) The posterior wall of the systemic venous baffle in this case is developed with a patch of pericardium and sutured anterior to the left sided pulmonary veins and posterior to the left atrial appendage. (e) The incision anterior to the right pulmonary veins has been made.*

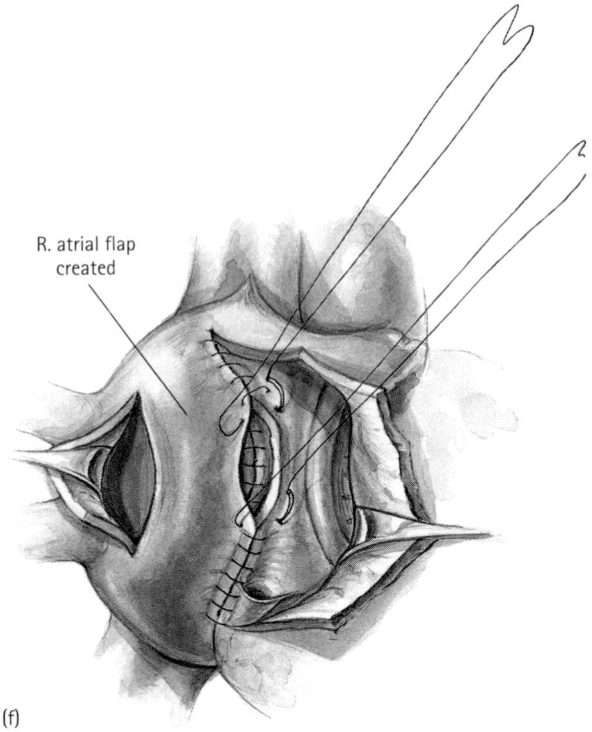

(f)

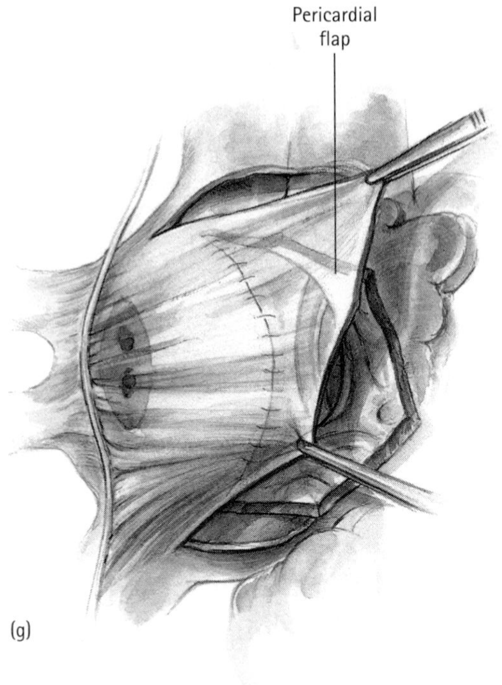

(g)

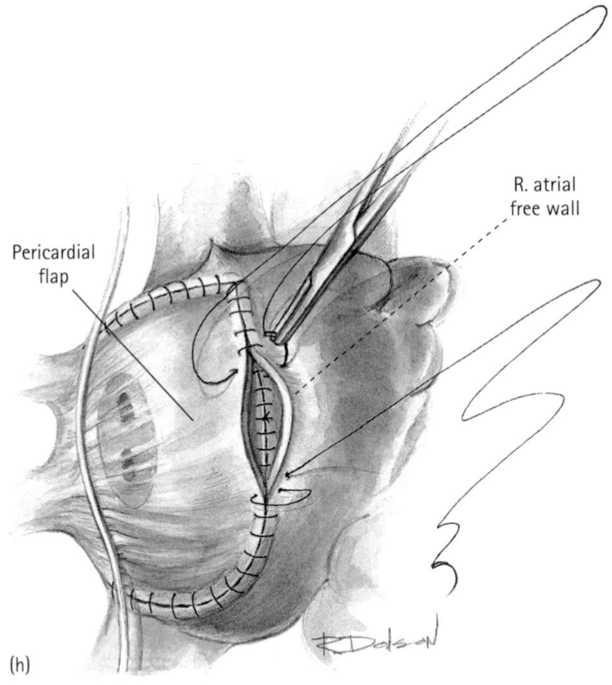

(h)

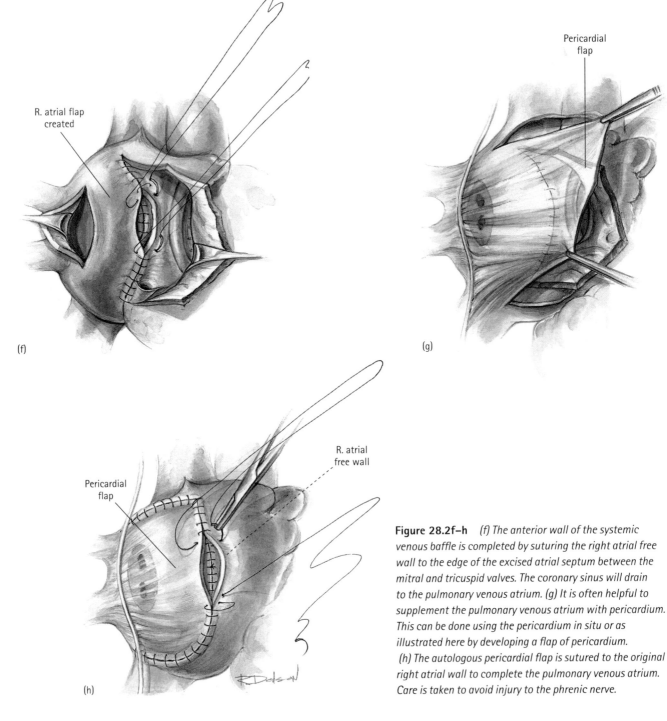

Figure 28.2f–h *(f) The anterior wall of the systemic venous baffle is completed by suturing the right atrial free wall to the edge of the excised atrial septum between the mitral and tricuspid valves. The coronary sinus will drain to the pulmonary venous atrium. (g) It is often helpful to supplement the pulmonary venous atrium with pericardium. This can be done using the pericardium in situ or as illustrated here by developing a flap of pericardium. (h) The autologous pericardial flap is sutured to the original right atrial wall to complete the pulmonary venous atrium. Care is taken to avoid injury to the phrenic nerve.*

ventricular septum in the posterior and inferior corner as for VSD closure with a standard d-loop. Upon completion of VSD closure the main pulmonary artery is divided proximal to its bifurcation. A Lecompte maneuver is performed bringing the pulmonary bifurcation anterior to the ascending aorta. The coronary arteries are reimplanted into the neoaorta at the sites which were carefully marked at the onset of the procedure as previously described for the arterial switch procedure for d-transposition (see Chapter 15). Accurate marking sutures for coronary transfer are a critically important part of this procedure as they are for an isolated arterial switch procedure. The aortic anastomosis is fashioned using continuous polypropylene suture. The coronary donor areas in the neopulmonary artery are filled with a single bifurcated patch of autologous pericardium using continuous 6/0 Prolene. At this stage the left heart is allowed to fill with blood and air is vented through a small vent site created in the ascending aorta. The aortic cross clamp is released with this vent site bleeding freely. Satisfactory perfusion of all areas should be noted confirming the accuracy of the coronary

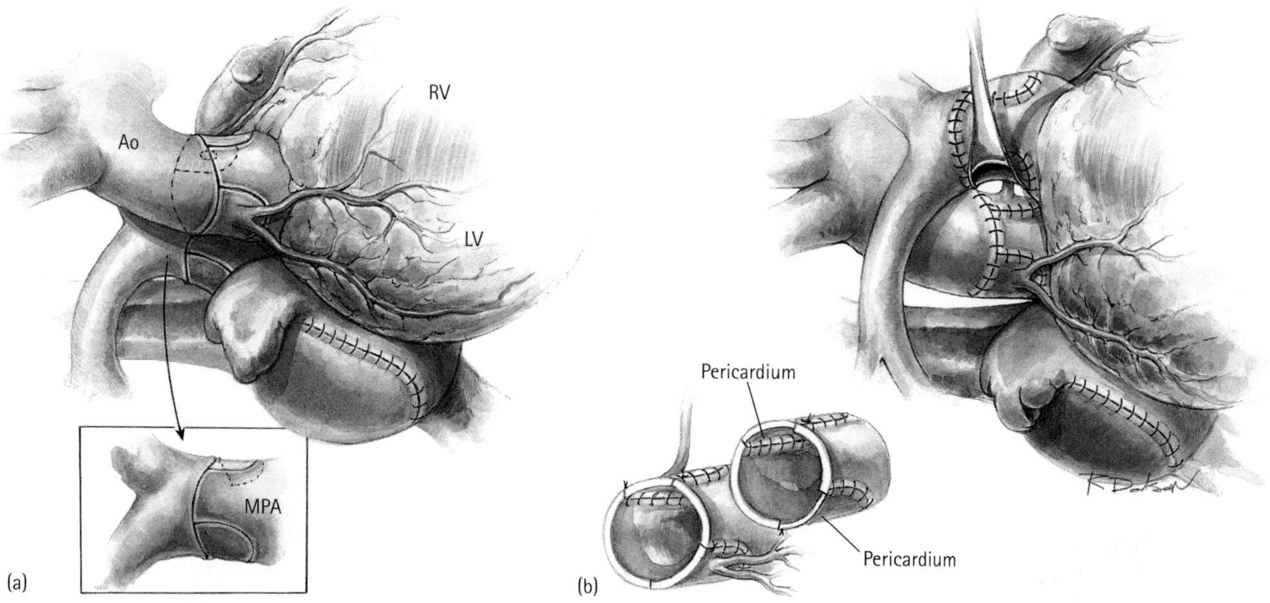

Figure 28.3 *Arterial switch procedure for congenitally corrected transposition as one component of the double switch procedure. (a) The ascending aorta is divided at its midpoint opposite the pulmonary bifurcation. The coronary buttons are developed in the usual fashion. Inset: appropriate U shaped areas of tissue are excised from the proximal main pulmonary artery for implantation of the coronary buttons. It is essential that marking sutures be placed before bypass is established in order to identify the sites for reimplantation of the coronary arteries. (b) A Lecompte maneuver has been performed and the pulmonary anastomosis has been completed. Inset demonstrates that the coronary donor areas are closed with autologous pericardium.*

transfer. During warming the pulmonary anastomosis is fashioned using continuous 6/0 Prolene. The left atrial vent is replaced in the original right atrial appendage with a monitoring catheter. Two atrial and two ventricular pacing wires should be placed. Consideration should be given to placement of a permanent ventricular pacing wire though in view of the duration and complexity of the procedure we generally avoid this if a child appears to be in stable sinus rhythm. A pulmonary artery monitoring line is inserted through the morphological right ventricle. With rewarming completed the child should wean from bypass with low to moderate dose dopamine support. Transesophageal echocardiography is useful to exclude baffle pathway obstruction, great vessel anastomotic obstruction or regional wall motion abnormalities secondary to a coronary transfer problem. Monitoring catheters including a central venous catheter are useful in particular to exclude the possibility of a gradient across the superior vena cava.

MUSTARD PROCEDURE

A number of factors may dictate that a patient is not suitable for a Senning procedure in which case a Mustard procedure must be performed. There may be adhesions from previous palliative procedures which render the atrial wall unsuitable for a Senning procedure. Patients with dextrocardia frequently have a poorly developed right atrium, particularly if there is associated left juxtaposition of the right atrial appendage. Thus there may be inadequate right atrial free wall to perform the Senning procedure. The atrial septal remnants are completely excised (Figure 28.4b). A baffle of autologous pericardium is sutured into the atria as shown in Figure 28.4c. The suture line runs anterior to the left pulmonary veins, around both the superior vena and inferior vena cava before completion to the atrial septal remnant (Figure 28.4c).

ATRIAL SWITCH/RASTELLI

The presence of important fixed left ventricular outflow tract obstruction contraindicates a double switch procedure. However, it is still possible to perform an 'anatomical' correction so long as left ventricular outflow can be baffled through the VSD to the aorta. It is not uncommon that at least two anatomical factors will increase the difficulty of an atrial switch/Rastelli so that a fallback option must be carefully planned. This fallback option will almost always be a Fontan procedure which we consider to be preferable to the traditional surgical management described above. Thus care must be taken in sequencing the procedure that the Fontan option is prepared for both preoperatively and in the early intraoperative steps. In particular a ventriculotomy should be avoided until it is clear that a biventricular approach will be used. Preoperatively, cardiac catheterization should be undertaken to assess suitability for a Fontan procedure with particular attention to measurement of pulmonary resistance, distortion of the pulmonary arteries and ventricular compliance.

The factors which may preclude an atrial switch/Rastelli are firstly the location of the VSD in the inlet septum, particularly if there are multiple tricuspid chords across the VSD.

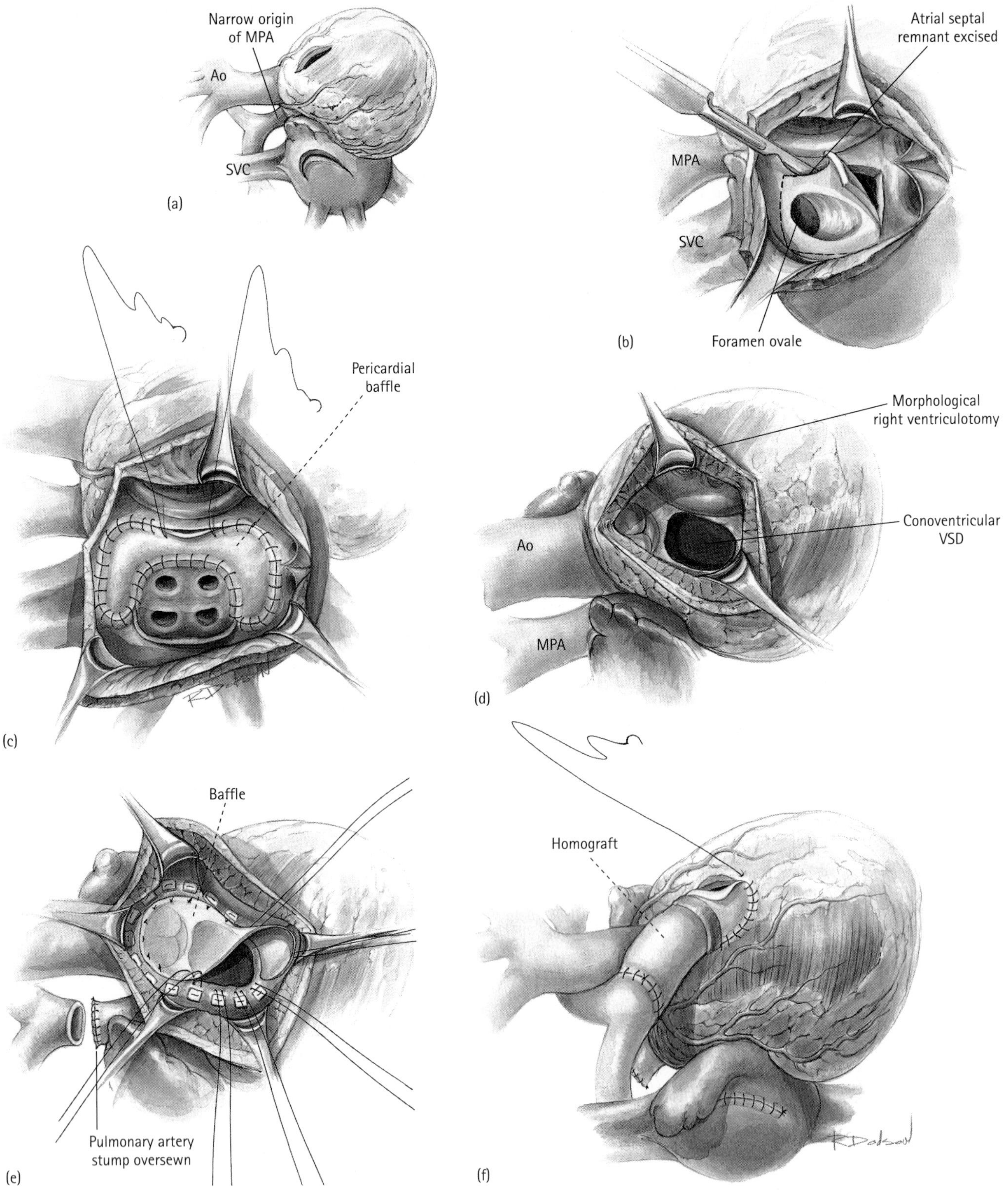

Figure 28.4 *Mustard plus Rastelli procedure for corrected transposition with VSD and pulmonary stenosis. (a) The atrial incision for the Mustard procedure is shown. A vertical incision is made in the infundibulum of the left sided morphological right ventricle for the Rastelli component. This ventriculotomy will allow VSD closure on the right ventricular aspect of the septum and is also used for the proximal conduit anastomosis. (b) The Mustard procedure requires complete excision of any atrial septal remnants. (c) An autologous pericardial baffle is sutured into the atria so as to direct IVC and SVC blood through the left sided tricuspid valve. (d) The conoventricular VSD is exposed through an infundibular incision in the morphological right ventricle. The length of the ventriculotomy has been exaggerated in this figure to allow complete visualization of the VSD. (e) Working through the right ventriculotomy VSD sutures are placed in the right ventricular aspect of the ventricular septum. The baffle will direct left ventricular blood to the aorta. (f) A homograft conduit is anastomosed between the distal divided main pulmonary artery and the right ventriculotomy. The proximal anastomosis is supplemented with a hood of autologous pericardium. The proximal divided main pulmonary artery has been oversewn.*

The other common factor is the presence of dextrocardia with associated underdevelopment of the right atrium. The latter will increase the difficulty of achieving a satisfactory Senning procedure while dextrocardia per se will often place a right ventricle to pulmonary artery conduit in an immediate retrosternal location where it is at risk of sternal compression.

Cannulation should be undertaken as described for the double switch procedure, preferably with the upper venous cannula in the left innominate vein. Following establishment of cardiopulmonary bypass, cooling to deep hypothermia, application of the aortic cross clamp and infusion of cardioplegia solution, an incision is made in the right atrial free wall that is suitable for a Senning procedure but which also would allow construction of a lateral tunnel Fontan baffle. Working through the right sided mitral valve the anatomy of the VSD is carefully examined. A decision must be made at this point regarding the suitability of the VSD for baffling to the aorta. It is unwise to make an incision in the morphological right ventricle and then subsequently to choose the Fontan option since the morphological right ventricle will function with the left ventricle at systemic pressure as a systemic ventricle if the Fontan option is selected. Assuming that a decision has been made that the conoventricular VSD is suitable for baffling to the aorta, a vertical incision is made in the morphological right ventricular free wall towards the base, i.e. in the infundibulum (Figure 28.4d). The site for the ventriculotomy should be carefully selected to minimize injury to the coronary arteries and to avoid injury to the anterior papillary muscle of the tricuspid valve. Working through the right ventriculotomy VSD sutures are placed which will baffle the left ventricle to the aorta (Figure 28.4e). A Dacron baffle is usually satisfactory through consideration may be given to using autologous pericardium treated with glutaraldehyde. The Senning or Mustard component of the procedure is now undertaken. An appropriate cryopreserved homograft is then thawed and cut to length. The proximal main pulmonary artery is divided, the pulmonary valve is excised and the proximal main pulmonary artery is oversewn. The distal end of the homograft is anastomosed to the distal divided main pulmonary artery (Figure 28.4f). The homograft may more appropriately lie to the right side of the ascending aorta when there is even a relatively mild degree of dextrocardia or mesocardia. However, ideally the homograft will be routed to the left of the left sided ascending aorta because this will allow it to lie well away from the sternum. It is often useful to perform the anastomosis with the homograft temporarily lying to the right side of the ascending aorta. It is then passed behind the aorta and the proximal anastomosis of the homograft to the right ventriculotomy is fashioned. Under these circumstances, mobilization of the right pulmonary artery into the hilum is useful. The proximal anastomosis of the homograft should be near to complete before the left heart is allowed to fill with blood and air is vented through the cardioplegia site. The aortic cross clamp is released with the cardioplegia site bleeding freely. When cardiac action is regained the proximal homograft anastomosis may be completed having previously served the function of venting systemic venous return that was not picked up by the cannulas. The pulmonary venous vent is also removed and replaced with a left atrial monitoring catheter. A pulmonary artery monitoring catheter is inserted into the conduit through the right ventricle. The same considerations apply regarding placement of a permanent epicardial wire as for a two stage arterial switch, i.e. it is rare that we place a permanent wire in view of the length and complexity of the procedure when sinus rhythm is stable.

FONTAN PROCEDURE

If a decision is made following the right atriotomy that it will not be possible to baffle the VSD to the aorta a standard lateral tunnel fenestrated Fontan is performed including a double cavopulmonary anastomosis. The superior vena cava is divided at the level of the right pulmonary artery. The azygous vein is doubly ligated and divided. The procedure is undertaken as described in Chapter 20. No incisions are made in either ventricle.

RESULTS OF SURGERY

Traditional surgery: VSD closure and conduit placement

The disappointing results of traditional surgical management of l-loop transposition were documented in a review of the experience at Children's Hospital Boston by Hraska et al.[27] A total of 123 patients with corrected transposition and two functional ventricles were managed by traditional surgery or the Fontan procedure between 1963 and 1996. Actuarial survival was 84% at one year, 69% at 10 years and 56% at 20 years. Risk factors for death by multivariate analysis were tricuspid valve replacement, right ventricular dysfunction, complete heart block after surgery and need for reoperation. Seventeen patients who underwent Fontan procedures had satisfactory outcomes.

A large multi-institutional study by Graham et al published in 2000[31] documented the long-term outcome in adults with congenitally corrected transposition. The authors reviewed 182 patients from 19 institutions. Risk factors for systemic ventricular dysfunction and congestive heart failure were examined. In general the authors found that patients either without any surgery or with traditional surgical management did poorly. By age 45, 67% of patients with associated lesions such as a VSD and pulmonary stenosis had congestive heart failure while 25% of patients without lesions had failure. Risk factors for systemic right ventricular dysfunction and congestive heart failure were older age, the presence of associated cardiac lesions, history of arrhythmia, previous pacemaker implantation as well as prior traditional surgery particularly surgery which included tricuspid valvuloplasty or tricuspid valve replacement. Aortic regurgitation was found to be relatively common.

In 1999, Voskuil et al[32] described the long-term clinical outcome for 73 patients followed for a mean of 12.7 years after traditional surgical management of congenitally corrected transposition. Survival of patients was significantly below normal. Overall mortality rate was 11%. Right ventricular function and tricuspid valve function deteriorated more frequently in patients following intracardiac operation compared with patients undergoing either palliative interventions or no surgery. In a recent report by Beauchesne et al from the Mayo Clinic,[33] 44 adult patients without previous surgery presenting between age 20 and 79 years were followed for up to 12 years. Systemic atrioventricular valve regurgitation developed in 59% of patients. Thirty of the 44 patients eventually underwent surgical intervention including tricuspid valve replacement. Although early mortality was zero the mean ejection fraction of the systemic right ventricle decreased significantly postoperatively with four patients eventually requiring cardiac transplantation. In an interesting study by Hornung et al from Sydney, Australia,[34] 20 patients with congenitally corrected transposition underwent myocardial perfusion studies. The authors found perfusion defects at rest in the right ventricle in all 20 patients involving five of a total of 12 segments. The extent of the resting perfusion defects correlated inversely with the right ventricular ejection fraction.

Results of the double switch and atrial switch/Rastelli

The double switch concept was introduced by Ilbawi et al in 1990.[26] In 2002 Ilbawi et al updated their results for the double switch procedure.[35] Ten patients had a Mustard procedure combined with a Rastelli procedure while two patients underwent a Mustard procedure with arterial switch. There was one hospital death in a patient who needed ventricular septal defect enlargement. One patient required a pacemaker and one patient developed SVC obstruction. After a mean follow-up of 7.6 years all patients are asymptomatic. Exercise testing was normal in the three oldest patients. Brady-tachyarrhythmias developed in four patients. Conduit replacement was required in five patients after a mean interval of 5.3 years. Mean systemic left ventricular fractional shortening was 39% and mean ejection fraction was 61%. The authors concluded that these are encouraging intermediate term results. The largest series of double switch procedures has been described by Imai et al from Tokyo Japan.[36] In 2001 they reported their latest follow-up on 76 patients who had undergone either a double switch ($n = 14$) or atrial switch/Rastelli procedures ($n = 62$). Overall hospital mortality was 7.9%. Four patients died late over a mean follow-up period of approximately five years. Three patients required reoperation, one for SVC obstruction one month postoperatively and two for residual shunts. At last follow-up 64 patients were in NYHA class 1 with two patients in class 2.

In 2002 Blume et al[37] presented the results of anatomical correction of corrected transposition at Children's Hospital Boston. Between 1992 and 2002, 28 patients underwent anatomical correction, 24 for l-loop transposition and four for IDD transposition. Eight patients had an associated VSD only and 12 patients had a VSD with pulmonary stenosis while seven patients had a VSD with pulmonary atresia. Twenty patients had a Senning procedure and eight had a Mustard procedure. There were two early deaths and one patient underwent heart transplantation. Six patients had pacemakers placed for complete heart block. At a median follow-up of 1.2 years, one homograft conduit had required replacement and two patients required surgical revision for pulmonary venous obstruction. A number of catheter interventional procedures were performed including balloon dilation of systemic venous obstruction in three, homograft dilation in four and device closure of a baffle leak in two.

Reddy et al[38] described 17 patients with congenitally corrected transposition who were managed in San Francisco between 1993 and 1996. Eleven of these patients underwent anatomical repair. Senning procedures were performed in seven patients and Mustard procedure in four. In seven of the 11 procedures a Rastelli procedure was performed. There was one early death and no patient developed surgical complete atrioventricular block. At a median follow-up of 22 months there were no late deaths and echocardiography revealed normal biventricular function in all patients.

In a report by Sharma et al from the All India Institute in Delhi, India,[39] 14 patients with congenitally corrected transposition underwent anatomical repair between 1994 and 1998. Seven of these patients had pulmonary stenosis and underwent a Rastelli type repair while the seven patients without pulmonary stenosis underwent an arterial switch procedure. There was one death in each group. At follow-up the mean left ventricular ejection fraction was 65% in the arterial switch patients and 52% in the Rastelli patients. All patients are in sinus rhythm.

Left ventricular retraining for double switch

The largest experience with retraining of the left ventricle to prepare a patient for a double switch procedure has been accumulated by Mee at the Cleveland Clinic. In the report by Poirier and Mee in 2000[40] a total of 84 patients, 45 with congenitally corrected transposition, underwent retraining of the left ventricle in preparation for a double switch procedure. The overall mortality for the retraining program was 15.4% with all deaths occurring in patients with d-transposition who had undergone a prior atrial switch procedure. A total of 91% of survivors showed normal left ventricular function at follow-up echocardiography. The authors conclude that left ventricular retraining produces good results in pre-pubescent patients but the response in older patients is less predictable and associated with a higher early and late mortality.

Complications of surgery

COMPLETE HEART BLOCK

If closure of the VSD is performed either through the left sided semilunar valve as in the double switch procedure or through a morphological right ventriculotomy in the atrial switch/Rastelli procedure the incidence of complete heart block should be quite low. Nevertheless spontaneous complete heart block can occur in up to 30% of patients with or without surgery and traction and repeated doses of cardioplegia also can result in temporary complete heart block. If sinus rhythm is not re-established within seven to eight days a dual chamber epicardial pacemaker system should be inserted. It is probably not wise to place a transvenous pacemaker system in a new Senning systemic venous baffle because this will increase the risk of baffle thrombosis.

SYSTEMIC VENOUS BAFFLE OBSTRUCTION

Systemic venous baffle gradients as low as 3 or 4 mm can result in important symptoms. Most commonly the superior limb of the baffle will be obstructed. This often becomes manifest as persistent pleural effusions. The head and face will appear engorged and there may be prominent veins on the anterior chest wall that develop over a week or two. It is important to visualize the baffle pathways by transesophageal echocardiography intraoperatively. However, it is also important to understand that the original right atrium is often quite small so that the baffle pathways will also appear small following the Senning procedure. Careful measurement of pressure above and below the baffle pathway is a useful supplement to echo examination.

PULMONARY VENOUS BAFFLE OBSTRUCTION

If the right upper and lower pulmonary veins lie one in front of the other this will necessarily result in quite a narrow pulmonary venous pathway where the pulmonary venous return passes around the systemic venous baffle to get to the tricuspid valve. Furthermore transesophageal echocardiography can be misleading because of compression of the posterior wall of the pulmonary venous chamber by the echo probe within the esophagus. It is usually not difficult to pass the left atrial catheter which has been inserted through the original right atrial appendage across the 'neck' of the pulmonary venous pathway and to obtain a pullback pressure tracing. A gradient of more than 4 or 5 mm may be important. Consideration should be given to use of the in situ pericardium technique or a free patch of pericardium to maximize the size of the pulmonary venous pathway in the area of the right pulmonary vein incision.

RESIDUAL VSD

The baffle pathway from the VSD to the aorta can be quite long and difficult to expose through the very left sided incision in the morphological right ventricle. The pulmonary artery line should provide useful information regarding the absolute pulmonary artery saturation, any stepup between right atrial saturation and pulmonary artery saturation as well as absolute pulmonary artery pressure that will help to determine the functional significance of any residual VSD identified by echocardiography.

CONDUIT OBSTRUCTION

If there is dextrocardia and the conduit is placed immediately retrosternally sternal closure may be associated with important conduit compression and obstruction. It may be necessary to leave the sternum open in order to avoid any conduit compression in the critical early postoperative hours. Other maneuvers that we have found useful in this setting have been to remove the posterior table of the sternum. Suspension of the sternum with large traction sutures emerging from the skin and supported by an overhead traction system thereby lifting the sternum off the homograft conduit has also been found to be a useful maneuver for the first 24–48 hours postoperatively. Usually it is possible to release the traction system after this time and conduit compression does not acutely recur.

REFERENCES

1. Fyler DC. 'Corrected' transposition of the great arteries. In Fyler DC (ed). *Nadas' Pediatric Cardiology*, Philadelphia, Hanley and Belfus, 1992, p 701.
2. DiDonato RM, Wernovsky G, Jonas RA, Mayer JE, Keane JF, Castaneda AR. Corrected transposition in situs inversus: Biventricular repair of associated cardiac anomalies. *Circulation* 1991; **84**:193–199.
3. McKay R, Anderson RH, Smith A. The coronary arteries in hearts with discordant atrioventricular connections. *J Thorac Cardiovasc Surg* 1996; **111**:988–997.
4. Allwork SP, Bentall HH, Becker AE et al. Congenitally corrected transposition of the great arteries: Morphologic study of 32 cases. *Am J Cardiol* 1976; **39**:910–923.
5. Anderson RH, Becker AE, Gerlis LM. The pulmonary outflow tract in classicially corrected transposition. *J Thorac Cardiovasc Surg* 1975; **69**:747–757.
6. Losekoot TG, Anderson RH, Becker AE, Danielson GK, Soto B. *Congenitally Corrected Transposition*. New York, Churchill Livingstone, 1983.
7. Castaneda AR, Jonas RA, Mayer JE, Hanley FL. *Cardiac Surgery of the Neonate and Infant*. Philadelphia, WB Saunders, 1994, p 439.
8. Krongrad E, Ellis K, Steeg CN, Bowman FO, Malm FR, Gersony WM. Subpulmonary obstruction in congenitally corrected transposition of the great arteries due to ventricular membranous septal aneurysms. *Circulation* 1976; **54**:679–683.
9. Levy MJ, Lillehei CW, Elliott LP, Carey LS, Adams P, Edwards JE. Accessory valvar tissue causing subpulmonary stenosis in corrected transposition of the great vessels. *Circulation* 1963; **27**:494.
10. Williams WG, Suri R, Shindo G, Freedom RM, Morch JE, Trusler GA. Repair of major intracardiac anomalies associated with atrioventricular discordance. *Ann Thorac Surg* 1981; **31**:527–531.

11. Anderson KR, Danielson GK, McGoon DC, Lie JT. Ebsteins anomaly of the left sided tricuspid valve. Pathological anatomy of the valvular malformations. *Circulation* 1978; **58**(suppl I):I87.
12. Anderson RH, Arnold R, Wilkinson JL. The conducting tissue in congenitally corrected transposition. *Lancet* 1973; **1**:1286–1288.
13. Anderson RH, Becker AE, Arnold R, Wilkinson JL. The conducting tissues in congenitally corrected transposition. *Circulation* 1974; **50**:911–923.
14. Dick M, Van Praagh R, Rudd M, Folkerth T, Castaneda AR. Electrophysiologic delineation of the specialized atrioventricular conduction system in two patients with corrected transposition of the great arteries with situs inversus (IDD). *Circulation* 1977; **55**:896–900.
15. Thiene C, Nava A, Rossi L. The conduction system in corrected transposition with situs inversus. *Eur J Cardiol* 1977; **6**:57–70.
16. Wilkinson JL, Smith A, Lincoln C, Anderson RH. Conducting tissues in congenitally corrected transposition with situs inversus. *Br Heart J* 1978; **40**:41–48.
17. Bharati S, McCue C, Tingelstad JB, Mantakas M, Shiel F, Lev M. Lack of connection between the atria and the peripheral conduction system in a case of corrected transposition with congenital atrioventricular block. *Am J Cardiol* 1978; **42**:147–153.
18. Anselmi G, Munoz S, Machado I, Blanco P, Espino-Vela J. Complex cardiovascular malformations associated with the corrected type of transposition of the great vessels. *Am Heart J* 1963; **66**:614–621.
19. Lieberson AD, Schumacher RR, Childress RH. Genovese PDI. Corrected transposition of the great arteries in a 73 year old man. *Circulation* 1969; **36**:96–100.
20. Carey LS, Ruttenberg HD. Roetgenographic features of congenitally corrected transposition of the great vessels. *AJR* 1964; **92**:623.
21. von Rokintansky CF. *Die Defekte der Scheidewande des Herzens.* Vienna, Wilhelm Braumuller, 1875.
22. Monckeberg JG. Zur Entwicklungsgeschichte des Atrioventrikularsystems. *Verh Dtsch Pathol* 1913; **16**:228.
23. Anderson RC, Lillehei CW, Lester RG. Corrected transposition of the great vessels of the heart. *Pediatrics* 1957; **20**:626.
24. de Leval MR, Bastos P, Stark J, Taylor JF, Maccartney FJ, Anderson RH. Surgical technique to reduce the risks of heart block following closure of ventricular septal defects in atrioventricular discordance. *J Thorac Cardiovasc Surg* 1979; **78**:515–526.
25. Lev M, Fielding RT, Zaeske D. Mixed levocardia with ventricular inversion (corrected transposition) with complete AV block. *Am J Cardiol* 1963; **12**:875.
26. Ilbawi MN, Deleon SY, Backer CL et al. An alternative approach to the surgical management of physiologically corrected transposition with VSD and pulmonary stenosis. *J Thorac Cardiovasc Surg* 1990; **100**:410–415.
27. Hraska V, Duncan BW, Mayer JE, Freed M, del Nido PJ, Jonas RA. Long-term outcome of surgically treated patients with corrected transposition of the great arteries. *J Thorac Cardiovasc Surg*, in press.
28. Castaneda AR, Jonas RA, Mayer JE, Hanley FL. *Cardiac Surgery of the Neonate and Infant.* Philadelphia, WB Saunders, 1994, p 430.
29. Lacour-Gayet F, Rey C, Planche C. [Pulmonary vein stenosis. Description of a sutureless surgical procedure using the pericardium in situ] *Arch Mal Coeur Vaiss* 1996; **89**:633–636.
30. Lacour-Gayet F, Zoghbi J, Serraf AE et al. Surgical management of progressive pulmonary venous obstruction after repair of total anomalous pulmonary venous connection. *J Thorac Cardiovasc Surg* 1999; **117**:679–687.
31. Graham TP Jr, Bernard YD, Mellen BG et al. Long-term outcome in congenitally corrected transposition of the great arteries: a multi-institutional study.*J Am Coll Cardiol* 2000; **36**:255–261.
32. Voskuil M, Hazekamp MG, Kroft LJ et al. Postsurgical course of patients with congenitally corrected transposition of the great arteries. *Am J Cardiol* 1999; **83**:558–562.
33. Beauchesne LM, Warnes CA, Connolly HM, Ammash NM, Tajik AJ, Danielson GK. Outcome of the unoperated adult who presents with congenitally corrected transposition of the great arteries. *J Am Coll Cardiol* 2002; **40**:285–290.
34. Hornung TS, Bernard EJ, Celermajer DS et al. Right ventricular dysfunction in congenitally corrected transposition of the great arteries. *Am J Cardiol* 1999; **84**:1116–19, A10.
35. Ilbawi MN, Ocampo CB, Allen BS, Barth MJ et al. Intermediate results of the anatomic repair for congenitally corrected transposition. *Ann Thorac Surg* 2002; **73**:594–599.
36. Imai Y, Seo K, Aoki M, Shin'oka T, Hiramatsu K, Ohta A. Double-switch operation for congenitally corrected transposition. *Semin Thorac Cardiovasc Surg Pediatr Card Surg Annu* 2001; **4**:16.
37. Blume ED et al. Anatomic repair of corrected transposition of the great arteries. Presented at the 2002 Scientific Sessions of the American Heart Association, 2002.
38. Reddy VM, McElhinney DB, Silverman NH, Hanley FL. The double switch procedure for anatomical repair of congenitally corrected transposition of the great arteries in infants and children. *Eur Heart J* 1997; **18**:1470–1477.
39. Sharma R, Bhan A, Juneja R, Kothari SS, Saxena A, Venugopal P. Double switch for congenitally corrected transposition of the great arteries. *Eur J Cardiothorac Surg* 1999; **15**:276–281.
40. Poirier NC, Mee RB. Left ventricular reconditioning and anatomical correction for systemic right ventricular dysfunction. *Semin Thorac Cardiovasc Surg Pediatr Card Surg Annu* 2000; **3**:198–215.

29

Vascular rings, slings, and tracheal anomalies

The development of the mediastinal great vessels, including the aortic arch and descending thoracic aorta, is a fascinating demonstration of embryological mechanisms.[1,2] The multiple paired branchial arches and paired dorsal aortae generally (but not always) fuse and resorb in the embryo in a predictable sequence to result in the usual left aortic arch and left descending aorta. Failure of resorption will result in any one of a number of vascular rings or a pulmonary artery sling, which, from a cardiovascular point of view, are generally quite benign. However, their tendency to constrict the trachea, the esophagus, or both, may result in important obstructive airway or esophageal symptoms, thereby necessitating division of the ring or relocation of the sling.

VASCULAR RING

EMBRYOLOGY

The evolution over millions of years of complex organisms is often mirrored in various stages of embryological development. Early in embryogenesis simple modules from less complex organisms are assembled. The embryo then utilizes the process of programmed cell death, similar to apoptosis, to eliminate redundant and unnecessary components.[3,4] The multiple branchial arches in the human embryo are an excellent example. They represent the blood supply of gill breathing organisms which lie in our phyllogenetic past. They are transiently present during human development but either partially or completely disappear as the pulmonary circulation develops and connects with the heart. Only a few useful segments usually remain. When unnecessary segments persist anomalies such as vascular rings result.

The paired (right and left) dorsal aortae, one of which will eventually become the descending thoracic aorta, are present in the embryo by approximately the 21st day of intrauterine life (Figure 29.1). Subsequently the first to sixth branchial arteries form bilaterally, each with its own aortic arch communicating from the aortic sac to the dorsal aortas. At this point in development therefore multiple vascular rings are present. The first and second arches largely resorb and contribute only to minor facial arteries, while the third arches form the carotid arteries. The left fourth arch forms the distal aortic arch and aortic isthmus from the origin of the left common carotid artery to the origin of the descending thoracic aorta, which itself represents a persistence of the left dorsal aorta.[5] Proximally, septation of the conotruncus produces the ascending aorta, which joins with the fourth left arch. The right dorsal aorta ultimately contributes to the right subclavian artery but otherwise resorbs.

ANATOMICAL VARIANTS

Dominant right aortic arch

By far the majority of vascular rings consist of a dominant right arch. The surgical relevance of this fact, as will be

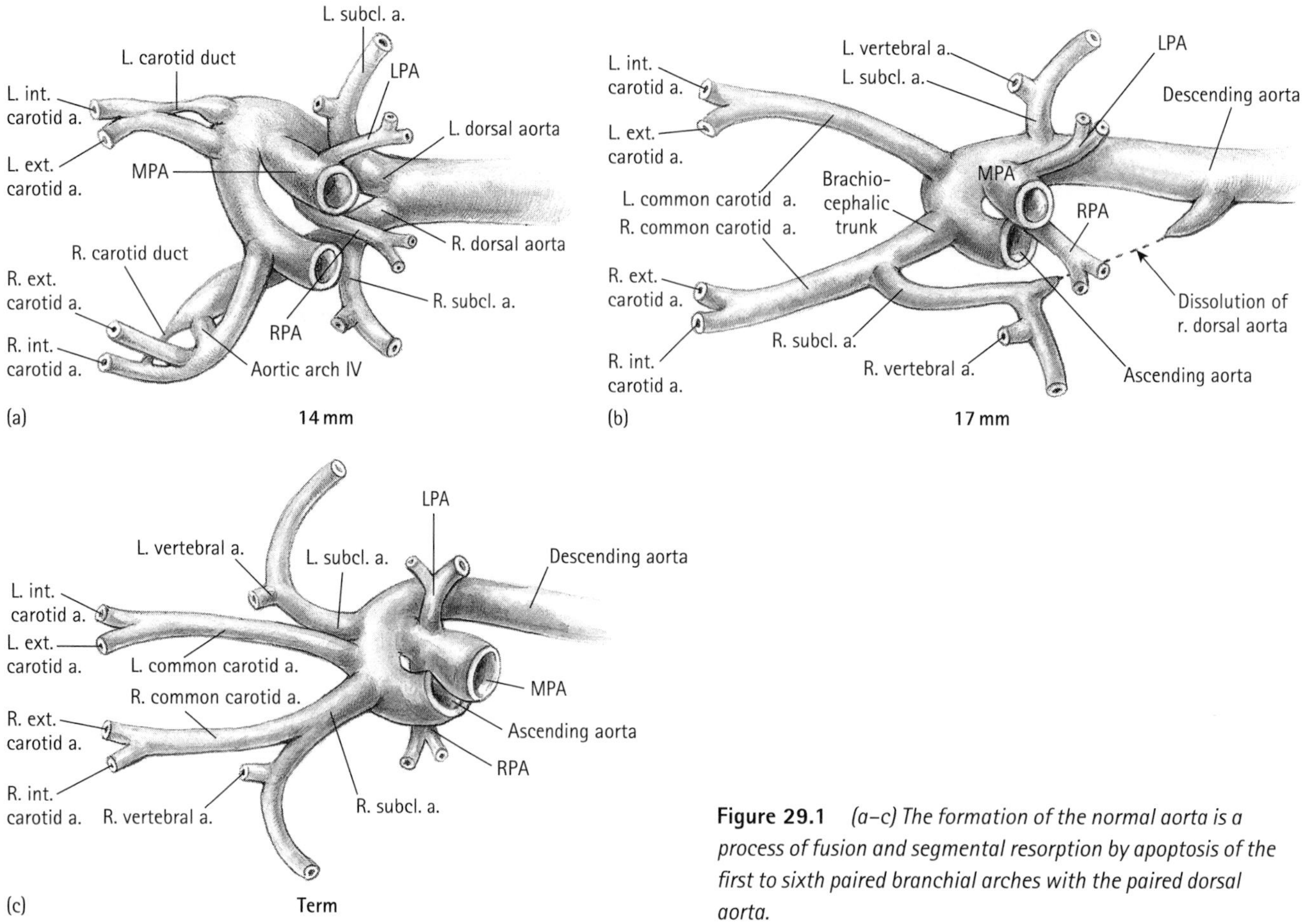

Figure 29.1 *(a–c) The formation of the normal aorta is a process of fusion and segmental resorption by apoptosis of the first to sixth paired branchial arches with the paired dorsal aorta.*

discussed later, is that almost all vascular rings are most safely and conveniently approached through a left thoracotomy.

DOUBLE AORTIC ARCH

As the name implies, this anomaly consists of two aortic arches, an anterior and leftward arch and a posterior and rightward arch[6] (Figure 29.2). Generally the descending aorta is left sided although it may be right sided or in the midline. The right arch is generally dominant and gives rise to the right common carotid and right subclavian arteries either as an innominate artery or as two separate vessels. The left arch gives rise to the left common carotid and left subclavian arteries. It may be hypoplastic or atretic beyond the origin of either the left common carotid or left subclavian artery, being little more than a fibrous cord. In the latter case, the fibrous cord joins the descending aorta, where the aorta emerges from behind the esophagus to become the left sided descending aorta near the insertion of the ligamentum arteriosum. This anomaly represents persistence of the right dorsal aorta with incomplete resorption of the left. Note that the right recurrent laryngeal nerve must pass around the right aortic arch, rather than being in its usual location around the right subclavian artery.

RIGHT AORTIC ARCH, ABERRANT LEFT SUBCLAVIAN ARTERY, AND LEFT LIGAMENTUM

With this form of vascular ring there is a right aortic arch that gives off, in sequence, the left common carotid, the right common carotid, the right subclavian, and the left subclavian arteries. The left subclavian passes behind the esophagus and then gives rise to the ligamentum arteriosum, which passes anteriorly to connect to the left pulmonary artery, thereby completing the vascular ring. This anomaly represents persistence of the right fourth aortic arch with resorption of the left fourth aortic arch.

RIGHT AORTIC ARCH, MIRROR-IMAGE BRANCHING, AND RETROESOPHAGEAL LIGAMENTUM

With this form of vascular ring there is a right aortic arch that gives off, in sequence, the left innominate artery (left common carotid with left subclavian), the right common carotid, and the right subclavian artery.[7] The final branch, often arising from a prominent ductus diverticulum, the diverticulum of Koumeroll, is a ligamentum that passes leftward, behind the esophagus, and then anteriorly to attach to the left pulmonary artery. This anomaly also represents persistence of the fourth right aortic arch with resorption of the fourth left

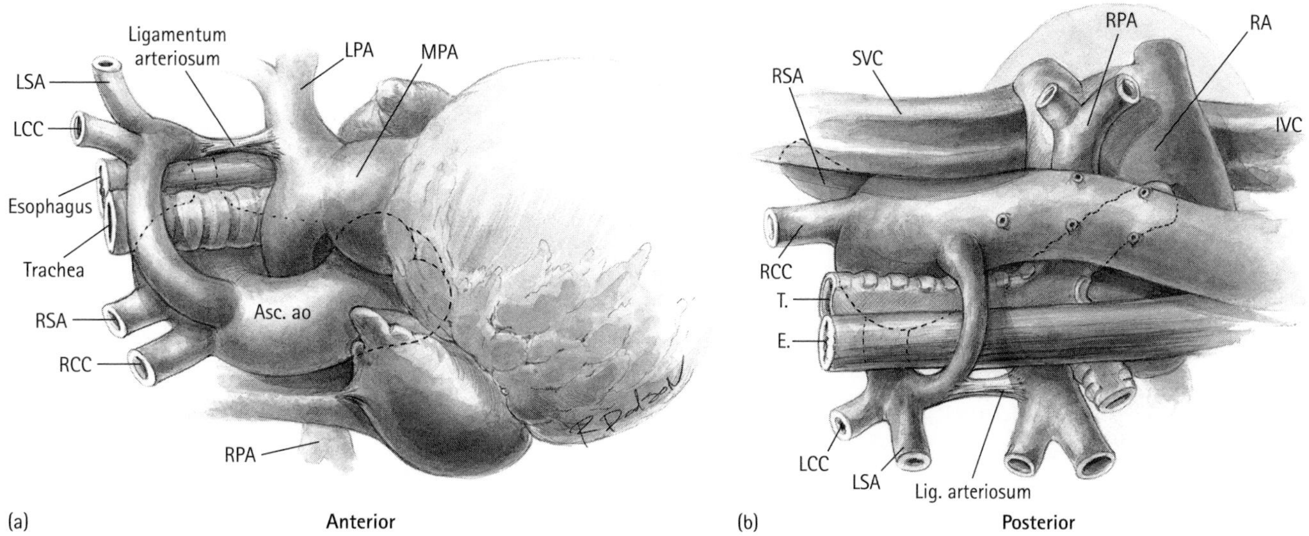

Figure 29.2 *A double aortic arch is a form of vascular ring in which there is usually a dominant right posterior arch with a hypoplastic or atretic left anterior arch. The ligamentum arteriosum contributes to secondary tracheoesophageal compression and should be divided together with the left anterior arch. (a) Anterior view; (b) posterior view.*

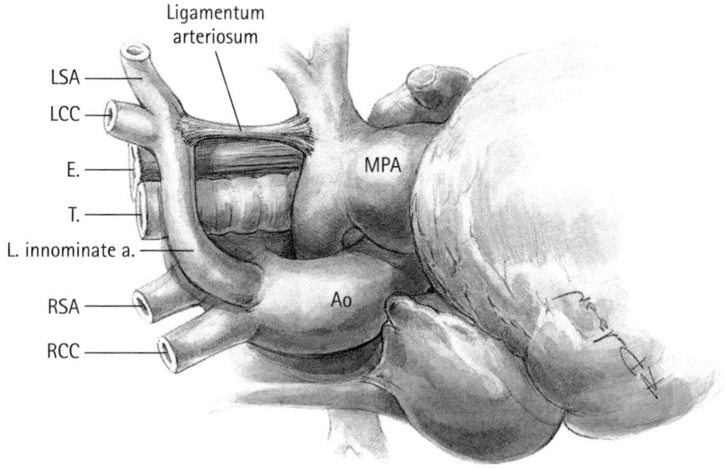

Figure 29.3 *When there is a right aortic arch with mirror-image branching and the ligamentum arteriosum arises from the innominate or left subclavian artery, no vascular ring is formed.*

aortic arch. A short segment of the distal end of the left fourth arch persists as an aortic diverticulum, which gives rise to the ligamentum. Note that the aortic diverticulum has been reported as the site of origin of aortic dissection. Also note that when there is mirror-image branching, if the ligamentum arteriosum arises from the innominate artery to pass to the origin of the left pulmonary artery rather than from the diverticulum of Koumeroll, this does not result in a vascular ring (Figure 29.3).

Dominant left aortic arch

A dominant left aortic arch is extremely rare but should be recognized, because the best approach for surgical division is through a right thoracotomy.[8]

LEFT AORTIC ARCH, MIRROR-IMAGE BRANCHING, RIGHT DESCENDING AORTA, AND ATRETIC RIGHT AORTIC ARCH

With this rare form of vascular ring (Figure 29.4), the arch vessels arise normally from the normal-size left aortic arch. The right arch is atretic.

LEFT AORTIC ARCH, RIGHT DESCENDING AORTA, AND RIGHT SIDED LIGAMENTUM ARTERIOSUM TO RIGHT PULMONARY ARTERY

The branching sequence from the left aortic arch is the right common carotid, left common carotid, left subclavian, and, finally, right subclavian as a fourth branch from the proximal descending aorta (Figure 29.5).

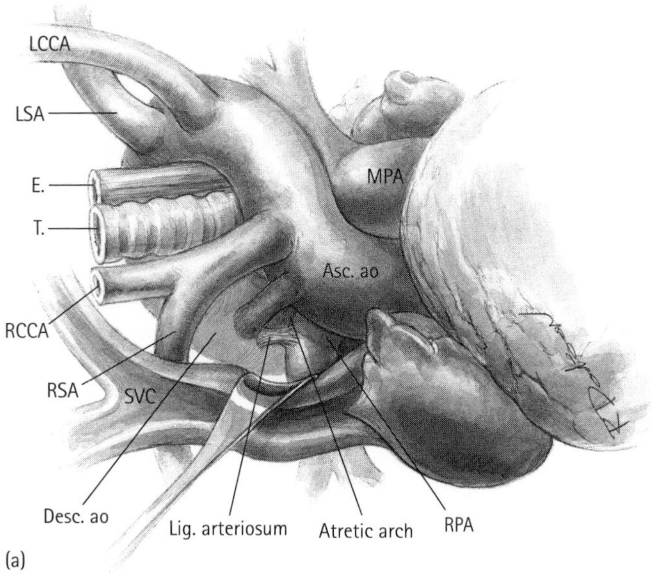

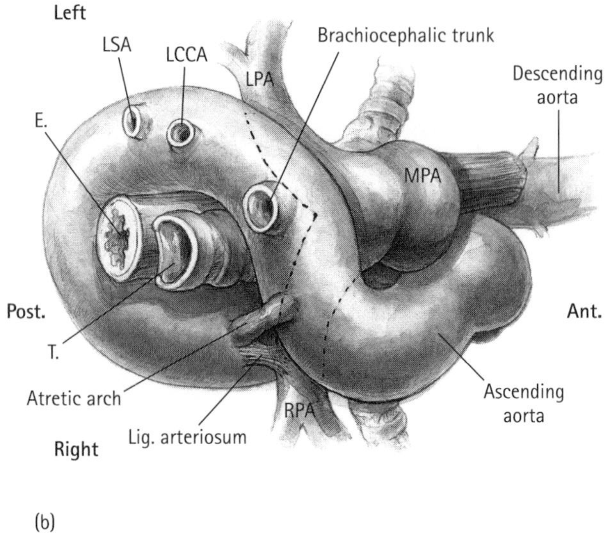

Figure 29.4 *In the rare case in which the left aortic arch is dominant and the right arch is atretic but forms a vascular ring, the surgical approach should be via a right thoracotomy. (a) Anterior view; (b) view from above.*

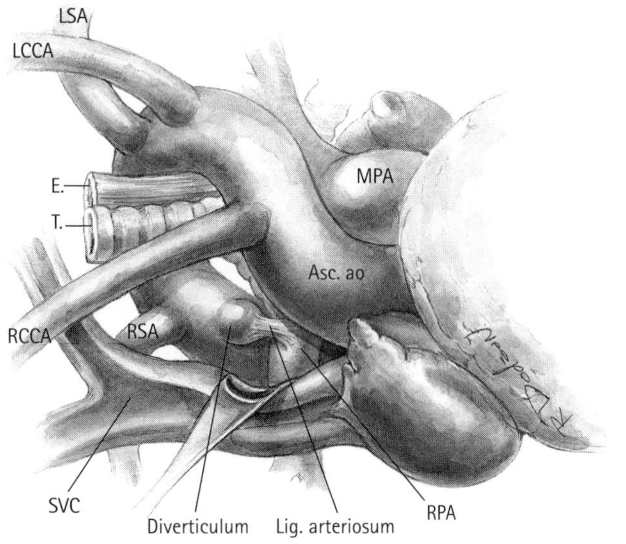

Figure 29.5 *A right thoracotomy is necessary for correction of the rare case of a dominant left arch with a right descending aorta and a right sided ligamentum arteriosum passing to the right pulmonary artery.*

PATHOPHYSIOLOGY

Vascular rings, in contrast to a pulmonary artery sling, encircle both the esophagus and trachea and, therefore, may result in obstructive symptoms of both. Nevertheless, the mere presence of a ring does not guarantee that there will be compression; indeed, rings may remain asymptomatic for life and not require any intervention.[9] It is very rare that there is vascular obstruction and therefore a hemodynamic reason for intervention in both arches of a double arch[10] or of the patent arch if there is a vascular ring with a nonpatent component.

CLINICAL PRESENTATION

If compression is severe, the child presents in the neonatal period with stridor or even respiratory distress, although the latter is rare. In the first months of life feeding may be slow. As the child progresses to solids, there is increasing difficulty with feeding. Reflux and respiratory infections are common. Vascular obstruction of both aortic arches must be exceedingly rare. At Children's Hospital Boston, we have managed one such child in whom coarctations were present in each of her two aortic arches; this was in a setting of Shone's syndrome.[10]

DIAGNOSTIC STUDIES

Many different types of diagnostic study are available for assessing the child with a vascular ring. Careful consideration should be given to the cost effectiveness of various studies before embarking on multiple imaging tests.

Barium swallow

A simple barium swallow, combined with an echocardiogram to exclude intracardiac anomalies, should suffice for most children suspected of having a vascular ring. Unlike the pulmonary artery sling, which produces an anterior indentation of the esophagus, vascular rings invariably produce a posterior indentation. An experienced radiologist can usally distinguish a double arch from the retroesophageal subclavian or ligament, based on the angulation of the esophageal impression.[11]

Echocardiography

The aortic arch is usually invested by thymus in the neonate and young infant, so in this age group it is generally possible to determine accurately the anatomy of a vascular ring, particularly when imaging is combined with color flow Doppler. Although there is acoustic shadowing as a result of air in the trachea, transesophageal echocardiography assists accurate imaging in this area when it is combined with transthoracic imaging. Echocardiography alone will not be able to reveal the presence of an atretic segment of aortic arch, but the general contours of the arch and branches in the context of an esophageal impression seen by barium swallow will almost always allow accurate diagnosis.

Computed tomography, magnetic resonance imaging

These expensive studies can generate spectacular images but are rarely an essential part of the diagnostic workup. Sometimes they can be useful for determining arch patency if a video-assisted, minimally invasive surgical approach is going to be used for management. Computed tomography involves exposure to radiation and the risk of intravenous contrast dye. Both CT and MRI usually require general anesthesia which is often undesirable in the small child who has obstructed airway symptoms. They also do not demonstrate the nonpatent ligamentous component of a vascular ring. Nevertheless CT and MRI are particularly useful when assessing the site and severity (particularly the length) of congenital tracheal stenoses and in the planning of tracheal resection and reconstructive procedures,[12,13] but this is almost never necessary for first-time management of a vascular ring.

Bronchoscopy

The same comments made for the CT scan and MRI also apply to bronchoscopy: it is expensive, involves additional risks, and although it is not useful for a simple vascular ring, it is an essential part of the workup for congenital tracheal stenosis.

Aortography

Expensive, invasive, and carrying additional risk for the patient, aortography is rarely justified for the diagnosis of a vascular ring. In addition, if there is an atretic segment, such a study may not be diagnostic.

MEDICAL MANAGEMENT

The general philosophy at present is that if either respiratory or dysphagic symptoms are present, surgical division of the ring is indicated. If the child is asymptomatic, surgery may be deferred. Preoperatively the child should be given maximal nutritional support as well as general respiratory care, including chest physiotherapy and appropriate treatment of respiratory infection. Surgery should not be unduly delayed because of the presence of a respiratory infection, as division of the ring, which allows more adequate clearing of respiratory secretions, is the most effective treatment of infection.

INDICATIONS FOR AND TIMING OF SURGERY

The presence of symptoms is an indication for surgery. Symptoms may include stridor, wheezing, frequent respiratory infections, dysphagia, reflux, and failure to thrive. Very mild symptoms appearing for the first time in the older infant may improve with time as the child grows, in which case it may be possible to defer surgery. Nevertheless, because the risks of surgery are extremely small, the child should undergo surgery within a reasonably short time from diagnosis. The maximal delay until surgery should be determined by the severity of the symptoms.

SURGICAL MANAGEMENT

History

The surgical management of double aortic arch was pioneered by Gross at Children's Hospital Boston in 1945,[14] the same year that he undertook the first surgical procedure in the United States for coarctation and seven years after his first operation for patent ductus arteriosus. Gross and Ware subsequently described surgical management of the various other forms of vascular ring.[15] The diagnosis of vascular ring by careful interpretation of the plain chest radiograph and barium swallow was described at about the same time by Neuhauser, also at Children's Hospital Boston.[11] The first description of the use of video-assisted thoracoscopic surgery (VATS) for surgical division of a vascular ring was by Burke et al from Children's Hospital Boston.[16]

Technical considerations

TRADITIONAL OPEN SURGERY

Preoperative studies must not only establish the presence of a vascular ring, but also confirm that the optimal approach will be through a left thoracotomy, which will be true in more than 95% of cases. If a double aortic arch is present, it is important to be aware preoperatively which of the arches is dominant. In the majority of cases, it will be the right aortic arch. Nevertheless, in cases of double patent arches it is useful to place pulse oximeter probes on both hands and one foot so that temporary occlusion of the arch branches will allow confirmation of the anatomy. Furthermore, blood pressure cuffs placed on one leg and both arms will confirm the absence of a pressure gradient when the intended point of division of the double arch is temporarily occluded. Because the point of division will be the narrowest segment of the ring, there should be no pressure gradient with occlusion.

The child is placed in a full right lateral decubitus position, and a left posterolateral thoracotomy is performed that is more posterior than lateral. The chest is entered through the fourth intercostal space, and the left lung is retracted anteriorly. Palpation in the area of the ring will reveal a taut, ligamentous structure in the case of a ring with an atretic left arch. If a double arch is present, it is generally visible to some degree through the mediastinal pleura. The vagus nerve, giving off the left recurrent laryngeal nerve (which then passes around the ligamentum arteriosum), is a useful landmark. The mediastinal pleura is reflected from the area of the left arch and ligamentum. Test occlusions of the arch vessels may be performed at this time to confirm the anatomy. The segment to be divided, if patent, should be controlled with clamps. After division the vessel ends are oversewn with a continuous Prolene suture. If the segment to be divided is clearly atretic, it suffices to doubly ligate the cord and divide it. After division the ends generally retract briskly, indicating the tension with which the ring has been surrounding the esophagus and trachea. In all cases it is particularly important that the ligamentum arteriosum should also be divided. There may be additional fibrous strands passing across the esophagus, and these should be divided. Final palpation in the area should reveal complete relief of the taut band that was present previously. The mediastinal pleura is approximated, a single chest tube is placed, and the thoracotomy is closed in a routine fashion, using absorbable pericostal suture together with absorbable suture to the muscle layers, with subcutaneous and subcuticular absorbable suture completing wound closure.

In the rare case requiring approach through a right thoracotomy, the same principles are applied. The right recurrent laryngeal nerve will pass around the right sided ligamentum arteriosum and should be carefully visualized and preserved.

VIDEO-ASSISTED TECHNIQUE OF MANAGEMENT OF VASCULAR RING

This has become the method of choice for all vascular rings unless preoperative studies suggest that there is a patent segment of a double arch that is more than 2 or 3 mm in diameter. The patient is placed in the right lateral decubitus position following single lumen endotracheal intubation. Four thoracostomies (3 mm in length) are made in the posterolateral chest wall to admit from medial to lateral a grasping forceps, a lung retractor, a videoscope and an L-shaped cautery probe. Exposure is achieved by retracting the inflated left upper lobe inferiorly and medially. The mediastinal pleura is incised over the left subclavian artery which leads to the other components of the vascular ring. The ring is dissected free from the esophagus and surrounding structures. The atretic segment of the vascular ring and ligamentum are identified. Clips are placed and the ring and ligamentum are divided between clips. Fibrous bands over the esophagus are divided. A small chest tube is placed under direct vision and the wounds are closed with steri strips.

POSTOPERATIVE MANAGEMENT

In the young infant with severe respiratory symptoms, there is likely to be an element of tracheomalacia associated with the long-standing compression by the ring during in utero development. Therefore, it should be anticipated that not all respiratory symptoms will be relieved immediately; in fact it may be several months before the child is free of stridor. However, there should be complete and immediate relief of any difficulty with feeding.

RESULTS OF SURGERY

Traditional thoracotomy approach

One of the largest reports of vascular anomalies causing tracheoesophageal compression is a report by Backer et al from Children's Memorial Hospital in Chicago published in 1989.[17] The authors described 204 infants and children with a mean age of 13 months who had undergone surgical procedures for tracheoesophageal obstruction. Of these, 113 patients had a vascular ring, 61 with a double aortic arch and 52 with a right aortic arch and left ligamentum. The operative mortality rate was 4.9% with a 3.4% late mortality rate. However, there no operative deaths over the most recent 28 years. At a mean follow-up of 8.5 years, 92% of patients were essentially free of symptoms.

In 1994, Cordovilla Zurdo et al[18] from Madrid, Spain described another series of traditional surgery for vascular ring. Of the 43 patients 42% had a double aortic arch, 32% an anomalous right subclavian artery and 25% a right aortic arch with left sided ligament. There was one hospital death and one late death. Over a mean follow-up of 11 years, 90% of patients were asymptomatic. In a similar report from Anand et al from Atlanta, Georgia,[19] 44 patients underwent surgery for either vascular ring or pulmonary artery sling between 1977 and 1990. Nineteen patients had a double aortic arch, 13 had a vascular ring with right arch and anomalous origin of the left subclavian artery and eight patients had innominate artery compression of the trachea. There were four patients with a pulmonary artery sling. Patients who died had complex associated congenital heart disease. Over a mean follow-up of 3.6 years 70% of the patients were asymptomatic though 30% of patients continue to have upper and lower respiratory symptoms at late follow-up. In 1993 Van Son et al[20] described the experience with vascular rings at the Mayo Clinic. Between 1947 and 1992, 37 patients underwent traditional surgery for relief of tracheoesophageal obstruction caused by vascular rings. Of the 37 patients, 18 had a double aortic arch, 11 had a right aortic arch with aberrant left subclavian, four had a left aortic arch with aberrant right subclavian and two had a pulmonary artery sling. The usual symptoms were stridor, recurrent respiratory infections and dysphagia. In 31 patients approach was through a left thoracotomy, in four through a right thoracotomy and in two through a median sternotomy. There was one early postoperative death and no late deaths. At long-term follow-up three patients had residual symptomatic tracheomalacia, one of whom required right middle and lower lobectomy for recurrent pneumonia. The authors suggest that MRI is the imaging technique of choice for accurate delineation of vascular and tracheal anatomy. A similar conclusion was drawn by Bakker et al who described 38 children diagnosed with vascular ring between 1981 and 1996 in Rotterdam, the Netherlands.[21] The delay between onset of symptoms and diagnosis of a vascular ring without associated anomalies ranged from 1 to 84 months. Associated anomalies were found in 53% of cases and in 80% these anomalies were cardiovascular. Barium swallow was a very useful diagnostic technique when a vascular ring was suspected. Echocardiography was not helpful in diagnosing the ring itself but was essential to exclude associated cardiovascular malformations. Of six patients who died, five had co-existent tracheal deformities. Only 43% of patients were free of symptoms immediately after surgery and at four years 57% were free of symptoms.

Results of video-assisted division of vascular ring

In 1995 Burke et al[22] described the first series of patients who had undergone video-assisted division of vascular ring at Children's Hospital Boston. Eight patients with a median age of five months underwent the procedure. Four had a double aortic arch with atretic left arch and four had a right arch with aberrant left subclavian and a left ligamentum. All eight patients had successful ring division with symptomatic relief and no mortality. In three patients a limited thoracotomy was performed to divide vascular structures. The eight patients who had a VATS approach were compared with a historical cohort of eight patients who had vascular ring division by conventional thoracotomy. The two groups did not differ in age, weight, ICU or postoperative hospital stay, duration of ntubation or thoracostomy tube drainage or hospital charges. Total operating room time was longer for the VATS group.

PULMONARY ARTERY SLING

ANATOMY

In a patient with a typical pulmonary artery sling the left pulmonary artery arises from the right pulmonary artery and passes leftward between the trachea and esophagus (Figure 29.6).[23] The ligamentum arteriosum passes posteriorly from the origin of the right pulmonary artery where it arises from the main pulmonary artery to the undersurface of the aortic

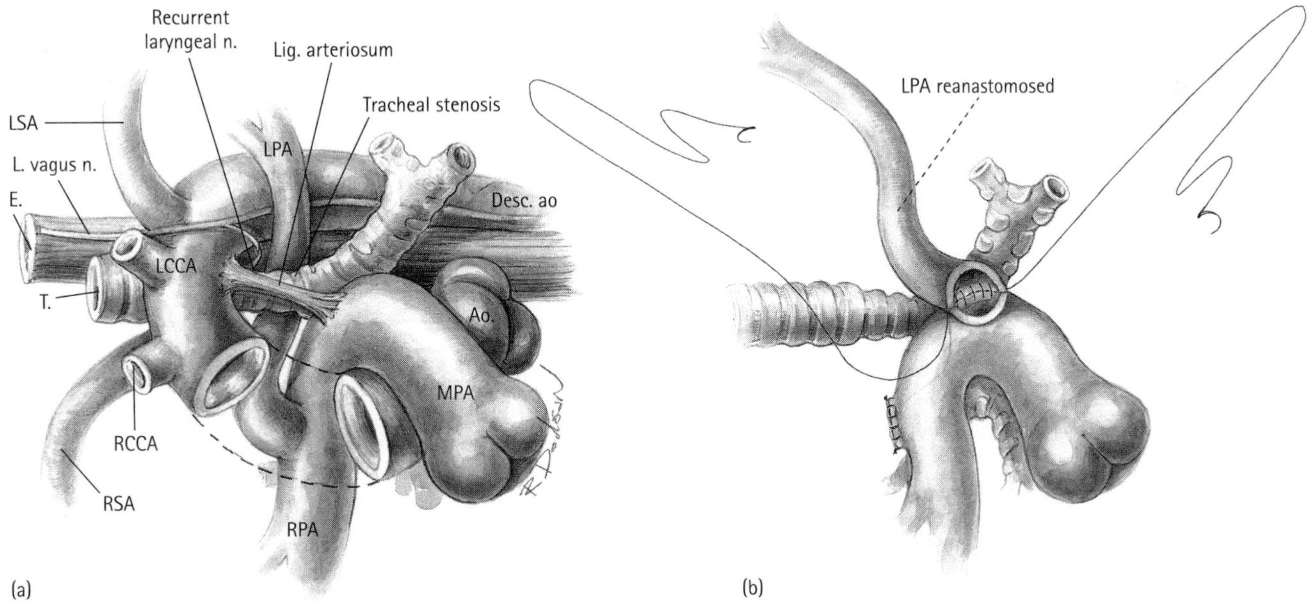

Figure 29.6 *Pulmonary artery sling. (a) Anatomy of a pulmonary artery sling. The left pulmonary artery, often hypoplastic, arises from the distal right pulmonary artery and passes leftward between the trachea and esophagus. The ligamentum arteriosum arises from the junction of the main pulmonary artery and the right pulmonary artery and passes posteriorly to the undersurface of the aortic arch, thereby creating what is effectively a vascular ring. (b) Traditional management of a pulmonary artery sling consists of division of the left pulmonary artery and reanastomosis of the left pulmonary artery to the side of the main pulmonary artery in front of the trachea. The procedure is best performed through a median sternotomy employing cardiopulmonary bypass. This technique does not deal with associated tracheal stenosis.*

arch effectively creating a vascular ring surrounding the trachea but not the esophagus. The left pulmonary artery is often relatively hypoplastic and considerably smaller than the right pulmonary artery, which itself appears larger than normal and almost like a direct extension of the main pulmonary artery. The small size of the left pulmonary artery may help to explain the high incidence of anastomotic problems that have been observed in the past with attempts to reimplant it.

ASSOCIATED TRACHEAL ANOMALIES

At least 50% of patients with a pulmonary artery sling have complete tracheal rings, i.e. the posterior membranous component of the trachea is absent, and the tracheal cartilages, rather than being U-shaped, are O-shaped.[24,25] The presence of complete rings does not imply that important stenosis necessarily will be present, although the trachea is often narrower than normal. The complete rings may be localized to the region where the sling passes around the trachea, although often they extend for the entire length of the trachea. Severe stenosis can involve the carina and extend for a considerable distance into one or both mainstem bronchi.

In the area where the sling passes around the trachea, there may be tracheal compression resulting in important functional stenosis, even if there is not an underlying anatomic stenosis. However, tracheal compression by the low pressure pulmonary artery is probably not the more important mechanism of tracheal stenosis as suggested by the following experience. Several years ago we managed a child at Children's Hospital Boston with a pulmonary artery sling in which the sling passed around the trachea *above* a very high 'pig bronchus' (bronchus suis, i.e. origin of the right upper lobe bronchus from the distal trachea rather than from the right main bronchus, is an association of pulmonary artery sling). Interestingly, in this child there was a tight, localized stenosis consisting of complete rings *below* the pig bronchus and extending to the carina, although the sling lay entirely above this area. There was no narrowing secondary to compression in the region where the sling passed around the trachea.

PHYSIOLOGY AND CLINICAL PRESENTATION

Respiratory symptoms predominate because of the direct tracheal compression, with or without congenital tracheal stenosis, and are essentially the same respiratory symptoms as those described for vascular rings. Symptoms of esophageal compression are rarely present.

DIAGNOSTIC STUDIES

Definition of the vascular anatomy may be made in the same fashion as described for vascular rings. However, unlike vascular rings, which produce a posterior indentation of the esophagus evident on barium swallow, pulmonary artery slings produce an anterior esophageal indentation, which can also be demonstrated on barium swallow. This was first described by Wittenborg et al at Children's Hospital Boston in 1956.[26] Echocardiography can usually confirm the vascular anatomy.

Assessment of the trachea

Because of the high incidence of tracheal anomalies other than simple compression by the sling, it is important to undertake a complete assessment of the trachea in all patients who are diagnosed to have a sling. This should include bronchoscopy (recorded on videotape or DVD) and at least one other mode of imaging to delineate the severity and extent of tracheal stenosis. We generally prefer CT assessment of the trachea, although the role of MRI is currently being defined.[27] CT allows accurate quantitation of the tracheal luminal diameter and area at various levels and demonstrates the presence of complete rings, which will also have been noted at bronchoscopy.[28] A well-penetrated plain chest X-ray is often extremely useful in defining the extent of the tracheal and bronchial stenosis. Bronchography can produce spectacular imaging of tracheal stenoses[29] but is generally reserved for children who are also undergoing angiography for definition of vascular anatomy, if this is not clear from echocardiography alone, or for definition of associated cardiac problems.

MEDICAL MANAGEMENT

General supportive respiratory care should be given before proceeding to surgery. As described for vascular rings, respiratory infection may be difficult to clear completely before surgery because of the difficulty in adequately clearing secretions.

INDICATIONS FOR SURGERY

Because pulmonary artery sling is a rare entity, its natural history remains poorly defined. Fortunately it is extremely rare for the anomaly to be diagnosed in the absence of symptoms because at present it remains unclear if surgery is indicated in the absence of symptoms. In most centers, however, current practice would probably dictate surgical intervention even in the absence of symptoms. Preoperative studies should define whether there is simple compression stenosis of the carinal region, which may be relieved by translocation of the left pulmonary artery; localized anatomic stenosis of the trachea (generally associated with complete tracheal rings in this area), which is best dealt with by tracheal resection and anterior translocation of the left pulmonary artery; or, finally, diffuse severe narrowing of the trachea related to complete tracheal rings, which may necessitate an extensive tracheoplasty procedure in addition to relocation of the left pulmonary artery.

SURGICAL MANAGEMENT

History

In 1954 Potts and associates described the approach to a pulmonary artery sling using a left thoracotomy with division of the left pulmonary artery, followed by translocation anterior to the trachea and reimplantation.[30] Potts performed reimplantation at the original site of origin of the left pulmonary artery, but Hiller and Maclean, in 1957, using the same operation, performed reimplantation into the side of the main pulmonary artery.[31] In this early description of what was to become the traditional operation for pulmonary artery sling, these authors also reported for the first time the complication that was to be commonly seen: namely, occlusion of the left pulmonary artery demonstrated by postoperative angiography.[32,33] Mustard and colleagues recognized the importance of the ligamentum arteriosum in effectively completing a vascular ring as part of this anomaly, and in 1962 they described simple division of the ligament as management of a pulmonary artery sling.[7] This operation has not been widely practiced.

Repair of a pulmonary artery sling through a median sternotomy with reimplantation of the left pulmonary artery (i.e. while the patient is on cardiopulmonary bypass) was described in 1986 by Kirklin and Barratt-Boyes.[34] None of the techniques described up to that time had dealt directly with the associated tracheal stenosis that was often present. These operations were based on the premise that the problem was primarily one of tracheal compression; although this was true in some cases, it was certainly not universally true. Although primary repair of the tracheal anomaly had been suggested previously, it had not been attempted because of fear of early and late tracheal anastomotic problems in the infant. Improved cardiopulmonary bypass techniques (which allowed cumbersome intraoperative airway intubation techniques to be avoided); improved sutures, such as absorbable monofilament polydioxanone; and greater familiarity with microvascular techniques have decreased the risk of tracheal anastomosis in the infant. We initially reported the successful application of cardiopulmonary bypass, tracheal resection, and anastomosis in a 2.6 kg neonate with very severe congenital tracheal stenosis[35] and have subsequently undertaken similar tracheal resections for a wide variety of tracheal problems in infants since the late 1980s.[12,13] Success with this technique led us, in 1989, to apply tracheal resection as an integral part of the repair of pulmonary artery sling when the sling is associated with important localized tracheal stenosis.[36] More recently we have found the slide tracheoplasty technique to be particularly useful for long-segment tracheal stenosis.

Technical considerations

DIVISION AND REIMPLANTATION OF THE LEFT PULMONARY ARTERY

Although the traditional approach has been through a left thoracotomy, we currently prefer to undertake a median sternotomy and use cardiopulmonary bypass (Figure 29.6b). Cardiopulmonary bypass should be undertaken with an ascending aortic arterial cannula and a single straight venous cannula in the right atrium. A nearly full-flow perfusion rate is used, with the heart beating throughout the procedure at a systemic temperature of 32°C to 34°C.

The approach through a median sternotomy with cardiopulmonary bypass has the advantage of allowing complete mobilization of the main and right pulmonary arteries as well as of the left pulmonary artery, thereby decreasing tension on the anastomosis. Furthermore, a side-biting clamp does not have to be applied for the anastomosis, because cardiopulmonary bypass is employed. The left pulmonary artery can be carefully and completely mobilized where it passes around the trachea, allowing maximal length for reimplantation. Care must be taken when dissecting posterior to the trachea, particularly when complete rings are not present, as there may be an intimate association between the left pulmonary artery and the membranous component of the trachea. When complete tracheal rings are present, the dissection is less likely to injure the trachea and in any event it is likely that this segment of trachea will be excised. The vascular anastomosis is constructed with continuous 6/0 or 7/0 Prolene sutures.

SHORT SEGMENT TRACHEAL RESECTION AND ANASTOMOSIS WITH ANTERIOR RELOCATION OF THE LEFT PULMONARY ARTERY

The approach is exactly as described for reimplantation of the left pulmonary artery through a median sternotomy, including the use of cardiopulmonary bypass with a single venous cannula and with the heart beating at a systemic temperature of 32°C to 34°C (Figure 29.7). The aorta is retracted to the left. The main pulmonary artery is traced to the origin of the left pulmonary artery, which is then dissected free where it passes behind the trachea. The stenotic segment of trachea, as defined by preoperative studies, is dissected free. The trachea is divided transversely through the center of the stenotic segment (Figure 29.7a). The left pulmonary artery is brought anteriorly between the two ends of the divided trachea (Figure 29.7b). Serial sections are taken of the two ends of the trachea until a satisfactory luminal area is found; this is often no longer than three to four tracheal rings. This amount of resection allows anastomosis with little tension (Figure 29.7c). It is important not to compromise the amount of resection, thereby leaving important residual stenosis because of concern regarding tension at the anastomosis. In fact up to 50% of the trachea can be resected with direct reanastomosis so long as the trachea and bronchi are widely

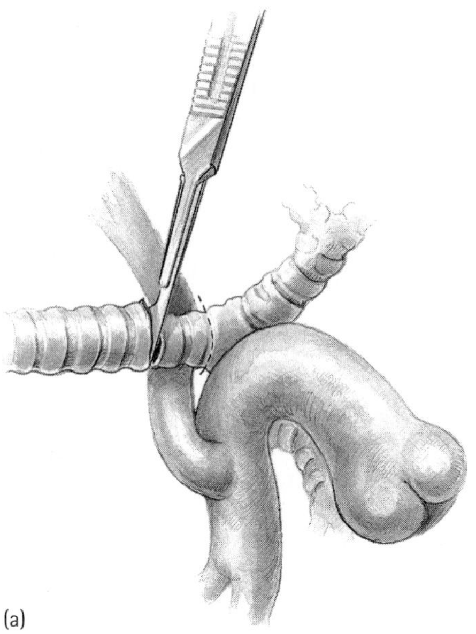

(a)

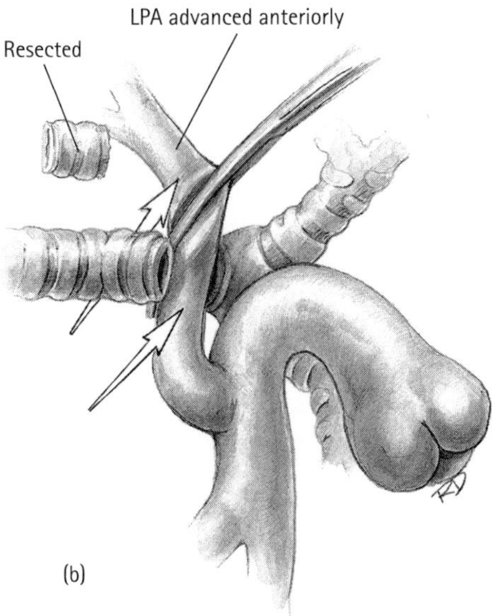

(b)

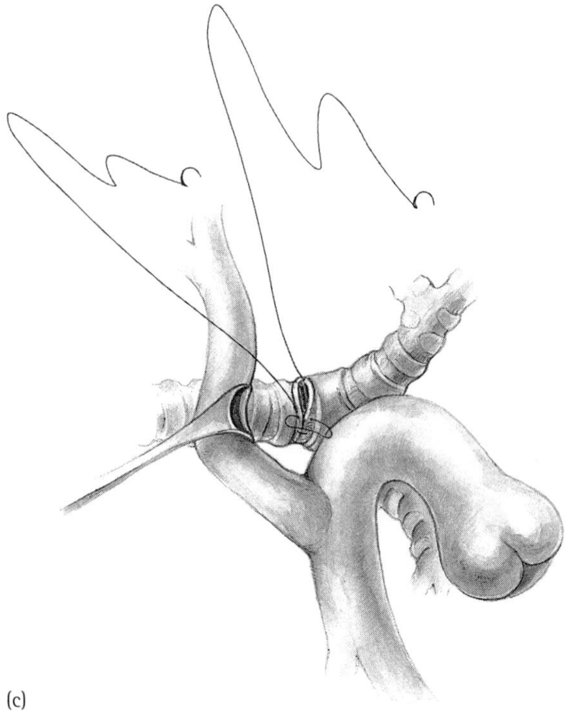

(c)

Figure 29.7 *The recommended technique for surgical management of pulmonary artery sling associated with localized tracheal stenosis usually secondary to the presence of hypoplastic complete tracheal rings. (a) A localized segment of stenotic trachea, e.g. two to three tracheal rings, is excised. (b) The left pulmonary artery is translocated anterior to the trachea. (c) The trachea is repaired by direct anastomosis using continuous polydioxanone or Maxon sutures.*

mobilized, though application of the slide tracheoplasty method has essentially eliminated the need for long-segment resection. The concern regarding devascularization which is important in adults and has been emphasized by Grillo appears not to be relevant in children who have an excellent mediastinal blood supply. Great care of course should be taken during mobilization of the trachea to avoid injury to the left recurrent laryngeal nerve.

The tracheal anastomosis is undertaken with a continuous 5/0 or 6/0 polydioxanone or Maxon suture. (A laboratory study in growing sheep at Children's Hospital Boston suggested that continuous polydioxanone suture results in a greater luminal area at a tracheal anastomosis than the previously recommended technique using interrupted polyglactin [Vicryl] sutures).[37] The anastomosis is not difficult because of the absence of an endotracheal tube through the anastomotic area, the absence of clamps, and the strength of the tracheal cartilages. In fact, the presence of complete tracheal rings simplifies the anastomosis because of the strength of the tracheal cartilages. If a membranous component is present posteriorly in the trachea, great care must be taken in this area allowing the tension to be absorbed by suture bites through cartilage. When the anastomosis has been completed, the trachea is pressurized to 40 cmH_2O to test for air leaks. The anastomosis is then wrapped with a flap of pedicled autologous pericardium, generally based on the right side of the pericardium, anterior to the right phrenic nerve.

The lie of the left pulmonary artery in its new location should be carefully observed. Because it arises more distally than normal, there is some risk of kinking at its origin. In approximately one third of patients with pulmonary artery sling who have undergone tracheal resection, we reimplanted the left pulmonary artery more proximally into the main pulmonary artery. In one case this was related to the fact that the child had absence of the right lung with a marked mediastinal shift to the right.

VERY-LONG-SEGMENT TRACHEAL RECONSTRUCTION WITH REIMPLANTATION OF THE LEFT PULMONARY ARTERY

Stenosis of a very long segment of the trachea in association with a pulmonary artery sling is usually related to the presence of complete tracheal rings over virtually the entire length of the trachea.[38] It is important to recognize that the presence of complete tracheal rings per se is not an indication for surgical intervention in that area of the trachea. Generally, stenosis of the trachea in a young infant does not become critical until the minimal diameter is between 1.5 and 2 mm. Although there is a direct relationship between the length of the stenotic segment and airway resistance, the relationship to luminal diameter is to the fourth power, so this should be the overriding factor in determining need for surgical intervention. The natural history for most airway problems, such as tracheomalacia and minimal compression from a vascular ring, is for improvement with age. Therefore it is relatively rare that it is necessary to intervene surgically for very-long-segment tracheal stenosis.

Several surgical methods have been described previously, including a posteriorly placed longitudinal incision with direct suturing to the anterior wall of the esophagus[39] as well as an anterior longitudinal incision with placement of a longitudinal rib cartilage graft (as is commonly applied for reconstruction of subglottic stenosis).[40] The largest series describing anterior tracheoplasty has been described by Backer and associates, who used a longitudinal incision placed along the full length of the trachea with the child on cardiopulmonary bypass.[38] An autologous pericardial patch was sutured into this anterior defect. The pulmonary artery sling was managed by division of the origin of the left pulmonary artery, with implantation into the main pulmonary artery. The patients were usually ventilated for at least two weeks, with the endotracheal tube functioning as a stent.

SLIDE TRACHEOPLASTY FOR LONG-SEGMENT TRACHEAL STENOSIS

This is our procedure of choice for long-segment tracheal stenosis.[41] The trachea is divided transversely at the midpoint of the narrow segment. If the carina is involved affecting equally the takeoff of the right and left main stem bronchi, a longitudinal incision should be made anteriorly in the distal segment of trachea with the incision extending to the inferior wall of the carina. A longitudinal incision is made on the posterior wall of the proximal trachea. Before beginning the anastomosis the left pulmonary artery is brought forward to its new location anterior to the trachea and is retracted with a silastic vessel loop while the anastomosis is performed. The posterior part of the anastomosis is performed first as this is more difficult. A continuous PDS or Maxon technique is used. The loops are not pulled tight until several bites have been taken so as to decrease the tension on each loop. Because the bites are in cartilage, however, considerable tension can be applied with little risk that the sutures will tear out. The anastomosis is carried inferiorly around the carina and is completed on the right side of the mid-trachea. It is particularly important that the anastomosis be performed as an everting suture line along its entire length. This is best achieved by suturing from the outside of the lumen. If the suture line is inverting it will result in an unacceptable ledge of cartilage within the lumen of the trachea.

If the tracheal stenosis extends into one or other of the right or left main stem bronchi, the slide incisions can be performed laterally such that the inferior incision extends onto the superior surface of the appropriate narrow bronchus. Although a lateral slide is considerably more easy to suture, it is not as effective for symmetrical enlargement of the carina as the anterior/posterior slide as described.

RESULTS OF SURGERY

In 2002, Backer et al summarized their results of surgery for 19 patients with congenital tracheal stenosis is associated with pulmonary artery sling.[42] These patients were part of a cohort of 54 infants with complete tracheal rings and congenital tracheal stenosis who underwent surgery at Children's Memorial Hospital in Chicago between 1982 and 2001. All procedures were performed with the use of cardiopulmonary bypass. A number of different procedures were performed including pericardial tracheoplasty, tracheal autograft, tracheal resection and slide tracheoplasty. The latter two procedures had shorter periods of hospitalization relative to the two former procedures. The authors suggest that tracheal resection should be limited to patients with eight or fewer rings of tracheal stenosis. Also in 2002, Grillo et al[41] described the application of slide tracheoplasty in eight pediatric patients and in three patients who underwent resection and anastomosis for congenital tracheal stenosis. Three of these patients had an associated pulmonary artery sling. There were no deaths. All patients were extubated within eight days of surgery. Long-term airway growth was satisfactory after slide tracheoplasty in four infants and small children. In 1999 Cotter et al from Children's Hospital Boston[43] described 17 infants with congenital tracheal stenosis who underwent surgery between 1986 and 1996. Six patients underwent resection and anastomosis and eight patients underwent tracheoplasty.

There was one death. The authors concluded that short segment (less than five rings) tracheal stenosis is best managed by resection and reanastomosis while longer segment tracheal stenosis can be managed by slide tracheoplasty or the castellation technique.

INNOMINATE ARTERY COMPRESSION OF THE TRACHEA

Innominate artery compression of the trachea was first described by Gross and Neuhauser from Children's Hospital Boston in 1951.[44] In this anomaly tracheal compression occurs at the level of the thoracic inlet because of a more distal than usual origin of the innominate artery. As the innominate artery passes rightward and superiorly it compresses the anterior and leftward aspect of the trachea. The trachea is usually malacic at this point over a distance of at least 2–3 rings.

Innominate artery compression of the trachea causes stridor during infancy. During respiratory infections the child may have an acute increase in stridor which may be sufficiently severe to cause the child to have apneic or syncopal episodes. Breathing is particularly noisy during feeding and crying but there is usually no difficulty with swallowing.

The diagnosis of innominate artery compression of the trachea is made by a combination of bronchoscopy with CT or MRI. At bronchscopy there is characteristic pulsatile compression of the anterior and leftward aspect of the trachea at the level of the thoracic inlet.

The treatment of innominate artery compression of the trachea as first described by Gross[44] consists of an aortopexy procedure which lifts both the arch of the aorta as well as the innominate artery origin in an anterior and leftwards direction. Approach is through a limited left anterolateral thoracotomy through the second intercostal space. The left lobe of the thymus which is often very large is excised. The aorta and innominate artery are not separated from underlying tissue. In fact adventitial tissue between the great vessels and the trachea is probably helpful in lifting the tracheal lumen open. Three or four horizontal mattress Teflon pledgetted 3/0 Ethibond sutures are placed partial thickness in the aortic arch and origin of the innominate artery similar to an aortic cannulation purse-string suture in depth. The curved needles are straightened and are then passed through the second costal cartilage and leftward edge of the sternum. When tied these sutures can pull the arch and innominate artery a considerable distance anteriorly and leftwards. Bronchoscopy should be performed before and after the procedure and usually documents an extremely impressive improvement in the appearance of the tracheal lumen. The child can be extubated either immediately following the procedure or within hours of arriving in the intensive care unit. There is usually a dramatic decrease in the amount of stridor though because of long standing tracheomalacia the child will continue to experience stridor and an exacerbation of symptoms during respiratory infections. Beyond infancy as the tracheal cartilages improve in strength symptoms usually resolve. In fact some have argued that the majority of patients with innominate artery compression should be managed conservatively[45] but in patients who have suffered syncopal or apneic episodes this approach carries significant risk.

REFERENCES

1. Edwards JE. Anomalies of the derivatives of the aortic arch syndrome. *Med Clin North Am* 1948; **32**:925.
2. Stewart J, Kincaid O, Edwards J. *An Atlas of Vascular Rings and Related Malformations of the Aortic Arch System.* Springfield IL, Charles C Thomas, 1964, pp 3–155.
3. Horvitz HR. Genetic control of programmed cell death in the nematode Caenorhabditis elegans. *Cancer Res* 1999; **59**:1701s–1760s.
4. Molin DG, DeRuiter MC, Wisse LJ et al. Altered apoptosis pattern during pharyngeal arch artery remodelling is associated with aortic arch malformations in Tgfbeta2 knock-out mice. *Cardiovasc Res* 2002; **56**:312–322.
5. Hiruma T, Hirakow R. Formation of the pharyngeal arch arteries in the chick embryo. Observations of corrosion casts by scanning electron microscopy. *Anat Embryol (Berl)* 1995; **191**:415–423.
6. Ekstrom G, Sandblom P. Double aortic arch. *Acta Chir Scan* 1951; **102**:183.
7. Mustard WT, Trimble AW, Trusler GA. Mediastinal vascular anomalies causing tracheal and esophageal compression and obstruction in childhood. *Can Med Assoc J* 1962; **87**:1301–1311.
8. Berman W, Yabek SM, Dillon I, Neal JF, Ake B, Burnstein J. Vascular ring due to left aortic arch and right descending aorta. *Circulation* 1981; **63**:458–460.
9. Godtfredsen J, Wennevold A, Efsen F, Lauridsen P. Natural history of vascular ring with clinical manifestations. A follow-up study of 11 unoperated cases. *Scan J Thorac Cardiovasc Surg* 1977; **11**:75–77.
10. Singer ST, Fellows KE, Jonas RA. Double aortic arch with bilateral coarctations. *Am J Cardiol* 1988; **61**:196–197.
11. Neuhauser EBD. The roentgen diagnosis of double aortic arch and other anomalies of the great vessels. *Am J Roentgenol* 1946; **56**:1.
12. Healy GB, Schuster SR, Jonas RA, McGill TJ. Correction of segmental tracheal stenosis in children. *Ann Otol Rhinl Laryngol* 1988; **97**:444–447.
13. Jonas RA. Invited letter concerning: Tracheal operations in infancy. *J Thorac Cardiovasc Surg* 1990; **100**:316.
14. Gross RE. Surgical relief for tracheal obstruction from a vascular ring. *N Engl J Med* 1945; **233**:586–592.
15. Gross RE, Ware PF. The surgical significance of aortic arch anomalies. *Surg Gynecol Obstet* 1946; **83**:435.
16. Burke RP, Chang AC. Video-assisted thoracoscopic division of a vascular ring in an infant: a new operative technique. *J Card Surg* 1993; **8**:537–540.
17. Backer CL, Ilbawi MN, Idriss FS, DeLEon SY. Vascular anomalies causing tracheoesophageal compression. Review of experience in children. *J Thorac Cardiovasc Surg* 1989; **97**:725–731.
18. Cordovilla Zurdo G, Cabo Salvador J, Sanz Galeote E, Moreno Granados F, Alvarez Diaz F. [Vascular rings of aortic origin: the surgical experience in 43 cases] *Rev Esp Cardiol* 1994; **47**:468–475.
19. Anand R, Dooley KJ, Williams WH, Vincent RN. Follow-up of surgical correction of vascular anomalies causing tracheobronchial compression. *Pediatr Cardiol* 1994; **15**:58–61.

20. van Son JA, Julsrud PR, Hagler DJ et al. Surgical treatment of vascular rings: the Mayo Clinic experience. *Mayo Clin Proc* 1993; **68**:1056–1063.
21. Bakker DA, Berger RM, Witsenburg M, Bogers AJ. Vascular rings: a rare cause of common respiratory symptoms. *Acta Paediatr* 1999; **88**:947–952.
22. Burke RP, Wernovsky G, van der Velde M, Hansen D, Castaneda AR. Video-assisted thoracoscopic surgery for congenital heart disease. *J Thorac Cardiovasc Surg* 1995; **109**:499–507.
23. Wolman IJ. Congenital stenosis of the trachea. *Am J Dis Child* 1941; **61**:1263.
24. Jue KL, Raghib G, Amplatz K, Adams P, Edwards JE. Anomalous origin of the left pulmonary artery from the right pulmonary artery. Report of 2 cases and review of the literature. *AJR* 1965; **95**:598.
25. Berdon WE, Baker DH, Wung JT et al. Complete cartilage ring tracheal stenosis associated with anomalous left pulmonary artery: The ring-sling complex. *Radiol* 1984; **152**:57–64.
26. Wittenborg MH, Tantiwongse T, Rosenberg BF. Anomalous course of left pulmonary artery with respiratory obstruction. *Radiology* 1956; **67**:339.
27. Soler R, Rodriguez E, Requejo I, Fernandez R, Raposo I. Magnetic resonance imaging of congenital abnormalities of the thoracic aorta. *Eur Radiol* 1998; **8**:540–546.
28. van Son JA, Julsrud PR, Hagler DJ, Sim EK, Puga FJ, Schaff HV, Danielson GK. Imaging strategies for vascular rings. *Ann Thorac Surg* 1994; **57**:604–610.
29. Capitanio MA, Ramos R, Kirkpatrick JA. Pulmonary sling. Roentgen Observations. *Am J Roentgenol Radium Ther Nucl Med* 1971; **112**:28–34.
30. Potts WJ, Holinger PH, Rosenblum AH. Anomalous left pulmonary artery causing obstruction to right main bronchus. Report of a case. *JAMA* 1954; **155**:1409.
31. Hiller HG, Maclean AD. Pulmonary artery ring. *Acta Radiol* 1957; **48**:434.
32. Castaneda AR. Pulmonary artery sling. *Ann Thorac Surg* 1979; **28**:210–211.
33. Sade RM, Rosenthal AM, Fellows K, Castaneda AR. Pulmonary artery sling. *J Thorac Cardiovasc Surg* 1975; **69**:333–346.
34. Kirklin JW, Barratt-Boyes BG. *Cardiac Surgery*. New York, John Wiley, 1986.
35. Benca JF, Hickey PR, Dornbusch JN, Koka BV, McGill TJ, Jonas RA. Ventilatory management assisted by cardiopulmonary bypass for distal tracheal reconstruction in a neonate. *Anesthesiology* 1988; **68**:270–271.
36. Jonas RA, Spevak PJ, McGill T, Castaneda AR. Pulmonary artery sling: Primary repair by tracheal resection in infancy. *J Thorac Cardiovasc Surg* 1989; **97**:548–550.
37. Freidman E, Perez-Atayde A, Silvera M, Jonas RA. Growth of tracheal anastomoses in lambs: Comparison of PDS and Vicryl suture and interrupted and continuous techniques. *J Thorac Cardiovasc Surg* 1990; **100**:188–193.
38. Backer CL, Idriss FS, Holinger LD, Mavroudis C. Pulmonary artery sling: Results of surgical repair in infancy. *J Thorac Cardiovasc Surg* 1992; **103**:683–691.
39. Ein SH, Friedberg J, Williams WG, Rearon B, Barker GA, Mancer K. Tracheoplasty – a new operation for complete congenital tracheal stenosis. *J Pediatr Surg* 1982; **17**:872–878.
40. Oue T, Kamata S, Usui N, Okuyama H, Nose K, Okada A. Histo-pathologic changes after tracheobronchial reconstruction with costal cartilage graft for congenital tracheal stenosis. *J Pediatr Surg* 2001; **36**:329–333.
41. Grillo HC, Wright CD, Vlahakes GJ, MacGillvray TE. Management of congenital tracheal stenosis by means of slide tracheoplasty or resection and reconstruction, with long-term follow-up of growth after slide tracheoplasty. *J Thorac Cardiovasc Surg* 2002; **123**:145–152.
42. Backer CL, Mavroudis C, Holinger LD. Repair of congenital tracheal stenosis. *Semin Thorac Cardiovasc Surg Pediatr Card Surg Annu* 2002; **5**:173–186.
43. Cotter CS, Jones DT, Nuss RC, Jonas R. Management of distal tracheal stenosis. *Arch Otolaryngol Head Neck Surg* 1999; **125**:325–328.
44. Gross RE, Neuhauser EBD. Compression of the trachea or esophagus by vascular anomalies. *Pediatrics* 1951; **7**:69–83.
45. Fearon B, Shortreed R. Compression tracheo-bronchique par anomalies vascularies congenitales chez l'enfant. Syndrome d'apnee. *Ann Otol* 1963; **72**:949–969.

30

Anomalies of the coronary arteries

INTRODUCTION

Various abnormalities of the coronary arteries can be important complicating factors for a number of the congenital cardiac anomalies. For example, pulmonary atresia with intact ventricular septum is frequently complicated by coronary artery fistulas with or without coronary artery stenoses. Transposition of the great arteries can be complicated by unusual coronary ostial distribution and branching patterns. Patients with hypoplastic left heart syndrome who have the anatomical variant of aortic atresia with mitral stenosis also have a high incidence of coronary artery fistulas to the left ventricle. At least 5% of patients with tetralogy of Fallot have an anomalous anterior descending coronary artery arising from the right coronary artery. These various coronary problems are covered in the relevant chapters for the major anomaly. This chapter will focus on anomalies in which the coronary artery problem is the principal lesion.

ANOMALOUS LEFT CORONARY ARTERY FROM THE PULMONARY ARTERY

Anomalous left coronary artery from the pulmonary artery differs from almost all other congenital cardiac anomalies in that there is often profound depression of myocardial function at the time of initial presentation and this cannot be reversed by any resuscitative measures. In the past it was frequently confused with cardiomyopathy but in the current era with the availability of color Doppler imaging this should be unusual.

Anomalous left coronary artery from the pulmonary artery (ALCAPA) is a rare lesion with an estimated incidence of between 1 in 30 000 and 1 in 300 000.[1] It is not a duct dependent lesion in the sense that ductal closure is inevitably followed by death but nevertheless it is frequently lethal in early infancy with some reports suggesting a mortality rate as high as 90% in the first year of life.[2] Before color Doppler was available, diagnosis even with excellent quality two-dimensional imaging was difficult. False dropout often suggested normal aortic origin of the left coronary artery and there also could be misinterpretation of the transverse sinus as the left main coronary artery leading to failure of early diagnosis in many cases.[3] Fortunately, surgical advances in the management of neonatal coronary arteries make this an eminently correctable lesion as long as surgery is performed sufficiently early in life.

EMBRYOLOGY

Normal development of the coronary arteries requires a connection between buds that arise from the aortic sinuses of Valsalva and the arterial plexus which forms epicardially. The epicardial arterial plexus communicates with the intramyocardial plexus, which is derived from venous structures. Buds also grow out from the pulmonary trunk as part of normal development, but these usually regress. In the case of ALCAPA, there is a failure of normal communication between the left aortic bud and the epicardial arterial plexus.[4]

ANATOMY

The anomalous ostium of the left main coronary artery can be situated almost anywhere in the main pulmonary artery or in its proximal branches. The most common location is the leftward and posterior sinus of the pulmonary root (Figure 30.1a) followed by the rightward and posterior sinus, the posterior wall of the main pulmonary artery trunk, and the origin of the right pulmonary artery posteriorly.[5] An anteriorly placed origin of the anomalous coronary from the main pulmonary artery is exceedingly rare.

There is often though not always development of collateral vessels, particularly between the right coronary artery and the left anterior descending coronary through the circle of Vieussens. In older patients, these vessels can become very dilated. There have been several reports of a conal coronary artery arising anteriorly from the aorta, separate from the right coronary artery and giving rise to collateral vessels to the anomalous left coronary artery system.[6] There may be fibrosis and scarring of the left ventricle depending on the age of the patient, degree of dominance of the left coronary artery, and amount of collateral formation.[5] Endocardial fibroelastosis is prominent in some patients,[7] and the left ventricle is often very dilated, sometimes massively, unlike in patients with obstructive left heart problems who have endocardial fibroelastosis. Left ventricular dilatation and papillary muscle dysfunction are responsible for the mitral regurgitation that is frequently present. Structural abnormalities of the mitral valve are unusual.

ASSOCIATED ANOMALIES

The association of ALCAPA with other anomalies is particularly rare, although such an association may be functionally important. For example, surgical ligation of a persistently patent ductus arteriosus[8] or closure of a ventricular septal defect[7] (both of which direct more oxygenated blood to the ALCAPA) without preoperative recognition of the associated ALCAPA is likely to lead to a fatal outcome. ALCAPA has also been reported in association with tetralogy of Fallot[9] and pulmonary valve stenosis.[7]

PATHOPHYSIOLOGY AND CLINICAL FEATURES

In 1964, Edwards[10] proposed the pathophysiologic mechanism that accounts for the common clinical presentation of young infants at approximately six weeks of age, a presentation that includes evidence of angina associated with feeding or an established infarct, massive left ventricular dilatation, and mitral regurgitation. During in-utero development, pulmonary artery pressure and aortic pressure are similar because of ductal patency, and there is adequate perfusion of the anomalous left coronary artery, albeit at a slightly reduced oxygen saturation. Following ductal closure postnatally, pulmonary artery pressure and, consequently, left coronary artery perfusion progressively decline as pulmonary vascular resistance decreases. Normally during the first weeks of life, hyperplasia and hypertrophy of myocytes, as well as coronary angiogenesis, are able to maintain appropriate wall stress as the left ventricle grows. With inadequate coronary perfusion, these things cannot happen, so the left ventricle becomes progressively dilated and thin walled.[11] Left ventricular dilatation, as well as papillary muscle dysfunction or infarction, result in functional mitral regurgitation. These events are modified by the relative dominance of the right and left coronary arteries, as well as the rapidity with which collateral vessels form between the two coronary trees.

If the infant survives this early crisis, there may be continuing collateral development that eventually results in an important left to right shunt secondary to retrograde flow through the anomalous coronary into the main pulmonary artery. Under such circumstances, diagnosis becomes more simple as color flow mapping or angiography demonstrates flow into the pulmonary artery, and an oxygen stepup can be measured. Such patients may be asymptomatic for several years, but as teenagers or young adults they may suffer from arrhythmias, angina, or sudden death.

DIAGNOSTIC STUDIES

The young infant who is brought to the cardiologist with dilated left ventricular cardiomyopathy must undergo exhaustive exclusion of ALCAPA. Often there is classic electrocardiographic evidence of left ventricular ischemia and infarction. Mitral regurgitation, as shown by two-dimensional echocardiography, can be massive, as is the left ventricular end-diastolic volume. For example in a group of six infants

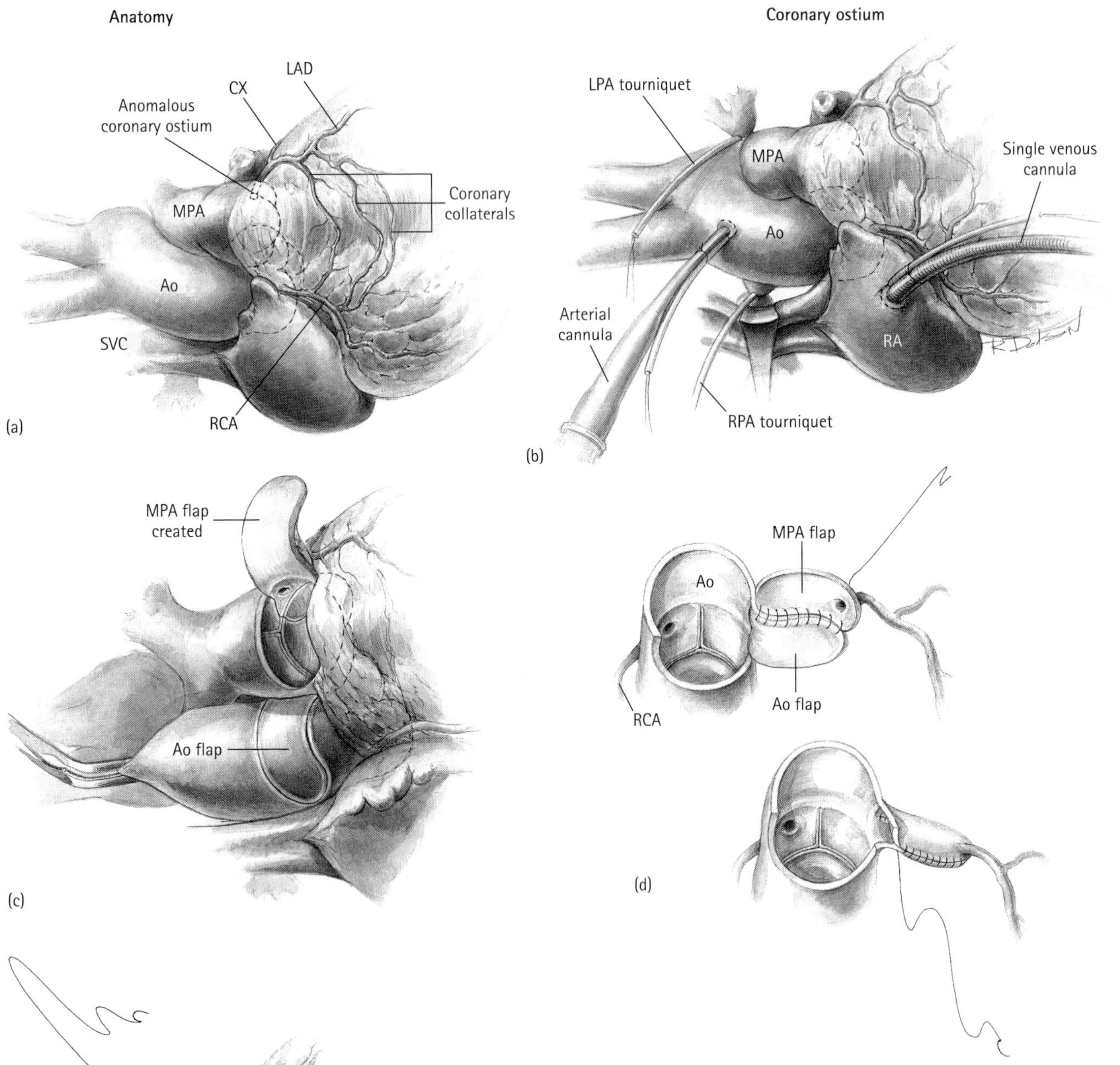

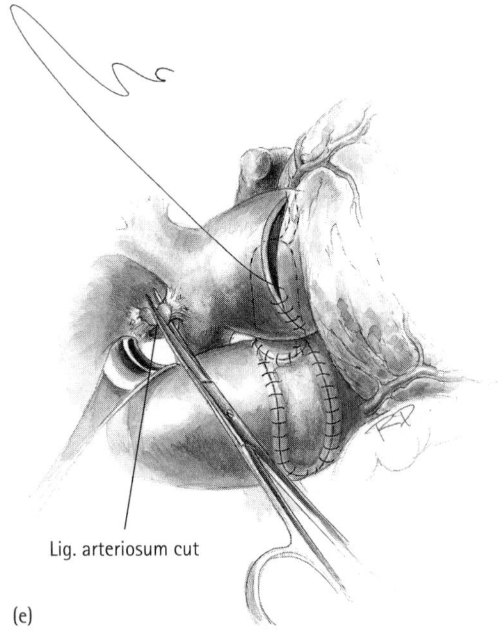

Figure 30.1 *(a) An anomalous left coronary artery from the pulmonary artery most commonly arises from the leftward and posterior sinus of the pulmonary root. In time coronary collateral vessels become prominent and cross the infundibulum of the right ventricle from the right coronary system to the left coronary system. (b) A very important step in the surgical management of anomalous left coronary artery from the pulmonary artery is to tighten tourniquets around the right and left pulmonary artery immediately after commencing bypass. This will prevent a steal of blood from both the right and left coronary systems into the pulmonary artery. It will also reduce left heart distention, though placement of a left ventricular vent is also important. (c) In order to avoid excessive tension on the reimplanted left coronary artery flaps can be developed from the anterior main pulmonary artery wall and ascending aorta as indicated. (d) The aortic and pulmonary artery flaps are sutured together to form a tube extension for the left coronary artery which is thereby implanted in the ascending aorta. (e) It is often preferable to completely transect the main pulmonary artery to facilitate reconstruction. The ductus or ligament is divided and the branch pulmonary arteries are mobilized as for an arterial switch procedure. The main pulmonary artery is reconstructed by direct anastomosis.*

described by Rein and coworkers,[11] the mean left ventricular end-diastolic volume was four times normal. Various indices of left ventricular function are profoundly depressed. As noted above visualization of the anomalous ostium may be difficult and may be complicated by false dropout when the pulmonary artery lies close to the aorta suggesting aortic origin. There also may be misinterpretation of the transverse pericardial sinus as a left main coronary artery passing posterior to the main pulmonary artery. However, modern color Doppler should allow accurate diagnosis of the anomalous ostium. Even if there is false dropout by imaging there should be no evidence of antegrade flow from the aorta. Color Doppler will also frequently but not always demonstrate retrograde flow from the anomalous coronary into the pulmonary artery. It should rarely if ever be necessary to perform cardiac catheterization to confirm the diagnosis. These babies are frequently severely compromised by very poor ventricular function. Invasive diagnostic cardiac catheterization will further compromise the condition of these children before surgery and should be avoided if at all possible.

MEDICAL AND INTERVENTIONAL THERAPY

There is no place for medical therapy for this anomaly. Diagnosis should be made as early in life as possible followed by surgery as soon as it is practical. Even in asymptomatic older children and adults the risk of a gradual deterioration of left ventricular function as well as the risk of sudden death justify creation of a dual coronary system following diagnosis.

Like medical therapy there is no role for interventional therapy in the management of anomalous left coronary artery from the pulmonary artery.

INDICATIONS FOR SURGERY

The diagnosis alone should be the indication for surgery in all patients with the aim to preserve as much myocardium as possible. It is possible that an extremely small subset of patients with profoundly depressed ventricular function and massive mitral regurgitation may be better served by heart transplantation than by corrective surgery. With early diagnosis and application of the techniques described below this should rarely if ever be necessary.

SURGICAL MANAGEMENT

History of surgery

Many surgical techniques have been described for both palliation and correction of ALCAPA after the first description of this anomaly by Bland and coworkers in 1933.[12] The aim of early palliative operations was to increase pulmonary artery pressure and thereby increase coronary perfusion pressure. Banding of the main pulmonary artery, as well as creation of an aortopulmonary window, were attempted. Another palliative approach was to decrease the myocardial steal. This was achieved by ligation of the anomalous left coronary artery, although there was a tendency for the ligated coronary to recanalize.[13] Physiologically corrective techniques have included creation of a dual coronary system with bypass grafting using the left subclavian artery, left common carotid artery, internal mammary artery and saphenous vein.

In 1979, Takeuchi and colleagues described creation of an aortopulmonary window and an intrapulmonary artery baffle to direct aortic blood to the anomalous ostium.[14] However, this procedure was subsequently found to suffer from a number of late complications and has been abandoned. The increasing experience with manipulation of neonatal coronary arteries as part of the neonatal arterial switch procedure has led most centers to use an anatomically and physiologically corrective procedure, i.e. direct reimplantation of the left coronary artery to the aorta.[15]

Technical considerations

ALCAPA is one of the few congenital heart anomalies in which myocardial function is likely to be profoundly compromised preoperatively, before the additional insult of intraoperative myocardial ischemia. In addition, the unusual anatomic and physiologic circumstances require that some extremely important changes be made in conducting cardiopulmonary bypass as well as in the techniques of myocardial protection. However, to the child's advantage, the postoperative circulation will be essentially a normal, in series, biventricular circulation, albeit with a variable degree of mitral regurgitation. It may well be appropriate in the case of the most severely compromised children to plan an elective period of postoperative left ventricular assistance with whatever system the surgical team is most familiar.

Approach is by a median sternotomy, with high arterial cannulation of the ascending aorta and a single venous cannula in the right atrium. Immediately after commencing bypass, the tourniquets that have been placed around the right and left pulmonary arteries should be tightened (Figure 30.1b). This very important step was first described relatively recently and serves several important functions.[16] First, there is always some collateral flow between the two coronary systems. If runoff is allowed into the pulmonary arteries which are decompressed by the act of going on bypass, there will be a steal away from and therefore compromised perfusion of both the right and left coronary systems. In addition, blood passing into the left coronary system and pulmonary artery will pass through the pulmonary veins into the left atrium and left ventricle. The compromised left ventricle will be unable to cope with this left heart return, resulting in serious left heart distention as well as pulmonary edema. Distention of the heart must be assidiously avoided during the procedure. A vent should be inserted through the right superior pulmonary vein across the mitral valve into the left ventricle. If there is any difficulty achieving this an alternative is to amputate the tip of the left atrial appendage.

During cooling to deep hypothermia the main pulmonary artery and its branches should be mobilized after carefully visualizing the external course of the anomalous coronary. At a rectal and tympanic membrane temperature of less than 18°C bypass flow is reduced to 50 ml/kg per minute and the ascending aorta is clamped. Cardioplegia solution is infused into the root of the aorta only. Although some have recommended simultaneous infusion of cardioplegia solution into the pulmonary artery root, we have observed satisfactory blanching of the left ventricle using aortic delivery of cardioplegia only. In fact, the pulmonary artery root is soon seen to fill with clear cardioplegia solution and equilibrate with aortic root pressure, the latter phenomenon also having been observed during the cooling phase on bypass. This anomaly may also represent an appropriate situation for retrograde infusion of cardioplegia solution into the coronary sinus. If adequate visualization is not achieved at any time during the procedure because of collateral return, deep hypothermic circulatory arrest may be established.

CORONARY REIMPLANTATION

The surgeon should have carefully studied the preoperative echocardiogram so as to have a clear idea of the exact location of the anomalous ostium relative to the pulmonary valve. If the ostium is close to the aortic side of the pulmonary artery it may be possible to simply rotate the button and with an appropriate short aortic flap (appropriately based to minimize rotation of the coronary button) proceed to direct reimplantation. However, the ostium often lies towards the leftward edge of the main pulmonary artery and is therefore a considerable distance, i.e. the width of the main pulmonary artery from the ascending aorta. The ostium is also not uncommonly below the tops of the commissures of the pulmonary valve. Therefore flaps of aortic and pulmonary artery wall should be developed in order to allow a tension free anastomosis to the aorta using a coronary extension developed from the aortic and pulmonary artery flaps (Figure 30.1c). The reconstructed left main coronary artery will run posterior to the reconstructed main pulmonary artery. An initial transverse incision in the main pulmonary artery is made a millimeter or two above the anticipated level of the anomalous ostium. A long flap of anterior main pulmonary artery wall is developed, similar to the flap that used to be used for the Takeuchi procedure (Figure 30.1c). However, for the reimplantation procedure a button is excised. If the ostium lies below the top of the leftward commissure of the pulmonary valve it may be necessary to detach this commissure and subsequently to reattach it to reconstruct the pulmonary valve. It is generally best to divide the main pulmonary artery completely at the level that the flap has been developed in order to minimize distortion of the pulmonary artery following reconstruction (as is also the case for truncus arteriosus). A flap of aortic wall based on the leftward and posterior aspect of the ascending aorta and consisting of the anterior wall of the ascending aorta is developed and rotated 180° leftward. This will form the posterior wall of the coronary artery extension. It is important that the initial transverse incision be the higher of the two so that the tops of the commissures of the aortic valve are identified and carefully preserved. The two flaps, i.e. the anterior pulmonary artery wall flap and the posterior aortic wall flap, are sutured together using continuous 7/0 Prolene (Figure 30.1d). It should not be necessary to mobilize any more than 2–3 mm of the actual left main coronary artery, which is frequently surrounded by enlarged venous and arterial collateral vessels that can be an important source of bleeding if they are divided as part of the mobilization.

PULMONARY ARTERY RECONSTRUCTION

In the neonate it is generally possible to reconstruct the divided main pulmonary artery by direct reanastomosis. This necessitates double suture ligation and division of the ductus as well as mobilization of the branch pulmonary arteries as for an arterial switch procedure. A direct anastomosis is fashioned using continuous 6/0 Prolene (Figure 30.1e). If a pulmonary valve commissure has been detached it must be resuspended using fine 7/0 Prolene sutures.

Careful venting of the left heart throughout the rewarming period is just as important as during the cooling phase. When cardiac action is re-established, generally coincident with the administration of calcium, venting may be cautiously discontinued, with monitoring of left atrial pressure. Appropriate inotropic support, generally with dopamine, should already be established. If the left ventricle is unable to handle the left heart return on bypass, as indicated by a progressive increase in left atrial pressure, venting should be re-established, and arrangements should be made to assist the left ventricle. Likewise, if weaning from bypass is only possible with very high levels of inotropic support and high left atrial pressure, left ventricular assistance should be seriously considered.

If extracorporeal membrane oxygenation (ECMO) is used for left ventricular assistance it is essential that a left ventricular vent be connected into the venous drainage system to ensure that the left heart remains decompressed. Remarkable improvement in left ventricular function can be observed within 48–72 hours at which time the left heart vent can be clamped and then removed. Following a further period of general support with right atrial to aortic ECMO the patient can gradually be weaned from ECMO and support discontinued. In general this should be possible within five to six days at most.

RESULTS OF SURGERY

The technique of repair of the anomalous left coronary artery by reimplantation in the aorta was introduced by Neches et al in 1974.[17] In 1995 Turley et al[15] described a number of innovative methods for achieving aortic implantation of the anomalous left coronary artery in 11 patients. There were no operative or late deaths. Follow-up for a mean period of 46 months revealed no new angina or infarction, improved ventricular function and decreased mitral regurgitation. Patency in the reconstructed coronary systems was demonstrated by echocardiography and angiography. The authors conclude – as noted in the title of their article – that 'aortic implantation is possible in all cases of anomalous origin of the left coronary artery to the pulmonary artery'.

In 2003, Azakie et al from the Hospital for Sick Children in Toronto, Canada[18] described the results of aortic implantation in 47 patients with anomalous left coronary artery. Median age at repair was 7.7 months. Hospital survival was 92%. Five children required ECMO postoperatively for a median of four days. The mean follow-up was 4.7 years with no late deaths. Freedom from reoperation was 93% at 10 years. At late follow-up echocardiography demonstrated significant improvement in mean ejection fraction from 33% preoperatively to 64% postoperatively. Normalization of ejection fraction and left ventricular function occurred within one year of repair. Improvement in mitral regurgitation lagged behind normalization of ejection fraction and left ventricular dilation.

Isomatsu et al from Tokyo Women's Medical College[19] also described excellent results with direct aortic implantation. Among 29 patients operated on between 1982 and 2000, 19 had direct aortic implantation and 10 had the Takeuchi procedure. Actuarial survival was 93% at 10 years. Left ventricular shortening z score was not normal at discharge but was normalized at a mean follow-up of 100 months.

Others reports have also documented excellent results, including Backer et al who described 16 consecutive children undergoing aortic implantation between 1989 and 1999.[20] No child required a ventricular assist device or ECMO. All patients survived.

Ando et al from the Cleveland Clinic[21] described 12 patients who underwent aortic implantation using a trap door flap method from the ascending aorta to reduce tension on the anastomosis as originally described by Turley et al.[15] There were no deaths among 12 patients operated on at a median age of 3.9 years.

Recovery of ventricular function

In 1987, Rein et al from Children's Hospital Boston[11] published the first comprehensive report demonstrating recovery of ventricular function following repair of anomalous left coronary artery. In patients who were able to achieve a true coronary circulation, almost all patients recovered to a normal end diastolic volume reaching near normal values by 7–22 months after surgery. In a follow-up report from Children's Hospital, Schwartz et al[22] analysed recovery of left ventricular function in greater depth. The authors concluded that the degree of preoperative mitral regurgitation was predictive of outcome whereas the severity of preoperative cardiac dysfunction and ventricular dilation were not. Similar results were described by Jin et al from Berlin.[23] However, Lambert et al from Paris[24] reviewed 39 consecutive patients with anomalous coronary artery, 34 of whom had direct aortic implantation with a 13% hospitality mortality. At last follow-up at a mean of 40 months postoperatively left ventricular shortening fraction was normal in 86% but left ventricular dilation persisted in 73% of patients and 39% had abnormal regional wall motion of the left ventricle. It is important to note that the median age at surgery in this series was 18.5 months.

Use of ventricular assist device

In 1999, del Nido et al from Children's Hospital Boston[25] described 31 children who underwent repair of anomalous left coronary artery between 1987 and 1996. Twenty six patients were infants, all but two of whom had severe left ventricular dysfunction and eight had moderate to severe mitral regurgitation. Seven patients were placed on mechanical left ventricular support using a centrifugal pump with support ranging from 2.2 to 71 hours. Two of the seven patients died. However, all five survivors had significant improvement in left ventricular function though two required late mitral valve repair. In contrast to this experience, Backer et al[20] emphasize that ventricular assist devices were not required for their series of 16 patients.

Associated anomalies

There are a number of case reports in which an anomalous left coronary artery from the pulmonary artery has been associated with other anomalies. For example, McMahon et al[26] described an association of anomalous left coronary artery with aortopulmonary window and interrupted aortic arch. Similar to the report by Kilic et al[27] who described a patient with patent ductus arteriosus and pulmonary hypertension, it is apparent that associated anomalies that raise pulmonary artery pressure and particularly those that also increase pulmonary artery saturation are likely to be associated with an improved natural history relative to patients with normal pulmonary artery pressure and saturation.

One particularly unusual and challenging variation of anomalous left coronary artery was described by Barbero-Marcial from Brazil.[28] The authors describe an intramural course of the anomalous left coronary artery after its origin from the pulmonary artery. This rare variation requires particularly careful preoperative diagnosis and surgical management.

Complications following the Takeuchi procedure

The innovative Takeuchi procedure[14] was first described in 1979. Although early results with this procedure were encouraging[29] many groups including our own have found a high incidence of late problems including supravalvar pulmonary stenosis and baffle leaks.

Review of results

Dodge-Khatami et al[30] have published a comprehensive review of the results of surgery for anomalous left coronary artery from the pulmonary artery in 2002.

CONCLUSION

The regenerative capacity of immature myocardium by hyperplasia in the first months of life mandates early diagnosis and establishment of a dual coronary system for ALCAPA. Coronary artery translocation with aortic implantation is today the procedure of choice. Technical details to optimize myocardial protection are of paramount importance to the success of surgery for this rare anomaly.

CORONARY FISTULAS

Isolated congenital coronary fistulas are exceedingly rare. Today they are usually dealt with in the interventional catheterization laboratory. However, occasionally large fistulas have a difficult origin and may present particular challenges to the interventional catheterization team and may require surgical management.

PATHOLOGIC ANATOMY

Isolated fistulas arise from both the right and left coronary arteries, probably with similar frequency, but terminate much more commonly in the right heart or pulmonary artery than in the left heart (Figure 30.2a,b). Lowe and associates[31] reported drainage to the right ventricle in 39%, to the right atrium in 33% and to the pulmonary artery in 20%; only 2% drained to the left ventricle. In a report in 1983 from the Texas Heart Institute,[32] 58 patients with coronary artery fistulas were described. In five, the fistulas drained into the right atrium from an anomalous artery to the sinus node. In 84% of patients there was a single fistula, while the remainder had multiple fistulas. Thirty seven patients had coronary artery fistulas as their only anomaly, while 21 had associated lesions, including coronary artery disease in nine, mitral regurgitation in two, aortic stenosis in two, and double outlet right ventricle, pulmonary stenosis, patent ductus arteriosus, tricuspid regurgitation, aortic stenosis with mitral regurgitation, and mitral valve prolapse each occurring in one patient.

Coronary artery fistulas are an important component of pulmonary atresia with intact ventricular septum, in which they can be associated with proximal coronary artery stenoses. In this setting, the fistulas may provide the only blood supply (derived from the hypertensive right ventricle) to a significant portion of the left ventricle. Sauer and coworkers[33] suggested that a similar situation may be present in children with mitral stenosis and aortic atresia as part of the hypoplastic left heart syndrome. Both of these conditions, including the significance of associated coronary artery fistulas, are discussed in greater detail in other chapters. Bogers and associates[34] described four patients with tetralogy of Fallot and pulmonary atresia in whom the pulmonary artery circulation was dependent on a fistula from the left main coronary artery. We also encountered this anomaly in several patients, always in the setting of severe hypoplasia of the true pulmonary arteries and dependency on multiple aortopulmonary collaterals.

PATHOPHYSIOLOGY AND CLINICAL FEATURES

The flow of blood through a coronary artery fistula into a low pressure right heart chamber causes myocardial ischemia, both by producing a coronary steal and by imposing a volume load on the left ventricle. Patients seen after the age of 25 years are almost always symptomatic with angina, congestive heart failure, or palpitations. Shear-induced intimal damage, caused by the high flow in the coronary artery supplying the fistula, may result in premature development of atherosclerosis, as well as aneurysmal dilatation of that artery. The fact that there are acquired as well as congenital aspects of coronary artery fistulas, including the slowly progressive enlargement of fistulas with time, may be responsible for the rarity with which this anomaly is seen during infancy.

Preoperative signs and symptoms are dependent on the volume of runoff through the fistula and are unlikely to be impressive in the infant. A continuous murmur is the classical physical finding.

DIAGNOSTIC STUDIES

The electrocardiogram may be normal though in 16 of the 58 patients reported by the Texas Heart Institute[32] there was evidence of myocardial ischemia or recipient chamber overload (atrial or ventricular hypertrophy). Even asymptomatic patients usually have an abnormal cardiothoracic ratio on plain chest X-ray. Two dimensional echocardiography with color Doppler is very sensitive in defining coronary artery fistulas. However, coronary angiography with assessment of a left to right shunt by oximetric data remains the gold standard. The specific details of the coronary artery are very important for designing an operation that will not place at risk a large area of viable myocardium supplied by the affected coronary artery distal to the fistula. This is particularly true of coronary fistulas found in association with pulmonary atresia with intact ventricular septum.

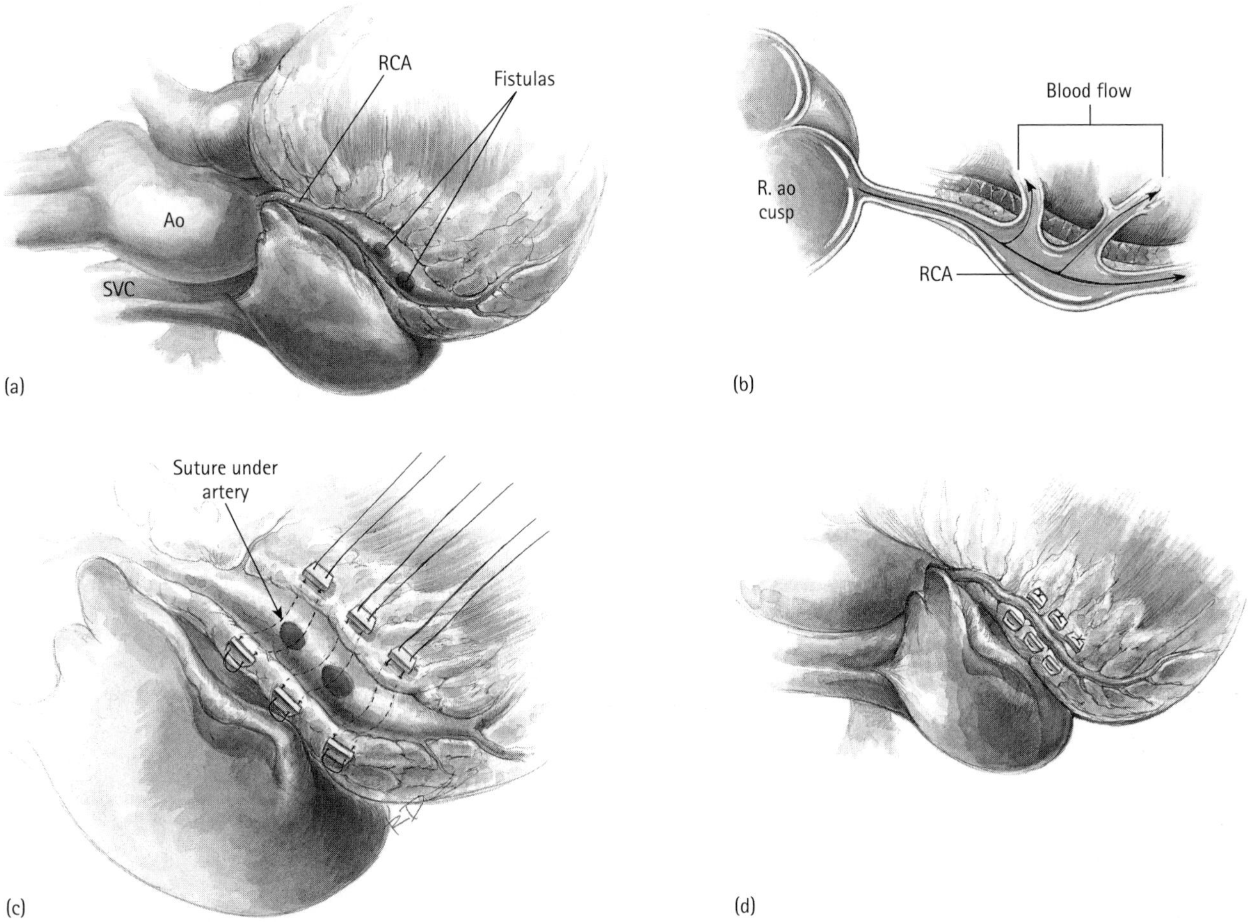

Figure 30.2 *(a,b) Isolated coronary fistulae can arise from either the right or left coronary artery but most commonly terminate in the right heart. The overlying coronary artery is often aneurysmally dilated. (c,d) Coronary fistulas arising from the distal right coronary artery can sometimes be managed by suture ligation without cardiopulmonary bypass. Pledgetted horizontal mattress sutures are placed underneath the coronary artery at the site of the fistulas. Digital palpation should confirm obliteration of the thrill.*

MEDICAL AND INTERVENTIONAL THERAPY

There is no specific medical therapy for coronary artery fistulas other than management of congestive heart failure, which may have developed secondary to the volume load with or without associated myocardial ischemia. Such therapy should be temporary and should simply optimize the patient's condition before surgical management. Undoubtedly there is a role for interventional catheter techniques, specifically embolization methods.[35]

INDICATIONS FOR SURGERY

It is extremely unusual for coronary artery fistulas to be diagnosed early in life before a significant left to right shunt has developed. Thus, the natural history of this lesion is not well known. Lowe and associates[31] described follow-up of one patient for 31 years before surgery was undertaken. During this time he underwent five cardiac catheterizations and progressed from being asymptomatic to having disabling angina and congestive heart failure. The presence of any symptoms or documentation of a measurable left to right shunt should almost certainly be an indication for surgery. However, the role of surgery for the patient who is asymptomatic and who has an immeasurable shunt by oximetry remains to be defined.

SURGICAL MANAGEMENT

History of surgery

The first report of surgical correction of a coronary artery fistula was by Biorck and Crafoord in 1947.[36] Cardiopulmonary bypass was first employed in conjunction with closure of a fistula as described in the 1959 report by Swan and coworkers.[37]

Technical considerations

Careful preoperative angiographic definition of the fistula, including its relationship to the coronary artery distal to the fistula, the presence of aneurysmal dilatation of the coronary artery, and the site of entry of the fistula into the heart, is essential. Several surgical options for management are available.

SUTURE LIGATION WITHOUT CARDIOPULMONARY BYPASS

If the fistula arises very distally (e.g. from the distal acute marginal branch of the right coronary artery entering the apex of the right ventricle), it can simply be oversewn. Digital pressure on the fistula before suturing will confirm operative assessment that no myocardium is at risk and that the thrill can be readily abolished. Intraoperative echocardiography may be useful in confirming that the fistula has been obliterated.

Suture ligation has also been successfully employed when the fistula arises laterally from a main coronary trunk. Pledgetted horizontal mattress sutures can be placed under the coronary artery in the area where the thrill is localized (Figure 30.2c,d).

TRANSCORONARY ANEURYSM SUTURE LIGATION WITH CARDIOPULMONARY BYPASS

If a large aneurysm is present, it is advisable to perform an aneurysmorrhaphy simultaneously with closure of the fistula (Figure 30.3). Before establishing bypass, the site of origin of the fistula should be confirmed by digital pressure. After bypass is begun, care must be taken to avoid excessive runoff through the fistula. A short period of aortic cross clamping is necessary, during which time a longitudinal incision is made in the aneurysm of the fistula (Figure 30.3a). The fistula is oversewn from within the aneurysm (Figure 30.3b), which is then appropriately tailored during closure (Figure 30.3c).

TRANSCARDIAC CHAMBER CLOSURE WITH CARDIOPULMONARY BYPASS

If an important area of myocardium is supplied distal to the origin of a fistula, particularly if external identification of the

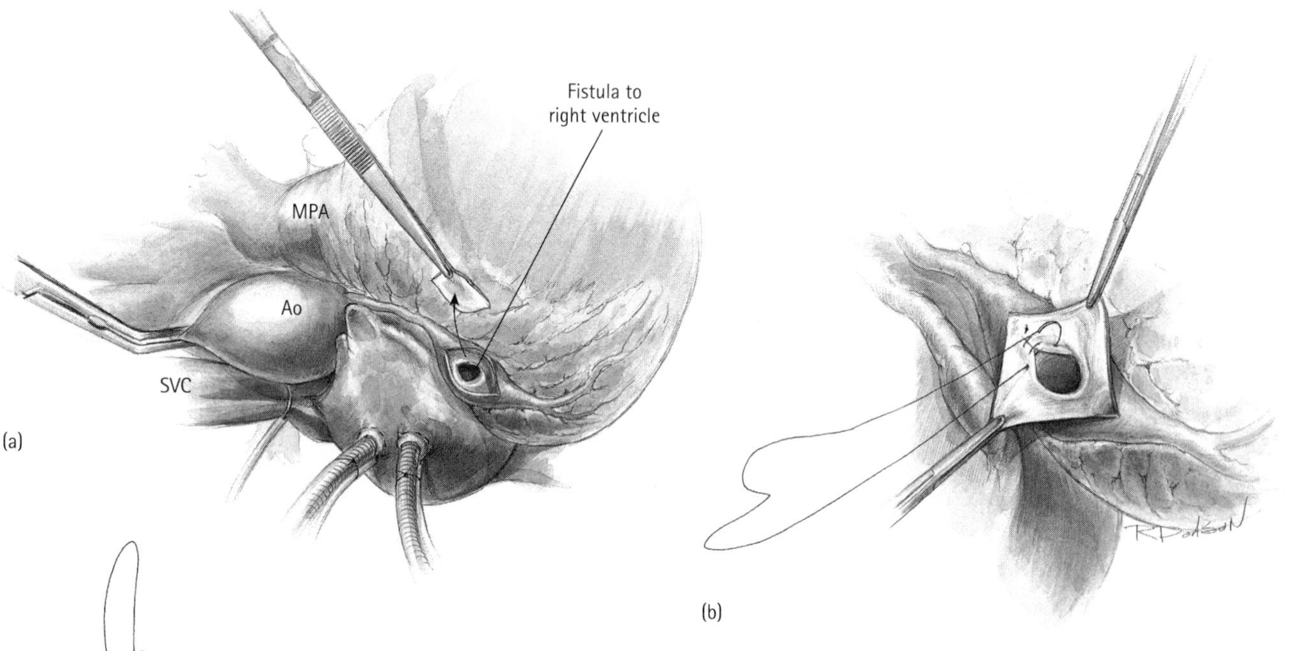

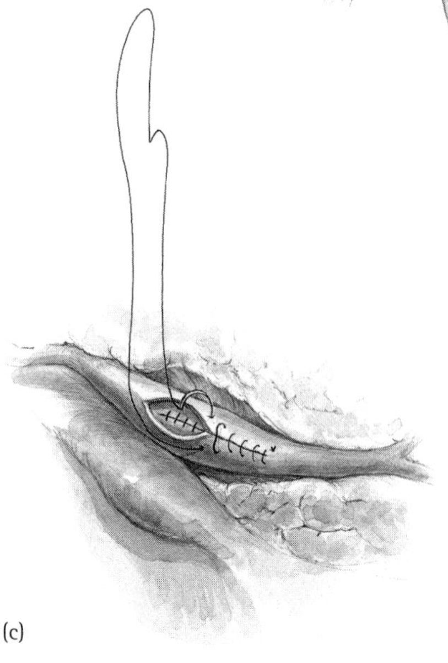

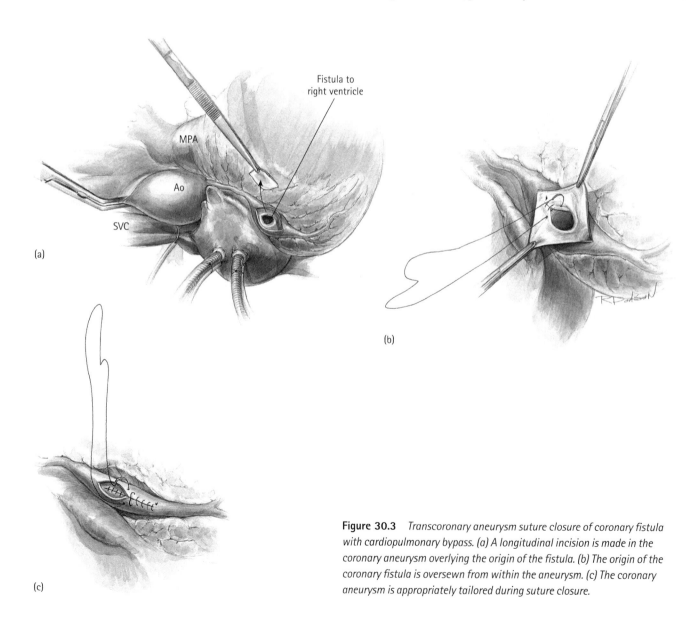

Figure 30.3 *Transcoronary aneurysm suture closure of coronary fistula with cardiopulmonary bypass. (a) A longitudinal incision is made in the coronary aneurysm overlying the origin of the fistula. (b) The origin of the coronary fistula is oversewn from within the aneurysm. (c) The coronary aneurysm is appropriately tailored during suture closure.*

fistula is difficult or there are multiple fistulas, approach from within the appropriate cardiac chamber is indicated. Identification of the fistulous orifice can be confirmed by delivery of cardioplegic solution. Likewise, the security of the closure, generally by pledgetted horizontal mattress sutures, can be confirmed by release of the aortic cross clamp. Some prefer not to clamp the aorta but prefer to rely on blood flow through the fistula to identify it.

SUMMARY

Color doppler echocardiography has become a sensitive tool for diagnosis of coronary artery fistulas. Interventional catheter techniques for embolization of coronary artery fistulas are now highly developed and can be utilized for the majority of fistulas. Occasionally large fistulas still must be managed surgically.

RESULTS OF SURGERY

The majority of reports describing management of coronary artery fistulas refer to catheterization techniques for fistula closure. For example, Armsby et al[38] described 33 patients who underwent transcatheter closure of coronary artery fistulas at Children's Hospital Boston between 1988 and 2000. Coils were used in 28, umbrella devices in six and a Grifka vascular occlusion device in one. Complete occlusion was achieved in 19, trace residual flow in 11 and small residual flow in five. Ultimately complete occlusion was accomplished in 82% of patients. There were no deaths or long-term morbidity.

Excellent results for the surgical management of coronary artery fistulas have been described by several groups particularly from Asia. For example, Wang et al[39] described 52 patients who underwent surgical management of coronary artery fistulas in Beijing, China. Cardiopulmonary bypass was used for all patients. An arteriotomy was made in the anomalous coronary artery in 10 patients. There were no deaths. In 1997, Mavroudis et al[40] described a 28-year surgical experience at Children's Memorial Hospital in Chicago with 17 patients who underwent surgical management of coronary artery fistulas. Cardiopulmonary bypass was used in eight patients. There were no operative or late deaths. There was no evidence of recurrent or residual fistula. The authors believe these results should stand as a gold standard against which transcatheter management should be measured. In 2002, Kamiya et al[41] from Kanazawa University, Japan reviewed 25 patients who underwent surgical management of congenital coronary artery fistulas. There were no deaths. One patient had slight residual flow. After an average follow-up time of 9.6 years all patients were asymptomatic. The authors also reviewed literature regarding surgical management of congenital coronary artery fistula.

ANOMALOUS CORONARY OSTIUM, INTRAMURAL CORONARY ARTERY AND CORONARY ARTERY BETWEEN AORTA AND PULMONARY ARTERY WITH NORMAL INTRACARDIAC ANATOMY

INTRODUCTION

Many anatomic variants of aberrant left coronary artery have been described.[42,43] In the past it was thought that the only important coronary anomalies of this type were those in which the left main coronary artery passed between the aorta and main pulmonary artery. There were several reports of sudden death associated with exercise in patients with such anatomy. However, more recent reports suggest that an oblique coronary ostium which is often associated with an intramural segment of left main coronary artery may in itself carry an increased risk of death even if it does not pass between the aorta and main pulmonary artery.[44–46]

PATHOLOGIC ANATOMY

A number of anatomical variants have been identified. Most commonly the left main coronary artery arises from an ostium that is close to the intercoronary commissure but still within the left coronary sinus (Figure 30.4). The coronary artery passes intramurally often deep to the top of the intercoronary commissure and subsequently passes between the aortic root and the pulmonary root. In another variation the left main coronary artery arises as a single trunk with the right coronary artery from the anterior sinus of Valsalva. It then passes posteriorly and leftward between the pulmonary artery and the aorta before dividing into the circumflex and left anterior descending coronary artery. In this variation also a segment of the left main coronary artery may be intramural.[47]

PATHOPHYSIOLOGY AND CLINICAL FEATURES

Several authors have suggested that the increased cardiac output associated with exercise results in compression of the left coronary artery between the aorta and pulmonary artery thereby causing left ventricular ischemia. For patients with a slit-like ostium or an intramural component of the left main coronary artery, dilation of the aorta associated with exercise may result in the slit-like ostium being occluded by a flap-like closure of the orifice. Patients may complain of angina during exercise. Unfortunately initial presentation is not infrequently cardiac arrest associated with exercise.

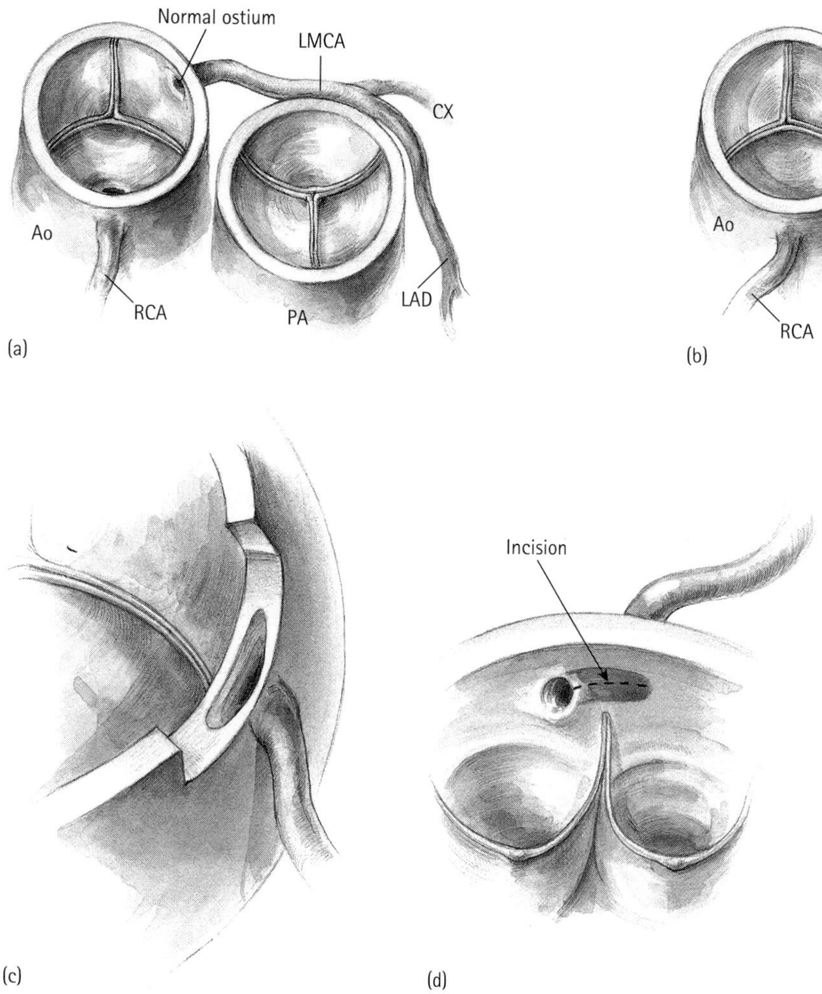

Figure 30.4 *Isolated intramural left coronary artery. (a) The normal left coronary artery arises centrally from the left coronary sinus perpendicular to the wall of the aorta. (b) An intramural left coronary artery often arises from the slit-like ostium that is close to the intercoronary commissure of the aortic valve. It passes intramurally between the aorta and main pulmonary artery and emerges externally from what appears to be the right coronary sinus. (c) Intramural segment of an anomalous left coronary artery. (d) Surgical management of the intramural left coronary artery involves unroofing of the intramural segment.*

DIAGNOSTIC STUDIES

A combination of echocardiography and cardiac magnetic resonance imaging is usually helpful in defining the proximal anatomy of the coronary arteries. Coronary angiography may be necessary to exclude the presence of distal coronary disease.

MEDICAL AND INTERVENTIONAL THERAPY

No medical therapy or interventional catheter therapy has been described for this anomaly. Perhaps coronary stenting may be useful if a surgical approach is not feasible.

INDICATIONS FOR SURGERY

The indications for surgery for this anomaly are difficult to define if the patient has been free of symptoms. Unfortunately however the anomaly is often not detected until a patient has suffered a cardiac arrest associated with exercise.[48,49] If there is no evidence of idiopathic hypertrophic subaortic stenosis, which is a more common cause of unheralded cardiac arrest in a young person, a very careful assessment should be undertaken for an anomalous ostium, intramural segment, or segment of coronary artery between the aorta and main pulmonary artery. If one of these anomalies is identified surgery is indicated. In the asymptomatic patient who is found to have one of these same anomalies, the patient should undergo exercise stress testing. If exercise stress testing including exercise perfusion scans are normal it may be reasonable to do no more than warn the patient to avoid competitive sports. However, if the ostium clearly appears compromised then consideration should be given to undertaking surgery even in the absence of symptoms or tests supporting the occurrence of myocardial ischemia.

SURGICAL MANAGEMENT

History of surgery

Although anomalous origin of the left coronary artery from the aorta has been described as a benign anomaly in several reviews of coronary anatomy,[50,51] case reports in the 1960s[52,53] suggested that such an anomaly could be the cause of sudden death in young people. In 1974 Cheitlin and coworkers[54] described 51 patients in whom both coronary arteries arose from the same sinus of Valsalva. In 33 of these, both coronaries arose from the anterior sinus and passed between the aorta and the pulmonary artery. Nine of these patients died suddenly between the ages of 13 and 36 years; death was generally related to exercise. They also described surgery in a 14 year old boy who had been successfully resuscitated from ventricular fibrillation. In 1974 he underwent enlargement of a slit-like orifice of the left coronary artery; others have recommended coronary artery bypass surgery for this anomaly.[55,56]

Technical considerations

It is unusual to diagnose this anomaly in the infant or neonate. In older children it is usually possible to perform an unroofing procedure of the intramural segment which is usually also the segment between the aorta and the main pulmonary artery. Usually the intramural segment runs immediately superior to the intercoronary commissure and therefore the intramural segment can be unroofed into the lumen of the aorta without injuring the aortic valve (Figure 30.4d). If the intramural segment runs behind the intercoronary commissure it may be possible to unroof the segment but spare the valve commissure by opening a second ostium into the segment from within the right coronary sinus. If necessary very fine tacking sutures can be placed if the incision extends outside the lumen of the coronary artery and aorta.

RESULTS OF SURGERY

Other than a few case reports[57,58] there is little information regarding management of patients with a congenitally anomalous ostium of a coronary artery or anomalous course between the aorta and pulmonary artery. Gulati et al[59] recently described a series of 12 patients with anomalous coronary artery from the wrong coronary sinus. The mean age of the patients was 10 years. Seven patients had an anomalous left coronary artery arising from the right sinus of Valsalva and five patients had an anomalous right coronary from the left sinus. Six of the 12 patients were symptomatic with angina occurring in all and syncope in two. Seven patients underwent unroofing or fenestration of the intramural component of the anomalous coronary artery and three patients had reimplantation. One patient had pulmonary artery translocation as previously described by Rodefeld.[57] One patient had a Lecompte maneuver to prevent pulmonary artery compression of the coronary artery. There were no operative deaths. One patient who had undergone pulmonary artery translocation developed complete heart block and required a pacemaker. One patient required heart transplantation six months postoperatively.

At Children's Hospital Boston five patients were noted to have anomalous origin of the right coronary artery from the left sinus. In all cases the intramural segment was unroofed. There were no operative or late deaths.

ACQUIRED CORONARY ANOMALIES

OCCLUDED CORONARY ARTERIES FOLLOWING THE ARTERIAL SWITCH PROCEDURE OR ROSS PROCEDURE

Introduction

A very small percentage of children have been identified following the arterial switch or Ross procedure to have occluded or severely stenotic coronary arteries.[60,61] The occlusion is usually at the ostium and presumably represents kinking, twisting or stretching of the coronary artery segment at the time of reimplantation. Usually the coronary artery is nondominant and may be quite small supplying a limited area of myocardium. Interestingly the myocardium supplied by such occluded coronary arteries is usually normal and functions normally, presumably reflecting excellent neonatal collateralization. On the other hand occluded coronary arteries have also been associated with sudden death and symptoms including angina.

Indications for surgery

Unfortunately there is not yet a sufficiently large experience to know the optimal treatment for the asymptomatic child who has been demonstrated to have a coronary artery occlusion following an arterial switch or Ross procedure. Perhaps a reasonable approach would be to determine the amount of myocardium supplied by the occluded coronary artery. If this is extensive enough to be life threatening if acute ischemia were in some way to occur then consideration should be given to placing an internal mammary graft. Exercise stress testing should also be undertaken. Placement of an internal mammary graft is definitely indicated for the child who is symptomatic because of an occluded or stenosed coronary artery subsequent to an arterial switch or Ross procedure.

CORONARY ANEURYSM ASSOCIATED WITH KAWASAKI DISEASE

Introduction

Although the coronary artery aneurysms resulting from Kawasaki disease are acquired rather than congenital nevertheless it is the pediatric cardiologist and cardiac surgeon who are most likely to be called upon to manage this entity. In the United States, Kawasaki disease is more commonly the cause of noncongenital heart disease in children than acute rheumatic fever. It usually occurs in young children with a peak incidence occurring in the second year of life. Eighty five percent of cases occur before five years of age.[62] The cause of Kawasaki disease remains unknown although it seems very likely that an infectious agent of some sort plays an important initiating role.

Pathologic anatomy

Kawasaki disease in its acute stage is characterized by a vasculitis of microvessels and small arteries. In 15–25% of children who do not receive intravenous gamma globulin, coronary artery aneurysms will develop. Dilation of coronary arteries can be detected within seven days of the onset of fever with coronary dilation usually peaking around four weeks after the onset of the illness.[63] Coronary artery aneurysms are at risk of thrombosis with subsequent myocardial infarction.

Clinical features

Kawasaki in Japan described the following clinical features in 1967:

- fever lasting five or more days
- bilateral conjunctivitis
- fissured lips, inflamed pharynx or 'strawberry tongue'
- erythema of the palms or soles, edema of the extremities
- polymorphous exanthem
- acute cervical lymphadenopathy.

None of the clinical features of Kawasaki disease is pathognomic so that other illnesses such as streptococcal infection must be carefully excluded.

Diagnostic studies

Laboratory findings confirm a generalized systemic inflammation but there is no specific biochemical or immune marker since the etiological agent remains unidentified.

Echocardiography is a sensitive and specific method for imaging the proximal right and left coronary arteries where aneurysms are most likely to develop. Selective coronary arteriography is useful for visualizing coronary artery stenoses or distal coronary lesions that are difficult to define by two-dimensional echocardiography. Coronary artery aneurysms can be subclassified according to their shape and the number of segments of the coronary arteries affected. Coronary aneurysms in early Kawasaki disease usually occur in the proximal segments of the major coronary vessels; aneurysms that occur distally are almost always associated with proximal coronary abnormalities.[64]

Medical and interventional therapy

The specific details of the medical therapy of Kawasaki disease are beyond the scope of this book. However, in summary high dose intravenous gamma globulin therapy in the acute phase of the disease reduces the prevalence of coronary aneurysms by three- to fivefold and has become the standard of care.[65] Steroids may also be beneficial in some patients. Aspirin and warfarin are also used to reduce the risk of coronary thrombosis. The role of interventional catheter therapy for the coronary abnormalities resulting from Kawasaki disease remains poorly defined. In older children coronary artery stents have been successfully placed. However, regular coronary angioplasty has not proven to be as effective in children with Kawasaki disease as it is in adults with atherosclerotic coronary disease.

Surgical management

The greatest experience with surgical management for Kawasaki disease is in Japan. Kitamura has reported the largest series of greater than 100 patients.[66] The usual procedure has been internal mammary artery grafting for obstructive lesions. Although the indications for coronary bypass procedures have not been well established, there is general agreement that surgery should be performed in patients with symptoms of ischemic heart disease or reversible ischemia on stress testing. Arterial grafts are definitely to be preferred relative to saphenous vein grafts which tend to shorten over time.

Results of surgery

In children younger than seven years of age graft patency at 90 months after surgery has been reported to be 70% in arterial grafts. In patients greater than eight years of age arterial graft patency has been reported to be 84%. Survival has been excellent with 98.7% of Kitamura's patients alive eight years after internal mammary artery grafting to the left anterior descending coronary artery.[66]

REFERENCES

1. Askenazi J, Nadas AS. Anomalous left coronary artery originating from the pulmonary artery. Report on 15 cases. *Circulation* 1975; **51**:976–987.
2. Vouhe PR, Baillot-Vernant F, Trinquet F et al. Anomalous left coronary artery from the pulmonary artery in infants. *J Thorac Cardiovasc Surg* 1987; **94**:192–199.
3. Menahem S, Venables AW. Anomalous left coronary artery from the pulmonary artery: A 15 year sample. *Br Heart J* 1987; **58**:378–384.
4. Becker AE, Anderson RH. *Pathology of Congenital Heart Disease.* London, Butterworths, 1981, p 369.
5. Smith A, Arnold R, Anderson RH et al. Anomalous origin of the left coronary artery from the pulmonary trunk. *J Thorac Cardiovasc Surg* 1989; **98**:16–24.

6. Tyrrell MJ, Duncan WJ, Hayton RC. Bharadwaj BB. Anomalous left coronary artery from the pulmonary artery: Effect of coronary anatomy on clinical course. *Angiology* 1987; **38**:833–840.
7. Cottrill CM, Davis D, McMillen M, O'Connor WN, Noonan JA, Todd EP. Anomalous left coronary artery from the pulmonary artery: Significance of associated intracardiac defects. *J Am Coll Cardiol* 1985; **6**:237–242.
8. Ortiz E, deLeval M, Somerville J. Ductus arteriosus associated with an anomalous left coronary artery arising from the pulmonary artery. Catastrophe after duct ligation. *Br Heart J* 1986; **55**:415–417.
9. Masel LF. Tetralogy of Fallot with origin of the left coronary from the right pulmonary artery. *Med J Aust* 1960; **1**:213.
10. Edwards JE. The direction of blood flow in coronary arteries arising from the pulmonary trunk. *Circulation* 1964; **29**:163.
11. Rein AJ, Colan SD, Parness IA, Sanders SP. Regional and global left ventricular function in infants with anomalous origin of the left coronary artery from the pulmonary trunk: Preoperative and postoperative assessment. *Circulation* 1987; **75**:115–123.
12. Bland EF, White PD, Garland J. Congenital anomalies of the coronary arteries: report of an unusual case associated with cardiac hypertrophy. *Am Heart J* 1933; **8**:787.
13. Midgley FM, Watson DC, Scott LP et al. Repair of anomalous origin of the left coronary artery in the infant and small child. *J Am Coll Cardiol* 1984; **4**:1231–1234.
14. Takeuchi S, Imamura H, Katsumoto K et al. New surgical method for repair of anomalous left coronary artery from pulmonary artery. *J Thorac Cardiovasc Surg* 1979; **78**:7–11.
15. Turley K, Szarnicki RJ, Flachsbart KD, Richter RC, Popper RW, Tarnoff H. Aortic implantation is possible in all cases of anomalous origin of the left coronary artery from the pulmonary artery. *Ann Thorac Surg* 1995; **60**:84–89.
16. Castaneda AR, Jonas RA, Mayer JE, Hanley FL. *Cardiac Surgery of the Neonate and Infant.* Philadelphia, WB Saunders, 1994, p 303.
17. Neches WH, Mathews RA, Park SC et al. Anomalous origin of the left coronary artery from the pulmonary artery. A new method of surgical repair. *Circulation* 1974; **50**:582–587.
18. Azakie A, Russell JL, McCrindle BW et al. Anatomic repair of anomalous left coronary artery from the pulmonary artery by aortic reimplantation: early survival, patterns of ventricular recovery and late outcome. *Ann Thorac Surg* 2003; **75**:1535–1541.
19. Isomatsu Y, Imai Y, Shin'oka T, Aoki M, Iwata Y. Surgical intervention for anomalous origin of the left coronary artery from the pulmonary artery: the Tokyo experience. *J Thorac Cardiovasc Surg* 2001; **121**:792–797.
20. Backer CL, Hillman N, Dodge-Khatami A, Mavroudis C. Anomalous origin of the left coronary artery from the pulmonary artery: Successful surgical strategy without assist devices. *Semin Thorac Cardiovasc Surg Pediatr Card Surg Annu* 2000; **3**:165–172.
21. Ando M, Mee RB, Duncan BW, Drummond-Webb JJ, Seshadri SG, Igor Mesia CI. Creation of a dual-coronary system for anomalous origin of the left coronary artery from the pulmonary artery utilizing the trapdoor flap method. *Eur J Cardiothorac Surg* 2002; **22**:576–581.
22. Schwartz ML, Jonas RA, Colan SD. Anomalous origin of left coronary artery from pulmonary artery: recovery of left ventricular function after dual coronary repair. *J Am Coll Cardiol* 1997; **30**:547–553.
23. Jin Z, Berger F, Uhlemann F et al. Improvement in left ventricular dysfunction after aortic reimplantation in 11 consecutive paediatric patients with anomalous origin of the left coronary artery from the pulmonary artery. Early results of a serial echocardiographic follow-up. *Eur Heart J* 1994; **15**:1044–1049.
24. Lambert V, Touchot A, Losay J et al. Midterm results after surgical repair of the anomalous origin of the coronary artery. *Circulation* 1996; **94**:II38–43.
25. del Nido PJ, Duncan BW, Mayer JE Jr, Wessel DL, LaPierre RA, Jonas RA. Left ventricular assist device improves survival in children with left ventricular dysfunction after repair of anomalous origin of the left coronary artery from the pulmonary artery. *Ann Thorac Surg* 1999; **67**:169–172.
26. McMahon CJ, DiBardino DJ, Undar A, Fraser CD Jr. Anomalous origin of left coronary artery from the right pulmonary artery in association with type III aortopulmonary window and interrupted aortic arch. *Ann Thorac Surg* 2002; **74**:919–921.
27. Kilic A, Elshershari H, Ozkutlu S. Anomalous left coronary artery from the main pulmonary trunk: physiologic and clinical importance of its association with patent ductus arteriosus and pulmonary hypertension. *Turk J Pediatr* 2002; **44**:363–365.
28. Barbero-Marcial M, Tanamati C, Atik E, Ebaid M, Jatene A. Anomalous origin of the left coronary artery from the pulmonary artery with intramural aortic route: diagnosis and surgical treatment. *J Thorac Cardiovasc Surg* 1999; **117**:823–825.
29. Bunton R, Jonas RA, Lang P, Rein AJ, Castaneda AR. Anomalous origin of left coronary artery from pulmonary artery. Ligation versus establishment of a two coronary artery system. *J Thorac Cardiovasc Surg* 1987; **93**:103–108.
30. Dodge-Khatami A, Mavroudis C, Backer CL. Anomalous origin of the left coronary artery from the pulmonary artery: collective review of surgical therapy. *Ann Thorac Surg* 2002; **74**:946–955.
31. Lowe JE, Oldham HN, Sabiston DC. Surgical management of congenital coronary artery fistulas. *Ann Surg* 1981; **194**:373–380.
32. Urrutia-S CO, Falaschi G, Ott DA, Cooley DA. Surgical management of 56 patients with congenital coronary artery fistulas. *Ann Thorac Surg* 1983; **35**:300–307.
33. Sauer U, Gittenberger-deGroot AC, Gieshuaser M, Babic R, Buhlmeyer K. Coronary arteries in the hypoplastic left heart syndrome. *Circulation* 1989; **80** (Suppl I):168–176.
34. Bogers AJJC, Rohmer J, Wolsky SA. Quaegebeur JM, Huysmans HA. Coronary artery fistula as source of pulmonary circulation in pulmonary atresia with ventricular septal defect. *Thorac Cardiovasc Surg* 1990; **38**:30–32.
35. Perry SB, Rome J, Keane JF, Baim DS, Lock JE. Transcatheter closure of coronary artery fistulae. *J Am Coll Cardiol* 1992; **20**:205–209.
36. Biorck G, Crafoord C. Arteriovenous aneurysm on the pulmonary artery simulating patent ductus arteriosus botalli. *Thorax* 1947; **2**:65.
37. Swan H, Wilson JH, Woodwark G et al. Surgical obliteration of a coronary artery fistula to right ventricle. *Arch Surg* 1959; **79**:820.
38. Armsby LR, Keane JF, Sherwood MC, Forbess JM, Perry SB, Lock JE. Management of coronary artery fistulae. Patient selection and results of transcatheter closure. *J Am Coll Cardiol* 2002; **39**:1026–1032.
39. Wang S, Wu Q, Hu S et al. Surgical treatment of 52 patients with congenital coronary artery fistulas. *Chin Med J (Engl)* 2001; **114**:752–755.
40. Mavroudis C, Backer CL, Rocchini AP, Muster AJ, Gevitz M. Coronary artery fistulas in infants and children: a surgical review and discussion of coil embolization. *Ann Thorac Surg* 1997; **63**:1235–1242.
41. Kamiya H, Yasuda T, Nagamine H et al. Surgical treatment of congenital coronary artery fistulas: 27 years' experience and a review of the literature. *J Card Surg* 2002; **17**:173–177.
42. Yamanaka O, Hobbs RE. Coronary artery anomalies with 126,595 patients undergoing coronary arteriography. *Cath Cardiovasc Diag* 1990; **21**:28–40.

43. Fernandes ED, Kadivar H, Hallman GL, Reul GJ, Ott DA, Cooley DA. Congenital malformations of the coronary arteries. The Texas Heart Institute Experience. *Ann Thorac Surg* 1992; **54**:732–740.
44. Virmani R, Chun PK, Goldstein RE, Robinowitz M, McAllister HA. Acute takeoffs of the coronary arteries along the aortic wall and congenital coronary ostial valve-like ridges: association with sudden death. *J Am Coll Cardiol* 1984; **3**:766–771.
45. Iyer RS, Huu NK, deLeval MR. Anomalous origin of the left coronary artery. *Asian Cardiovasc Thorac Ann* 1996; **4**:184–185.
46. Davis JA, Cecchin F, Jones TK, Portman MA. Major coronary artery anomalies in a pediatric population: Incidence and clinical importance. *J Am Coll Cardiol* 2001; **37**:593–597.
47. Massih TA, Clur SA, Bonhoeffer P. Exertional pulmonary edema revealing anomalous origin of the left coronary artery from the right coronary aortic sinus. *Cardiol Young* 2002; **12**:78–80.
48. Basso C, Corrado D, Thiene G. Congenital coronary artery anomalies as an important cause of sudden death in the young. *Cardiol Rev* 2001; **9**:312–317.
49. Basso C, Maron BJ, Corrado D, Thiene G. Clinical profile of congenital coronary artery anomalies with origin from the wrong aortic sinus leading to sudden death in young competitive athletes. *J Am Coll Cardiol* 2000; **35**:1493–1501.
50. Laurie W, Woods JD. Single coronary artery. *Am Heart J* 1964; **67**:95.
51. Ogden JA. Congenital anomalies of the coronary arteries. *Am J Cardiol* 1970; **25**:474–479.
52. Benson PA, Lack AR. Anomalous aortic origin of left coronary artery. *Arch Pathol* 1968; **86**:214–216.
53. Cohen LS, Shaw LD. Fatal myocardial infarction in an 11 year old boy associated with a unique coronary artery anomaly. *Am J Cardiol* 1967; **19**:420–423.
54. Cheitlin MD, DeCastro CM, McAllister HA. Sudden death as a complication of anomalous left coronary origin from the anterior sinus of Valsalva. *Circulation* 1974; **50**:780–787.
55. Liberthson RR, Dinsmore RE, Fallot JT. Aberrant coronary artery origin from the aorta. *Circulation* 1979; **59**:748–754.
56. Scully RE (ed). Case Records of the Massachusetts General Hospital. Case 22–1989. *N Eng J Med* 1989; **320**:1475.
57. Rodefeld MD, Culbertson CB, Rosenfeld HM, Hanley FL, Thompson LD. Pulmonary artery translocation: a surgical option for complex anomalous coronary artery anatomy. *Ann Thorac Surg* 2001; **72**:2150–2152.
58. Kaza AK, Tribble CG, Crosby IK. Repair of an anomalous left coronary artery. *Cardiovasc Surg* 2002; **10**:276–278.
59. Gulati R, Hanley FL, Helston G, Suleman S, Reinhartz O, Reddy VM. Avoiding sudden death? Repair of the anomalous coronary artery arising from the wrong coronary sinus. Presented at the 10th Biennial Meeting of the Castaneda Society of Pediatric Cardiovascular Surgery, Boston, May 3 2003.
60. Bonhoeffer P, Bonnet D, Piechaud JF et al. Coronary artery obstruction after the arterial switch operation for transposition of the great arteries in newborns. *J Am Coll Cardiol* 1997; **29**:202–206.
61. Tanel RE, Wernovsky G, Landzberg MJ, Perry SB, Burke RP. Coronary artery abnormalities detected at cardiac catheterization following the arterial switch operation for transposition of the great arteries. *Am J Cardiol* 1995; **76**:153–157.
62. Allen R. Kawasaki disease. *RCH Report* 1995; **11**:1–3.
63. Kuramochi Y, Ohkubo T, Takechi N, Fukumi D, Uchikoba Y, Ogawa S. Hemodynamic factors of thrombus formation in coronary aneurysms associated with Kawasaki disease. *Pediatr Int* 2000; **42**:470–475.
64. Suzuki A, Kamiya T, Kuwahara N et al. Coronary arterial lesions of Kawasaki disease: cardiac catheterization findings of 1100 cases. *Pediatr Cardiol* 1986; **7**:3–9.
65. Newburger JW, Takahashi M, Beiser AS et al. A single intravenous infusion of gamma globulin as compared with four infusions in the treatment of acute Kawasaki syndrome. *N Engl J Med* 1991; **324**:1633–1639.
66. Yoshikawa Y, Yagihara T, Kameda Y et al. Result of surgical treatments in patients with coronary-arterial obstructive disease after Kawasaki disease. *Eur J Cardiothorac Surg* 2000; **17**:515–519.

Index

Notes: Page numbers in **bold** refer to figures; page numbers in *italics* refer to tables. To save space in the index, the following abbreviations have been used: ALCAPA – anomalous left coronary artery from the pulmonary artery; ASD – atrial septal defect; CHD – congenital heart disease; CPB – cardiopulmonary bypass; VSD – ventricular septal defect; *vs.* indicates a comparison or differential diagnosis

W

X

Y